Head [obscured by label] omy

A Self-Instructional Program

Head & Neck Histology and Anatomy

A Self-Instructional Program

Sarah Kay Smith, DDS
Owens Community College
Toledo, Ohio

Nancy Shobe Karst, CDA, RDH, MS
Missouri Southern State College
Joplin, Missouri

Appleton & Lange
Stamford, Connecticut

Notice: The authors and the publisher of this volume have taken care to make certain that the doses of drugs and schedules of treatment are correct and compatible with the standards generally accepted at the time of publication. Nevertheless, as new information becomes available, changes in treatment and in the use of drugs become necessary. The reader is advised to carefully consult the instruction and information material included in the package insert of each drug or therapeutic agent before administration. This advice is especially important when using, administering, or recommending new or infrequently used drugs. The authors and publisher disclaim all responsibility for any liability, loss, injury, or damage incurred as a consequence, directly or indirectly, of the use and application of any of the contents of this volume.

www.appletonlange.com

99 00 01 02 03 / 10 9 8 7 6 5 4 3 2 1

Prentice Hall International (UK) Limited, *London*
Prentice Hall of Australia Pty. Limited, *Sydney*
Prentice Hall Canada, Inc., *Toronto*
Prentice Hall Hispanoamericana, S.A., *Mexico*
Prentice Hall of India Private Limited, *New Delhi*
Prentice Hall of Japan, Inc., *Tokyo*
Simon & Schuster Asia Pte. Ltd., *Singapore*
Editora Prentice Hall do Brasil Ltda, *Rio de Janeiro*
Prentice Hall, *Upper Saddle River, New Jersey*

Library of Congress Cataloging-in-Publication Data
Smith, Sarah K.
Head and neck histology and anatomy : a self-instructional program / Sarah Kay Smith, Nancy Shobe Karst.
p. cm.
Companion v. to: Dental anatomy / Nancy Shobe Karst. Sarah K. Smith. 10th ed. ©1998.
Includes bibliographical references and index.
ISBN 0-8385-3652-2 (pbk. : alk. paper)
1. Teeth—Anatomy—Programmed instruction. 2. Teeth—Anatomy—Atlases. 3. Head—Anatomy—Programmed instruction. 4. Head—Histology—Programmed instruction. 5. Neck—Anatomy—Programmed instruction. 6. Neck—Histology—Programmed instruction.
I. Karst, Nancy Shobe. II. Title.
[DNLM: 1. Head—anatomy & histology programmed instruction. 2. Neck—anatomy & histology programmed instruction. WE 18.2 S659h 1999]
RK280.K37 1998 Suppl.
611′.91—dc21
DNLM/DLC
For Library of Congress 98-32396

Acquisitions Editor: Kimberly A. Davies
Editorial Assistant: Nicole R. Cooper
Production Editor: Lisa M. Guidone
Manager of Art Services: Eve Siegel
Art Coordinator: Pamela Carley
Art Studio: ElectraGraphics
Designer: Janice Barsevich Bielawa
Cover: Libby Schmitz

ISBN 0-8385-3652-2

PRINTED IN THE UNITED STATES OF AMERICA

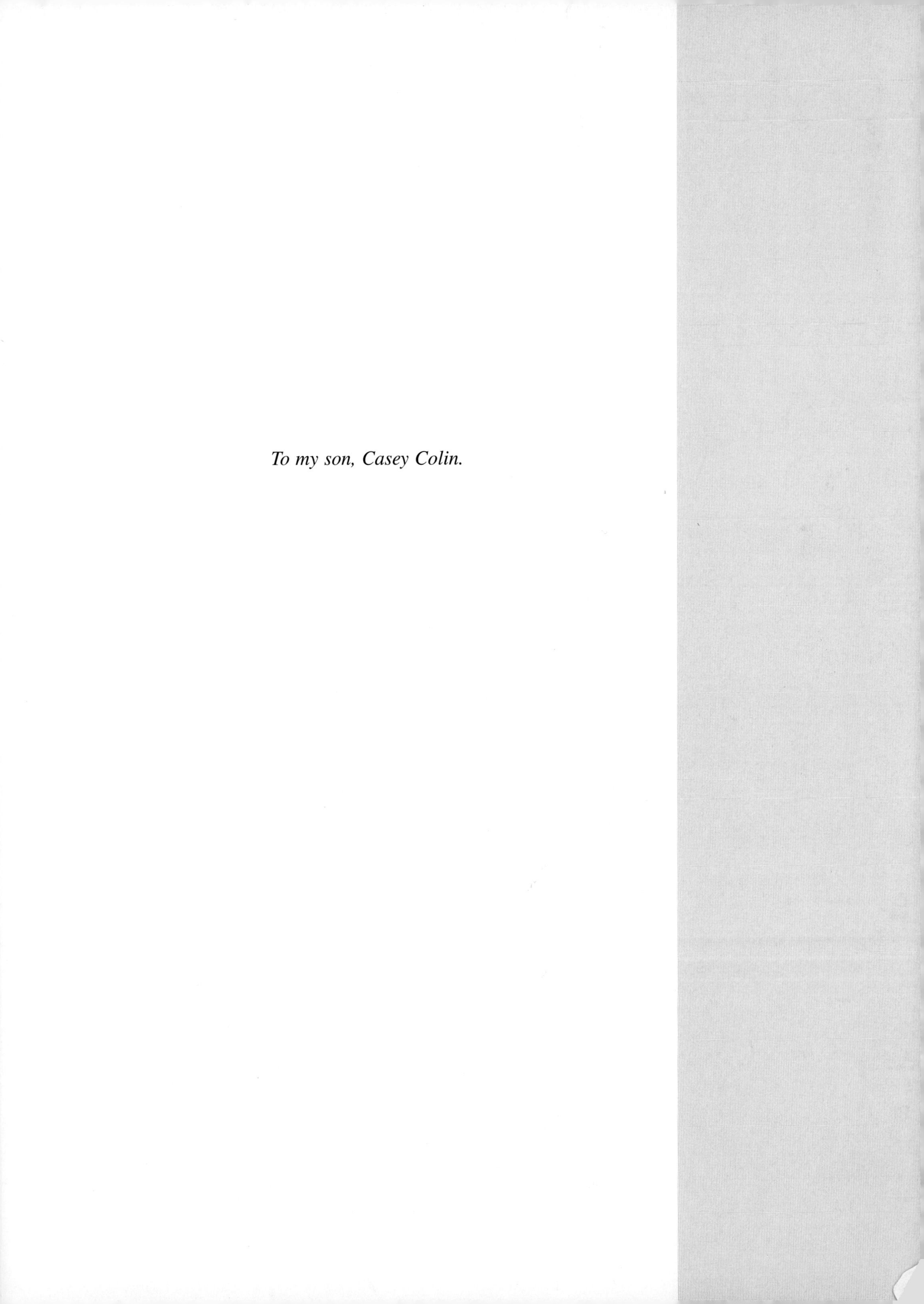

To my son, Casey Colin.

CONTENTS

Chapter 3 Tooth Development 89

Chapter 4 Dental Histology 137

Chapter 5 Periodontal Tissues 185

Chapter 6 Mucosa and Other Oral Tissues 221

Chapter 7 Skeletal System 299

Chapter 8 Muscular System 375

Chapter 9 Nervous System 453

PREFACE

Head and Neck Histology and Anatomy: A Self-Instructional Program can be used either as a self-instructional textbook or as a required text in the dental curriculum. Many dental, dental hygiene, and dental assisting instructors require incoming students to purchase and work through the book prior to the beginning of their professional education. Mastery of the information will give the student a head start in the dental profession.

The book is organized into two major sections: *histology* and *anatomy.* The histology section also covers the topics of *embryology* and *tooth development.* Self-instructional questions within the body of the text allow for better retention of facts and concepts as the student progresses through the book. Also, the end-of-chapter *review tests* aid in reinforcing concepts already learned. Anatomic and histologic drawings that can be labeled by the student for further practice are included both within and at the end of each chapter.

Head and Neck Histology and Anatomy is meant to be a companion book to *Dental Anatomy: A Self-Instructional Program* (Appleton & Lange, 1997, Karst and Smith), as these two subjects are often combined or taught simultaneously in most dental programs. The same methods of self-instruction and self-testing are included in both texts.

ACKNOWLEDGMENTS

This text is the result of 15 years of anatomy instruction at Owens Community College in Toledo, Ohio, and the resulting feedback to personal instructional materials used. Materials and illustrations are both drawn from that experience, as is an expressed desire by the students for a self-instructional text much like that of *Dental Anatomy* (Appleton & Lange, 1997). I also acknowledge the medical anatomy program of the Medical College of Ohio at Toledo, from which I gained considerable knowledge and experience with instructional and cadaver materials, as well as research in head and neck anatomy.

DIRECTIONS FOR THE STUDENT

The objective of this text is to help you master the terminology and facts of head and neck histology and anatomy. It has been demonstrated that when students use the text according to directions and diligently answer the embedded questions and review tests, they effectively learn head and neck histology and anatomy.

In addition to reading, you will be answering questions that are "embedded" in the text. Answers appear in the margin.

1. As you read the text, use the *answer mask* provided to cover the answer column on each page. Begin with the entire column covered.
2. As you read down the page, answer the questions by writing the answer either on the blank line, or on a separate sheet of paper.
3. Uncover the answer, which will appear below the dotted line in the shaded column.
4. Continue down the page. If you miss one or more answers, repeat the section until you have mastered it.
5. You are given *review tests* to complete at the end of each chapter. Check your answers in the appendix. Repeat if necessary.
6. The text and *review tests* contain unlabeled histologic and anatomic drawings. You can label these in the book with pencil (to correct if needed). Also, some sections may ask you to use colored pencil to define certain structures.

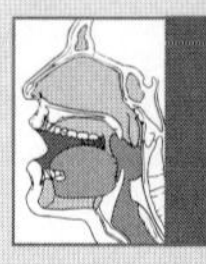

1

General Histology

BASIC HISTOLOGY 1.0

All living organisms are built from those "blocks" of organized living matter that we call **cells.** Cells are the smallest, self-contained units of life. They group together, sharing the jobs of living, for example, respiration, nutrition, and replication, in many forms, with certain cells assuming shapes better suited to specific jobs. We will first look at an individual, average cell and then at similar cells that band together to do a similar job or function called a **tissue. Histology** is the study of tissues.

The cell shown illustrates many characteristics of cells in general, but remember each cell may not have all of these parts or may have others to perform its function.

The **nucleus** is the "command center" of the cell, containing instructions for its growth, function, and reproduction within the DNA of its chromosomes. Find it on the drawing. Also find the outer limit of the cell, the **cell membrane,** and the clear gellike protein, the **cytoplasm,** which contains all of the cell's parts or **organelles.**

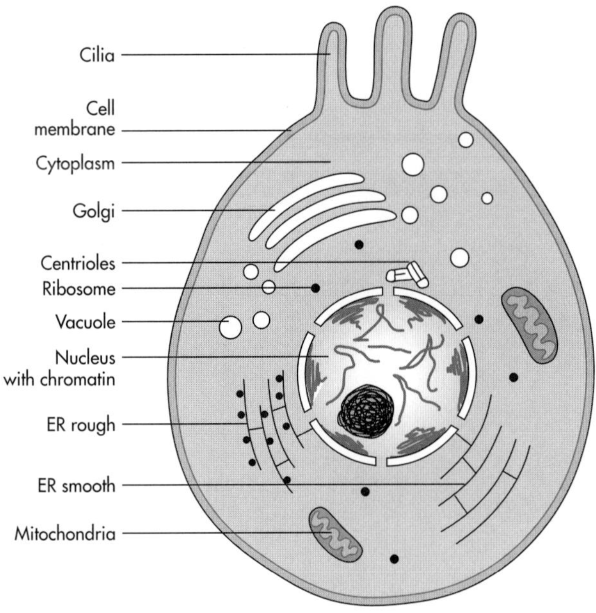

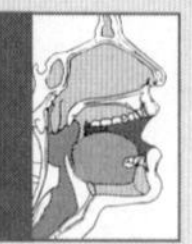

Other organelles of importance are the connecting tubule system within the cytoplasm or **endoplasmic reticulum** (ER); the **ribosomes,** which line the ER or are found free-floating; and the **mitochondria,** a peanut-shaped organelle responsible for creating energy for the cell. Find them on the drawing.

Another interesting organelle is the **Golgi apparatus.** These membranous plates are producing a **cell product,** which will be secreted via the **vacuoles** that bud off from it.

Cell product that is secreted by the cell and remains around the cell, often becoming the "house" or environment within which it resides, is called its **matrix.**

nucleus, golgi apparatus

Label the cell parts shown on the blank drawing. Check your answer with the previous drawing. The command center of the cell is its ______________, and the organelle responsible for the creation of secretory products is the ______________.

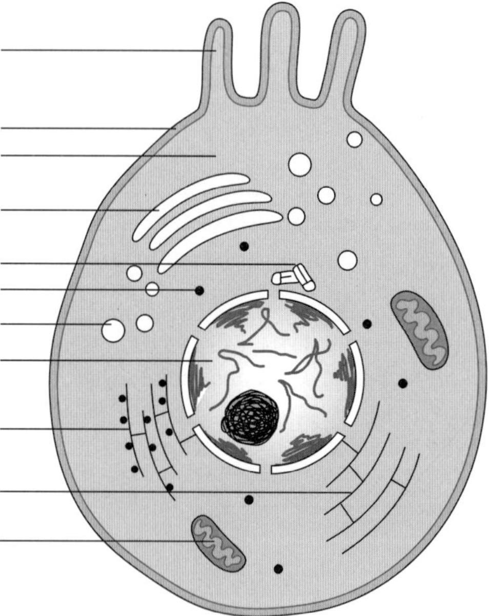

tissue

Similar cells that group together to perform a similar function are called a(n) ______________.

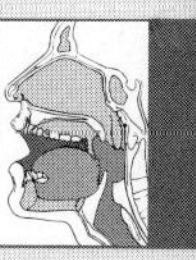

Tissues can be classified into four basic groups according to the shape of the cells, the amount of matrix surrounding them, and the function they perform:

1. Epithelium
2. Connective
3. Muscle
4. Nervous

The first group of tissue types we will study is epithelium. The other three tissue types are _______________, _______________, and _______________.

connective, muscle, nervous

EPITHELIUM 2.0

Epithelium is a basic tissue type composed of many cells that do the job or function of covering or lining body parts. Epithelial tissue contains many cells and little matrix. It does not contain blood vessels and is therefore **avascular.**

Epithelium can be described or classified by the shapes of its cells. Epithelium with flat cells is called **squamous epithelium.** Epithelium with cube-shaped cells is called **cuboidal epithelium.** Epithelium with tall cells is called **columnar** epithelium. In the illustrations of these three types of epithelium, which is which?

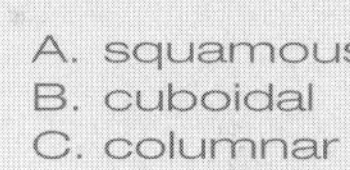

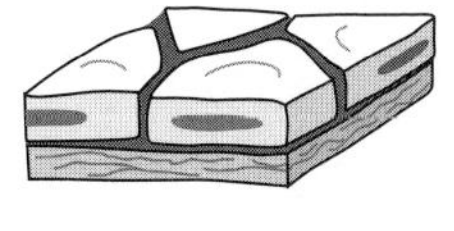

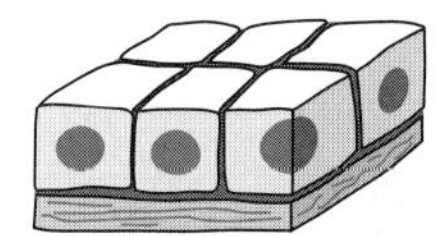

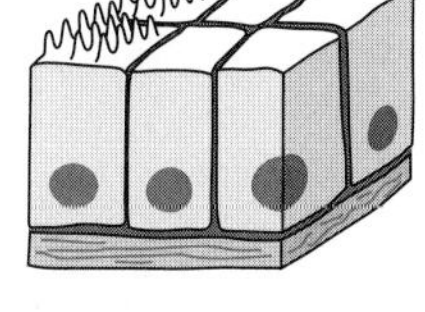

A _______________ B _______________ C _______________

Epithelium is also classified by the number of layers it has. If an epithelium is composed of only one layer of cells, it is a **simple epithelium.** If it has multiple layers, it is a **stratified epithelium.** Label the simple and stratified epithelia in the illustrations.

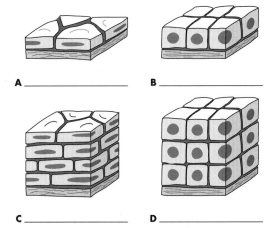

A. simple
B. simple
C. stratified
D. stratified

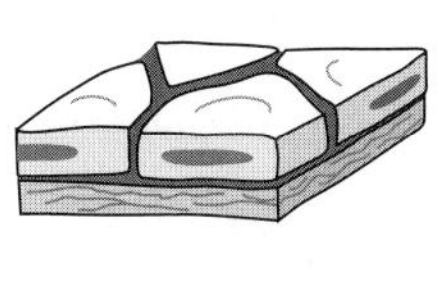

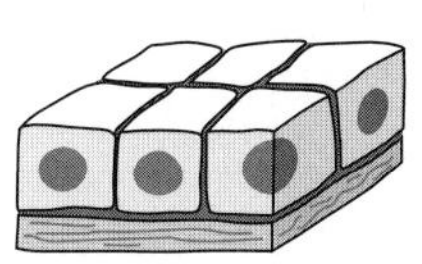

A _______________ B _______________

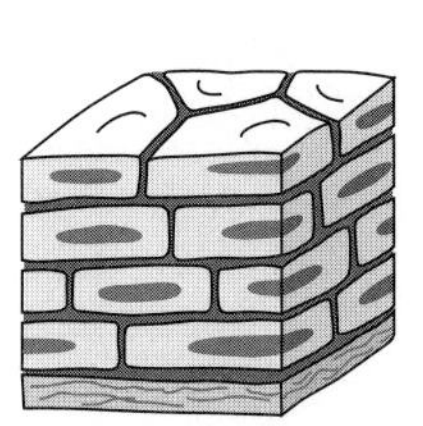

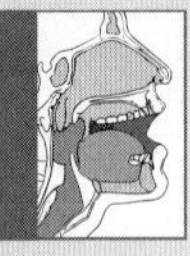

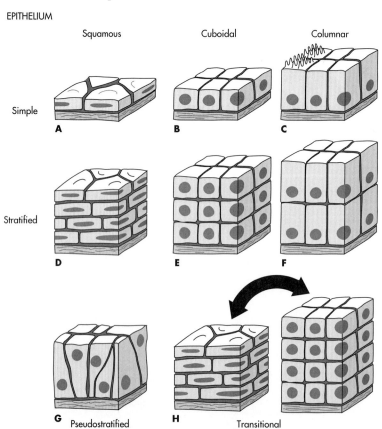

stratified cuboidal

Putting both terms together we can describe any epithelium. For example, an epithelium that is made of many layers of flat cells is called a **stratified squamous epithelium.** An epithelium composed of one layer of tall cells would be a **simple columnar epithelium.** What would an epithelium made up of many layers of cube-shaped cells be called?

In the accompanying diagram of all the varieties of epithelium, you will note two exceptions. **Pseudostratified epithelium** is actually one layer of cells that looks like many because of the uneven levels of nuclei present. Pseudostratified epithelium often has projections on its cells called **cilia.** Pseudostratified epithelium is a tissue type found often within the lining of the respiratory system.

Transitional epithelium refers to the epithelium of the bladder, which, when stretched out, looks like stratified squamous and, when relaxed, looks like stratified cuboidal.

Examples of the types of epithelium are as follows:

A. Simple squamous: peritoneum
B. Simple cuboidal: ducts of glands
C. Simple columnar: digestive tract lining
D. Stratified squamous: epidermis, mucosa
E. Stratified cuboidal: liver
F. Stratified columnar: glands
G. Pseudostratified: respiratory epithelium
H. Transitional: bladder epithelium

EPITHELIUM

Squamous
Cuboidal
Columnar
Simple
A
B
C
Stratified
D
E
F
G Pseudostratified
H Transitional

Identify the types of epithelium in the diagram. Check your answers with the previous diagram.

Epithelium, then, is a ______________ or ______________ tissue with ______________ cells and little ______________. It has no blood vessels and is ______________.

lining, covering, many, matrix, avascular

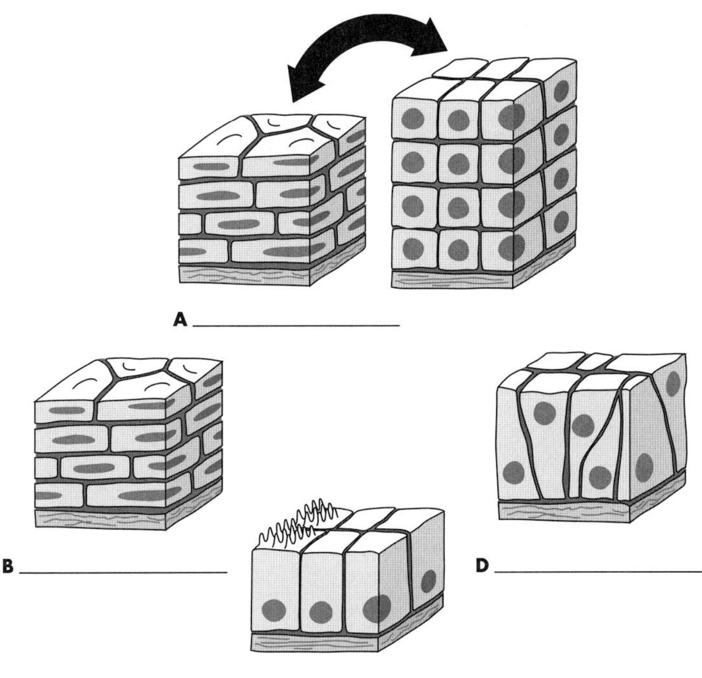

A. transitional
B. stratified squamos
C. simple columnar
D. pseudostratifed

Glands

2.1

Glands fall under the classification of epithelium because of the way in which they develop. They develop from the epithelial surfaces of the embryo, as shown in the illustration. Epithelial cells grow downward into the future connective tissue and develop saclike shapes connected to the surface by tubes. The sacs formed, which will be covered in connective tissue, are the **secretory units** of the gland. This is where the cells lining the unit will dump their cell product to be stored. The tubes leading away from them are the glands **ducts.** These ducts help lead the cell product out of the gland to the surface of the epithelium. Not all glands have ducts. Those that do are call **exocrine glands** and those that do not are called **endocrine glands.** Ductless glands, or ______________ glands, simply expel their product or secretion out into their surroundings, usually near blood vessels.

endocrine

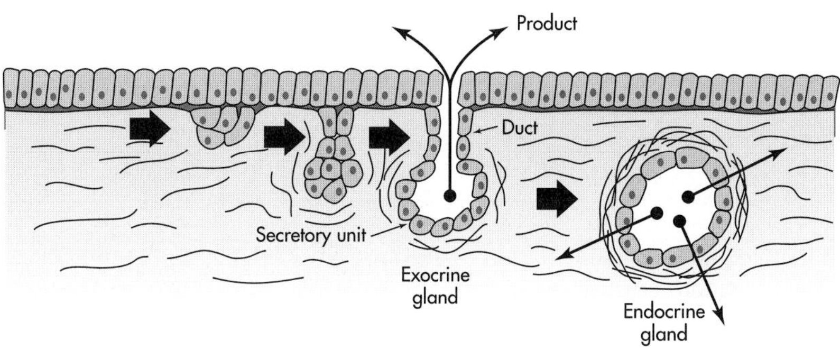

secretory unit, exocrine

The working part of the gland, producing a cell product is called its ______________. If it has a duct it is a(n) ______________ gland.

Glands are classified by the shape and number of secretory units. A gland with units shaped like Figure A is called an **acinar gland.** A gland with units shaped like Figure B is a **tubular gland.**

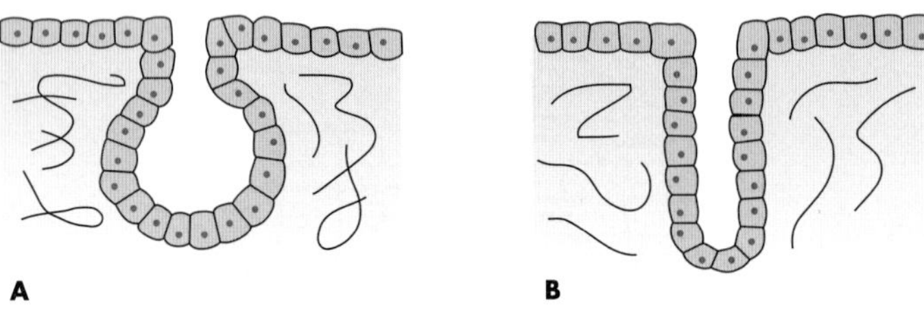

---

compound acinar

Glands with only one secretory unit are called **simple glands.** Glands with multiple units are called **compound glands.** Figure B is an example of a sweat gland. It is a simple tubular gland. Figure A is a salivary gland. It is a ______________ gland.

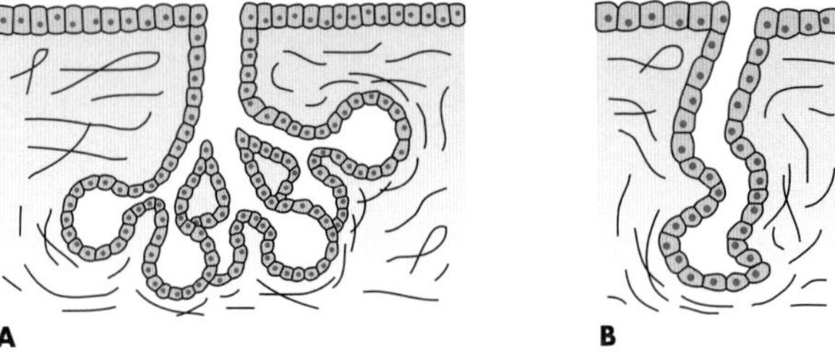

3.0 MUSCLE TISSUE

The second type of tissue is **muscle tissue.** It is the only tissue that can contract: it is **contractile.** It is made up of cells that are built to contract when stimulated. That type of tissue is composed of **muscle fibers,** which are, in turn, composed of contractile protein rods, which, when stimulated, will slide into or past each other as shown.

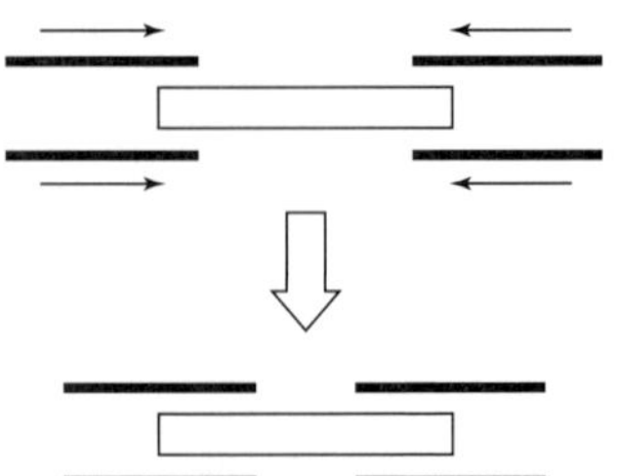

Muscle tissue is found in the body in one of three types: (1) skeletal muscle, (2) cardiac muscle, or (3) smooth muscle.

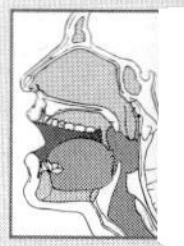

Skeletal muscle tissue forms the bulk of the muscles of the body that voluntarily move all the limbs of the body and head and trunk. It is composed of very long bundles of cells, so long that each cell or fiber needs many nuclei to operate. Skeletal muscle is multinucleate. Skeletal muscle shows evidence of its contractile proteins in the form of bands or stripes. Striping in muscle tissue is called striations: skeletal muscle is striated. The diagram shows what skeletal muscle looks like under the microscope.

Skeletal

Cardiac muscle is striated also, but its cells are smaller and connected together, appearing as many interconnected branches. The connections between cells are called **intercalated disks** and are important to the quick communication between cells and their subsequent simultaneous response. This action is important, as this type of muscle is found in the heart.

Cardiac muscle is operated on an **involuntary** level. You do not have to consciously think about making your heart beat. The diagram shows what it looks like under the microscope.

Cardiac

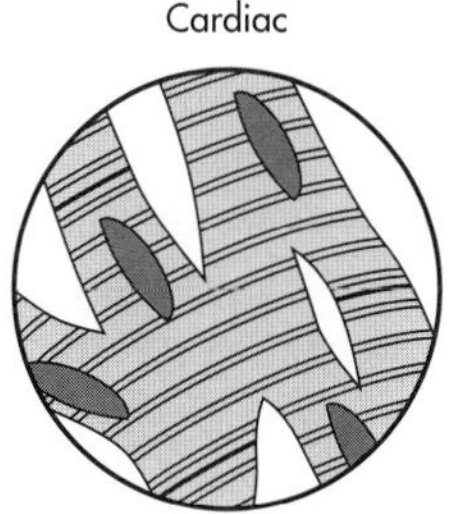

The third type of muscle tissue is **smooth muscle.** It has contractile proteins, but they are not as readily visible so this cell is not striated. The cells are comparatively small and spindle-shaped and have only one nucleus per cell.

Smooth muscle is found within the walls of many organs and glands, helping to operate them. Smooth muscle, therefore, is also involuntary. The diagram shows what it looks like under the microscope.

Smooth

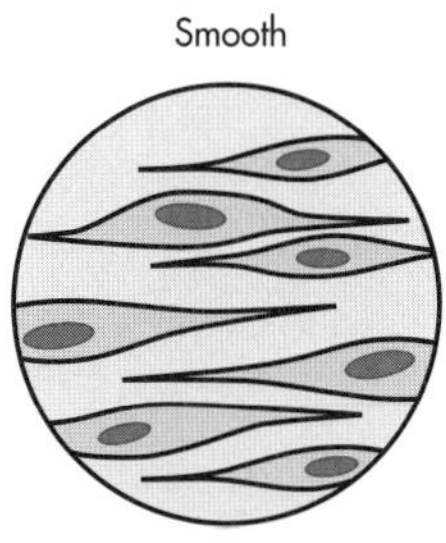

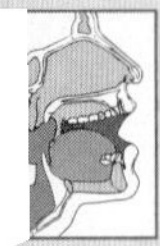

A. smooth
B. cardiac
C. skeletal

Identify the types of muscle tissue in the drawing and discuss what makes them different from each other. Consult the previous pages for your answers.

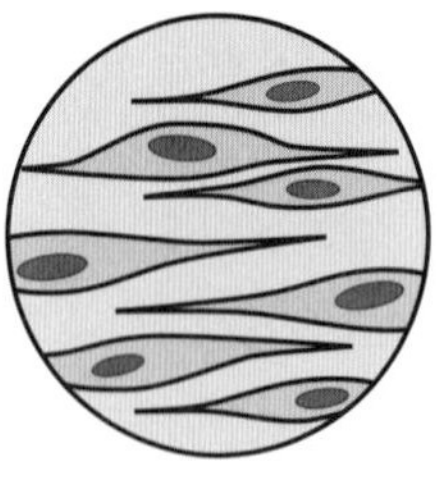

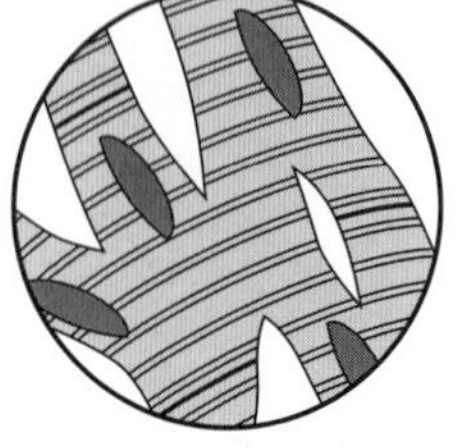

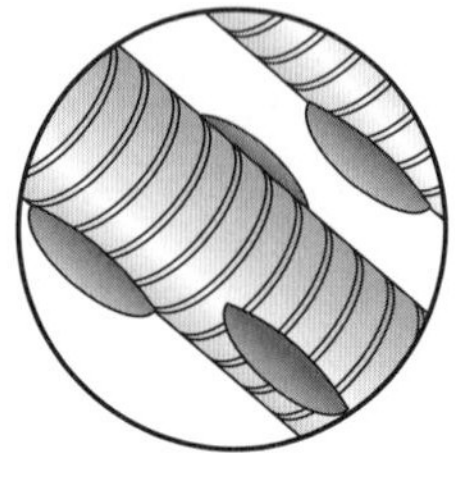

A ________________ B ________________ C ________________

4.0 NERVOUS TISSUE

The third type of tissue is called nervous tissue. It is also excitable like muscular tissue but does not contract. Nervous tissue is capable of generating an electrochemical signal that is passed along from one cell to the next.

The two types of cells of which nervous tissue is composed are neurons and supporting cells. **Neurons** are the basic functioning unit of the nervous system and are the cells that actually transmit messages throughout the body. **Supporting cells,** or **neuroglia,** are the cells that nourish and maintain the neurons.

The neuron looks, in general, like the diagram shown. There are many types of neurons with differently shaped cell bodies and **processes,** that is, the spidery extensions off of the main cell body. Processes fall into two categories: processes that receive signals, or **dendrites,** and processes that send out signals, or **axons.** Axons may or may not be insulated or have a **myelin sheath.**

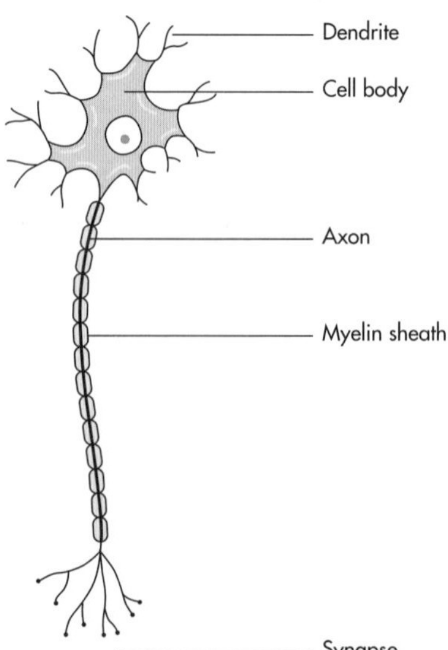

What types of tissue are illustrated by the accompanying diagrams?

A. epithelium
B. muscle
C. nervous

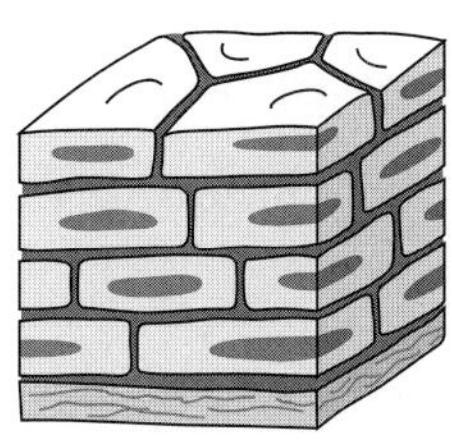

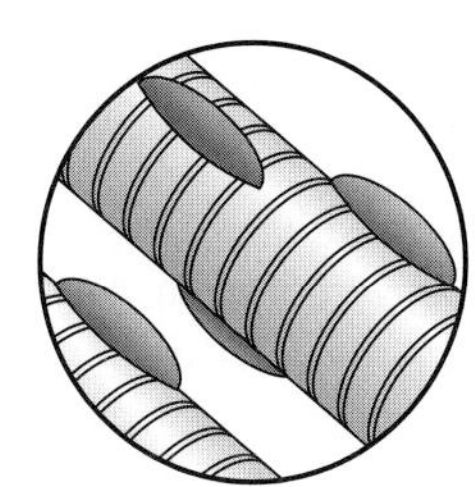

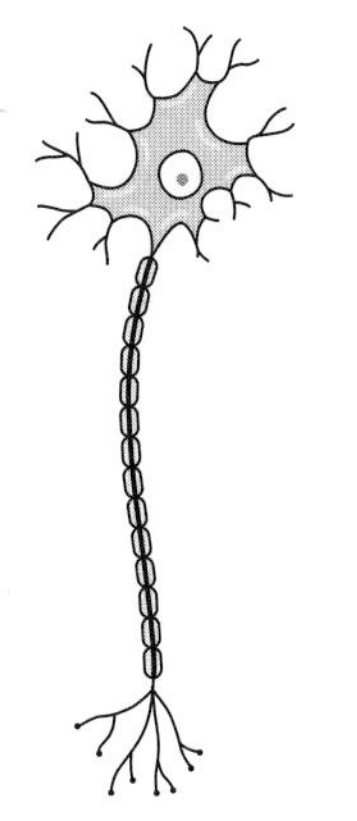

A ________________ B ________________ C ________________

This cell is a ______________. Label its dendrites, axon, and cell body. The jump that a nerve signal has to make between cells is called a **synapse.**

neuron

A. dendrite
B. cell body
C. axon
D. myelin sheath
E. synapse

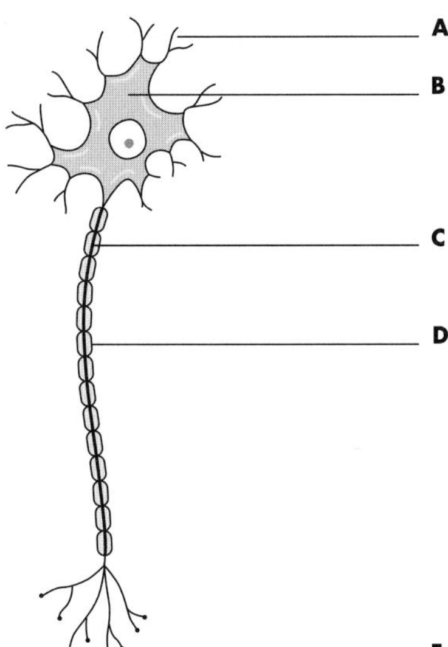

CONNECTIVE TISSUE 5.0

The fourth or last type of tissue is called **connective tissue.** Connective tissue is the largest group and contains a wide variety of seemingly different types. The thing they all have in common is that connective tissue has few cells and lots of matrix. That is, the cells of connective tissue surround themselves with their own cell products. All connective tissues begin with a **fibrous matrix.**

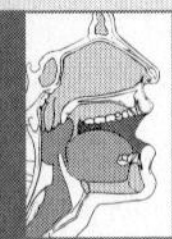

The fibers of connective tissue are made by cells called **fibroblasts** and are of three types in general: reticular fibers, collagen fibers, and elastic fibers.

Reticular fibers are actually an immature form of collagen fibers, being very thin, irregular versions of the latter.

Collagen is a tough, resilient protein that forms fibrils, which band together to make larger collagen fibers. These fibers are the most common type and form one of the basic building blocks of the body, usually in the form of nets or sheets or bundles.

Elastic fibers are formed from a different protein called elastin, and although they are smaller, they function differently than collagen. Where collagen gives strength and support, elastic fibers have spring and allow a tissue to have some "give" or spring back when pressure is removed. All three fibers are diagrammed as they appear under the microscope.

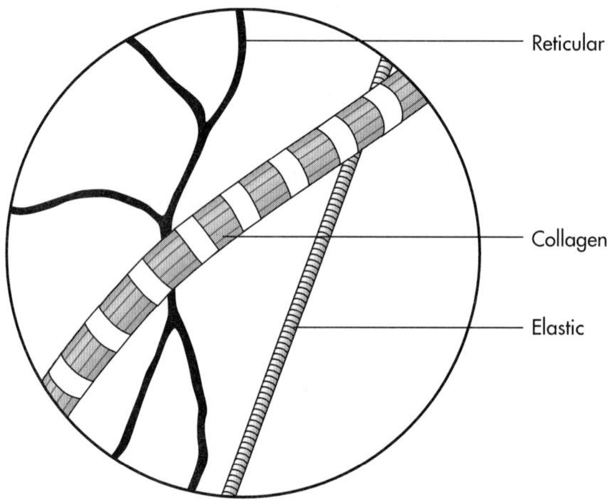

reticular, collagen, elastic

What are the three types of connective tissue fibers?

5.1 Generalized Connective Tissue

Connective tissue may be grouped into two major types: **generalized connective tissue** and **specialized connective tissue.**

Generalized connective tissue is the main "glue" of the body. It is found between and surrounding all organs of the body. It is made mainly of cells and fibrous matrix.

Generalized connective tissue is classified by its appearance or structure. If the fibers are tightly packed, it is a **dense connective tissue.** If the fibers are loosely packed, it is a **loose connective tissue.**

If the fibers are arranged in parallel rows, the connective tissue is called **regular;** if the fibers are randomly arranged it is called **irregular.**

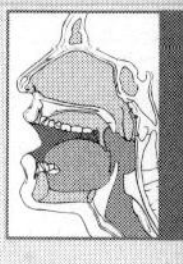

Four types of generalized connective tissue are diagrammed here: (1) **dense regular,** (2) **dense irregular,** (3) **loose regular,** and (4) **loose irregular.**

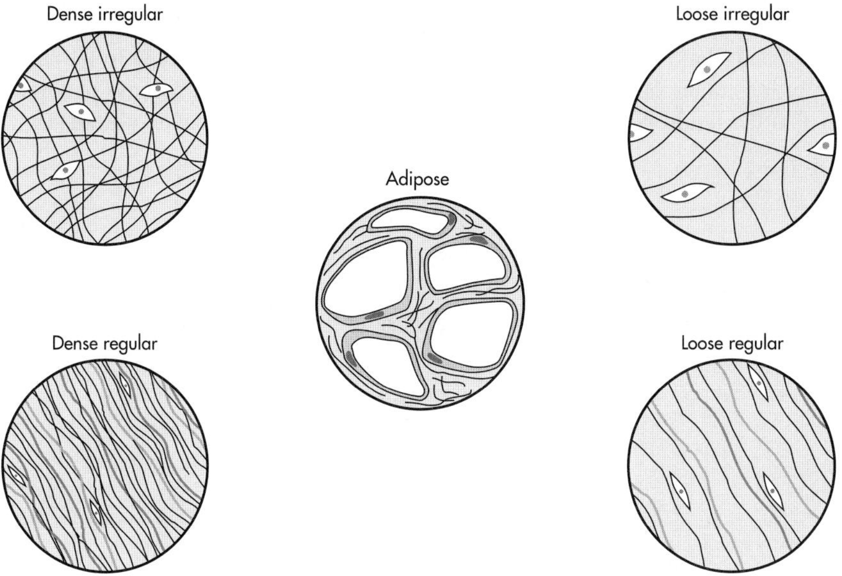

A fifth "type" shown in the middle is **adipose** or fatty tissue. It has very large **fat cells,** which contain a large fat dropule that squeezes the rest of the cell and nucleus to the outside. A few fibers are found between the cells.

Generalized connective tissue examples are as follows:

1. Dense regular: tendons and ligaments
2. Dense irregular: capsules
3. Loose regular: fascia
4. Loose irregular: fascia

Which type of generalized connective tissue is illustrated here? What type of fibers are found in this tissue? Where might one find this type of tissue? Does it have many or few cells?

dense regular, collagen, tendons and ligaments, few

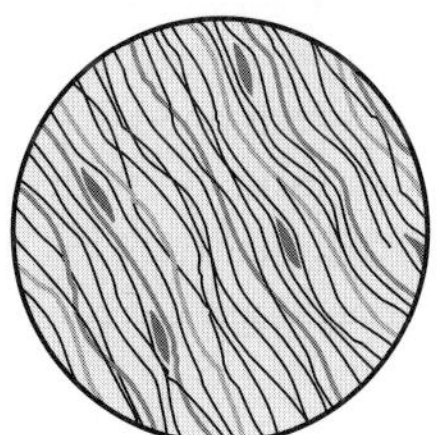

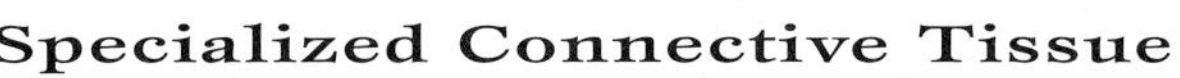

Specialized Connective Tissue

5.2

All other connective tissue is called **specialized.** It is so named because both cells and matrix are very unique and perform a very specialized function. Remember that all connective tissue has few cells and lots of ______________ and that matrix contains fibers.

matrix

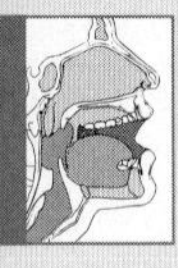

BLOOD

The first type of specialized connective tissue is **blood.** At first, this may not appear to be a connective tissue, that is, few cells in a fibrous matrix. The matrix is liquid, or **serum.** Many red and white cells travel within this matrix. If blood is exposed to the air, the fibrous portion can be observed. The serum develops fibers, or **clot,** because of several factors within the liquid portion and with the aid of pieces of cells called **platelets.**

The cells of blood fall into two categories: (1) red cells or **erythrocytes** and (2) white cells or **leukocytes.** Diagrammed here is a sample of blood as seen under the microscope. Leukocytes are the larger cells and erythrocytes are the smaller disk-shaped cells, which predominate.

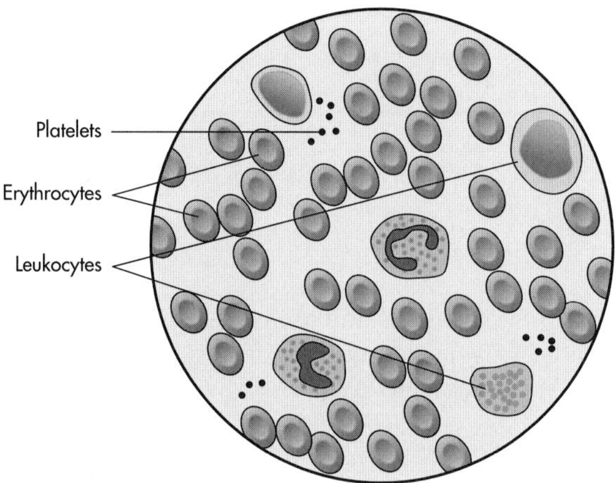

Erythrocytes

_______________ are biconcave disk-shaped cells that have no nuclei when mature. Their primary function is the transportation of oxygen (O_2) and carbon dioxide (CO_2) in the body. They pick up O_2 at the lungs and distribute it to cells and pick up waste CO_2 and take it back to the lungs for disposal.

Leukocytes

_______________ or white cells fall into two major types: granulocytes and agranulocytes. **Granulocytes** comprise three types of white cells with large packets of chemicals within their cells or granules. They are named by their color on staining and are (1) **eosinophils** (red), (2) **basophils** (blue), and (3) **neutrophils** (both). Granulocytes are defense cells of the blood, using their chemically laden granules and cell bodies to fight off foreign invaders, that is, bacteria, viruses, grafts, cancer cells. They either use a chemical attack or engulf and digest the invaders.

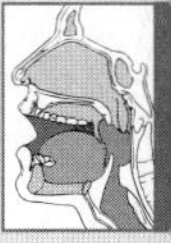

The other type of white cells without large granules are the lymphocytes and monocytes. Both have large nuclei and little cytoplasm. **Monocytes** are the larger of the two and may be found outside the circulatory system. **Lymphocytes** are smaller cells that reside mainly in the lymphatic and blood systems, but can travel anywhere when needed to launch a chemical attack against invaders. There are two types of lymphocytes: **B lymphocytes** and **T lymphocytes** (which originally came from the thymus).

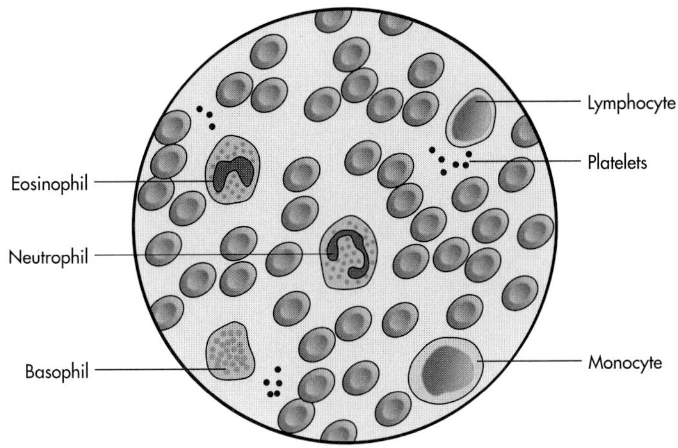

In the diagram of the blood, label the various cell types. Explain the function of each. Refer to the preceding text and diagram for explanations.

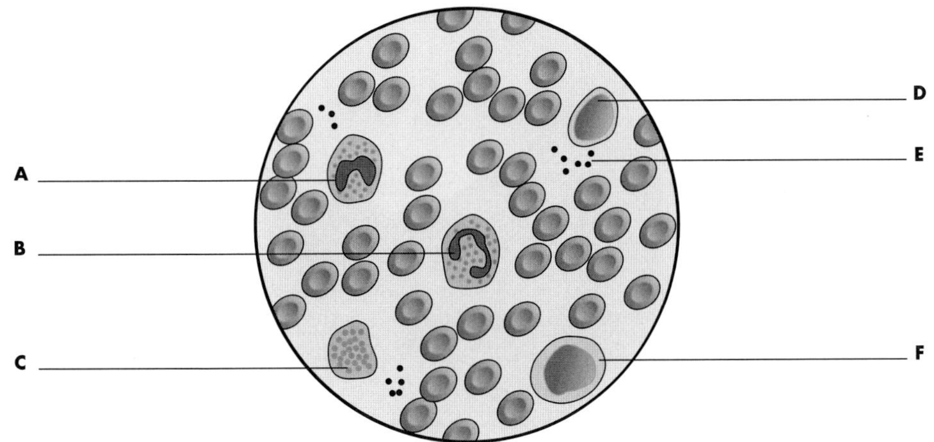

A. eosinophil
B. neutrophil
C. basophil
D. lympocyte
E. platelets
F. monocyte

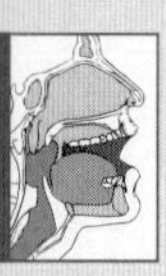

CARTILAGE

The cells of cartilage are called **chondrocytes.** They have created a stiff, gelatinous matrix around themselves, called **cartilage.** This tissue is a resilient yet firm type of connective tissue, found in areas that need a strong cushion. The chondrocytes, when they are actively producing cartilage matrix, are called **chondroblasts.** Note the last portion of the word, "-blasts." This little word is part of the names of all cells of any hard tissue that is in the process of building matrix, or **deposition.** The opposite type of cell is called a **"-clast,"** and its function is different. It is a totally different cell that breaks down or "chews up" matrix. For example, **chondroclasts** tear down cartilage or resorb it. Which type of cell deposits matrix?

'blast cell

cartilage

Cartilage is diagrammed here as it appears under the microscope. Cartilage is avascular. Chondrocytes are often "nested" together in pairs or in rows of single cells, surrounded on all sides by an apparently clear ______________ matrix. What is not visible are the fibers within that matrix.

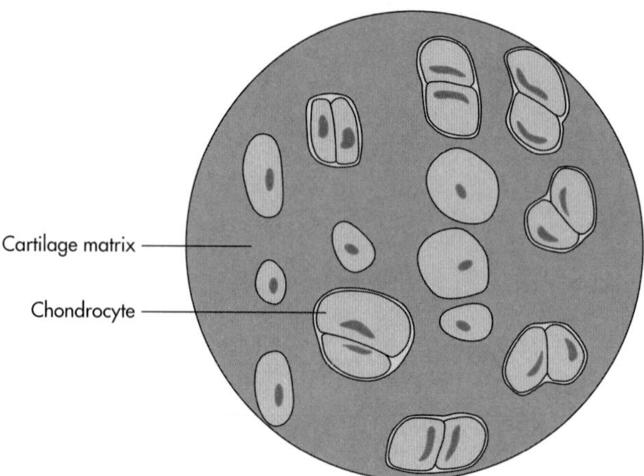

Cartilage is formed by a process that occurs in all hard tissues: calcification. **Calcification** is the process by which hard tissues become hard. It begins with the cells creating a fibrous matrix or network around themselves. This network serves as a pattern or template for the next step. Calcium salts from the bloodstream are attracted to this network and begin to line up on it.

Calcium salts are the building blocks of hard tissues. They develop bigger and more complex crystals within the network. One of the first types of crystals built is called **hydroxyapatite,** and this crystal is common to all the hard tissues. Further elaboration of hydroxyapatite produces the wide variety of hard tissue matrices: cartilage, bone, enamel, and so on.

3, 2, 1, 4

Place the steps leading to calcification in order:

_____ Crystallization of hydroxyapatite
_____ Attraction of calcium salts
_____ Creation of a fibrous matrix
_____ Crystallization of the specific matrix

Cartilage cells are called ______________ when they are actively making matrix and ______________ when they are at rest. The hard matrix, cartilage, is made by the process of ______________.

chondroblasts, chondrocytes, calcification

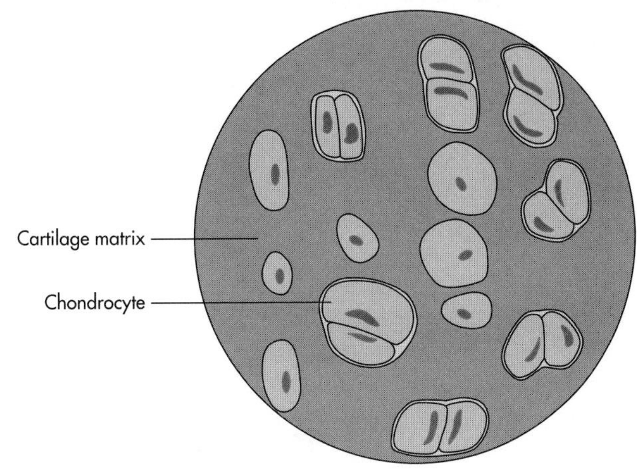

BONE

This hard tissue contains spider-shaped cells called **osteocytes.** Osteocytes, when actively creating bone tissue, are called **osteoblasts.** There are other giant, multinucleate cells around bone called **osteoclasts.** Remember that -blasts build and -clasts tear down. ______________ are responsible for the resorption of bone. In an adult, bone tissue reaches a balance between these two actions: **deposition** (building up) and **resorption** (tearing down). Osteoblasts continually lay down new bone, whereas osteoclasts get rid of old bone; so, bone tissue is in a constant state of turnover.

Osteclasts

Osteocytes create bone matrix around themselves, as do chondrocytes. But bone cells do not isolate themselves as do cartilage cells. Look at the diagram of an osteocyte. The cell body has several cell processes jutting off itself. These processes are like "fingers" that maintain contact with other bone cells, to communicate and to pass along nutrients and waste products. Bone cells act together as a community.

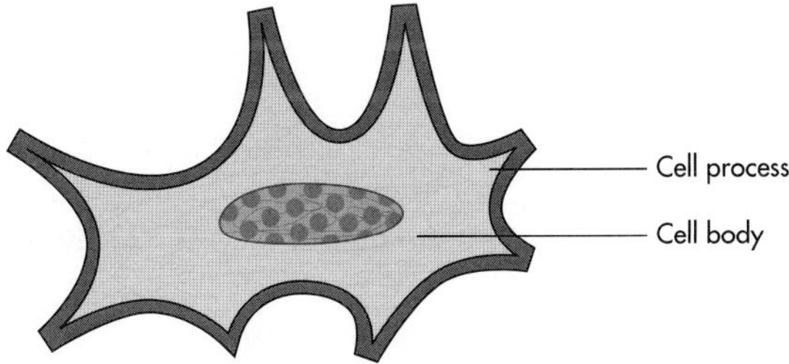

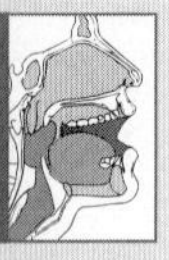

As the osteoblasts create bone matrix around themselves, the matrix follows the shape of the cells. There is a space within the bone for the cell body called a **lacuna** ("little lake") and a space around the process called a **canaliculus** ("little canal"). If you were to remove the cell from bone and leave the matrix, as many slide preparations do, it would leave a spider-shaped hole in the bone as shown.

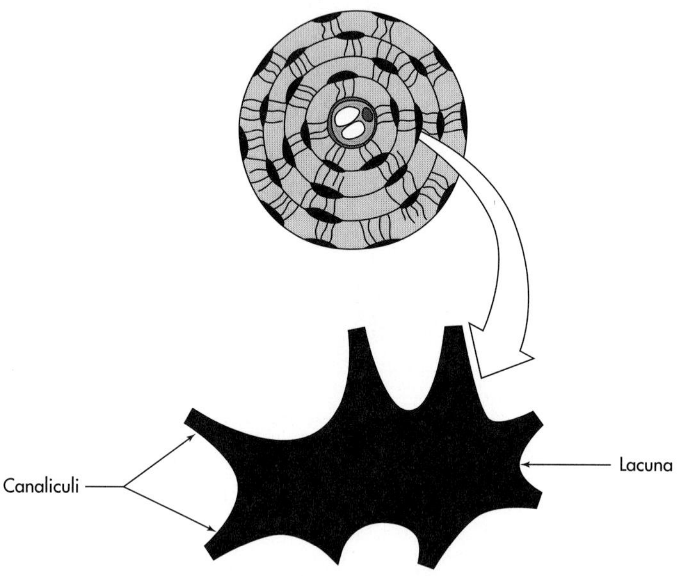

process in canaliculus, body in lacuna

Label the lacunae and canaliculi. Which part of the osteocyte fits in each?

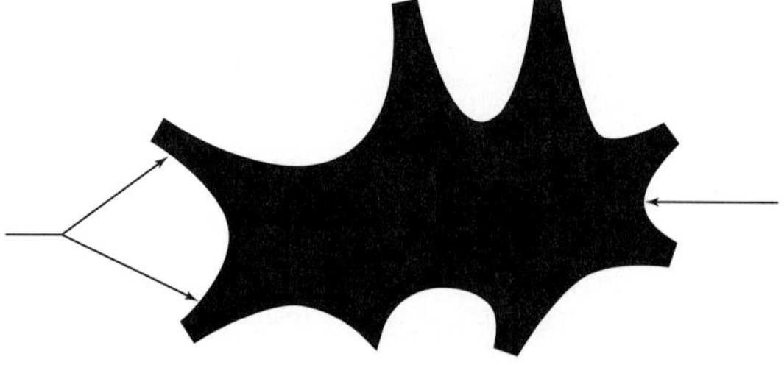

fibrous, calcium, Hydroxyapatite

Calcification of bone occurs in much the same way it does in other hard tissues. First, a ______________ matrix is laid down by the osteoblasts as a network on which to build. Second, ______________ salts are attracted from the bloodstream to the network and crystallization begins. ______________ crystals are built first, and eventually the more elaborate crystals of bone are finished. Bone matrix then surrounds the cell.

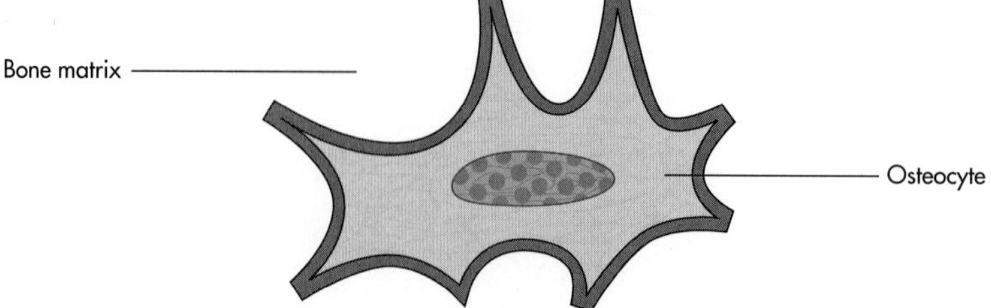

Bone is deposited by the bone cells in layers or **laminae.** In some areas the bone cells will lay down bone in circles, or rings, much the way a tree lays down rings of woody growth. The diagram illustrates a section through a piece of bone where this has happened. Each one of these "trees" with ring-shaped laminae is called an **osteon.** Within each osteon, in the middle, is a hollow area filled with blood vessels and nervous tissue. The vertical "tubes" are called **haversian canals** and the horizontal ones are **Volkmann's canals.**

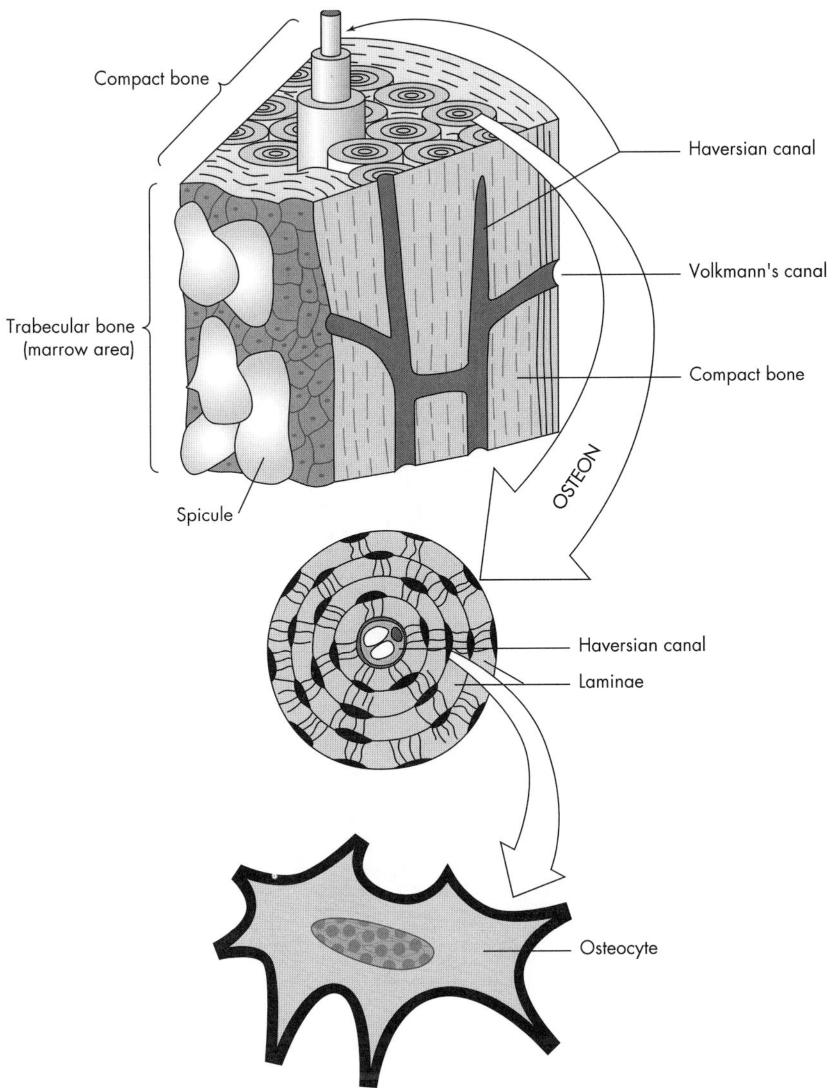

Several osteons are packed together to form this **compact** or cortigal bone. In other areas, such as in the **marrow area** of bone, the cells form more irregular layers and make looser-packed spicules or pieces of bone. This type of bone is called loose, spongy, or **trabecular bone.** Find the compact **bone** and trabecular **bone.**

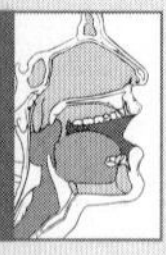

A. compact bone
B. trabecular bone
C. haversian canal
D. Volkmann's canal
E. laminae
F. cell process
G. osteocyte cell body

Label the parts of the diagrams shown here. Make reference to the preceding text and diagram for the correct answers.

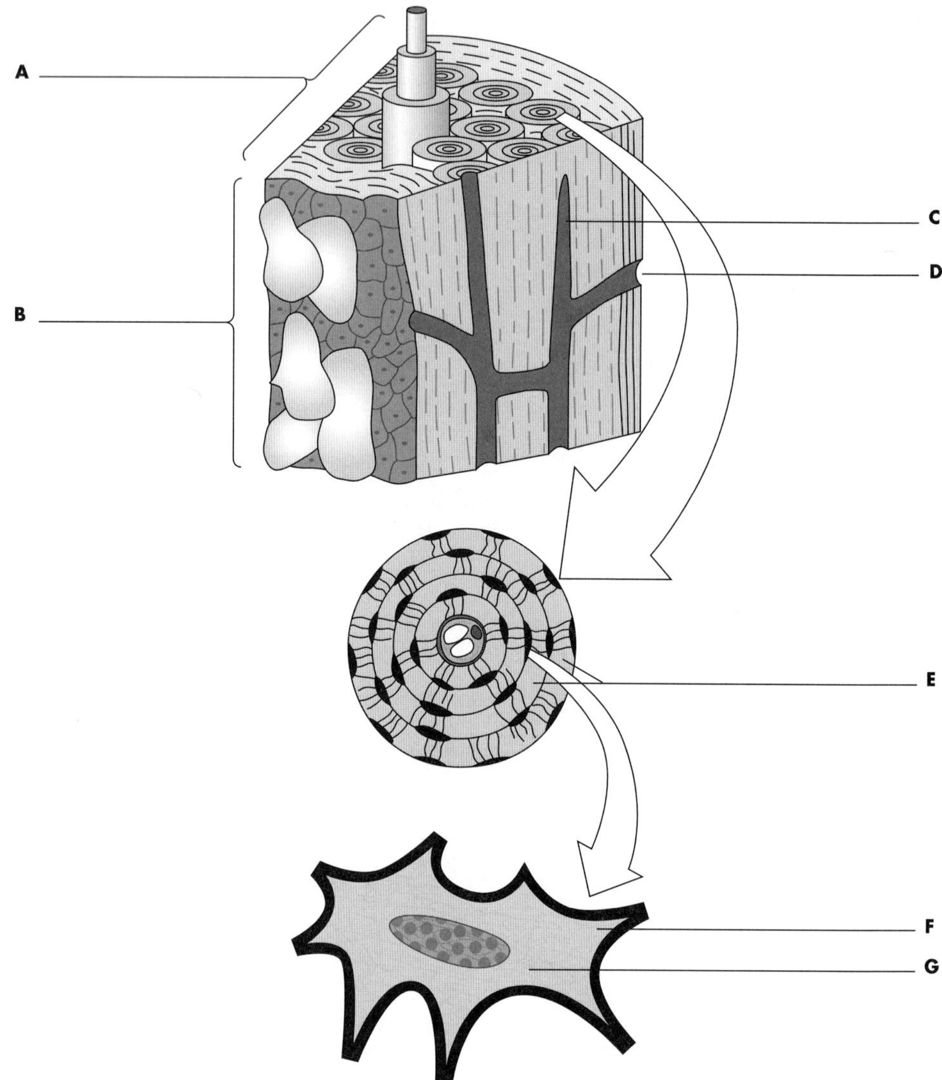

Bone originates from the osteoblasts creating the situation for bone matrix to form. In the developing human this can occur in one of two ways. First, bone can develop from an area that first has a membrane in that location. An example is the skull. The embryo needs to build large, yet flexible plates of bone to cover the brain. Membrane tissue first covers the top of the brain. As blood vessels invade the area, bone cells populate the membranous area and begin to build bone. This type of development is called **membranous bone development.**

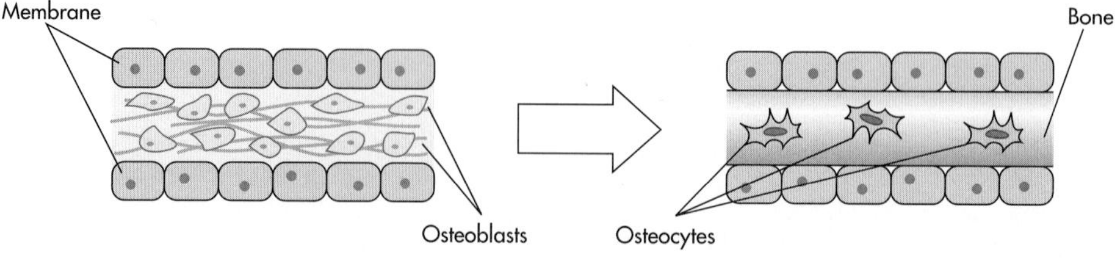

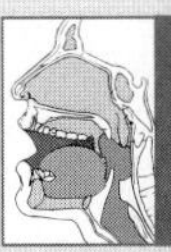

Below the brain, a strong support is needed immediately and a plate of cartilage is first developed to hold up the developing brain. As time goes on, more support is needed and bone tissue replaces the cartilage, in much the same shape. The bone cells use the cartilage they replace as a model or template, to build bone. The bone begins to replace the cartilage as soon as blood vessels invade, bringing the osteoblasts with them. This type of bone development is called **endochondral bone development.**

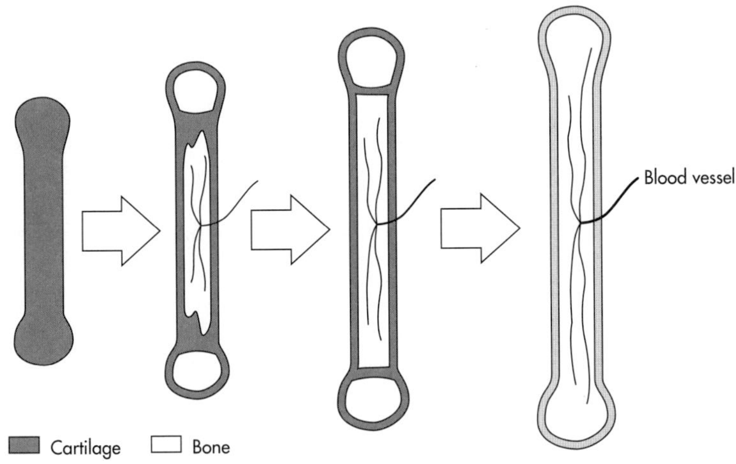

Most bones in the body are built by endochondral type development, but the skull is a unique area that shows both types of development.

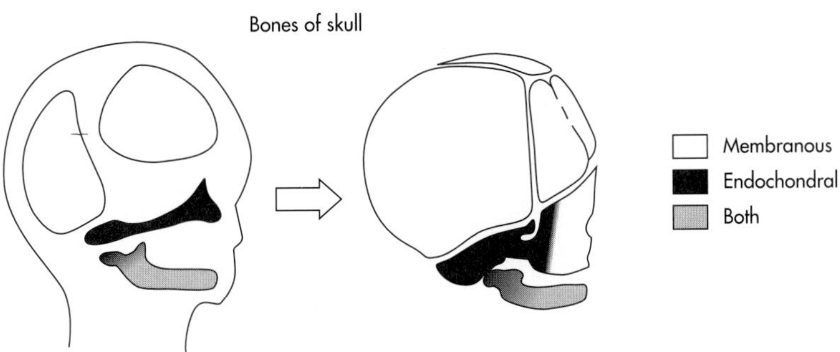

Which type of bone development is occurring here? Note the space between the bones; this space will remain there until a year or so after birth. It is called a **fontanel.** The "cracks" or smaller spaces between the bones will join together and may eventually fuse in old age. These joints or places where two bones meet are called **sutures.**

membranous

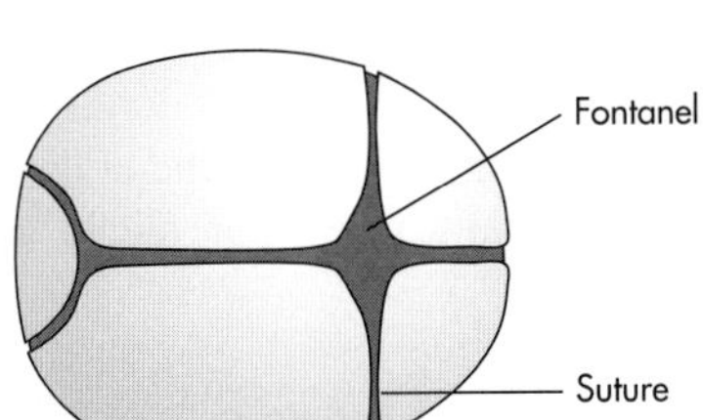

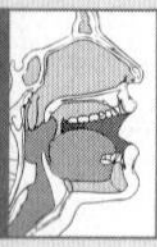

6.0 SKIN VERSUS MUCOSA

epithelium, muscle, nervous, connective

So far, we have looked at the four basic tissue types: ____________, ____________, ____________, and ____________. Now we will see how various parts of the head and neck are composed of the four tissues or how they are combined to make organs and systems.

epidermis

Epidermis is the outermost layer of the skin. It is classified as an epithelium because it is a tissue composed of lots of layers of flat cells, with no blood vessels and little matrix. Do not confuse the two words *epidermis* and *epithelium,* though they are similar! The top layer of the skin is ____________.

stratified squamous

Epidermis is a ____________-type epithelium, because it has many layers of flat cells.

The drawing illustrates a section of skin. It shows the **epidermis** as the topmost layer. Below the epidermis is the **dermis.** Dermis is classified as a connective tissue, because it contains lots of collagen fibers, blood vessels, and few cells. Together epidermis and dermis make up the **organ** skin, which has the job of covering and protecting the body.

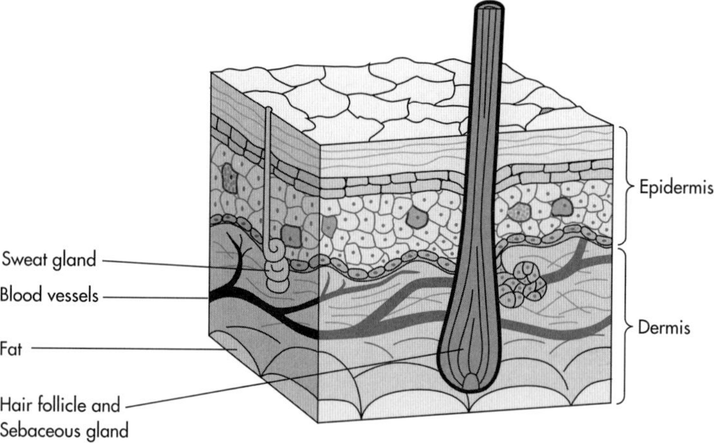

Note the large structure piercing both dermis and epidermis. It is a hair follicle. Attached to the base of the follicle is an oil or **sebaceous gland.**

A coiled tubular gland called a **sweat gland** is also located in the dermis layer.

A layer of fat cells or **adipose** lies at the bottom of the dermis.

stratified squamous epithelium

Skin is divided into two major layers: epidermis and dermis. Epidermis is further divided into four layers, depending on the stage of life of the cells. Epidermis grows new cells constantly from the base up. Old cells lose their nuclei and die and are then shed. Epidermis is a ____________.

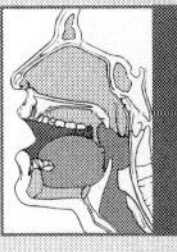

The first layer of growing cells is called **stratum basale.** Above this single layer of cells is **stratum spinosum,** named for the spiny appearance of the cells in this large layer. The "spines" are cell-to-cell connections. **Stratum lucidum** is an outer layer of clear cells that have lost their nuclei. **Stratum corneum** is the outermost layer of dying cells, which are shed as new cells grow beneath them. Find the layers in the accompanying diagram.

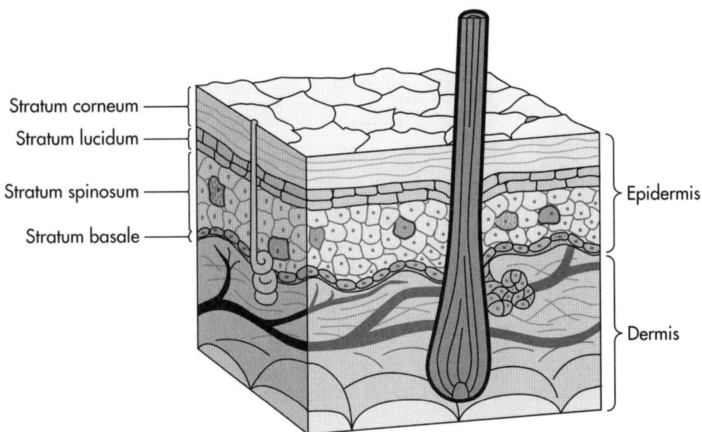

Melanocytes, keratinocytes

Within the four strata of the epidermis are specialized cells that give skin some of its characteristics. Pigment cells or **melanocytes** develop at the basal layers and release pigment, giving skin color and providing solar protection.

Keratinocytes are cells that produce a protein called **keratin.** Keratin acts as a waterproofing agent that makes this outer layer of the body resistant to the elements and to drying out. Although keratin is always found in skin and hair, it is sometimes found in mucosa where extra strength is needed. ______________ produce pigment that protects skin from light, and ______________ make skin waterproof and tough.

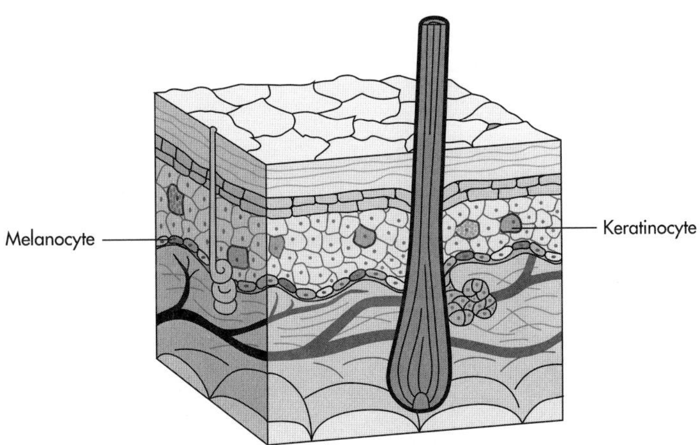

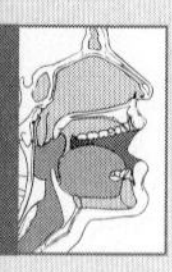

stratified squamous

The drawing illustrates **mucosa.** It is the equivalent of "internal skin," as it lines the oral cavity, pharynx, and all of the digestive tract in some form. In the oral cavity it appears in two layers: (1) many layers of flat cells (a ______________-type epithelium), and (2) a connective tissue base with many blood vessels. The epithelium is the **mucosa proper** and the connective tissue is the **lamina propria.** Compare these with the epidermis and dermis of the preceding drawing. Which structures are missing? Which are the same?

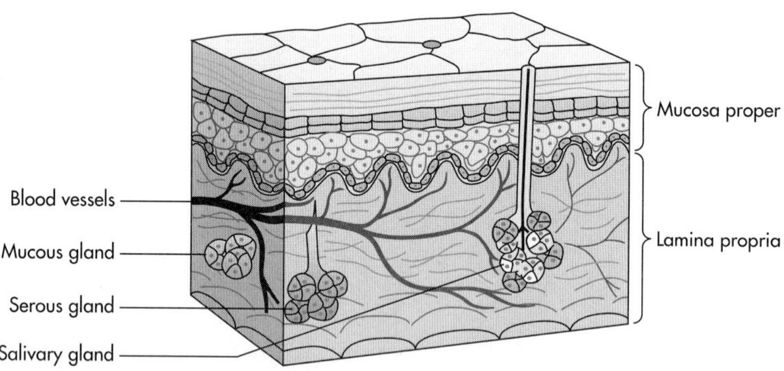

You should have noticed the salivary and mucous glands present in mucosa. Sweat glands, sebaceous glands, and hair are not present. Mucosa is also thinner, has more blood vessels, and must maintain a constantly moist surface. It does so with mucous and salivary glands.

Which of the drawings is mucosa and which is skin? Label the parts of each. Compare the characteristics of each. Refer to the previous text and diagrams for your answers.

A. skin thicker; has hair, sebaceous and sweat glands
B. mucosa thinner; has mucous and salivary glands

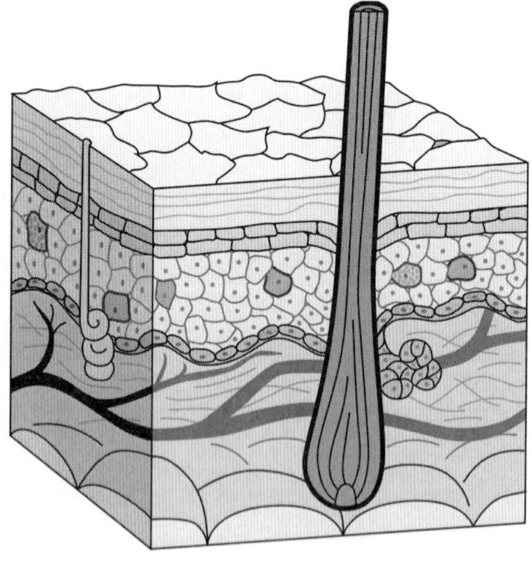

A ______________________________

____

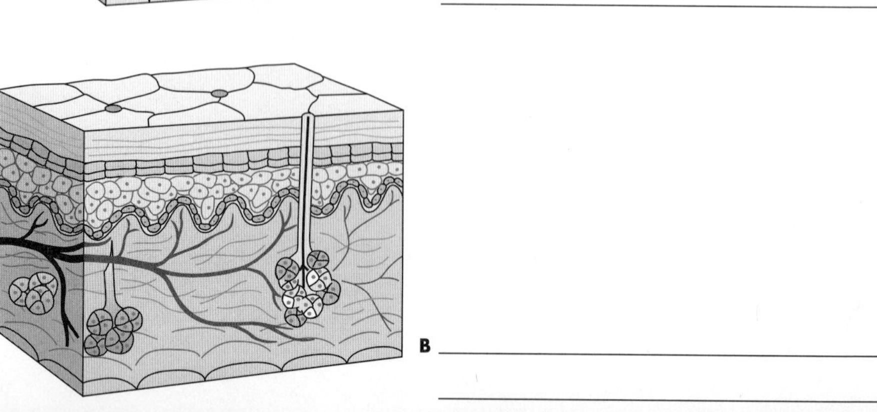

B ______________________________

____

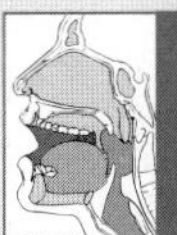

We now begin study of the specific oral tissues, but keep in mind that they are composed of the four basic tissues, just like skin and mucosa were. An example is the section through a lip and through a tooth. Which of the four tissue types might be found here?

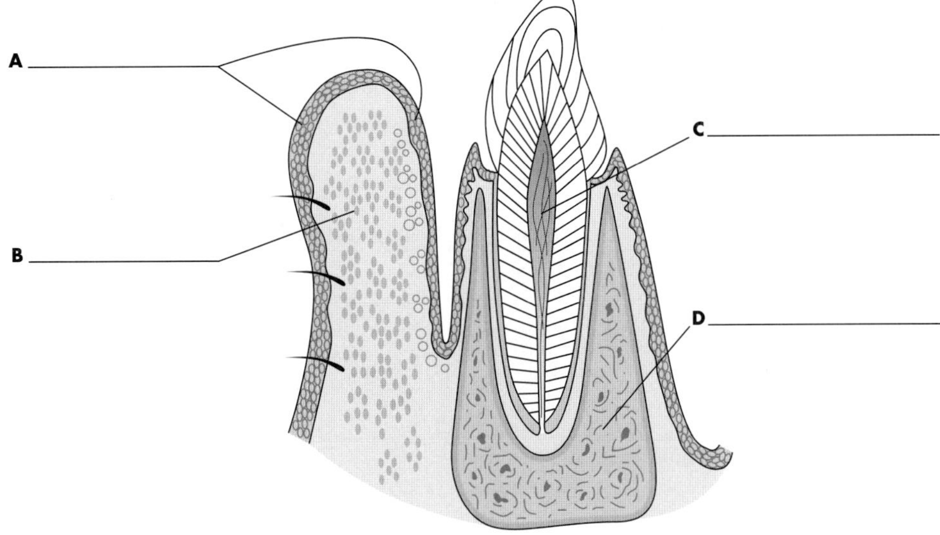

A. epithelium
B. muscle
C. nervous
D. connective

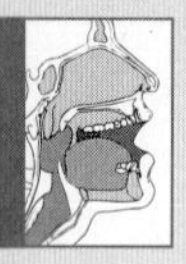

REVIEW TEST 1.1

SELECT THE CORRECT ANSWER.

1. All living organisms are built from those "blocks" of organized living material that we call
   a. nuclei
   b. organs
   c. cells
   d. tissue

2. A basic tissue type that is composed of cells with little matrix and no blood vessels and forms linings or coverings of the body is
   a. epithelium
   b. connective tissue
   c. muscle tissue
   d. nervous tissue

3. Glands belong to which basic tissue group?
   a. epithelium
   b. connective tissue
   c. muscle tissue
   d. nervous tissue

4. Blood is what type of basic tissue?
   a. epithelium
   b. connective tissue
   c. muscle tissue
   d. nervous tissue

5. A gland with multiple, sphere-shaped units is a ______________ type of gland.
   a. simple acinar
   b. simple tubular
   c. compound acinar
   d. compound tubular

6. A basic tissue type that is contractile when stimulated is ______________ tissue.
   a. epithelial
   b. connective
   c. muscle
   d. nervous

7. A basic tissue type that is excitable, but not contractile, is ______________ tissue.
   a. epithelial
   b. connective
   c. muscle
   d. nervous

8. A tissue type with large amounts of matrix and few cells in it is called ______________ tissue.
   a. epithelial
   b. connective
   c. muscle
   d. nervous

9. A generalized connective tissue with many tightly packed fibers arranged in random order is called ______________ connective tissue.
   a. dense regular
   b. loose regular
   c. dense irregular
   d. loose irregular

10. Tendons are made of ______________ connective tissue.
   a. dense regular
   b. loose regular
   c. dense irregular
   d. loose irregular

REVIEW TEST 1.2

SELECT THE CORRECT ANSWER.

1. The matrix portion of blood is its
   a. serum
   b. platelets
   c. leukocytes
   d. erythrocytes

2. Cartilage is vascular. True or false?

3. Rank the stages of calcification in order:

first ______________	a. attraction of calcium salts
second ______________	b. crystallization of hydroxyapatite
third ______________	c. crystallization of specific matrix
fourth ______________	d. creation of fibrous matrix

4. The building of hard connective tissues is called calcification or deposition; its destruction is called resorption. True or false?

5. Bone is a tissue undergoing constant cycles of deposition and resorption. True or false?

6. Bones of the skull are an example of endochondral formation only. True or false?

7. A joint in the top of the skull where two bones come together is called
   a. the TMJ
   b. a suture
   c. a fontanel

8. Which is not found in mucosa?
   a. mucous glands
   b. blood vessels
   c. salivary glands
   d. hair

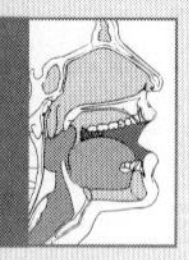

9. Skin is more suited to the outer body because
   a. it is thin
   b. it is very vascular
   c. it is moist
   d. it is thick and waterproof

10. Dermis is connective tissue. True or false?

REVIEW TEST 1.3

FILL IN THE CORRECT ANSWER(S).

1. The command center of the cell is its ______________.

2. A group of cells that perform a certain function together is called a(n) ______________.

3. The four basic tissue types are
   (a) ______________, (b) ______________, (c) ______________, and
   (d) ______________.

4. An epithelium composed of many layers of flat cells is a ______________-type epithelium.

5. ______________-type epithelium is found lining the respiratory system.

6. The working portion of a gland is called its ______________.

7. Three types of muscle are (a) ______________, (b) ______________, and (c) ______________.

8. The jump between neurons that its signal makes is called a(n) ______________.

9. Three types of fibers found in connective tissue are (a) ______________, (b) ______________, and (c) ______________.

10. Fat tissue is a type of generalized connective tissue and is called ______________ tissue.

REVIEW TEST 1.4

FILL IN THE CORRECT ANSWER(S).

1. Red cells of the blood are called ______________.

2. The cells of cartilage are called ______________. If they are actively producing cartilage they are called ______________.

3. The cells of bone at rest are called ______________. Cells that tear down bone are called ______________.

4. The "fingers" of the osteocyte that maintain contact with other cells are called ______________.

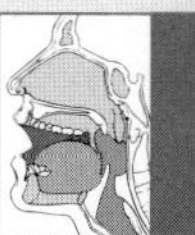

5. Areas where bone is laid down in concentric circles around blood vessels are called ______________.

6. A bone that originates from a cartilage model comes from ______________-type bone development.

7. The soft spot at the top of an infant's skull is called a(n) ______________ and is where the bony plates have not yet come together.

8. Epidermis is a ______________-type epithelium.

9. The four layers of epidermis are (a) ______________, (b) ______________, (c) ______________, and (d) ______________.

10. What is the protein formed in epidermis that rises to the top layers and creates "waterproofing" for the skin?

REVIEW TEST 1.5

LABEL THE DIAGRAMS.

1.

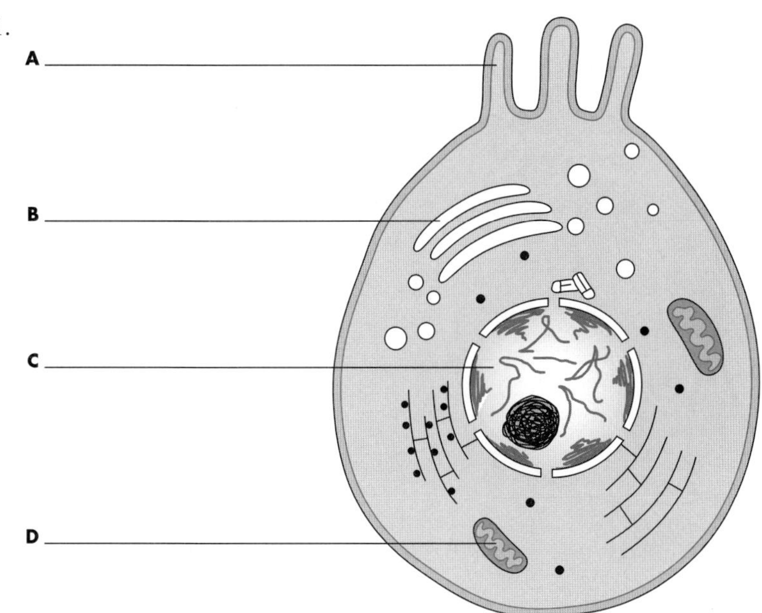

2.

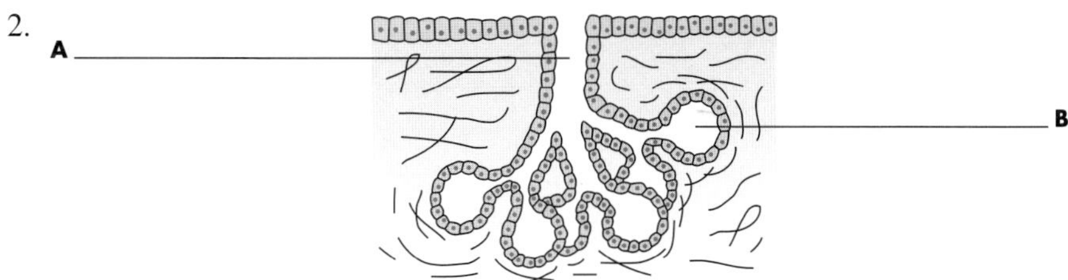

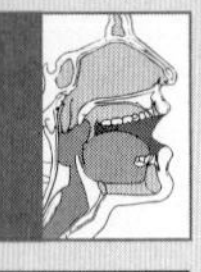

3.

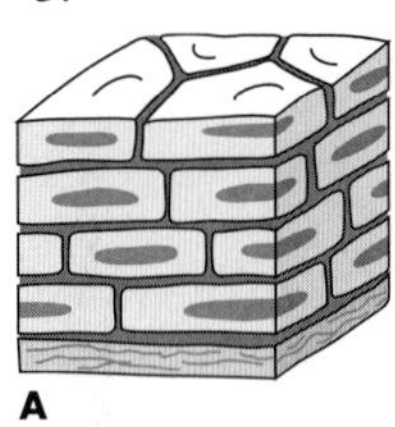
A ________________

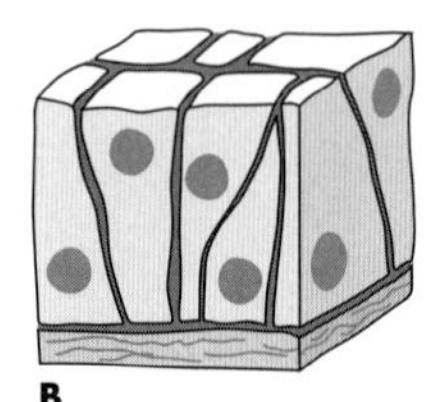
B ________________

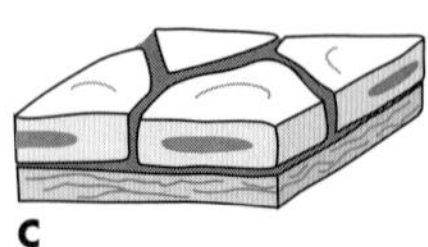
C ________________

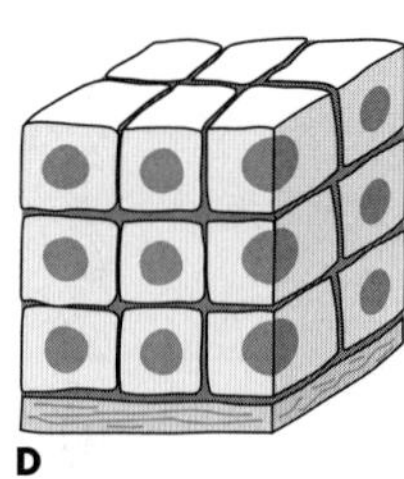
D ________________

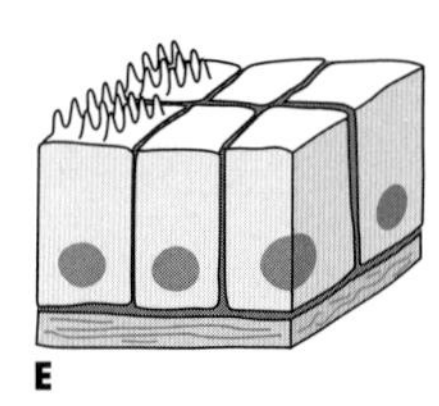
E ________________

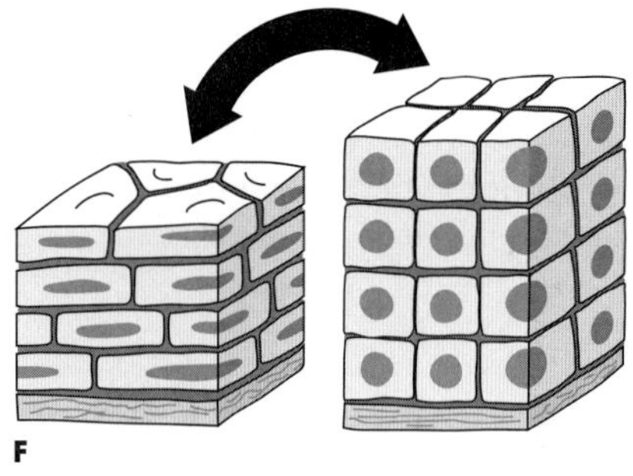
F ________________

4.

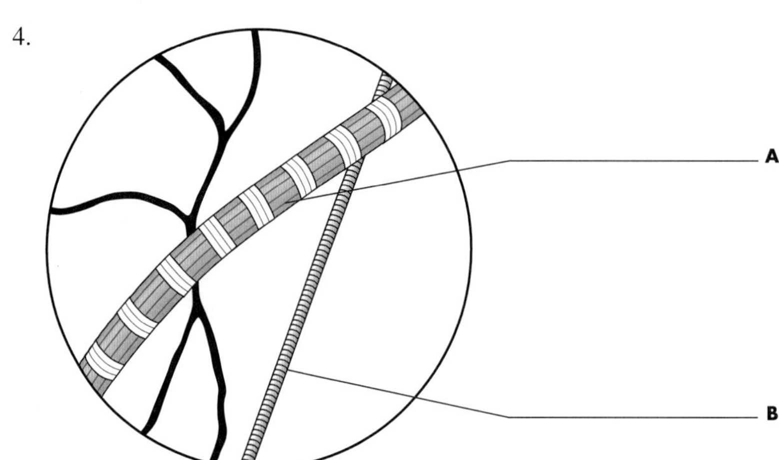

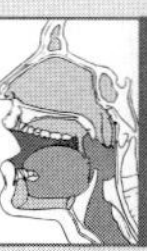

5.

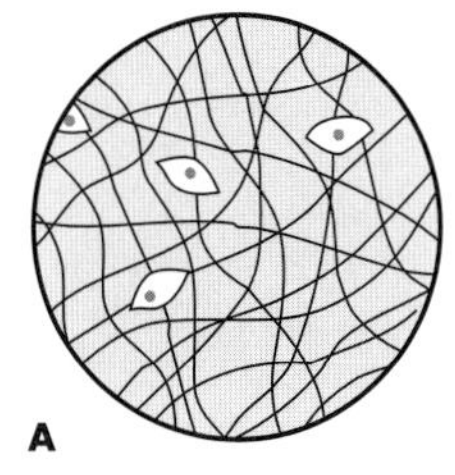

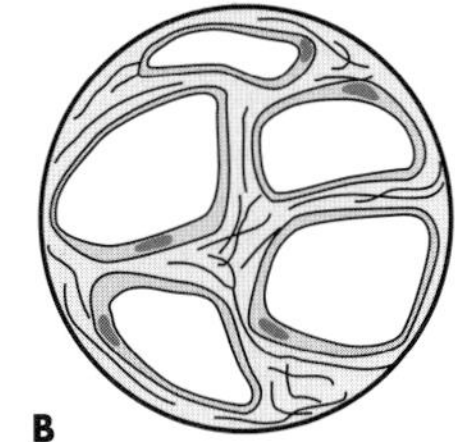

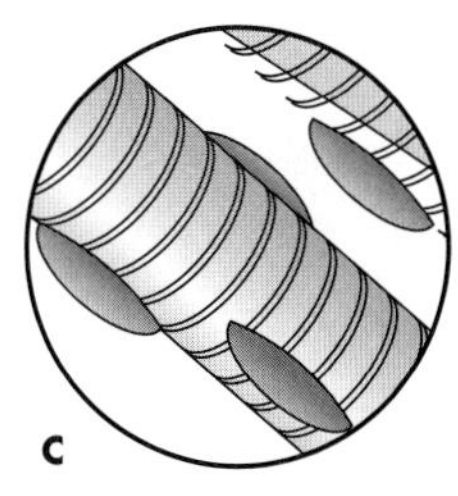

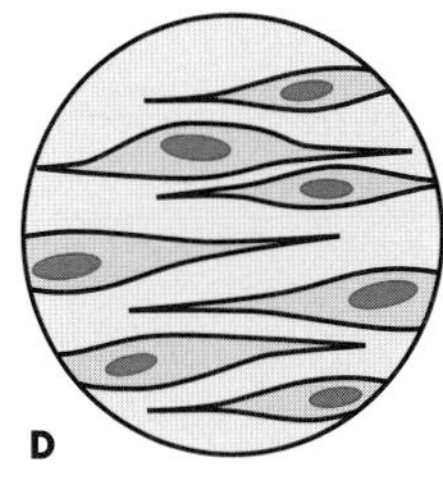

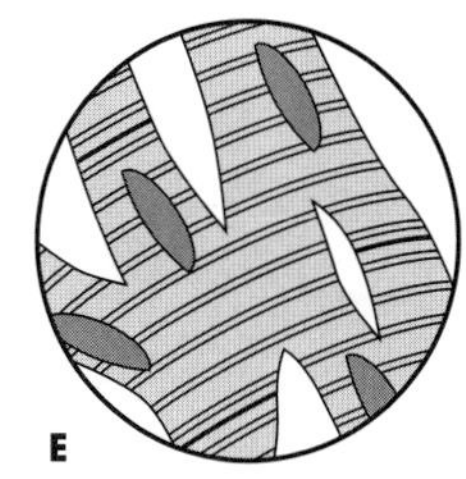

6.

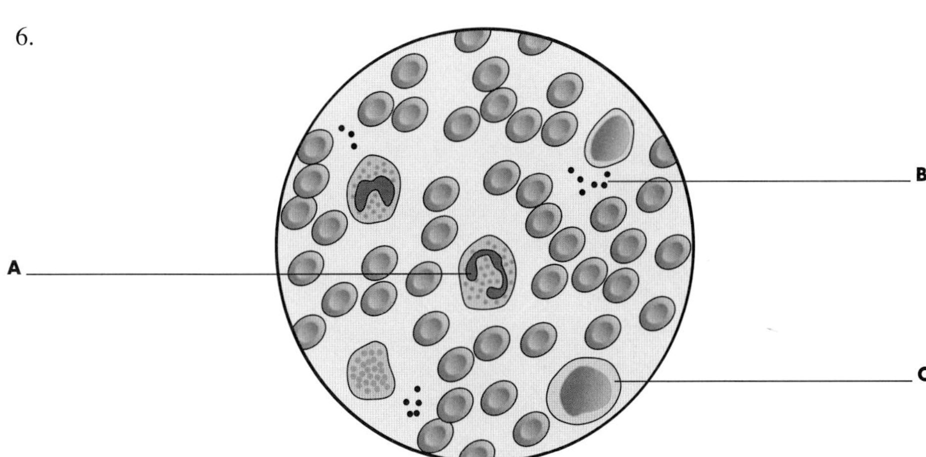

7.

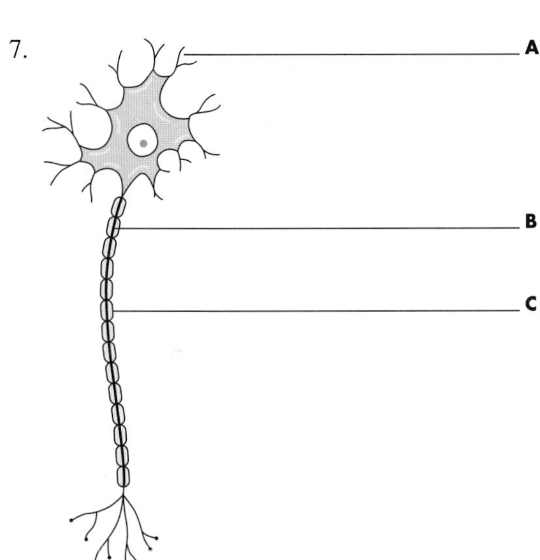

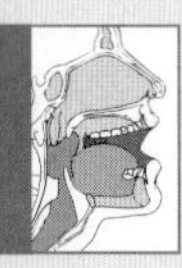

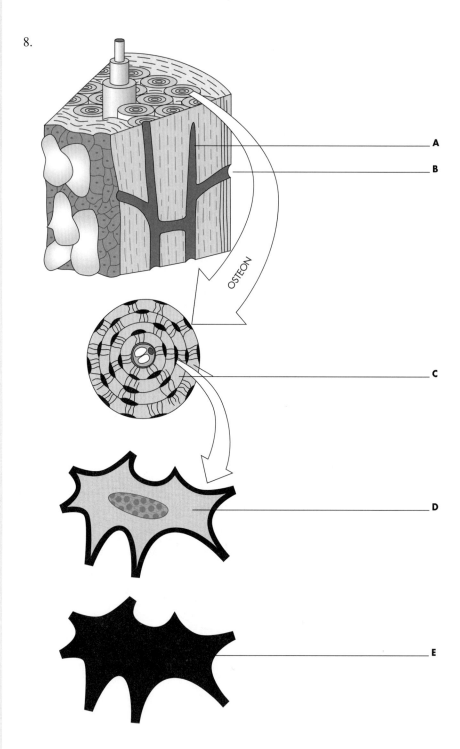

8.

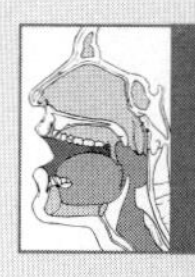

9.

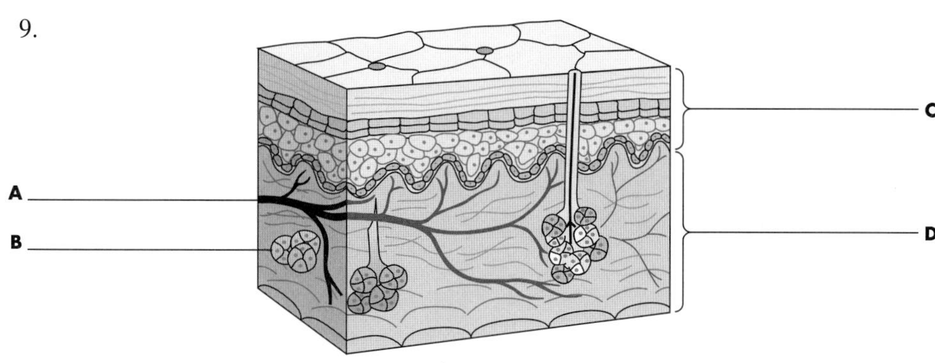

10.

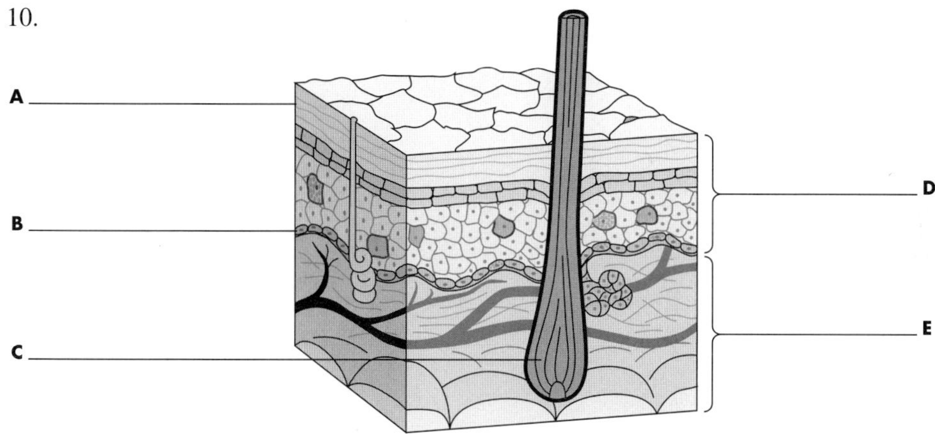

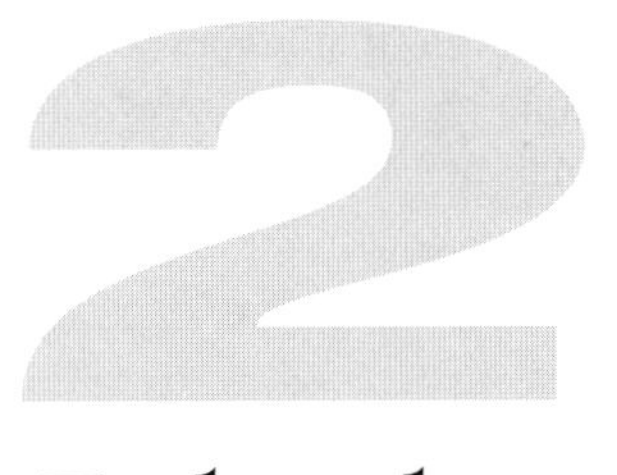

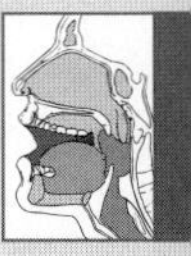

Embryology

GENERAL EMBRYOLOGY

1.0

All humans begin life from a single cell **(zygote)** that contains half of a nucleus from the mother **(egg cell)** and half of a nucleus from the father **(sperm cell).** These **gametes** or sex cells have only half of the normal cell's chromosome number, or 23 chromosomes. When gametes combine, or are **fertilized,** they produce the zygote with the full 46 chromosomes. Each chromosome contains genetic information not only to build the resulting new human being, but to regulate its future life-giving functions. And each genetic code is unique to each individual, though many of the patterns of growth and development are shared. We study those early patterns of growth and development of the human in **embryology** with a special focus on what occurs in the development of the head and neck region.

zygote

Fertilization occurs within the female when the egg is penetrated by sperm and the resultant combination of genetic material or chromosomes produces a single _______________. This act of fertilization usually occurs within the **fallopian tube** of the female and the zygote, then passes down into the uterus.

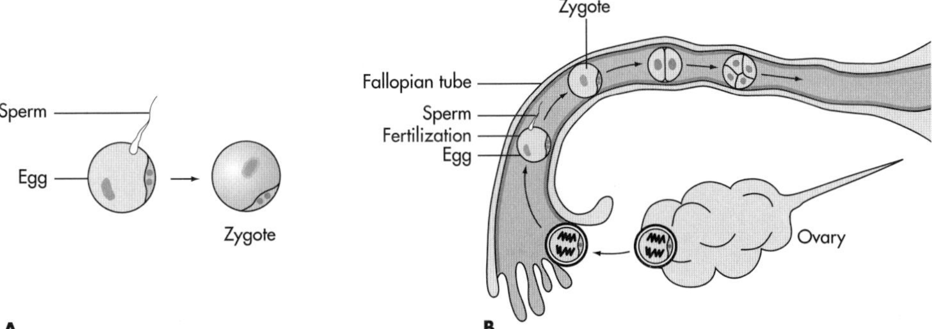

Differentiation

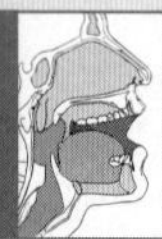

While it takes that journey, the zygote receives instructions from its chromosomes to divide into many copies of itself. Replication (cell division) is called **mitosis.** At first, the cells created look very much alike. Later, the cells will receive instructions to make cells that are different from each other. This type of mitosis is called **differentiation.** ______________ makes different cells.

The zygote, after dividing to make many cells, is no longer called a zygote. A grapelike cluster of cells is formed called a **morula.** The morula then arranges its cells to form a hollow ball called a **blastula.** The blastula continues to move into the uterus and will implant on the uterine wall, a favorable site, engorged with blood vessels. **Implantation** joins the mother to the growing child where it will be nourished as it grows and develops.

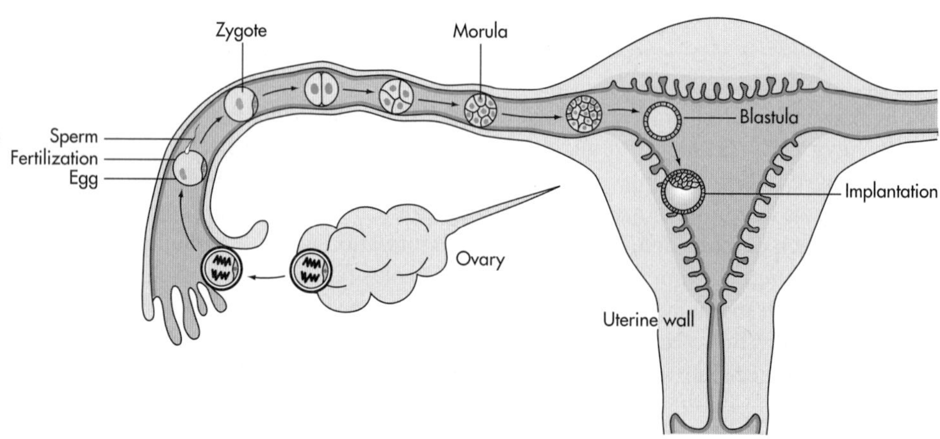

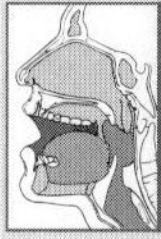

On implantation, the blastula has already begun to differentiate its cells to become the gastrula. One group of cells will migrate to a side of the ball and become the **supporting tissues** that surround the growing human, and the other group will migrate and cluster together to become the future embryo. The **embryo** is the group of cells that will develop into a human being.

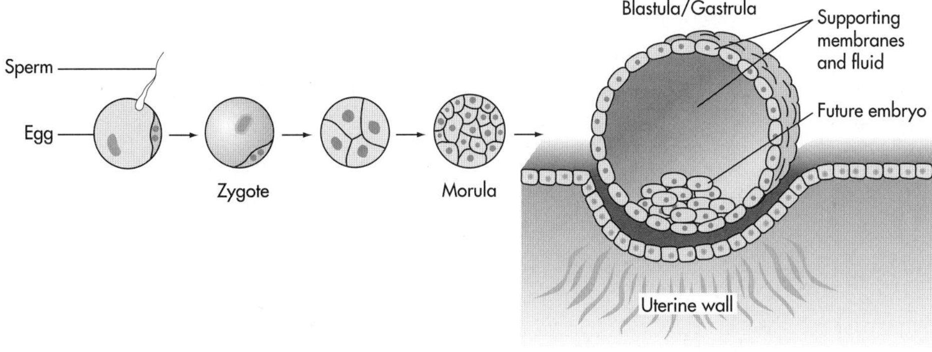

Label the stages of development in the accompanying diagrams.

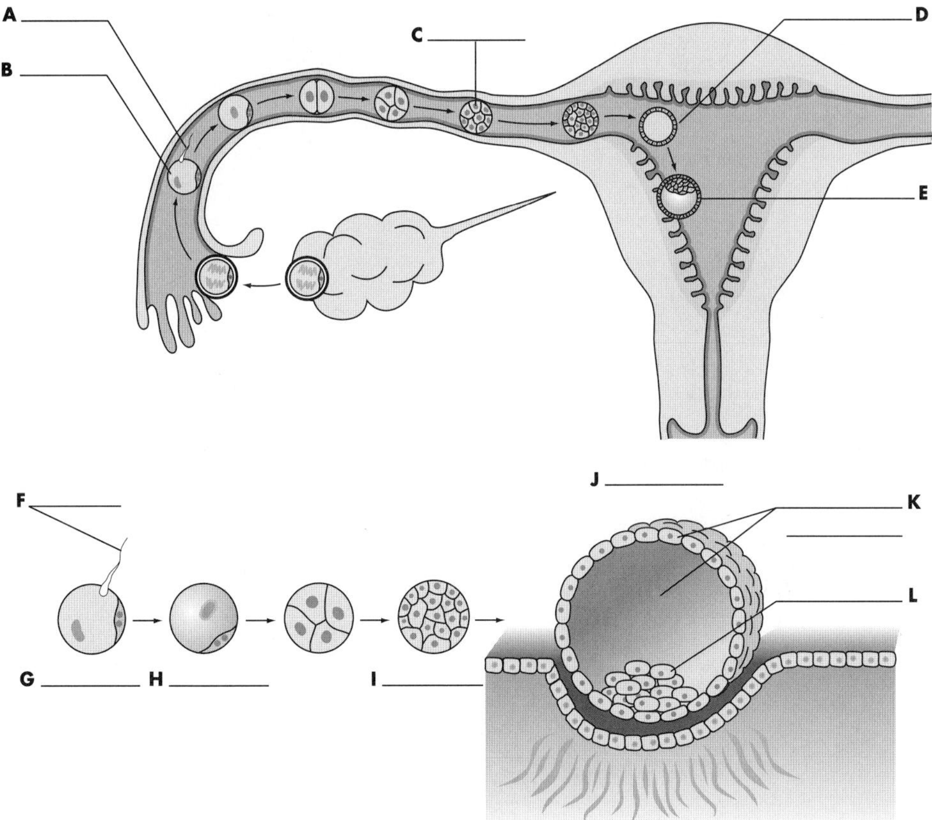

A. sperm
B. egg
C. morula
D. blastula
E. implantation
F. sperm
G. egg
H. zygote
I. morula
J. blastula/gastrula
K. supporting membranes and fluid
L. future embryo

embryonic

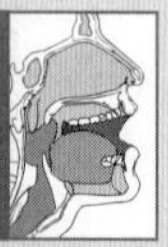

The embryo is a collection of cells differentiated to become, in this case, a human being. The **embryonic period** is the period from conception (fertilization) to the time the embryo becomes a fetus. This is from 8 to 10 weeks long or the first 2 to 3 months of pregnancy. Most of differentiation and development occurs during this first or _______________ period. The **fetal period** lasts 6 months and is a time for refinement of structures and weight gain. Birth then occurs at 9 months postconception. The diagrams summarize the development of the embryo and fetus.

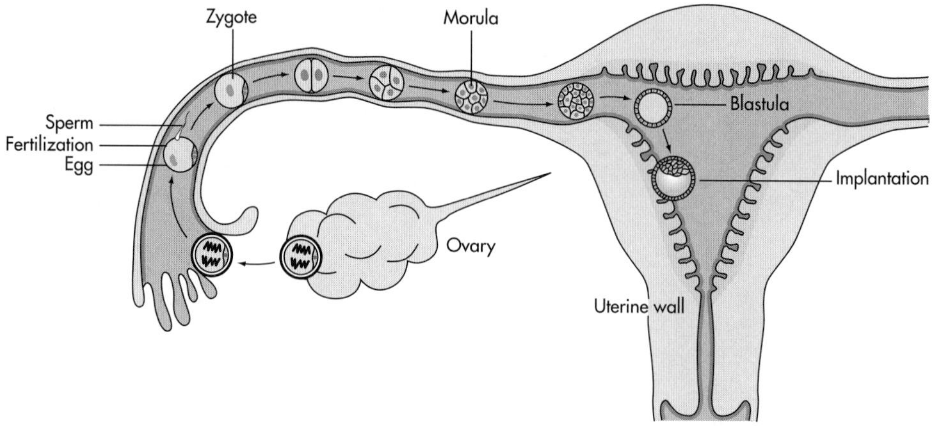

Zygote
Morula
Sperm
Fertilization
Egg
Blastula
Implantation
Ovary
Uterine wall

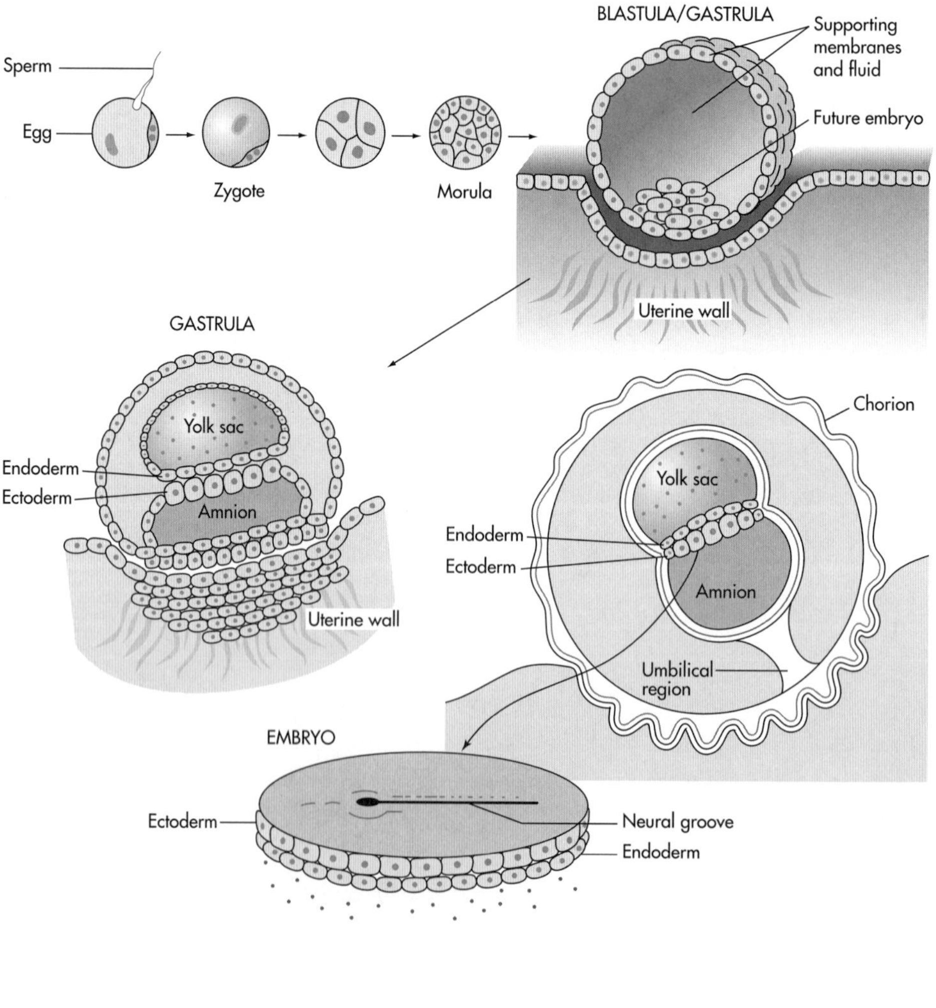

BLASTULA/GASTRULA
Supporting membranes and fluid
Future embryo
Sperm
Egg
Zygote
Morula
Uterine wall

GASTRULA
Yolk sac
Endoderm
Ectoderm
Amnion
Uterine wall

Chorion
Yolk sac
Endoderm
Ectoderm
Amnion
Umbilical region

EMBRYO
Ectoderm
Neural groove
Endoderm

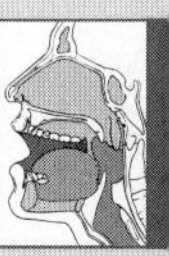

continued

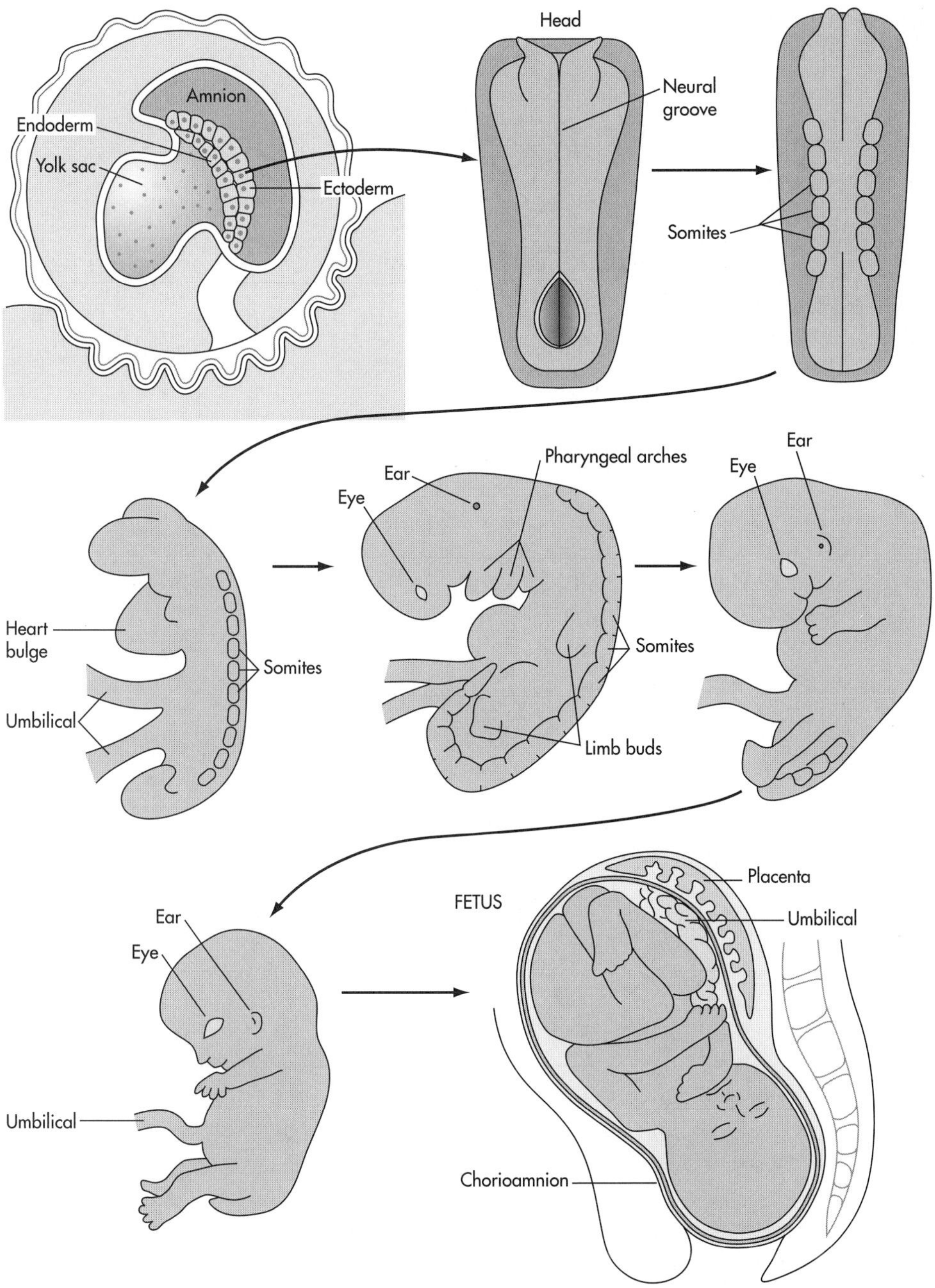

Amnion
Endoderm
Yolk sac
Ectoderm
Head
Neural groove
Somites

Heart bulge
Umbilical
Somites
Ear
Eye
Pharyngeal arches
Somites
Limb buds
Eye
Ear

Ear
Eye
Umbilical
FETUS
Placenta
Umbilical
Chorioamnion

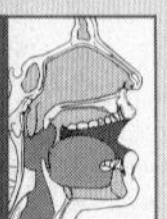

Note the group of cells that becomes the tissues that surround the embyro. They serve to protect the embryo or fetus as a fluid-filled sac and also to attach it to the mother (uterus) for nourishment. The fingerlike projections do this.

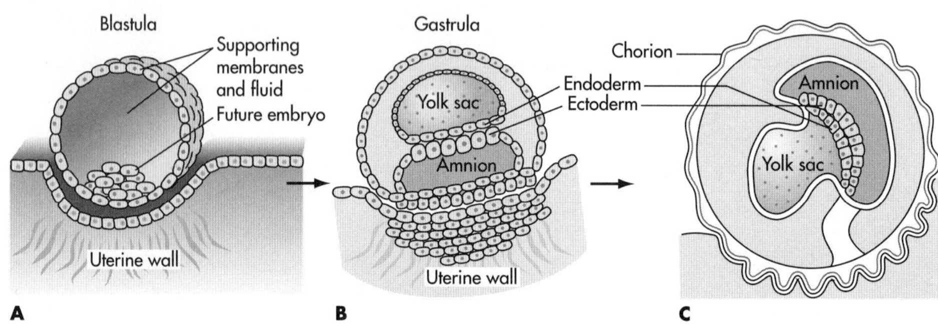

At first, nourishment for the embryo comes from a separate sac, the **yolk sac.** This disappears with time, as a cord of blood vessels takes its place. The **umbilical cord** is a collection of blood vessels going in and out of the embryo into the **placenta,** which exchanges blood products with the maternal uterine blood.

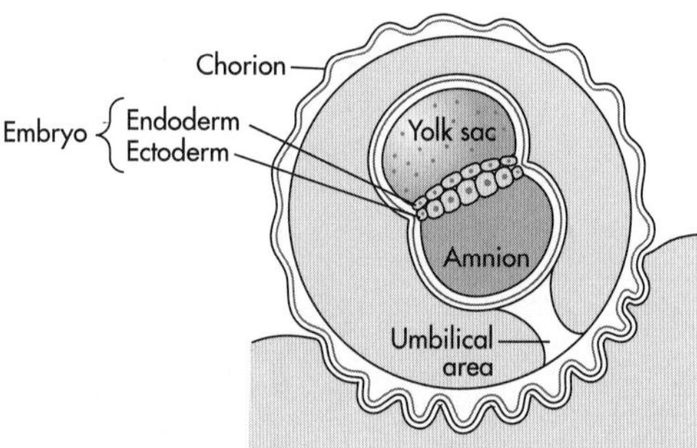

Label the yolk sac and umbilical area in the diagram.

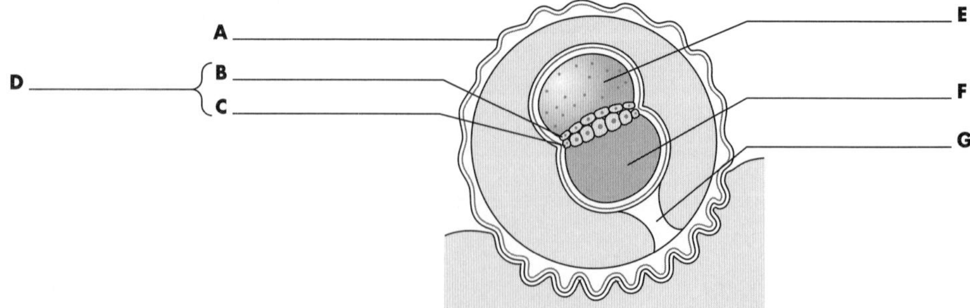

A. chorion
B. endoderm
C. ectoderm
D. embryo
E. yolk sac
F. amnion
G. umbilical area

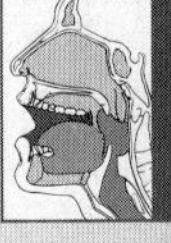

The supporting or surrounding tissues of the embryo/fetus are the amnion and chorion. They create a fluid-filled sac in which the embryo/fetus lies. As the fetus grows, the membranes come together to become one **chorioamnion.**

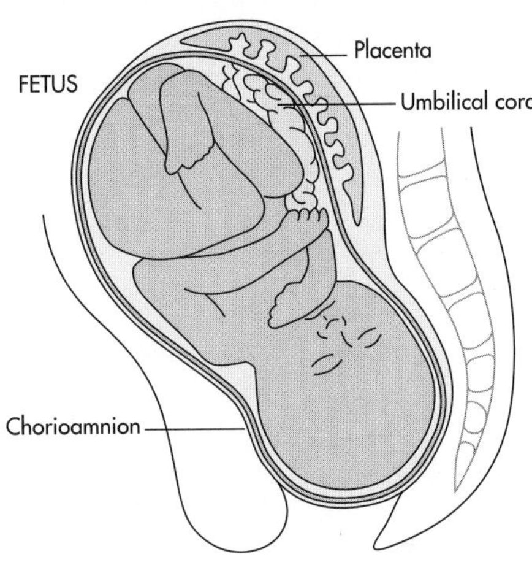

THE TRILAMINAR EMBRYO 2.0

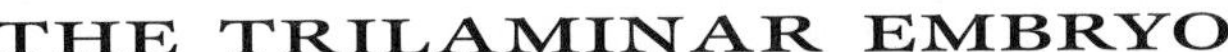

We look at the development of the embryo now, or **embryology.** As all development begins in this short period from the differentiation and development of cells it is very important.

ectoderm and endoderm

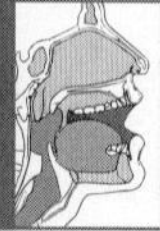

The embryo, as seen, begins as a ball of cells in the blastula stage that then forms a flat plate of cells in the **gastrula stage.** The cells differentiate into groups of cells that are different and will become different things. Cells of the embryo differentiate into three different layers **(trilaminar embryo)** that, in turn, develop into three different types of tissues and, eventually, organs. These three different germ (beginning) layers are called (1) **ectoderm** ("outer layer"), (2) **mesoderm** ("middle layer"), and (3) **endoderm** ("inner layer"). In the diagram you can see the mesoderm layer forming between which two layers?

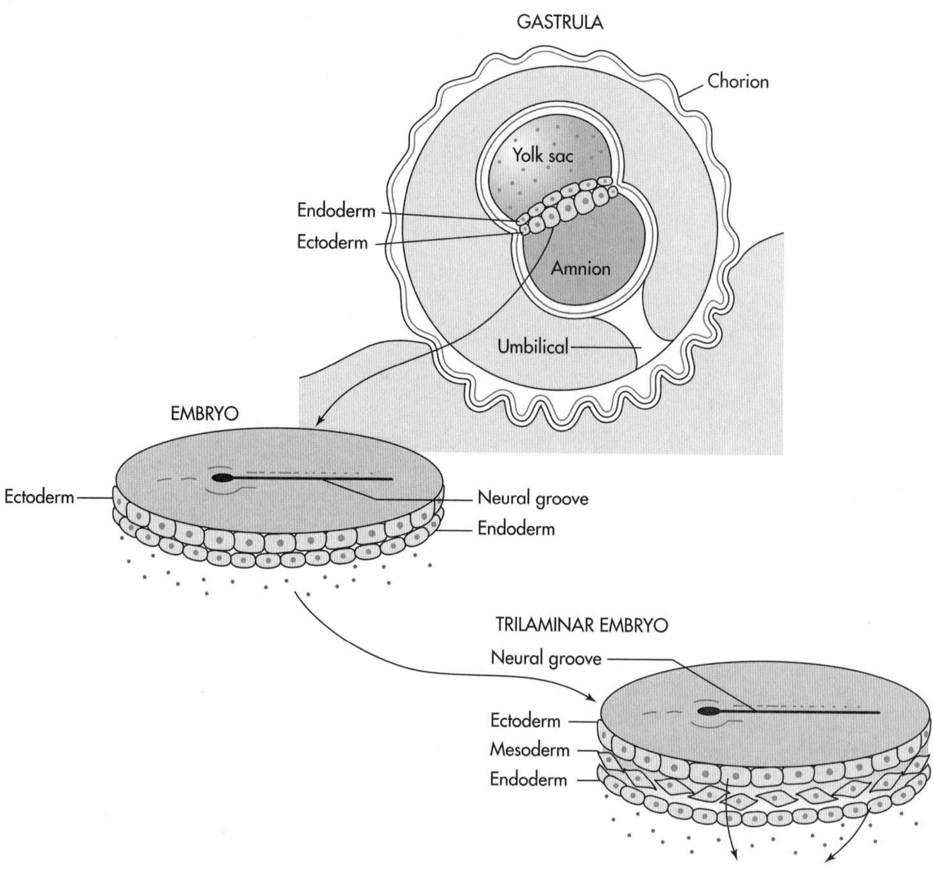

ectoderm, mesoderm, endoderm

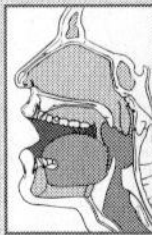

The three layers of cells of the embryo are ______________, ______________, and ______________. Traditionally, each layer in anatomy textbooks is colored a different color: blue for ectoderm, red for mesoderm, and yellow for endoderm. The illustrations in this book are made so that you may, if you wish, color them as an aide for memorization. Color the layers of the trilaminar embryo.

Ectoderm — Blue
Mesoderm — Red
Endoderm — Yellow

derivative

The cells in each type of layer have different fates; that is, they differentiate into specific structures (organs and systems). These future organs and systems that the three "derms" will build are called **derivatives.** For example, some of the cells from the mesoderm layer will derive the heart, so that the heart is a ______________ of mesoderm.

ectoderm, mesoderm, endoderm

Some of the cells of the mesoderm layer will migrate or move into the area where a heart is needed, differentiate into heart cells, and make a heart!

We now study the derivatives of the three germ layers: the organs and systems that come from ______________, ______________, and ______________.

Ectodermal Derivatives 2.1

The cells of the outermost layer have genetic instructions to derive certain structures. Let's follow what happens to ectoderm in the embryo. You may color all things that derive from ectoderm blue, if you wish, as we go along.

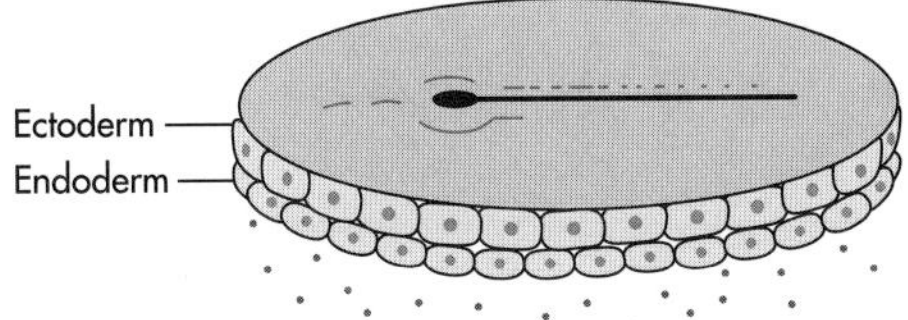

It remains on the outside of the embryo.

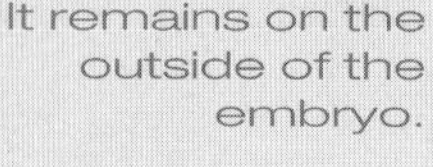

In the embryo in the diagram, as it ages note the change in its shape. It began, remember, as a flat disk of cells. It then folds up into a tubular shape (looking much like a hot dog in a bun!) and then later curves in on itself in a C-shape. What is happening to its ectoderm layer?

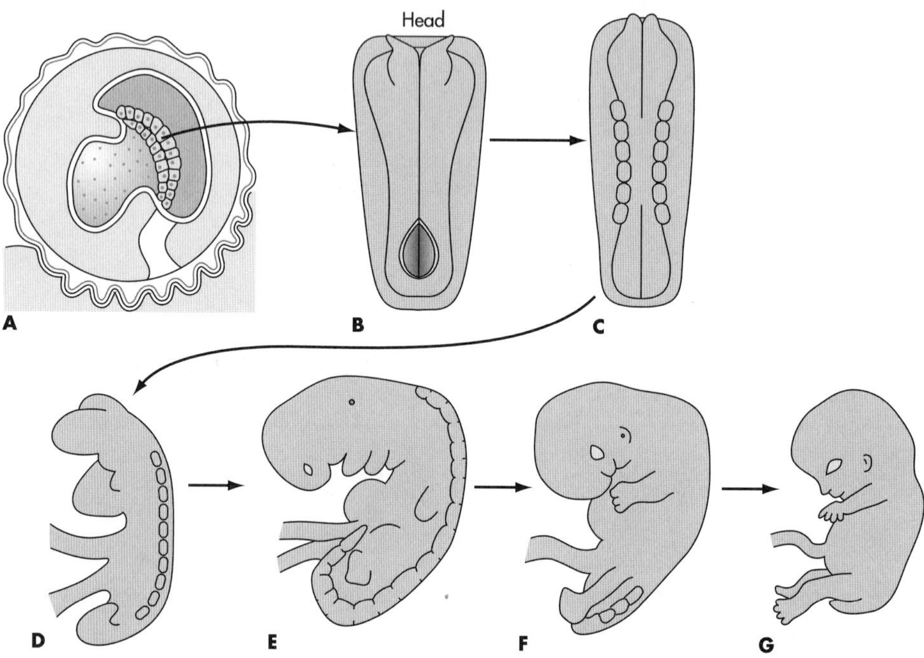

The ectoderm forms cells that cover the embryo with a protective outer layer, a sort of equivalent to the adult skin.

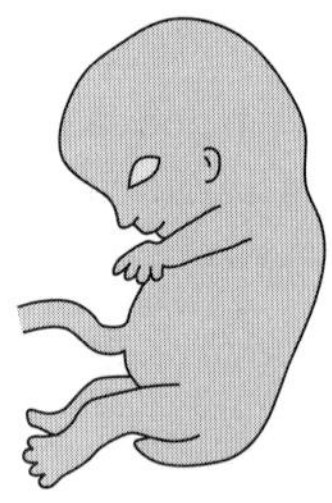

In truth the adult skin as seen in general histology is made of a layer of epidermis (epithelial tissue) and dermis (connective tissue). The epidermis of the adult skin is derived from ectoderm, but the second layer, the ______________, is not. The dermis is derived from underlying mesoderm instead.

dermis

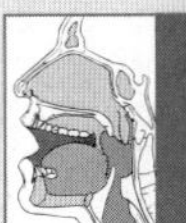

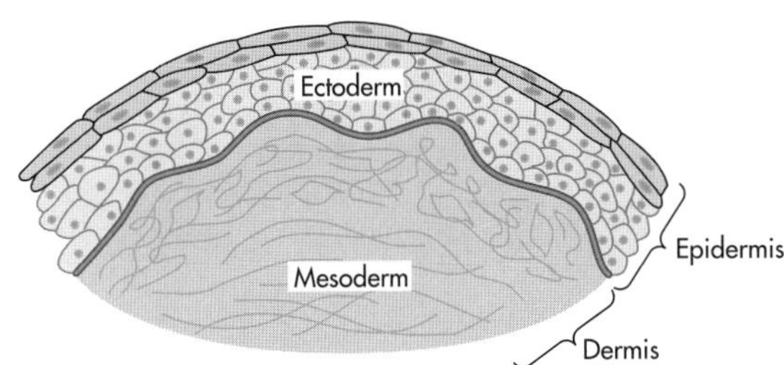

Follow the sequence for development of the skin. Color in red or blue for mesoderm and ectoderm.

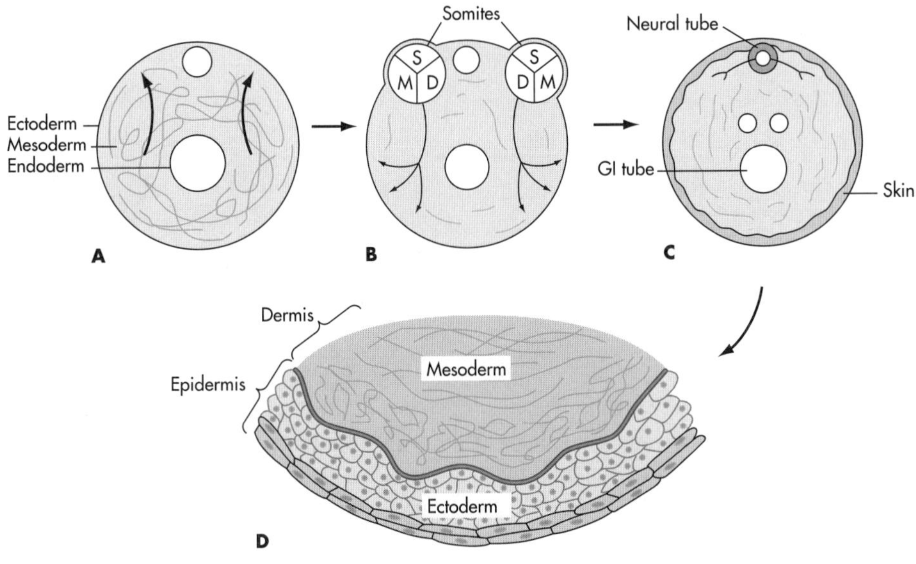

The first derivative of ectoderm, then, is the ______________ of the skin.

epidermis

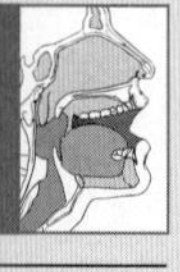

Other things are happening to the outer layer of the embryo, as seen by all the folding going on. It looks as though the outer "skin" is being folded and zipped together into a second tube, as shown.

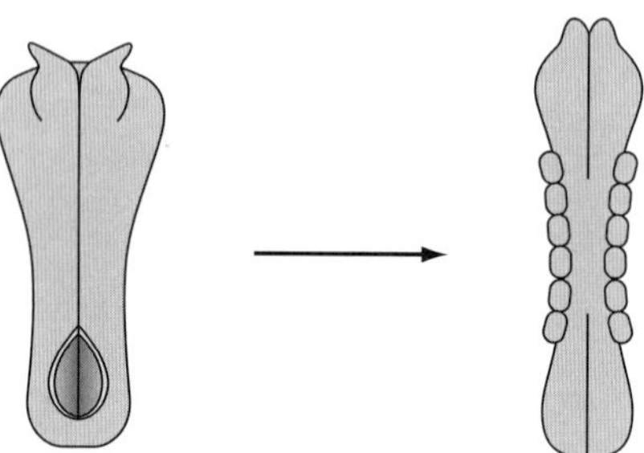

It may be easier to understand what is happening if we "slice" through the embryo and make a cross section.

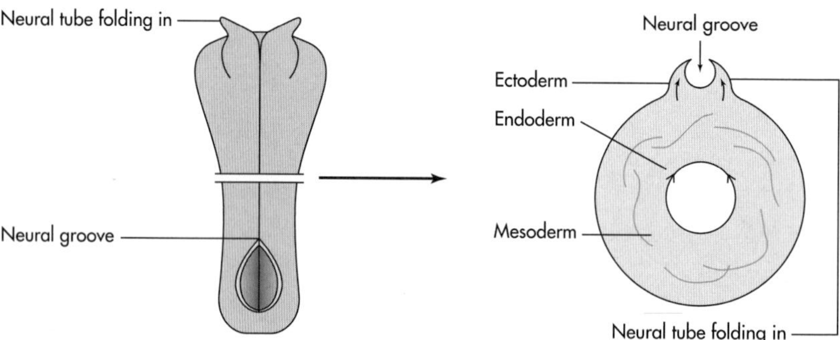

The cross section through the tube-shaped embryo shows the positions of the three germ layers now: ectoderm on the outside, mesoderm on the inside, and endoderm on the inside. Watch what happens to the ectodermal layer.

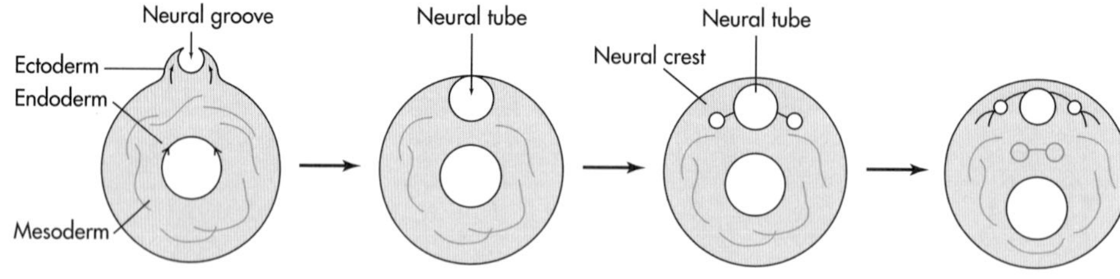

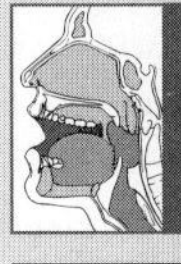

The ectodermal outer layer is folding up on itself, forming another long tube from end to end. The tube that is formed is called the **neural tube,** and it is the beginning definition of the head and tail of the embryo. It also shows where the back **(dorsum)** and belly **(ventrum)** of the embryo will be. Look at the neural tube's development both longitudinally and in cross section.

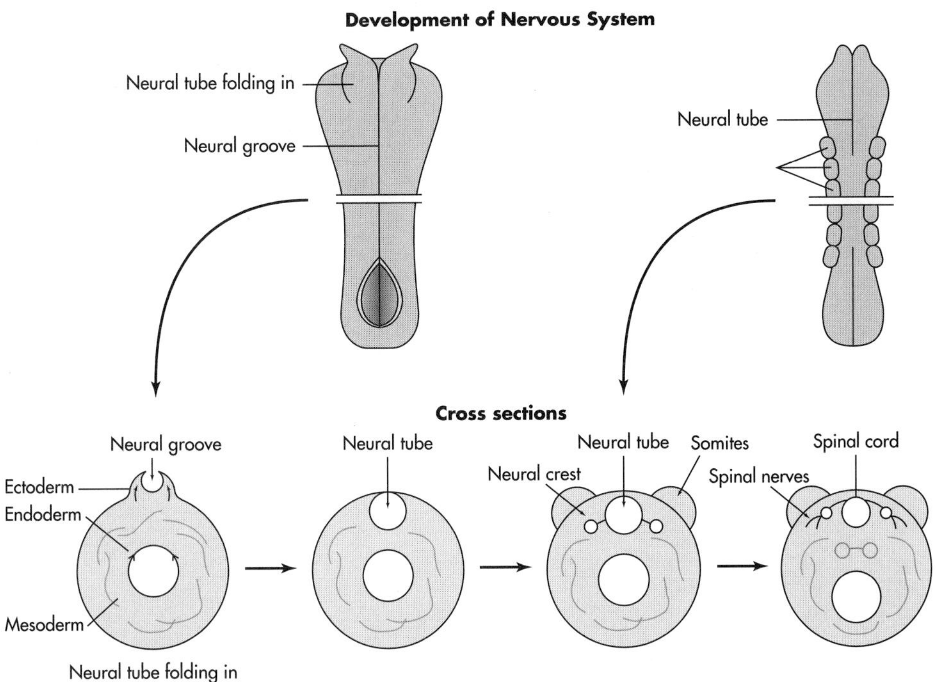

One end of the ______________ bulges out while the rest of the tube remains narrow. The bulged-out area will become the brain, and the rest of the tube becomes the spinal cord. These two parts of the central nervous system (CNS) are two more derivatives of ______________.

neural tube, ectoderm

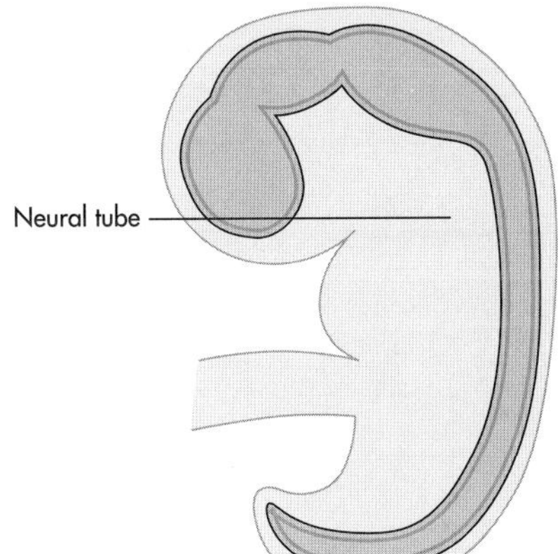

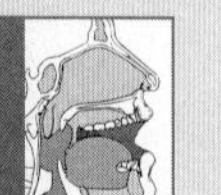

blue

Note that after the neural tube is formed, paired groups of cells branch off of it. These cells are called **neural crest cells** and come off in pairs from the future brain and spinal cord, connecting to it. Label neural crest in the drawing. All of these structures would be colored what?

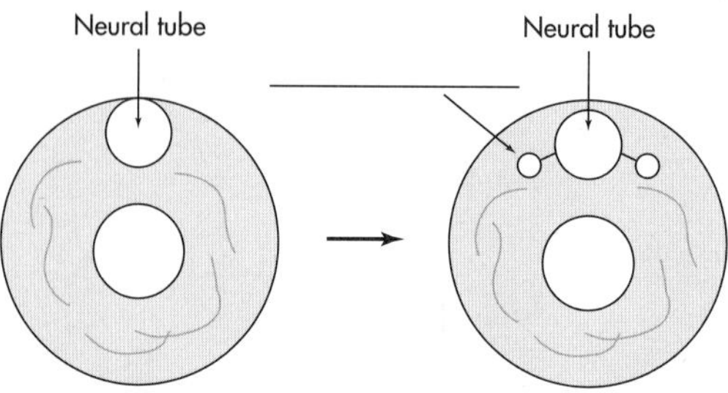

neural crest

The groups of cells pairing off of the neural tube are ______________ cells. These pairs coming off the future spinal cord will maintain their connection, as shown, and branch out into the body as paired **spinal nerves.** Label the spinal nerves.

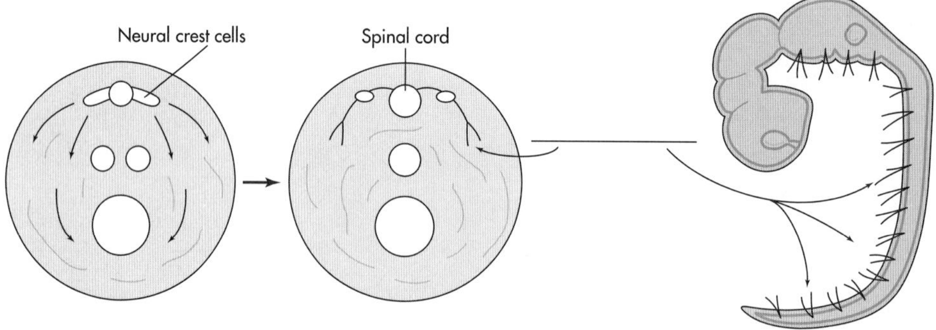

The neural crest of the head also develops paired nerves coming off of the future brain, called **cranial nerves.** Find the cranial nerves. Note that other tissue from the brain is developing the future eyes (sight) and ears (hearing) in areas called optic cup and otic placode.

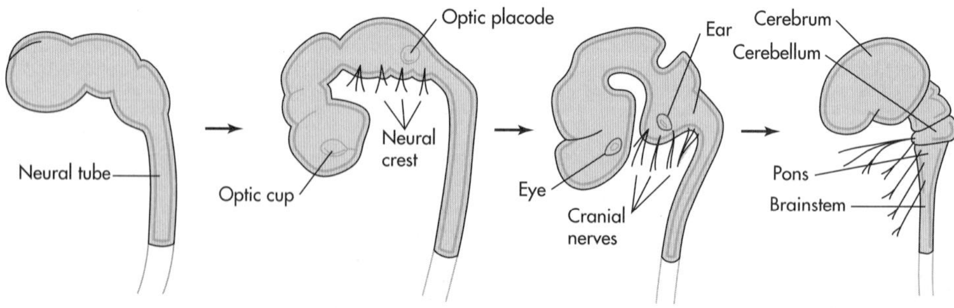

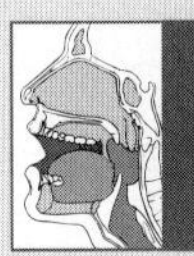

The **neural crest of the head** also develops into the ______________ nerves and into a special mesoderm of the facial region. This is ectoderm that becomes mesoderm! This is the only place in the embryo that such a thing happens. This mesoderm will become or derive the muscle, connective tissue, and bone of the face. Watch it travel out from the neural tube into the pharyngeal arches.

cranial

NEURAL CREST MIGRATION

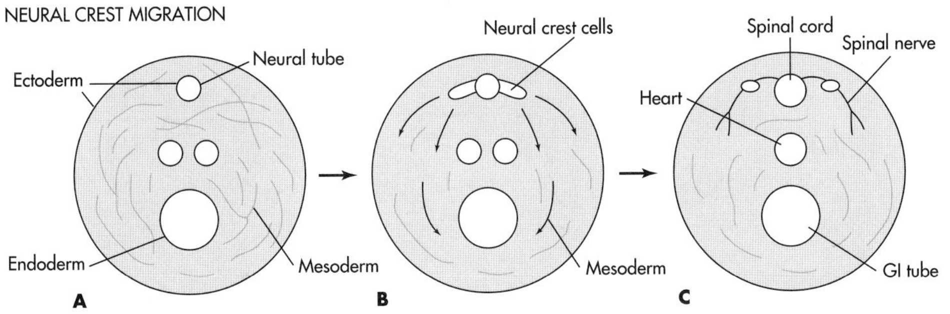

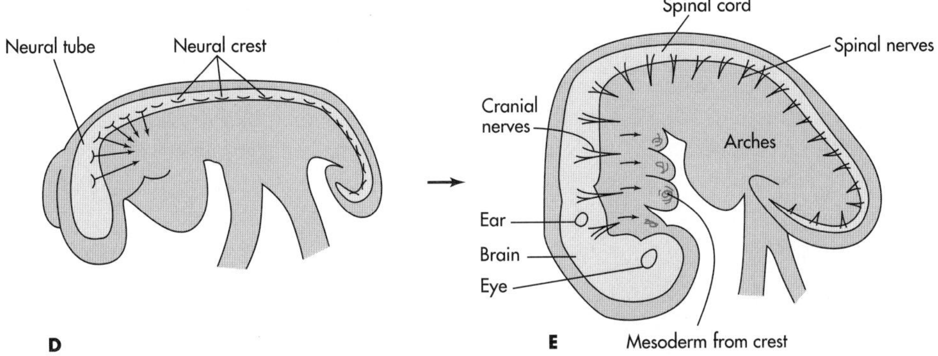

The derivatives of ectoderm, then, are the epidermis of the skin, the brain, the spinal cord, the nerves (the ______________ system), and the mesoderm of the face. What color have we used to symbolize ectoderm and its derivatives?

nervous, blue

Endodermal Derivatives 2.2

Endoderm is the innermost layer or lining of the embryo. Just as the ectodermal layer became the outer "tube" of the embryo, the endodermal layer will fold in to become the inner "tube."

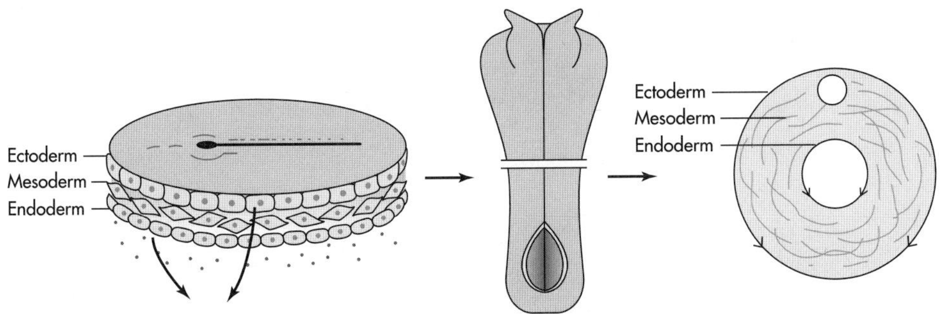

The embryo begins as a "tube within a tube." Let us follow the development of that tube by looking at sections of the embryo, longitudinal and cross.

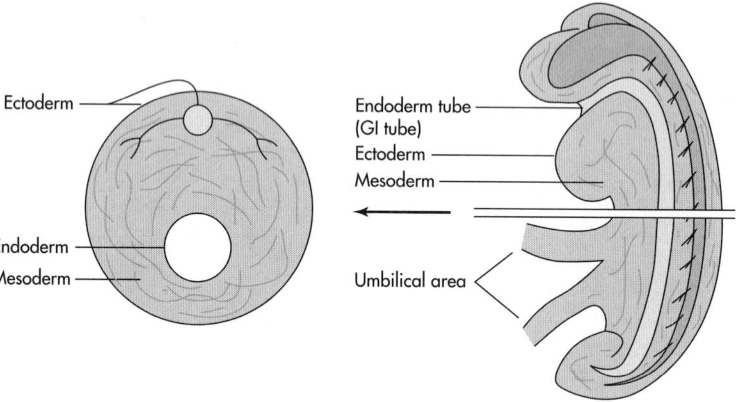

yellow, blue

To gain length the endodermal tube, as it develops, bends and folds. Some areas pouch out to form structures. The first part of the tube to form is the pharynx. It bulges out and develops four pouched areas within the neck area of the embryo, as shown. The color code for endodermal tissue is yellow. You may color in the portions of the embryo that are the endoderm ______________ and the ectoderm ______________.

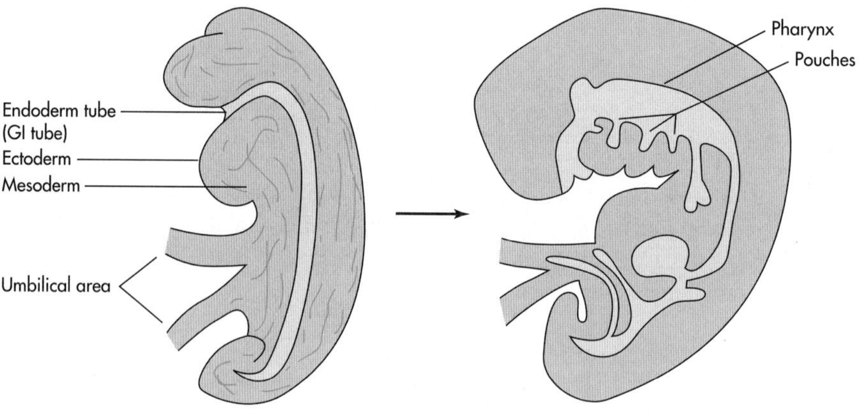

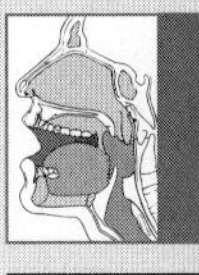

The tube narrows beyond the pharynx and becomes the future esophagus. It then bulges out and bends to develop the stomach. After the stomach the tube narrows again, making many coils. This is the intestine.

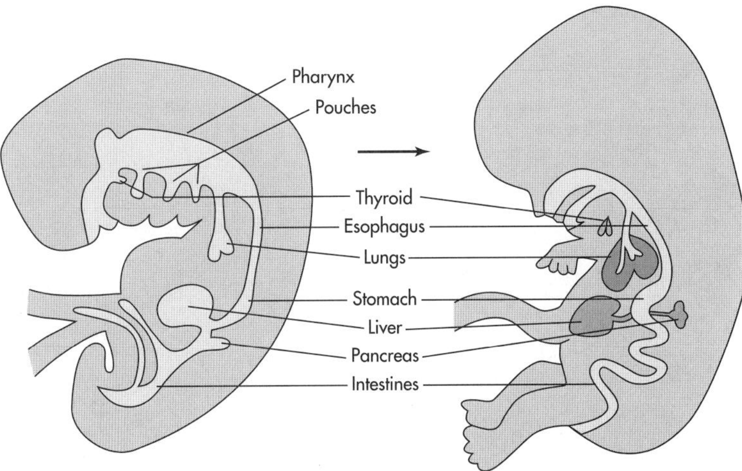

digestive system

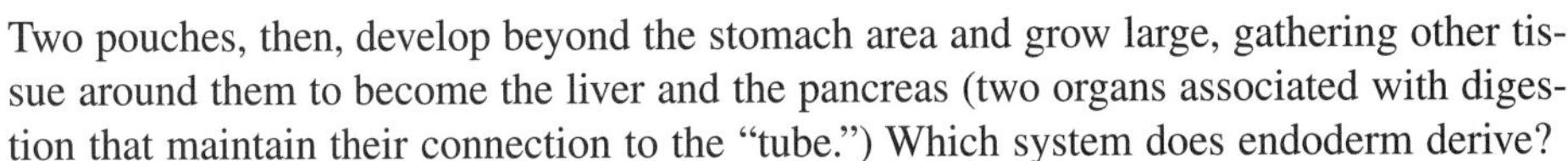

Two pouches, then, develop beyond the stomach area and grow large, gathering other tissue around them to become the liver and the pancreas (two organs associated with digestion that maintain their connection to the "tube.") Which system does endoderm derive?

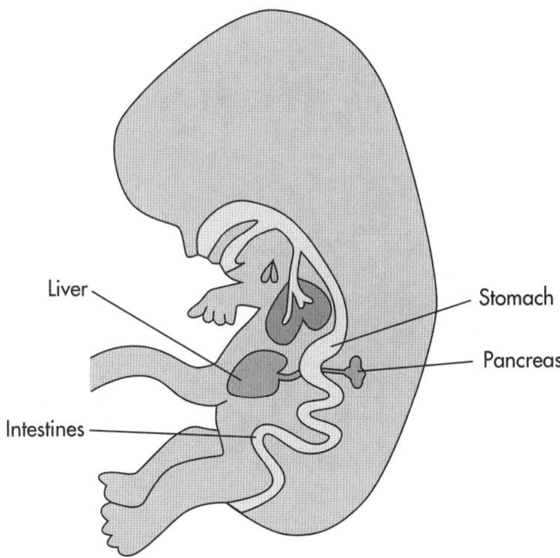

respiratory, yellow

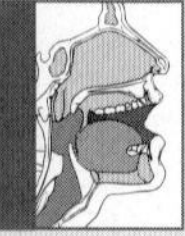

We will look more closely at the pharyngeal endoderm's development later. Note that from the floor of the pharynx, a double pouch develops, growing down from the neck into the embryonic chest cavity. These are the future lungs and trachea. Endodermal derivatives include two systems: the digestive system and the ______________ system. Which color is endoderm?

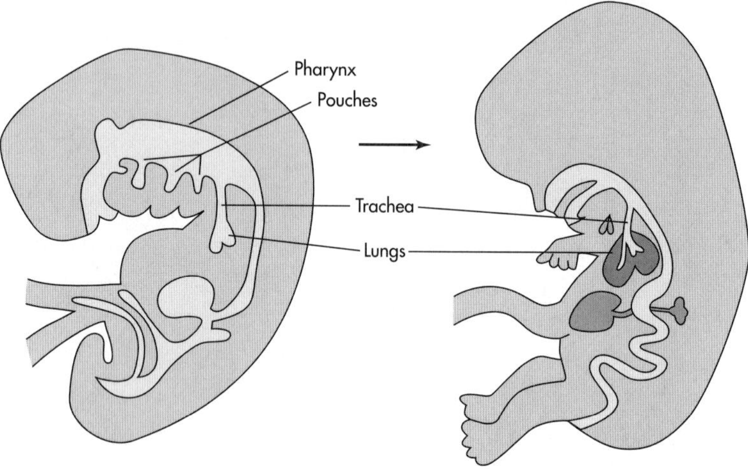

2.3 Mesodermal Derivatives

So far we have seen that ectoderm forms the outer layer of the embryo, and endoderm forms the inner layer or "tube." Mesoderm forms between the two and is the most versatile of the three germ layers with many derivatives. Look at the embryo cross section to locate mesoderm and color it red.

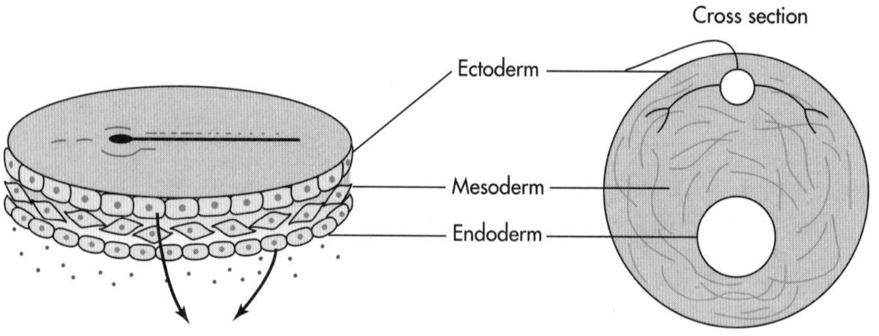

Mesoderm often occurs as star-shaped cells that can travel far within the embryo's body to regroup and form structures. We have already seen one type of mesoderm that came from neural crest cells that were originally ectodermal cells, which ended up in the face. Early in the embryo's development paired bumps of mesoderm gather under the "skin" on either side of the developing neural tube. They are called **somites.**

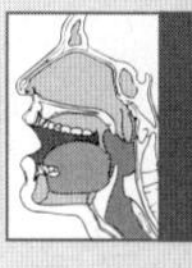

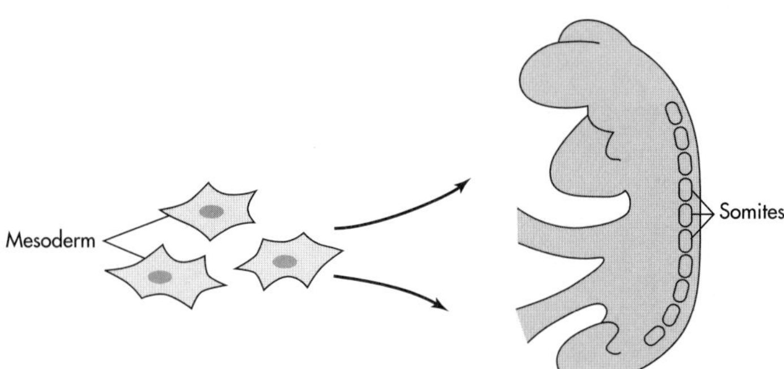

Somites look like a backbone, but they are not. They remain along the neural tube, next to the neural crest "bumps," for a short period. They then migrate or leave the area in three different groups. Label the somites. Remember each somite is covered by a layer of ectodermal skin. How would you color the picture? Do it.

Blue:
ectoderm and all outer embryo "skin," neural tube, spinal cord, spinal nerves
Yellow:
endoderm,
GI tube
Red:
all other structures

Somite Development

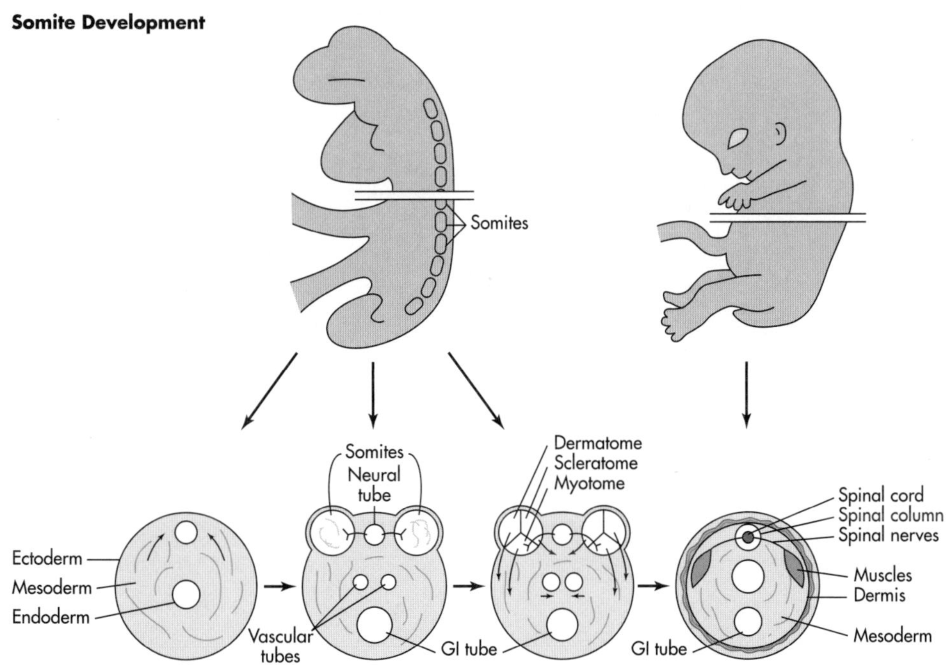

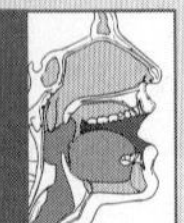

Each **somite** divides into three groups of cells that differentiate into different types of tissue. The **dermatome** portion travels to the underside of the embryonic "skin" or future epidermis to become the **dermis,** as shown. Color the portion of skin that comes from ectoderm blue and the portion that comes from mesoderm red.

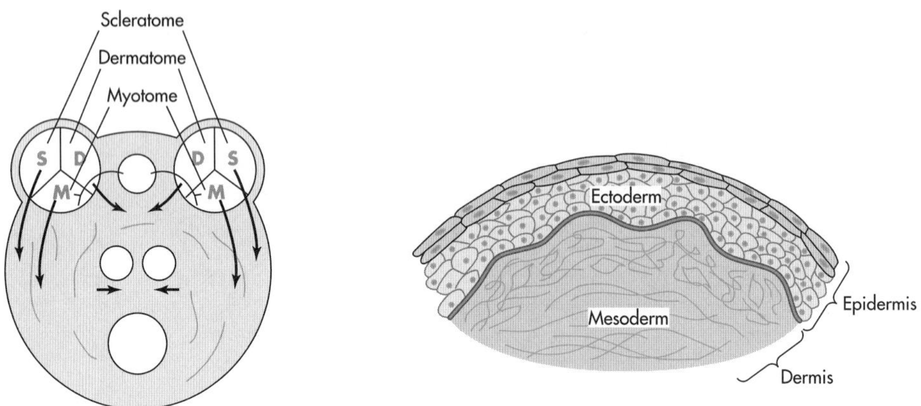

The second portion of the somite, the **sclerotome,** will send cells out to become **bone.** The area around the future spinal cord will become encircled in bone called the vertebrae, which together are called the spinal column. Don't confuse cord (nerve tissue from ectoderm) and column (bone from mesoderm). Other bones formed will be the skull, paired ribs, pelvis, and, later, the limbs.

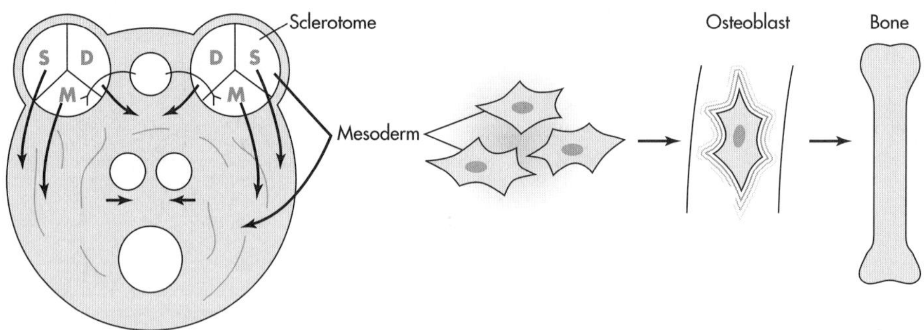

The last part of the mesodermal somite is the **myotome.** These mesodermal cells migrate out to form muscles to attach to the bones that are forming.

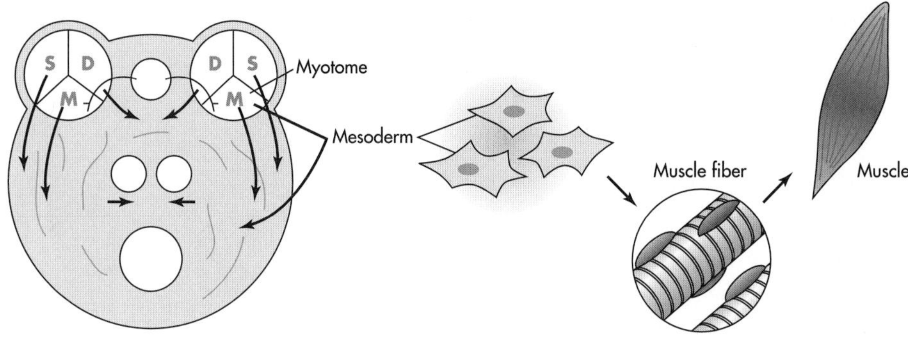

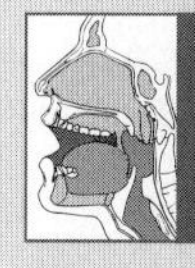

Other mesoderm will form the "packing" or in between tissues of the body, that is, connective tissue. All fascia, capsules, ligaments, and tendons come from mesoderm.

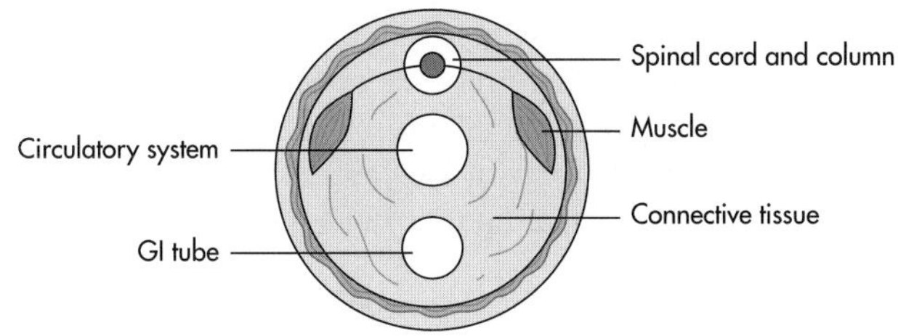

What are the derivatives of mesoderm so far?

muscles, bone, dermis

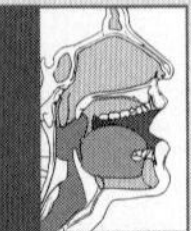

You will also note that pairs of tubes are formed around the endoderm tube from mesoderm. These tubes are the beginning of the circulatory system.

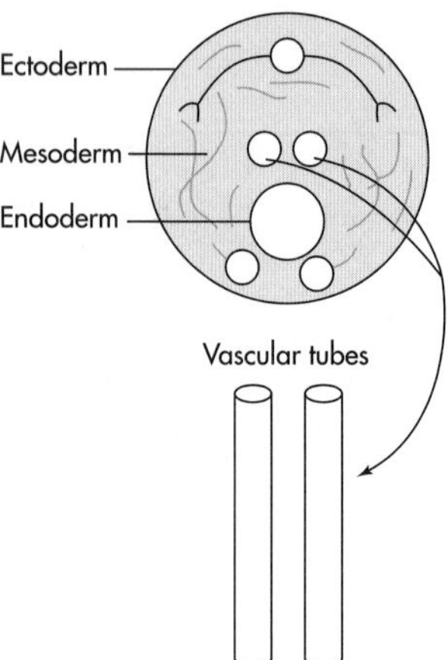

Tubes develop from mesoderm that run the length of the embryonic body. They begin to develop smaller and smaller connecting branches or blood vessels. Other mesoderm derives blood cells. In the chest, the double tube fuses and bends on itself to form a single heart, and it begins to pump or beat early in the embryo's life. In fact, the heart occupies a major portion of the embryo's body at first, as you can see in the diagram.

DEVELOPMENT OF CIRCULATORY SYSTEM

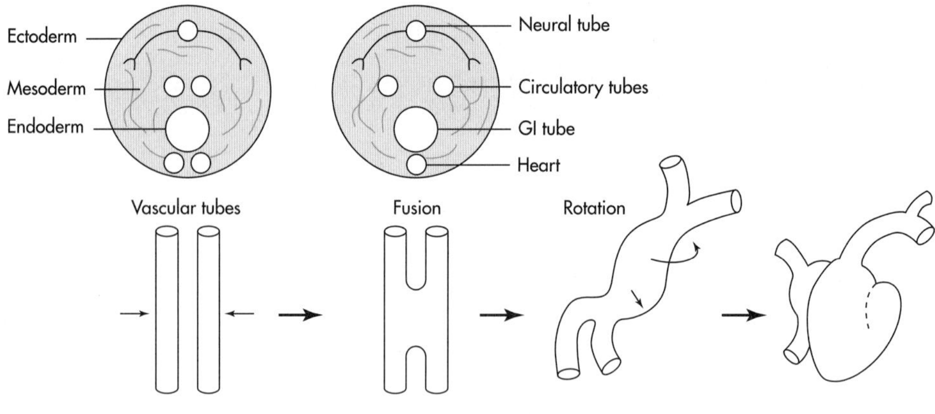

DEVELOPMENT OF HEART

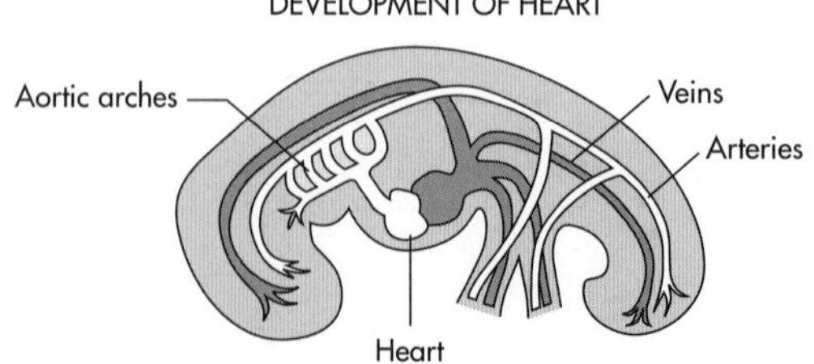

Which systems and structure does mesoderm derive?

What color symbolizes mesoderm?

skeletal, muscular, circulatory, dermis; red

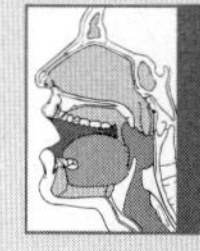

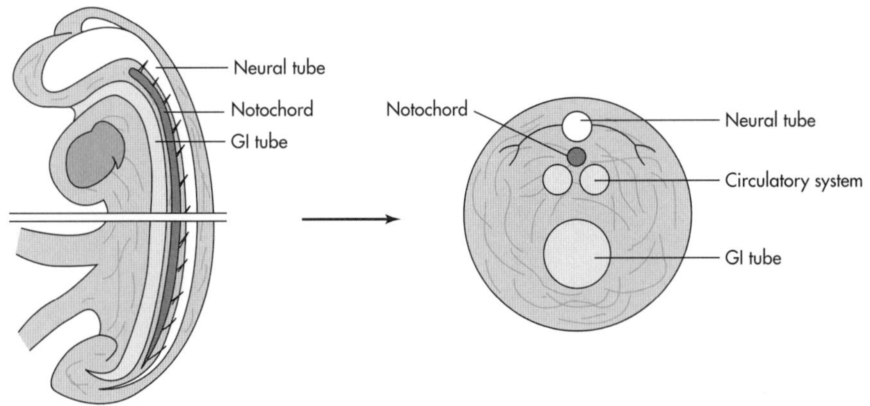

There is a structure in the embryo that comes from a distinct tissue (not ectoderm, mesoderm, or endoderm). It exists for only a short time and leaves only a small portion remaining in the adult, or a **remnant.** It is called the **notochord** and it is a temporary backbone under the neural tube until the spinal column is completed. See the diagram below.

There is also a temporary jawbone, which we will study later.

Reviewing the derivatives of the three germ layers, list in each column the organs or systems that come from each layer. Refer to the previous three sections for your answers.

Ectoderm	Mesoderm	Endoderm
______	______	______
______	______	______
______	______	
	______	

Ectoderm: epidermis, nervous system, mesoderm of face
Mesoderm: dermis, circulatory system, muscular system, skeletal system
Endoderm: respiratory system, digestive system

DEVELOPMENT OF THE PHARYNX 3.0

Now that you have traced the development of the embryo through its three major layers, ectoderm, mesoderm, and endoderm, we will take a closer look at the development of our particular area, the head and neck.

3.1 Arch, Pouch, and Groove

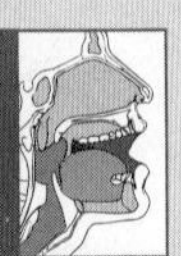

Look at the embryo. Can you tell which end is the head and neck? The head region develops first in the embryo, as it is more important. It is also larger than the "tail" region. From the outside of the future head and neck, you can see several paired bumps developing. These are the **pharyngeal arches.**

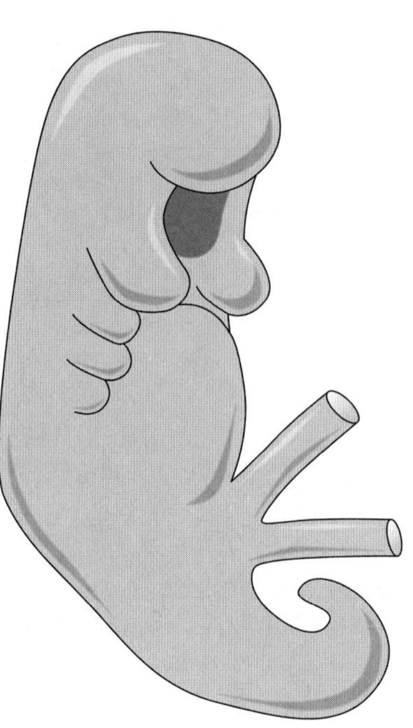

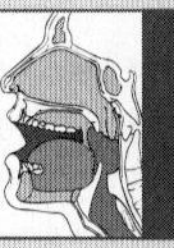

Each pair of arches is numbered with a roman numeral, that is, arch I, arch II, arch III, and arch IV. Find each arch on the drawing. Note that the arches seemed to be clustered around an opening. This is the place that will become the opening in the face known as the mouth or future oral cavity or **stomodeum.**

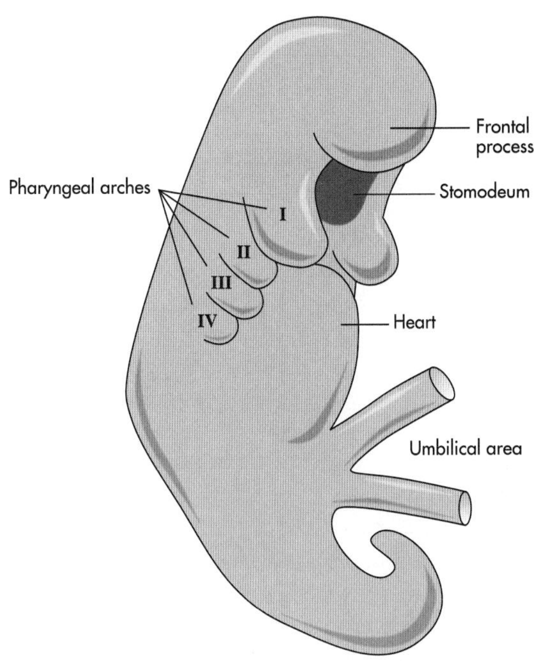

The embryo is covered with tissue from which of the three germ layers? This "skin" covers the outside of each arch. Note that between the arches there are spaces. Each space is called a groove and is numbered I through IV, just like the arches. Label grooves I, II, III, and IV.

ectoderm

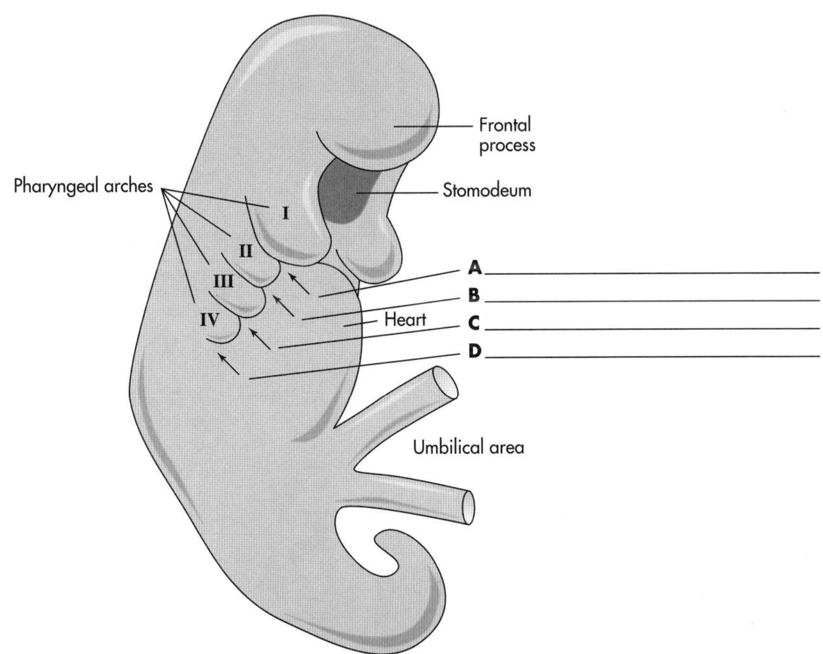

A. groove I
B. groove II
C. groove III
D. groove IV

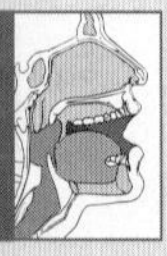

A. arch I
B. arch II
C. arch III
D. arch IV
E. groove I
F. groove II
G. groove III
H. groove IV

If you were to slice into the embryo through the pharyngeal area, it would look like the accompanying diagram. First, identify arches I, II, III, and IV. The outside of each arch is covered in ectoderm. Color that line blue that represents the outside covering or "skin." The arrows are pointing to the grooves. Label grooves I, II, III, and IV.

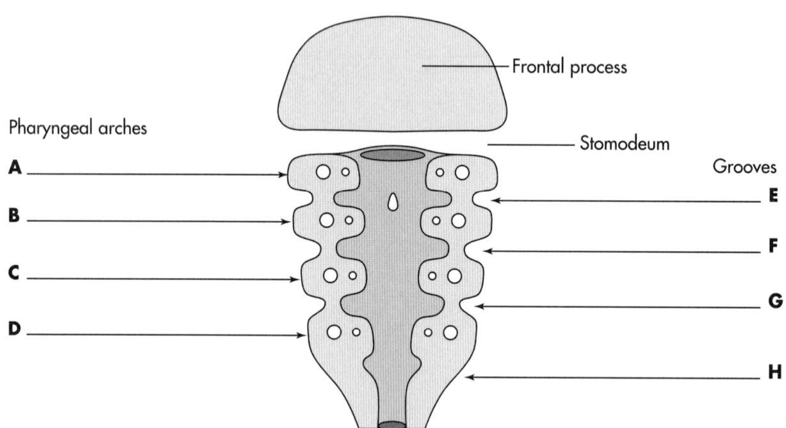

A. groove I
B. groove II
C. groove III
D. groove IV

Arches, pouches, and grooves are important because each turns into or derives something. The paired arches, in general, merge together or fuse to become the face and neck. Let's see first what will become of each groove. It begins with the four grooves on the outside of the embryonic face/neck. Label each groove.

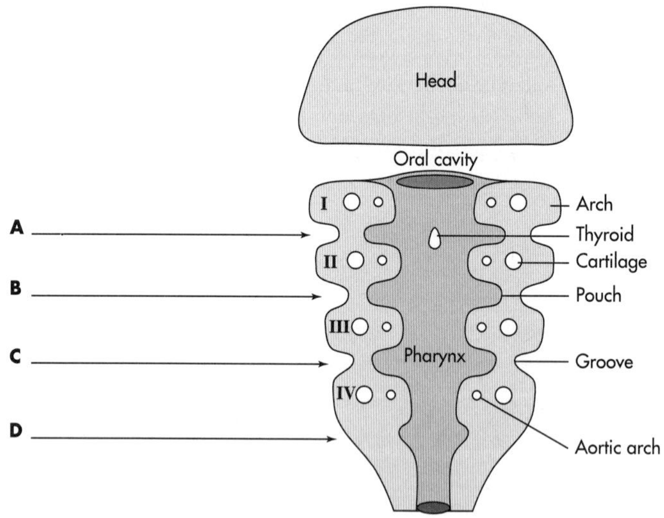

Later, **groove I** bulges into the head, forming an opening at the end of a tube. The tube ends in a pocket that touches pouch I. What is happening to **grooves II, III,** and **IV?**

Grooves II, III, and IV are disappearing.

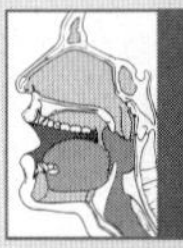

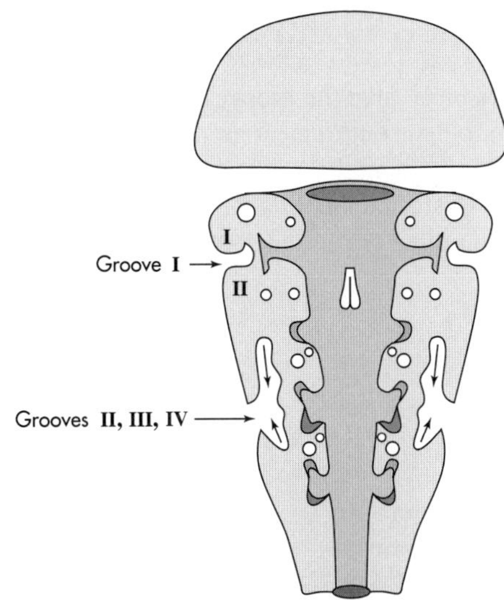

Inside the cutaway of the arches is the inner endoderm tube, the pharynx. Note how the pharynx bulges out directly opposite each groove. Each of these bulges is called a pouch, and these are numbered just like the arches and grooves. Label the drawing.

A. pouch I
B. pouch II
C. pouch III
D. pouch IV

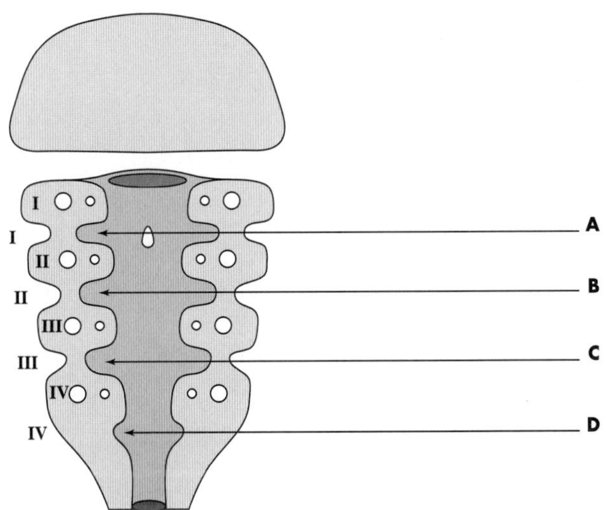

ectoderm, yellow

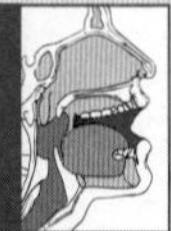

Each groove and pouch define the boundaries of an arch. The outside of the arch is covered with ______________, which you should color as a blue line, and the inside is covered with endoderm, which you can color ______________. The middle of each arch contains mesoderm, which can be colored red.

The pouches develop differently than the grooves. Each pair derives a different structure. **Pouch I,** as we have seen, bulges out to meet groove I. Besides creating the inner portion of the **eardrum,** it makes an opening into the pharynx known as the **Eustachian tube.** Also, the space before the Eustachian tube is the **middle ear cavity,** to which it connects. The middle ear contains the three small bones of the ear known as the **ossicles.**

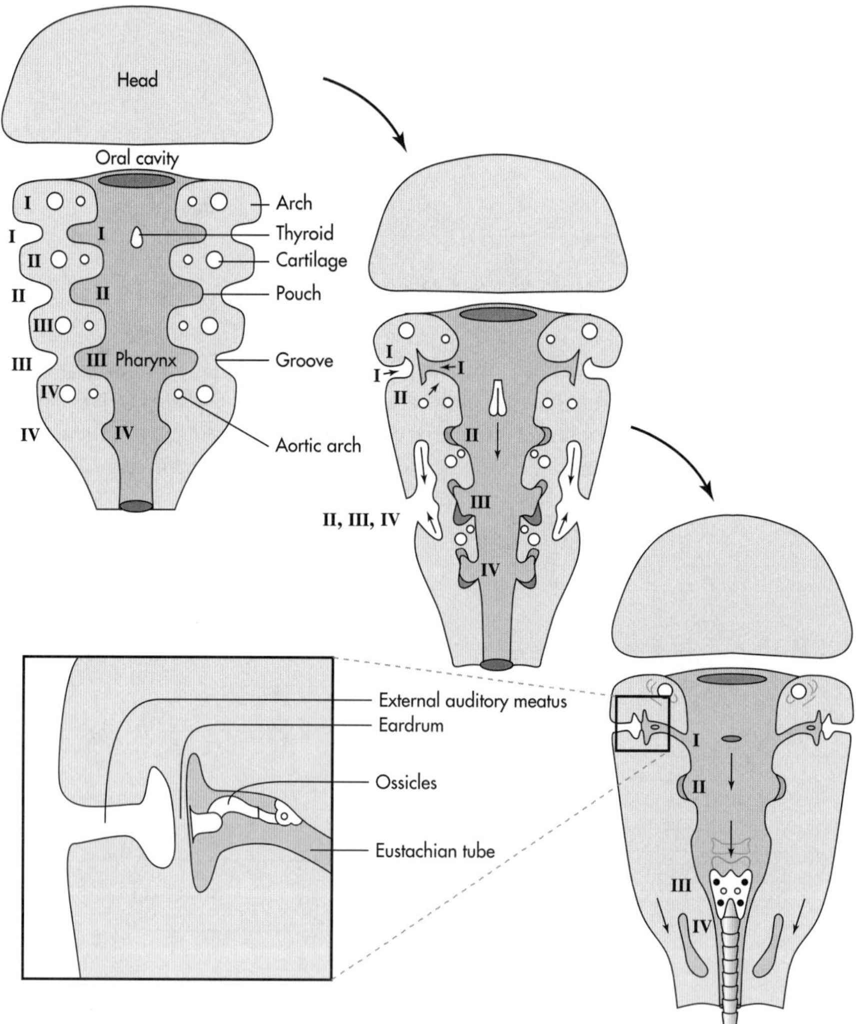

Follow what happens to **pouch II.** It bulges in by itself to form a gland in the pharynx called the **palatine tonsil.**

palatine tonsils

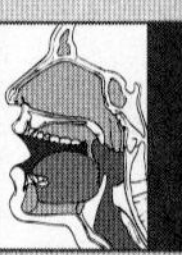

Pouches III and IV divide into two bulges each as shown before. These eight different areas develop into the glands known as the **parathyroids,** the **C cells of the thyroid,** and the **thymus gland.** All are migrating down the neck, where they relocate. What does pouch II derive?

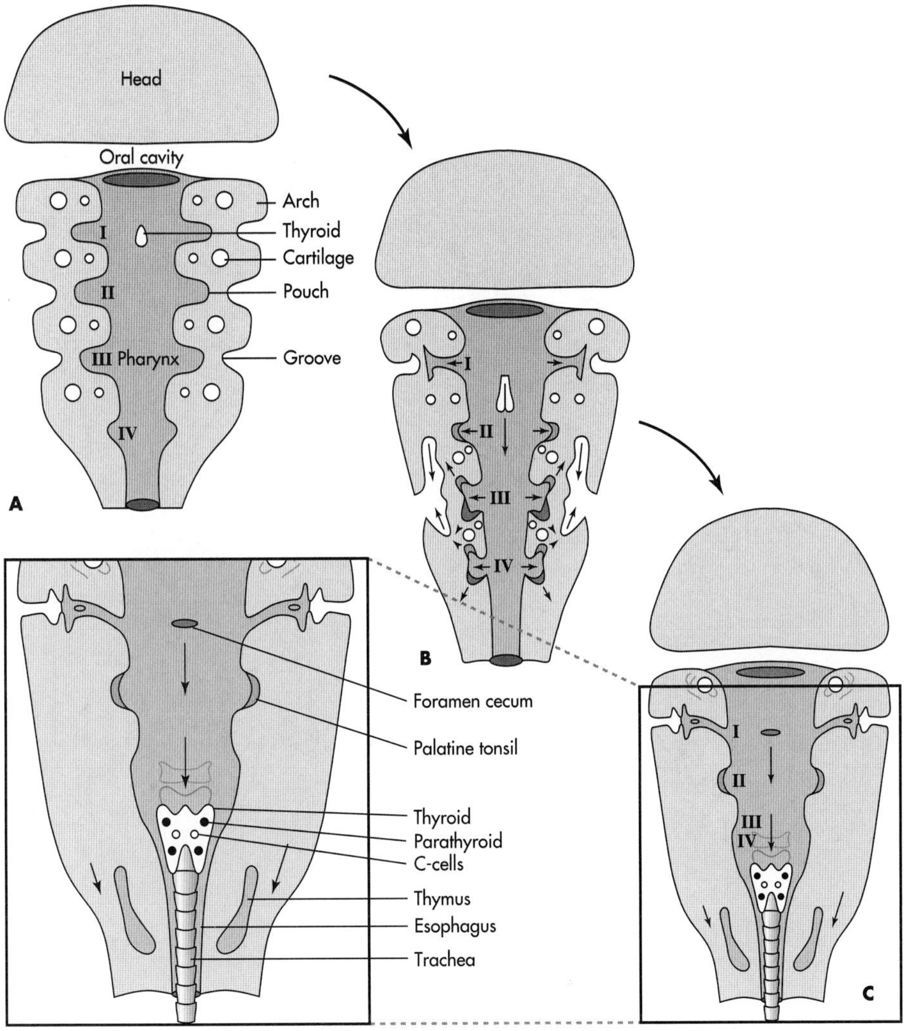

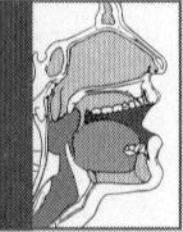

The mesoderm in each arch also has a special fate. Remember that this mesoderm came originally from the neural crest cells. Some of that mesoderm condenses into a rod of cartilage in each arch, also labeled cartilage I, II, III, and IV, although cartilage I and II are also named for scientists who discovered them. The rest of the mesoderm becomes the muscle, bone, and connective tissue of the face and neck.

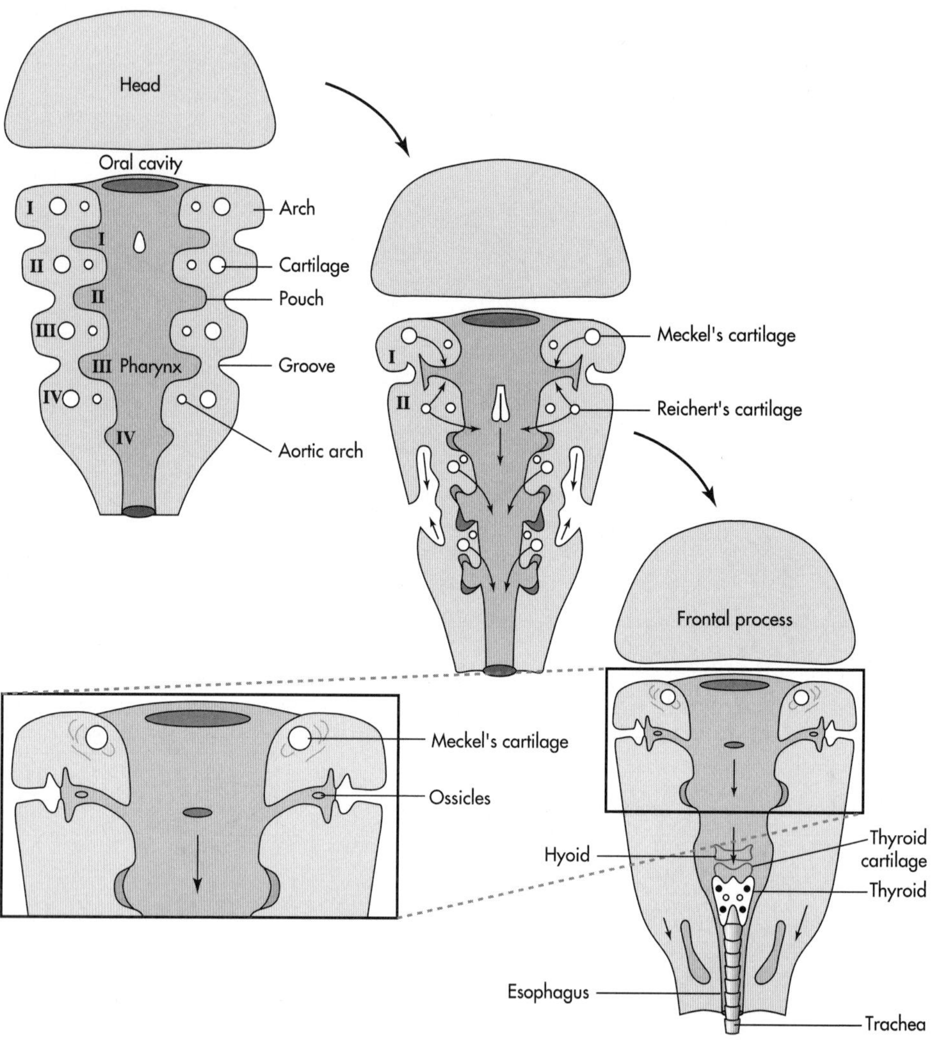

Meckel's cartilage

Cartilage I is more frequently called Meckel's cartilage and cartilage II is called Reichert's cartilage. What is arch I cartilage called?

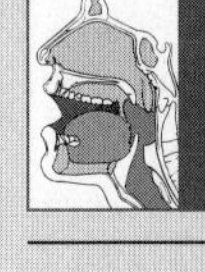

Meckel's cartilage persists in the embryo for a long time, but eventually disappears with bone development. Meckel's cartilage forms a temporary "jawbone" for the developing embryo by fusing together to form a single rod in the mandible. The very tip of this cartilage near the ear helps form the ossicles of the middle ear, and in the adult, a few derivatives of Meckel's cartilage persist as ligaments.

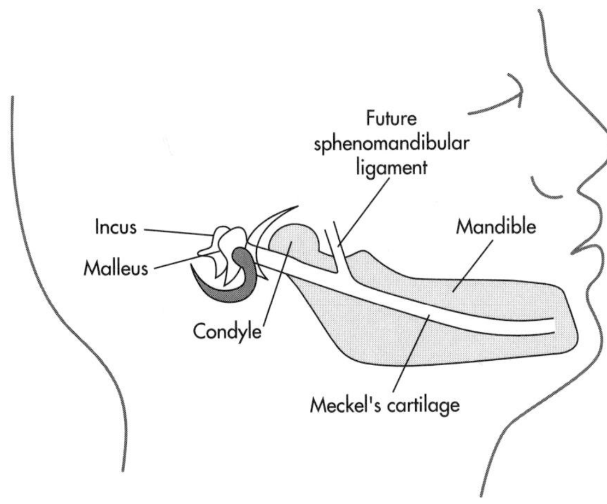

It becomes the temporary "jawbone" of the mandible, ossicles, and sphenomandibular ligament.

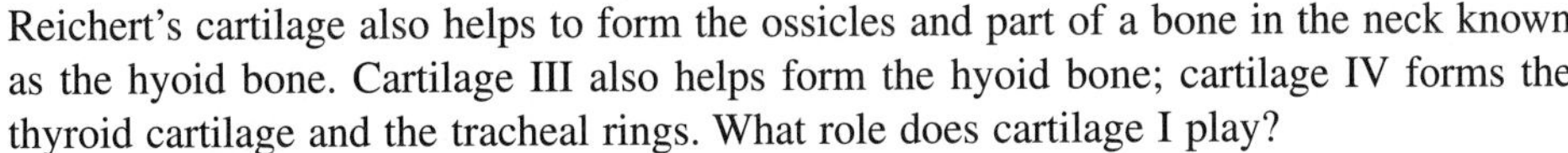

Reichert's cartilage also helps to form the ossicles and part of a bone in the neck known as the hyoid bone. Cartilage III also helps form the hyoid bone; cartilage IV forms the thyroid cartilage and the tracheal rings. What role does cartilage I play?

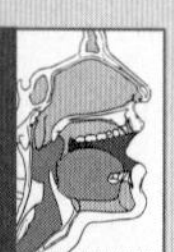

Groove I: external meatus, tympanic membrane
Groove II: disappears
Groove III: disappears
Groove IV: disappears
Pouch I: eustachian tube, tympanic membrane, middle ear cavity
Pouch II: palatine tonsils
Pouch III: parathyroid, thymus
Pouch IV: parathyroid, C cells
Meckel's cartilage: temporary jaw, ossicles
Reichert's cartilage: ossicles, hyoid
Cartilage III: hyoid
Cartilage IV: tracheal rings, thyroid cartilage

Each arch also contains a blood vessel from the mesoderm, called an aortic arch, but we will not follow them.

Review the derivatives of the pharyngeal arches by listing what they develop:

Groove I ____________________
Groove II ____________________
Groove III ____________________
Groove IV ____________________
Pouch I ____________________
Pouch II ____________________
Pouch III ____________________
Pouch IV ____________________
Meckel's cartilage ____________________
Reichert's cartilage ____________________
Cartilage III ____________________
Cartilage IV ____________________

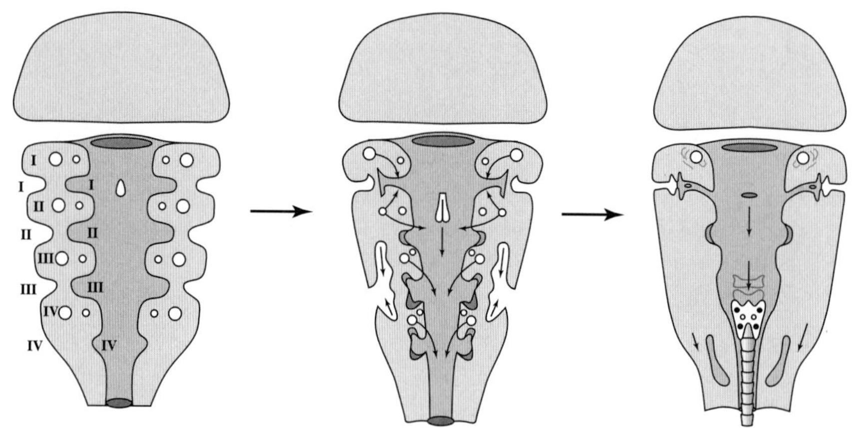

3.2 Stomodeum and Tongue

At the head end of the embryo we have seen something that looks like the diagram here.

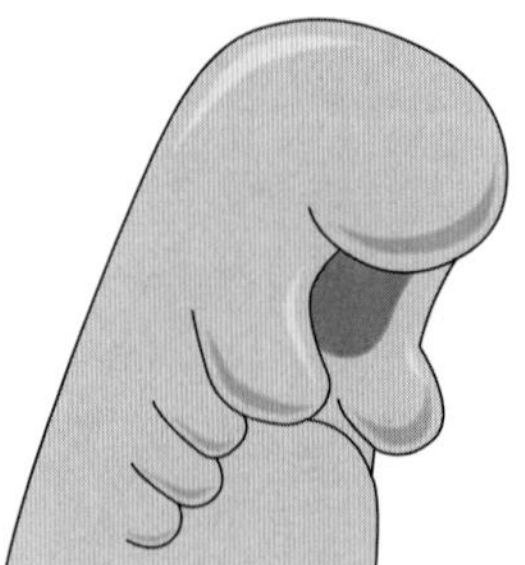

pharyngeal, ectoderm

Note the paired bumps or ____________ arches, named because they cluster around the pharynx. The outside of the head is covered with which embryonic germ layer?

The arches surround an apparent opening to the inside of the embryo. This area is called the **stomodeum,** or future mouth region. At first, the stomodeum is covered by a membrane called the **buccopharyngeal membrane.** This membrane eventually ruptures and disappears. What is the future mouth called?

stomodeum

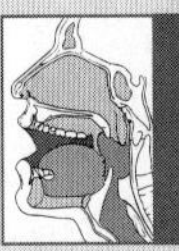

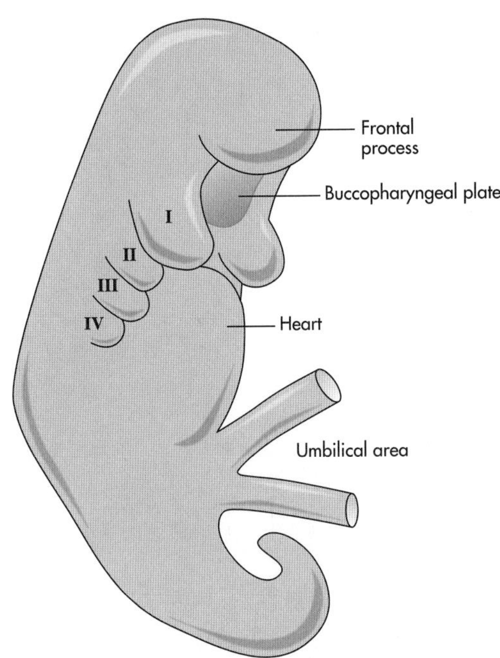

The stomodeum leads into the future digestive tube of the embryo, which is made of which embryonic layer? You can see both the inside and outside of the embryo in this picture.

endoderm

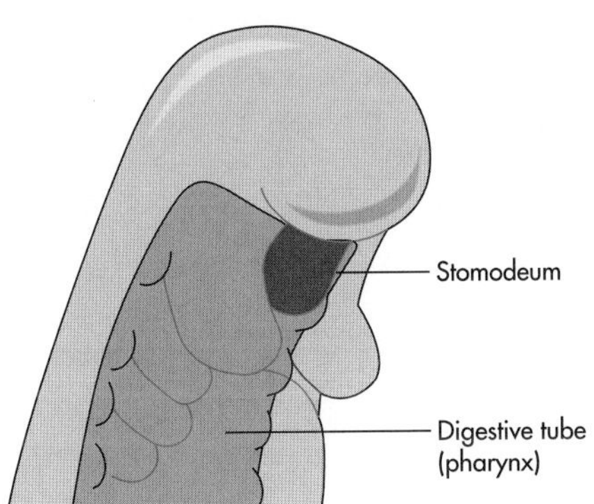

buccopharyngeal membrane

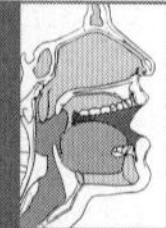

Note that Figure A is drawn with the temporary membrane; the _______________ is in place and it is gone in Figure B. Now look at the stomodeum in the floor of the future mouth or oral cavity. Tissue is beginning to bulge out in this area as shown in the next frame.

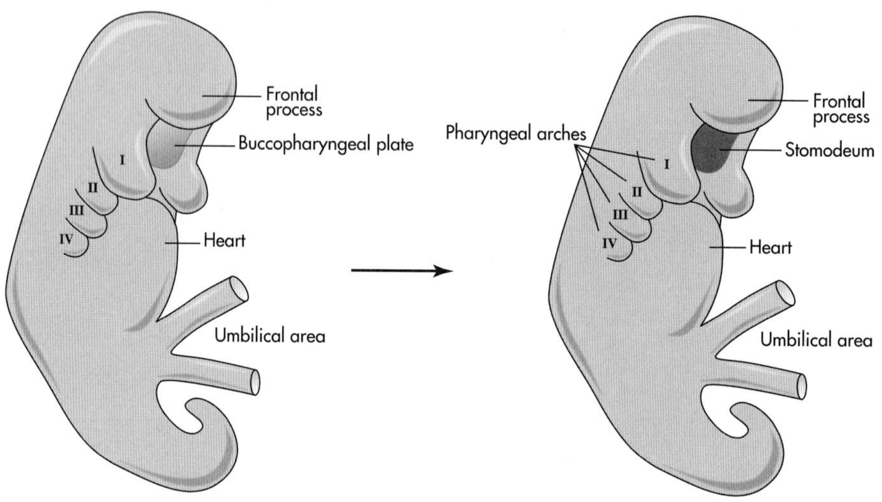

six

This is a different view of the floor or ventrum of the developing mouth. Find the pharyngeal arches. Figure A is a diagram of earlier development than Figure B. How many "bumps" are coming together to form the single "bump" known as the tongue?

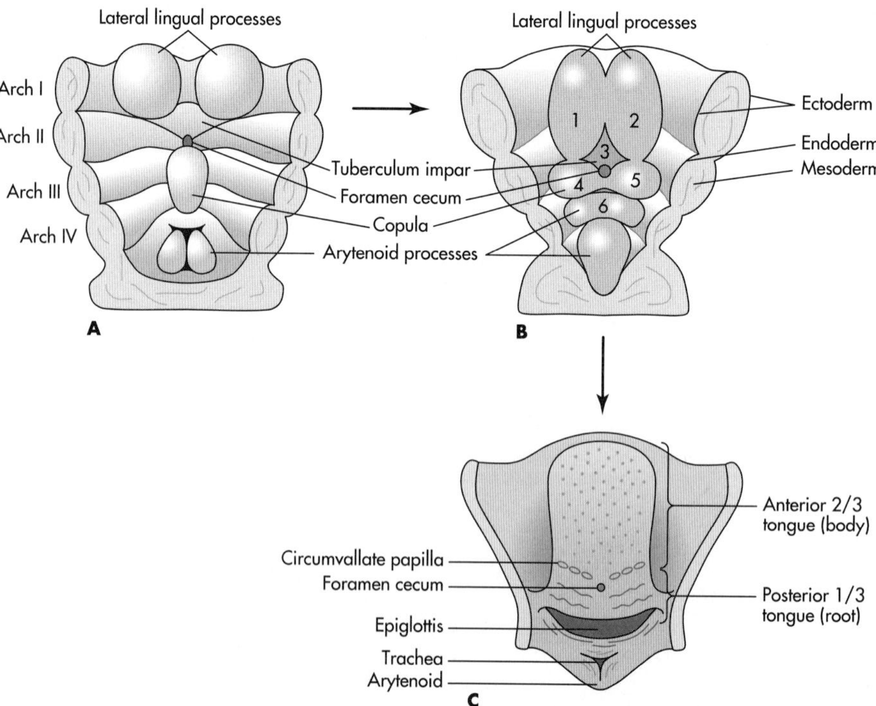

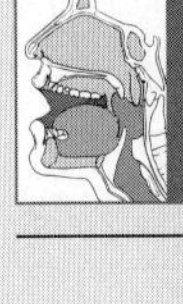

The front of the tongue is called the **anterior two thirds** of the tongue or the **body of the tongue.** Three "bumps" or **processes** come together to form the anterior two thirds of the tongue. They are the two **lateral lingual processes** and the **tuberculum impar.**

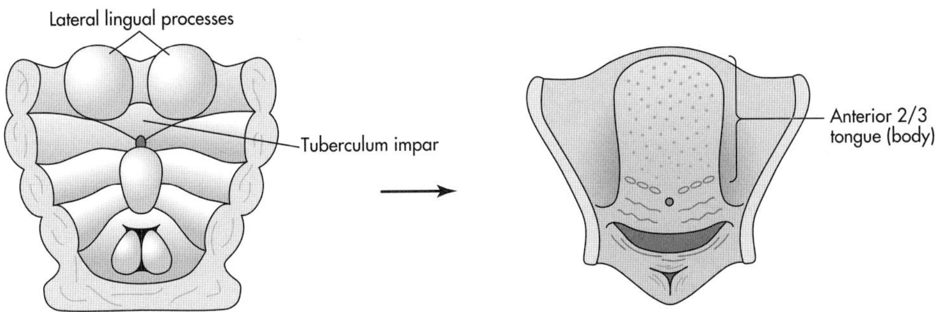

Look again at the development of the tongue from the side view or section through the embryo. Look at where the ectoderm and endoderm layers lie. They meet inside the future oral cavity and you can see that meeting place on the tongue. The border between the ectoderm and endoderm is also the border between the anterior two thirds and posterior one third of the tongue, where the **circumvallate papillae** and **foramen cecum** lie. Which three processes form the body of the tongue?

two lateral lingual processes plus tuberculum impar

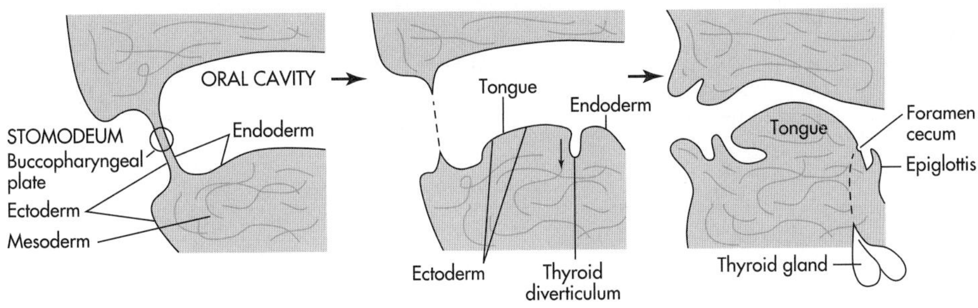

Ectoderm forms the covering tissue over the ______________ of the tongue, and endoderm covers the ______________. In the middle of the tongue are muscles that have been formed by the third embryonic germ layer or ______________. You may color these tissues red, blue, or yellow as needed.

anterior two thirds or body, posterior one third or root, mesoderm

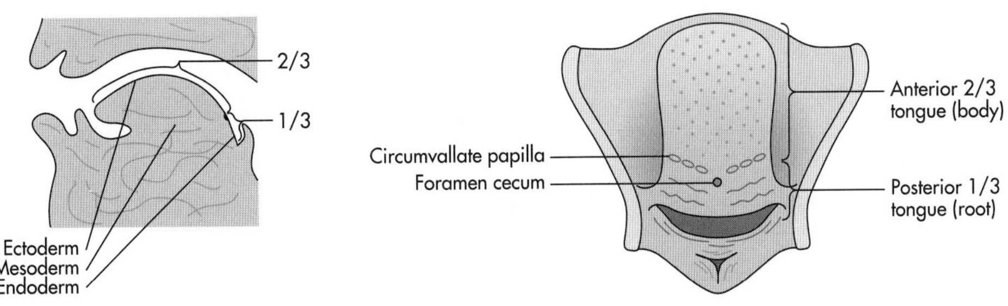

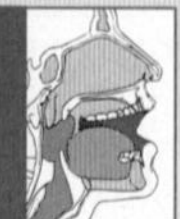

The posterior one third or root of the tongue is also formed by three processes coming together or **coalescing.** They are the **copula** and two parts of arch II.

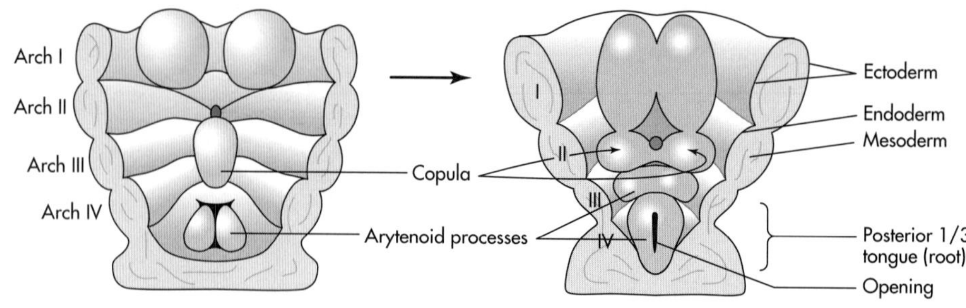

Note that there is a natural border between the anterior tongue and the posterior tongue created by a V-shaped row of circumvallate papillae and a bump or "hole" at the base of the V called the foramen cecum.

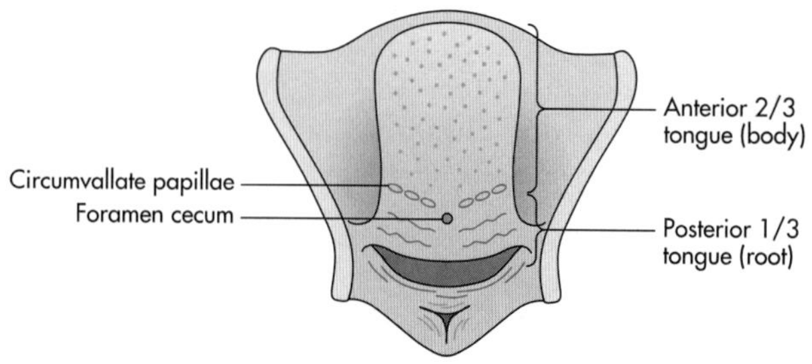

A. lateral lingual processes
B. tuberculum impar
C. foramen cecum
D. copula
E. arytenoid processes
F. circumvallate papillae
G. foramen cecum
H. epiglottis
I. trachea
J. anterior two thirds of tongue
K. posterior one third of tongue

Label the three diagrams of the tongue.

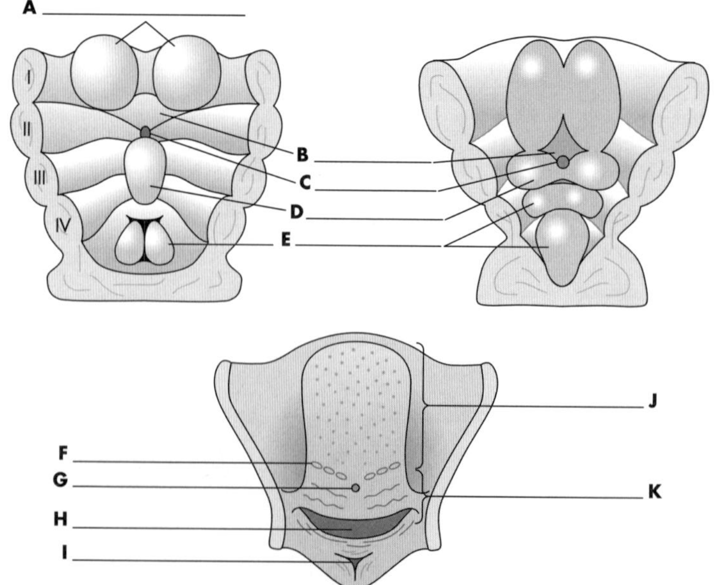

Lungs and Thyroid

3.3

thyroid diverticulum

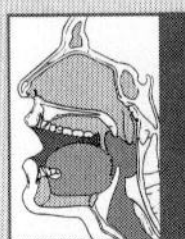

Next we see where the foramen cecum originates. Look again at a side or sagittal section of the embryo's head. Label and/or color where ectoderm, endoderm, and mesoderm are located. Find the area of the developing tongue and note the small pouch developing downward inside that tongue tissue. What is it called?

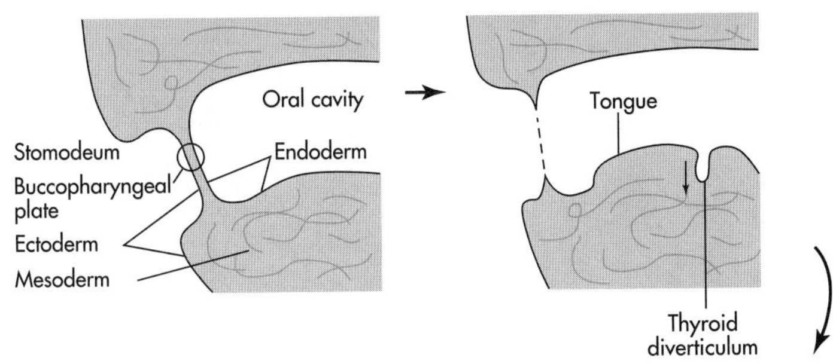

Watch as the pocket of tissue (endoderm) bulges downward, splits into two lobes, and travels away from the tongue, eventually separating from it. This is the development of the **thyroid gland.** The thyroid glad is a bilobed gland located in the anterior neck.

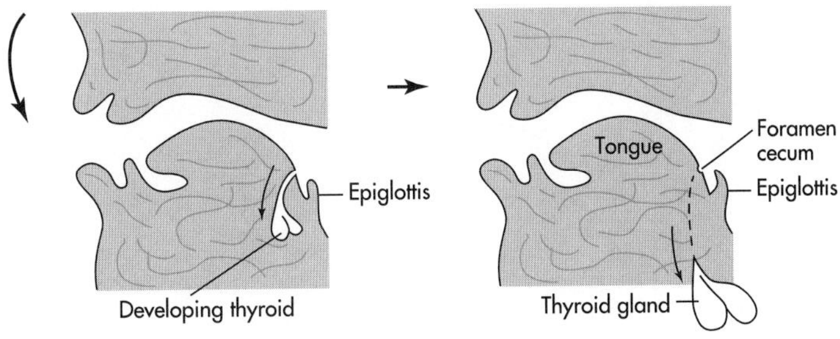

thyroid

After the _______________ gland is done developing, it leaves behind on the tongue some tissue that has no apparent function, the **foramen cecum,** a remnant. Label it in the diagram. Remember it is on the border between anterior and posterior tongue (or the border between the ectoderm and endoderm layers).

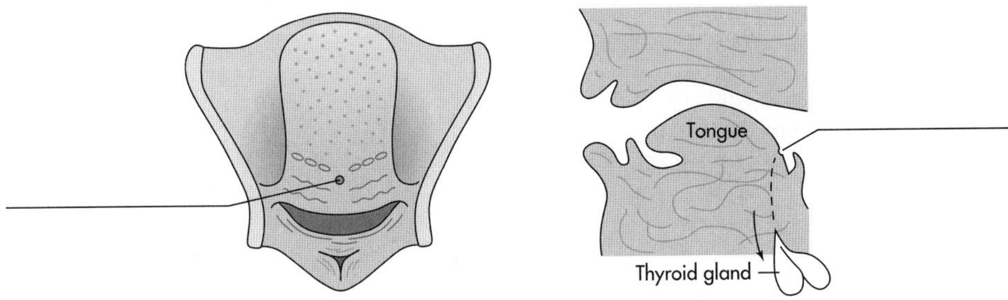

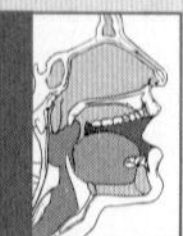

Look again at a sagittal section of the embryo's head. We assume that the tongue and thyroid are developed. Look at another pocket of tissue bulging out from the floor of the pharynx, behind the tongue and behind the thyroid bulge.

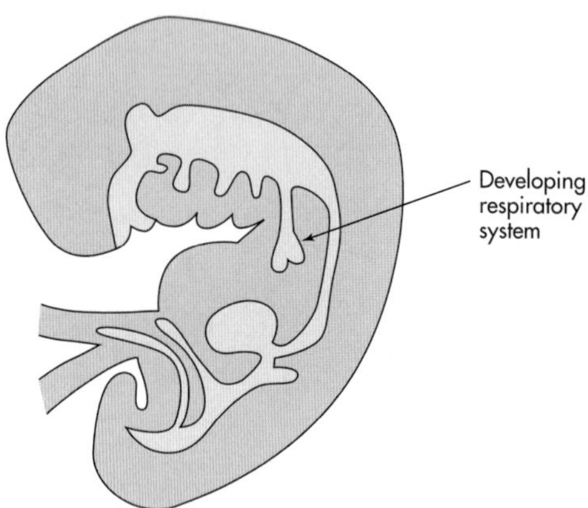

Watch as this endoderm tissue develops downward, dividing into two lobes. This tissue grows quite large as compared with the thyroid gland. These endodermal derivatives are the **trachea, bronchii,** and **lungs** of the **respiratory system.**

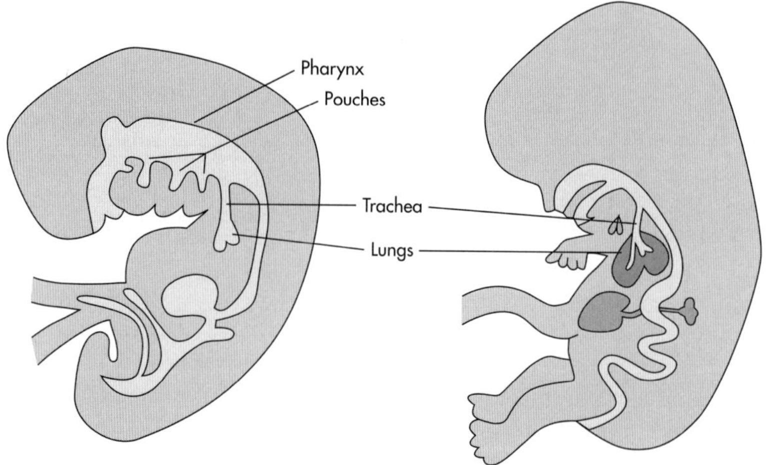

trachea (air)

Development of the trachea divides the single tube inside the embryo into two tubes: one for food (the pharynx) and one for air (the trachea). They lie next to each other in the neck. Which tube is more anterior?

FACIAL DEVELOPMENT

4.0

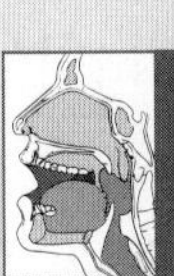

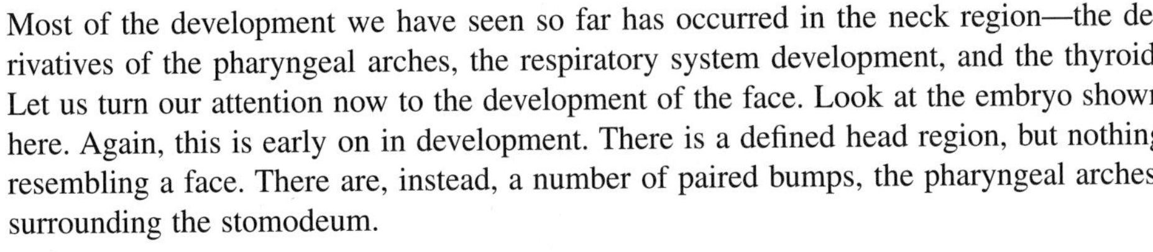

Most of the development we have seen so far has occurred in the neck region—the derivatives of the pharyngeal arches, the respiratory system development, and the thyroid. Let us turn our attention now to the development of the face. Look at the embryo shown here. Again, this is early on in development. There is a defined head region, but nothing resembling a face. There are, instead, a number of paired bumps, the pharyngeal arches, surrounding the stomodeum.

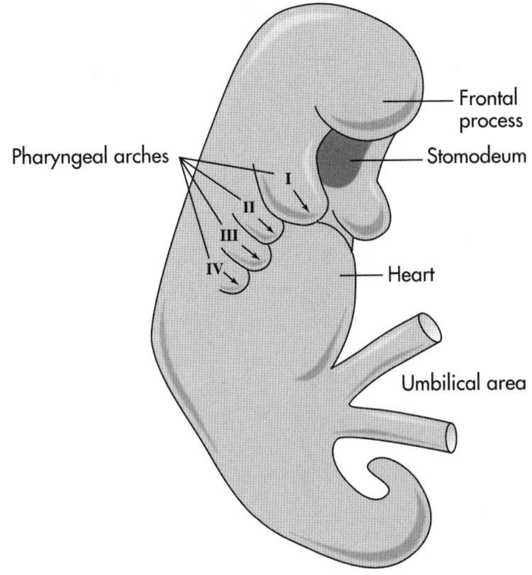

endoderm

The drawing is an interior view of the preceding embryo. Remember that the head is covered with ectoderm and has an inside tube made of ________________ with mesoderm filling all the spaces in between. Color them.

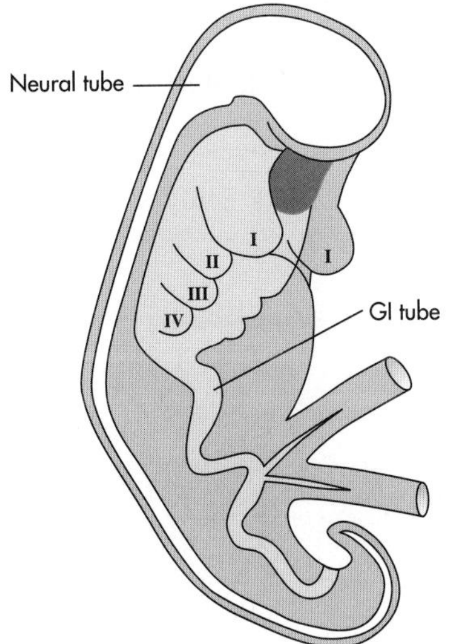

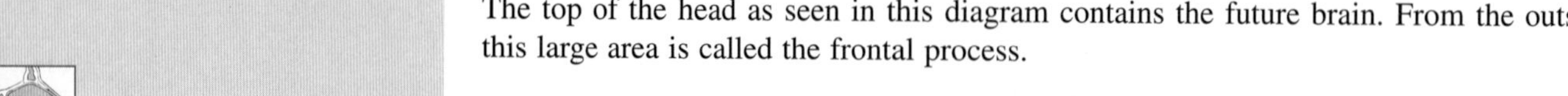

The top of the head as seen in this diagram contains the future brain. From the outside this large area is called the frontal process.

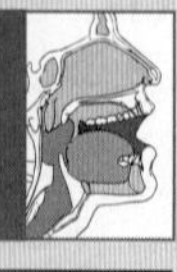

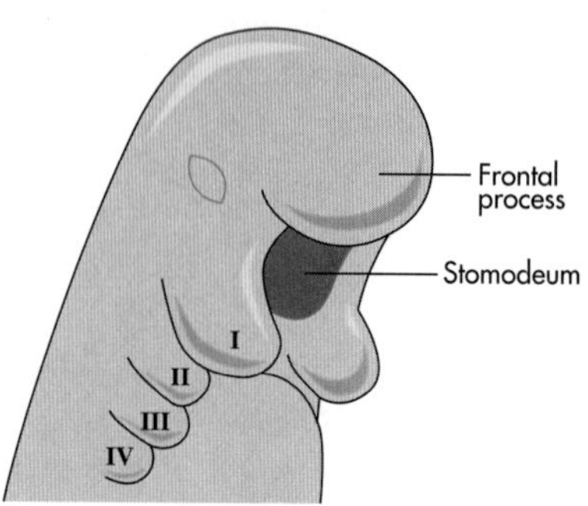

The **frontal process** is going to give rise to five other processes that will help form the face. Let us follow its development.

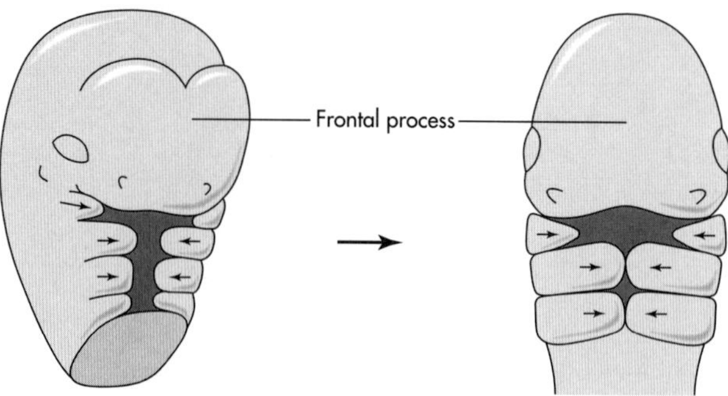

The frontal process grows down toward the stomodeum, developing a long extension down the middle of the face called the **globular process.** Follow its development below.

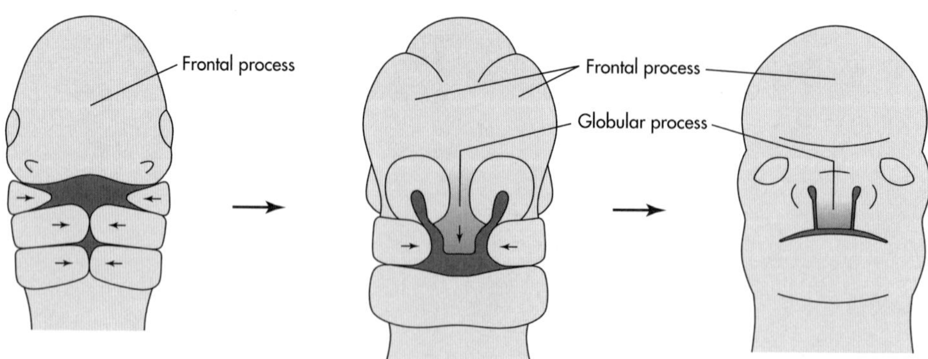

Beneath the surface of the face the globular process is growing into an area that will become the roof of the mouth or palate. Look under the mouth area to see that portion of the globular process becoming the **primary palate.** The primary palate is part of which process?

globular

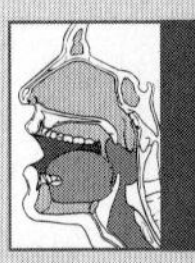

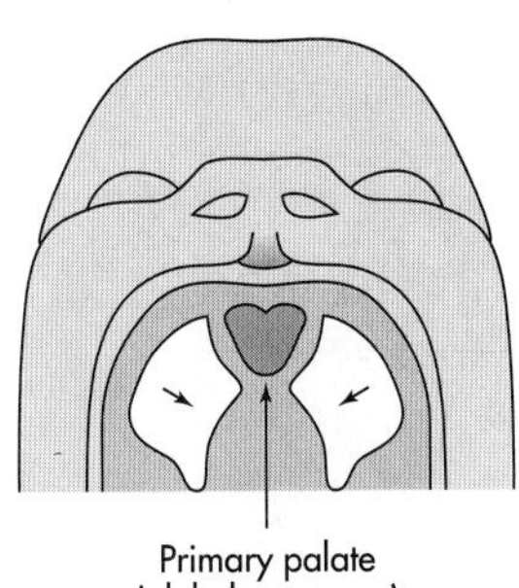

The frontal process also develops two semicircular areas or four processes in the middle face. The diagram shows the **lateral** and **median nasal processes** on both right and left sides.

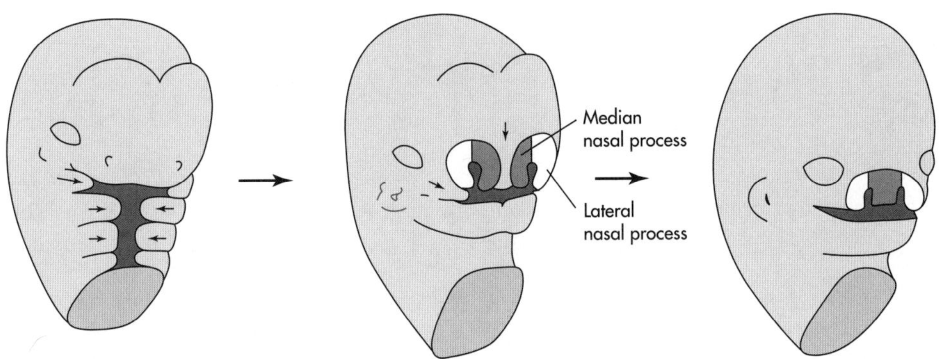

Note how the nasal area comes together, with the fusion of the median nasal processes forming the middle of the nose. The sides of the nose are formed by the lateral nasal processes, and the philtrum of the lip, by the ______________ process.

globular

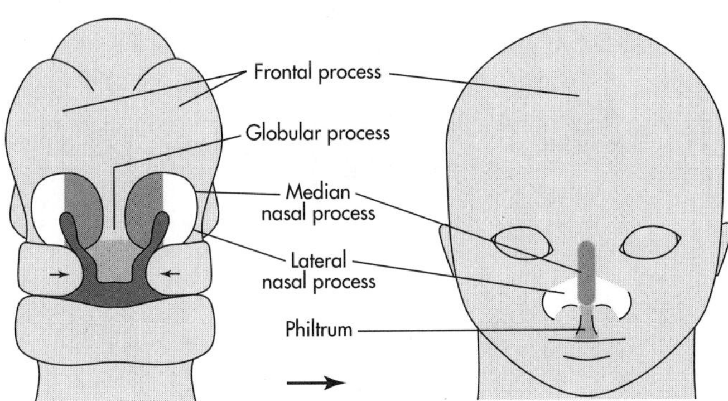

maxilla
and mandible

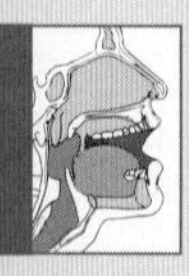

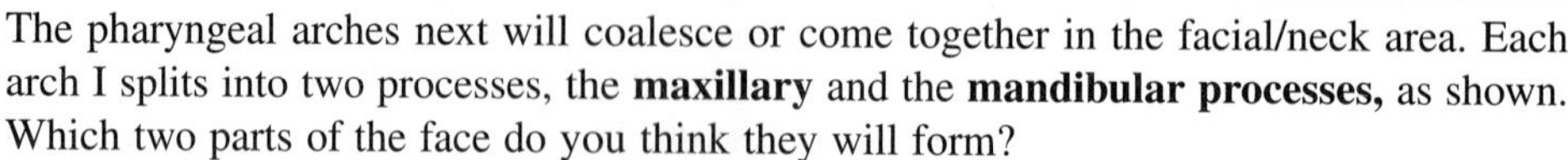

The pharyngeal arches next will coalesce or come together in the facial/neck area. Each arch I splits into two processes, the **maxillary** and the **mandibular processes,** as shown. Which two parts of the face do you think they will form?

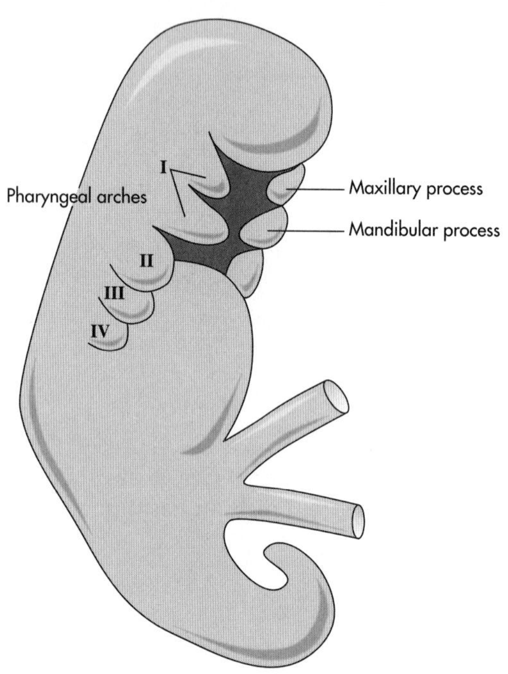

neural crest

Remember that each arch was covered in ectoderm and has a core of mesoderm. This mesoderm was special and came from the ______________ cells that used to be ectoderm.

Follow next the movement of the **maxillary processes** as they try to join together, but meet in the middle with the globular process.

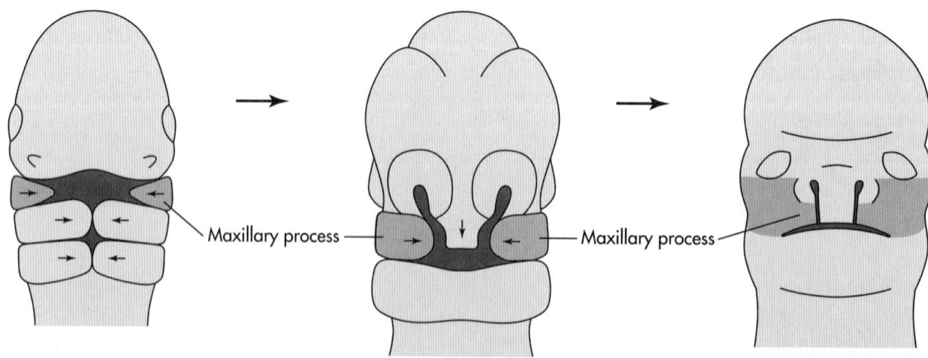

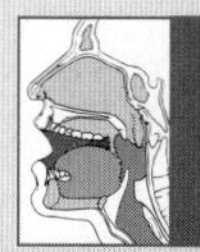

The maxillary processes form the maxilla and cheeks of the embryonic face and part of the lip. If you tip up the embryo to look in the mouth again, you will see the maxillary processes forming the sides of the palate or the **lateral palatine processes.**

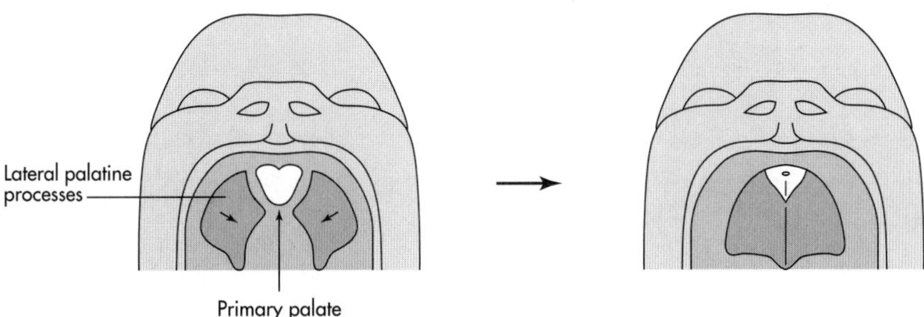

The palate, then, is formed by three processes coalescing: two maxillary processes (____________ palatine processes) and one globular process (____________ palatine).

lateral, primary

PALATAL DEVELOPMENT

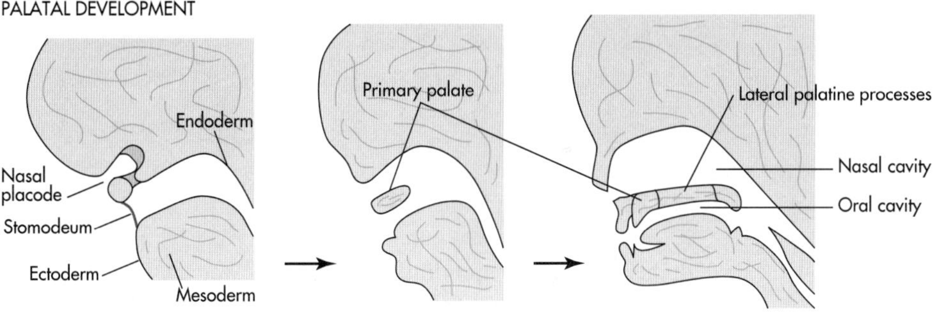

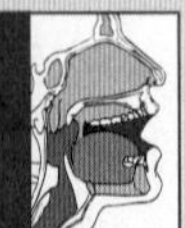

If processes do not come together properly, the embryo and child will have an anomaly or abnormality. When the globular and maxillary processes do not join properly, the result is either a **cleft lip** or a **cleft palate.** Either type of cleft may happen anywhere along the line of normal fusion.

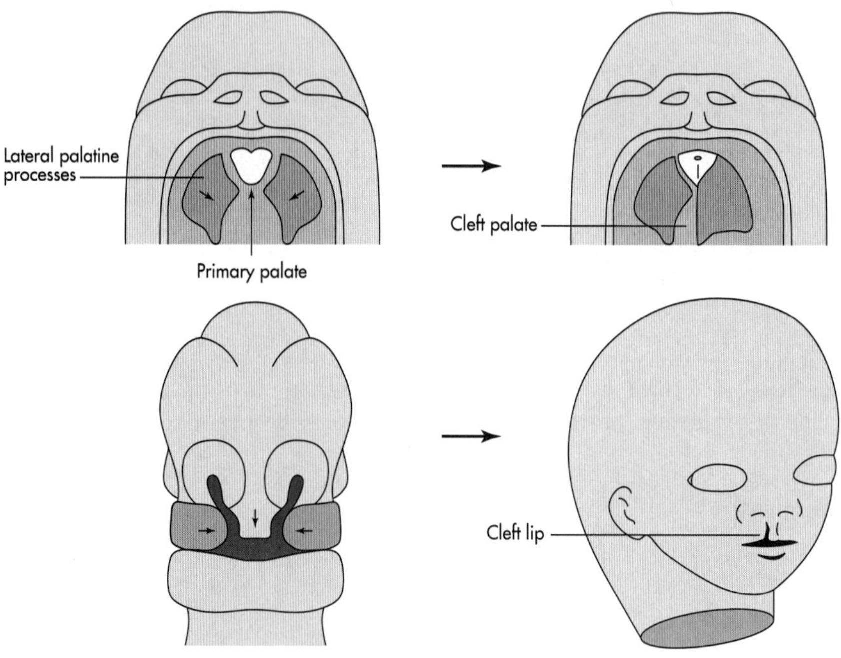

Lastly, follow the development of the two **mandibular processes.** Watch as they come together in the middle and fuse to become one process, the future lower jaw: the mandible.

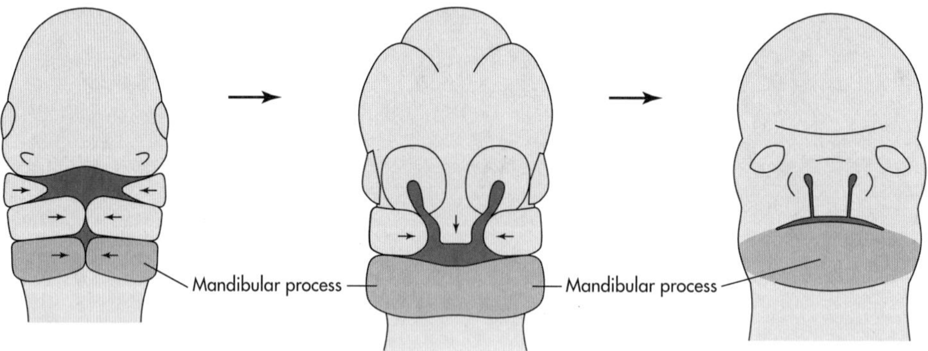

maxillary

Remember the mandibular processes were half of arch I. What facial process was the other half?

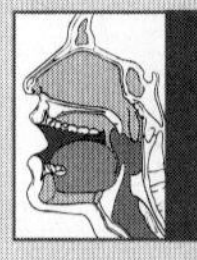

Remember also that inside of arch I, now located medial to the mandibular process, is a rod of cartilage that goes from one side to the other: **Meckel's cartilage.** This will act as a temporary "jawbone" until the bone of the mandible envelops it and most of it disappears.

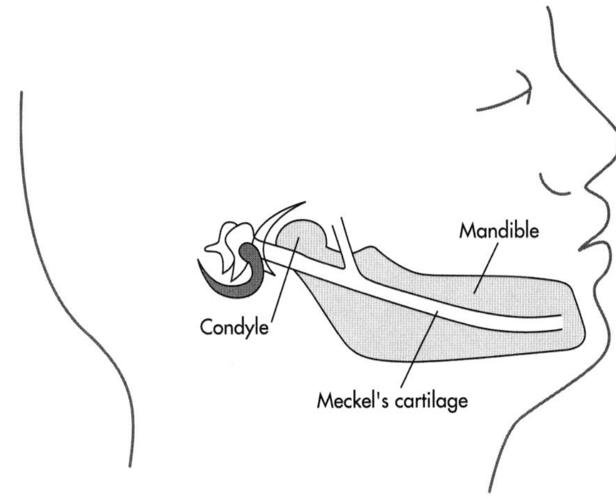

upward

Note the overall development of the face now: how the eyes begin on the outside of the face and move around toward the middle as the facial processes grow together. Also, the ears begin down low on the neck and move _______________ as the jaw grows larger.

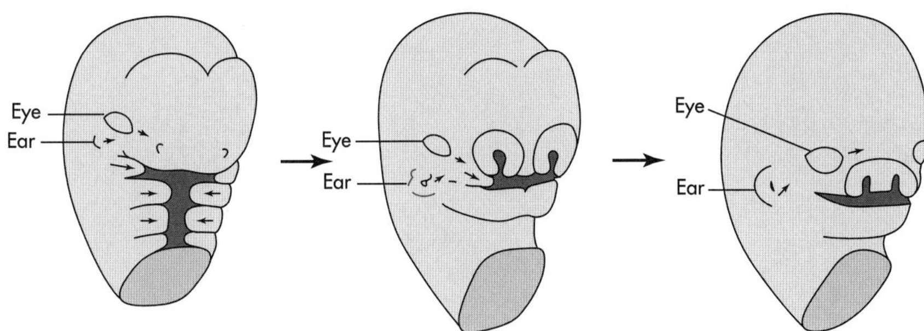

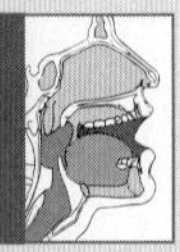

A. frontal
B. mandibular
C. globular
D. lateral nasal
E. median nasal
F. globular
G. philtrum
H. maxillary
I. maxillary
J. lateral nasal
K. mandibular
L. maxilla

Review the development of the face by labeling the processes.

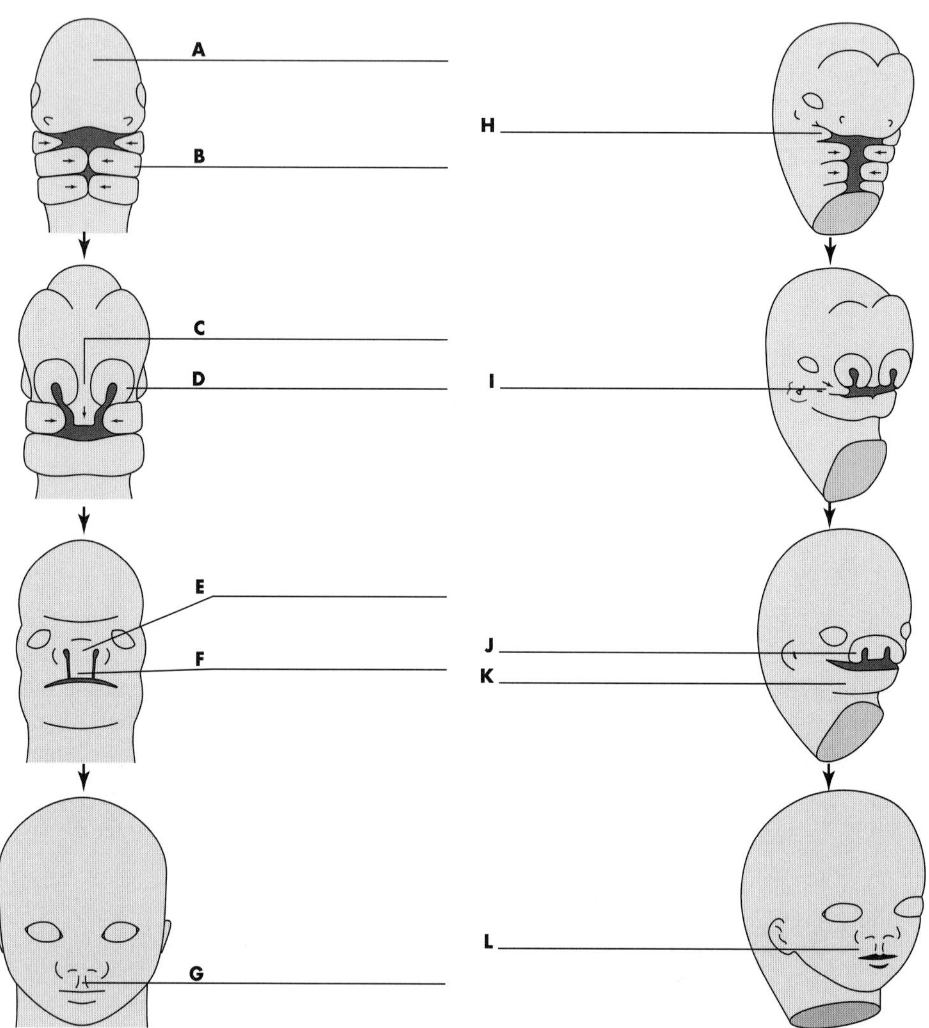

We have followed the development of the embryo, with special consideration of the fate of each of the three germ layers: ectoderm, endoderm, and mesoderm. If there is a section of the body's development you do not understand, review it at this time. In the next chapter we focus on the development of the teeth, which also ultimately come from the embryo and its layers of developing cells.

REVIEW TEST 2.1

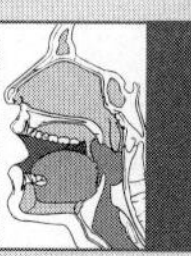

SELECT THE CORRECT ANSWER.

1. When gametes combine they form a(n)
   a. fetus
   b. morula
   c. zygote
   d. egg cell

2. Cell division that makes different types of cells from another cell is called
   a. mitosis
   b. meiosis
   c. differentiation

3. The hollow ball of cells formed from the zygote is the
   a. gamete
   b. blastula
   c. morula

4. A human 10 weeks of age from conception is a(n)
   a. embryo
   b. fetus

5. The embryo will attach and gain nourishment through fingerlike projections into the uterus. This area will develop into the ______________ and ______________ of the fetus.
   a. chorion, amnion
   b. placenta, umbilical cord

6. The embryo diffentiates into three primary ______________ layers.
   a. fetal
   b. chorionic
   c. germ

7. The future organs and systems built from the three germ layers are its
   a. remnants
   b. differentiations
   c. derivatives

8. The ______________ is the first derivative of ectoderm on the outer body of the embryo.
   a. skin
   b. epidermis
   c. dermis

9. Ectoderm that has been folded in from the surface and sunk below the surface as a tube from head to tail is called the
   a. groove
   b. neural tube
   c. somites
   d. neural crest

REVIEW TEST 2.2

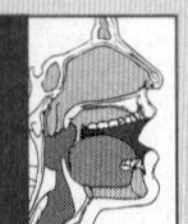

SELECT THE CORRECT ANSWER.

1. Cells that bud off of the neural tube in pairs are called
   a. somites
   b. neural crest

2. Pairs of neural crest cells coming off of the brain area will become the
   a. spinal nerves
   b. cranial nerves
   c. facial mesoderm
   d. b and c

3. The beginning portion of the developing endoderm tube is the ______________, which is a wide area that forms paired pouches.
   a. stomach
   b. pharynx
   c. intestine

4. The endoderm tube bulges out and bends just beyond the esophagus to form the
   a. stomach
   b. pharynx
   c. intestines

5. Paired bumps of mesoderm form along the sides of the neural tube and are called
   a. neural crest
   b. spinal nerves
   c. somites

6. Which is not a division of the somite?
   a. sclerotome
   b. myotome
   c. dermis
   d. dermatome

7. The circulatory system derives from paired tubes of endoderm. True or false?

8. Paired bumps growing along either side of the embryo's head and neck region are called the pharyngeal
   a. arches
   b. grooves
   c. pouches

9. The outside of an arch is covered with ______________; the pouch is made of
   a. endoderm, ectoderm
   b. mesoderm, endoderm
   c. ectoderm, endoderm

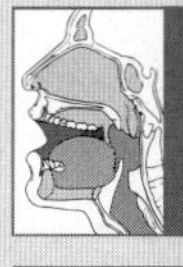

REVIEW TEST 2.3

SELECT THE CORRECT ANSWER.

1. Grooves I to IV eventually disappear. True or false?
2. Which does not derive from pouch I?
   a. external auditory meatus
   b. Eustachian tube
   c. middle ear cavity
   d. eardrum
3. What derives the palatine tonsils?
   a. groove I
   b. pouch I
   c. pouch II
   d. pouch III
4. The anterior two thirds of the tongue is called the
   a. root
   b. body
   c. epiglottis
5. The lateral lingual processes coalesce with the tuberculum impar to form the posterior tongue. True or false?
6. The V-shaped row of bumps on the tongue are the ______________, and they mark the border between anterior and posterior tongue.
   a. foramen cecum
   b. thyroid diverticulum
   c. copula
   d. circumvallate papillae
7. Which pharyngeal arch divides into the maxillary and mandibular processes?
   a. I
   b. II
   c. III
8. Which process does not come from the frontal process?
   a. maxillary process
   b. globular process
   c. median nasal process
   d. lateral nasal process
9. The globular process becomes the philtrum and the primary palate. True or false?

REVIEW TEST 2.4

FILL IN THE CORRECT ANSWER(S).

1. The combination of sperm and egg cells to form a zygote is called ______________, and it usually occurs in the fallopian tube.

2. ______________ is the embedding of the developing embryo into the maternal uterine wall.

3. The embryo is the group of cells that will differentiate into a human being. True or false?

4. The blastula contains cells that differentiate into the embryo and the ______________ and fluid.

5. Following development of the embryo, we begin with a flat plate of cells that fold up into a tube that then folds over as a C-shaped organism. True or false?

6. At first, nourishment for the embryo comes from a temporary fluid-filled sac called the ______________ sac.

7. The three embryonic germ layers are ______________, ______________, and ______________.

8. We have used the color ______________ for endoderm.

9. Ectoderm folding in along the length of the embryo is called the ______________ groove, and it becomes the ______________ tube.

10. Neural tube derives the ______________ and ______________ of the central nervous system.

11. Pairs of neural crest cells coming off the spinal cord will become the ______________ nerves.

12. The only place in the embryo where ectoderm will turn into mesoderm is in the tail. True or false?

13. The ______________ system consisting of the brain, spinal cord, and all the nerves derives from ectoderm.

14. The color code for ectoderm is ______________.

15. The ______________ and ______________ systems develop from the endodermal tube.

REVIEW TEST 2.5

FILL IN THE CORRECT ANSWER(S).

1. Mesoderm is color coded ______________.

2. Two systems that give structure and movement to the body are the ______________ and ______________ systems, and they derive from mesoderm.

3. A tissue that is "left over" from development with no particular function in the adult is called a(n) ______________.

4. The area of the embryo that will become the future mouth is called the ______________. It is covered for a short time by the ______________ membrane.

5. The cartilage of arch I is called ______________ cartilage.

6. The ossicles come from the cartilage of arch I (Meckel's) and arch II, also known as ______________ cartilage.
7. How many processes come together to form the tongue?
8. The remnant of the developing thyroid gland left on the surface of the tongue is called the ______________.
9. The facial process that becomes the forehead is called the ______________ process.
10. Which processes coalesce to become the hard palate?
11. Do the two maxillary processes ever come together?
12. If facial processes do not come together properly, a ______________ lip or palate may result.
13. The temporary "jawbone" in the mandibular arch is known as ______________.

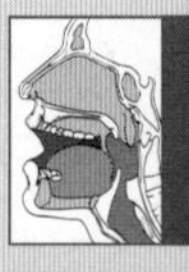

REVIEW TEST 2.6

MATCH THE STRUCTURE WITH THE GERM LAYER FROM WHICH IT IS DERIVED.

1. digestive system ______________
2. thyroid gland ______________
3. epidermis ______________
4. bones ______________
5. brain ______________
6. muscle ______________
7. respiratory system ______________
8. lining of anterior two thirds tongue ______________

a. ectoderm
b. mesoderm
c. endoderm

REVIEW TEST 2.7

MATCH THE ARCH/POUCH/GROOVE WITH THE STRUCTURE IT DERIVES.

1. Eustachian tube ______________
2. parathyroid glands ______________
3. Meckel's cartilage ______________
4. palatine tonsils ______________
5. eardrum ______________
6. external meatus ______________

a. groove I
b. arch I
c. arch II
d. pouch I
e. pouch II
f. pouches III and IV

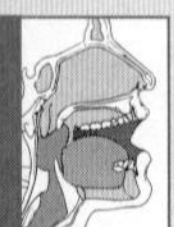

REVIEW TEST 2.8

MATCH THE PROCESS WITH THE STRUCTURE THAT IT BECOMES.

1. cheeks ______________
2. forehead ______________
3. mandible ______________
4. sides of nose ______________
5. philtrum ______________
6. sides of palate ______________
7. front of palate ______________

a. frontal
b. globular
c. lateral nasal
d. median nasal
e. maxillary
f. mandibular

REVIEW TEST 2.9

LABEL THE DIAGRAMS. COLOR IN RED, BLUE, OR YELLOW FOR MESODERM, ECTODERM, OR ENDODERM, WHERE INDICATED.

1.

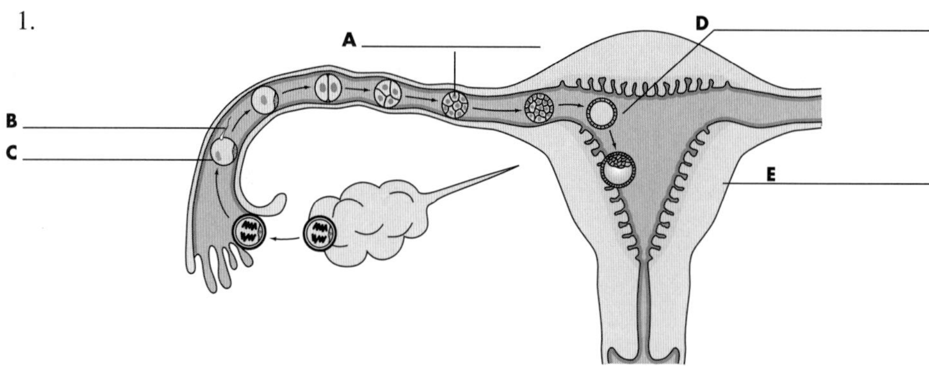

2.

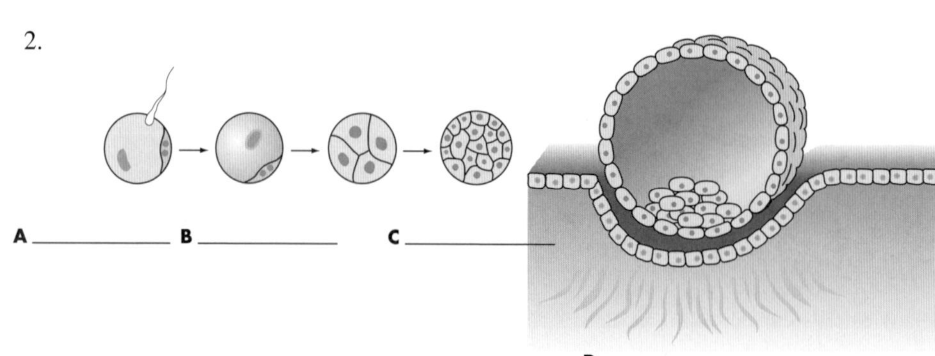

3.

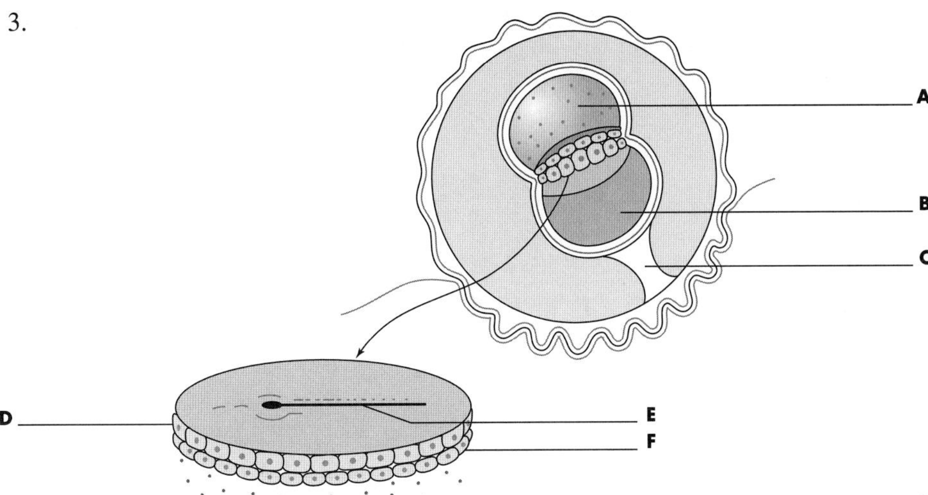

4. Color in.

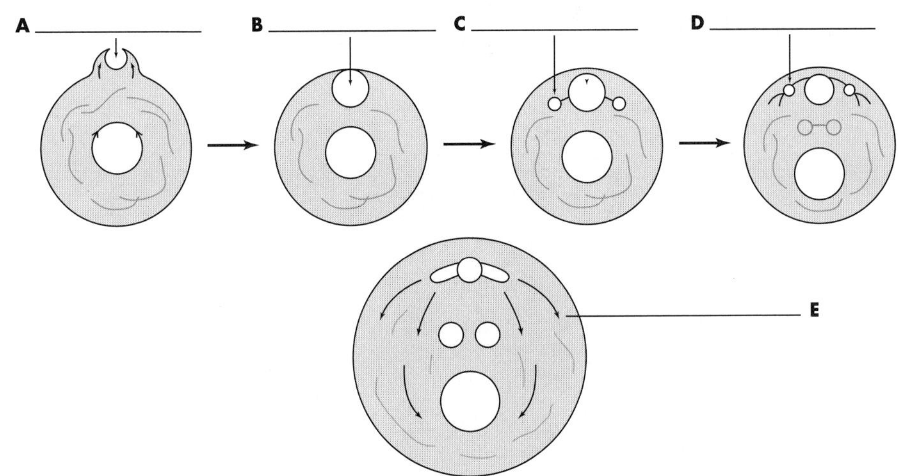

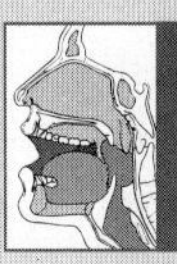

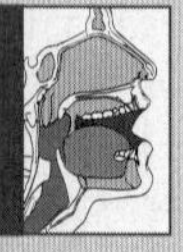

5.

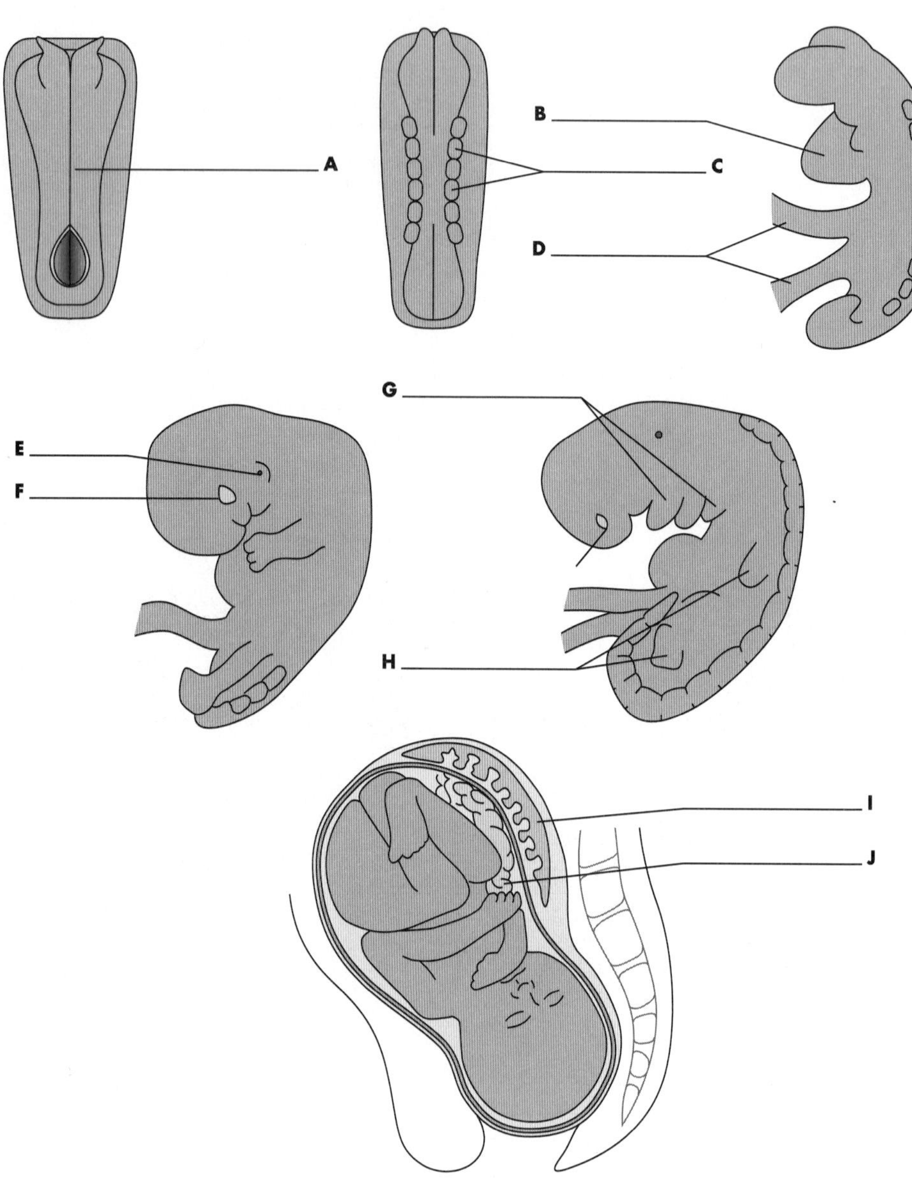

6. Color in.

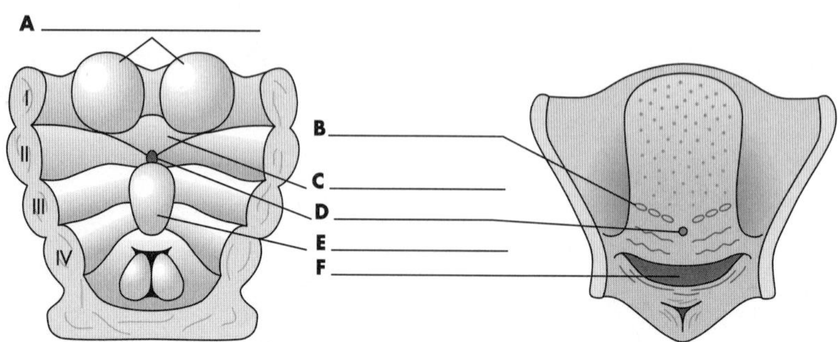

7. Color in.

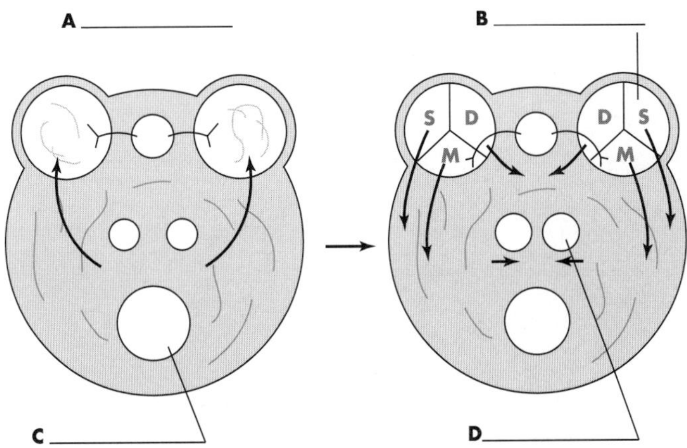

8. Color in.

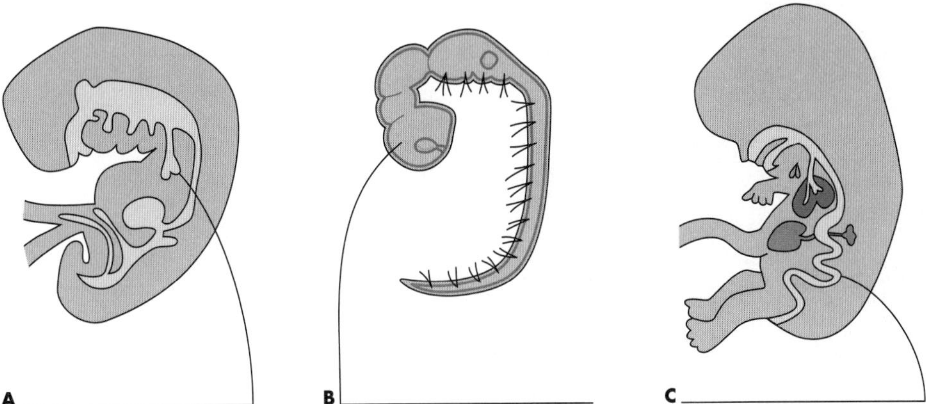

9. Color in.

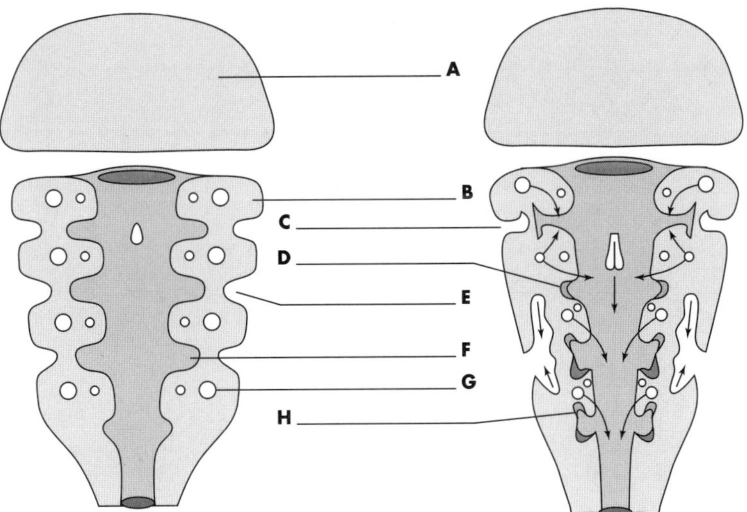

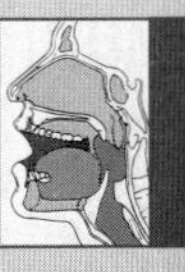

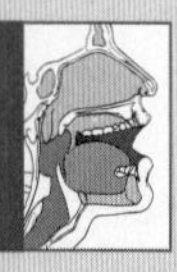

10.

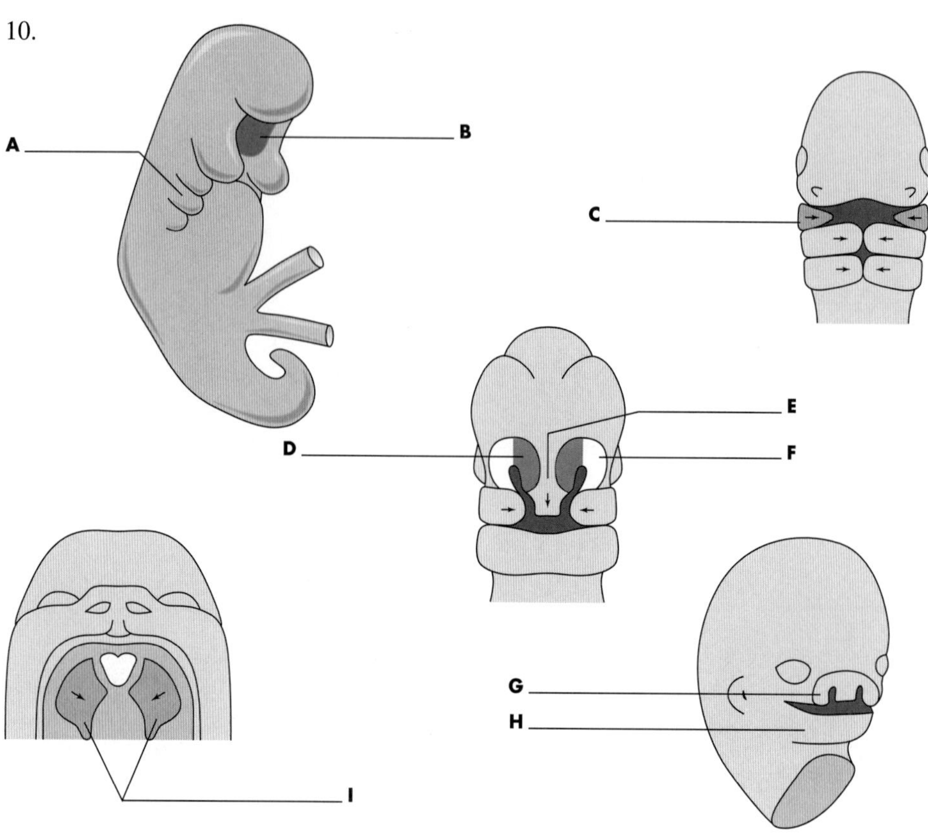

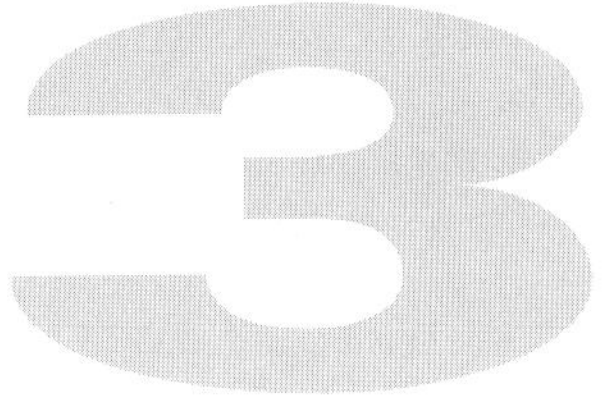

Tooth Development

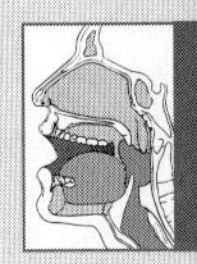

ENAMEL ORGAN

1.0

We followed the development of the head and neck in the embryo in the last chapter. We have seen how all the structures of the body originally came from three layers of germ cells called ______________, ______________, and ______________. In this chapter we follow the embryo a little further in the development of teeth in the mouth.

ectoderm, mesoderm, endoderm

Oral Ectoderm

1.1

Remember what the stomodeum or future mouth of the embryo looks like, surrounded by the coalescing pharyngeal arches.

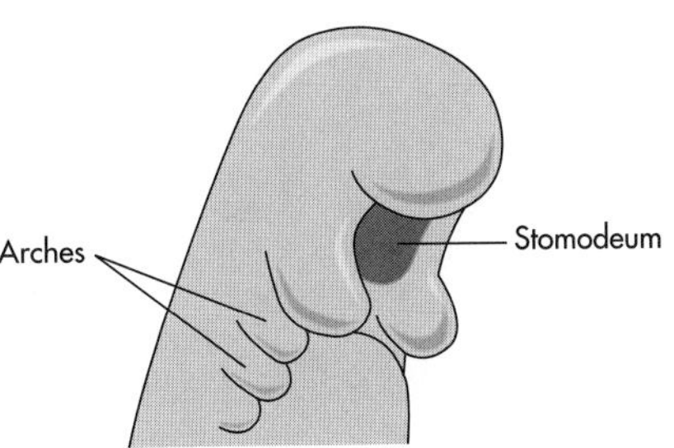

The outer layer or "skin" of the embryo is ______________. Remember, also, that the stomodeum was covered for a short time with the buccopharyngeal membrane. It ruptures and disappears.

ectoderm

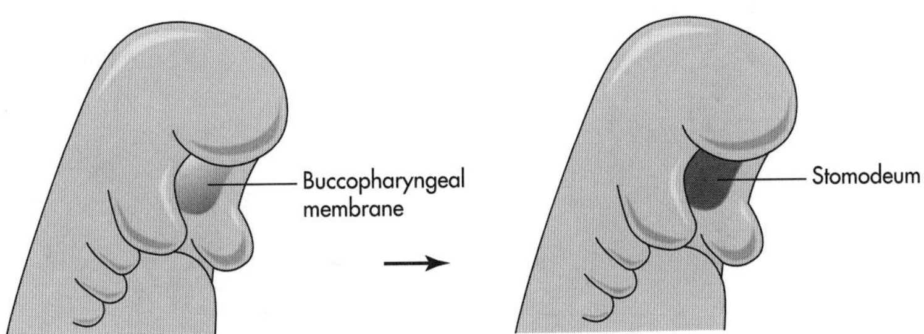

The inside tube of the embryo is made of which germ layer? The diagrams shows what it would look like if we were to slice through the embryo's head to see the inside and outside. In Figure A, the buccopharyngeal membrane is present; in Figure B, it is ruptured. You may color the ectoderm blue and the endoderm yellow.

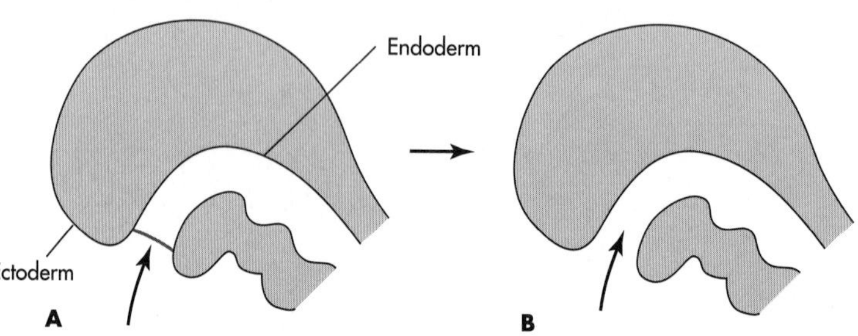

endoderm

With the membrane gone, the space between the mouth and digestive tube becomes continuous. The oral cavity is lined with ectoderm, and the pharynx is lined with ______________.

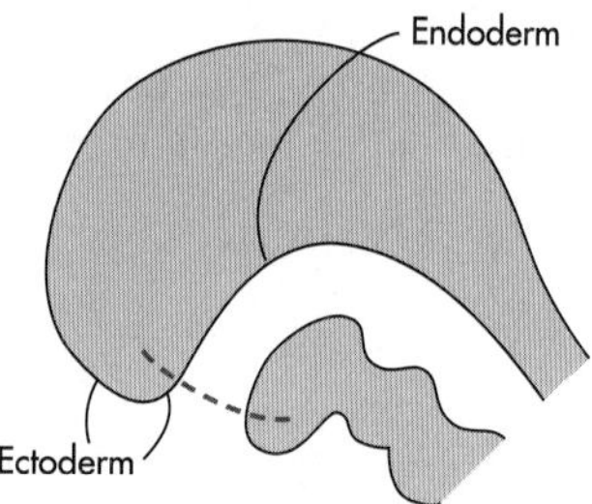

Don't forget that the "inbetween spaces," between ectoderm and endoderm, are filled with mesoderm.

The arches will come together developing a face and mouth.

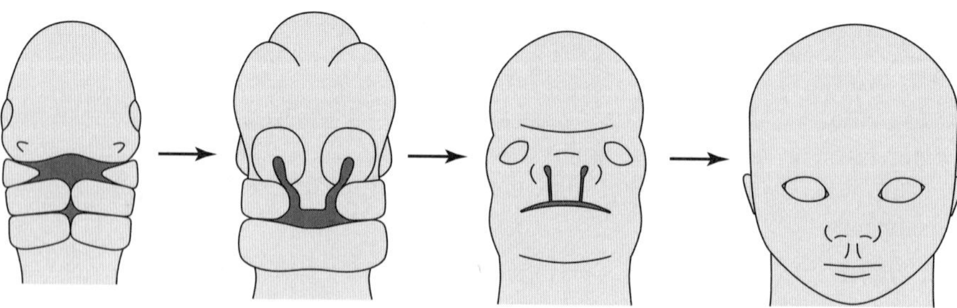

In the floor of the mouth the tongue will develop from six processes or "bumps." Here you can see the border between the lining tissue of ectoderm and endoderm along a V-shaped structure called the ______________.

circumvallate papillae

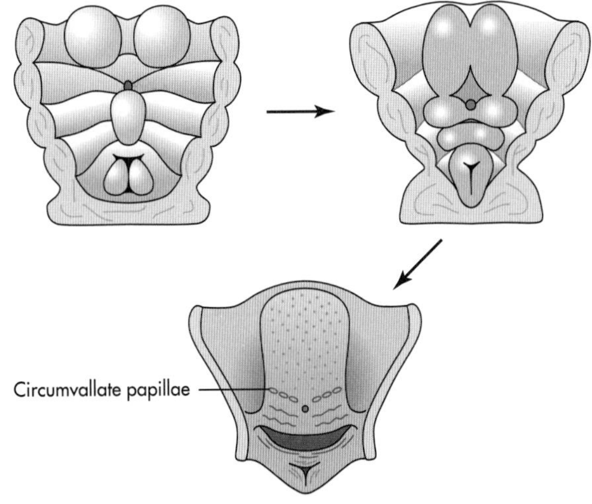

The rest of the oral cavity is covered in ectoderm—oral ectoderm.

The circumvallate papillae form the border between the ectoderm and endoderm coverings of the tongue. They also mark the division between the anterior two thirds or body of the tongue and the posterior one third or root.

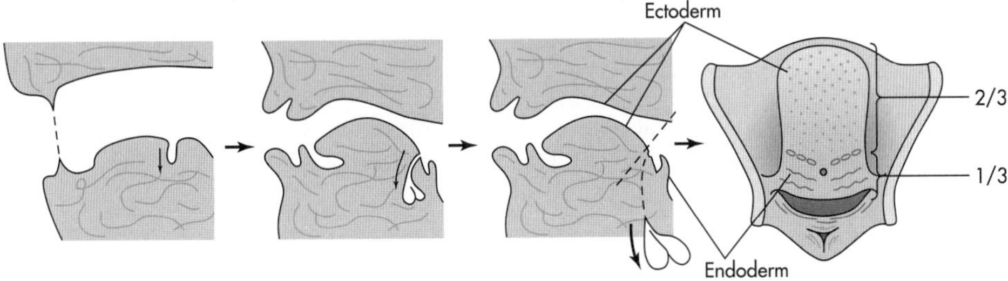

The pharynx is lined with ______________ and the oral cavity with ______________, except the posterior portion of the tongue. Color each area blue or yellow. Don't forget that below the surface of these two is tissue that originated from mesoderm! Color it red.

endoderm, ectoderm

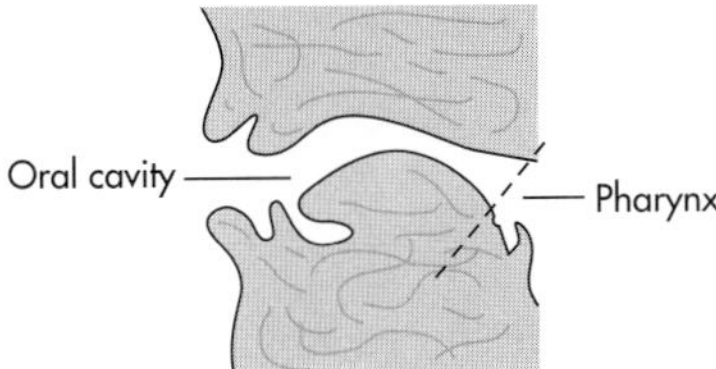

Oral ectoderm will become the mucosa of the mouth or oral cavity. It will become thick in some areas and thin in others.

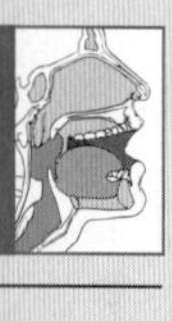

As the facial processes come together, we can see that the embryo has an upper "jaw" or maxilla and a lower "jaw" or mandible.

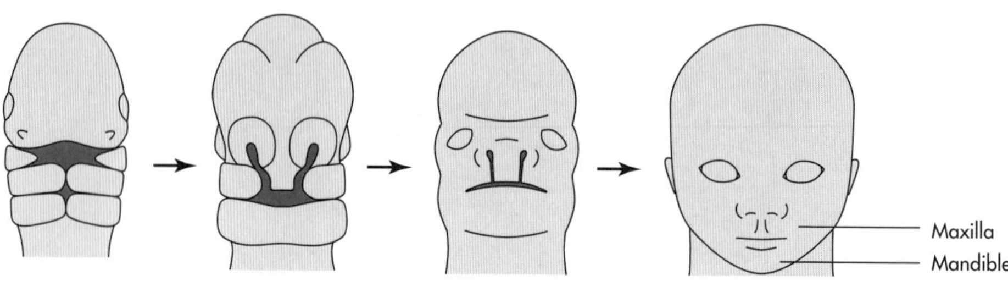

From the inside of the mouth the maxilla and mandible look like two horseshoe-shaped structures or arches.

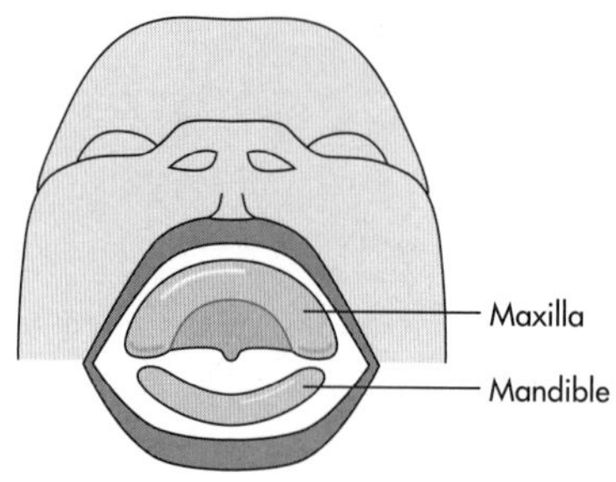

(oral) ectoderm

Which embryonic layer covers the maxillary and mandibular arches? This layer will become the type of mucosa known as gingiva or gum tissue.

To see what happens to the oral ectoderm of the maxillary and mandibular arches, we need to see beneath the surface or look at a cross section.

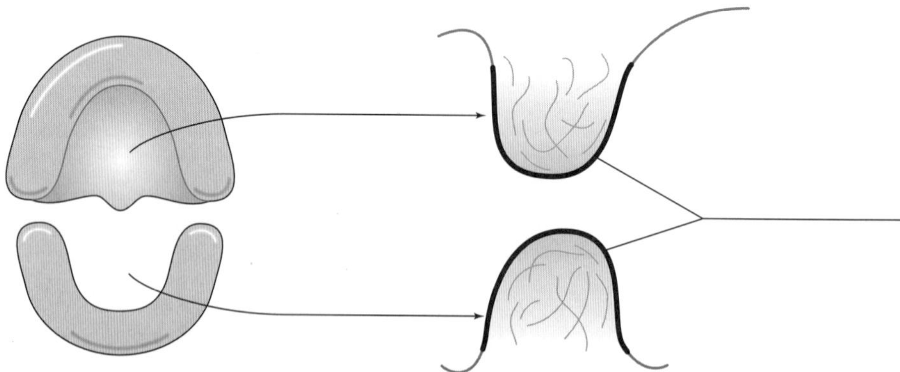

mesoderm

In this cross section through an embryo's maxillary arch, label the oral ectoderm layer. Beneath this, what germ layer do you find, constituting the bulk of the jaw?

You may color the appropriate areas blue or red.

Dental Lamina

1.2

In the cross section through the maxilla of the embryo, we see at first two layers of tissue: one is the outer covering or oral ectoderm, and below that is the mesoderm.

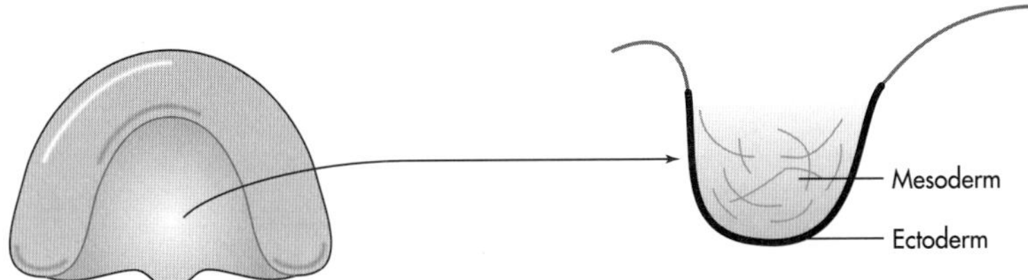

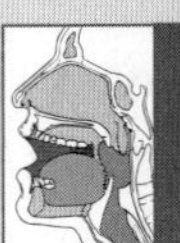

At 20 special places on top of the maxillary and mandibular arches in the oral ectoderm layer, something begins to occur at about 14 weeks of embryogenic age. In these areas the ectoderm begins to thicken.

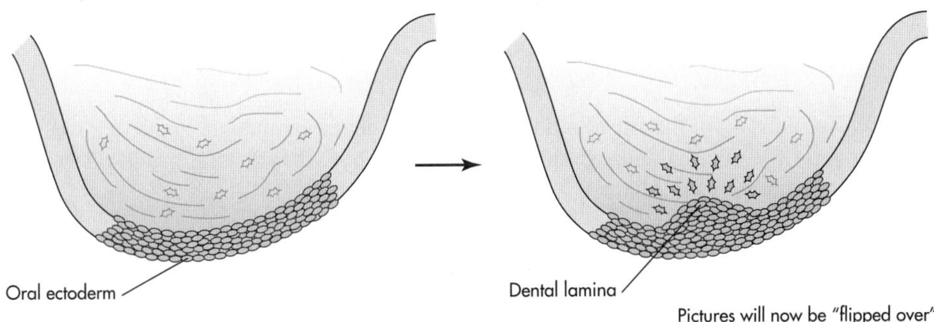

Pictures will now be "flipped over"

These 20 thickenings of ectoderm are called the dental lamina or the "tooth layer." What do you think will develop from these 20 places?

teeth

Let's see how teeth develop from these areas of "thickened skin" by looking again, at a cross section.

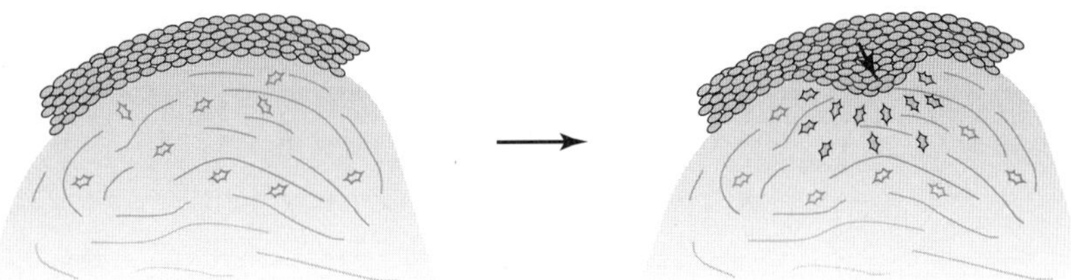

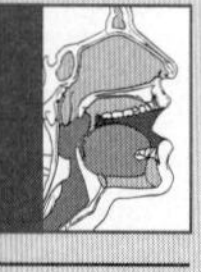

Note how cells of the dental lamina grow down from the oral ectoderm into the surrounding lower layer of mesoderm.

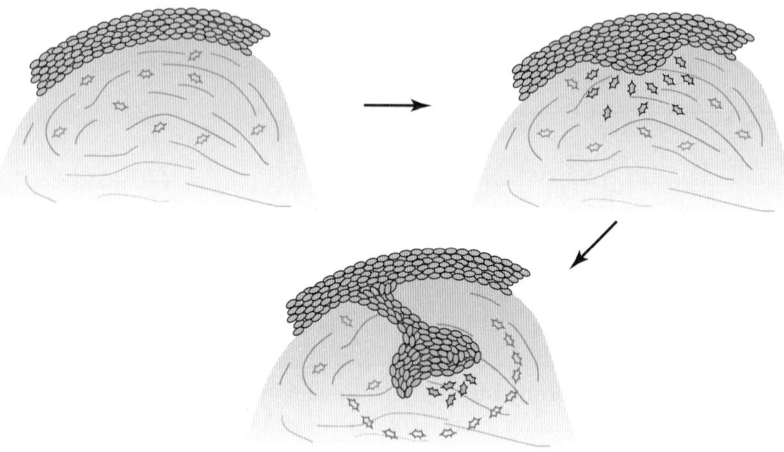

You may color the ectoderm blue and the mesoderm red.

The areas of mesoderm that surround the developing dental lamina are areas that will become bone of the maxilla and mandible as time goes by. We will look at mesoderm development in greater detail later.

As the dental lamina grows downward it takes the shape shown in Figure A. Later it takes the shape shown in Figure B.

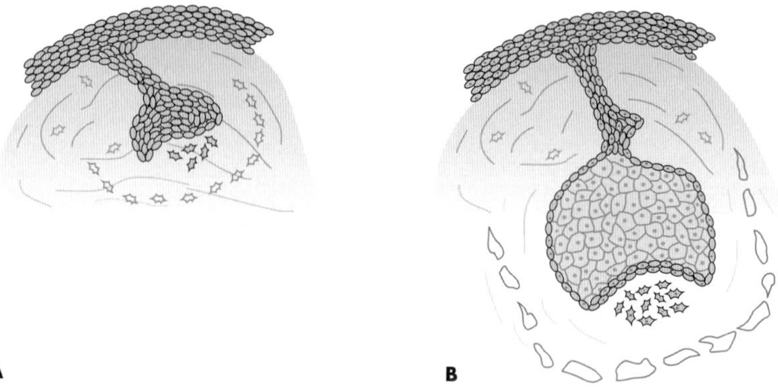

The structure forming from the dental lamina is called an **enamel organ.** Enamel organs are forming in 20 places along the maxillary and mandibular arches. Because they look like little "caps" and later like "bells," some scientists have called these the **cap stage** and **bell stage** of the enamel organ. Remember that these figures show a two-dimensional section as it would appear under the microscope. In three dimensions, enamel organs do look like "caps" or "bells."

Enamel Organ

1.3

At this stage of development, all the cells of the enamel organ look the same. They will soon differentiate into different layers of cells as shown below. Each layer has a different name. The top three layers serve a supportive function. Also note the continuing attachment of the organ to the surface ectoderm.

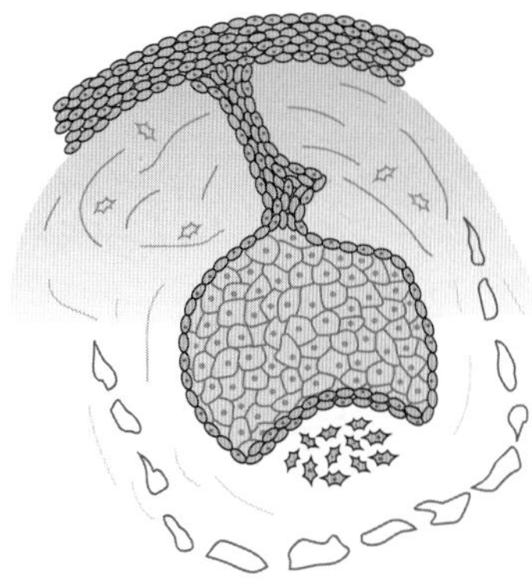

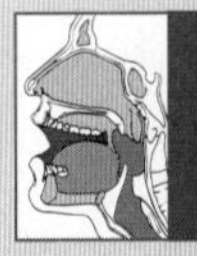

Remember that these diagrams are two dimensional or just a slice through a solid object.

The innermost layer, or **inner enamel epithelium,** has a special function. These cells will become **ameloblasts,** enamel-producing cells.

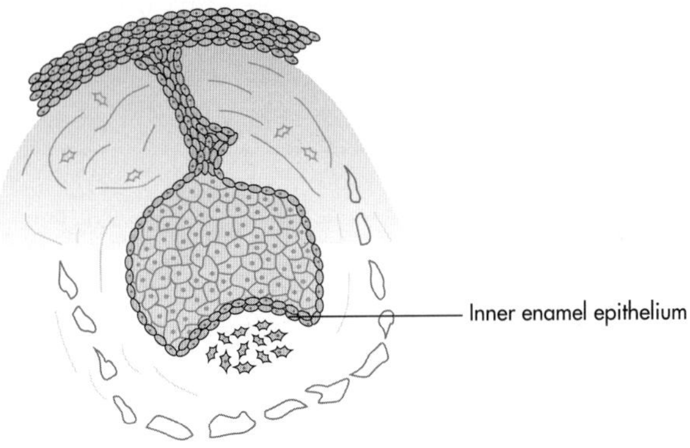

The inner enamel epithelium is the layer that will give rise to the ameloblasts. These cells are ultimately responsible for laying down the dental tissue called **enamel** by a process called **calcification.** It is very similar to the way we saw that bone was formed. We will look at calcification in detail soon.

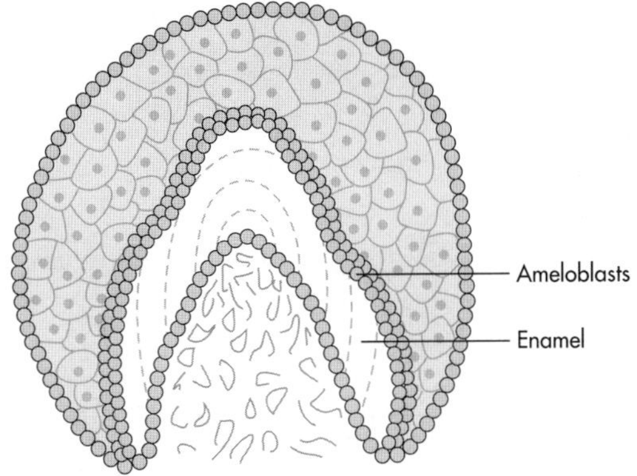

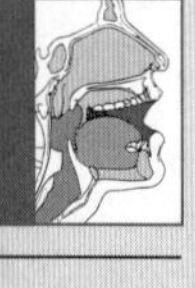

The other three layers are called the **stratum intermedium, stellate reticulum,** and **outer enamel epithelium.** It is not known exactly what the function of these layers is, but they may have a supportive role for the ameloblasts or have a part in the process and timing of development and eruption.

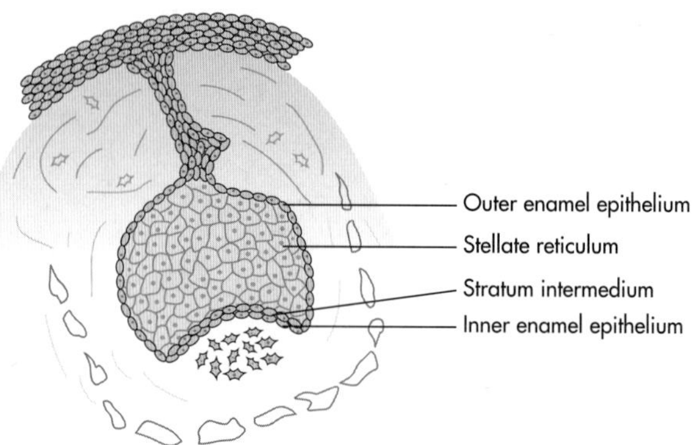

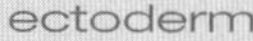

ectoderm

Label the layers of this enamel organ. Circle the layer that will become ameloblasts. Place an arrow where you think enamel might develop. Do you remember what the enamel organ originally came from: ectoderm, mesoderm, or endoderm?

A. outer enamel epithelium
B. stellate reticulum
C. stratum intermedium
D. inner enamel epithelium
ectoderm

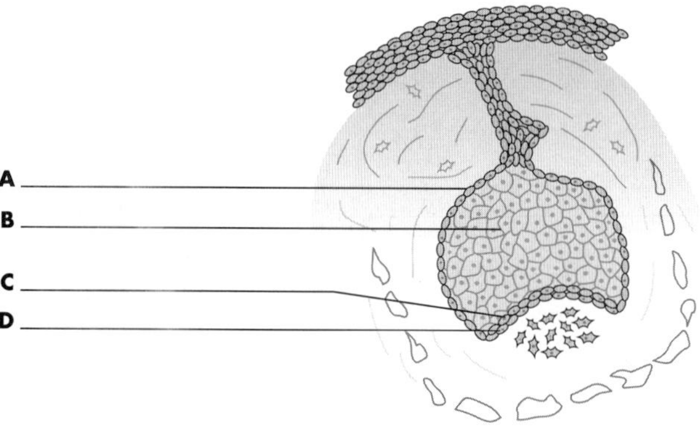

Let's look at the enamel organ as it develops. Look what happens to each of the four layers of cells. Where is a layer of enamel developing?

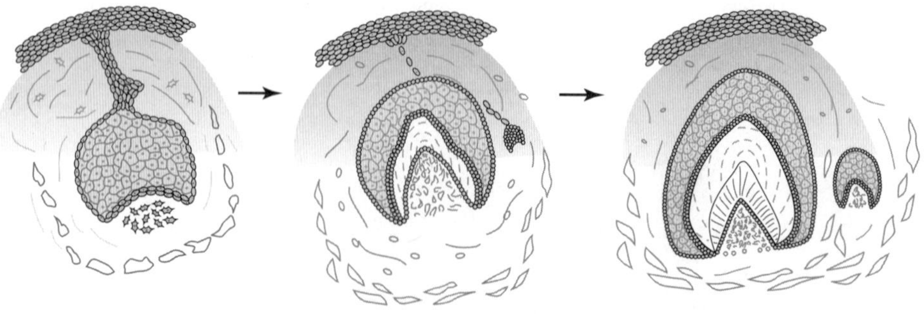

Look under the inner enamel epithelium (ameloblast) layer. This is where these cells will create or lay down **enamel.**

The outer three layers of the enamel organ will be pushed together to form the **reduced enamel epithelium.** Now these cells are not easy to distinguish. What happened to the attachment of the enamel organ to the oral ectoderm?

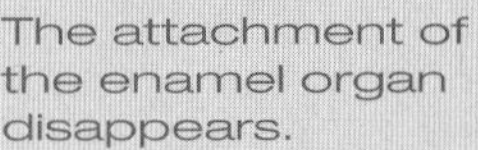
The attachment of the enamel organ disappears.

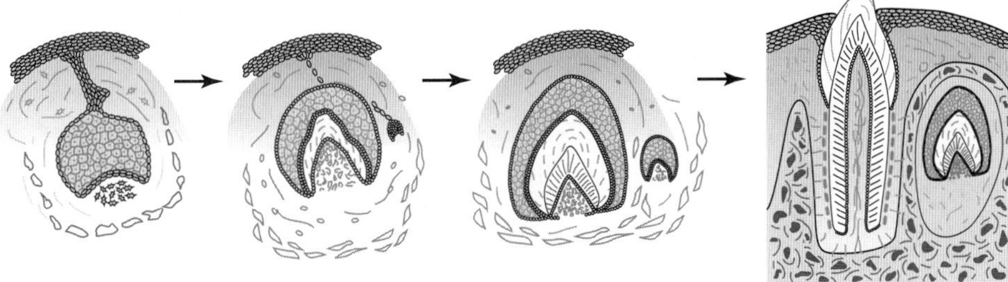

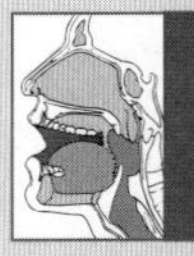

Look on the side of the enamel organ. As it develops, a bump of tissue begins to grow off and develop. What do you think it is?

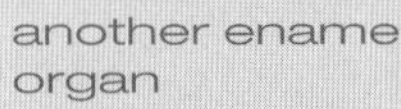
another enamel organ

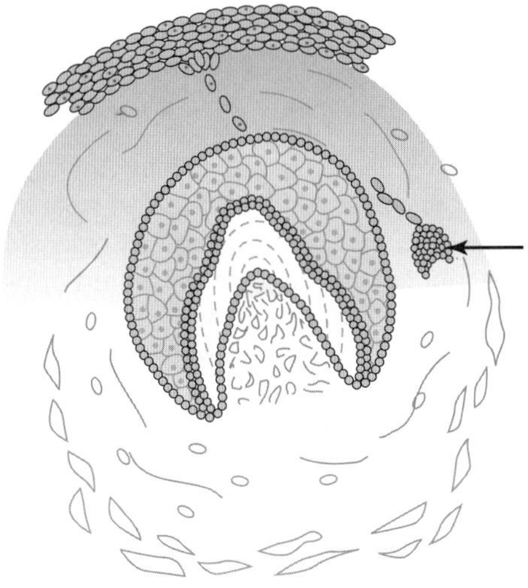

The permanent tooth is developing.

The enamel organ is actually making another, second enamel organ or **secondary dental lamina** or enamel organ. This will develop into a second tooth, but later. What is happening?

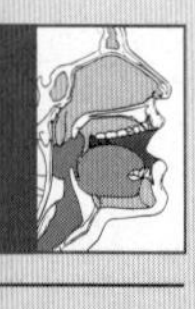

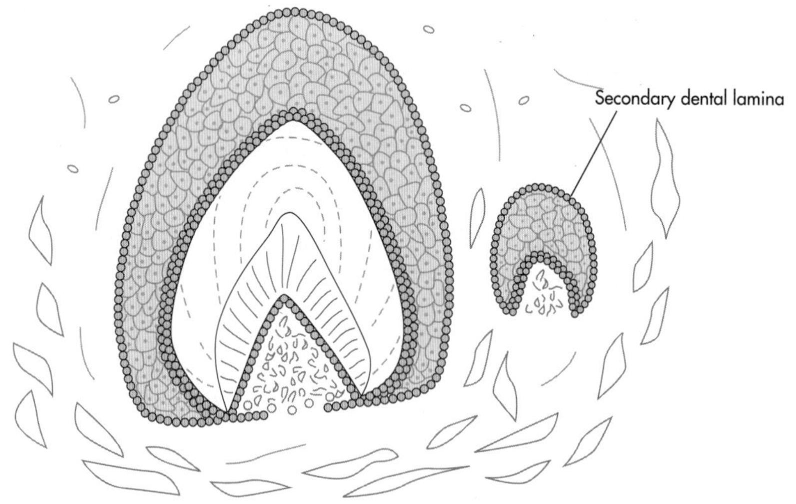

If you guessed that the secondary enamel organ will develop the secondary tooth (permanent tooth), you were right. Remember that the first set of teeth in a child are the **primary** or **deciduous** teeth. They are the first set of 20 enamel organs to develop. Later, below and to the side of them (inferior and lingual), the **secondary** or **permanent teeth** will develop from 20 enamel organs that budded off the first ones and will eventually develop and replace the primary teeth. These are the **succedaneous teeth.**

A. outer enamel epithelium
B. stellate reticulum
C. enamel
D. ameloblasts
E. secondary lamina

Label the parts of the enamel organ.

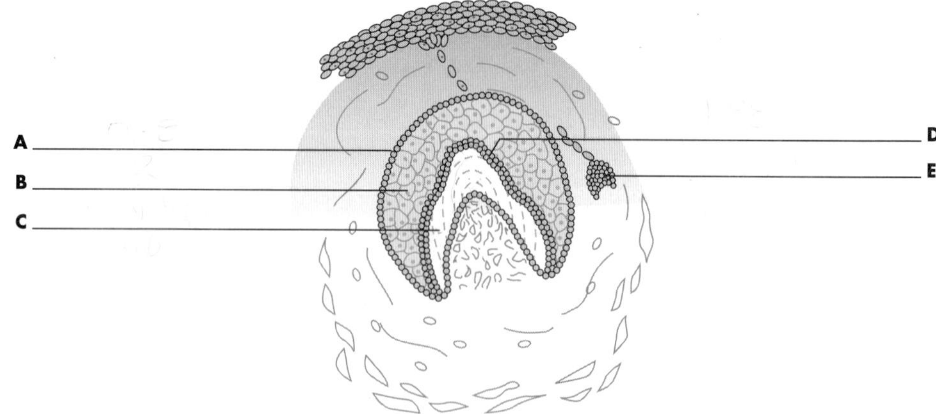

MESODERMAL DERIVATIVES 2.0

We have seen what happens to the ectoderm. It begins as the outer covering layer of the mouth and arches and develops 20 areas that will sink into the maxillary and mandibular "jaws" to become the enamel organs that will create the enamel of the teeth. But that's only part of the story. What about the rest of the tooth and its surroundings? What happens to the mesoderm into which the ectoderm (enamel organ) sinks?

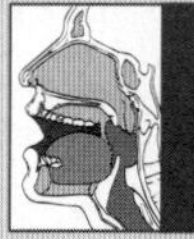

Dental Papilla 2.1

Let's go back to the beginning. Note the dental lamina growing into the mesoderm layer. Color each layer appropriately.

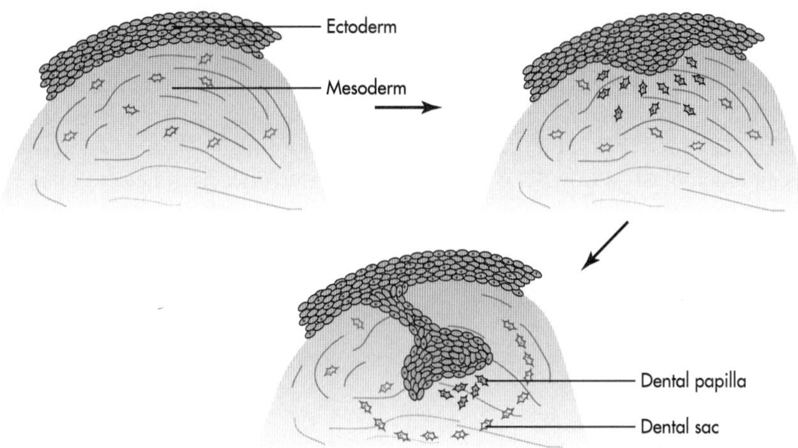

The mesoderm surrounding the enamel organ and the mesoderm that is trapped underneath it begin to condense (gather together) and differentiate.

The mesoderm that is trapped under the enamel organ is called the **dental papilla,** and the mesoderm that surrounds it is the **dental sac.**

Let's first follow the development of the dental papilla. Watch those cells under the enamel organ as they come together and differentiate.

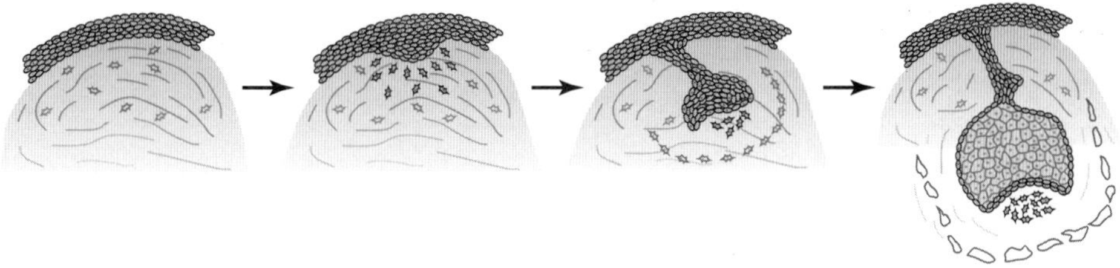

ameloblasts

Look at the cells directly under the enamel. These cells are called odontoblasts. Cells that form enamel are called ________________ and cells that will form dentin are called odontoblasts.

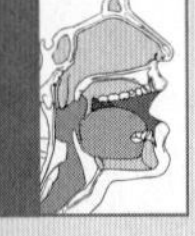

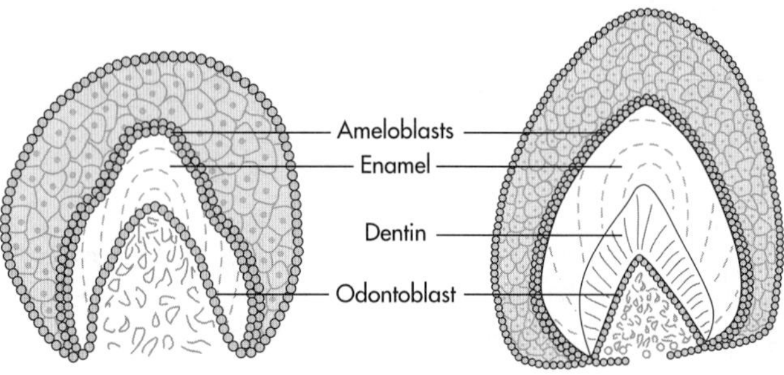

A. Odontoblast makes dentin.
B. Ameloblast makes enamel.

Odontoblasts are a very unique kind of cell. Not only do they help create the hard tissue **dentin** by calcification of their matrix, but they have a long "finger" or **odontoblastic process** that they leave behind in the dentin as it grows. Which cell is an odontoblast and which is an ameloblast—**A** or **B?** What hard tooth tissue does each help to make?

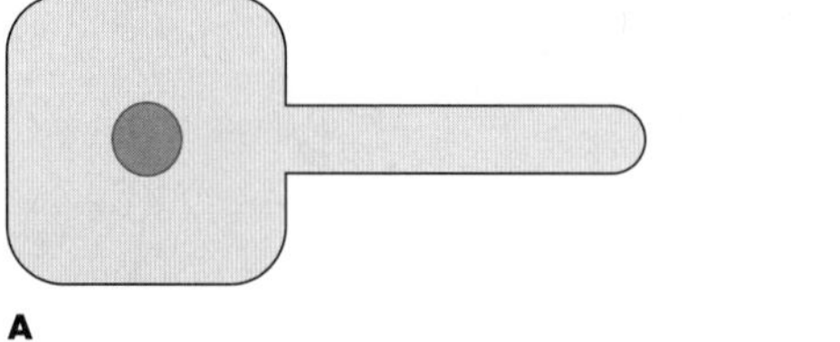

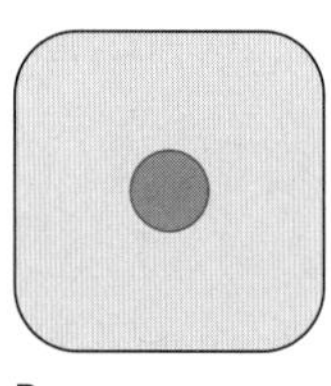

Follow the sequence of development as more and more dentin is laid down in layers on the inside of the tooth. Each new layer of enamel is laid down on the outside of the tooth and each new layer of dentin is laid down on the innermost side, so it looks like the ameloblasts are moving out while the odontoblasts are moving in.

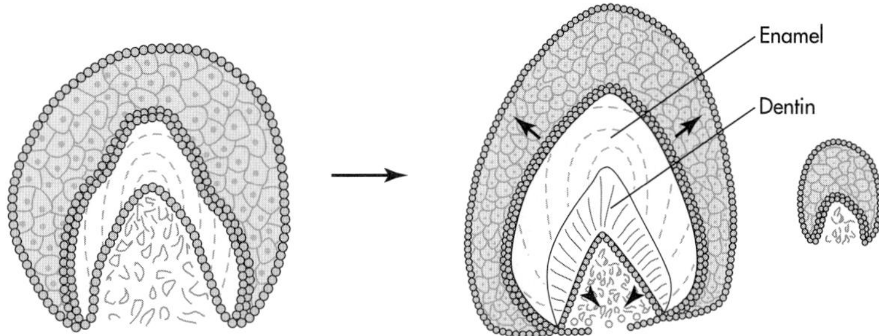

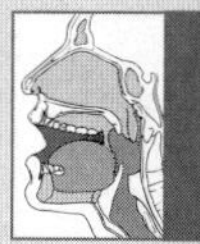

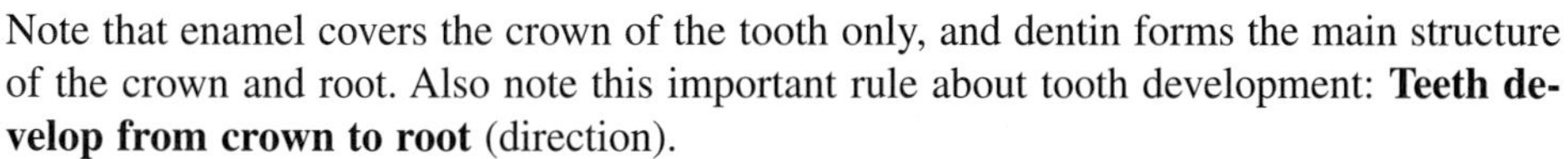
Note that enamel covers the crown of the tooth only, and dentin forms the main structure of the crown and root. Also note this important rule about tooth development: **Teeth develop from crown to root** (direction).

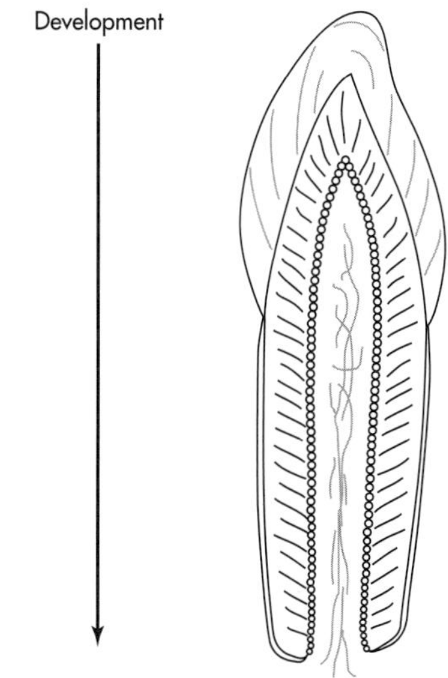

It becomes pulp.

What happens to the rest of the dental papilla? The other mesoderm cells differentiate into many types of cells: blood and blood vessels, connective tissue and fibers, and a gelatinous matrix called ground substance. This soft tissue area left in the center of the tooth is called the **pulp.**

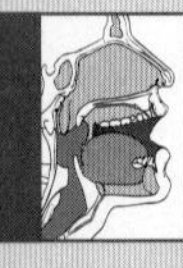

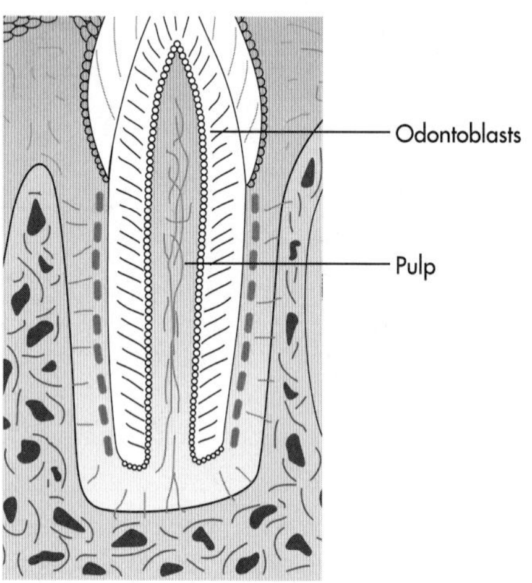

dentin and pulp

What two things are derived from the dental papilla?

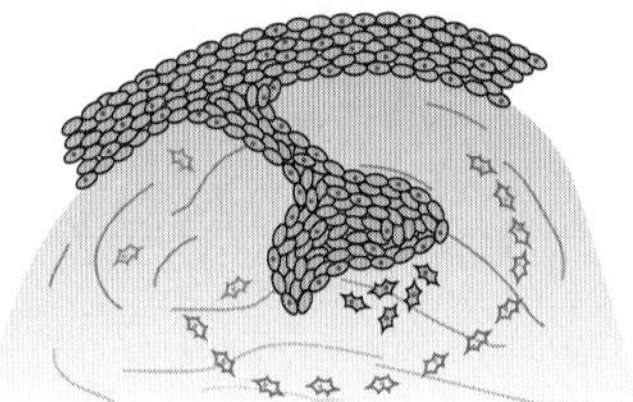

2.2 Dental Sac

Return to the beginning of the development sequence. Look at the mesoderm that is condensing around the enamel organ. This is called the **dental sac.** Several different structures will be derived from it, all originally from mesoderm: one dental tissue and the periodontal tissues.

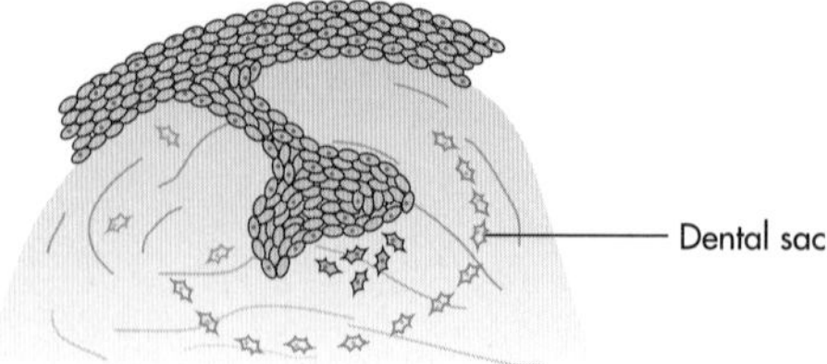

The word *periodontal* means "around the tooth."

The first large group of mesoderm condensing around the tooth is not part of the dental sac, but will blend together with it. It is the bony tissue of each jaw, the **maxilla** and **mandible.** Mesoderm cells are differentiating into osteoblasts (bone-forming cells).

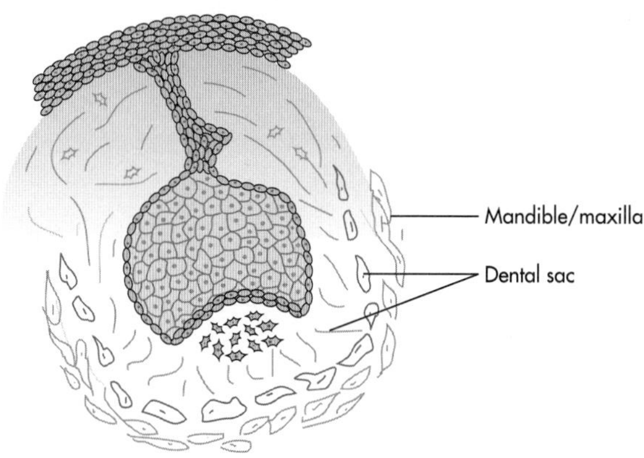

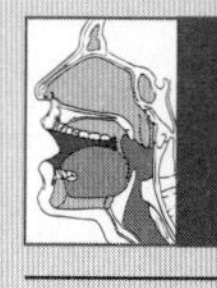

Follow the development of bone in this sequence. The portion of the bone closest to the surface and surrounding the future teeth is called **alveolar bone.** This bone is derived from the dental sac.

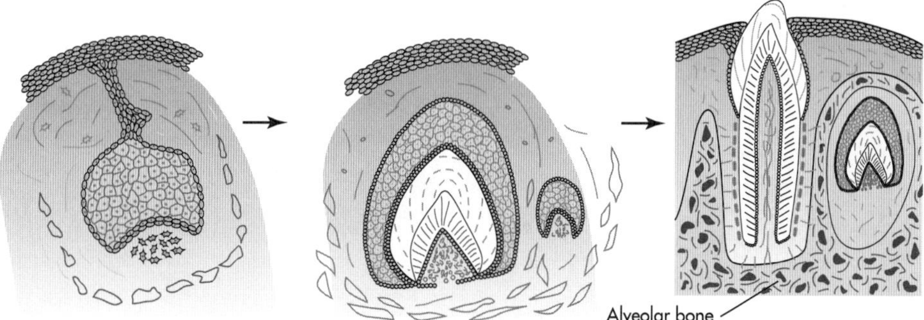

Something a little different occurs in the mandible, remember. Pictured below is a large circular area of cartilage within the developing bony area. This is Meckel's ______________. It is a temporary support or "jawbone" for the mandible, while the bony portion develops. What happens to it?

cartilage; It disappears.

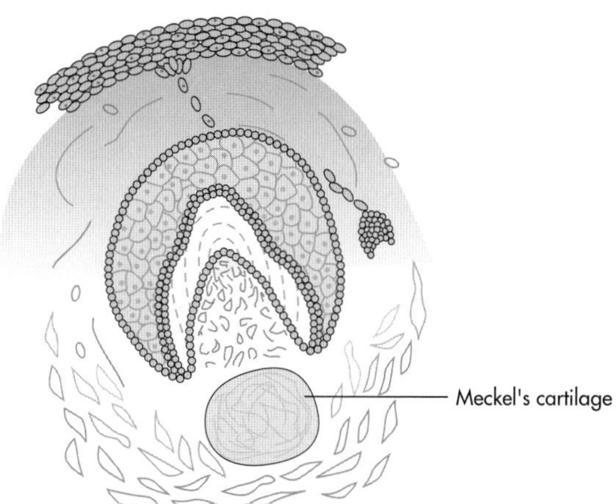

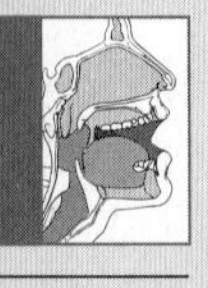

As the bone develops around the future tooth, a spherical space for the tooth is formed called a **crypt.** The enamel organ by now has lost all attachment to the surface.

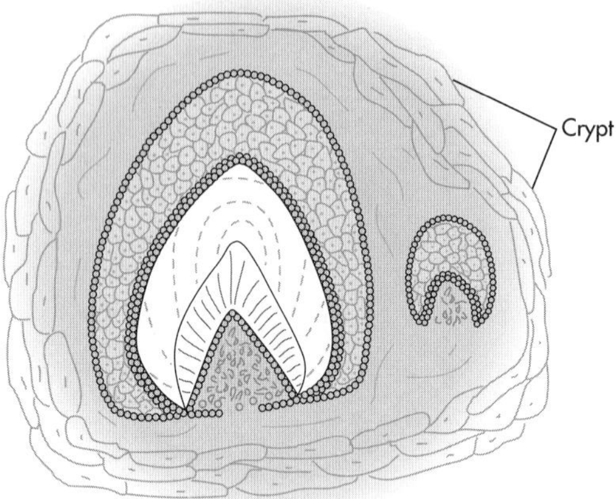

periodontal ligament fibers

Follow this sequence of development paying attention to the space between the developing root and bone. Large bundles of fibers are developing to attach the tooth to the bony socket. These are called the **periodontal ligament fibers.** Now we have two derivatives of the dental sac: the alveolar bone and the ______________.

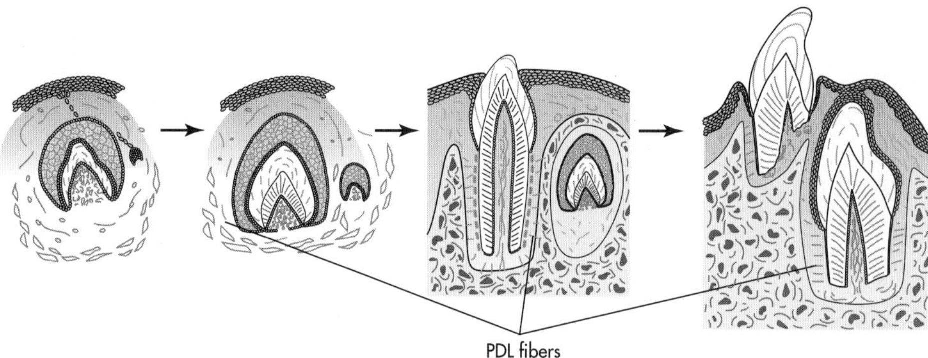

Periodontal ligament (PDL) serves the important function of attaching the tooth to the alveolar bone. It will provide support and attachment for the tooth. During development of the tooth it is the site of two other stages of differentiation. First, the tooth needs to know where to stop building its crown and where to start building a root. It does that in an area called the **diaphragm.**

diaphragm

Somehow the cells at the end of the enamel organ know where the end of the tooth is and will define the area with a layer of cells that grow out horizontally called the **diaphragm.** Also, other cells will come off of the enamel organ vertically, leaving a trail downward that will serve as a guide for other cells to follow to build the root. These cells are called **Hertwig's epithelial root sheath.** They come from the ______________.

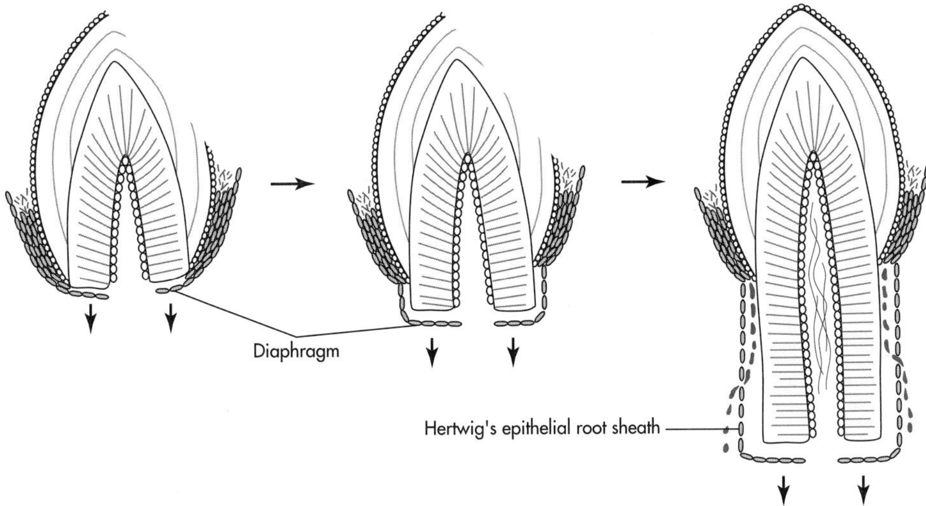

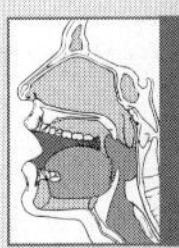

periodontal ligament

On one side of the sheath, odontoblasts will be attracted to form the dentin of the root. On the other side, a new kind of cell is recruited from the PDL to cover the outside of the root. These are **cementoblasts** and they make **cementum.** Where do cementoblasts come from originally?

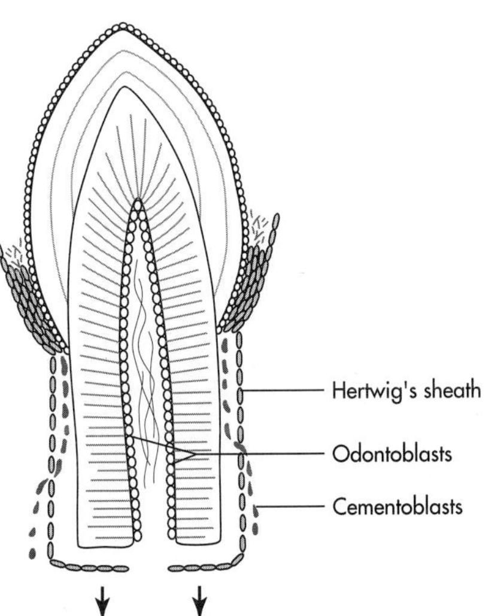

crown to root

So you can see that the root will be developed from the crown on down, with the apex being formed last. In what direction does tooth development proceed?

Looking at a closeup view of the cells of the PDL, look for Hertwig's epithelial root sheath cells, odontoblasts, and the cementoblasts.

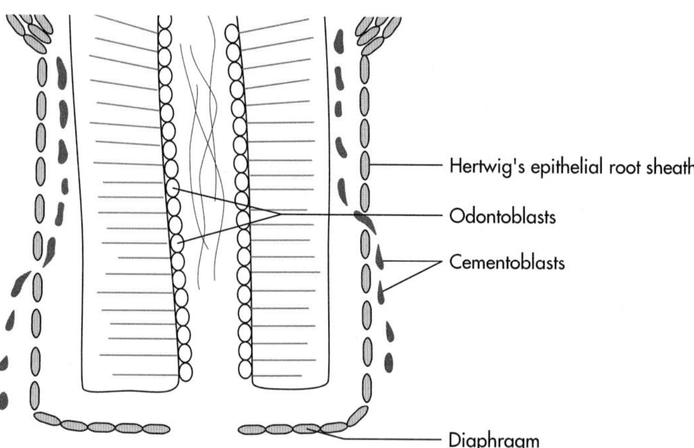

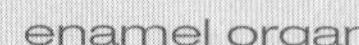

enamel organ

When development of the root is complete, most of Hertwig's sheath will have disappeared, but some small "islands" of cells will be left behind in the PDL. These are called the **rests of Malassez** and are epithelial remnants of the enamel organ. They have no apparent function. Where do the rests of Malassez derive from?

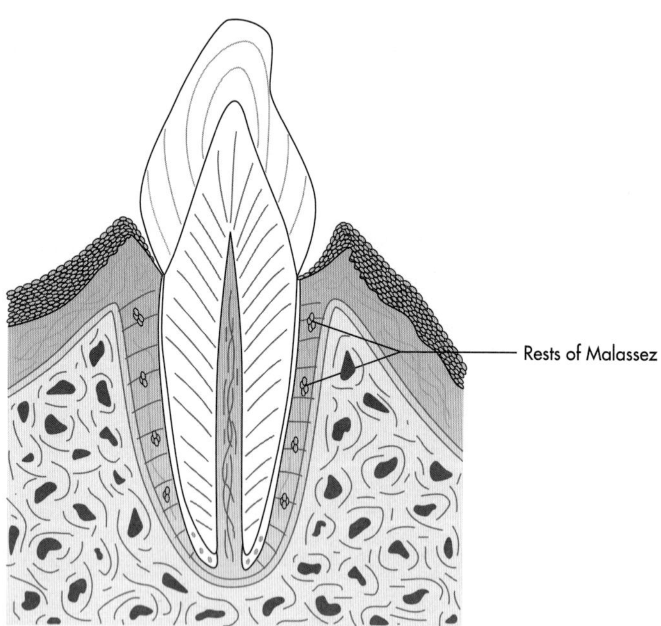

Which cells serve as a guiding trail for the development of the dentin and cementum of the root? Which cells are remnants of the enamel organ left behind in the PDL after root development?

Hertwig's epithelial root sheath, rests of Malassez

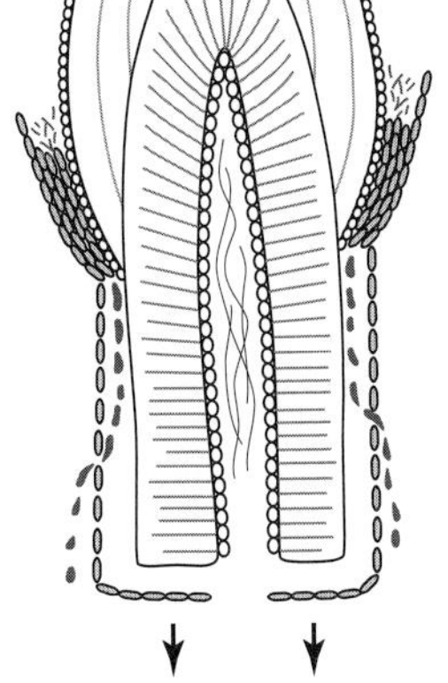

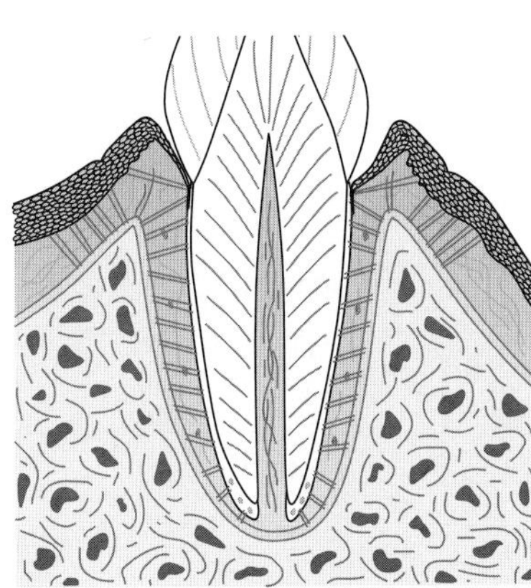

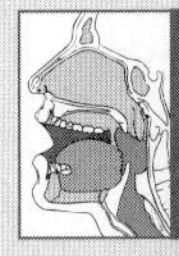

Now we have the last derivative of the dental sac, the **cementum.** The other two are the _______________ and the _______________.

alveolar bone, PDL

Cementum, the outer hard covering of the root, is made by the cementoblasts that came from the PDL. It is formed by calcification in much the same manner that bone is formed. In fact, under a microscope, cementum and bone look very much alike with lacunae, spider-shaped cells, and lamellae. Cementum, however, will, in all but the apical area, lose its cells.

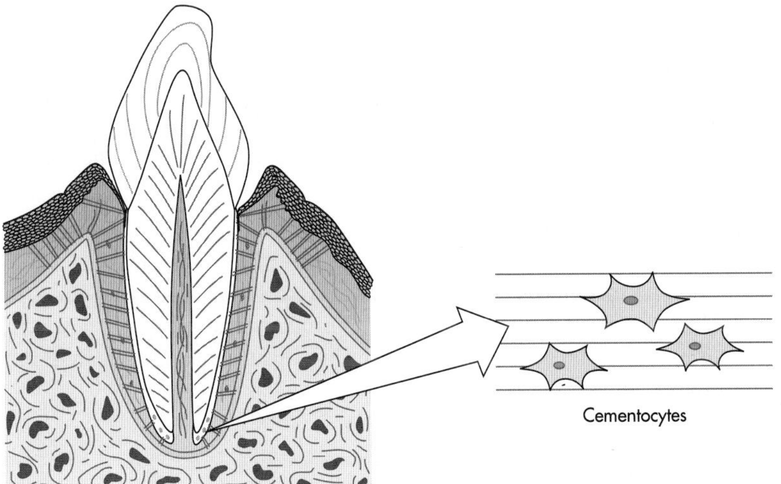

3.0

ERUPTION AND EXFOLIATION

The overall effect of root development "pushes" the tooth upward to the surface of each jaw. Eventually, the tooth breaks through the surface or erupts. It is not known exactly what causes **eruption,** but all the teeth erupt loosely following a timed sequence known as the eruption sequence.

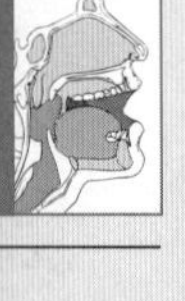

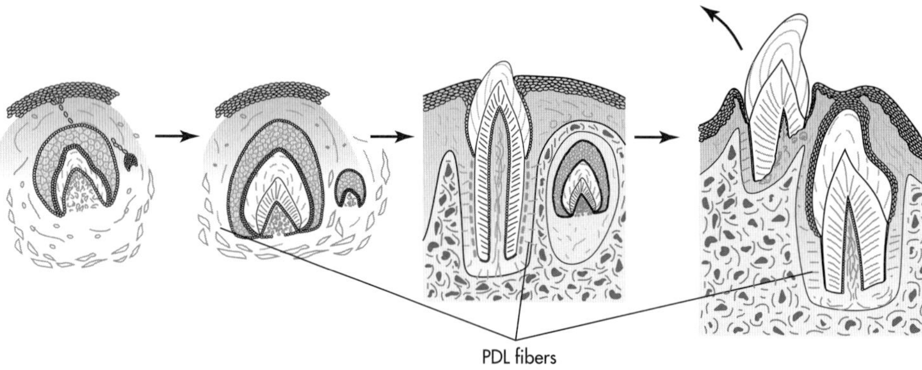

The eruption sequence of the primary teeth is reviewed in the table.

ERUPTION SEQUENCE AND DATES FOR PRIMARY TEETH

Maxillary and Mandibular	Range of Typical Eruption Dates
Central incisors	6 months–1 year
Lateral incisors	9–16 months
First molars	1–1.5 years
Canines	1.5–2 years
Second molars	2–3 years

succedaneous

The 20 primary teeth erupt first. This dentition is used by the child and starts to be replaced at about age 6. The resulting mixture of primary and permanent teeth is called **mixed dentition.** What are the permanent teeth called that will replace the primary teeth?

secondary lamina

From what do the permanent teeth develop? Twenty of the permanent teeth or **succedaneous teeth** develop from the extra "bud" off the primary enamel organ known as the **secondary dental lamina.** The other 12 permanent or nonsuccedaneous teeth develop from their own separate enamel organs.

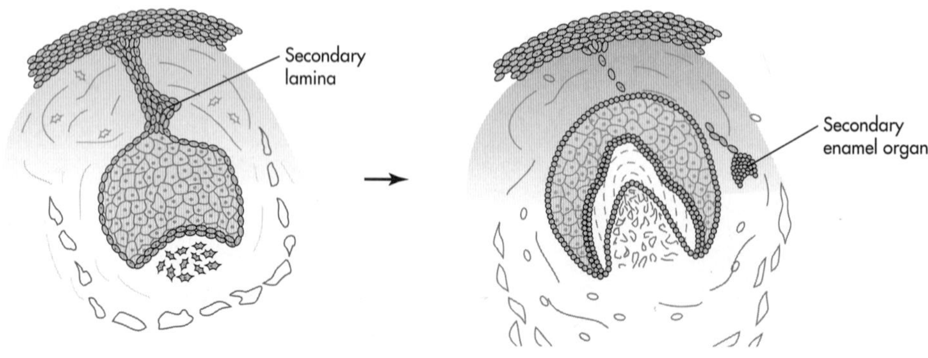

The succedaneous permanent teeth develop inferior to and lingual to the primary teeth. Permanent teeth often erupt lingual to their primary predecessor.

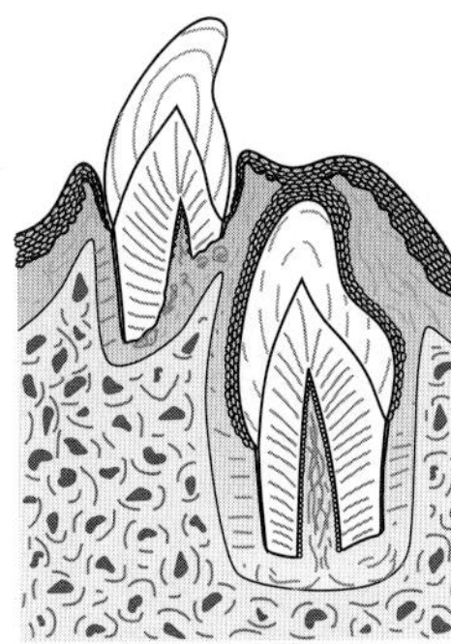

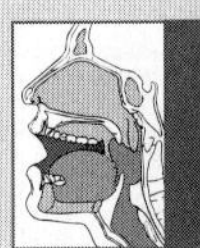

The eruption sequence for permanent teeth is reviewed in the table.

ERUPTION SEQUENCE AND DATES FOR PERMANENT TEETH

Typical Eruption Date (years)	Range	Eruption Sequence	
		Maxillary	*Mandibular*
6	6–7		First molar
6	6–7	First molar	
6	6–7		Central incisor
7	7–8	Central incisor	
7	7–8		Lateral incisor
8	8–9	Lateral incisor	
10	9–10		Canine
10	10–12	First premolar	First premolar
11	10–12	Second premolar	Second premolar
11	11–12	Canine	
12	11–13		Second molar
12	12–13	Second molar	
20	17–21	Third molar	Third molar

To replace the primary tooth the permanent tooth needs room, so the primary tooth must be shed or **exfoliated.** For a tooth to easily fall out, which part (that anchors the tooth) must be lost?

The root!

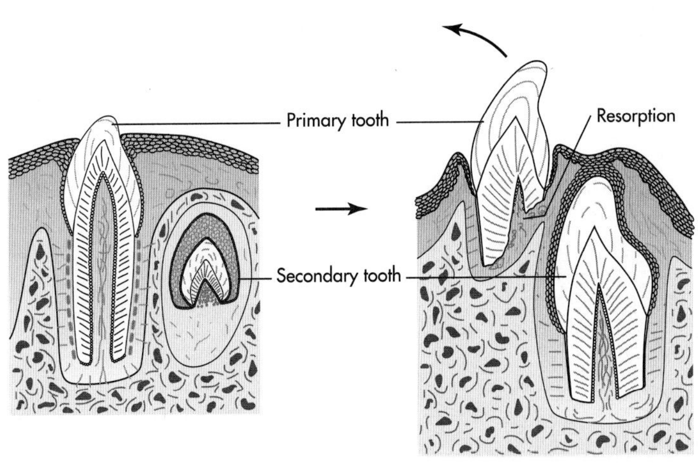

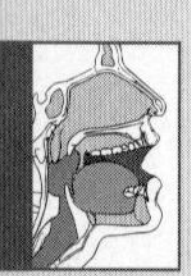

The root of the primary tooth is conveniently "dissolved away" by cells that "eat away" the hard tissue. These are 'clasts—cementoclasts and odontoclasts—and they chew away at the root when it is time for the permanent tooth to erupt. This dissolving of the root is called **root resorption** and right now, it is a normal process.

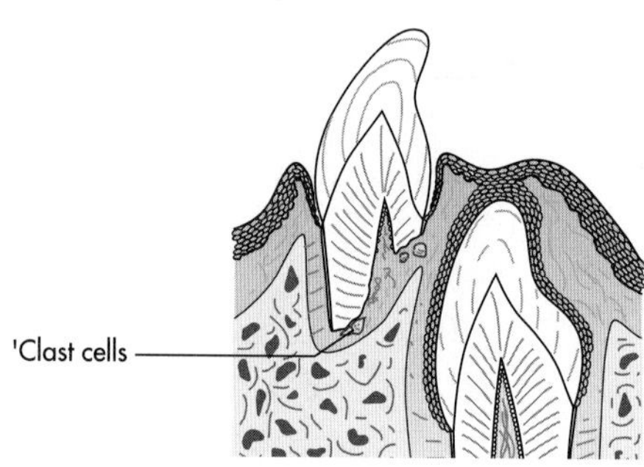

A. primary
B. permanent,
at primary apex

Which tooth pictured here is the primary tooth? Which is the permanent tooth? Where is root resorption taking place?

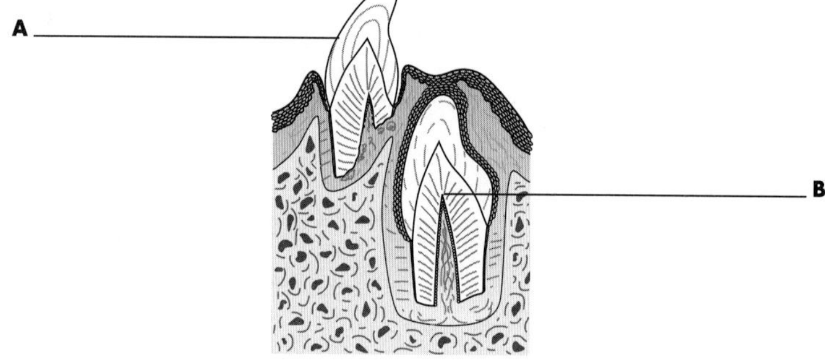

With the root gone, the primary tooth exfoliates and the permanent tooth erupts.

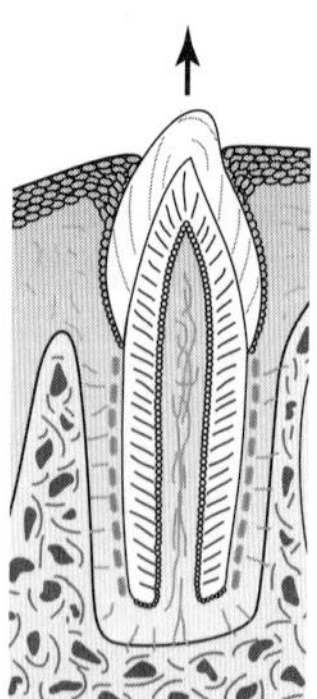

Let's look at the tissue surrounding the crown of the tooth as it erupts, as something special is occurring there.

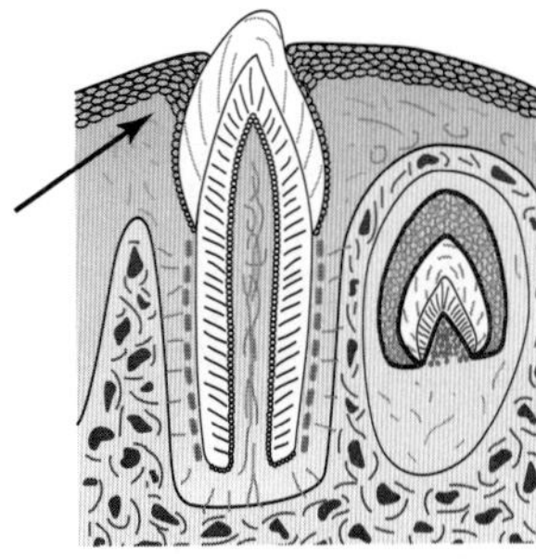

What has happened to the top three layers of the enamel organ?

They have come together.

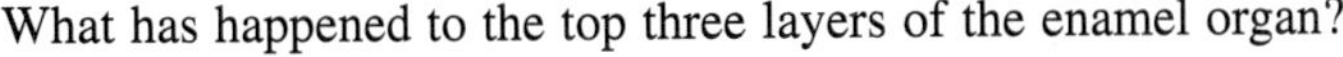

The layers of the enamel organ have been squeezed together as the new tooth erupts, becoming the **reduced enamel epithelium.** The bottom layer of the enamel organ, the inner enamel epithelium, became the ______________ that made the enamel, the diaphragm, and Hertwig's sheath.

ameloblasts

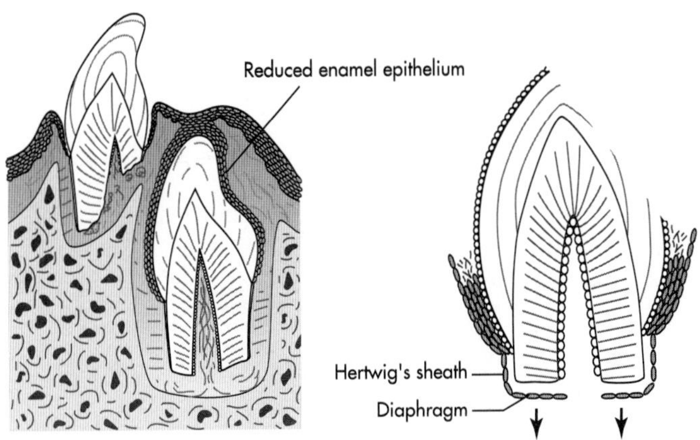

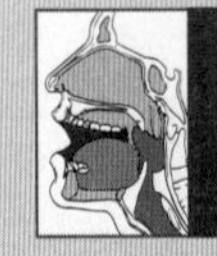

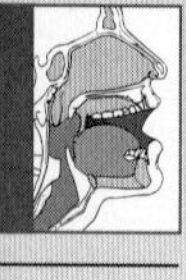

Most of the reduced enamel epithelium seems to be lost as the tooth erupts, except for the very last bit that remains attached to the tooth.

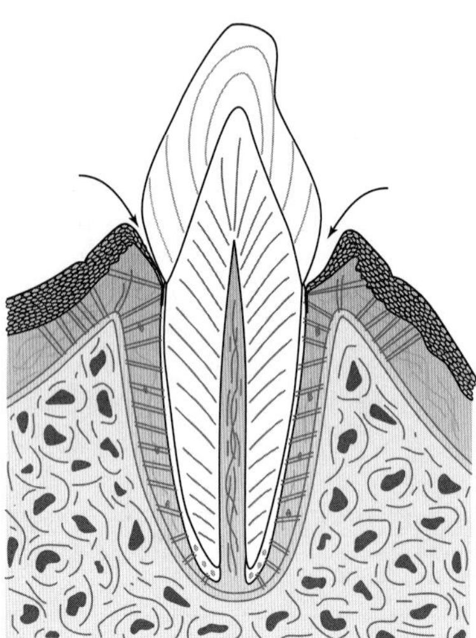

This last remnant of the reduced enamel epithelium becomes the attachment epithelium of the sulcus.

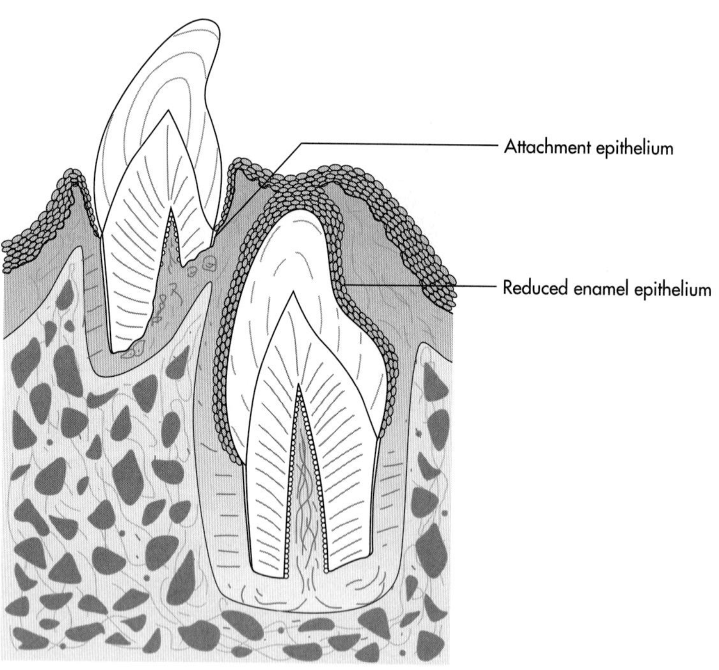

Label the structures in this development sequence.

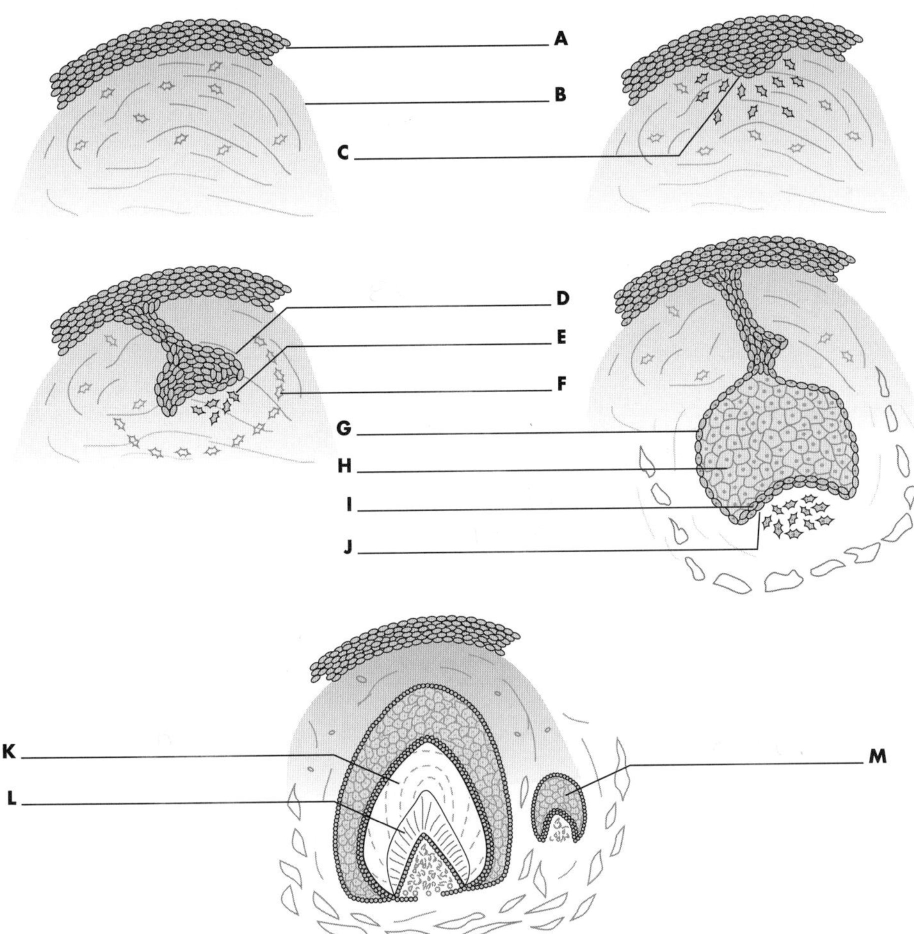

A. oral ectoderm
B. mesoderm
C. dental lamina
D. enamel organ
E. dental papilla
F. dental sac
G. outer enamel epithelium
H. stellate reticulum
I. stratum intermedium
J. inner enamel epithelium
K. enamel
L. dentin
M. secondary lamina

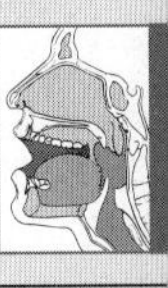

CALCIFICATION

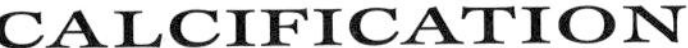

4.0

Let's look at a "cell's view" of the process of making hard tissue. That hard tissue can be bone, cartilage, enamel, dentin, or cementum; they are all made in a similar manner called **calcification.**

What did we call the products the cell made around itself like a "house" (see Chapter One)?

matrix

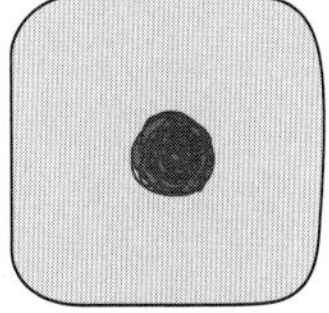

Matrix is the material made by the cell that surrounds the cell. This occurs, if you recall, in connective tissue. For example, bone is the matrix around bone cells (osteocytes) and cartilage is the matrix around cartilage cells (chondrocytes).

'clast cells

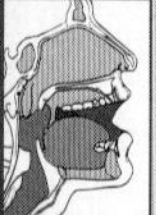

Cells that are actively producing matrix are called **-blasts;** for example, bone-producing cells are osteoblasts. Cells at rest are **-cytes,** and bone cells at rest are osteocytes. A kind of cell that "chews up" or tears down matrix is called a **-clast;** cells that tear down bone are osteoclasts. Remember that the building or laying down of any hard tissue is called **deposition,** and its destruction is called **resorption.** What type of cells resorb?

Deposition of all types of hard tissue matrix follows a similar pattern. The building of hard tissue matrix is called **calcification** and we will follow its four stages.

First the cell forms a matrix of **fibers.**

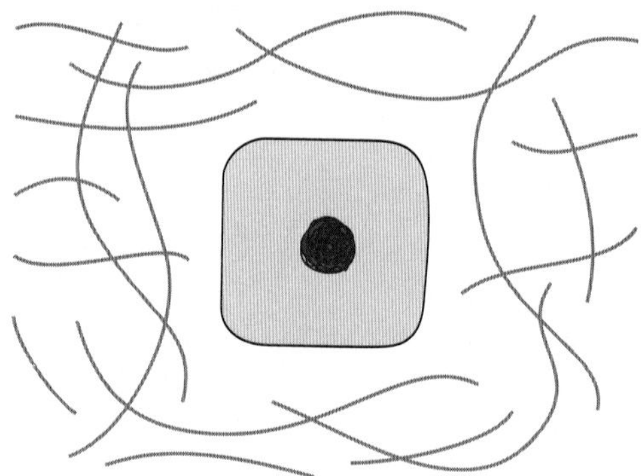

Second, **calcium salts** from the bloodstream are attracted to the fibrous matrix.

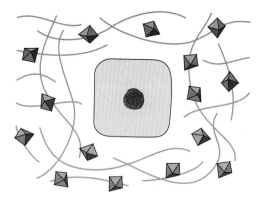

Third, those calcium salts are used to build larger crystals of a substance called **hydroxy-apatite,** the building blocks of all hard tissues.

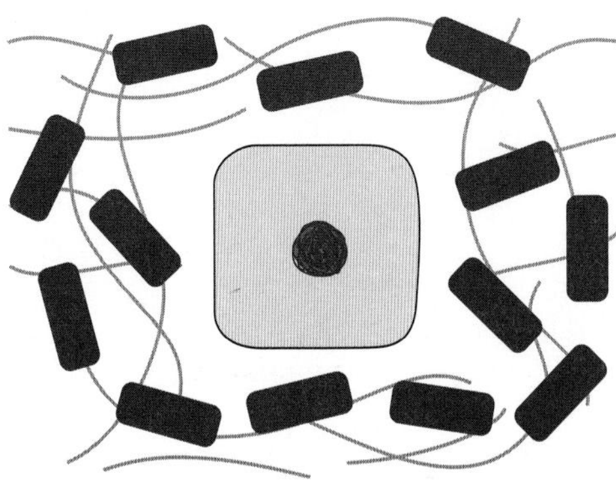

Fourth, a more complex crystalline structure is built depending on the type of tissue that will be the final result (bone, enamel, etc.)

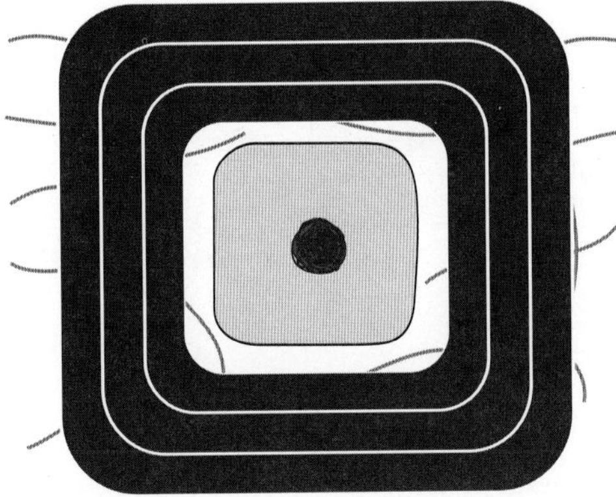

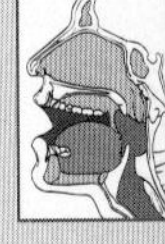

Describe the four stages of calcification in your own words. Look at the preceding text if you have difficulty.

Review now the formation of bone in Chapter One.

Enamel Formation

4.1

What type of cell "makes" enamel? These cells originally came from the inner enamel epithelium, which came from the enamel organ, which came from the dental lamina, which came from the oral ectoderm.

ameloblasts

fibrous

Diagrammed here is an **ameloblast.** It produces a ______________ matrix.

calcium

Next, ______________ salts are attracted to the fibers from the bloodstream.

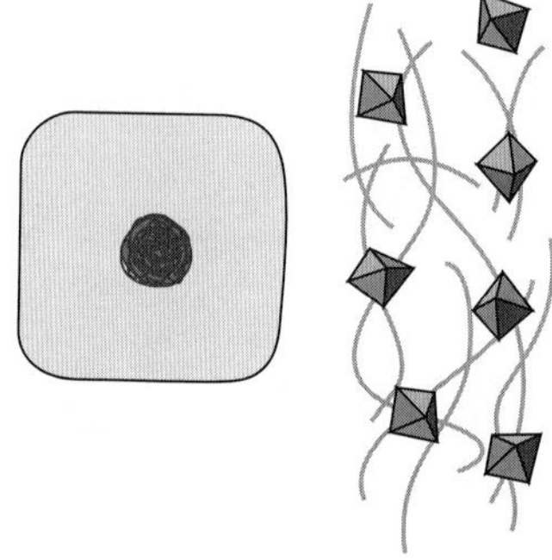

hydroxyapatite

Third, larger crystals of ______________ are formed from the calcium salts.

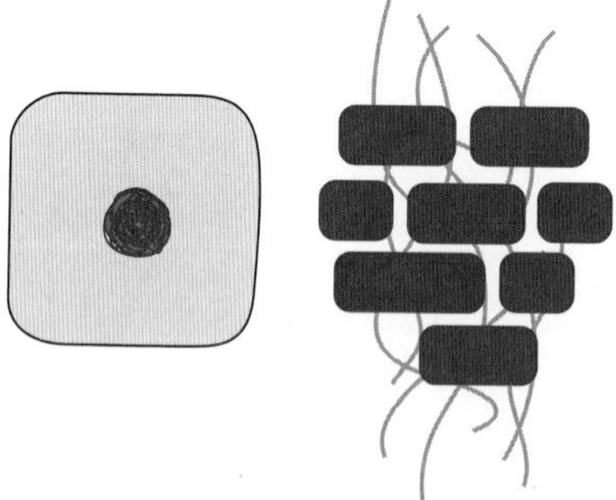

Last (this is the stage that is different for each hard tissue), larger crystals are formed from the smaller hydroxyapatite crystals.

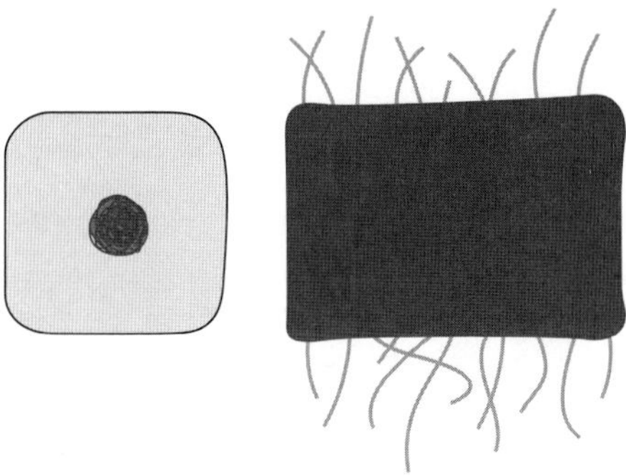

These "enamel crystals" are very dense and hard and are "keyhole shaped" so that they fit together tightly. These large enamel crystals are called **enamel rods.**

The ameloblasts keep laying down layer upon layer of enamel.

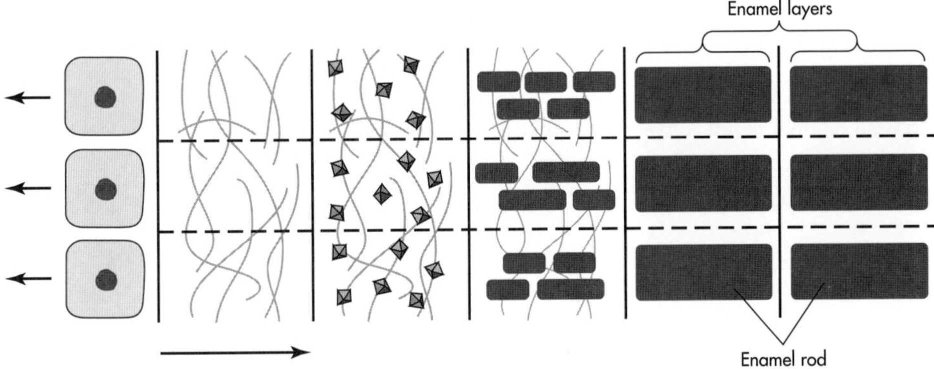

Look now at a smaller cross section through the crown of a tooth. Can you see the layers of enamel? The dark lines in the enamel between layers are called the **lines of Retzius.**

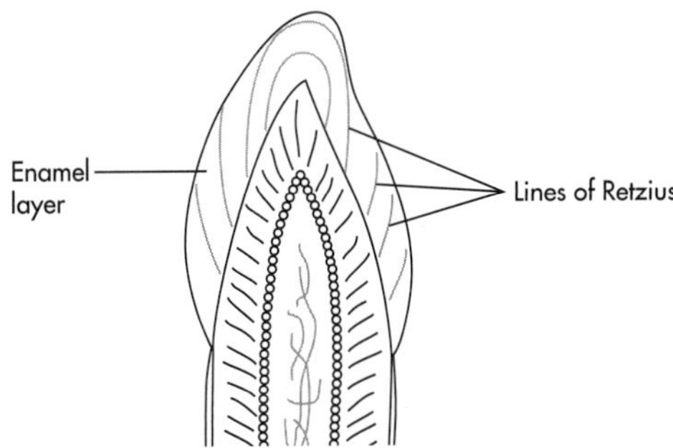

When the enamel of the crown is completed, the ameloblasts stop producing enamel.

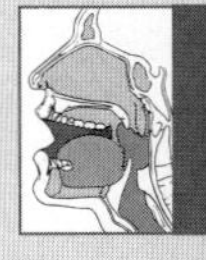

On eruption (moving into the oral cavity), the ameloblasts and the reduced enamel epithelium (i.e., most of the old enamel organ) are lost. After eruption, enamel has no live cells, only matrix.

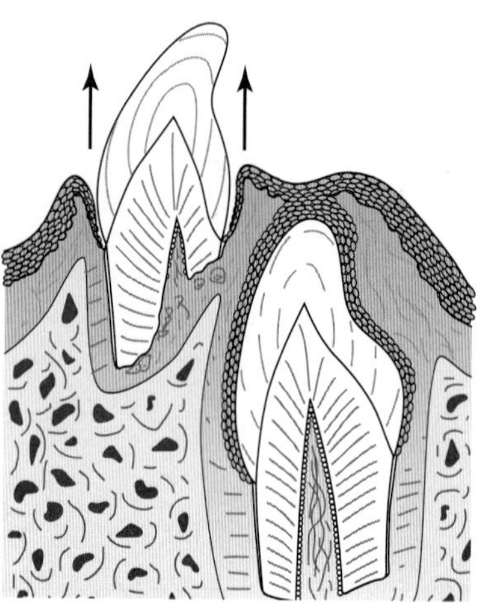

no, no

If enamel has no live cells after eruption, is it capable of more growth? Can it repair itself?

Erupted enamel is not a live tissue. It is not able to grow or repair itself, if damaged.

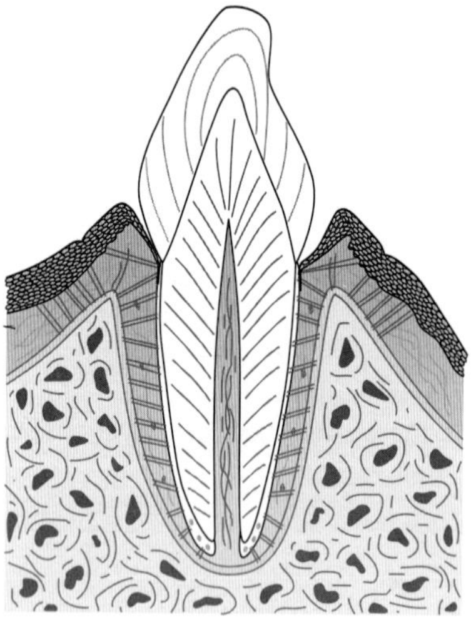

4.2 Dentin Formation

odontoblasts

What cells make dentin? While enamel formation begins, beneath it, dentin formation also starts.

The cell shown is an **odontoblast.** How is it different from the ameloblast? As calcification begins, the odontoblast forms a fibrous matrix.

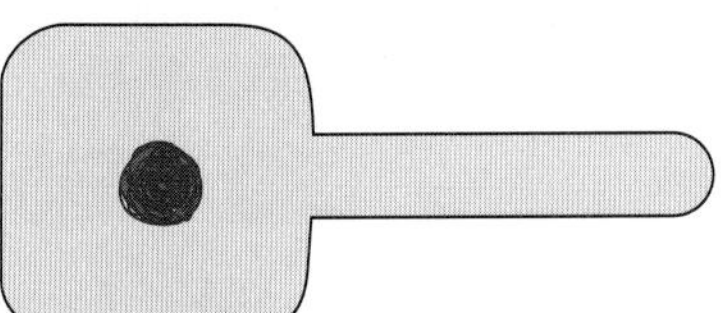

It has a process.

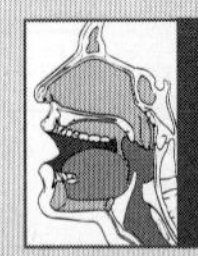

The odontoblast has a "finger" or **odontoblastic process** extending off its cell body. This process remains out in the matrix.

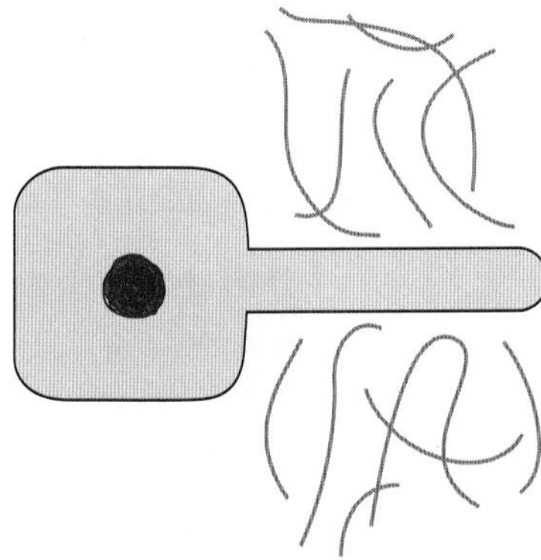

_______________ salts will be attracted to the fibers from the bloodstream.

Calcium

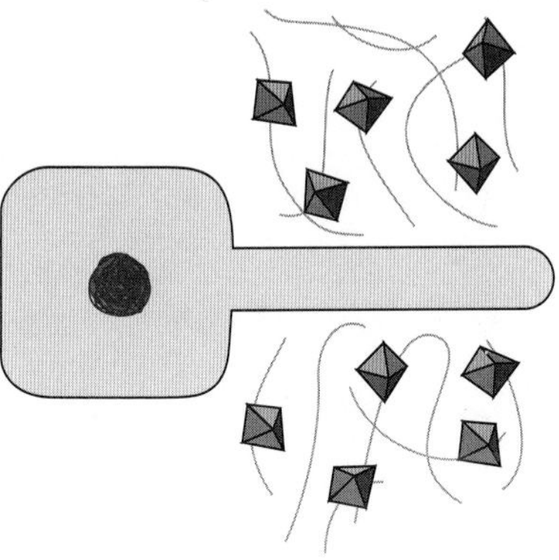

hydroxyapatite

The calcium salts form the larger ______________ crystals.

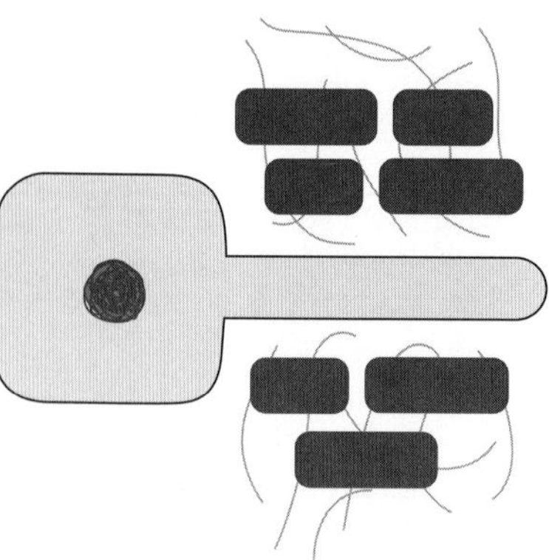

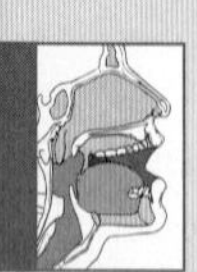

The hydroxyapatite crystals come together to form larger crystals of **dentin.** In the earliest stage of calcification, this matrix is called **predentin.**

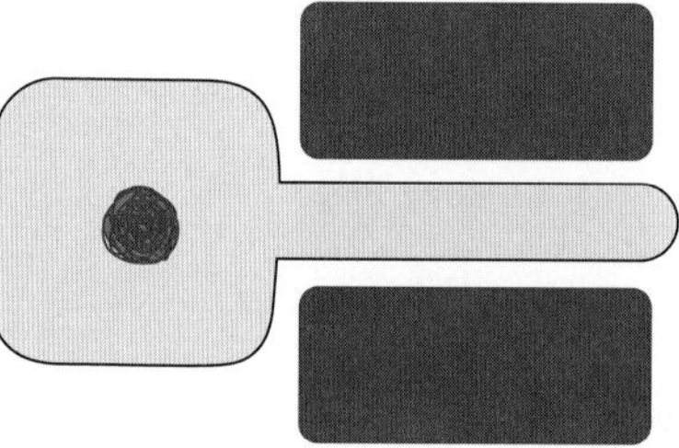

dentin

As the crystals become more tightly packed, the tissue is called ______________.

odontoblastic processes

Although it is dense, dentin is not as hard as enamel. What else is different about dentin?

As you can see, the odontoblastic process remains in the calcified dentin within spaces called **dentinal tubules.** It looks as though the processes stretched out as the dentin developed, layer after layer.

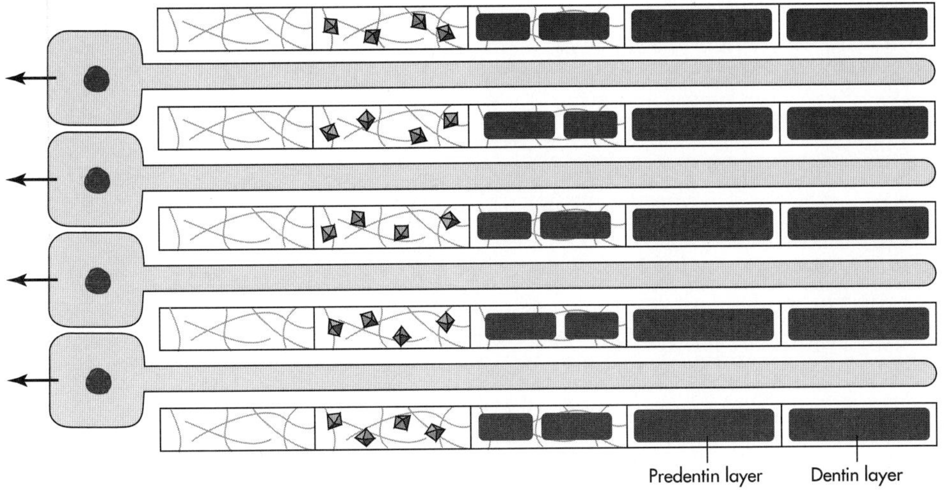

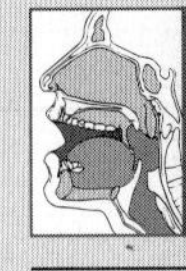

If you were to cut through the dentin at a right angle to the diagram, it would look like the section shown. Identify now the dentinal tubule with its odontoblastic process within. Dentin is a very unique looking tissue, like "Swiss cheese" when cut through the tubules. Why?

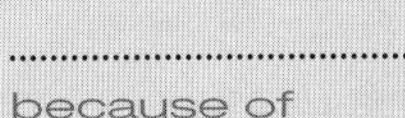
because of dentinal tubules

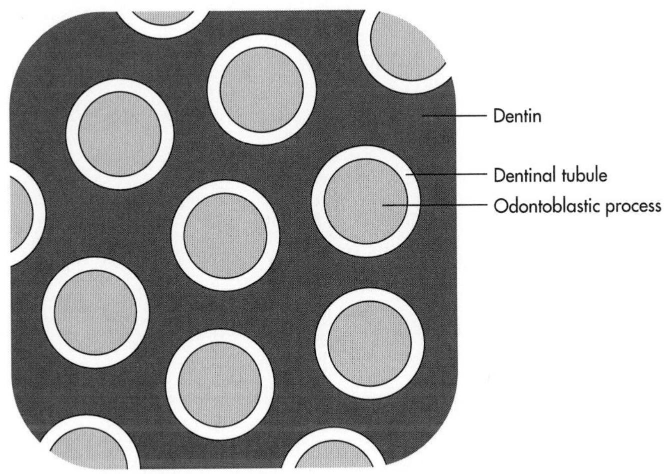

Looking at a long section through a tooth, can you see the layers of dentin as they were laid down by development? The dark lines separating the layers have no name. Don't confuse the growth lines with the tubules, which appear to radiate out.

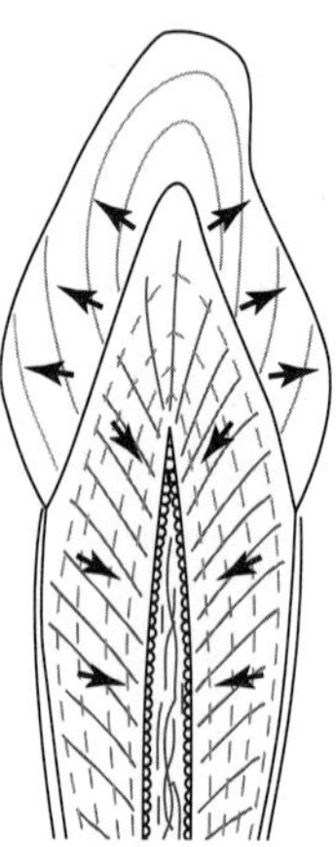

on the outer layer of the pulp

Dentin grows inward, toward that "hollow space" known as the **pulp.** The enamel grows outward in the opposite direction. Where are the odontoblastic cell bodies are located?

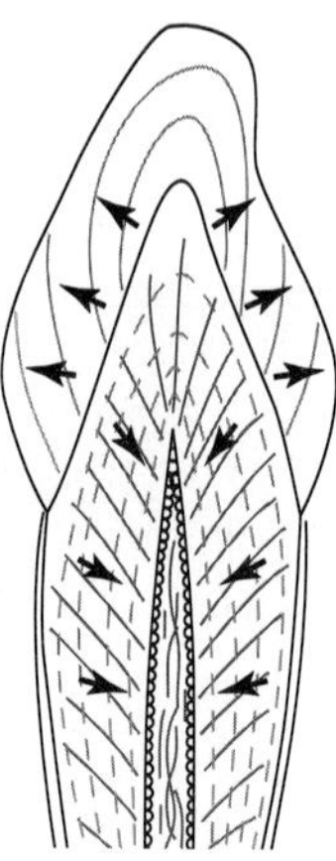

4.3 Cementum Formation

The last hard tissue of the tooth to form is **cementum.** Its formation is similar to that of bone. In fact, under the microscope, bone and cementum are hard to distinguish.

Remember in development that **cementoblasts** are recruited from the PDL to line up outside the developing dentin of the root and **Hertwig's epithelial root sheath.** The sheath tells the odontoblasts and cementoblasts where to form the root.

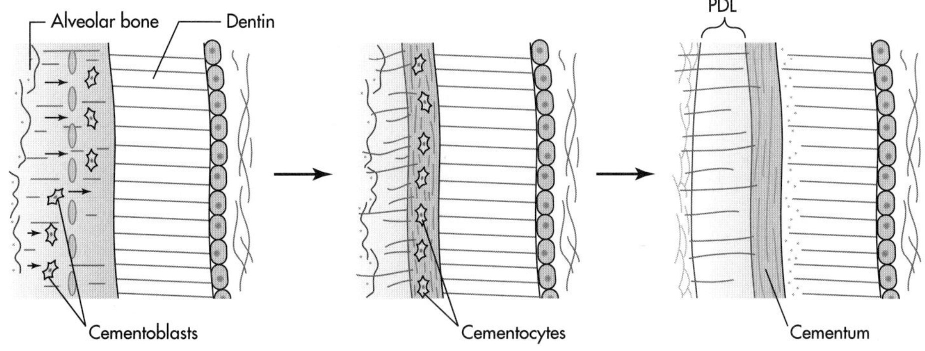

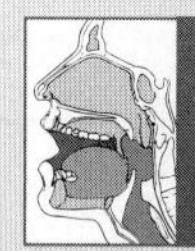

This is a **cementoblast.** First, it will form a fibrous matrix around itself.

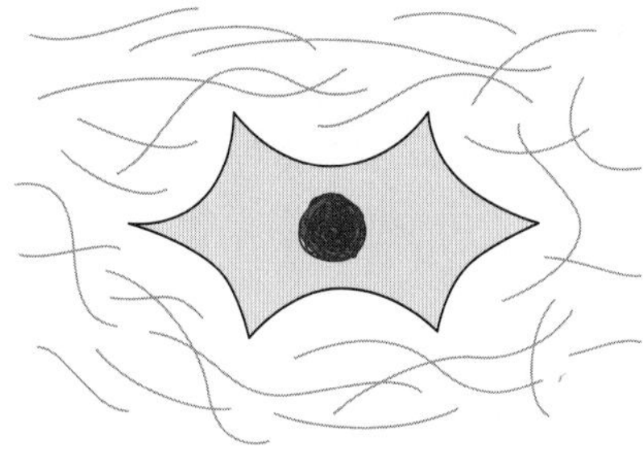

Second, _______________ will be attracted to the fibers from the bloodstream.

calcium salts

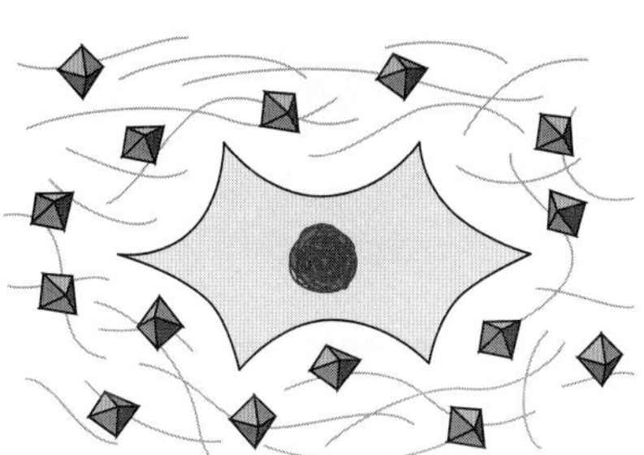

hydroxyapatite

Third, _______________ crystals will be formed from the salts.

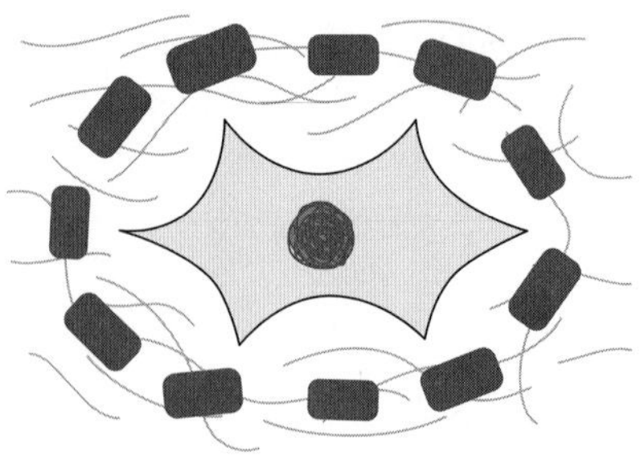

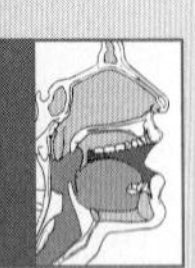

Last, larger crystals of cementum will be formed all around the cell.

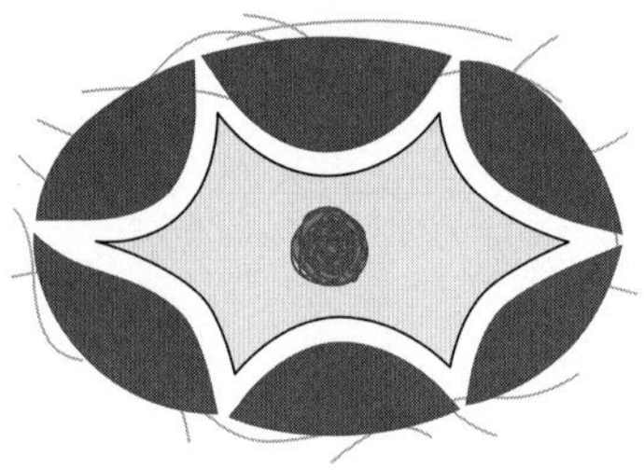

bone

The **cementocyte** will now be surrounded by cementum, housed within a space called a **lacuna.** It has a spidery shape with many cell processes, which keep in contact with other cementum cells. Each process lies in a space called a **canaliculus.** Cementum is laid down in layers around the root. What other tissue does cementum remind you of?

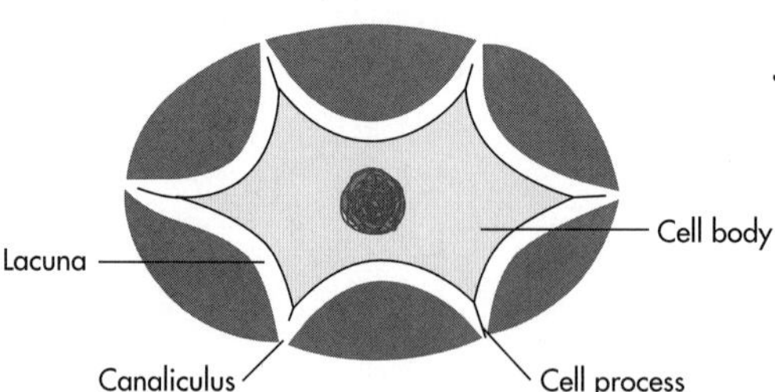

The cementum closest to the cervix of the tooth will eventually lose its cells and become **acellular cementum.** The cementum around the apex of the root will maintain its cells and is called **cellular cementum.**

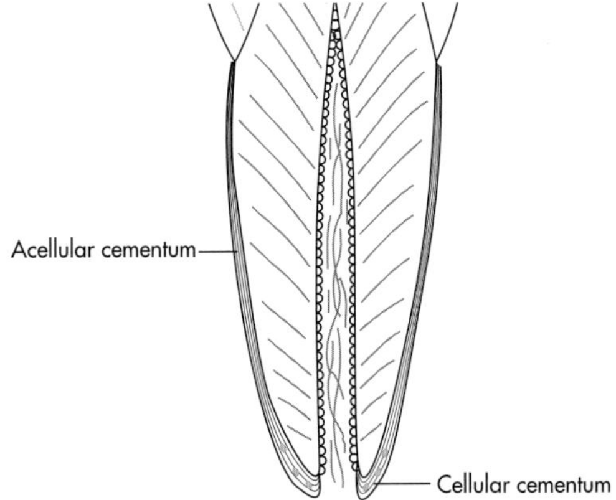

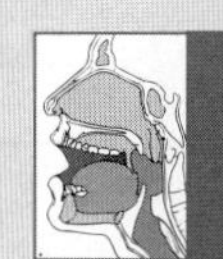

Is cementum a live tissue? Is it capable of growth and repair?

yes, at the apex; yes, at the apex

The outer layer of the pulp is where the odontoblastic cell bodies lie, with their processes poking up into the dentin. As dentin contains cells after it is formed, is it a live tissue? Is it capable of further growth and repair?

yes, yes

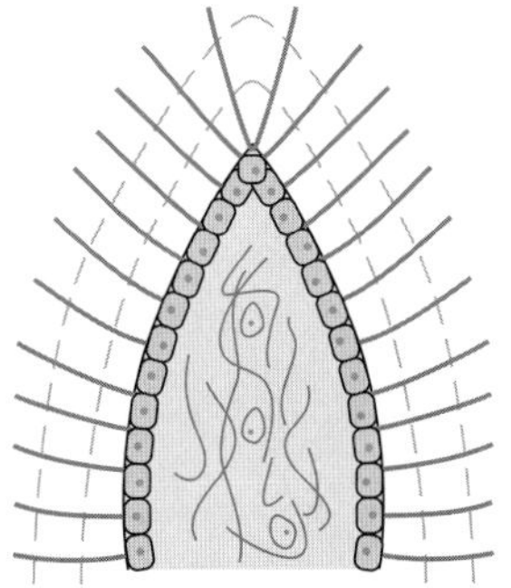

yes

Dentin is a live tissue, capable of growth and repair. It is also a sensitive tissue able to respond to stimuli such as hot and cold. Is this different than enamel?

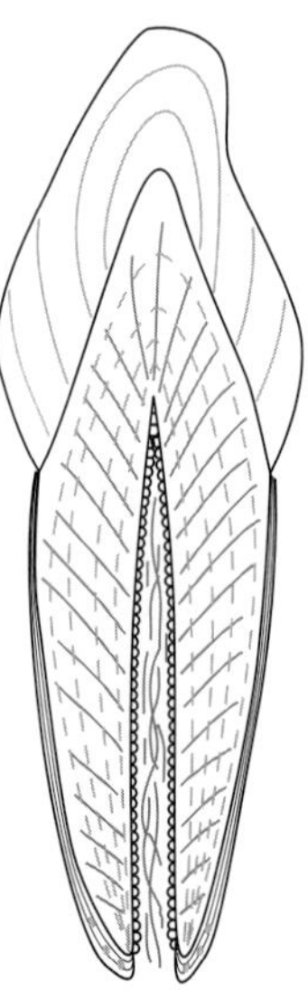

5.0 LOBES

So far we have been looking at the development of teeth in two dimensions, or in flat diagrams. Technically, these are called longitudinal sections of teeth. These diagrams gave us a good idea of what was occurring in the tooth, but not the entire picture. Compare, for example, these two-dimensional (Figure A) and three-dimensional (Figure B) diagrams of the enamel organ.

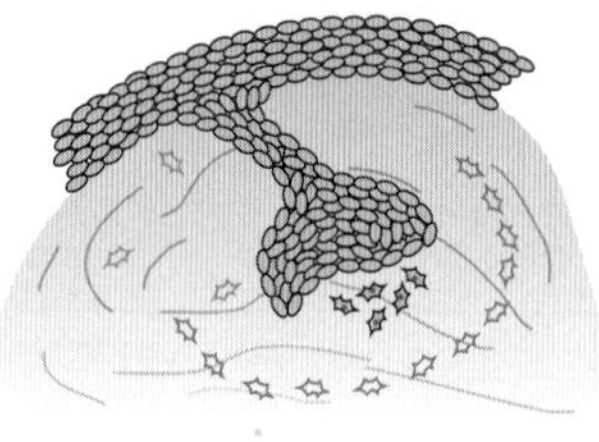

A

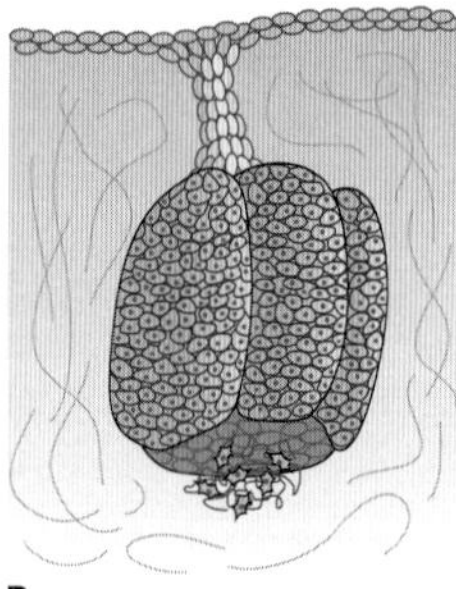

B

What we have not been able to see in sections is that the teeth are developing more in certain areas than others. In three dimensions, the teeth appear to develop in four or five "bumps" or areas called **lobes.** This is most evident in the crowns. Look at the developing crown of an incisor. How many lobes do you see?

four

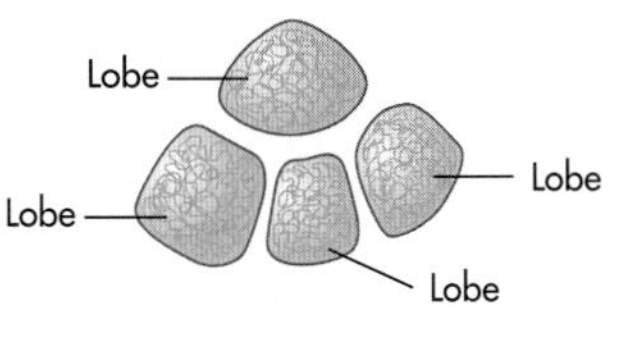

Incisal view

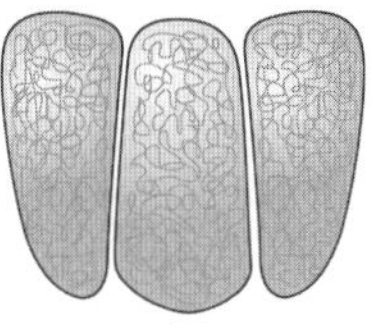

Facial view

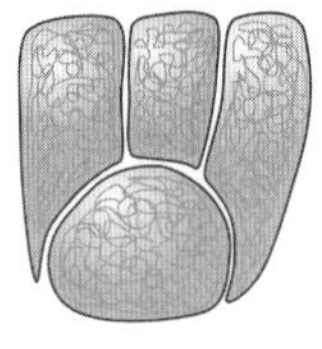

Lingual view

Lobes are areas of developing tooth that will eventually come together or **coalesce.** In the diagram, an incisor is coalescing from ______________ lobes.

four

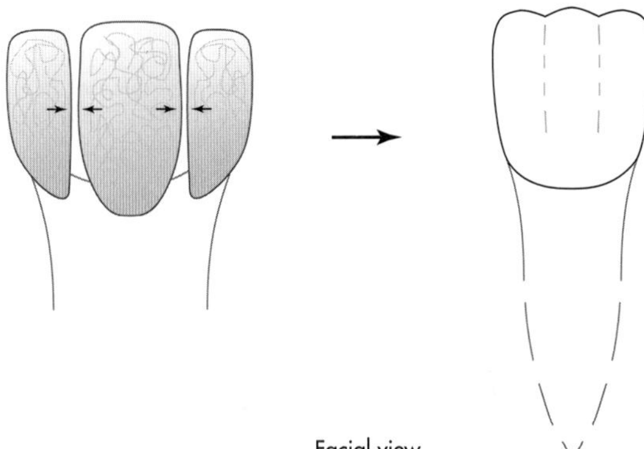

Facial view

In the next diagram a molar is coalescing from ______________ lobes.

five

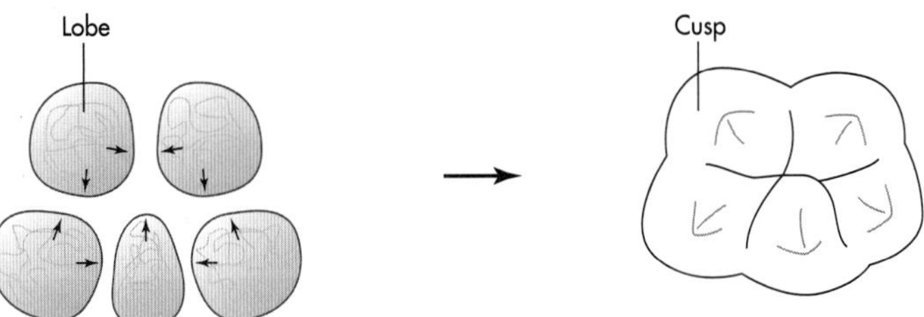

Occlusal view

Evidence of the coalescence of the four or five lobes that make up the tooth is found in the enamel of the crown. Look at the two vertical lines on the facial side of this incisor. They are called **developmental lines** or **grooves.** These lines divide the three facial lobes.

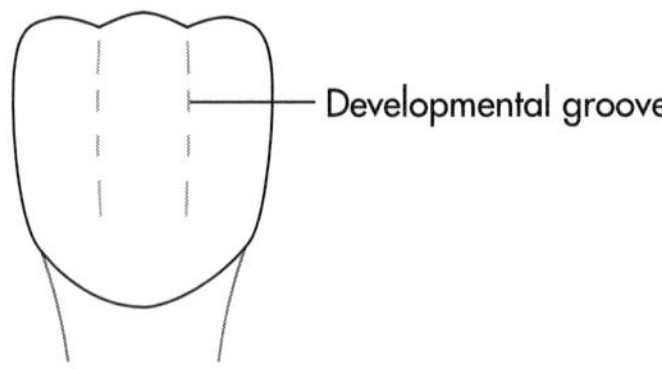

The developmental lines or grooves on molars are the lines between the cusps, as shown.

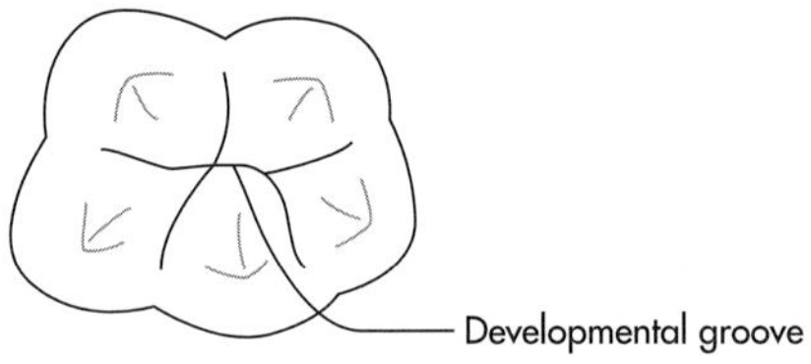

four or five, developmental lines or grooves

How many lobes coalesce to form a tooth? What remnant remains of the fully formed tooth to show evidence that the tooth once consisted of lobes?

REVIEW TEST 3.1

SELECT OR FILL IN THE CORRECT ANSWER.

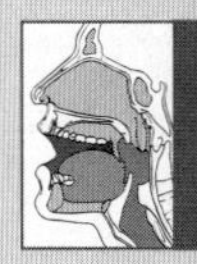

1. The 20 areas of oral ectoderm that thicken and grow down into the mesoderm of the developing jaws are called
   a. gingiva
   b. dental lamina
   c. crypts
   d. dental papilla

2. How many primary teeth develop from the dental lamina?
   a. 32
   b. 20
   c. 40

3. The enamel organ will capture mesoderm beneath it called the
   a. dental lamina
   b. dental sac
   c. dental papilla
   d. dentin

4. The innermost layer of the enamel organ is called the
   a. inner enamel epithelium
   b. stratum intermedium
   c. stellate reticulum
   d. outer enamel epithelium

5. Cells that make enamel are called ________________.

6. Cells that make dentin are called ________________.

7. Mesoderm that condenses around the enamel organ is called
   a. dental lamina
   b. dental papilla
   c. dental sac
   d. dentin

8. Which is not a derivative of the dental sac?
   a. dentin
   b. PDL
   c. cementum
   d. alveolar bone

9. Which hard tissue is not a live tissue after eruption?
   a. enamel
   b. dentin
   c. bone
   d. cementum

REVIEW TEST 3.2

SELECT THE CORRECT ANSWER.

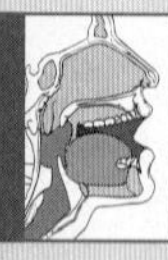

1. Which is the first stage of the process of calcification?
   a. attraction of calcium salts
   b. creation of a fibrous matrix
   c. formation of hydroxyapatite
   d. formation of the final hard matrix
2. Cells that are recruited from the PDL to line up along the developing root to make hard tissue are
   a. odontoblasts
   b. osteoblasts
   c. cementoblasts
3. The ______________ defines the end of the tooth while it is developing.
   a. ameloblasts
   b. Hertwig's sheath
   c. diaphragm
   d. rests of Malassez
4. ______________ is a trail of cells left by the enamel organ as a guide for root development.
   a. Ameloblasts
   b. Cementoblasts
   c. Rests of Malassez
   d. Hertwig's epithelial root sheath
5. The attachment epithelium is the only derivative of the
   a. enamel organ
   b. dental papilla
   c. dental sac
   d. reduced enamel epithelium
6. The tissue that most resembles bone is ______________.
   a. enamel
   b. dentin
   c. cementum
7. Enamel, dentin, cementum, and bone matrix are all laid down in layers by their cells. True or false?

REVIEW TEST 3.3

SELECT OR FILL IN THE CORRECT ANSWER.

1. The enamel organ develops from oral ______________.
2. The enamel organ will maintain attachment to the oral ectoderm for a short time. True or false?

3. An ectoderm "bud" grows off the primary enamel organ called the _______________, which will later develop into a second enamel organ.

4. The four cell layers of the enamel organ are the _______________, _______________, _______________, and _______________.

5. Cells of the inner enamel epithelium will become odontoblasts. True or false?

6. The long "finger" of the odontoblast is called its _______________.

7. The two derivatives of the dental papilla are _______________ and _______________.

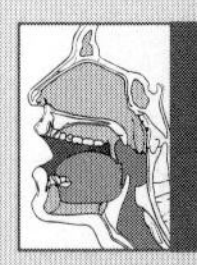

8. The making of hard tissue matrix is called _______________.

9. Cells that make hard tissue are called _______________ cells, and cells that break down hard tissue are _______________ cells.

10. Dentin has spaces in its matrix for the odontoblastic processes called _______________.

11. The _______________ are remnants of the enamel organ, left over in the PDL of the erupted tooth.

12. The largest crystals that enamel is finally made of are called enamel _______________.

13. Before it is totally calcified, dentin is called _______________.

REVIEW TEST 3.4

MATCH EACH STRUCTURE WITH THE TISSUE FROM WHICH IT DERIVES.

1. enamel _______________
2. dentin _______________
3. cementum _______________
4. PDL _______________
5. alveolar bone _______________

a. dental papilla
b. dental sac
c. enamel organ

MATCH EACH STRUCTURE WITH THE TISSUE FROM WHICH IT DERIVES.

1. ameloblasts _______________
2. odontoblasts _______________
3. dental papilla _______________
4. enamel organ _______________

a. ectoderm
b. mesoderm

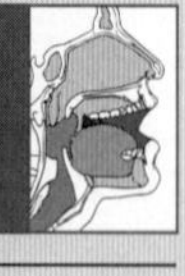

REVIEW TEST 3.5

LABEL THE DIAGRAMS.

1.

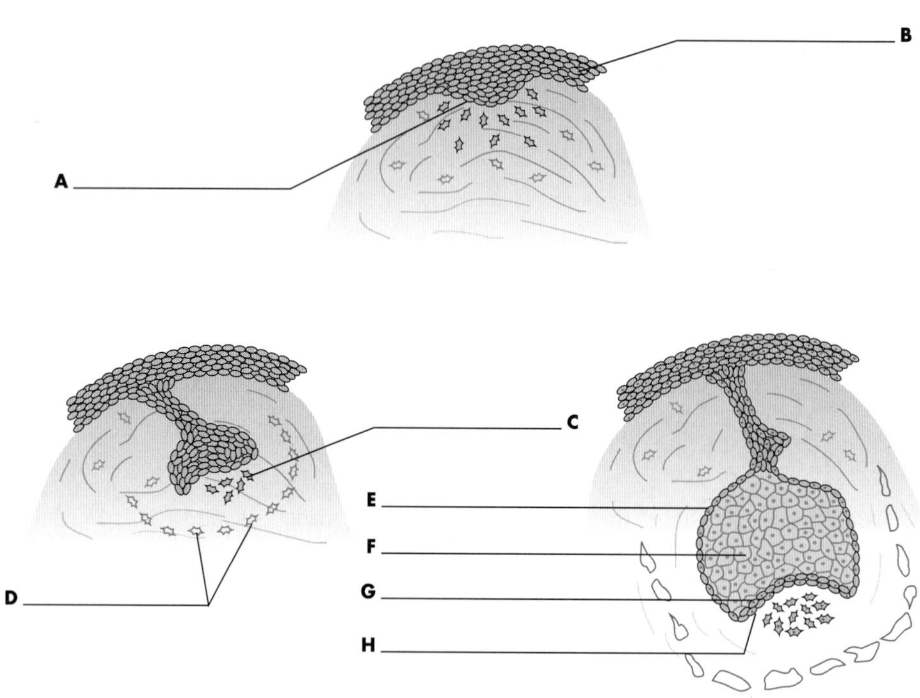

2.

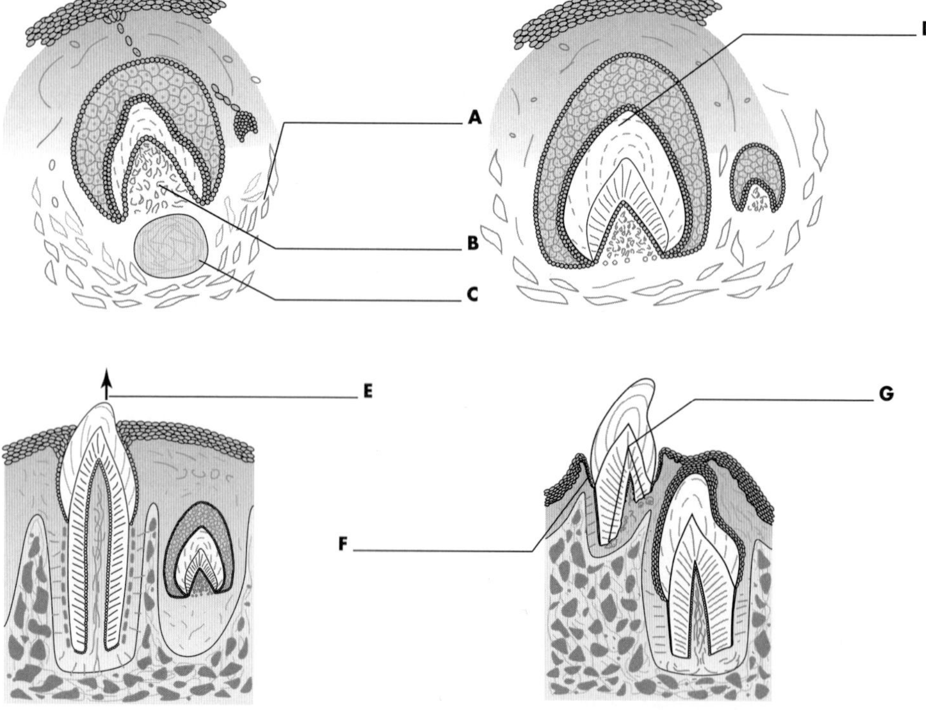

3.

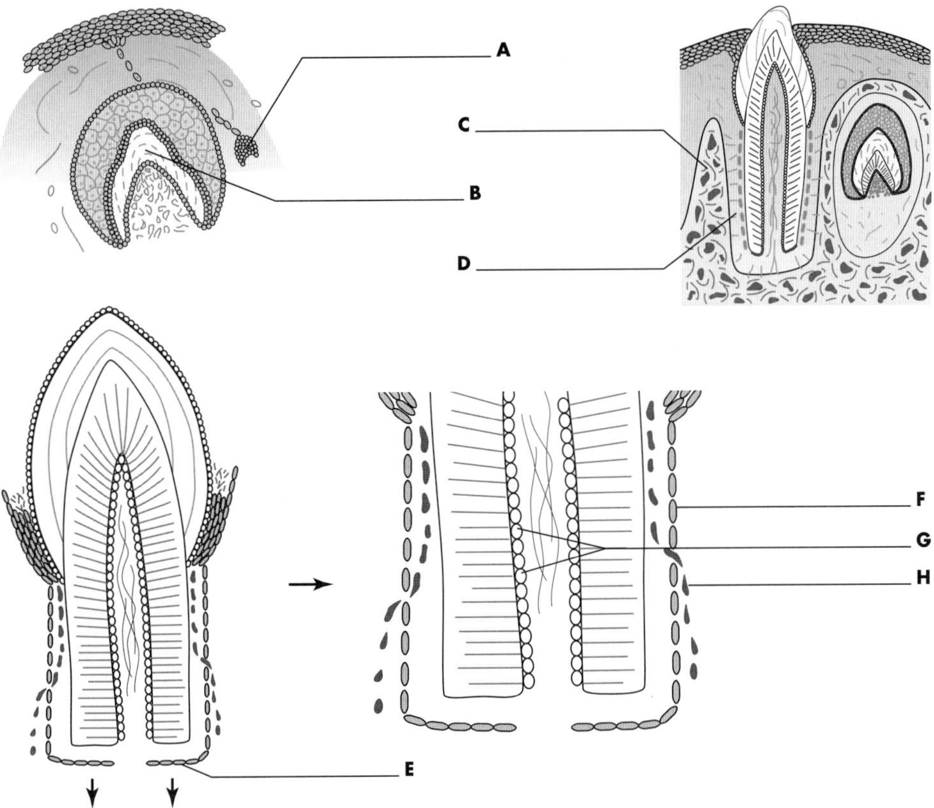

4.

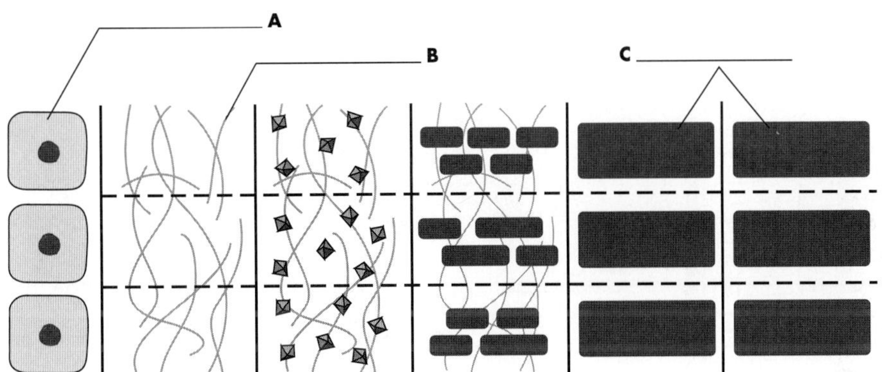

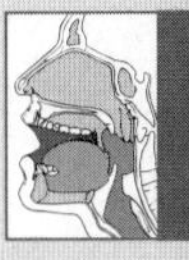

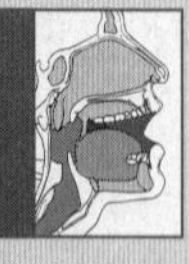

5.

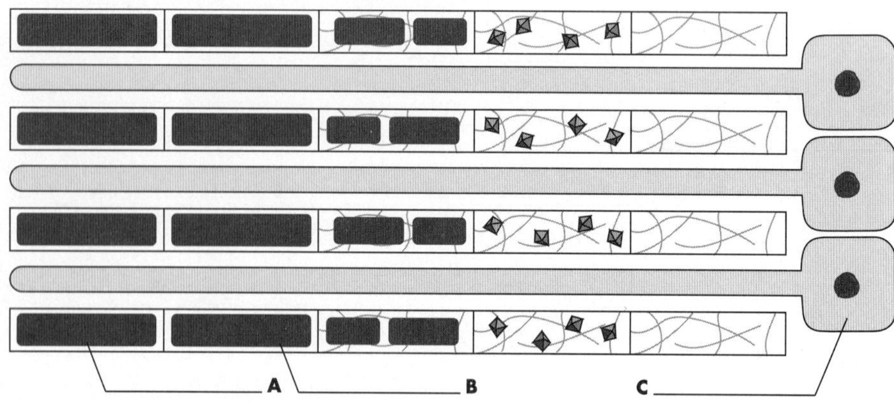

6.

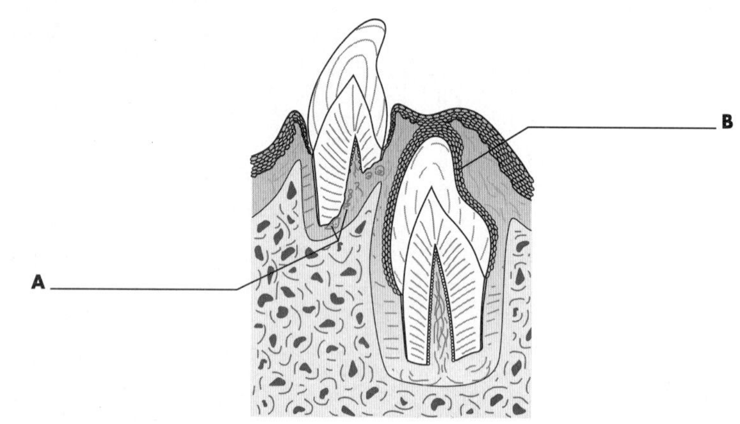

7.

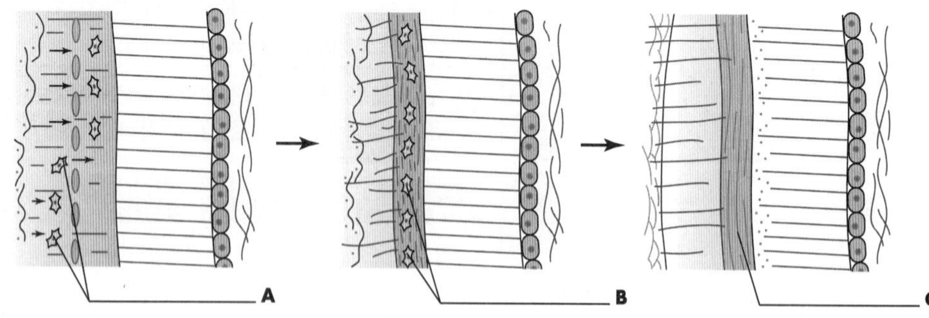

8.

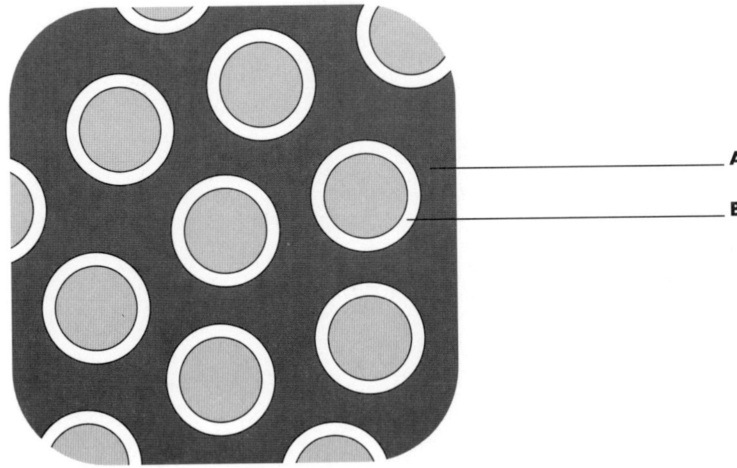

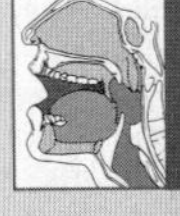

9.

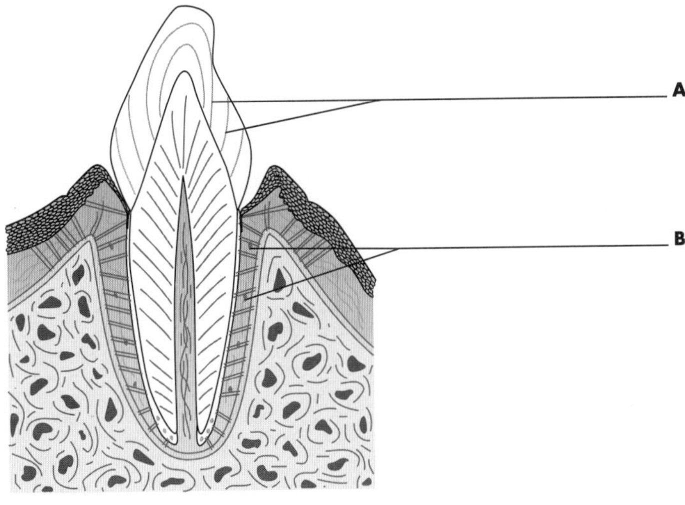

Dental Histology

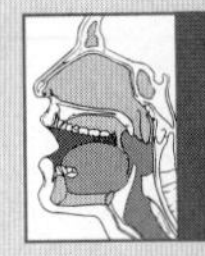

ENAMEL 1.0

Enamel is a dense, hard, white, crystalline tissue found covering the outer aspect of the **crown** of the tooth. It is, in fact, the hardest tissue found in the human body.

Consider its function: to provide a hard, protective outer layer on the teeth that will endure the forces of mastication over a lifetime. It must help to cut, pierce, and grind food without fracturing itself. The microstructure or histology of enamel will show us how this is accomplished.

As strong as it is, damage does occur to enamel. **Trauma** and fracture are accidental breakage of enamel structure. **Abrasion** is abnormal wear on enamel, whereas **attrition** is normal wear and tear. **Erosion** is chemical damage to enamel. **Caries** is a disease process that can cause damage to all tooth tissues.

Which one of the above modes of damage to enamel is caused by normal wear?

attrition

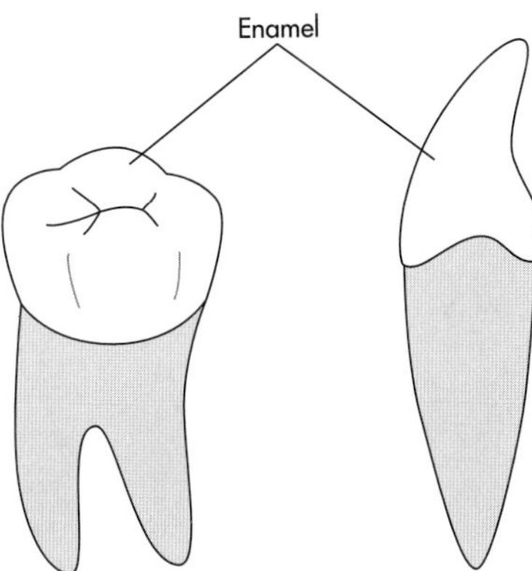

ameloblasts, lamina

Let's review how enamel is formed. Enamel is formed by ____________, which came from the inner enamel epithelial layer of the enamel organ. Remember that enamel organs came originally from oral ectoderm that lumped up in 20 places called the dental ____________.

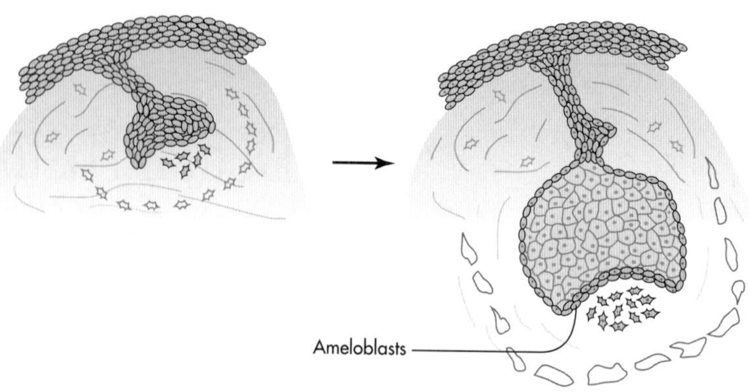

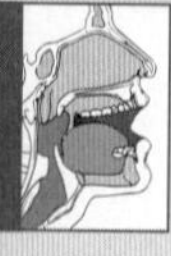

Ameloblasts make enamel by first forming a fibrous network, which will attract calcium salts from the bloodstream.

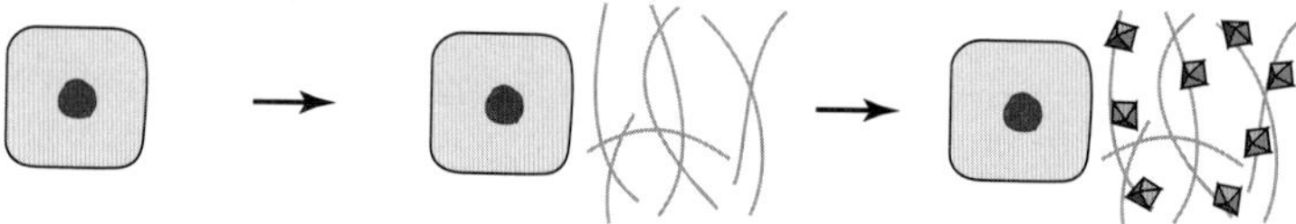

Then, larger and larger crystals will form, beginning with hydroxyapatite crystals and ending with enamel rods.

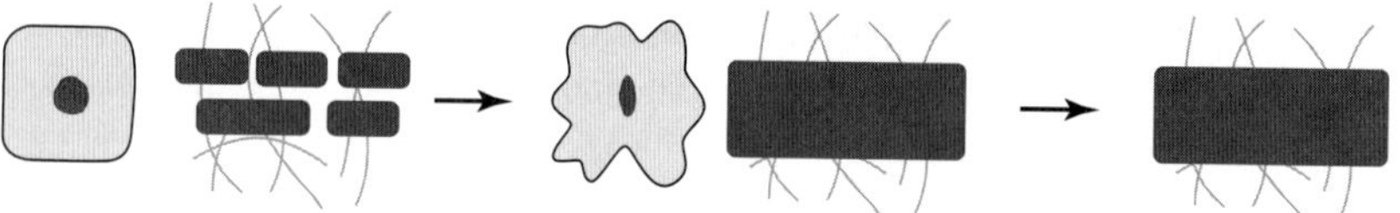

Enamel rods are keyhole-shaped crystals.

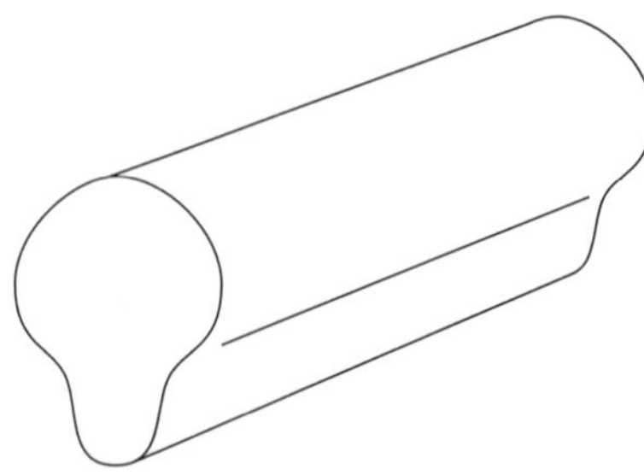

Enamel rods are shaped so that they will fit closely together.

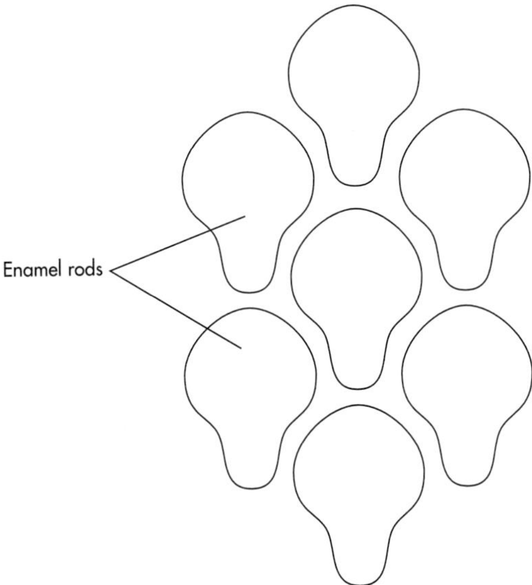

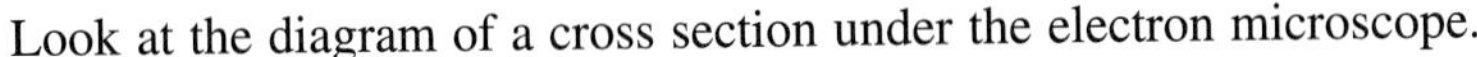

Look at the diagram of a cross section under the electron microscope.

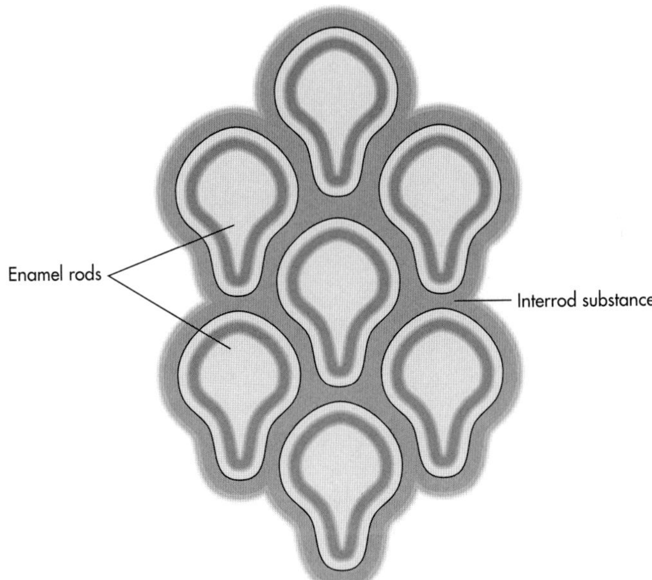

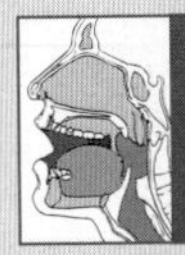

Note that there is some space between rods, and it is filled with an enamel-like material. It is called **interrod substance.** It is not as strong as enamel rods; therefore, it is weaker between rods.

hypocalcified

Areas of hard tissue that structurally are not as strong because of less tightly packed crystals are called **hypocalcified areas.** Interrod substance is a _______________ area.

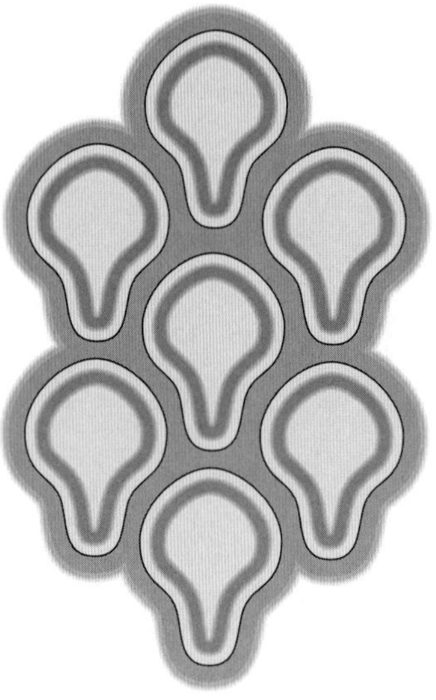

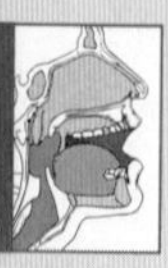

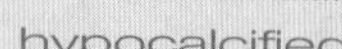

hypocalcified

Enamel is laid down in layers, from the inside toward the outside. The spaces between the layers (the dark lines on the picture) are not as strongly calcified; they are _______________ areas. These lines are called the **lines of Retzius.**

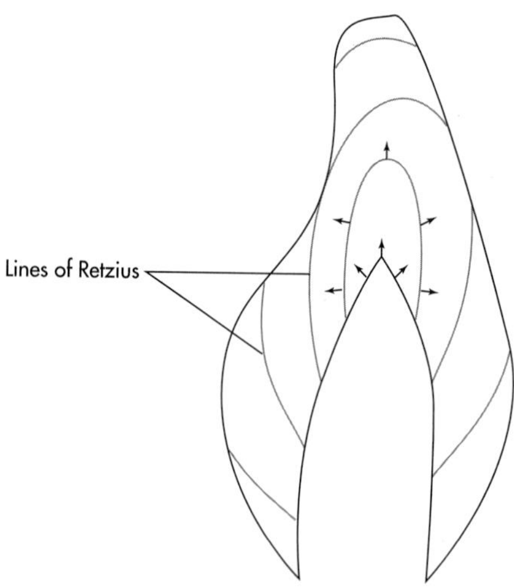

The lines of Retzius and the interrod substance are hypocalcified areas, or weaker, less structured areas that are more prone to damage. The crystalline structure in hypocalcified areas is less tightly packed. Where do you think enamel would break?

between rods or along lines of Retzius

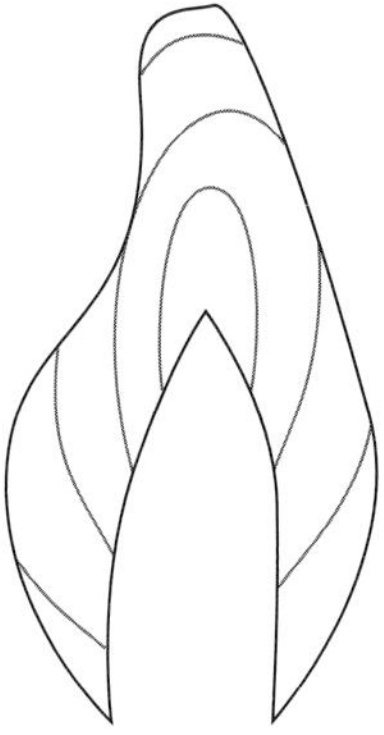

Enamel is a strong tissue, but it can break along its growth lines, the ______________, or between rods. It also is susceptible to acid attack in these areas.

lines of Retzius

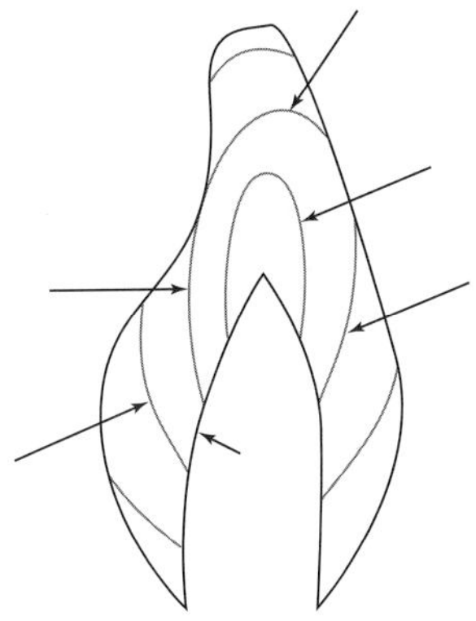

While examining slices of enamel under the microscope, a microscopist found that if polarized light was shown on the specimen, a second set of lines appeared. These lines appear as a series of dark and light bands and are called the **Hunter–Schreger bands.** They are not the same as the lines of Retzius. They are an optical phenomenon due to the crystalline structure of enamel, not growth lines.

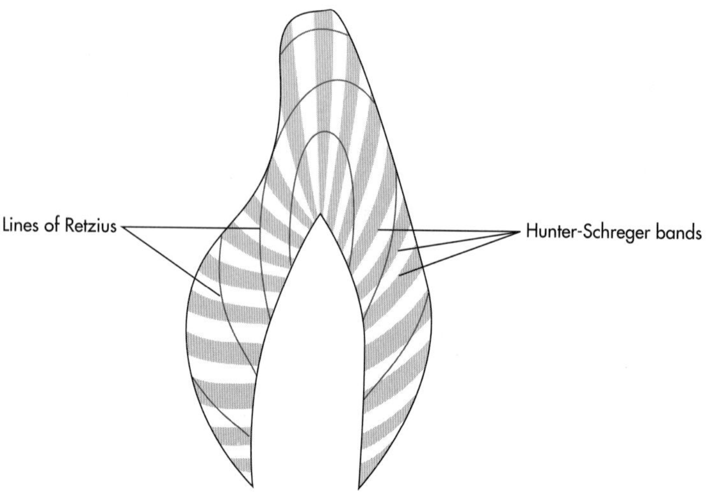

Label the growth lines or lines of Retzius on the crown in Figure A. Note that these lines continue to the outside surface of the crown, where they form a series of ridges on the enamel. These ridges are called **perikymata.** Lines between them are the **lines of imbrication.**

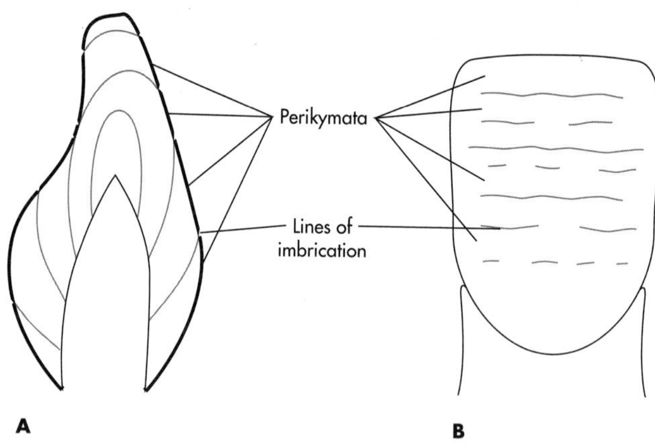

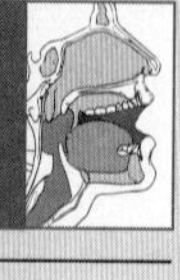

Label the perikymata on this tooth. What do they represent?

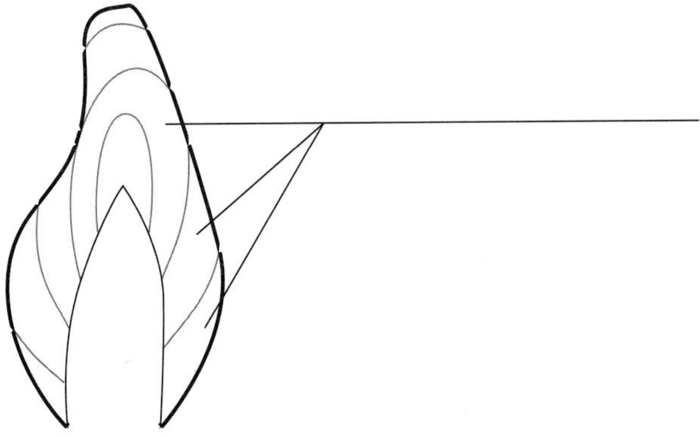

layers of enamel growth

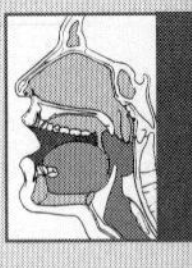

The perikymata are a series of ridges on the outside of the crown. They are more evident in the freshly erupted tooth, but are worn away with time.

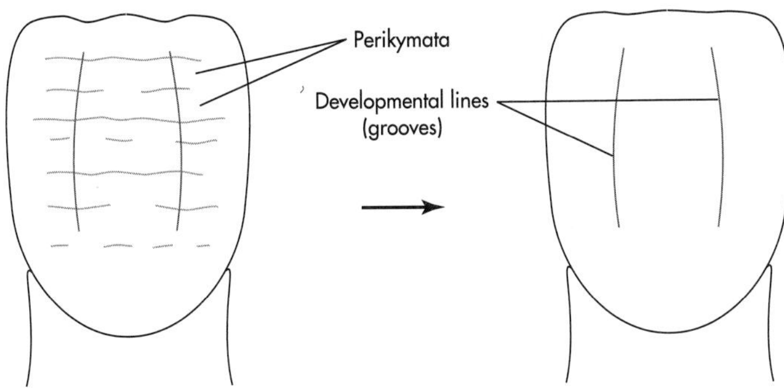

There are other vertical lines on the outside surface of the enamel, besides the horizontal lines of imbrication (growth) or perikymata. These are the lines left as remnants of the coalescence of lobes when the tooth is formed. They are called **developmental lines.**

On the diagram of the incisor, label the perikymata and the two labial developmental lines.

A. perikymata
B. developmental lines

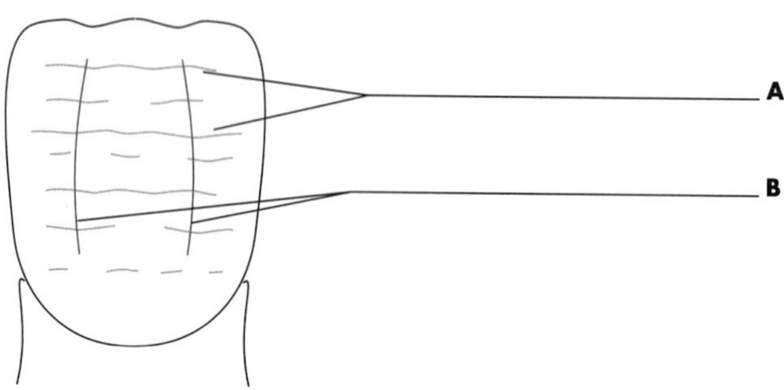

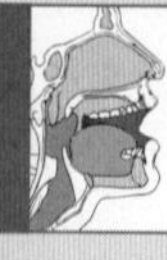

Developmental lines on posterior teeth enamel form grooves between the cusps. They may also be called **developmental grooves.** Label them on the molar. Remember that each cusp represents where a lobe used to be.

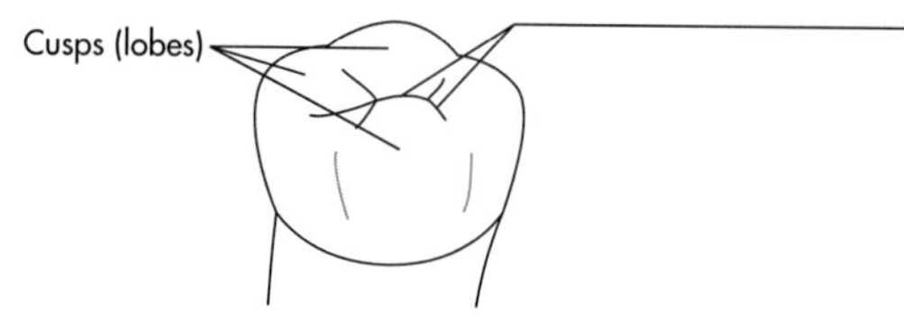

Another feature of incisor enamel is found on the incisal edge. A series of "bumps" called mamelons are also remnants of development. **Mamelons** are remnants of the three facial lobes that came together to form the incisor crown. Find them on the diagram.

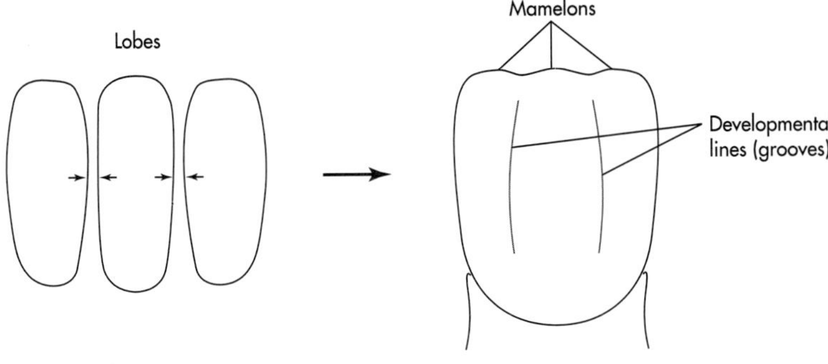

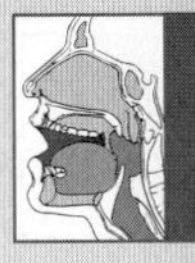

Mamelons

_______________ are usually present on freshly erupted teeth, but will wear away with years of chewing to a flat surface.

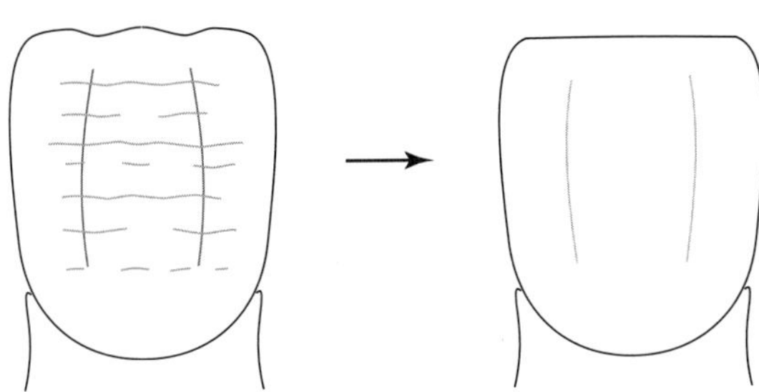

A. perikymata
B. Hunter–Schreger bands
C. lines of Retzius

Label the anatomic features of enamel.

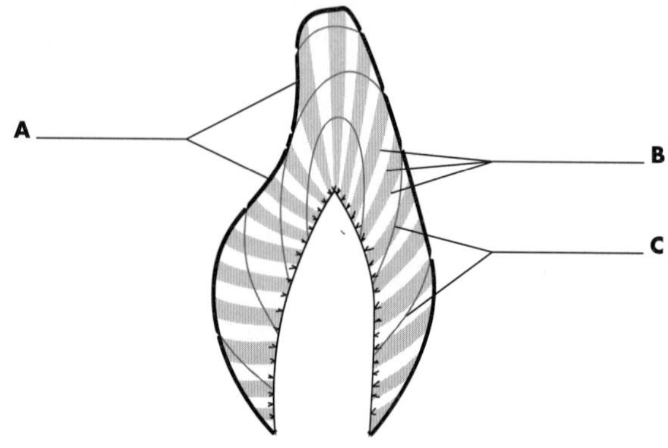

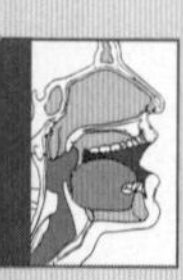

The border between enamel and dentin is called the **dentinoenamel junction (DEJ).**

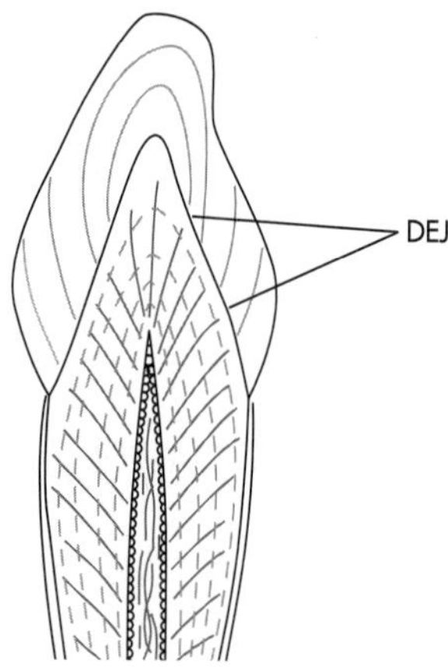

This is another hypocalcified area of the tooth. It is an especially weak area and is susceptible to damage.

Draw an arrow pointing to the DEJ. The dentinoenamel junction is a ____________ area that is susceptible to fracture and acid attack. Which two groups of cells used to lie along this junction before the tooth was formed?

hypocalcified, ameloblasts and odontoblasts

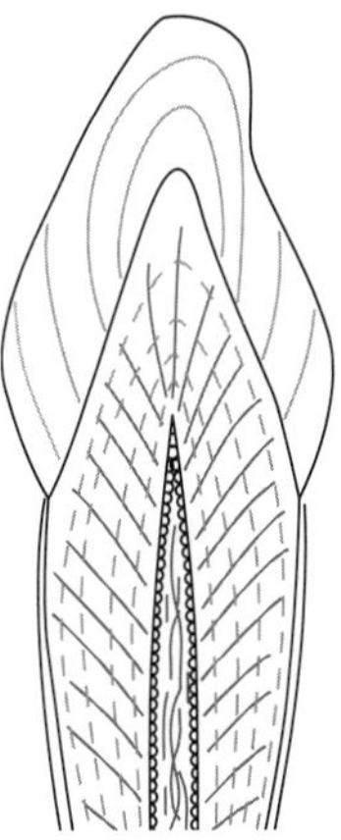

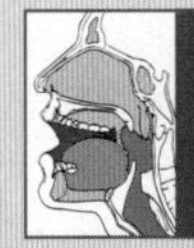

In this closeup view of the DEJ, one side is the dentin and one side is enamel. Look inside the enamel side. There are structures that look like the tips of paint brushes. These are hypocalcified areas called **enamel tufts and spindles** because of their appearance.

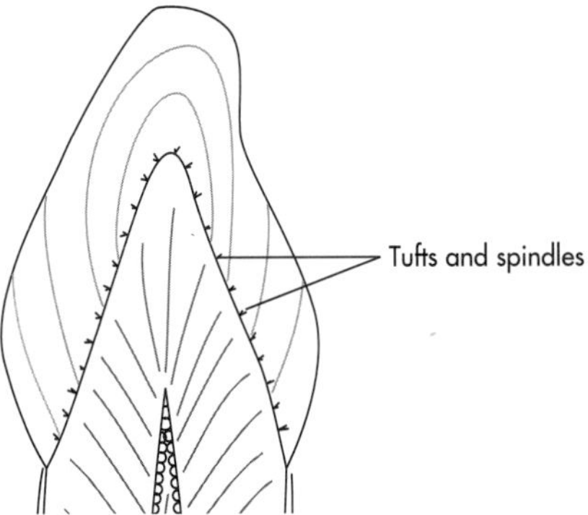

Place arrows indicating the location of enamel tufts and spindles. Are these weak areas? What lies in the tubules on the dentin side?

yes, odontoblastic processes

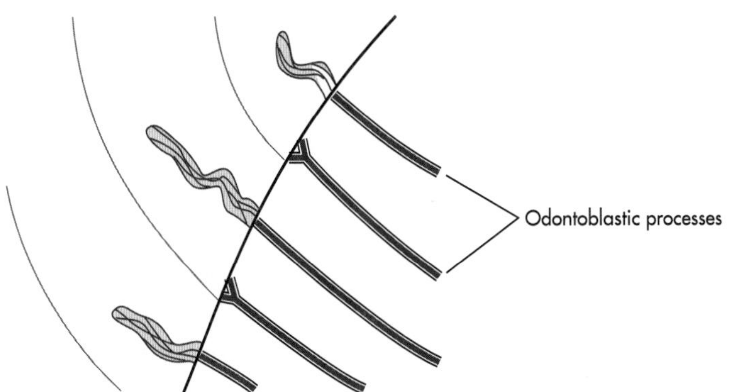

no, no

Is enamel a live tissue? Is it capable of growth or repair?

As enamel loses its cells after development (the ameloblasts) it is no longer a live tissue. Once it is damaged, it cannot repair itself. It also has no sensitivity.

80 year old

Enamel is worn down naturally by years of wear and tear from mastication and other normal forces. This normal wear on enamel is called **attrition.** Who would demonstrate more attrition on their teeth: an 8 year old or an 80 year old?

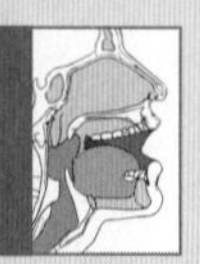

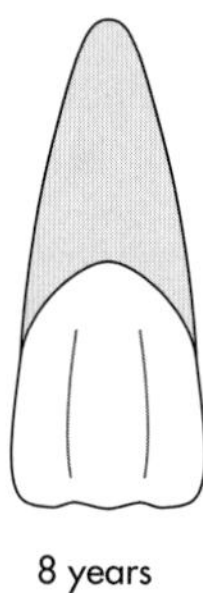

8 years

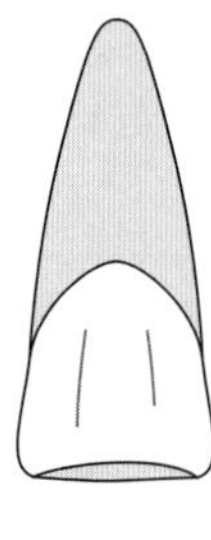

80 years

Attrition wears down the incisal edges of the anterior teeth and flattens the cusps of the posteriors. Another type of mechanical wear of enamel is abnormal and is called **abrasion.** An example is wear caused by overly vigorous toothbrushing.

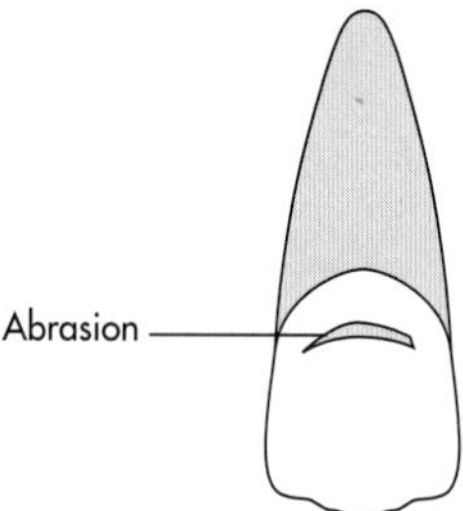

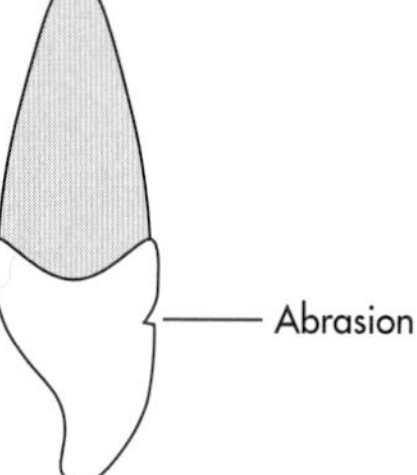

Abrasion can be caused by any poor oral habit that places excess wear on the enamel. ______________, however, is considered normal wear.

Attrition

Enamel is also susceptible to damage by acidic solutions, ingested or bacterial. This kind of chemical damage is called **erosion,** and it literally erodes or eats away enamel structure, creating smooth surfaces.

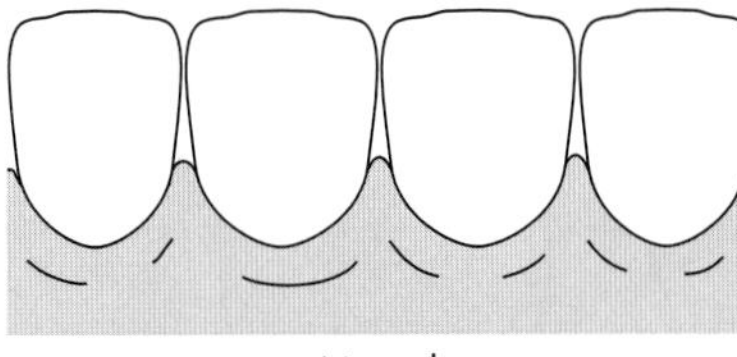

Normal

Lower anteriors

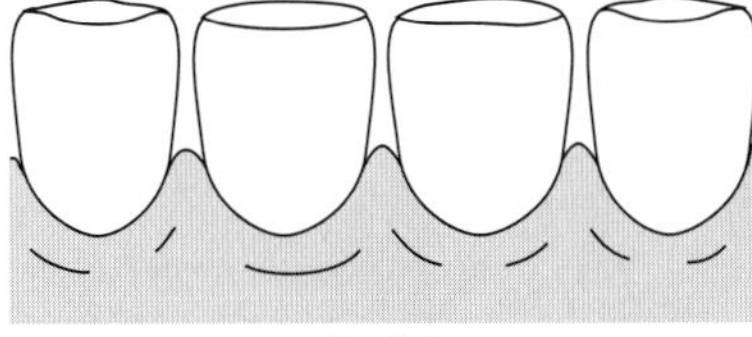

Eroded

So, the three types of wear and tear of enamel are attrition, abrasion, and erosion. Which is caused by acids? Which is caused by abnormal mechanical wear?

erosion, abrasion

DENTIN 2.0

The second hardest tissue in the body is dentin, the layer of hard tissue that constitutes the bulk of the tooth. It lies underneath the enamel and cementum layers and ends at the hollow area in the middle of the tooth known as the pulp.

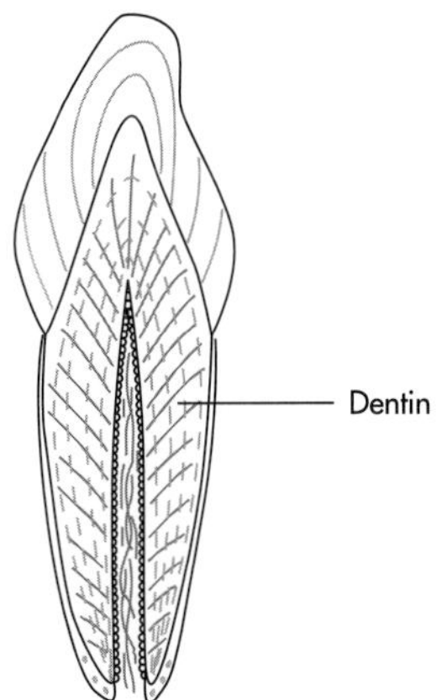

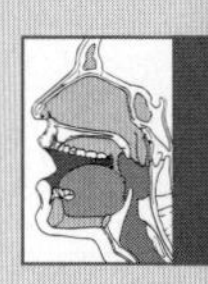

We have seen how dentin is developed from mesoderm of the dental papilla. Let's review that process.

dental papilla

Mesoderm condenses under the enamel organ and is called the ______________. The cells that line up at the outermost aspect are called odontoblasts.

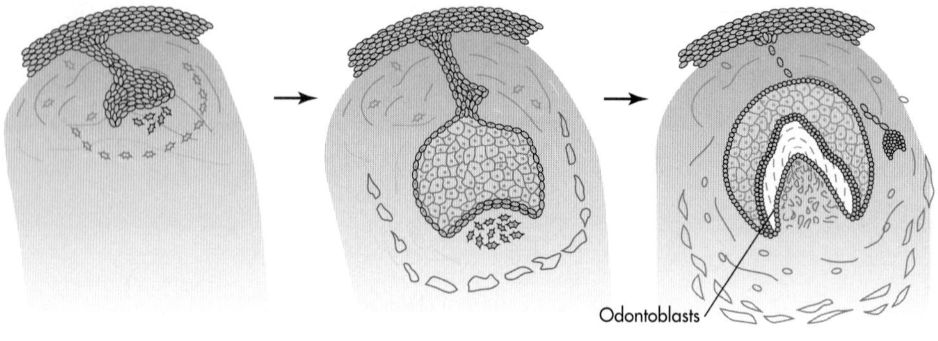

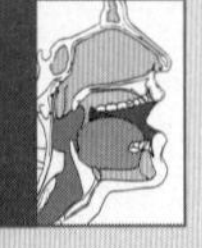

Ameloblasts

Odontoblasts form dentin by the process of calcification, under the enamel that has already begun forming. ______________ form the enamel. The first stage is for the odontoblasts to form a fibrous network.

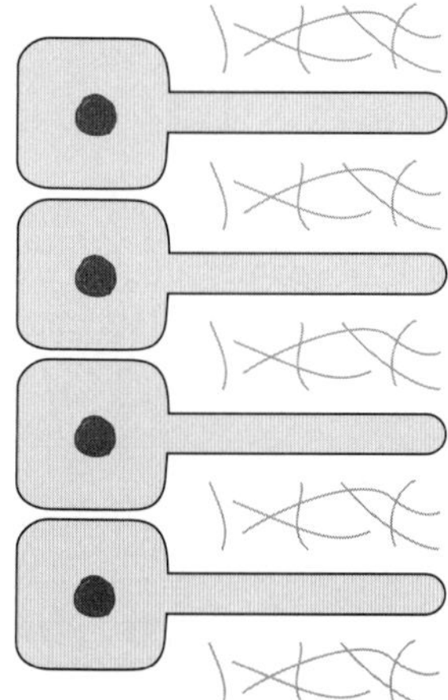

Next, calcium salts are attracted to the fibers and begin to grow larger and larger crystalline formations, the first of which is called hydroxyapatite crystals.

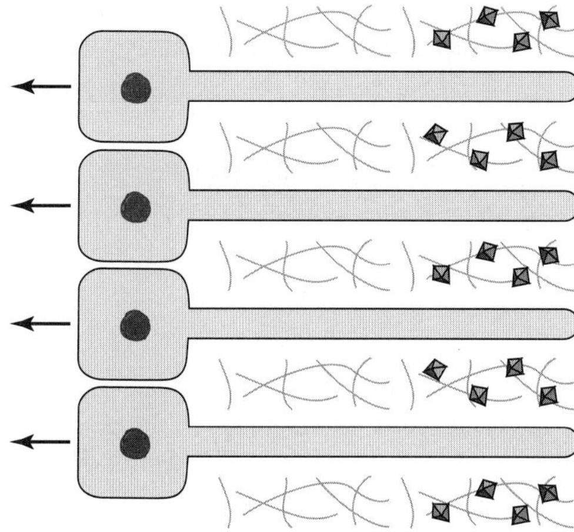

Last, dentin is formed from the crystalline structure, with the first stage of dentin or predentin.

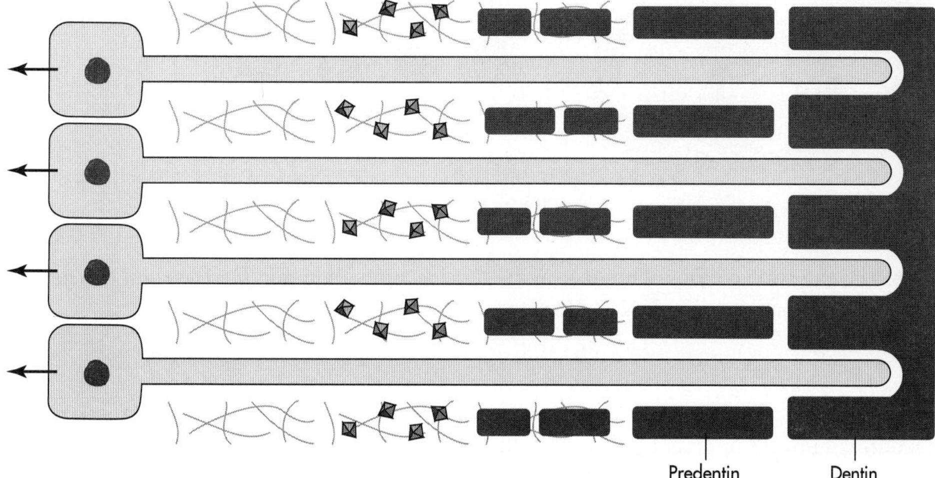

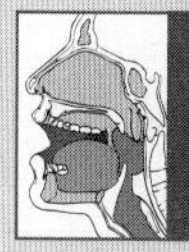

Dentin is finally formed, but remember the odontoblasts leave a long, fingerlike process in the dentin as it is formed in layers. Dentin surrounds the **odontoblastic processes,** making many **dentinal tubules,** or hollow spaces in which the processes reside.

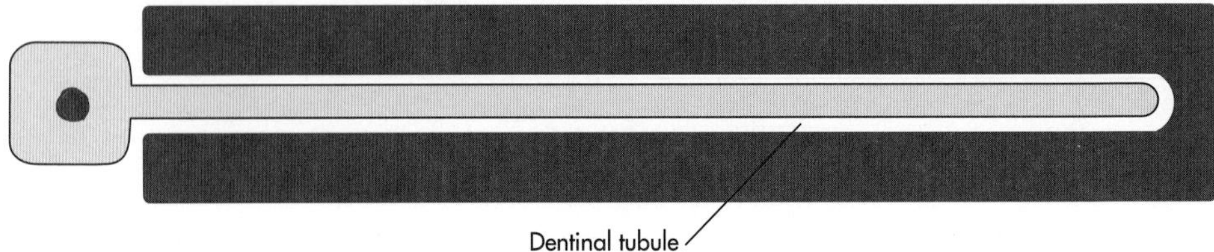

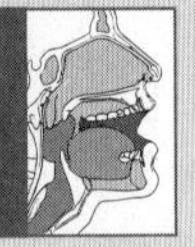

odontoblastic process

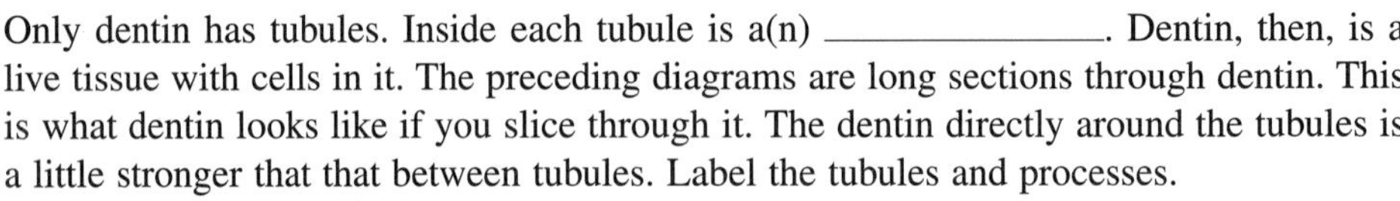

Only dentin has tubules. Inside each tubule is a(n) ______________. Dentin, then, is a live tissue with cells in it. The preceding diagrams are long sections through dentin. This is what dentin looks like if you slice through it. The dentin directly around the tubules is a little stronger that that between tubules. Label the tubules and processes.

A. odontoblastic process
B. tubule

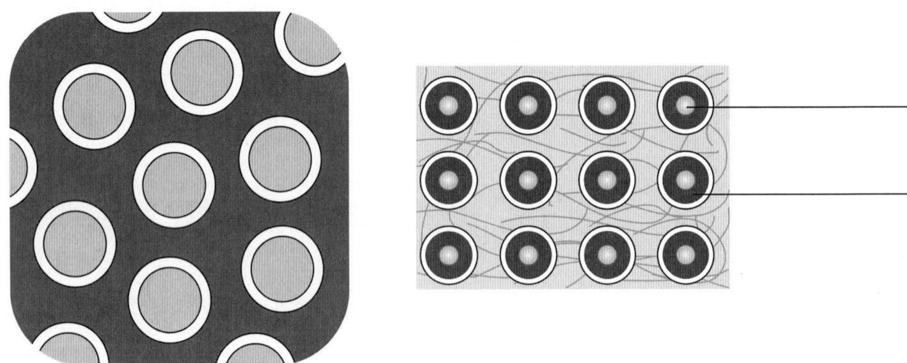

Compare the two sections. The one on the left is calcified dentin. On the right decalcified section, the fibrous network is visible.

cementum

Dentin is built up in layers underneath the crown or enamel and then is extended downward to form the bulk of the root. What hard tissue forms over the outside of the root to cover the dentin?

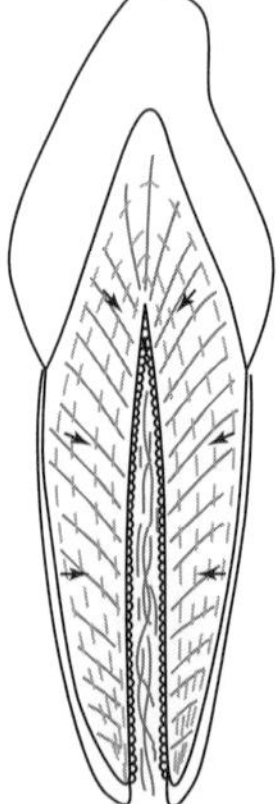

This is what the newly erupted tooth looks like. The dentin that has been formed so far is called **primary dentin.** It is the dentin that the tooth has on eruption. Note the size of the **pulp chamber.** Is it large or small?

large

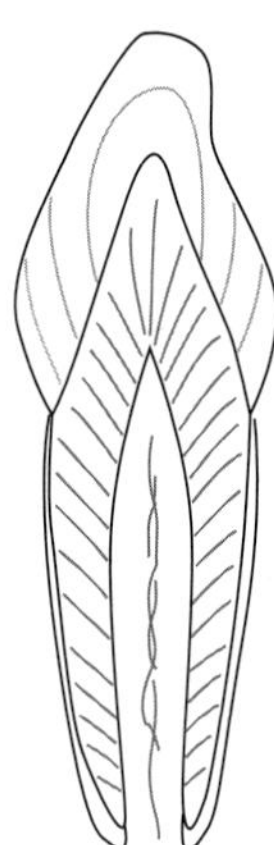

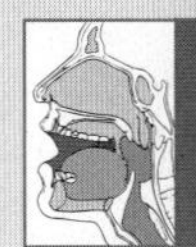

Dentin is laid down in layers, much like enamel. Can you see the growth lines between the layers in this drawing? There is no name for these **growth lines** as there is in enamel.

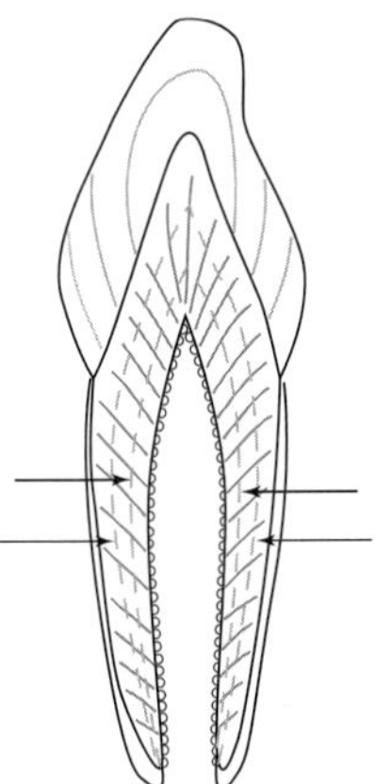

As you look at the layers of primary dentin, which layer was laid down first? Which layer last?

layer on DEJ first, layer on pulp last

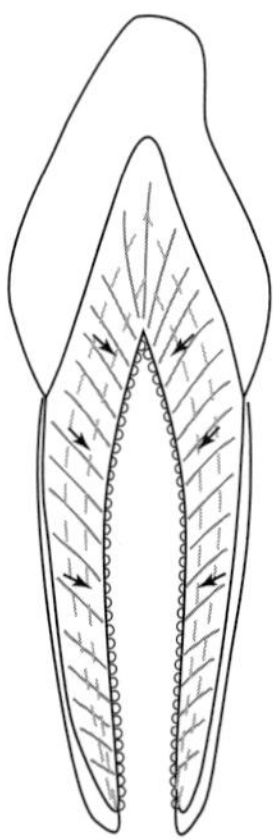

Dentin was laid down from the enamel border (DEJ) inward toward the pulp. After the tooth erupts and is functioning, more layers of dentin will be laid down on the pulpal side. This is called **secondary dentin.**

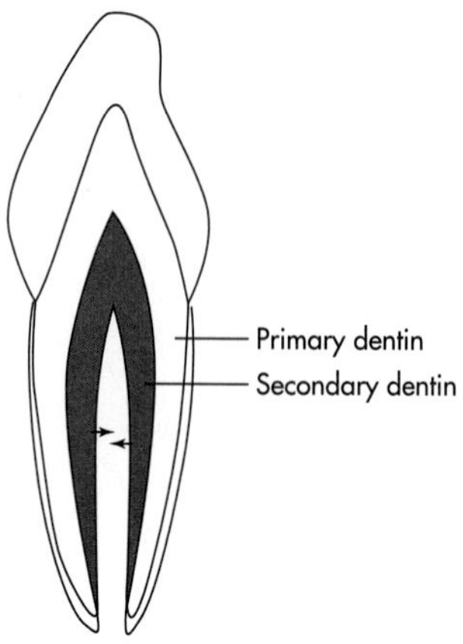

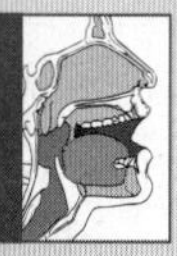

smaller

As more and more secondary dentin is laid down, will the pulp chamber become larger or smaller?

growth, secondary, B

Dentin is a live tissue capable of ______________ and repair. As time goes by, the amount of ______________ dentin increases and the pulp chamber gets smaller. Which tooth belongs to an elderly person—A or B?

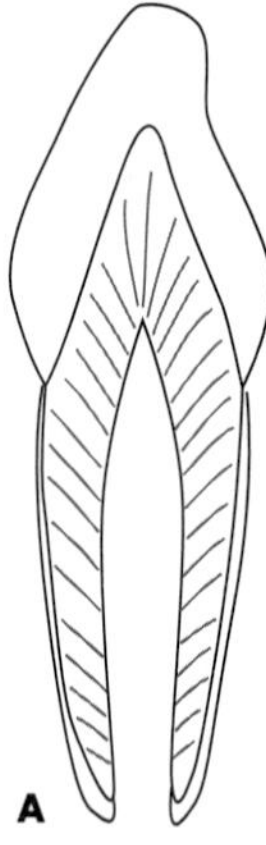

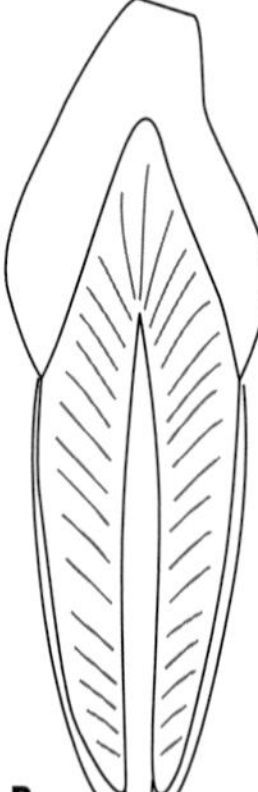

In the elderly, the pulp chamber may be totally obliterated by dentin.

As dentin is laid down in neat layers, an occasional "mistake" is made, forming an irregular area of dentin. These areas are called **globular dentin.** Find them in the diagram.

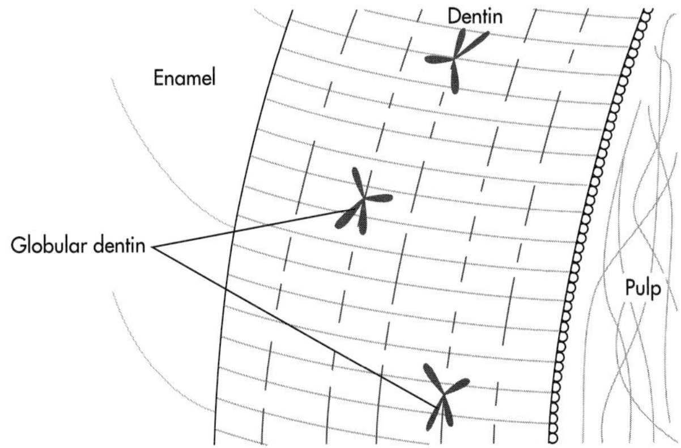

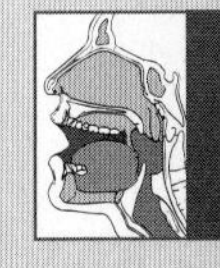

globular

Part of the dentin forms some small, irregular areas that look like grains of sand under the microscope. They are found only in the root dentin, on the surface next to the cementum as pictured. This dentin is called **Tome's granular layer.** The other decalcified areas in dentin are _______________ dentin.

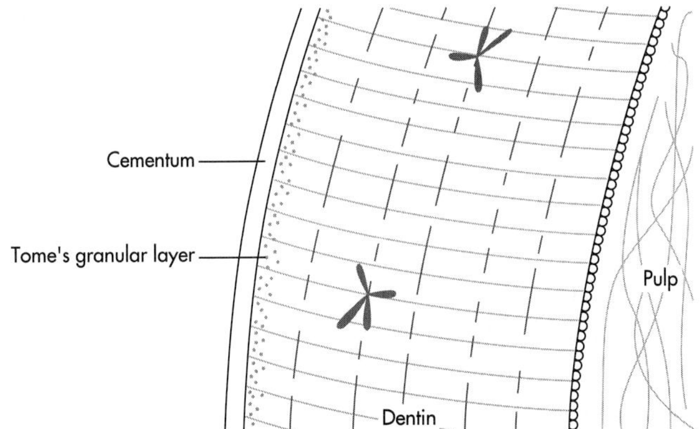

Tome's granular layer is a hypocalcified area in the dentin and is weaker. It is, in part, responsible for the sensitivity of roots, as is the sensitive structure of live dentin and the thinness of the cementum layer.

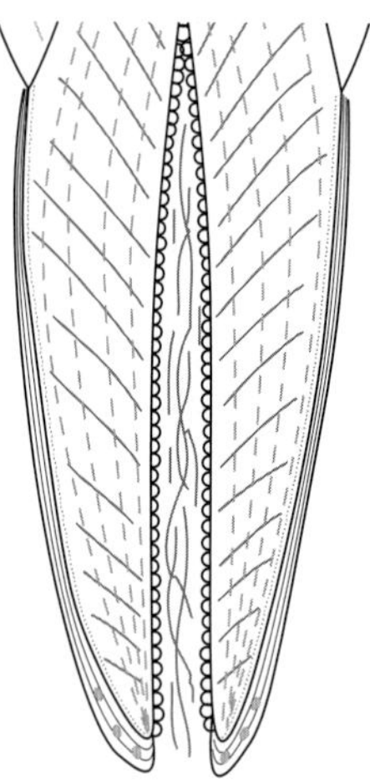

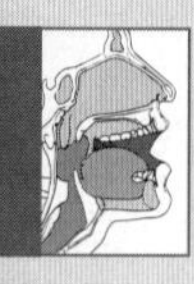

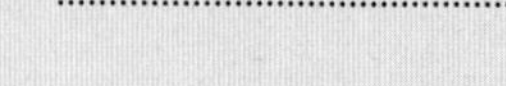

Label the anatomic structures found in dentin.

A. dentinal tubule
B. growth lines
C. Tome's layer
D. globular dentin
E. odontoblast

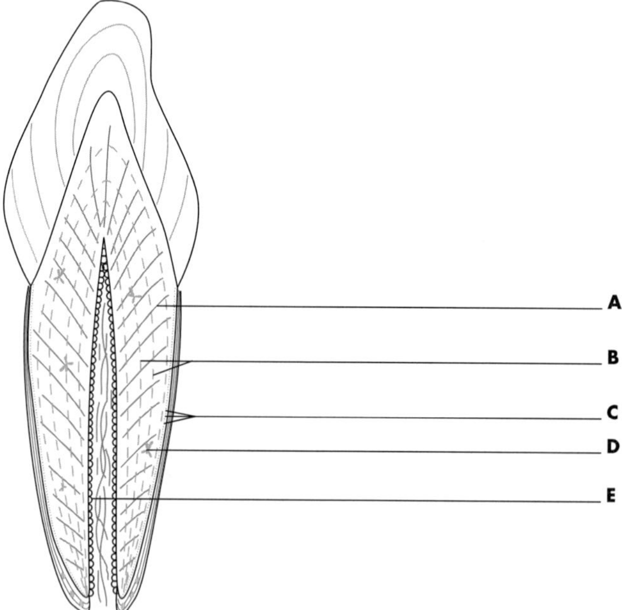

CEMENTUM

3.0

The third hardest tissue in the body is **cementum,** a thin layer that covers the roots of teeth.

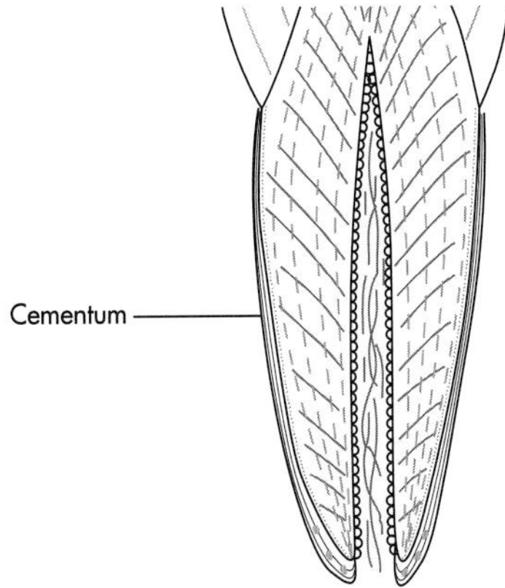

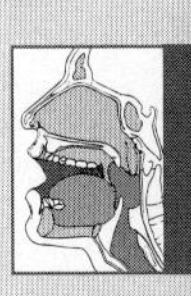

Cementum originates from cells recruited from the periodontal ligament (PDL) called **cementoblasts.** Cementoblasts line up along the trail of cells left by the enamel organ (Hertwig's epithelial root sheath).

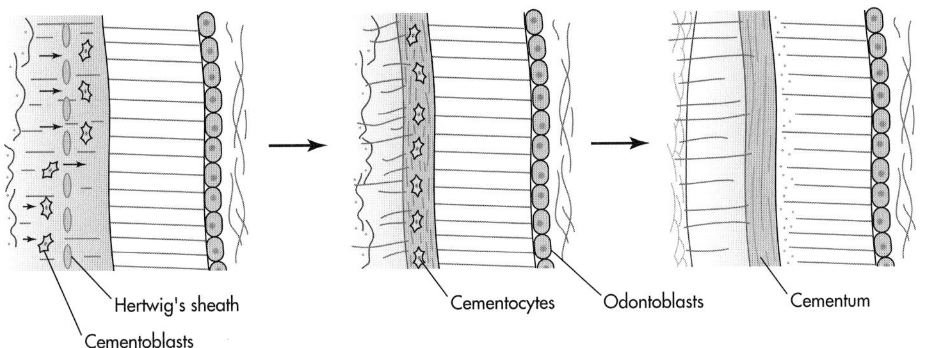

_______________ line up along the outside of the root dentin and begin making cementum by calcification.

Cementoblasts

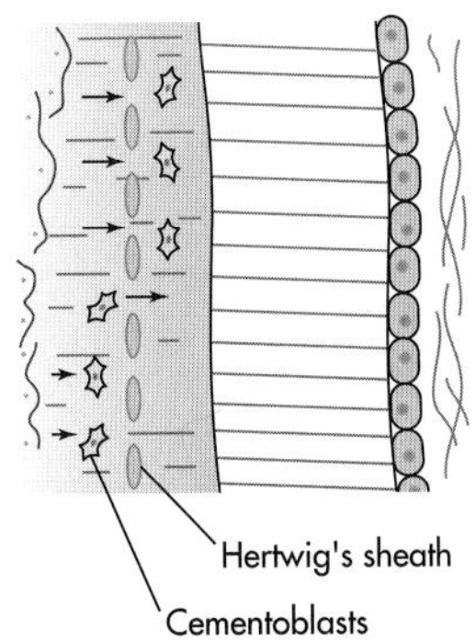

As in other types of calcification, the cementoblasts lay down a fibrous network, which then attracts calcium salts, which build larger and larger crystals.

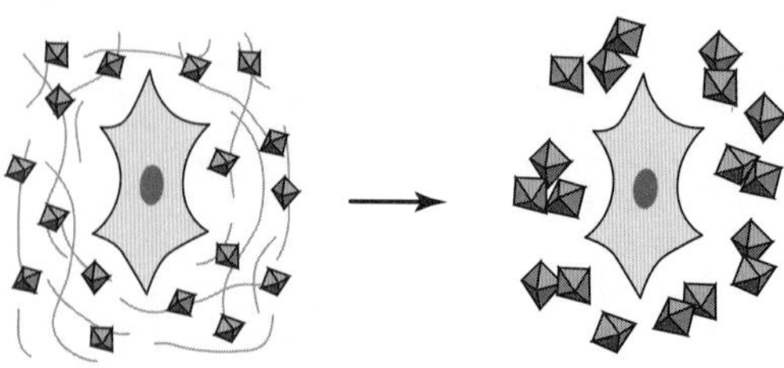

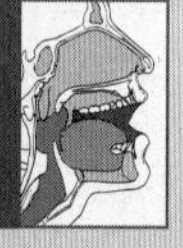

cementocyte

Layers or **laminae** of cementum are laid down by the cementoblasts until the root is covered and the cells are encased in hard tissue. At rest, the cementoblast is called a ______________.

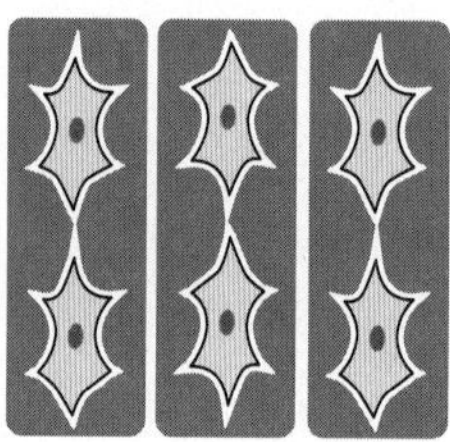

osteocyte

Which cell does the cementoblast (cyte) resemble?

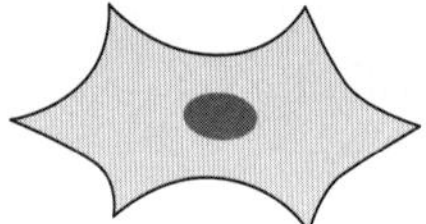

Cementum tissue is very similar to bone. The cementum cell is similar in shape to osteocytes with multiple cell processes, giving it a spiderlike appearance.

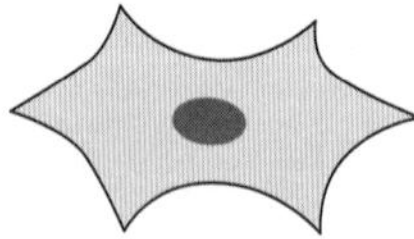

Cementocytes are encased in cementum, similar to bone, with their cell bodies lying in small spaces called **lacunae** and their processes lying in tubular spaces called **canaliculi.** What are these spaces called in bone?

the same

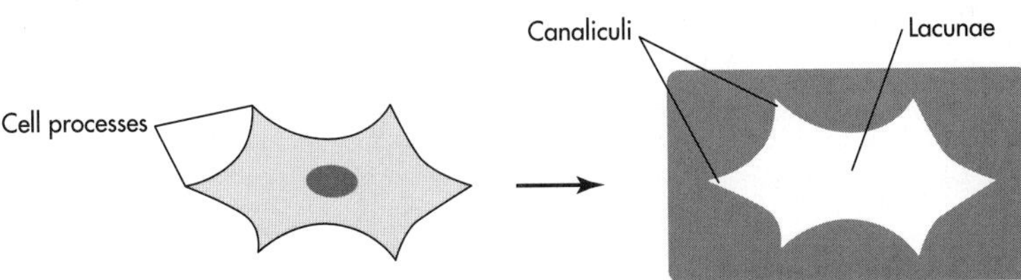

Cementum is laid down in layers, like a tree or onion, much like the layers of _______________ are laid down. These layers are called **laminae.**

bone

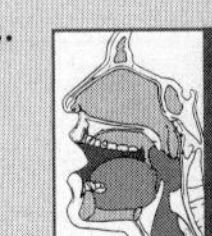

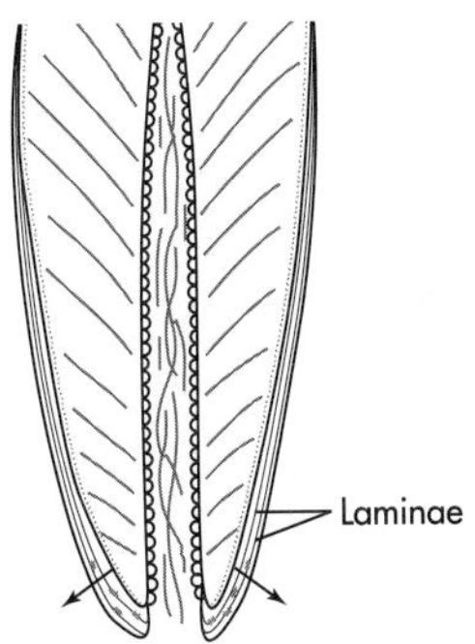

Overall, the cementum on the roots of teeth is a thin layer—thinner than enamel. The thinnest portion of the cementum layer lies around the **cervix** of the tooth, where it meets the enamel. This junction is called the **cementoenamel junction (CEJ).** This thin layer of cementum contains no cells and is called **acellular cementum.**

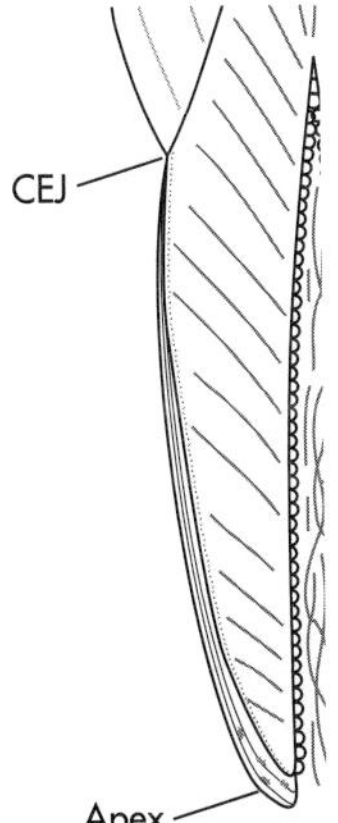

Cementum is thicker on the apex of the root. This type of cementum has cells and is called _______________.

cellular cementum

Acellular cementum is not a live tissue. Cellular cementum is.

Is cementum a live tissue? Before you answer that question, look at the diagram. The cementum of the cervical and middle portions of the root is covered in a thin layer of cementum that has no cells called the acellular cementum.

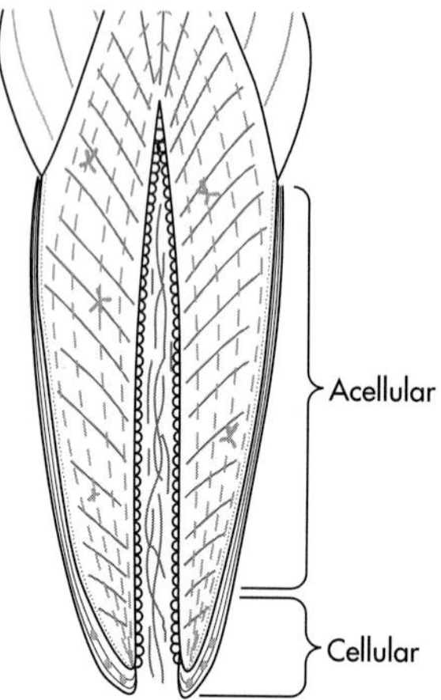

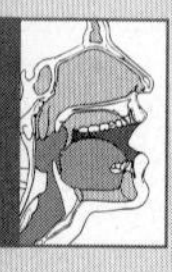

The apical portion of the root is covered in thick cementum with cells called the cellular cementum.

apical portion

Which portion of the cementum is capable of growth and repair?

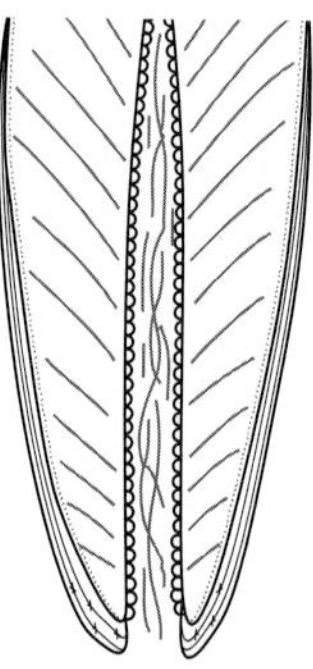

The portion of the cementum covering the apices of the roots can continue to grow throughout life, although it does so only moderately. In some pathologic conditions, an excessive amount of cementum grows, forming ball-shaped growths on the apices. This is called **hypercementosis.**

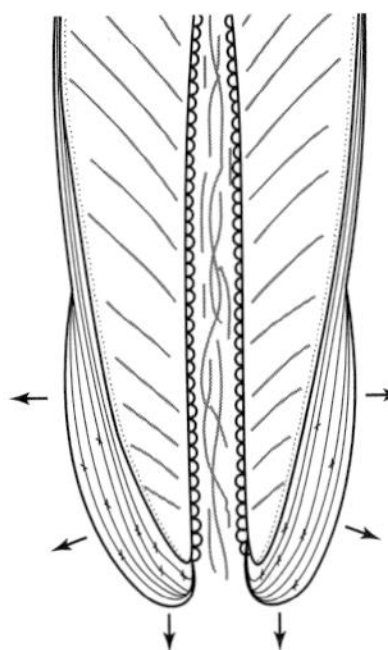

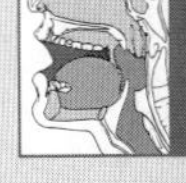

There are three ways that the CEJ can come together:

A. The enamel and cementum just meet.
B. The enamel and cementum do not meet, leaving a bare spot of dentin.
C. The cementum overlaps the enamel.

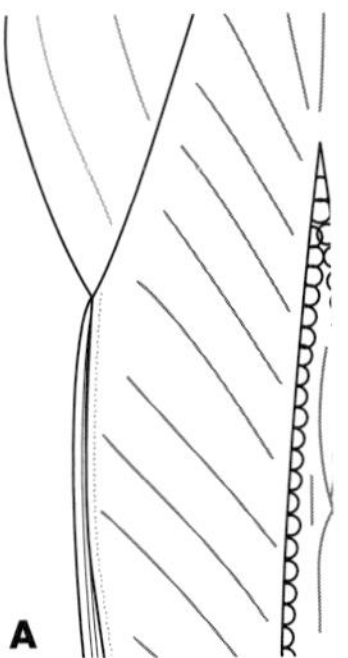

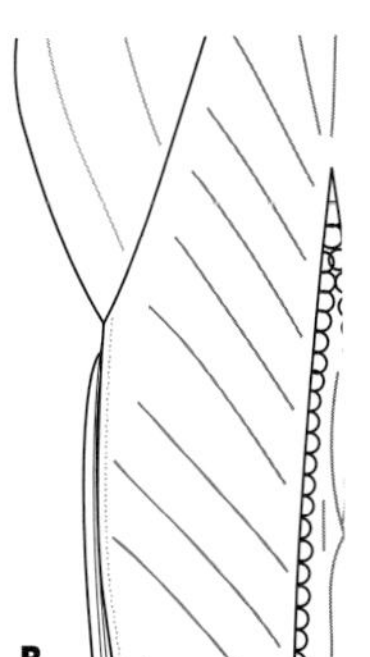

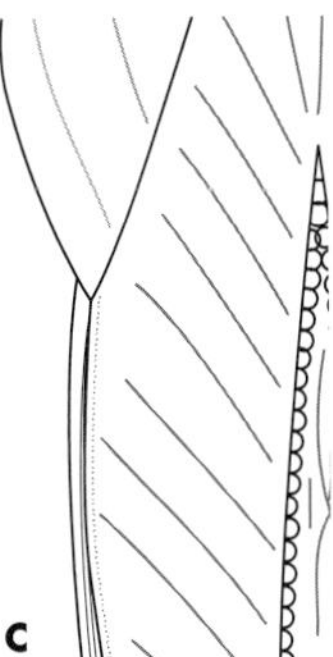

The junction between the two outer hard tissues of the tooth is called the ______________.

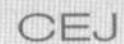

CEJ

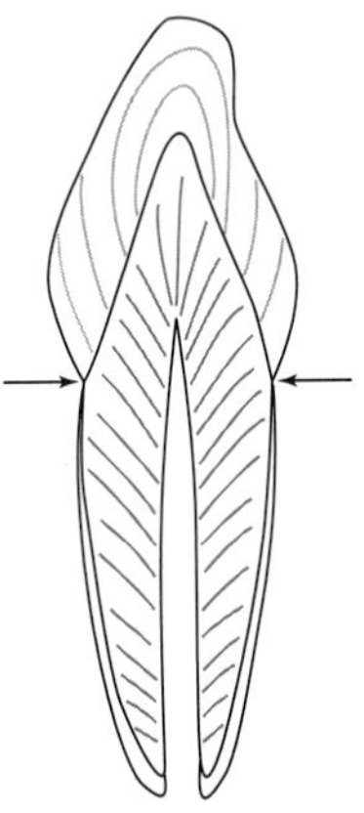

not alive

Cementum is a live tissue, as is dentin. What is enamel? Remember that not only is the cementum layer thin, it is a weaker tissue than even dentin. It does not provide the root dentin with much protection.

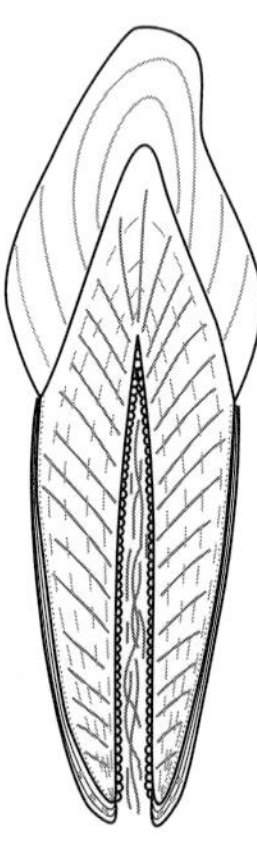

Tome's

Cementum is not usually exposed to the oral environment unless the periodontal tissues (bone and gingiva) have receded because of disease. Cementum, if exposed, is both an area susceptible to damage and a sensitive area. Beneath the thin layer of cementum is ______________ granular layer in the dentin, and dentin is a very sensitive tissue. Scaling procedures or root planing may become an uncomfortable process for many people.

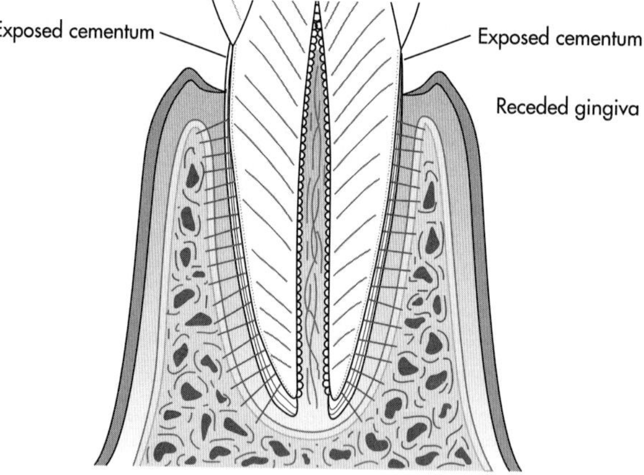

Label the anatomic features of cementum.

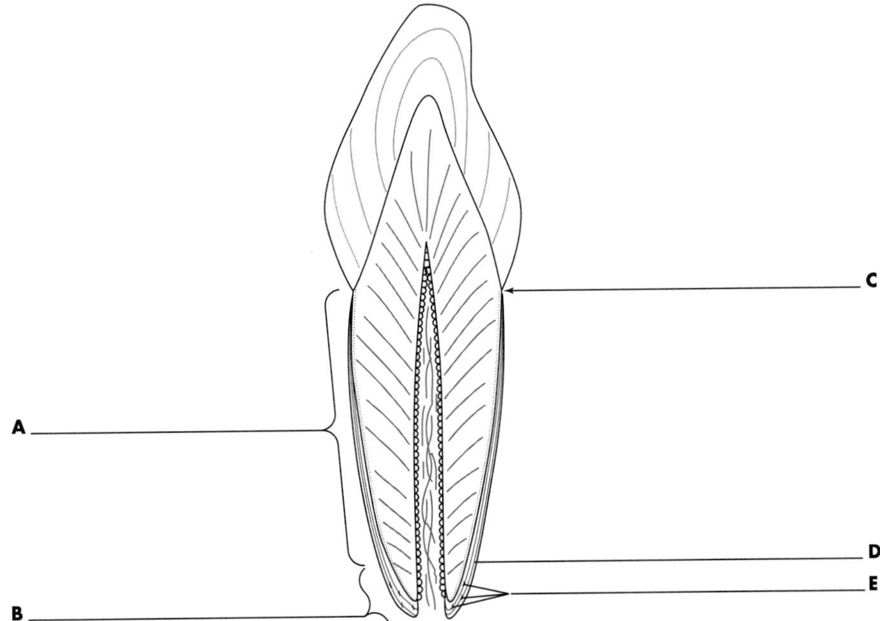

A. acellular cementum
B. cellular cementum
C. CEJ
D. laminae
E. cementocytes

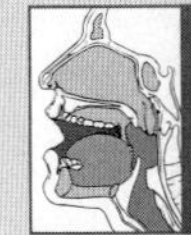

PULP

4.0

The innermost soft tissue occupying the hollowed out inner portion of the dentin is called the **pulp.** The space is called the **pulp chamber** and **root canals.**

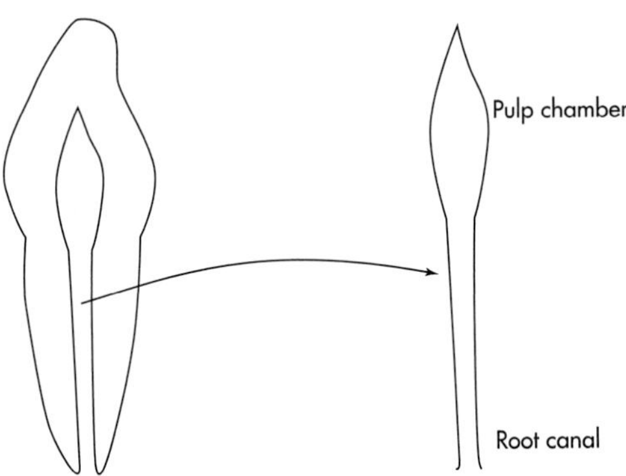

Review the terminology for the pulp chamber as found in *Dental Anatomy: A Self-Instructional Program.*

The **pulp chamber** is the main space found under the crown of the tooth. As it is shaped like a three-dimensional "room" it has a **roof, floor,** and four **walls.**

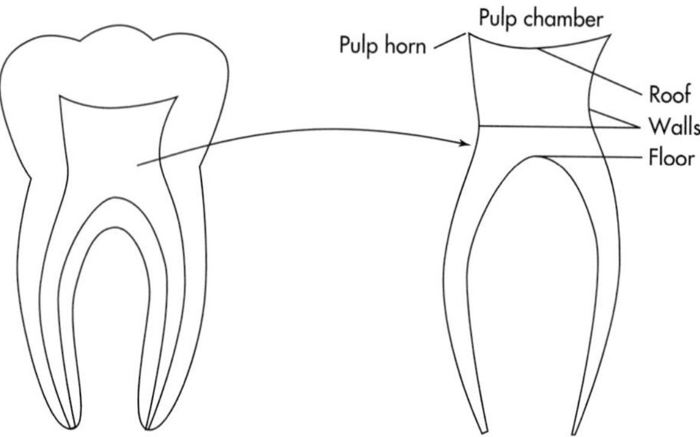

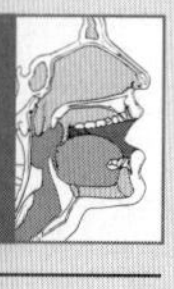

The roof of the pulp chamber comes to peaks underneath the incisal edge and under each cusp. These are called **pulp horns.**

The pulp chamber space leads directly down into tubular spaces within each root of the tooth. These are called **root canals.**

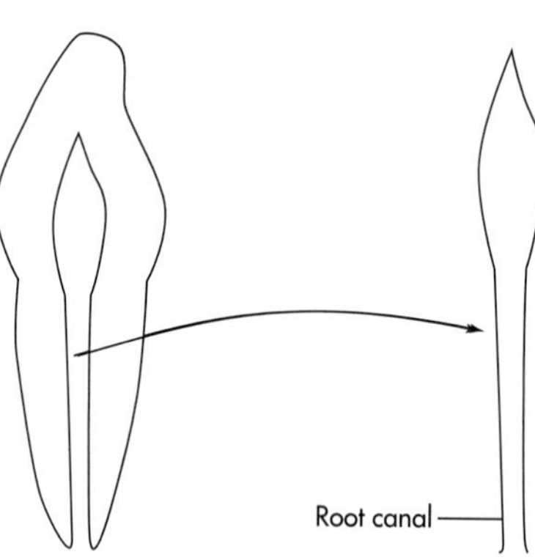

Each root canal continues the length of the root and ends with an opening out of the root called the **apical foramen.**

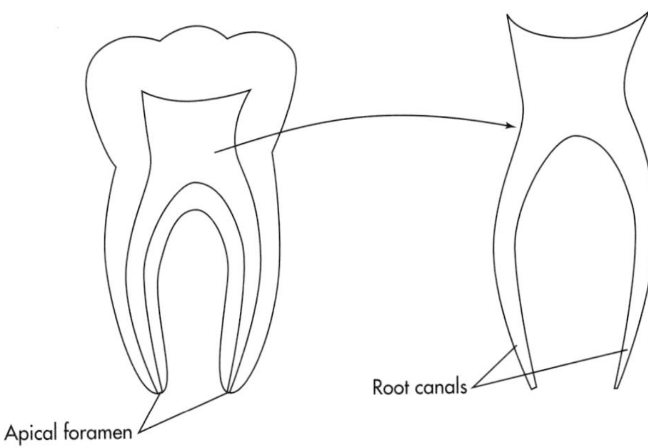

Label the parts of the pulp space. Check your answers in the preceding diagrams.

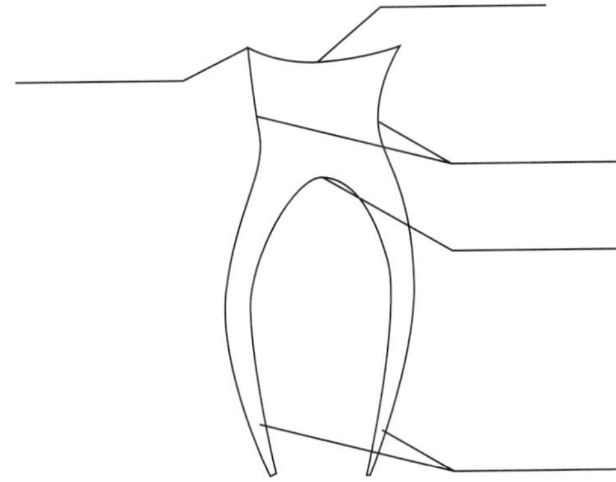

The pulp occupies the pulp chamber and the root canals. It is a soft connective tissue, meaning it has lots of matrix and few ______________.

cells

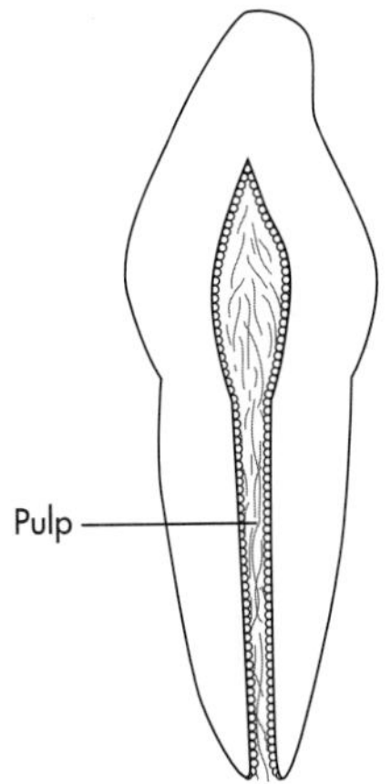

odontoblasts

The outer layer of the pulp, remember, comprises the cell bodies of the cells that made the dentin. They each have a cell process extending out into the dentin. These are called the _____________.

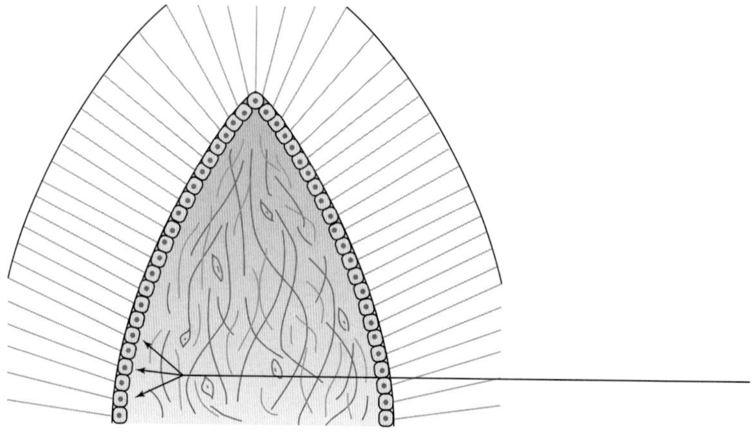

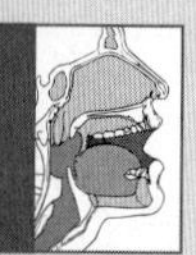

The odontoblast cell body layer makes up the outer layer of the pulp.

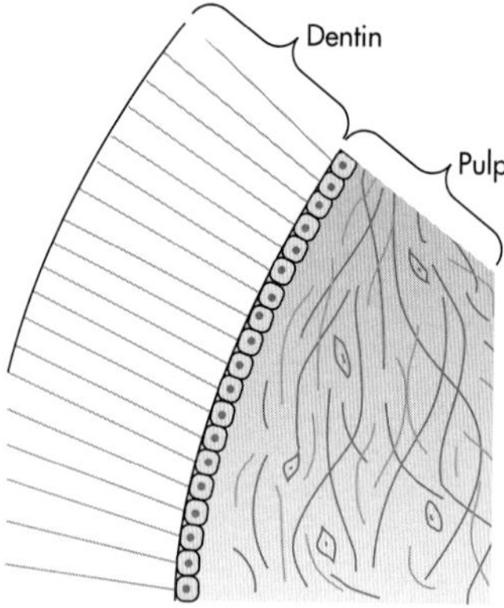

Deeper into the pulp we find cells and matrix. The matrix is a gelatinous mixture of proteins and water.

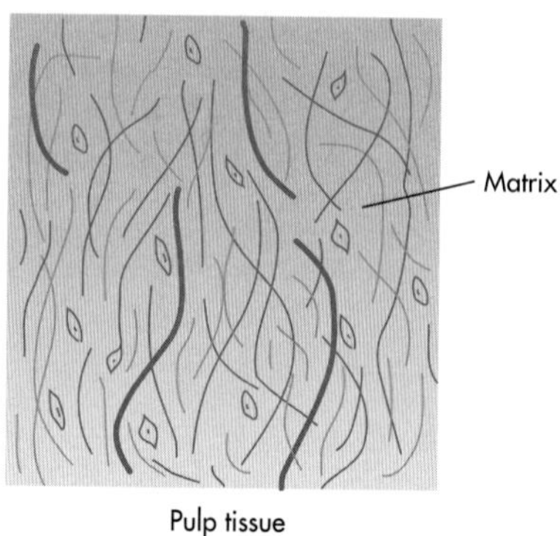

Pulp tissue

The cells are of various kinds. One of the main cell types found is the **fibroblast,** a fiber-producing cell common to all connective tissues. The main type of fiber produced is the collagen fiber.

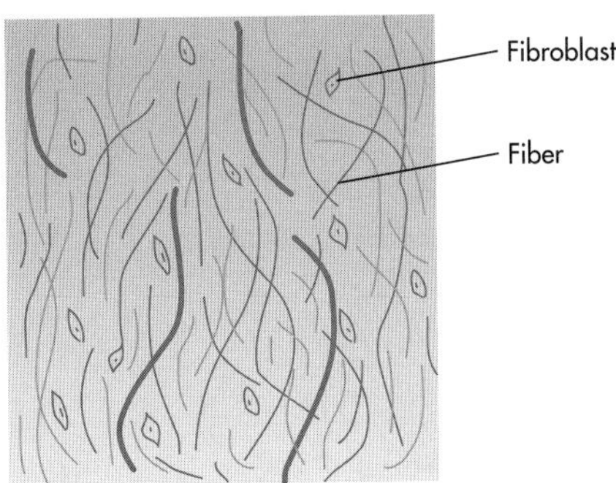

Blood vessels and blood cells are found in the pulp. This small loop of the circulatory system is there to provide nutrients and respiratory gases for all the cells of the pulp and the odontoblasts to keep them alive. A lymph vessel and lymph cells are also present for defense against foreign invaders like bacteria.

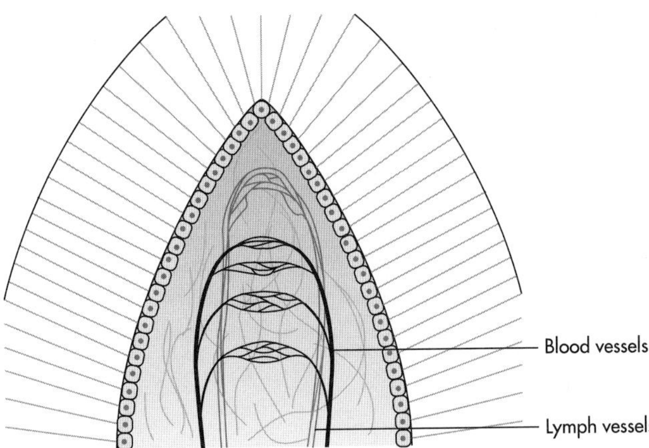

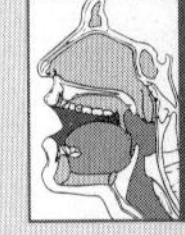

to provide nutrients and gases for pulp cells

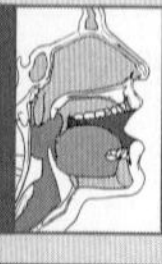

Why do we find blood vessels in the pulp? Nerve cells are found in the pulp also. Nerves regulate blood flow and sense changes in the pulp. The main sensory neurons of the pulp are pain fibers.

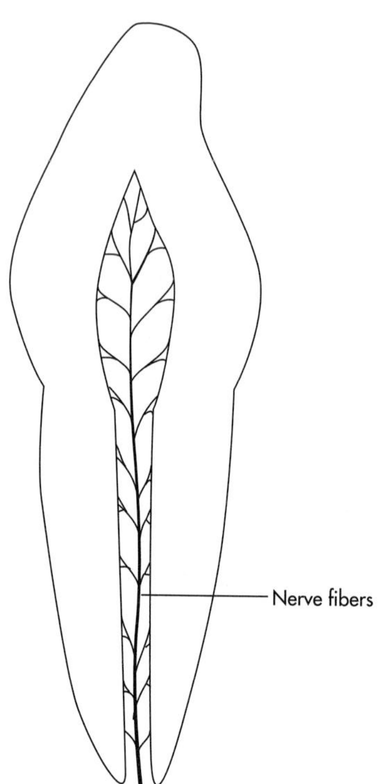

Pain is the chief reaction of the pulp of the tooth to any trauma, bacterial invasion, or heat or cold. This is due to the predominance of pain type fibers in the pulp. Some researchers have noted nerve fibers may extend even into the dentinal tubules, accounting for the sensitivity of live dentin.

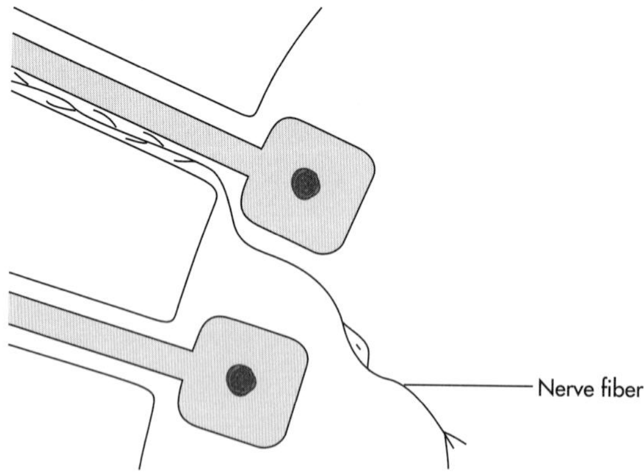

The pulp is a complex community of many different types of cells, fibers, and vessels. Name the components of the pulp. For the pulp to be vital, all of these elements must be alive and functioning.

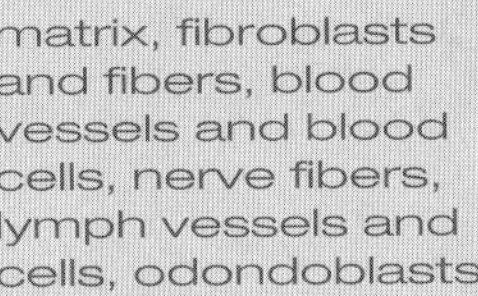
matrix, fibroblasts and fibers, blood vessels and blood cells, nerve fibers, lymph vessels and cells, odondoblasts

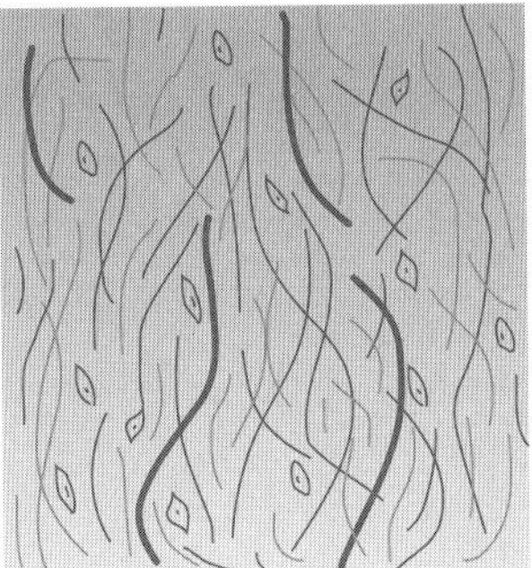

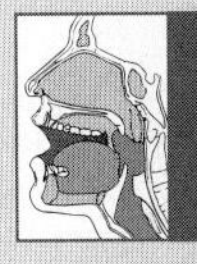

A nonvital pulp is a dead pulp with no live cells. This will often cause the cell to abscess. Would the dentin still be alive?

no

Sometimes odontoblasts break away from the walls of the pulp chamber and produce small "islands" of dentin inside the pulp. These are called **pulp stones** or **denticles.**

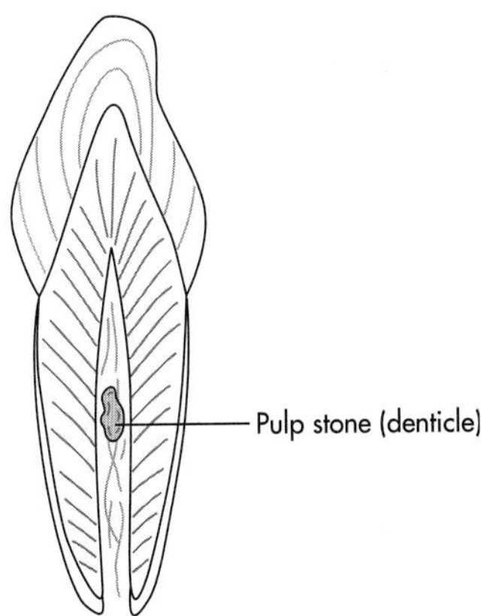

DENTAL TISSUE RESPONSES 5.0

Caries 5.1

Decay or **caries** is a disease caused by cariogenic bacteria and results in the invasion and destruction of dental tissues by acid damage and infection. Let's follow what happens to each dental tissue during the progressive stages of caries.

caries

Decay is called ______________. It begins on the outer surface of the tooth, usually on the enamel, but sometimes on the cementum. **Cariogenic bacteria** adhere to the teeth by way of a sticky substance called **plaque** and begin producing acids.

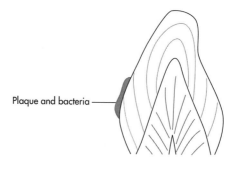

Plaque and bacteria

Plaque

______________ provides the initial sticky medium for bacterial growth. Even though it is an extremely hard substance, enamel will begin to dissolve under consistent acidic attack. It is most susceptible in weaker or hypocalcified areas.

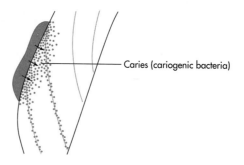

Caries (cariogenic bacteria)

interrod substance

Enamel rods are very resistant to decay but the areas between them are not as resistant. Between the rods we find ______________.

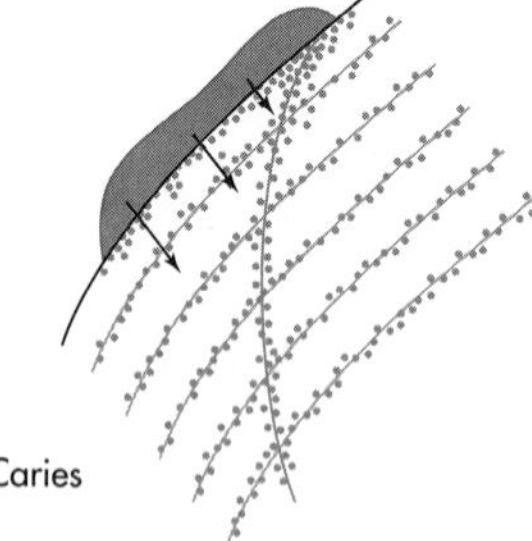

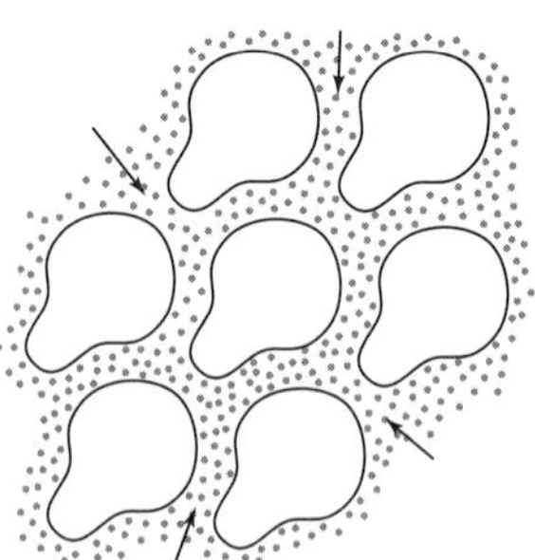

Also, between the layers of enamel we find the lines of ______________, which are another hypocalcified area, where acid damage may spread faster.

Retzius

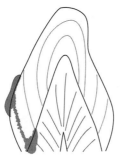

Caries

As caries penetrates the enamel it comes to the end or junction between the enamel and dentin called the ______________. Do you think this is a weak area?

DEJ, yes

In the last area of the enamel, near the DEJ, are the tufts and spindles, another ______________ area in the enamel where caries will spread faster. The DEJ itself, however, is one of the weakest areas in the tooth. Decay will actually mushroom out along and underneath it, because we have reached the weaker dentin.

hypocalcified

The arrows show the penetration and spread of cariogenic bacteria and acid. Where does it seem to spread quickly? Why?

at the DEJ, because it is weaker

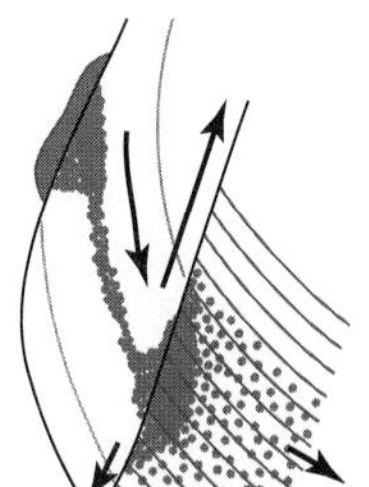

due to dentinal tubules, dentinal tubules

Why is dentin so weak? Think of the spaces in dentin that would cause no resistance to invasion. What are they?

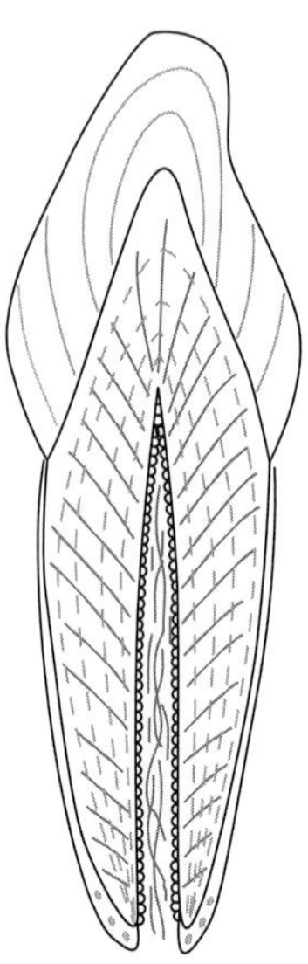

The dentinal tubules are hollow, cell-filled spaces that would be easy for the bacteria to invade. Dentin is full of them.

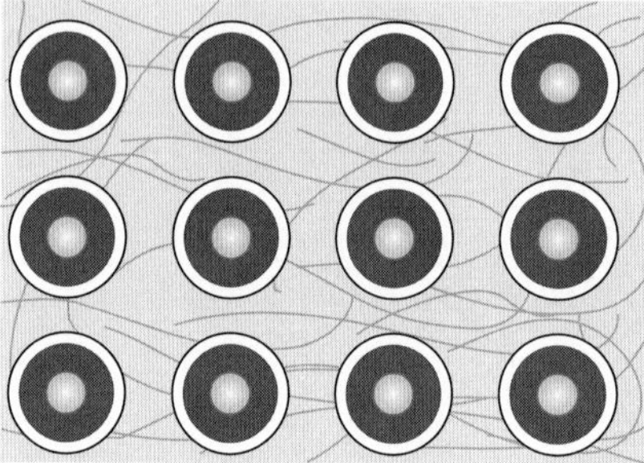

odontoblastic process

What lies in the dentinal tubules? Once bacteria have invaded the dentinal tubules the odontoblastic processes try to retreat into the pulp, leaving an empty tubule called a **dead tract.**

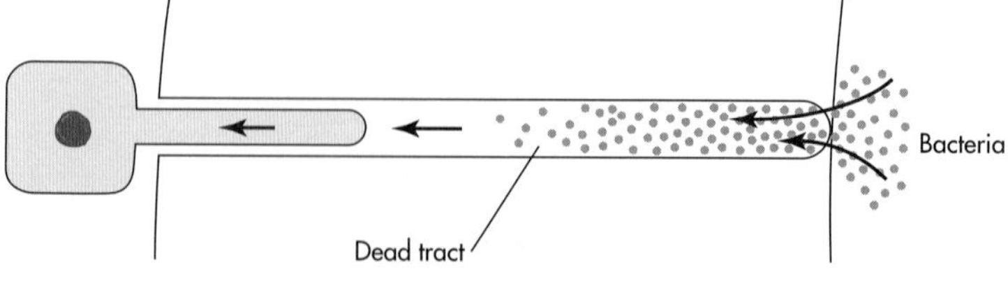

_______________ are empty dentinal tubules produced by retreating odontoblastic processes. If given enough time by the bacteria, dentin will also try to seal off the tubules from invasion. They create a kind of dentin that is rapidly laid down in an irregular pattern called **sclerotic** or **reparative dentin.**

Dead tracts

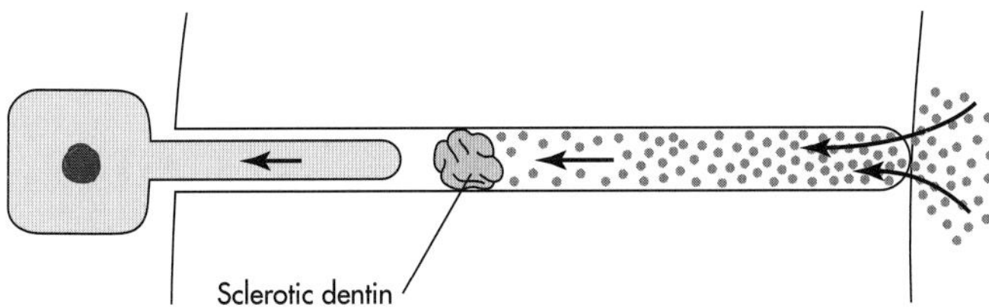

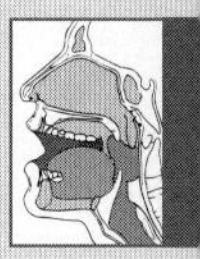

Sclerotic (reparative) dentin is a type of dentin made in response to invasion (or trauma) to try to seal off the dentinal tubules. Some sclerotic dentin is made within the tubules. Reparative dentin is also made opposite the lesion on the pulpal side of the dentin, as pictured.

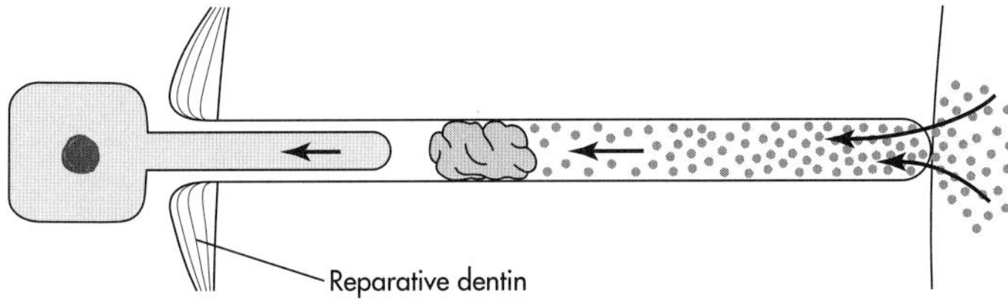

What type of dentin was made in neat layers, after the tooth erupted? Is dentin a live tissue?

secondary dentin, yes

As you can see, dentin is a live tissue capable of growth and repair in the case of insult by bacterial invasion of caries.

If the attempts of the dentin to ward off invasion do not work, the pulp is invaded by bacteria. This is a serious situation. The pulp will send out white blood cells (leukocytes) to fight off the invaders, but they are often overwhelmed and the pulp dies.

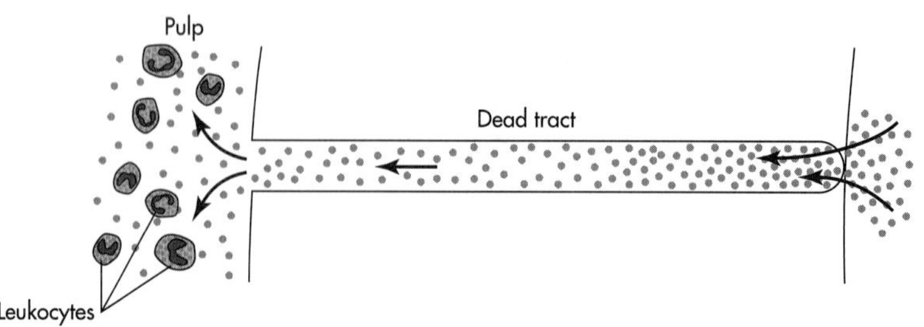

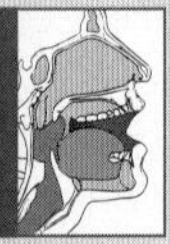

enamel

A nonvital pulp with bacteria causes the tooth to **abscess** and causes pain and infection. It must be treated. Only from the point of invasion of the dentin may the person be aware of the situation because all of the tooth tissues are alive except ______________.

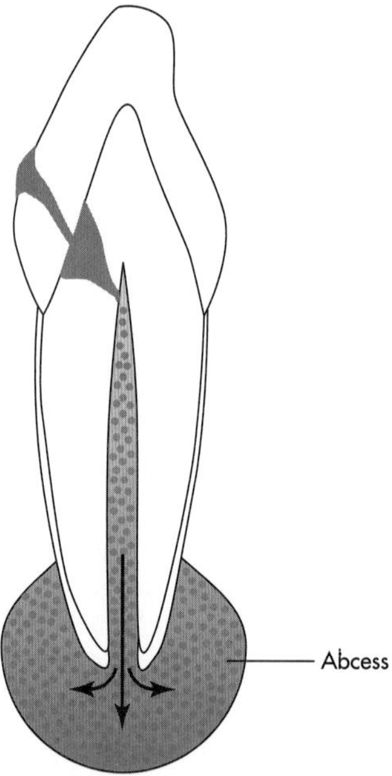

The same sequence of events may occur in the root, only faster because cementum is thinner and weaker than enamel. **Root caries** is a rapid process.

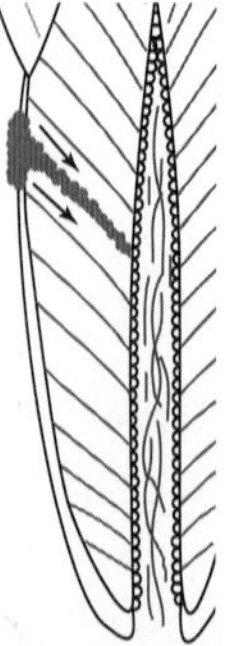

Label the different types of dentin.

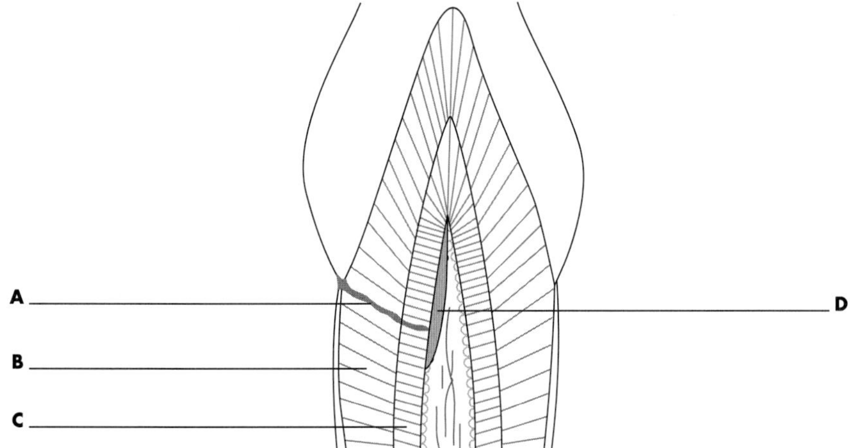

A. dead tract with sclerotic dentin
B. primary dentin
C. secondary dentin
D. reparative dentin

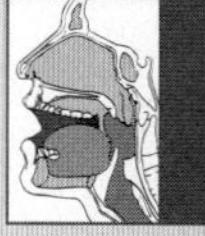

Trauma

5.2

The response of dental tissues to trauma, that is, an abnormal amount of force placed on the tooth, is very similar to its response to caries.

The arrow shows the direction of trauma, for example, continuous hard force on an incisal edge.

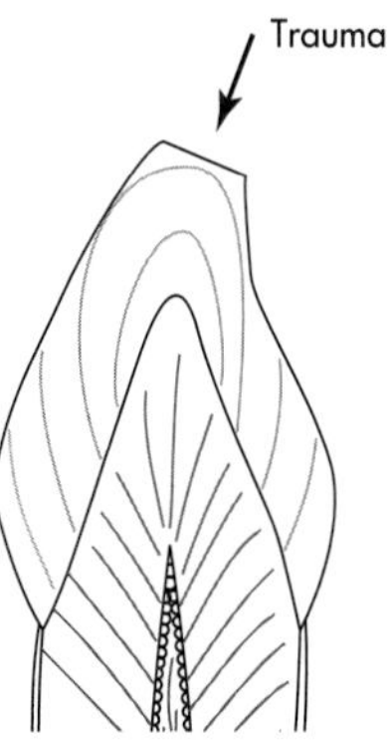

The response of the enamel is excessive mechanical wear. It will be smoothly worn down or suffer fractures. Where are the mechanically weak areas in enamel?

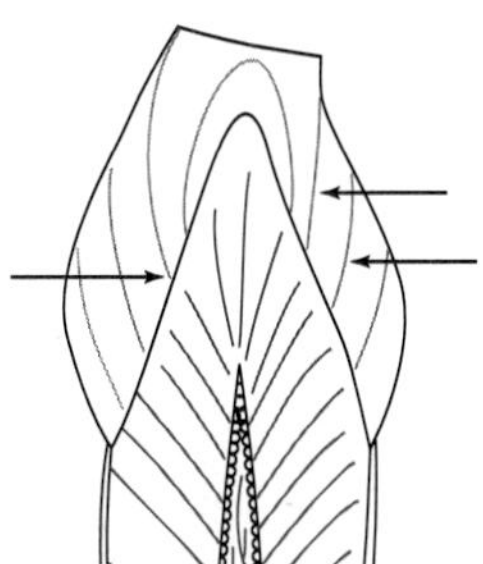

between rods (interrod substance), growth lines (lines of Retzius), DEJ, and tufts and spindles

Trauma can begin to break off or wear enamel at any of these hypocalcified areas and then break enamel rods themselves. Fractures usually occur between rods and growth layers.

empty dentinal tubules

Below the enamel, while trauma is occurring, the dentin responds by withdrawing sensitive odontoblastic processes, creating dead tracts. What are dead tracts?

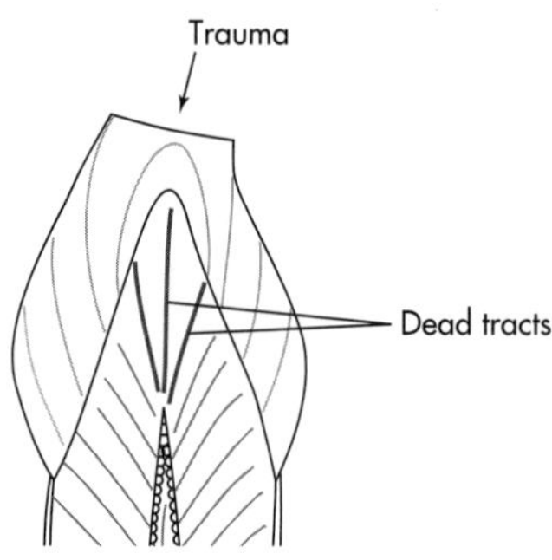

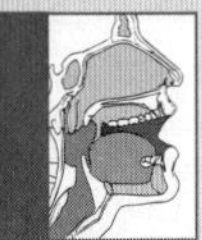

reparative or sclerotic

Odontoblasts try to thicken the barrier between the trauma and the pulp by creating new dentin, sclerotic dentin. They try to seal off the tubules and create an extra layer of _______________ dentin on the pulpal side of the dentin. If trauma is slow and moderate, dentin has time to protect the pulp. If trauma is severe or sudden, irreversible pulpal damage may occur, causing death and abscess of the pulp.

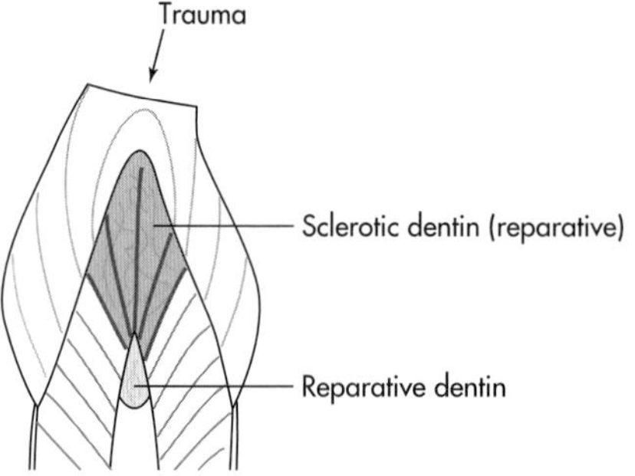

REVIEW TEST 4.1

FILL IN THE CORRECT ANSWER.

1. _______________ is the hardest tissue in the body.
2. The _______________ are growth lines found in enamel.
3. Enamel is created by cells from the enamel organ called _______________.
4. The matrix material found between enamel rods is called _______________.
5. An optical phenomenon of light and dark bands created by using polarized light under the microscope is called _______________.
6. An area of hard tissue that is weaker because of less organized structure is a(n) _______________ area.
7. Small brush-shaped structures of hypocalcified enamel along the DEJ are called _______________ and _______________.

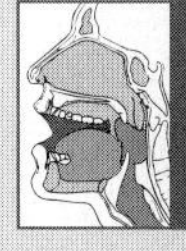

REVIEW TEST 4.2

FILL IN THE CORRECT ANSWER.

1. Cells that make dentin come from the dental papilla and are called _______________.
2. The second hardest tissue is _______________.
3. Dentin is a unique dental tissue, full of "holes" called _______________.
4. Within each dentinal tubule lies a(n) _______________.
5. Irregular areas of calcification within dentin are called _______________ dentin.
6. Dentin present on eruption is _______________ dentin.
7. Regular dentin that is laid down posteruption is _______________ dentin.
8. The hypocalcified area in root dentin, directly underneath the cementum, is called _______________.
9. The dental hard tissue most like bone is _______________.
10. Cementocyte cell bodies lie in spaces called _______________.
11. Cementum on the roots of the teeth is called _______________ cementum.
12. The outermost cell layer of the pulp is made of _______________ cells.
13. The peaks of the pulp chamber roof that occur under cusps are called _______________.

REVIEW TEST 4.3

SELECT THE CORRECT ANSWER.

1. Enamel is capable of repairing itself. True or false?

2. Enamel grows in layers from the DEJ outward. True or false?

3. Enamel may fracture
   a. between rods
   b. along the lines of Retzius
   c. on the DEJ
   d. all of the above
   e. none of the above

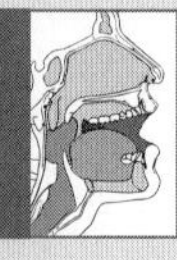

4. Which is not a hypocalcified area in enamel?
   a. tufts and spindles
   b. enamel rods
   c. interrod substance
   d. lines of Retzius

5. Caries will spread quickly
   a. between enamel rods
   b. along the DEJ
   c. in dentinal tubules
   d. all of the above
   e. none of the above

6. Which dental hard tissue develops in layers?
   a. enamel
   b. dentin
   c. cementum
   d. a and b only
   e. all of the above

REVIEW TEST 4.4

SELECT THE CORRECT ANSWER.

1. What type of dentin is formed in an attempt to seal off the dentinal tubules from the invasion of cariogenic bacteria?
   a. primary
   b. secondary
   c. globular
   d. sclerotic

2. Reparative dentin is dentin
   a. formed only in response to trauma
   b. formed around the dentinal tubules
   c. formed only in response to caries
   d. formed on the pulpal side of the dentin

3. Which tissue is not a live tissue?
   a. enamel
   b. dentin
   c. cementum
   d. pulp

4. The pulp provides nutrients, removes wastes, and acts as a sensor for teeth. True or false?

5. Dead tracts are
   a. lines of growth in dentin
   b. cell processes
   c. empty dentinal tubules
   d. cariogenic bacteria

6. Caries, on penetration of the dentin, spread rapidly at the DEJ into the enamel. True or false?

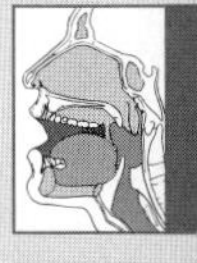

REVIEW TEST 4.5

LABEL THE DIAGRAMS.

1.

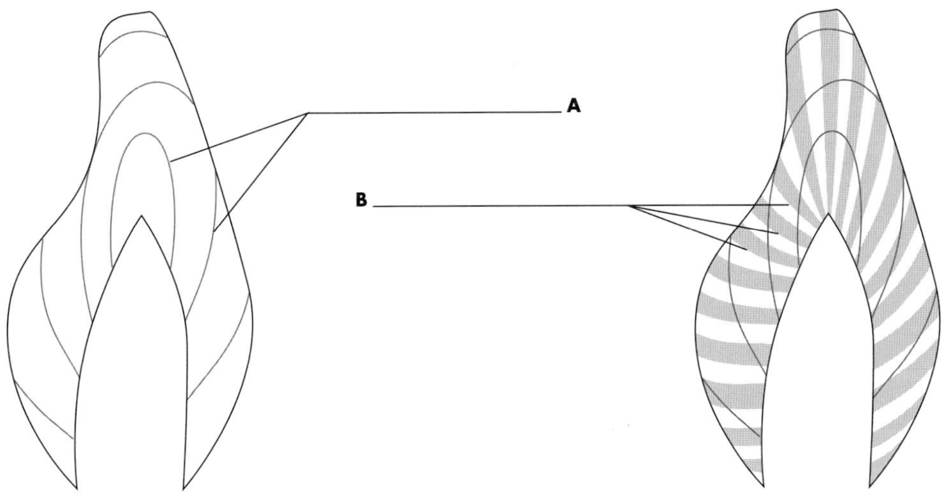

2.

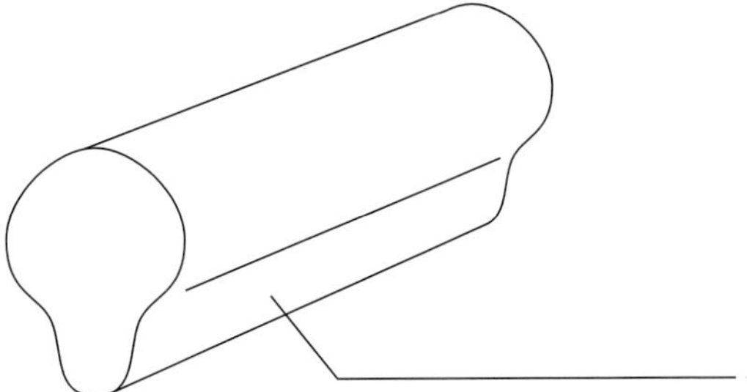

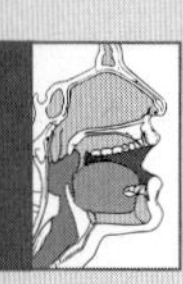

3.

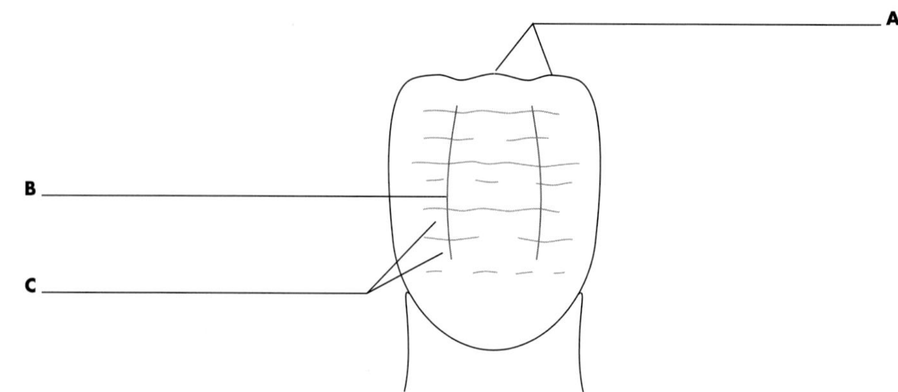

4.

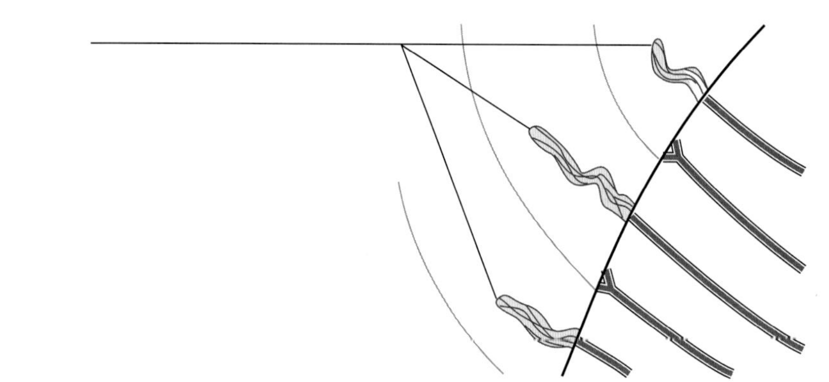

5.

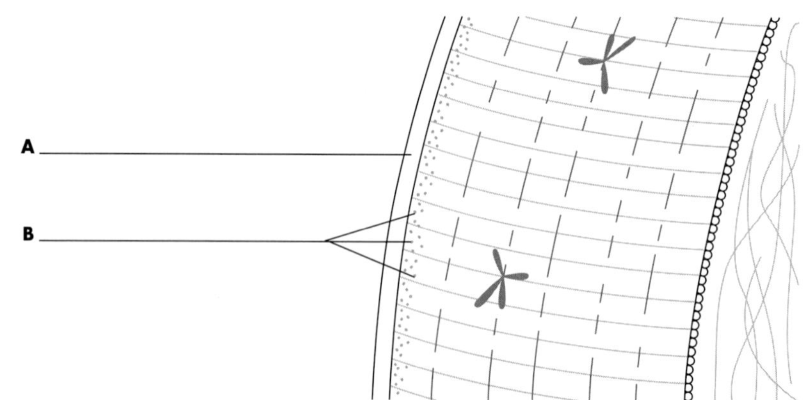

6.

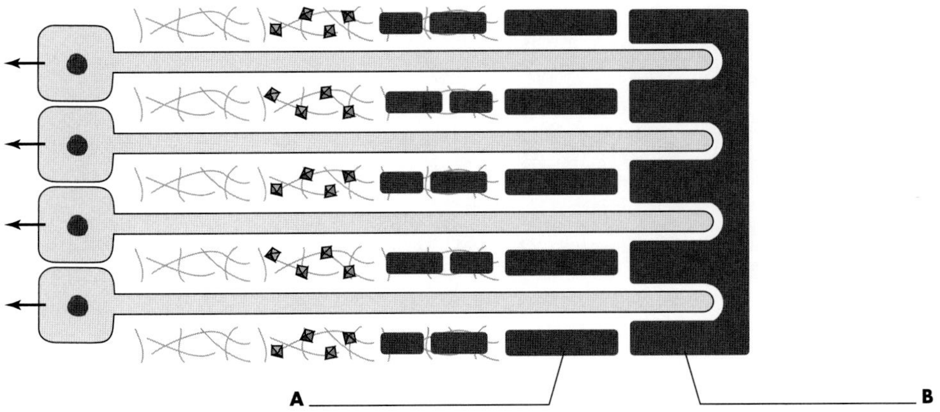

7.

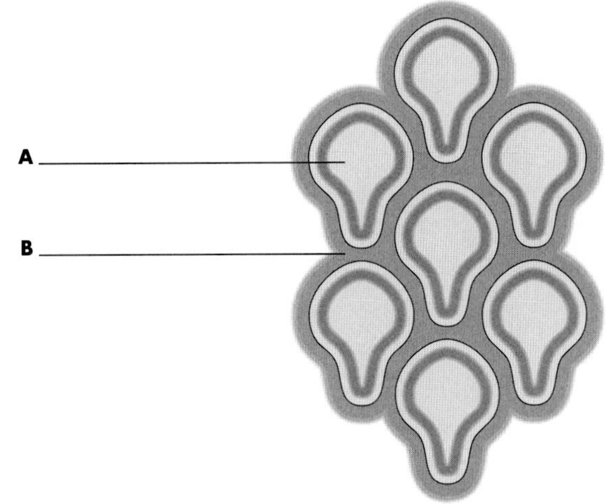

8.

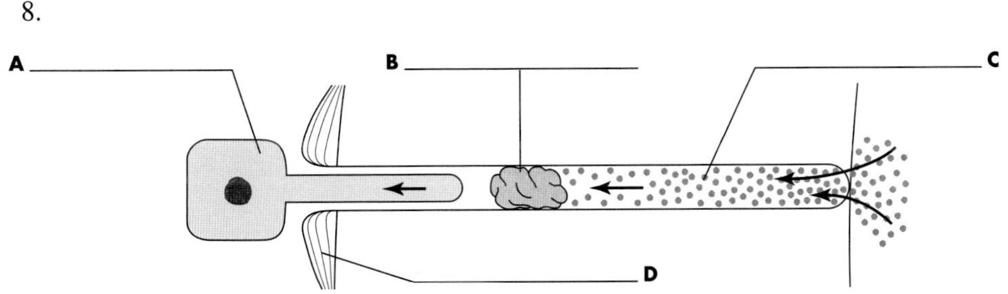

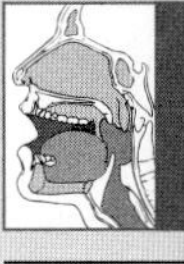

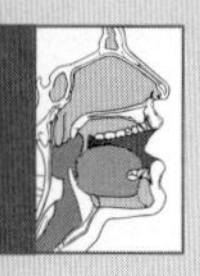

9.

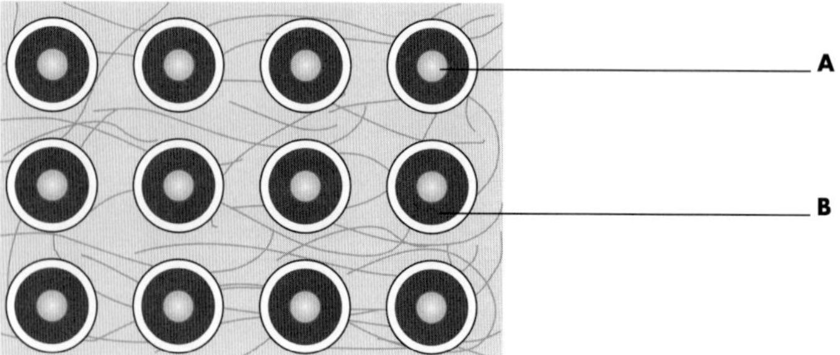

10.

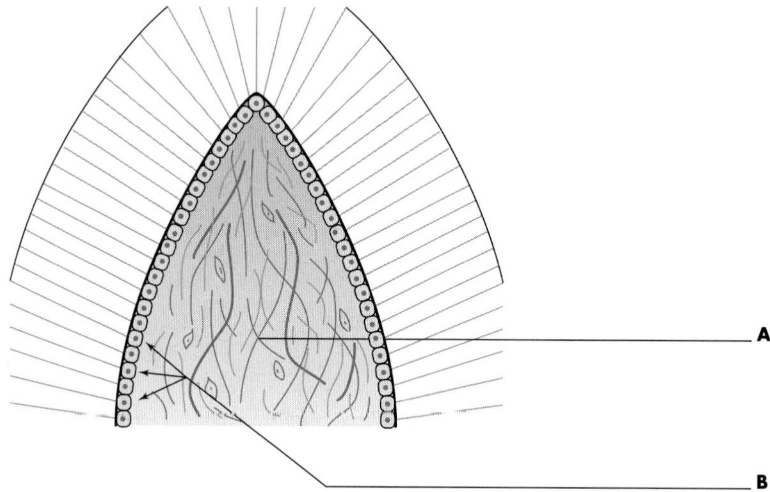

11.

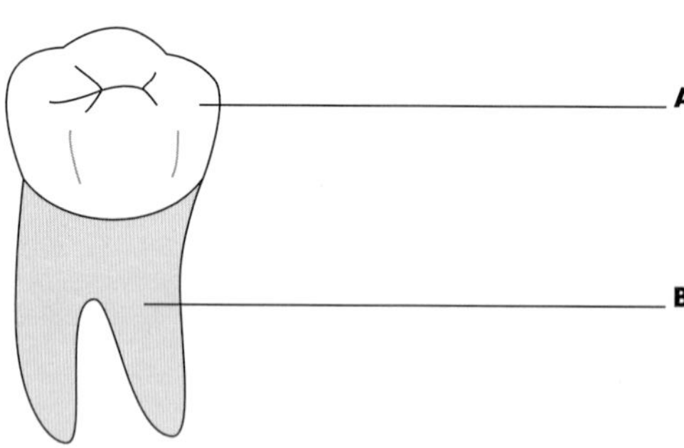

12.

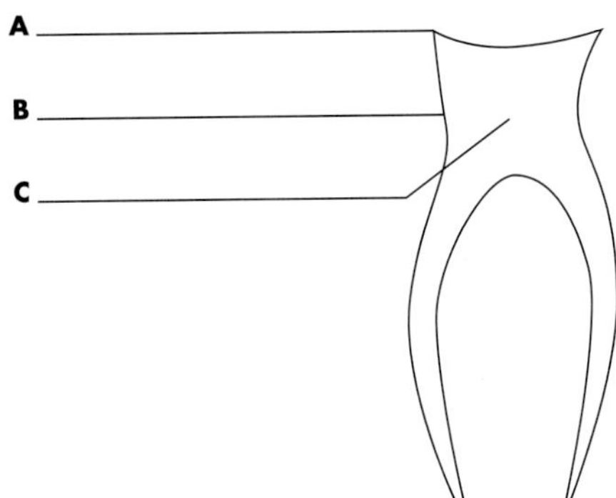

13.

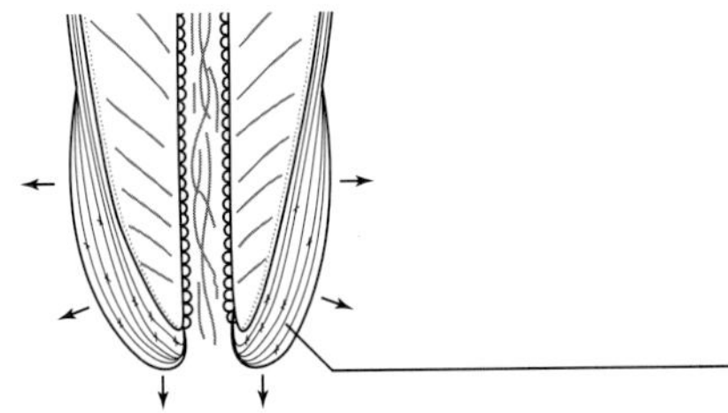

14.

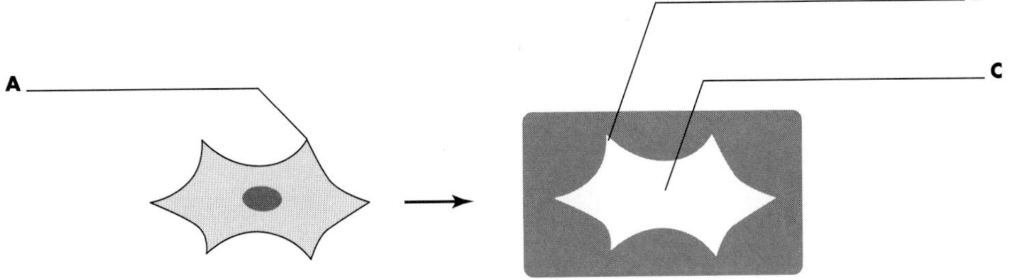

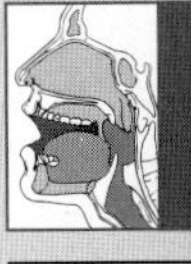

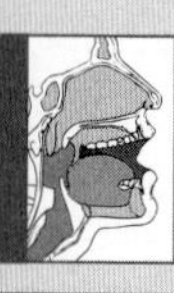

15.

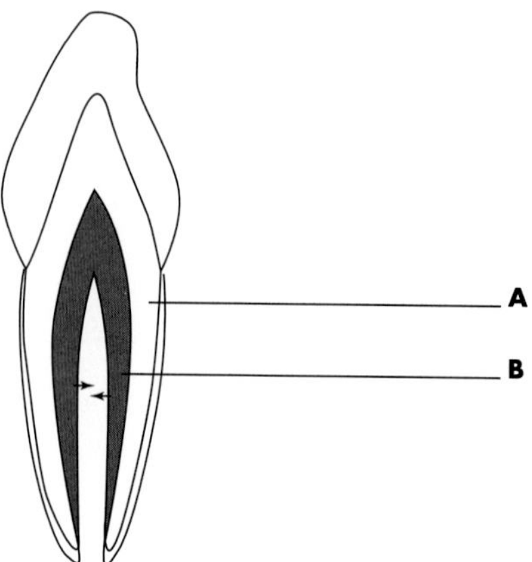

16.

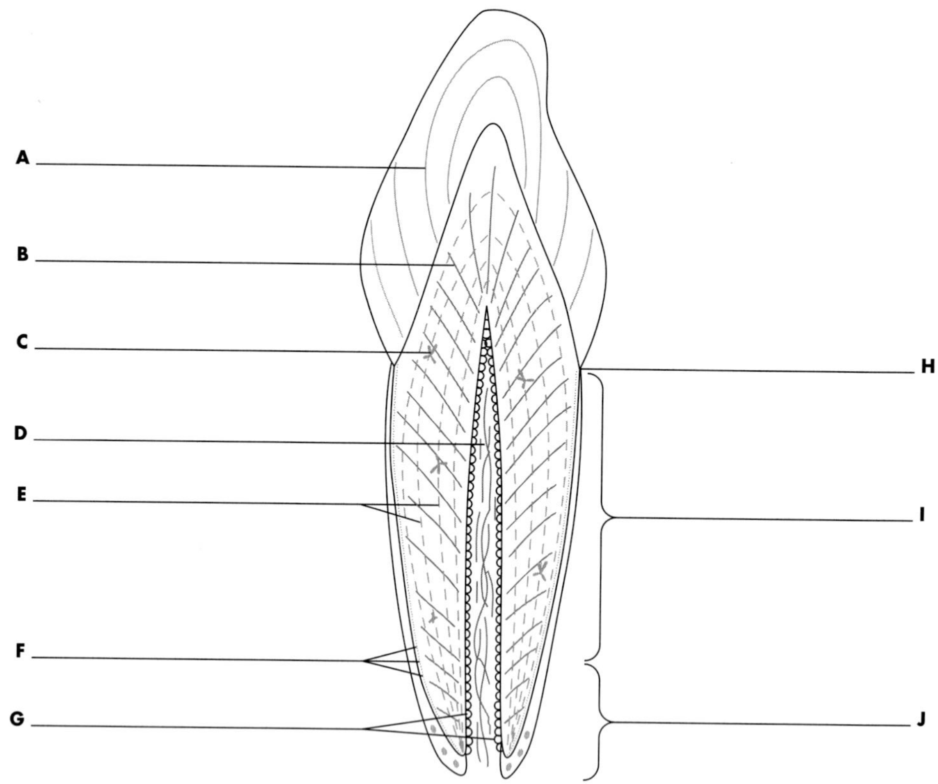

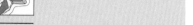

5

Periodontal Tissues

PERIODONTAL LIGAMENT

1.0

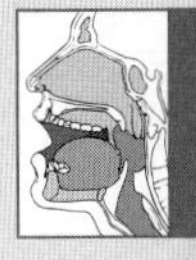

We have looked at the tissues or histology of the tooth—the dental tissues—in the previous chapter. In this chapter, we look at the tissues that surround the tooth—the periodontal tissues. The words *peri* and *dont* are stem words meaning "around the tooth."

periodontal tissues: gingiva, periodontal ligament, alveolar bone

So, looking at the diagram, what are the tissues that surround the tooth? This is a longitudinal section.

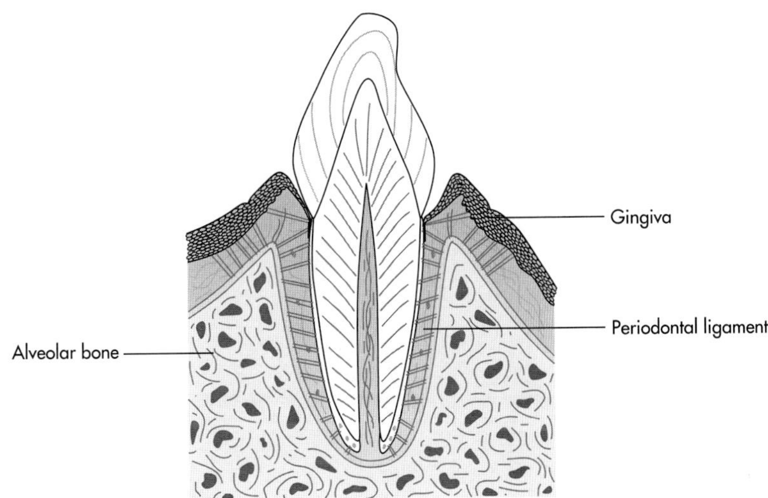

The bony socket or **alveolus** that holds the tooth is an obvious periodontal tissue, as is the "gum" tissue or **gingiva.** Not as obvious is a small "space" between the tooth and the socket that is not a space at all but rather a soft connective tissue. This is called the **periodontal ligament (PDL).**

Label the locations of the alveolus, the PDL, and the gingiva in the diagram.

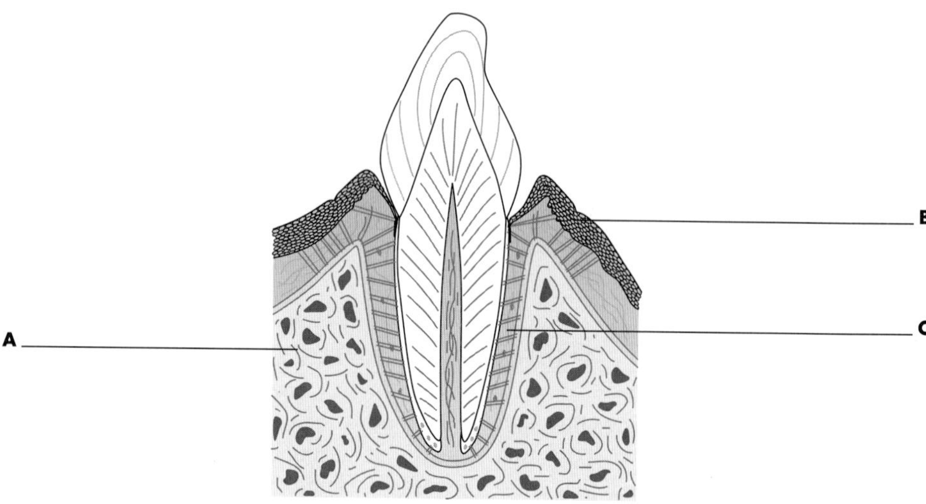

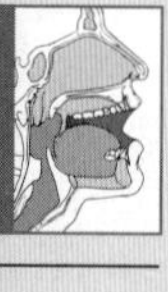

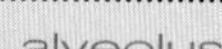

alveolus

The **PDL** is a soft connective tissue that is found between the ______________ and the tooth. It is a very small, thin tissue, but is very important for attaching the tooth to the alveolus and providing a cushion against trauma for the tooth.

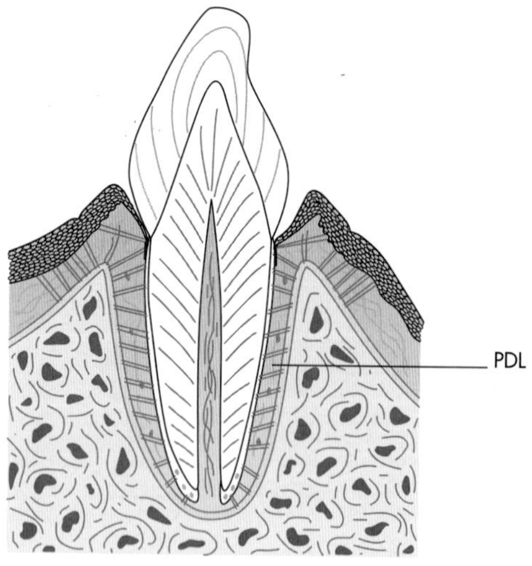

mesoderm

From what embryologic tissue did the PDL derive?

If you guessed that the PDL came from the mesoderm of the dental sac, you're right. If not, return to Chapter Three to review.

As the root of the tooth is being developed along the guiding path of Hertwig's epithelial root sheath next to the developing cementum, the PDL is organizing between it and the alveolar bone, as shown.

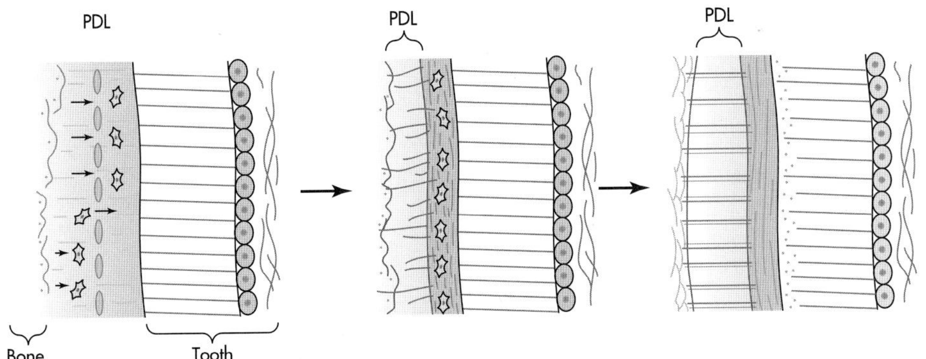

The fibroblasts of the PDL begin to make fibers, which will bridge the gap between the cementum and alveolar bone, embedding their ends on either side to attach the tooth to the socket.

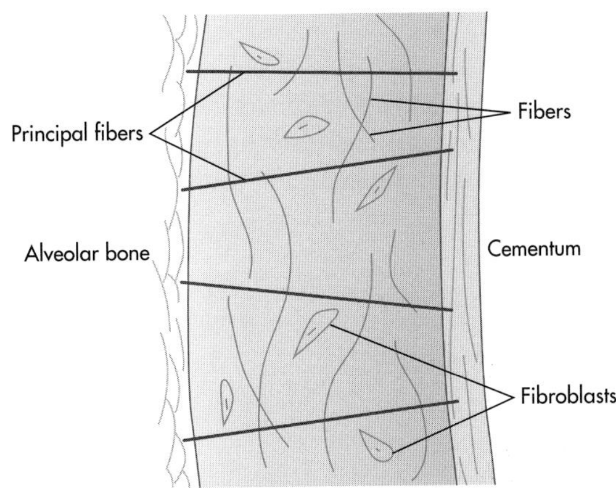

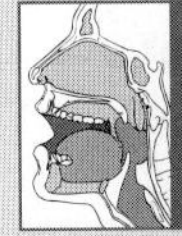

As the PDL is a connective tissue, which does it have more of, cells or matrix?

matrix

A lot of different cells and matrix components are found in the PDL. Of the tissues studied so far, it most resembles pulp. In the PDL, a great deal of **ground substance** (proteins and water) is found. What makes its matrix very different from that of the pulp is the presence of large amounts of fibers.

The cells of the PDL are many, but one of the predominant ones found is the **fibroblast.** From its name, can you tell what it produces?

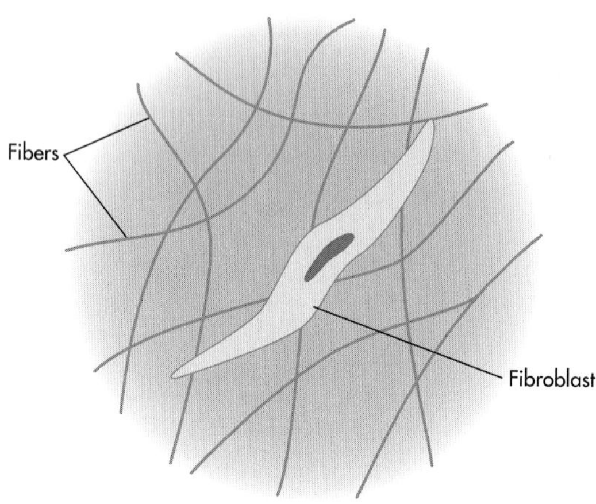

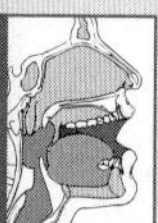

pulp

Also found in the PDL are the cells and vessels of the circulatory system, that is, blood cells and capillaries (important to nutrition of the ligament and waste removal) and lymph cells and vessels (important to the defense of the health of the ligament). This is similar to the ______________ tissue.

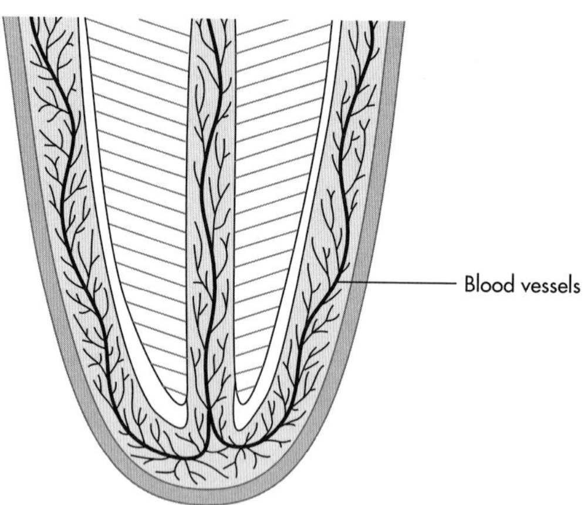

The PDL also contains nerve fibers as did the pulp. Though many of the nerve fibers are pain conduction fibers, some regulate blood flow and one type of sensory fiber is unique. These are **proprioceptive nerve fibers;** these fibers transmit information about the position of the jaw in space. When the teeth come together, nerve endings in the PDL fire, telling the brain that the teeth have come in contact. They are a kind of touch sensory neuron.

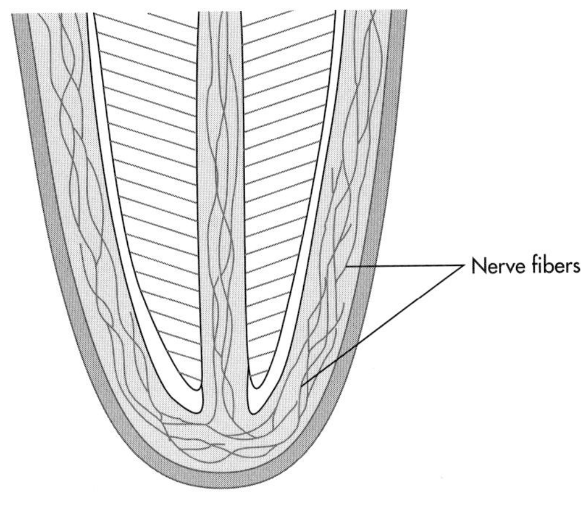

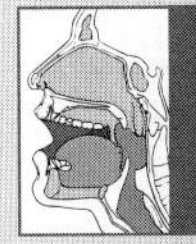

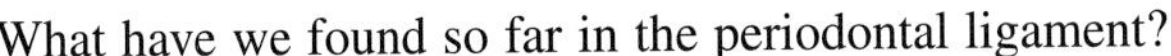

What have we found so far in the periodontal ligament?

ground substance, fibers and fibroblasts, blood cells and vessels, lymph cells and vessels, nerve fibers

And now for the "ligament" part of the periodontal ligament! One of the most important functions of the PDL is attachment of the tooth to the alveolus. This is accomplished by fibers. The fibroblasts of the PDL produce two major types of fibers: (1) collagen fibers and (2) elastic fibers.

Elastic fibers are a minor but important component of the PDL, forming a network around the root. Elastic fibers can stretch and then return to their original shape, much like a rubber band. The function of the elastic fibers in the PDL is to provide some "give" in the ligament or act as a cushion to traumatic forces on the teeth.

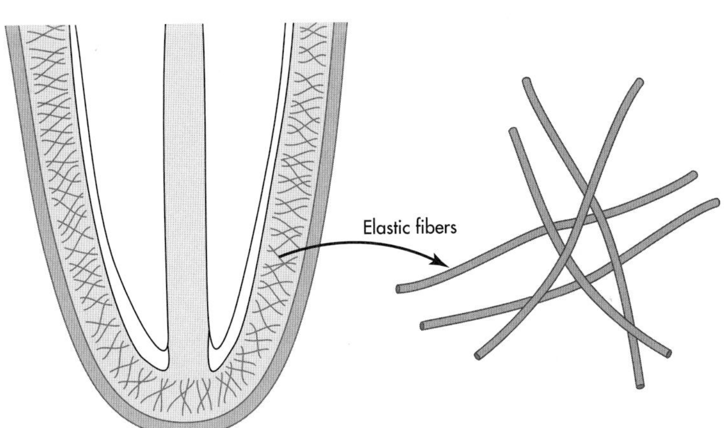

collagen

The second type of fibers is ______________ fibers. These fibers are tough and don't "give." They are the fibers used to support and attach the tooth in its bony socket.

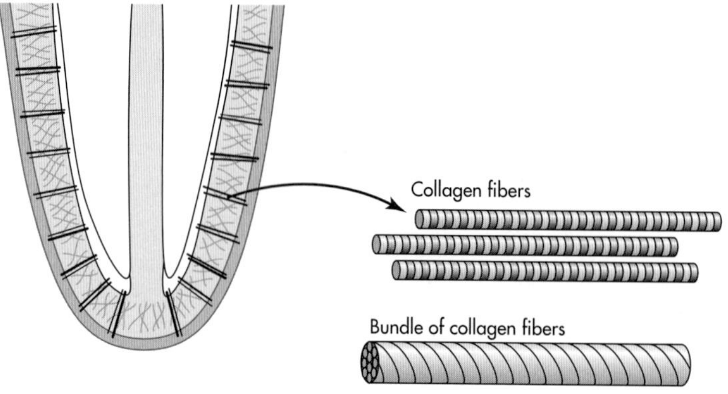

collagen, elastic

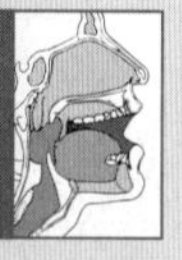

Review the difference between the two types of fibers, ______________ and ______________, as found in Chapter One. Note that the PDL is similar to a generalized type of connective tissue.

collagen, elastic

Which type of fiber is important to attachment of the tooth in the PDL? Which type gives a "cushioning" structure to the PDL?

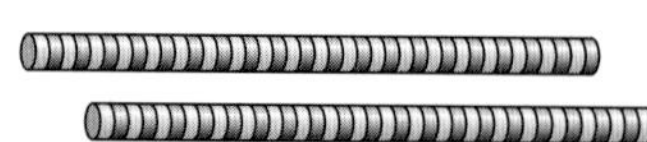

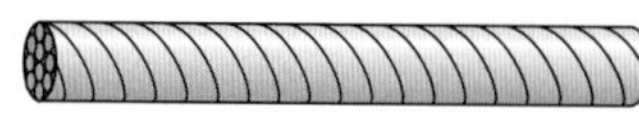

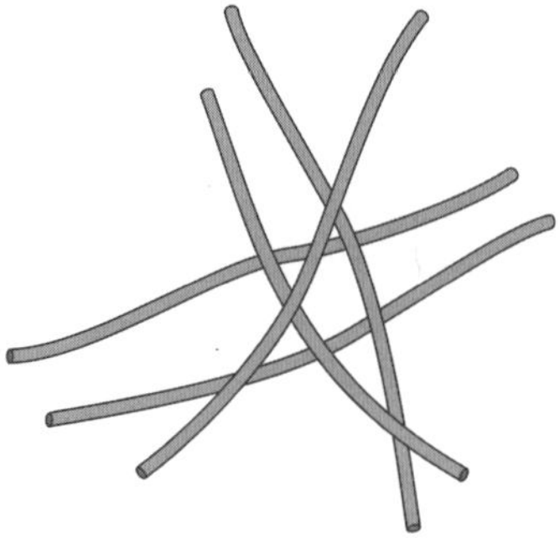

To what purpose are nerve fibers found in the PDL? What special function do they have?

to sense pain and to regulate blood flow, proprioception (position sense of jaw)

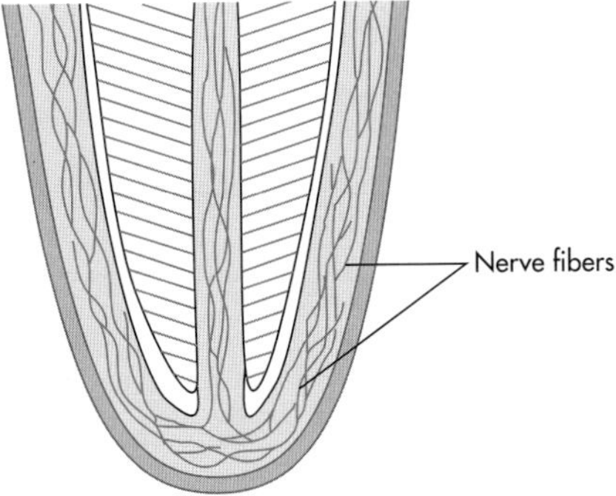

The collagen fibers form a network around the root, and also run from attachment sites in the cementum across the PDL space to attachment sites in the bone of the alveolus.

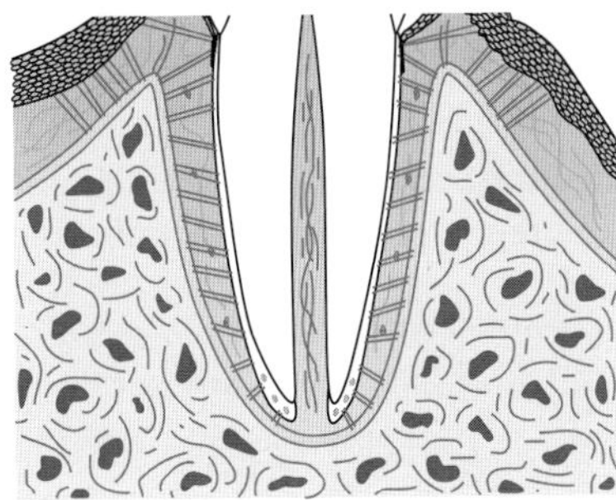

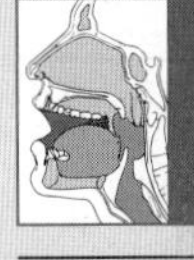

The collagen fibers are often braided together to form strong fiber bundles. These bundles traverse the PDL attaching to the cementum on one side of the PDL and to the alveolar bone on the other side. These large collagen fiber bundles that attach the tooth to the alveolus are called the **principal fibers.**

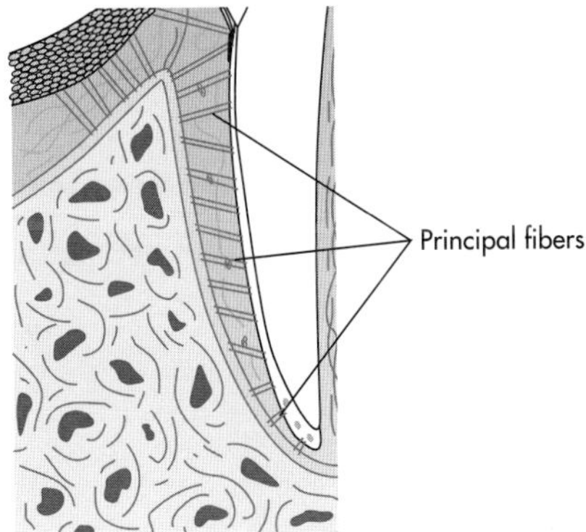

cementum on the right

In this enlarged view of the PDL, which side is the cementum and which is the alveolar bone? The very ends of the collagen fibers that are embedded within the hard tissue (cementum or bone) are called **Sharpey's fibers.**

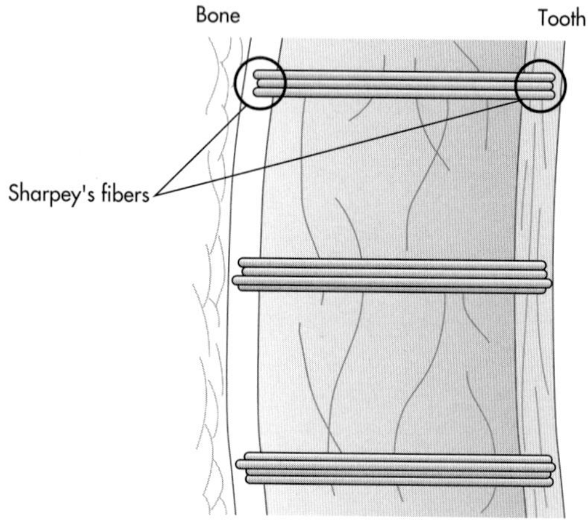

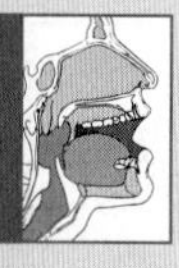

The principal fibers are located in specific locations within the PDL and have names according to their sites. Four different types of principal fibers are shown.

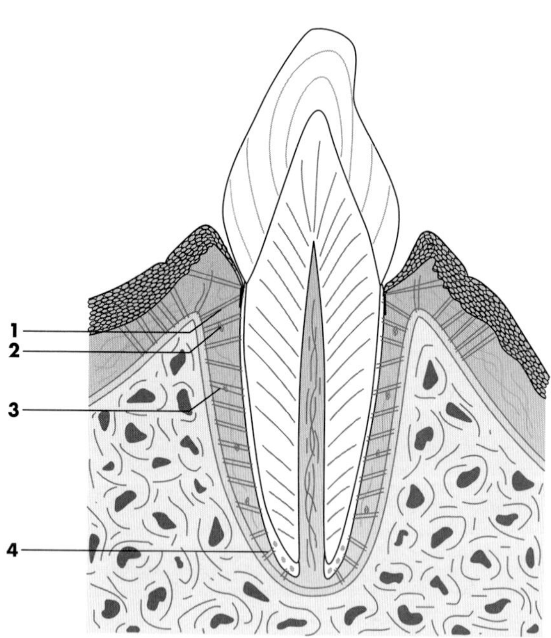

The **alveolar crest fibers** extend from the crestal bone to the cementum of the tooth.

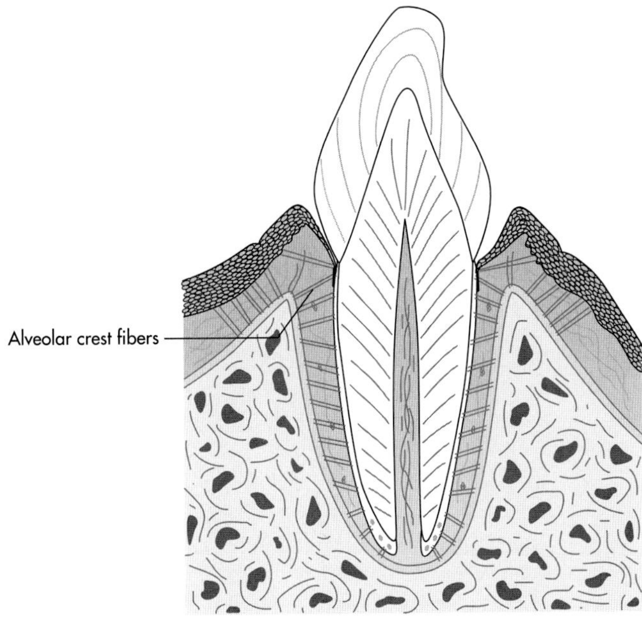

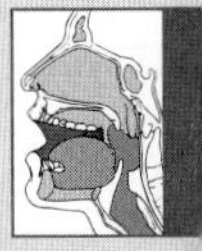

First **horizontal fibers,** then **oblique,** and lastly **apical fibers** run the length of the alveolus to attach on the opposite side, the cementum.

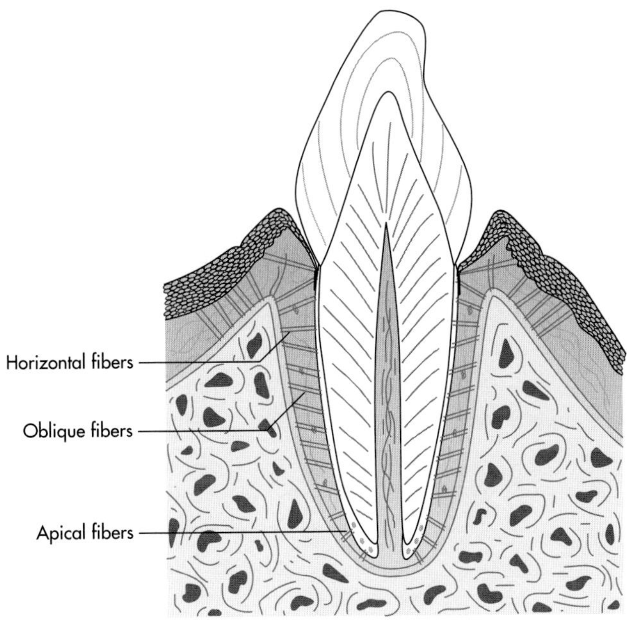

The alveoli of multirooted teeth are different as are the PDLs that inhabit them. There is a fifth type of principal fiber that exists between roots in the PDL, the **interradicular fibers.**

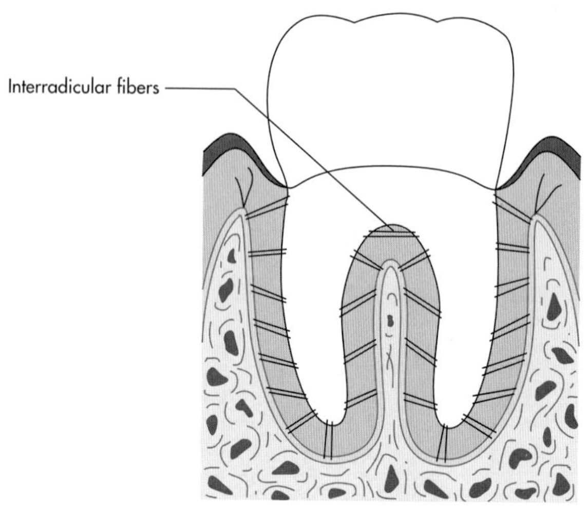

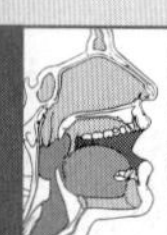

List the five types of principal fibers. Describe where they are located.

1. ______
2. ______
3. ______
4. ______
5. ______

Now show where these groups are in the diagram.

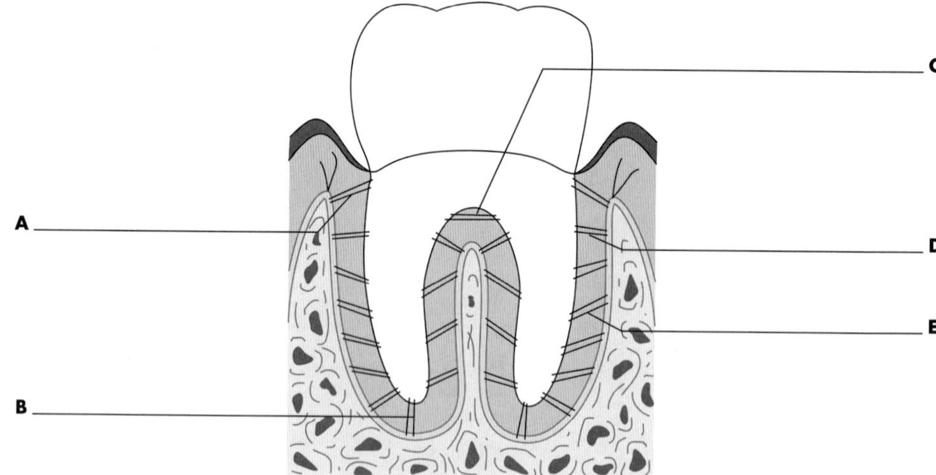

1. Alveolar crest: upper cementum to crestal bone
2. Horizontal: upper cementum to upper alveolus
3. Oblique: middle to lower cementum to same alveolus
4. Apical: root cementum to apical alveolus
5. Interradicular: root cementum to root cementum

A. 1
B. 4
C. 5
D. 2
E. 4

ALVEOLAR BONE

2.0

The **alveolus** or bony socket that contains the tooth is made up of **alveolar bone,** which is similar to all bone found throughout the body.

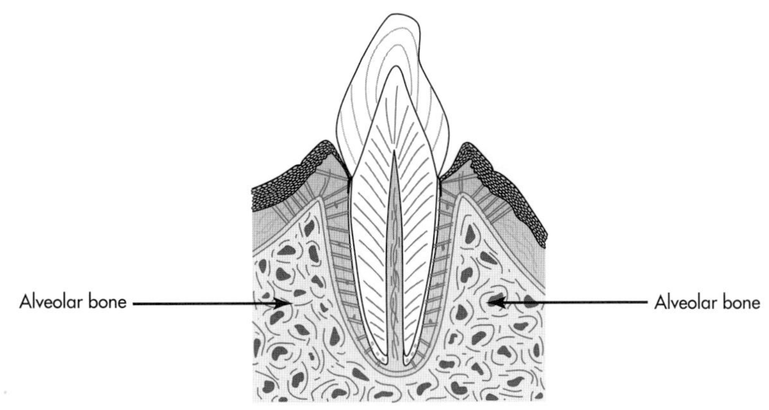

If you have forgotten what bone tissue looks like, please review Chapter One at this time.

From what embryologic tissue does the alveolar bone derive?

Mesoderm—dental sac

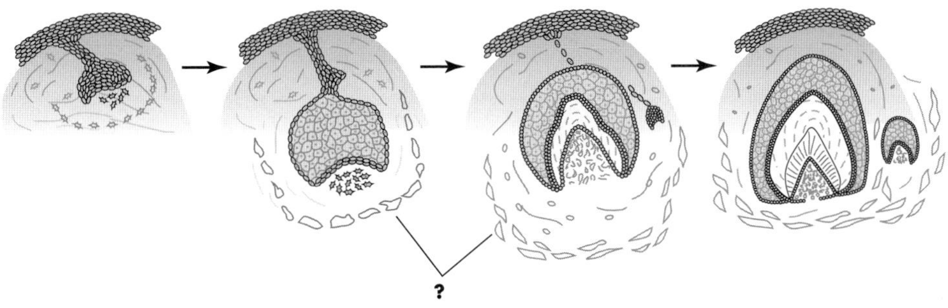

If you guessed the mesoderm of the dental sac, you're right! Mesoderm condenses all around the developing tooth, forming osteoblasts, which, in turn, form a bony shell around the tooth. At this time, the space in bone that contains the developing tooth is called the **crypt.**

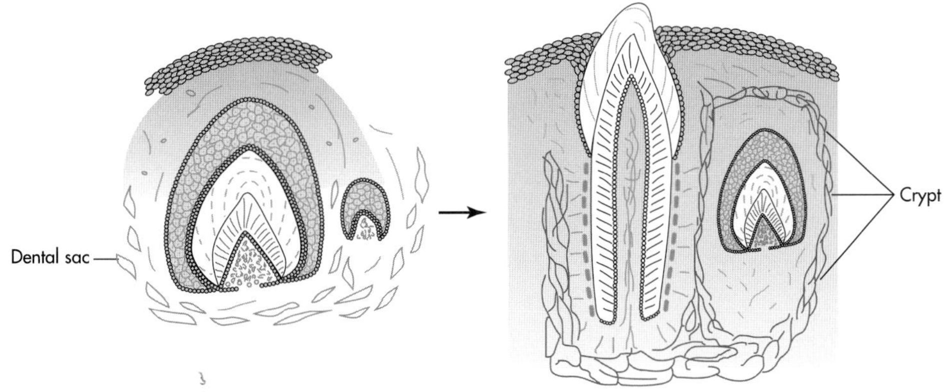

After the tooth erupts, the bone surrounding the tooth is called the **alveolus.** Remember that most of the diagrams we are looking at are two-dimensional ones or long sections through tooth and bone. In reality, the alveolar bone extends all the way around the tooth.

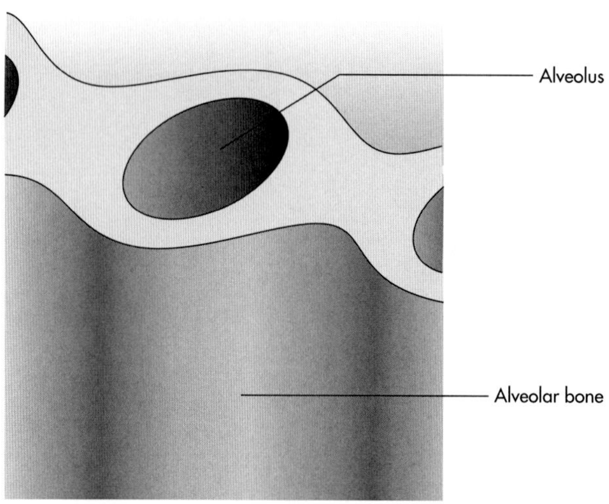

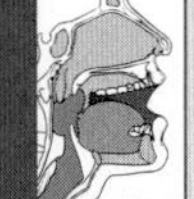

crypt

What is the space in bone that contains the developing tooth called?

The alveolar bone comes to peaks at the top of the alveolus. These peaks of bone that occur between the cervices of the teeth are called **crestal bone.**

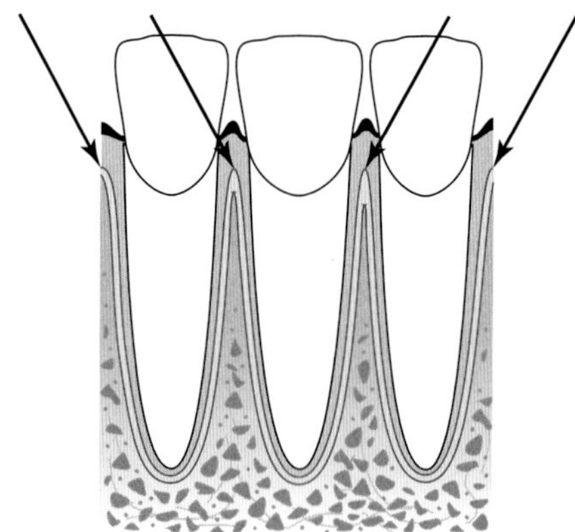

________________ is the bony peaks at the top of the alveolus found between teeth. If the bone is healthy these peaks are sharp and covered with compact bone. If the bone is diseased, they are blunted trabecular bone.

Crestal bone

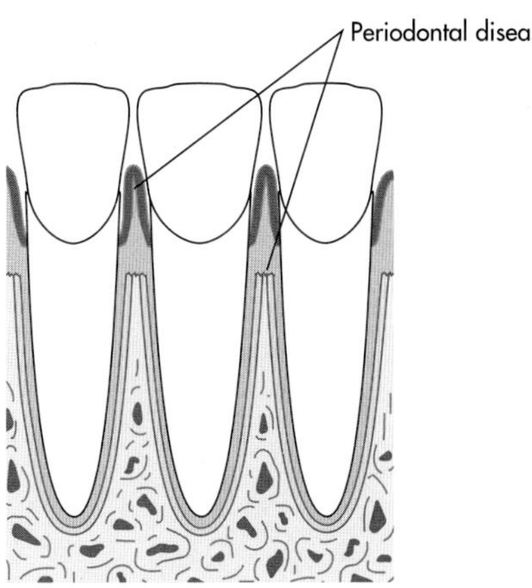

The bone of the alveolus is like any other bone. Lets look at the microstructure. First, remember that the cells of mature bone are called ________________. One is pictured. Bone cells are spider-shaped, with many processes coming off of their cell bodies.

osteocytes

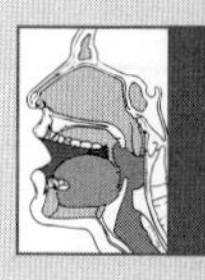

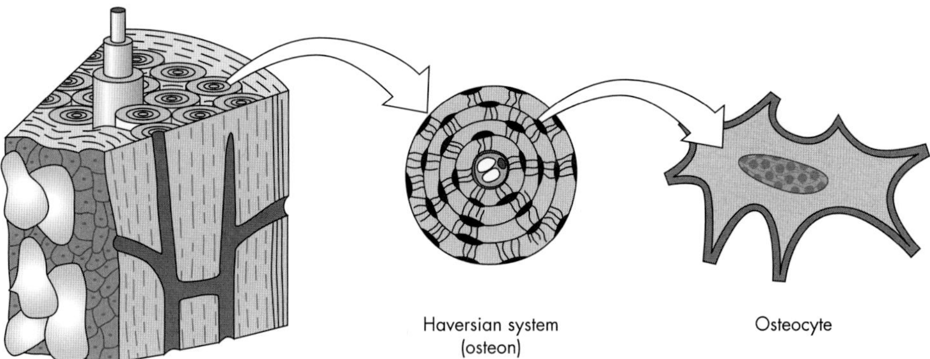

Osteocytes used to be ________________ before they formed a hard, bony matrix around themselves by calcification. The spaces they left for the mature cells are also spider-shaped, and there are different names for the space where the cell body lies and where the processes lie; these are the ________________ and the ________________.

osteoblasts, lacuna, canaliculi

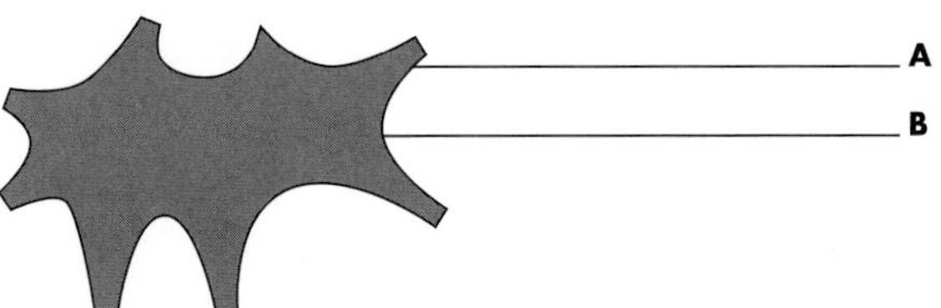

A. canaliculus
B. lacuna

both

Calcification forms the matrix of bone from calcium salts and is laid down by the osteoblasts in layers or laminae. Bone that is laid down in tightly packed layers is called **compact bone.** Bone laid down in loosely packed pieces (spicules or trabeculae), with spaces between each, is called **loose, spongy,** or **trabecular bone.** Which type of bone is alveolar bone?

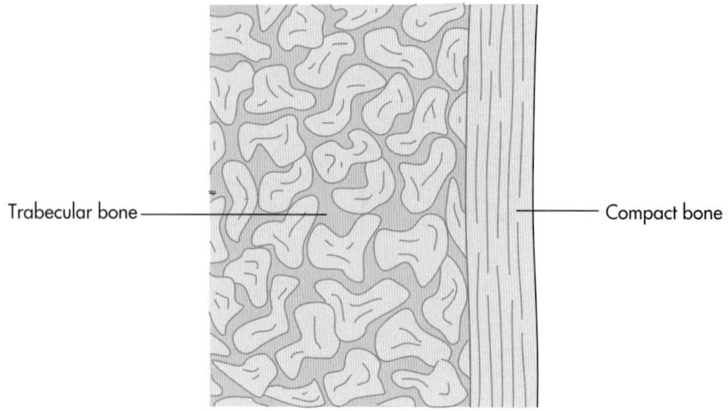

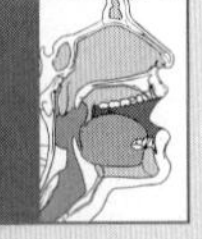

Most bones in the human body have a core of spongy bone covered by a thin hard layer of compact bone. Inside the spaces of the spongy bone are found blood-making cells called **marrow.** Alveolar bone is the same—a core of trabecular bone covered by a layer of compact bone. Note that the compact bone lines the socket, extends over the crest, and continues over the outside of each jaw.

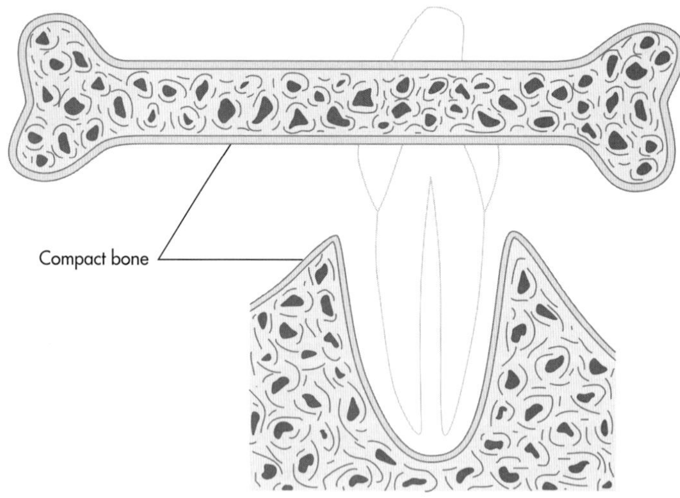

In the diagram of the alveolar bone, label with an arrow where the layer of compact bone is found.

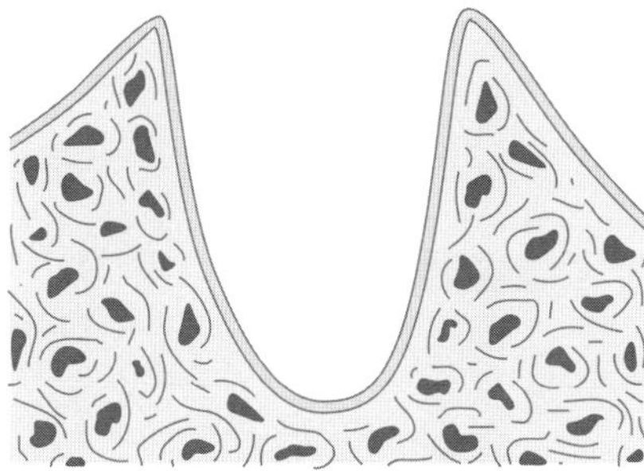

You should have found this layer of compact bone. It has been darkened in for you to see. Note how the layer is continuous over the top of the crests and into the socket area. The hard layer that lines the socket is called the **lamina dura.** The layer over the "peaks" covers **crestal bone.**

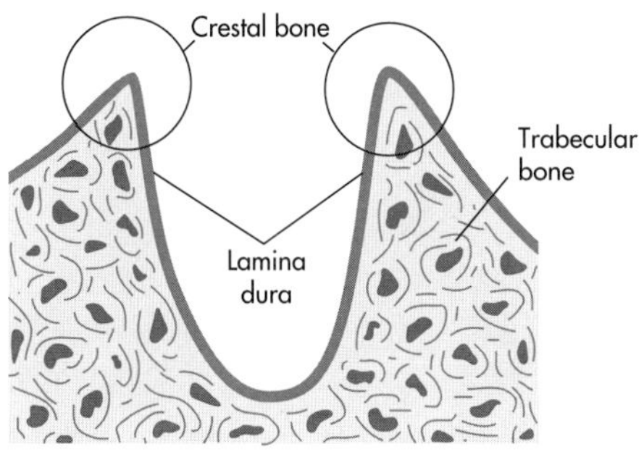

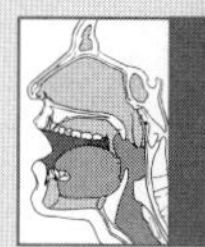

As bone is dense, it appears white on an x-ray, especially the compact bone. The white line that is the compact bony layer of the inner alveolar bone appears on this diagram of an x-ray. This is the lamina dura. Where is the PDL?

the dark line next to the tooth

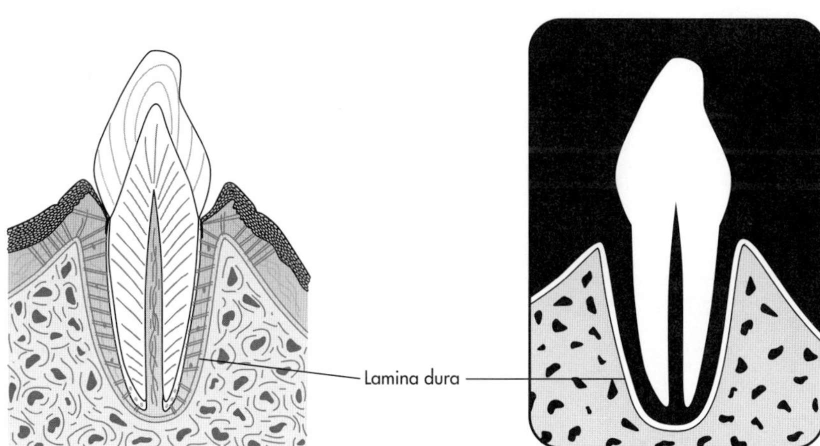

Sharpey's fibers

Remember that the PDL attaches on the compact bony surface of the alveolus, embedding its collagen fibers directly within the bone. These ends of the fibers, embedded in the bone, are called ______________.

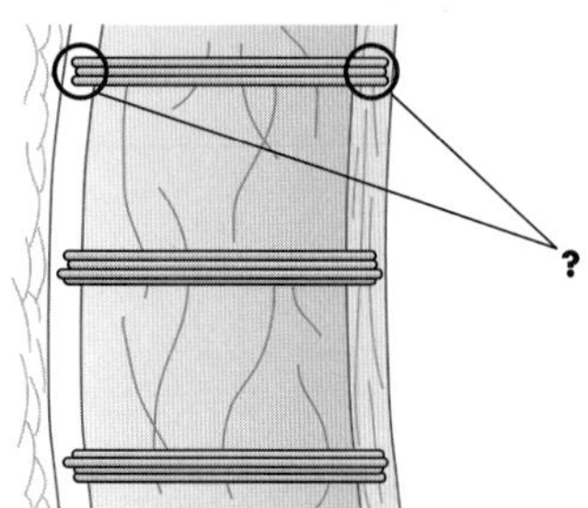

alveolar

Thus is the tooth attached by means of fibers of the PDL from its cementum to the ______________ bone. There are also fibers that attach the gingiva to alveolar bone.

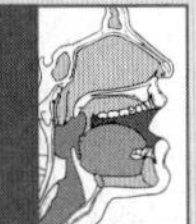

A, B. compact bone
C. crestal bone
D. trabecular bone

Label the parts of the alveolar bone. Check your answers in the previous text.

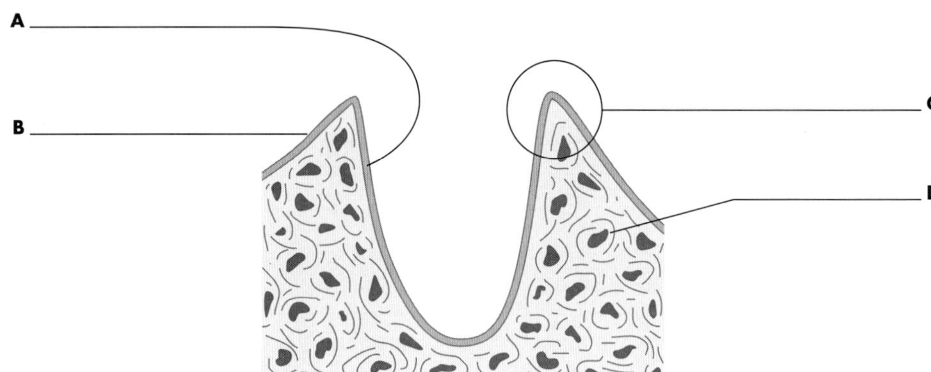

GINGIVA

3.0

The last periodontal tissue is the **gingiva.** It is the firm, coral pink tissue that surrounds each tooth and it is visible to the eye when looking in the mouth. See the accompanying diagrams of the surface and a long section of the gingiva.

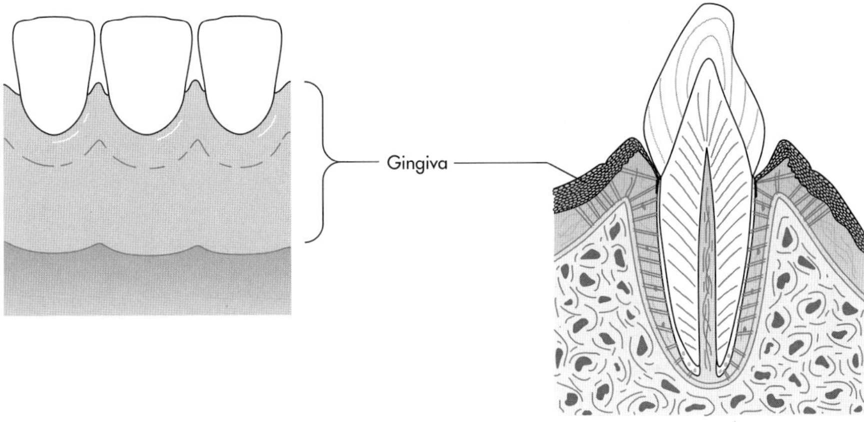

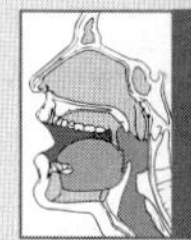

Gingiva or the gum tissue surrounds the teeth like a collar, dipping around each cervix of the teeth and attaching itself to the tooth in a small area. In the long section, you can see the gingiva as it creates a pocket around the tooth. This periodontal pocket or sulcus is created by the gingiva folding around the tooth like a collar.

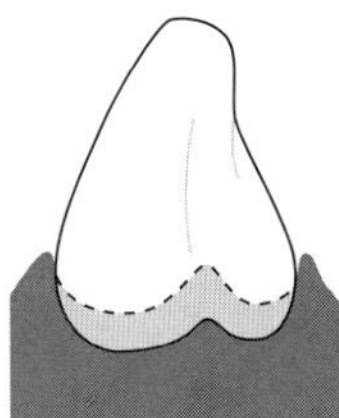

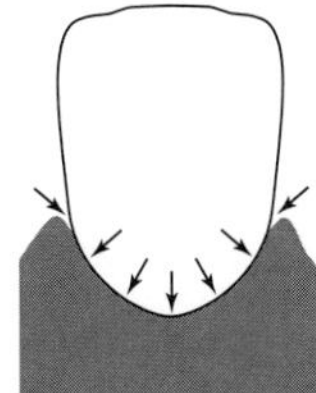

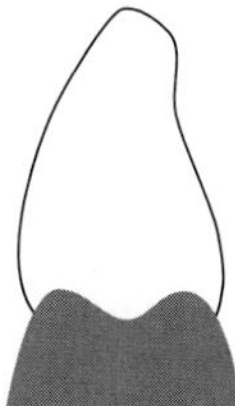

pocket

The **sulcus** or periodontal ________________ is a space or crevice created by the gingiva as it wraps around the tooth. Note where the gingiva is attached to the tooth, at the bottom of the sulcus. Remember that this is a section through the tooth and gingiva.

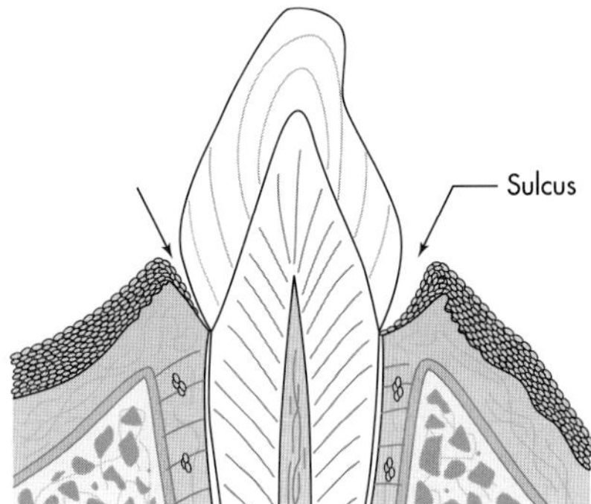

Let us look at the histology of the gingiva, that is, the cells that make up this type of oral tissue. Remember from Chapter One that gingiva is a type of **mucosa,** a lining tissue of the entire digestive tract. Mucosa is a kind of inside "skin" that we compared with the outside skin in Chapter One. Please review at this time.

mucosa proper, lamina propria

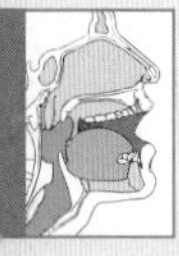

All mucosa is made up of an epithelial layer (the **mucosa proper**), a connective tissue layer below it (**lamina propria**), and sometimes a bottom muscular layer. Oral mucosa is diagrammed here. It has (1) a stratified, squamous epithelial layer called the ______________ and (2) a connective tissue layer called the ______________.

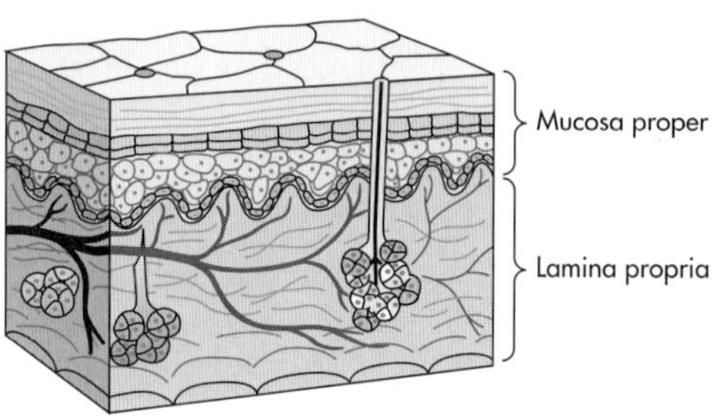

The epithelium of oral mucosa contains no hair and must be maintained in a constant moist state by its glands. The mucosa proper is thin and has fewer layers than skin, with a smaller stratum corneum with nucleated cells.

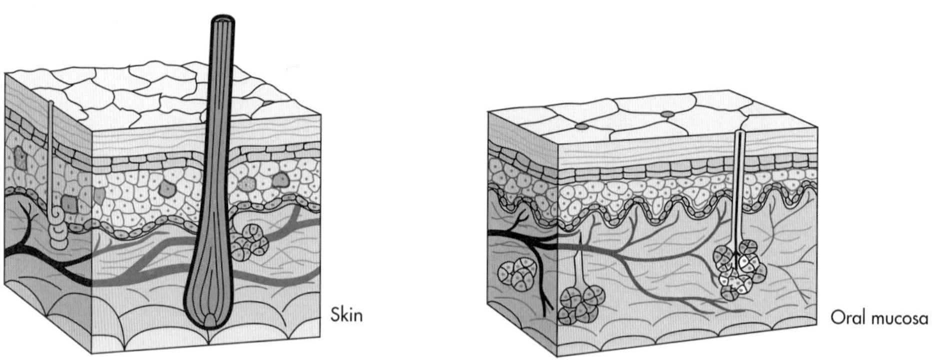

The connective tissue of oral mucosa contains many blood vessels, nerves, fibers, and two types of glands: salivary glands and mucous glands.

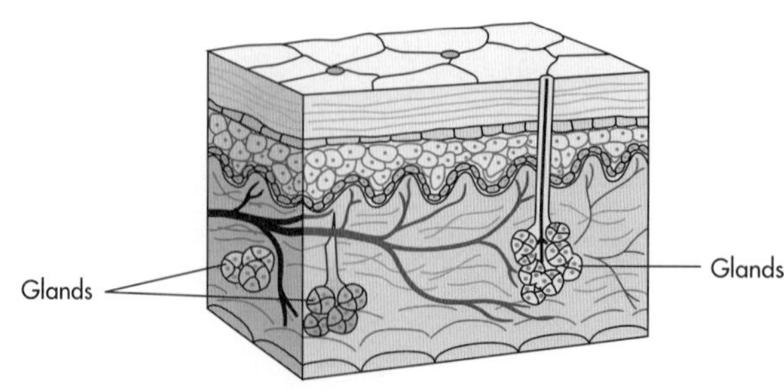

How is oral mucosa different from skin?

thinner; no hair, sebaceous, or sweat glands; has salivary mucous glands; very vascular

Mucosa proper may or may not be **keratinized,** which means it contains the protein keratin made by cells called keratinocytes. Keratin is added to mucosa when it needs to be extra tough.

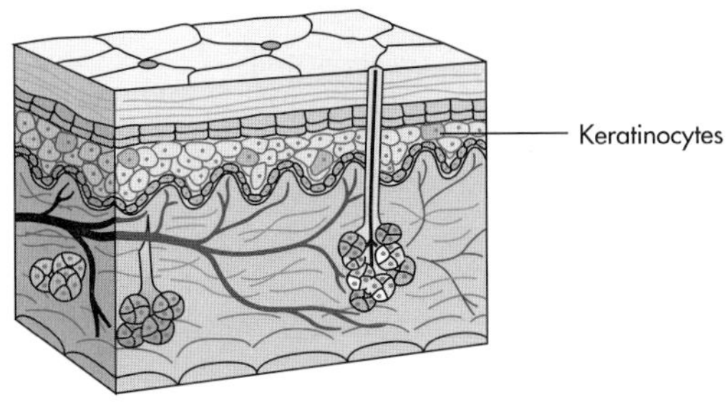

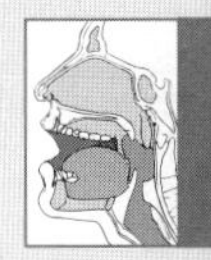

In oral mucosa are found the _______________ glands and _______________ glands. Both types of glands expel their product to the surface to create a constantly moist environment.

salivary, mucous

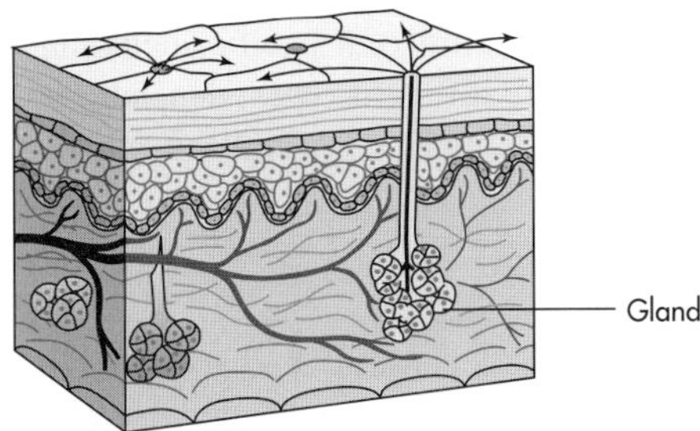

As you can see, mucosa is a thin, moist lining tissue of the mouth (and the rest of the digestive system) that is more fragile than skin. When damaged, mucosa bleeds a lot but repairs itself quickly because it has many blood vessels.

epithelial, connective, nervous, muscle

Mucosa is a tissue that is comprised of at least three and sometimes all four basic tissue types, which are ______________, ______________, ______________, and ______________.

mucosa proper, lamina propria

Mucosa, in general, is composed of an upper epithelial layer called the ______________ and a lower layer of loose, irregular connective tissue with blood vessels, nerves, and glands called the ______________. Find these two layers in the diagram.

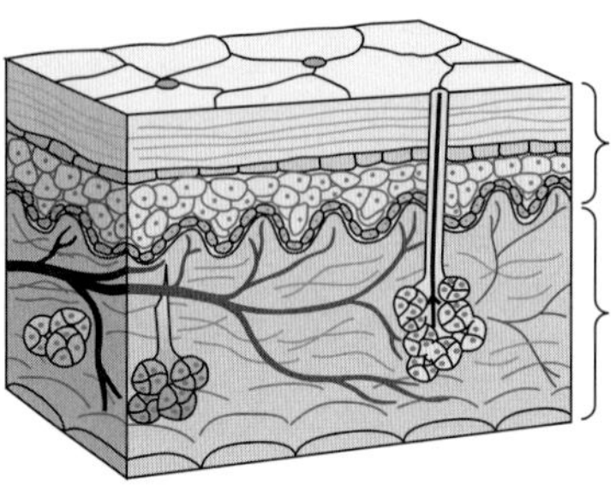

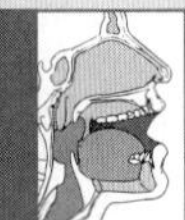

flat

Mucosa proper is a thin layer and in the mouth is composed of stratified squamous epithelium, which means many layers of ______________ cells.

Oral mucosa is found lining the entire oral cavity, including the tongue, cheeks, and oropharynx. It is divided into three different types, depending on its location: (1) **masticatory mucosa,** (2) **lining mucosa,** and (3) **specialized mucosa.**

Gingiva

Gingiva is a "masticatory mucosa" because it is adjacent to the teeth or chewing apparatus. ______________ is that soft tissue that surrounds the teeth.

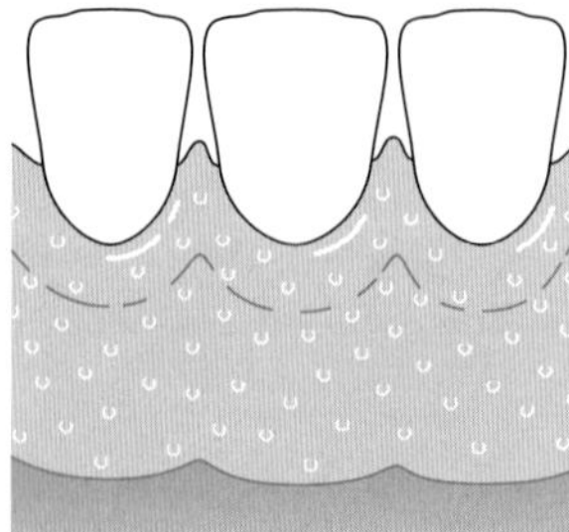

A diagram of a long section through the gingiva and tooth is shown. We have already seen that the gingiva surrounds the tooth like a collar, creating a space next to the tooth called the ______________.

pocket or sulcus

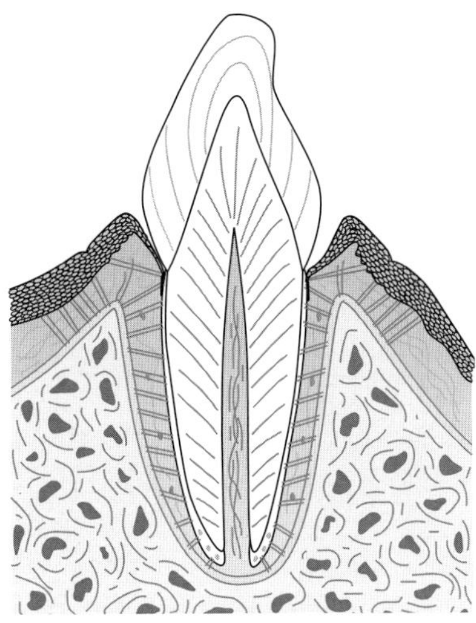

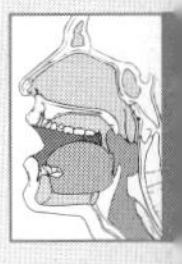

The gingiva attaches to the tooth at the bottom of the sulcus, to the enamel or cementum of the tooth. This part of the gingiva that attaches is called the **attachment epithelium.**

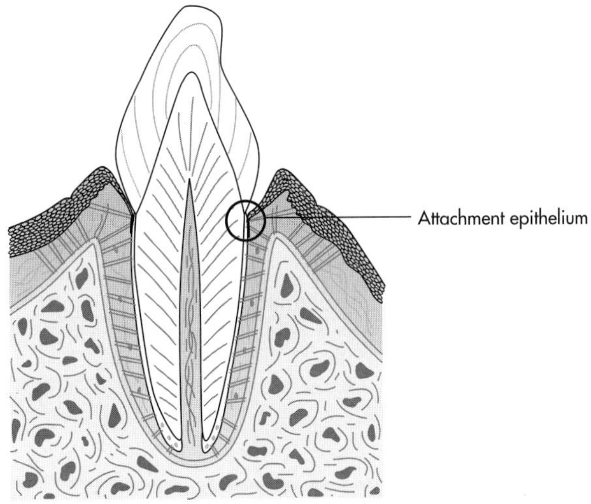

keratin

Attachment epithelium is a very thin, nonkeratinized epithelium. What is lacking in this tissue? This makes this tissue a weak, permeable area able to pass fluids back and forth from pocket to lamina propria and vice versa. Bacteria can easily overwhelm the lymphatic cells of the underlying lamina propria here.

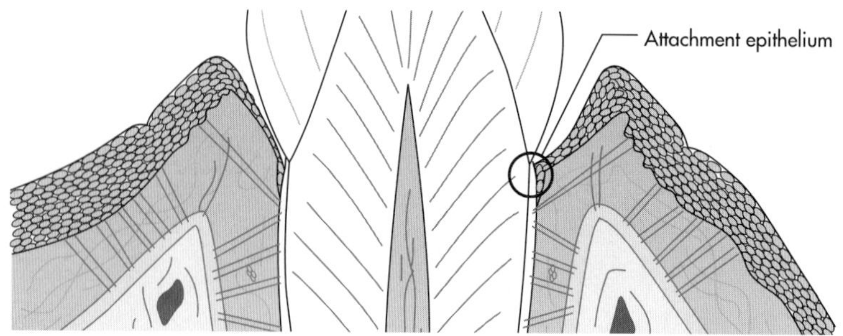

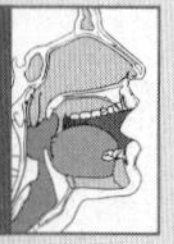

Attachment epithelium is part of the whole epithelium of the sulcus called **sulcular epithelium.** Again, none of the pocket epithelium is keratinized.

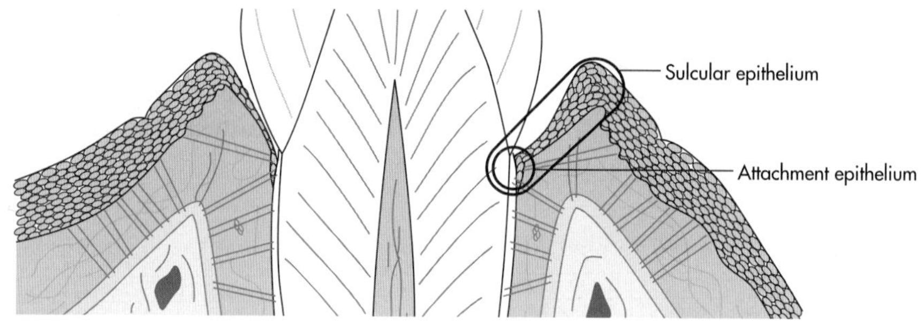

The next part of the gingiva occurs over the top of the pocket and is the gingiva that is visible in the mouth. You can't see the sulcular or attachment epithelium. You can only feel it with a periodontal probe, which is a sort of stick for measuring pocket depth.

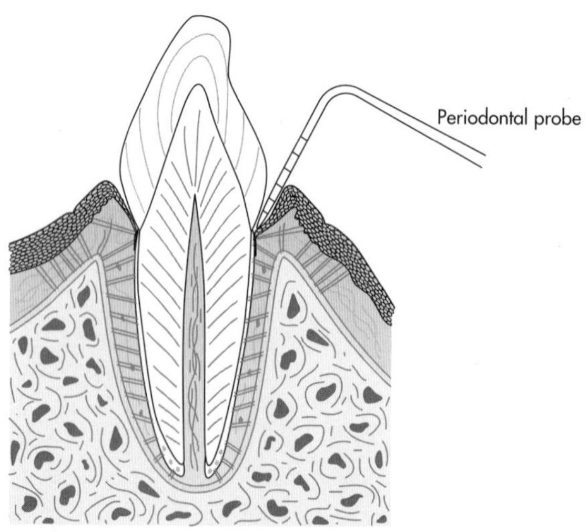

The gingiva outside the pocket instantly becomes thicker and stronger. It must be so to weather the forces of mastication. This portion of the gingiva is keratinized. Note that part of the gingiva is directly opposite the sulcular epithelium and is not attached to the underlying alveolar bone.

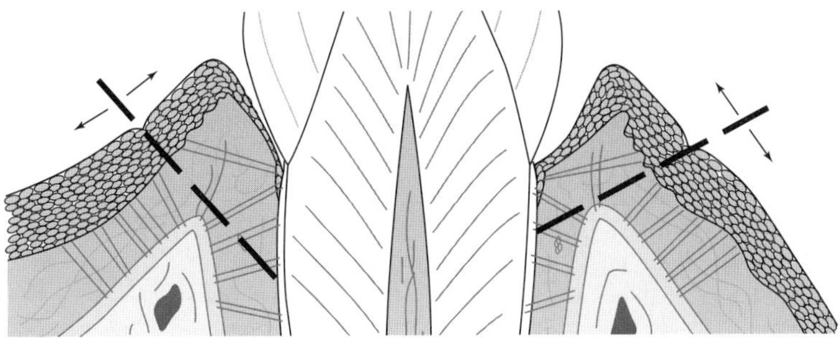

Gingiva that is not attached to the alveolar bone is called **free** gingiva. Two views of the **free** gingiva are shown.

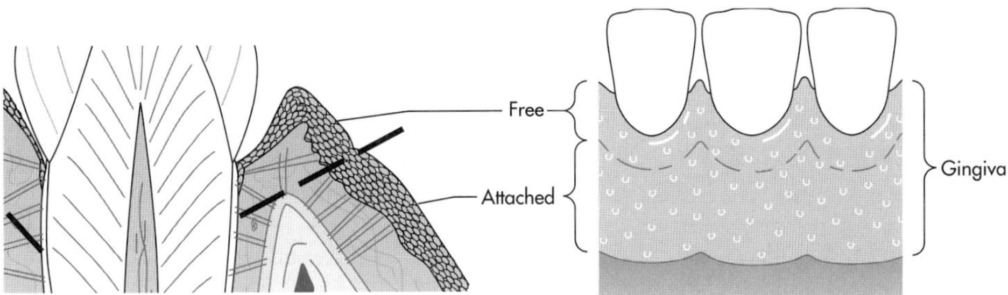

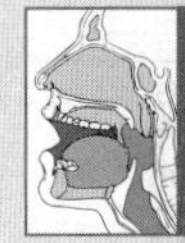

Look at the surface between the mucosa proper of the free gingiva and its lamina propria. Besides being thicker, what has happened to this epithelium?

appears folded

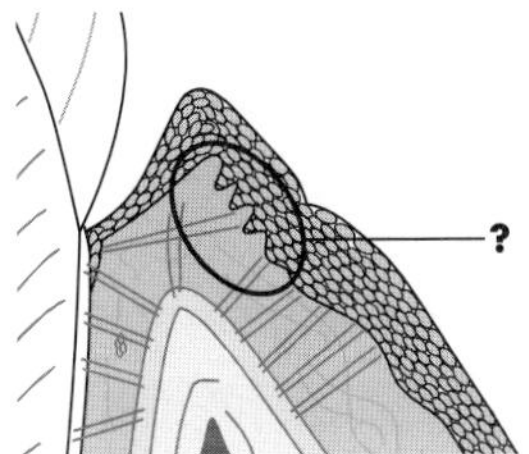

Those "folds" that appear in the mucosa proper–lamina propria border are actually "fingers" or ridges of epithelial tissue. They are called **rete pegs** or ridges and they help hold the two layers together to make the gingiva a strong tissue.

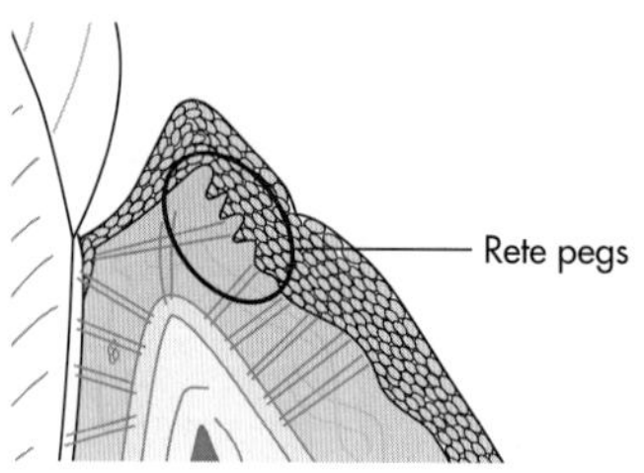

Rete pegs

_______________ are fingerlike extensions of epithelium into the lamina propria found in the free gingiva. Rete pegs and keratin are two ways to strengthen the gingiva.

gingiva

Collagen fibers bundled together as in the PDL are important to the strength and attachment of the gingiva. Fibers that attach gingiva to the teeth and alveolar bone are called **gingival fibers** and there are four types: (1) dentogingival, (2) alveologingival, (3) transeptal, (4) circular. They provide attachment for the _______________.

The **dentogingival fibers** run from the cervical tooth to surrounding gingiva, and are located in the free gingiva above the alveolus.

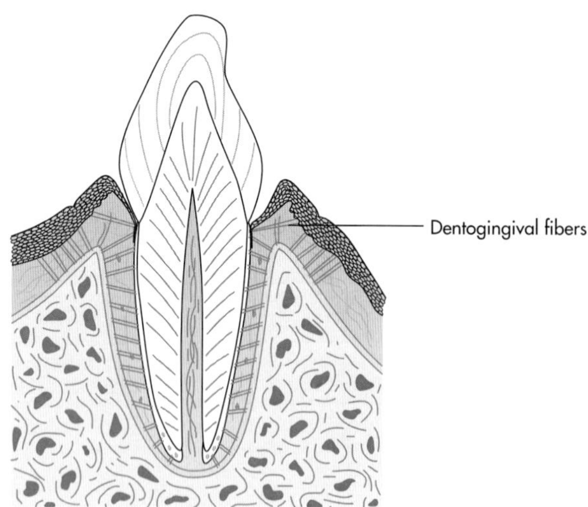

attached

Alveologingival fibers begin at the crestal bone and end at the bottom of the alveolar bone, attaching to the gingiva that covers this bone. They provide an especially strong attachment for the gingiva below the free gingival groove known as the ____________ gingiva.

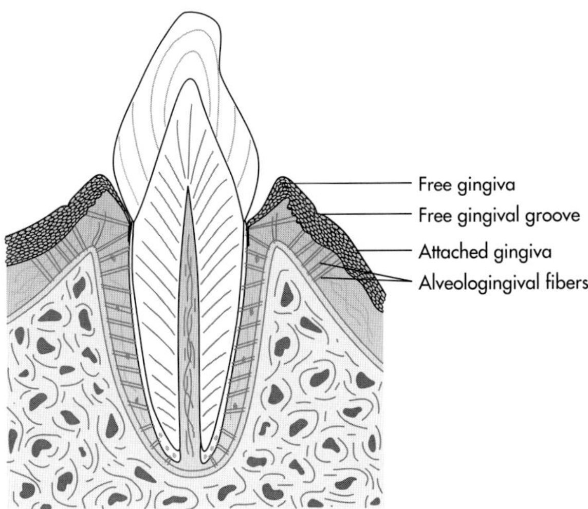

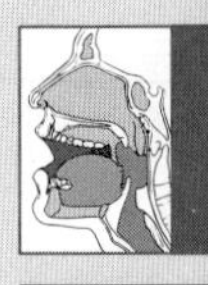

Transseptal fibers are a special group of fibers that run from cervix to cervix of the teeth, across the crestal bone as shown.

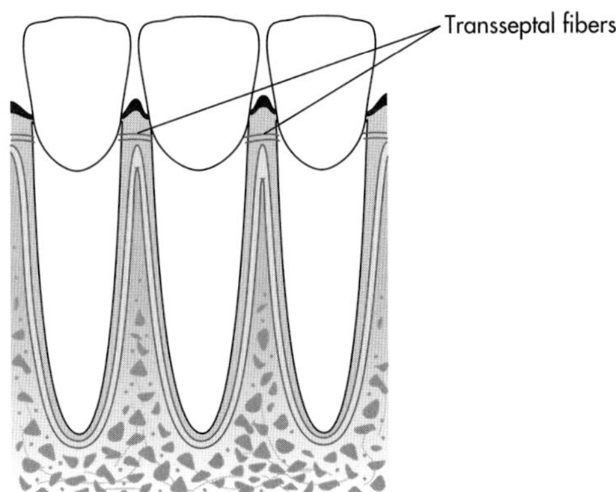

Last, there are groups of **circular fibers** shown encircling each tooth, giving support to the gingival collar.

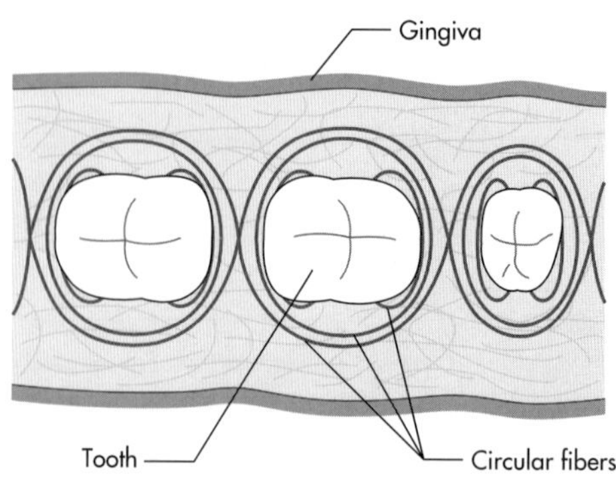

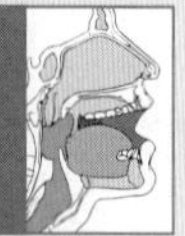

A. dentogingival fibers
B. alveologingival fibers
C. circular fibers

List three groups of gingival fibers and identify them on the diagram.

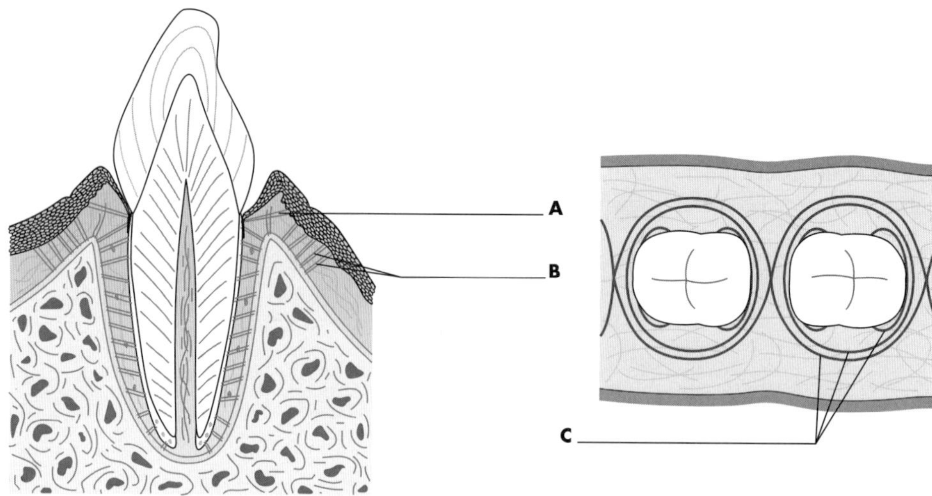

free

Below the _______________ gingiva is gingiva that is attached to the underlying alveolar bone. It is called **attached gingiva** and it is the last area of gingiva, extending down to a redder area of mucosa. Remember that healthy gingiva is a coral pink color.

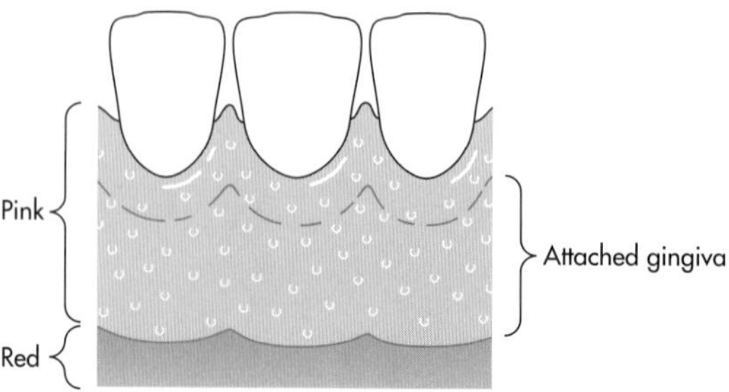

There is a natural dividing line between the free gingiva and the attached gingiva in the form of a scalloped indentation that follows the contour of the teeth. It is called the **free gingival groove.** Find it on the drawing and label free and attached gingiva.

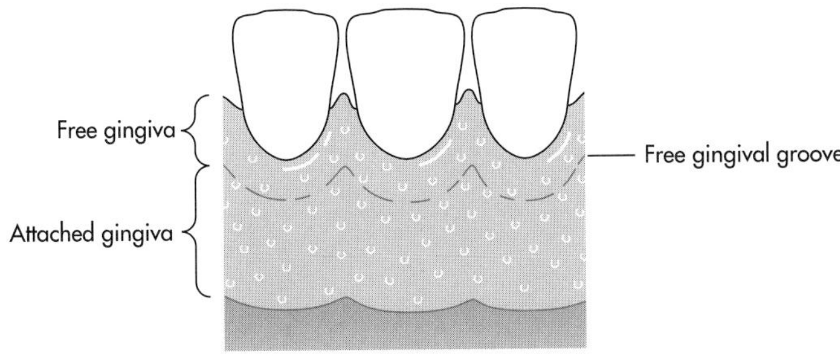

healthy

Healthy gingiva show the free gingival groove as it does a number of small round indentations. These indentations are called **stippling** and are present in ______________ gingiva.

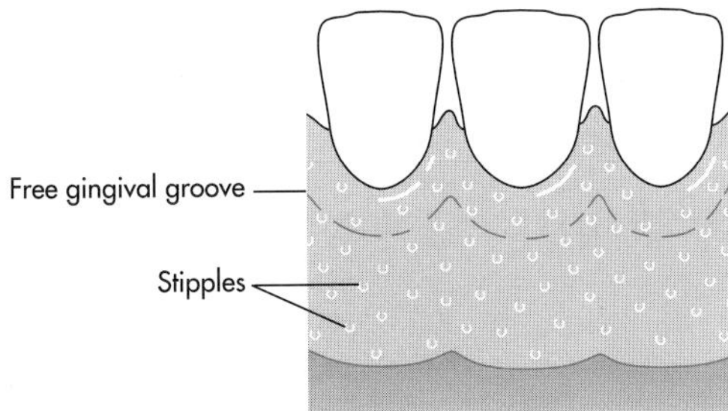

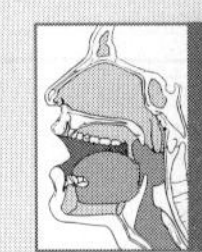

free gingiva, attached gingiva

The free gingival groove is a dividing line between the ______________ and the ______________.

In three dimensions the gingiva continues all around the tooth, peaking between the teeth. These peaks of free gingiva are called **papillae.** The balance of the encircling free gingiva is called **marginal gingiva.**

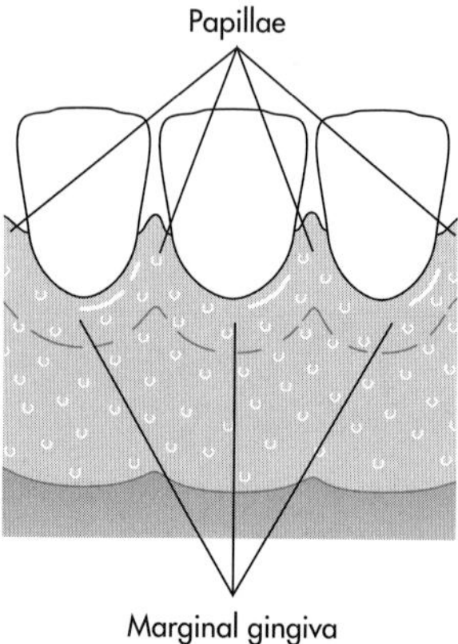

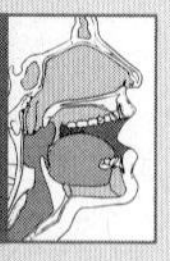

There are gingival papillae on both the facial and lingual sides of the tooth. From a different angle, the proximal or "in between" view of a tooth, we can see both papillae and a dip midway between them called the **coll.**

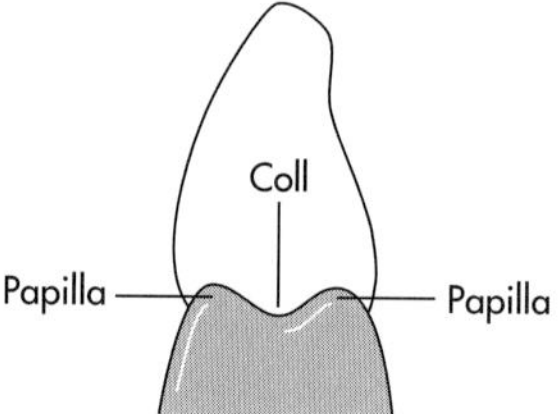

Label the various parts of the gingiva we have studied so far.

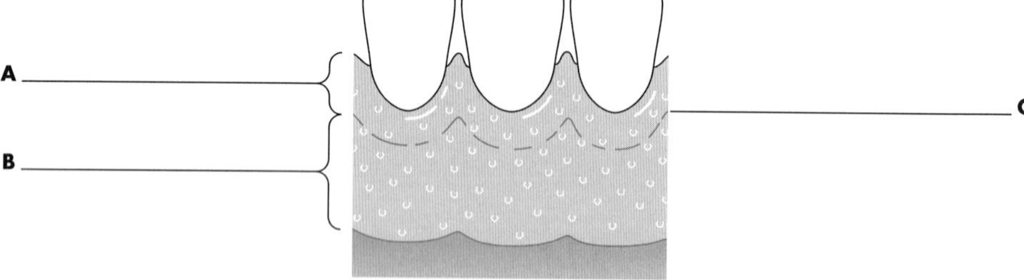

A. free gingiva
B. attached gingiva
C. free gingival groove

continued

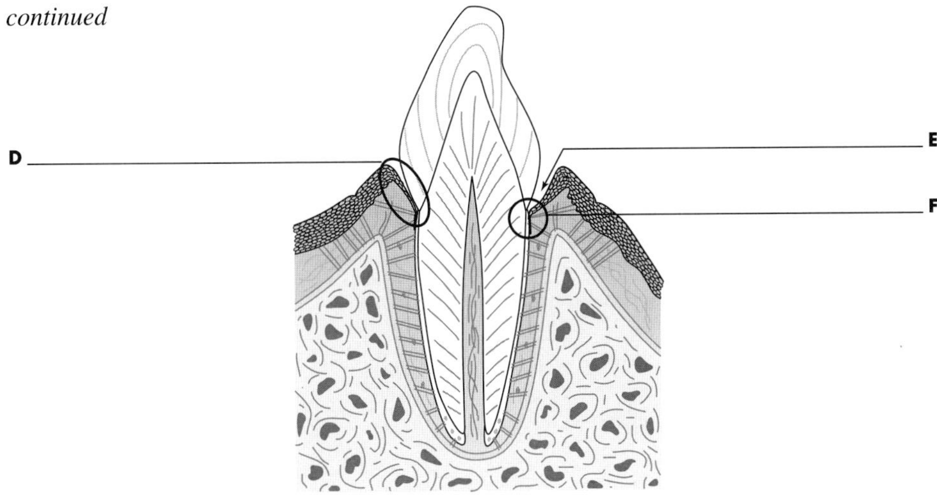

D. sulcular epithelium
E. sulcus
F. attachment epithelium

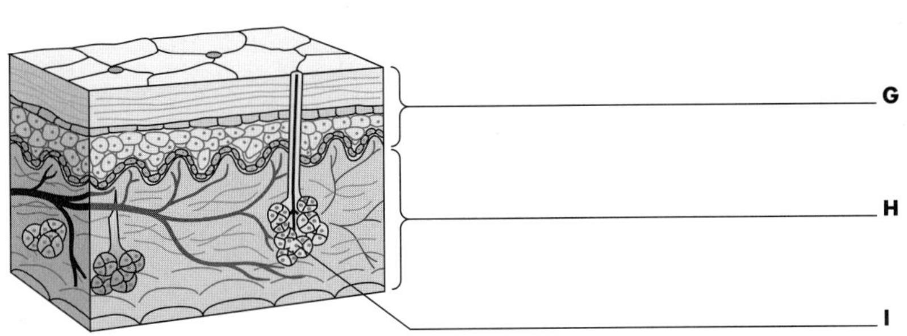

G. mucosa proper
H. lamina propria
I. gland

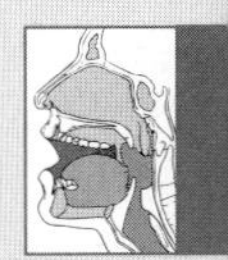

J

K

J. coll
K. papilla

REVIEW TEST 5.1

SELECT THE CORRECT ANSWER.

1. The three periodontal tissues are
   a. gingiva, PDL, cementum
   b. PDL, mucosa, alveolar bone
   c. gingiva, PDL, alveolar bone
   d. PDL, mucosa, gingiva

2. Which is not a component of the periodontal ligament (PDL)?
   a. collagen fibers
   b. nerve fibers
   c. blood vessels
   d. odontoblasts

3. The ends of collagen fibers of the PDL that are embedded in either alveolar bone or cementum are called
   a. collagen fiber bundles
   b. principal fibers
   c. elastic fibers
   d. Sharpey's fibers

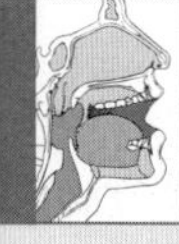

4. The primary function of the PDL is the attachment of the tooth to the alveolus. True or false?

5. Alveolar bone is covered with a thin layer of trabecular bone. True or false?

REVIEW TEST 5.2

SELECT THE CORRECT ANSWER.

1. The hard, thin layer of bone that lines the alveolus is called
   a. crestal bone
   b. alveolar bone
   c. lamina propria
   d. lamina dura

2. The points of bone found between the teeth are called
   a. papillae
   b. crestal bone
   c. alveolar bone
   d. lamina dura

3. That portion of the gingiva that attaches directly to the tooth is called
   a. sulcular epithelium
   b. attached gingiva
   c. attachment epithelium
   d. mucosa proper

4. Tissue that lines the periodontal pocket is called
   a. sulcular epithelium
   b. attached gingiva
   c. attachment epithelium
   d. mucosa proper

5. Gingiva directly adherent to alveolar bone is called
   a. gingiva proper
   b. free gingiva
   c. marginal gingiva
   d. attached gingiva

REVIEW TEST 5.3

SELECT OR FILL IN THE CORRECT ANSWER.

1. The bone that surrounds and holds the tooth is called the ______________.

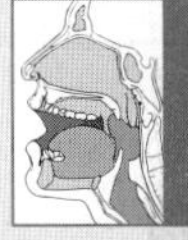

2. Attachment of the tooth to its bony socket is the main function of the ______________.

3. Alveolar bone comes to peaks between the teeth called ______________ bone.

4. The layer of compact bone that lines the alveolus is called the ______________.

5. Large bundles of collagen fibers that cross the PDL to provide attachment for the tooth are called ______________ fibers.

6. The ends of collagen fibers embedded in hard tissue (bone or cementum) are called ______________ fibers.

7. ______________ fibers provide a cushion for the tooth in its socket.

8. ______________ are cells that produce fibers.

9. ______________ is the firm, coral pink soft tissue that surrounds each tooth like a collar.

10. ______________ gingiva surrounds the cervices of the teeth and is not attached to bone.

11. ______________ gingiva is attached to and covers alveolar bone on its outer aspect.

12. Which tissue is not keratinized?
    a. attached gingiva
    b. attachment epithelium
    c. marginal gingiva
    d. free gingiva

13. ______________ epithelium lines the periodontal pocket.

14. ______________ epithelium attaches directly to the tooth.

REVIEW TEST 5.4

LABEL THE DIAGRAMS.

1.

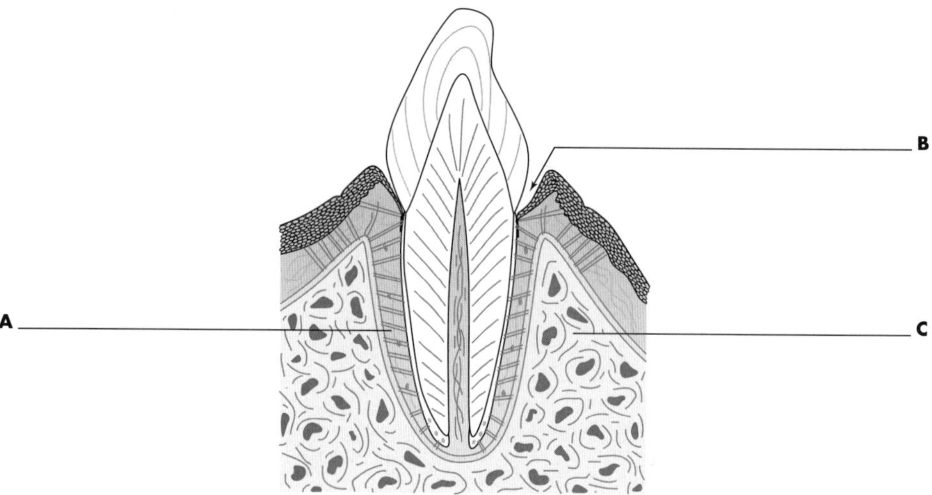

2.

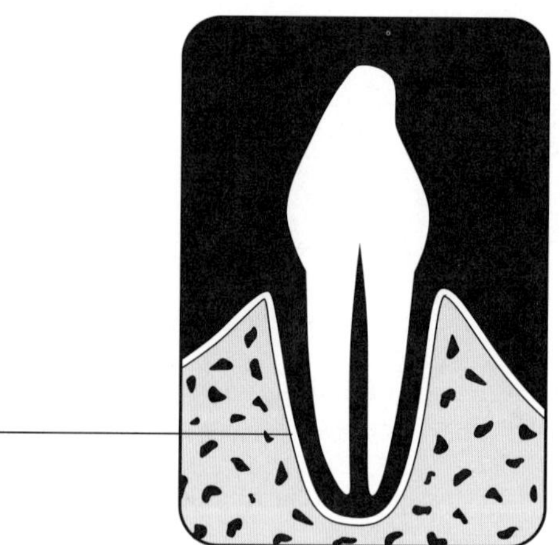

3.

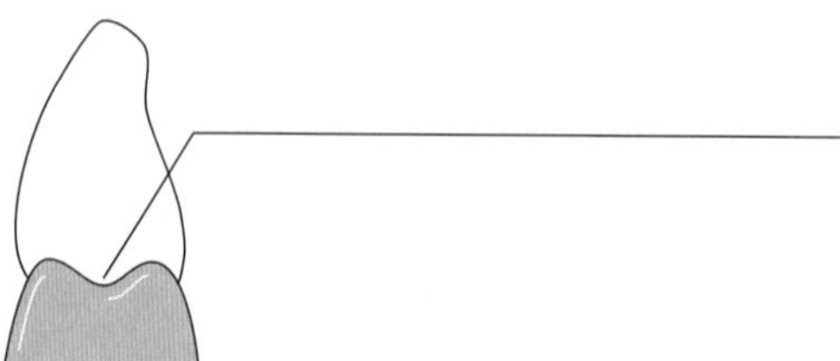

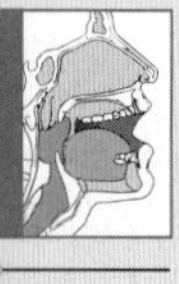

4.

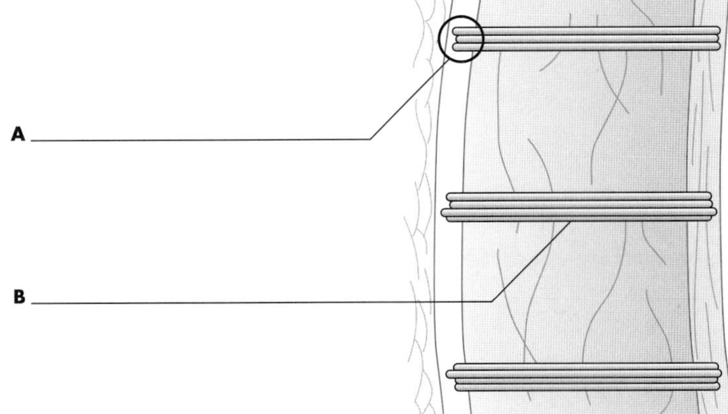

5.

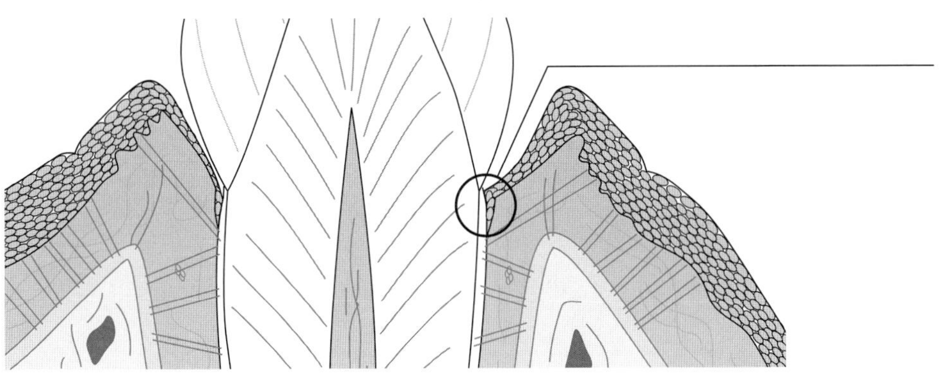

6.

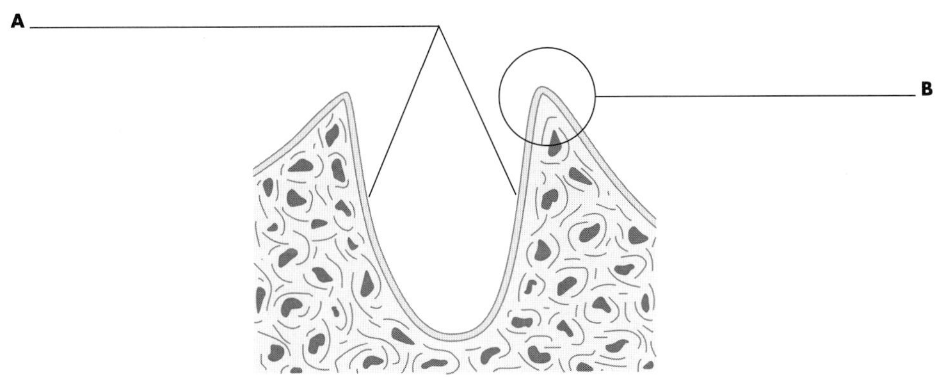

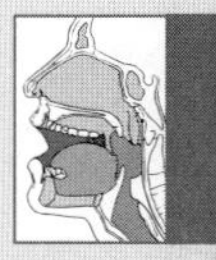

7.

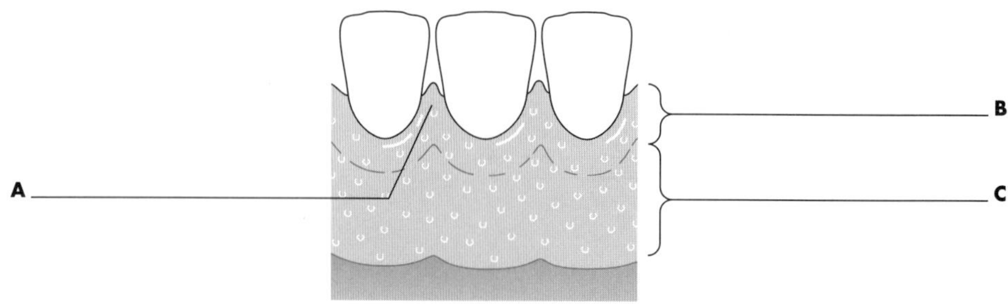

8.

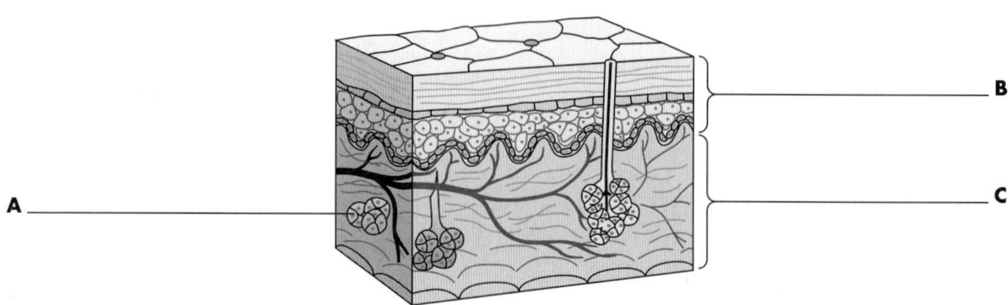

9.

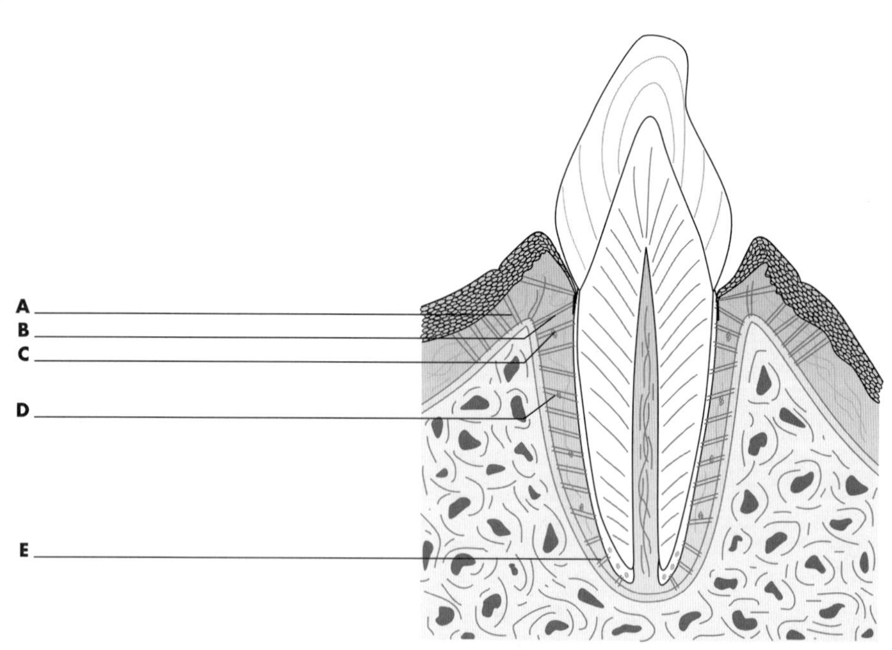

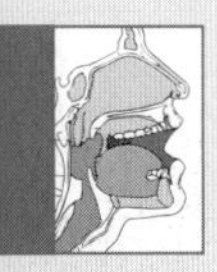

10.

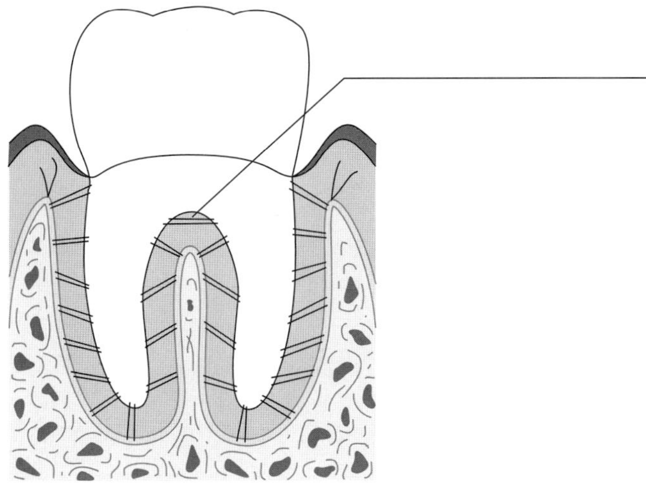

11.

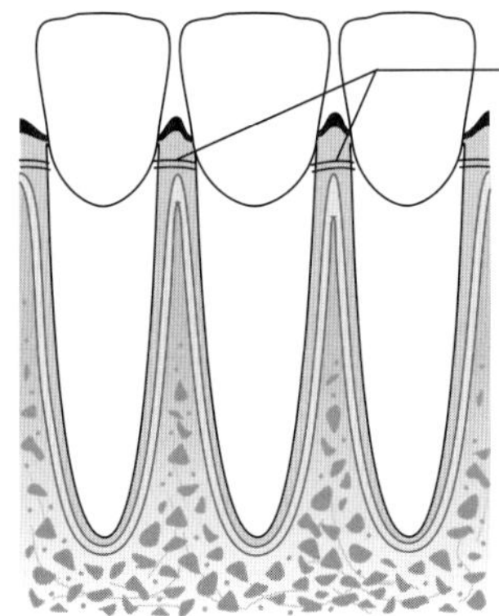

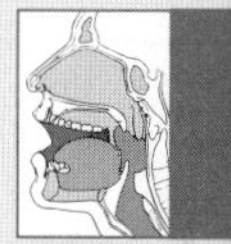

Mucosa and Other Oral Tissues

MUCOSA

1.0

Mucosa is the soft lining tissue of not only the oral cavity, but the entire digestive system. We briefly studied mucosa in Chapters One and Five. Let's review.

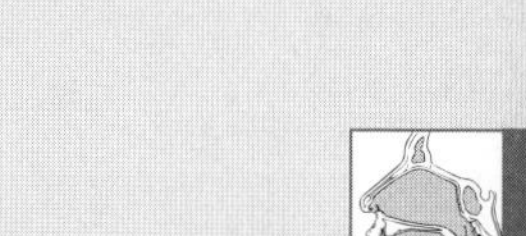

Mucosa, as stated, is a lining tissue. It is composed of three layers no matter where in the digestive tract it is found. The top or epithelial layer is called the **mucosa proper,** and the second or connective tissue layer is called the **lamina propria.** A third muscular layer is not present in the mouth.

mucosa proper, lamina propria

The oral mucosa is the mucosa of the mouth that lines the cheeks, tongue, maxillary and mandibular processes, and throat or pharynx. Oral mucosa is pictured here. It has two layers: the epithelial layer called the ______________ and the connective tissue layer called the ______________.

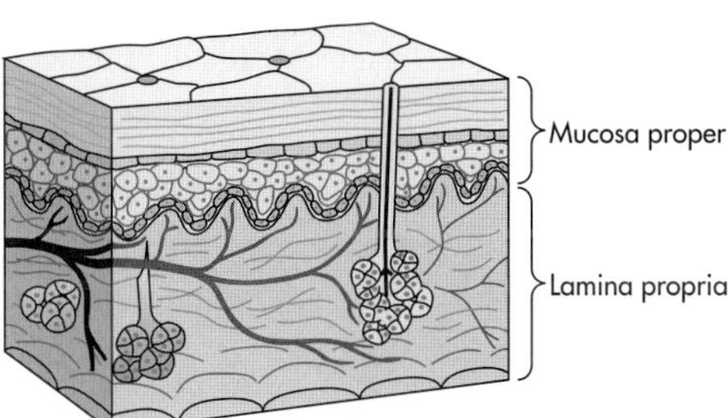

flat

Note that the oral mucosa resembles the skin. The mucosa proper is a stratified squamous epithelium or an epithelium with many layers of ______________ cells. Skin, however, has a thicker epithelium with many top layers of dead, keratinized cells called the stratum corneum.

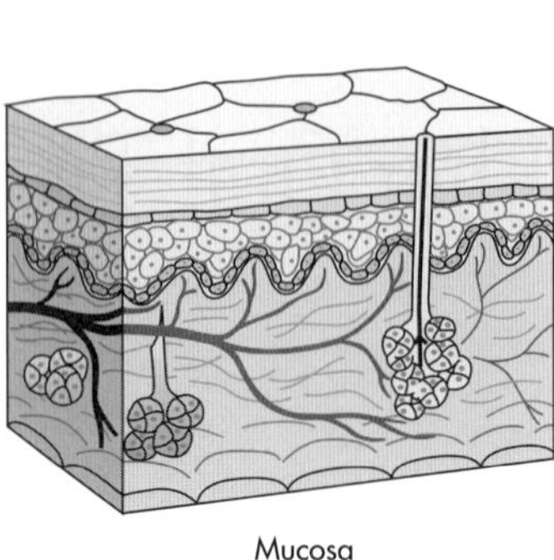

Mucosa

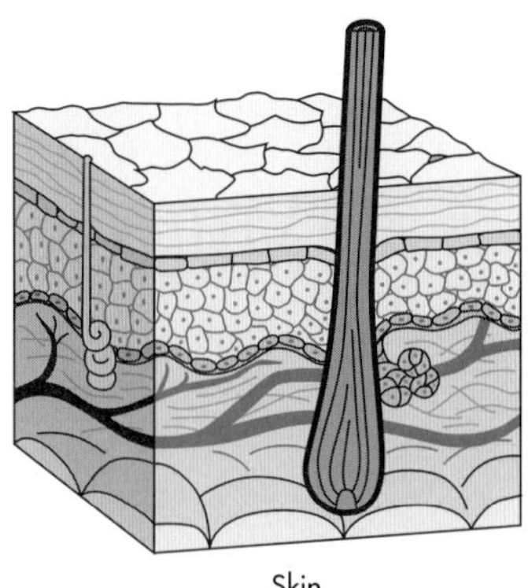

Skin

The mucosa proper of oral mucosa is a thin epithelium with mainly nucleated cells. In fact, the outermost layer of mucosa proper can easily be scraped off and placed on a slide showing the separate flat (squamous) cells.

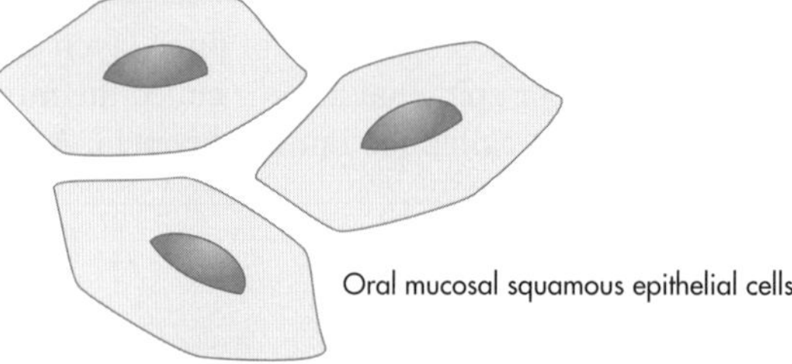

Oral mucosal squamous epithelial cells

lamina propria

The connective tissue layer is called the ______________ and contains many blood vessels as well as nerve fibers. Mucosa is a very vascular tissue compared with skin, meaning that it bleeds easily when damaged. Because of the abundance of vessels, it also heals quickly.

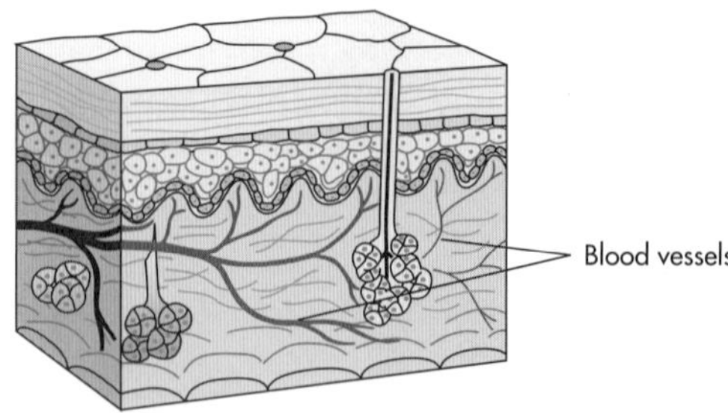

Fibers (mostly collagen) and fibroblasts are present in the lamina propria. They present in a dense, irregular pattern and provide a tough underlayer for the mucosa. The surface between mucosal epithelium and lamina propria is rippled to hold the two layers together.

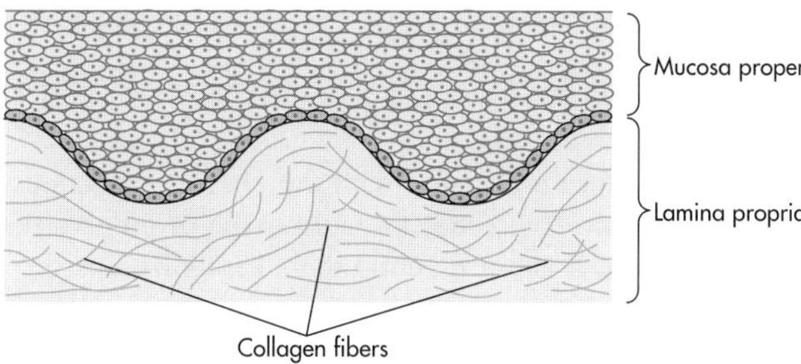

Glands may also be present in the lamina propria. In the case of oral mucosa these glands are salivary glands.

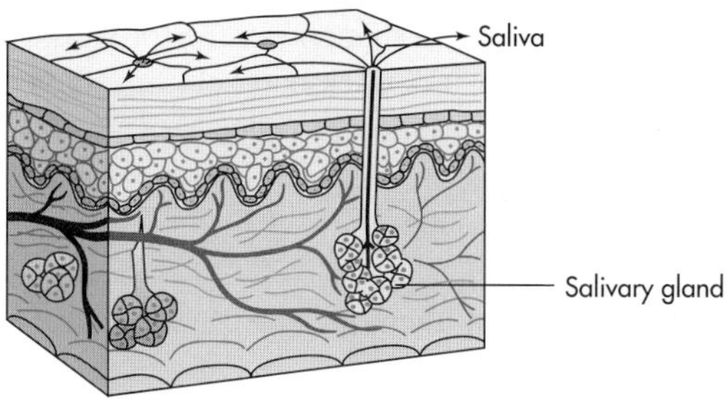

The surface of mucosa, unlike skin, must be maintained in a constantly moist environment. What structures help do this?

salivary glands

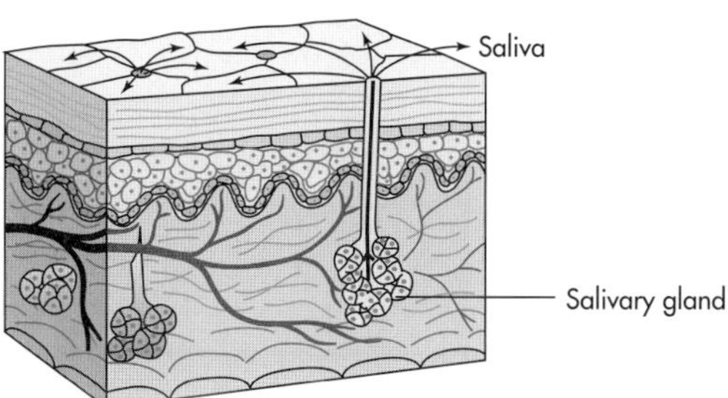

There are some regional differences in each type of oral mucosa and we will note them. One difference is that oral mucosa can be either **keratinized** (have the protein keratin in its epithelium) or **nonkeratinized.** Which type would be a stronger mucosa?

keratinized

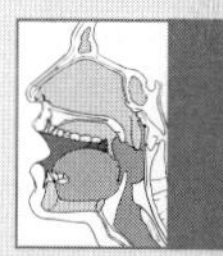

Categories of oral mucosa are labeled by their locations in the oral cavity:

1. masticatory mucosa
2. lining mucosa
3. specialized mucosa

Masticatory mucosa is mucosa associated with the chewing apparatus—the maxillary and mandibular jaws and teeth. It includes the gum tissue or **gingiva** that surrounds the teeth and the **palatal mucosa.** It is a firm, coral pink, keratinized tissue.

Lining mucosa is mucosa that lines the rest of the oral cavity, underside (ventrum) of the tongue, and back of the throat (pharynx). It is a reddish, thin, nonkeratinized tissue.

Specialized mucosa refers to the mucosa that covers the top of the tongue (dorsum). It is similar to masticatory mucosa in that it is thick and keratinized, but it contains very specialized cell structures to aid in the sensation of taste.

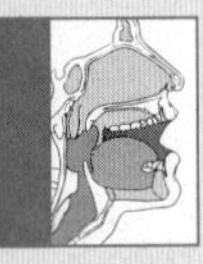

1. masticatory
2. lining
3. specialized

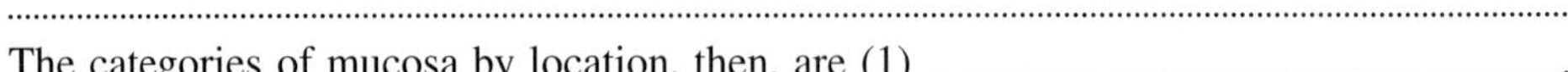

The categories of mucosa by location, then, are (1) ______________, (2) ______________, and (3) ______________. We further investigate each type.

1.1 Masticatory Mucosa

GINGIVA

We have already studied the gingiva in Chapter Five. Please review that material at this time.

Gingiva is the firm, coral pink soft tissue that surrounds each tooth like a collar. If healthy, it has a **stippled** surface. The gingiva creates a space between itself and the tooth called the **sulcus** or **periodontal** pocket.

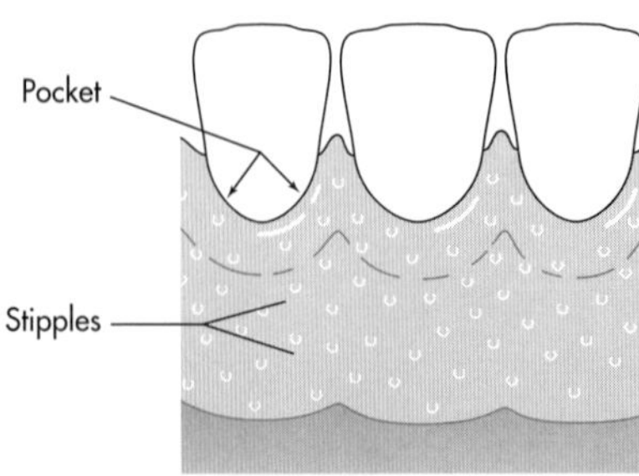

The gingiva either is attached to the alveolar bone that it covers **(attached gingiva)** or lies unattached around the tooth **(free gingiva).** Which type is keratinized?

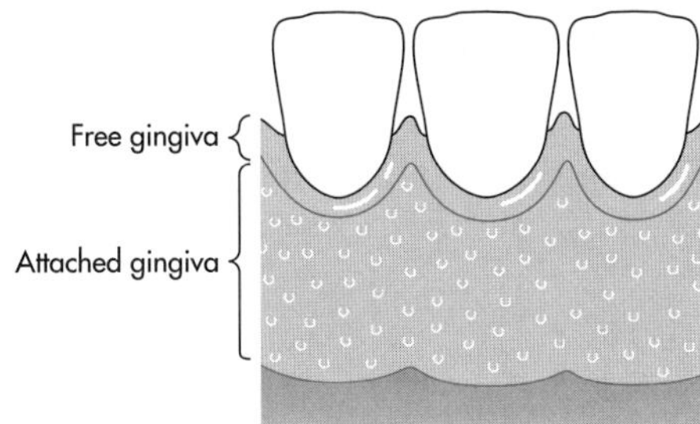

both

The **free gingiva** may also be divided into the **papillary gingiva** (the interproximal peaks of gingiva on both facial and lingual sides) and the **marginal gingiva,** which extends around the cervices of the tooth. What is below the free gingiva? What is the name of the line that divides them?

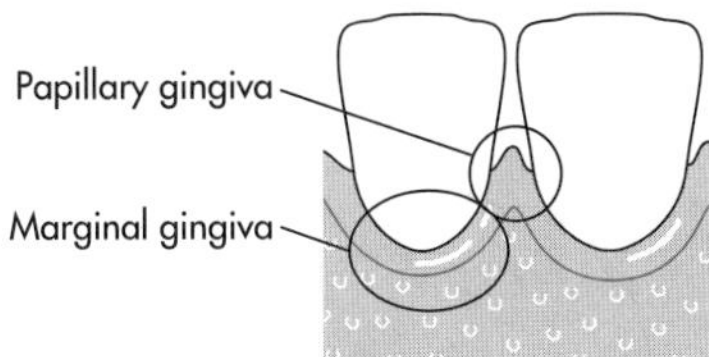

attached gingiva, free gingival groove

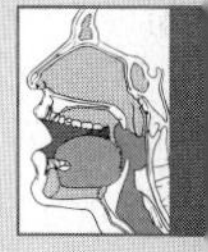

A section through the gingiva shows the free gingiva, the attached gingiva, the **free gingival groove,** and the epithelium of the sulcus or ______________.

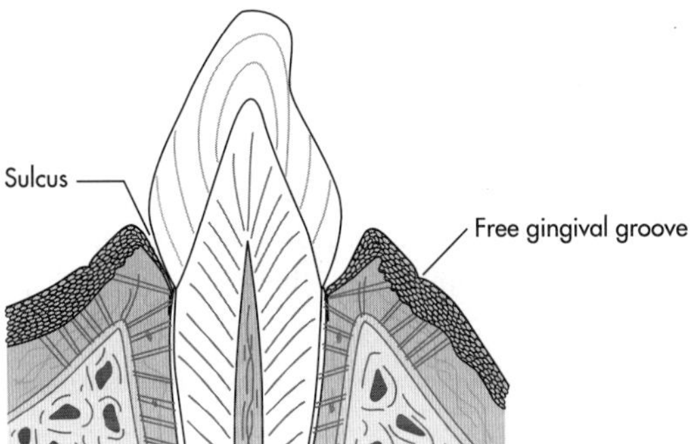

sulcular epithelium

rete pegs

Remember when looking at this section that the epithelial/connective tissue border of the gingiva is different from the rest of the mucosa. Follow it up from the pocket, where the border is relatively smooth, over the top and into the free gingiva, which has a highly scalloped border. This is caused by the extension of "fingers" of gingival epithelium into "fingers" of connective tissue of the gingival lamina propria. These are called ______________.

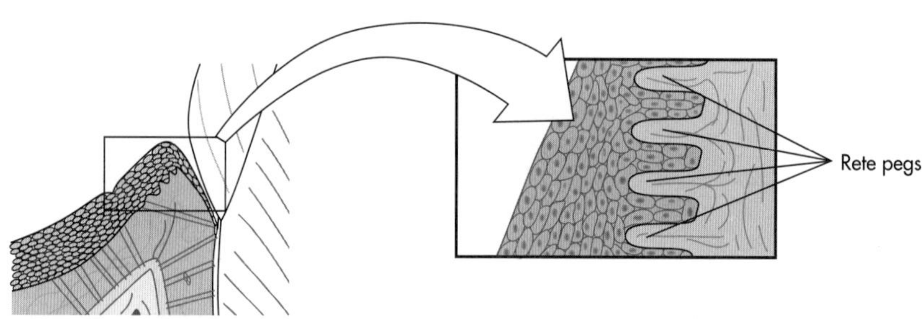

dentogingival, alveologingival, circular

Rete pegs are a device to strengthen the attachment of lamina propria to mucosa proper in this area, making gingiva a tough tissue to damage. There are collagen fibers in its lamina propria that attach to the the tooth and alveolar bone also. Name those fibers (see Chapter Five).

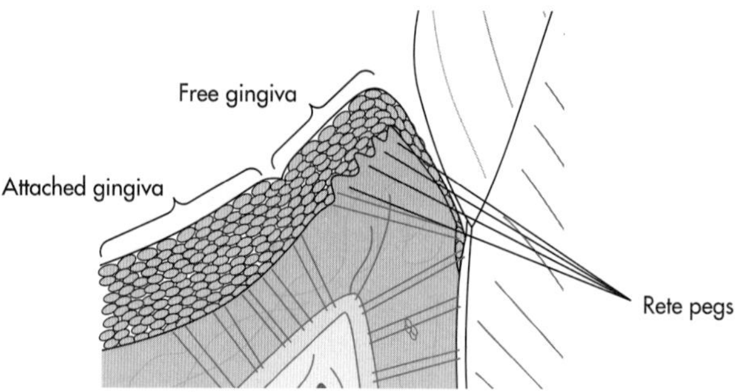

no

The **sulcular epithelium** is the gingival epithelium that lines the pocket. Is it keratinized? Remember that the very end of the epithelium that directly attaches to the tooth is called the **attachment epithelium** (a remnant of the enamel organ!).

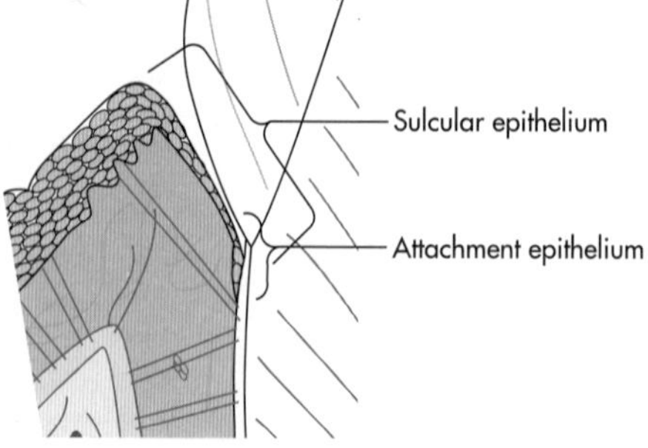

The sulcular epithelium is a thin, permeable tissue that is easily damaged. None of the sulcular epithelium is keratinized.

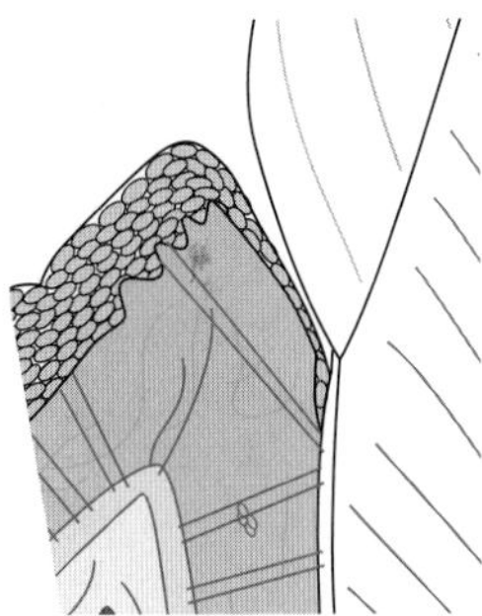

PALATAL MUCOSA

The mucosa of the palate, or roof of the mouth, is a continuation of the gingival tissue, so it resembles it in many aspects. It is also a firm, coral pink tissue, and because it takes a lot of wear and tear during mastication and swallowing, it is keratinized.

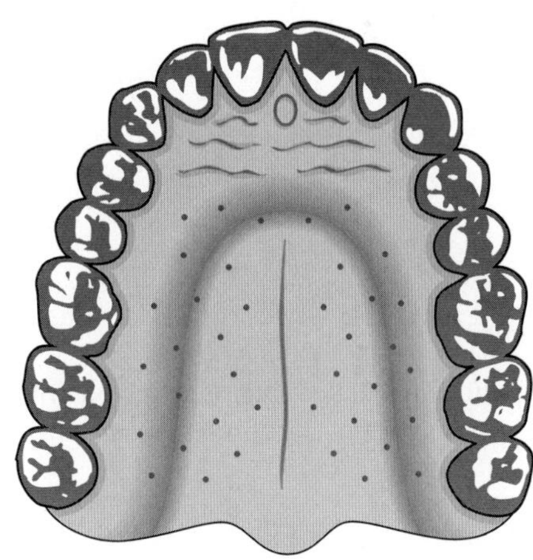

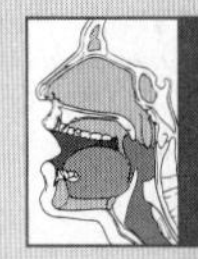

Palatal mucosa covers bone in an area called the hard palate. Beyond the hard palate is the soft palate, a "flap" of soft tissue that moves during swallowing to seal off the nasal cavity from the oral cavity. Beneath the mucosa covering the soft palate are cartilage, muscles, tendons, fat, and glands.

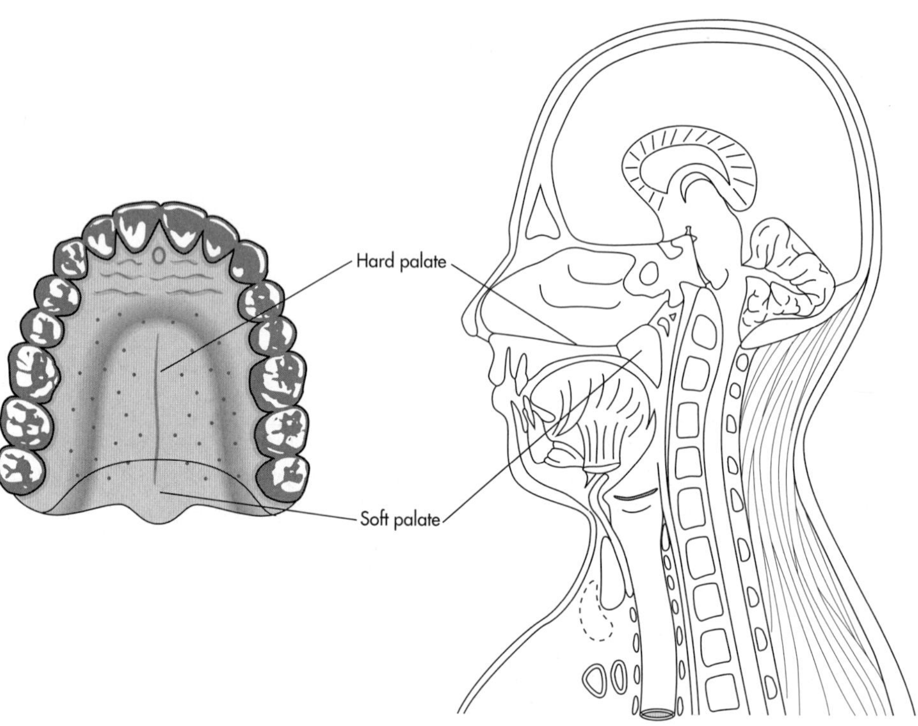

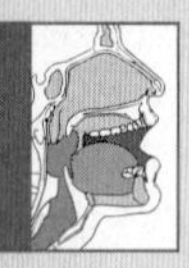

Palatal mucosa is thrown into folds called **rugae** in the anterior portion. Rugae are different in each individual and may serve in the breakdown of food masses during mastication.

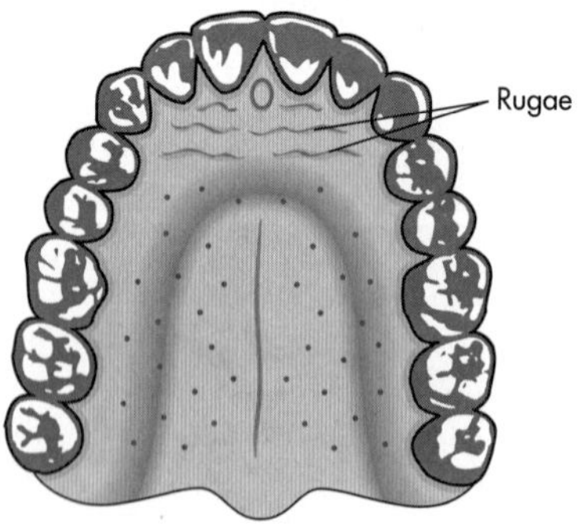

The folds are called ______________, but the bump anterior to and in the middle of these folds is a structure called the **incisive papilla.** It is an area where the mucosa covers a foramen with blood vessels and nerves that extend to the lingual anterior teeth.

rugae

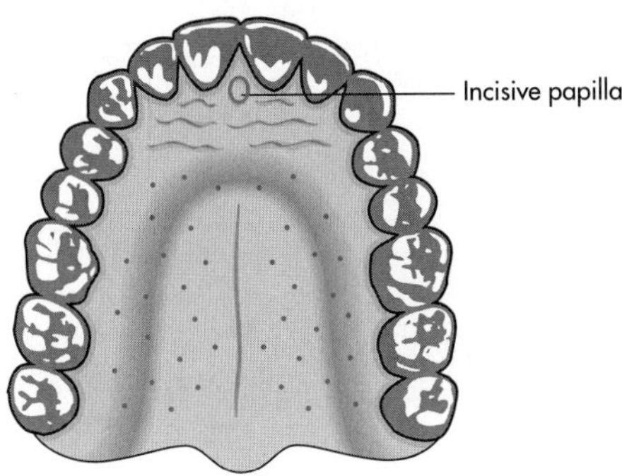

At the distal end of the palate lies a pendular structure called the **uvula.** It contains glandular tissue and is covered in palatal mucosa. The palatal mucosa also covers a bony joint in the midline called the **midpalatine suture.**

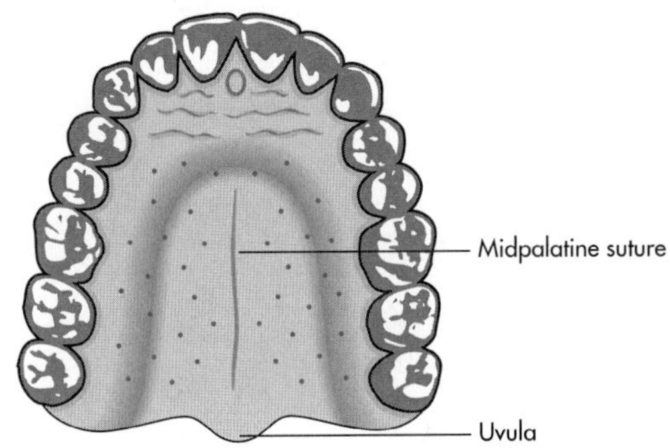

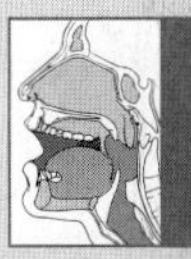

If we were to slice through the palatal mucosa, we would see a surface layer of epithelium (mucosa proper) and an underlying layer of connective tissue (lamina propria) resting on a layer of bone (hard palate bone). Superior to the bony layer is more lamina propria and the epithelial layer of the nasal cavity (which is quite different!).

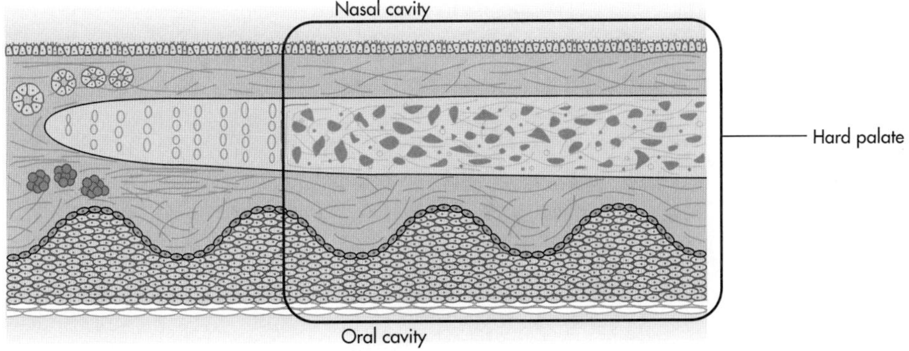

Bone is gone; different tissues are present.

A section taken further back in the soft palate area would resemble the diagram shown here. What is different?

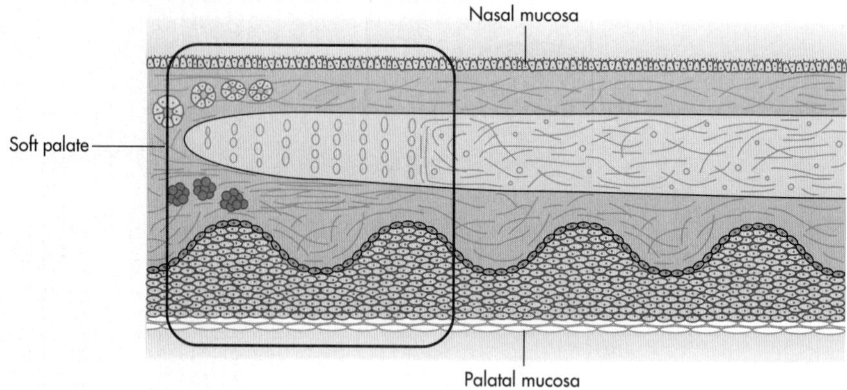

What is different about the layers? One layer is muscle and tendon. Cartilage replaces bone in the soft palate, and the lamina propria is filled with glands, mucous and salivary.

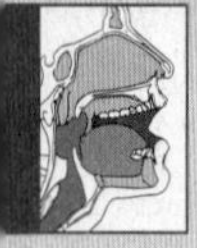

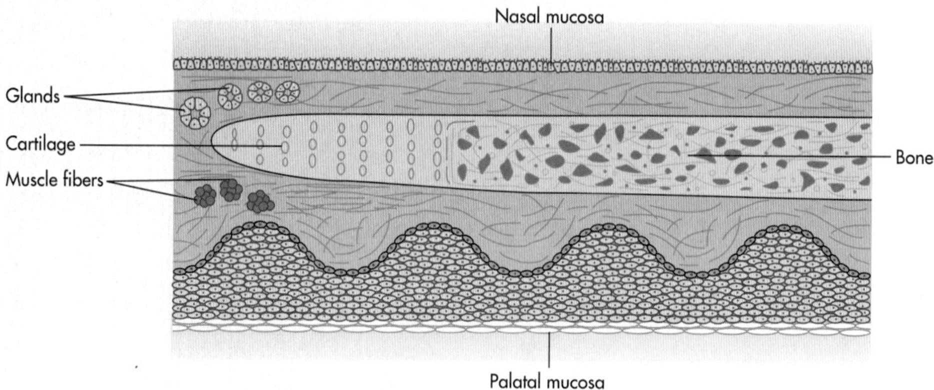

Scattered throughout the palatal mucosa are small, but distinguishable salivary glands called the minor salivary glands. You may be able to see them on the palate of patients as a series of dots. In smokers, these glands may stain a dark color.

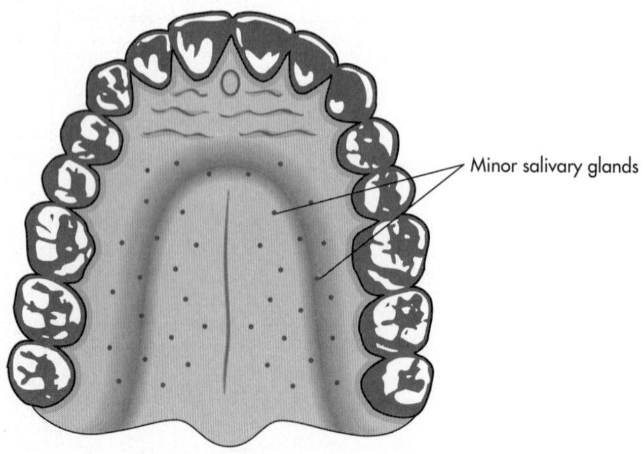

Label the areas of the masticatory mucosa we have studied so far.

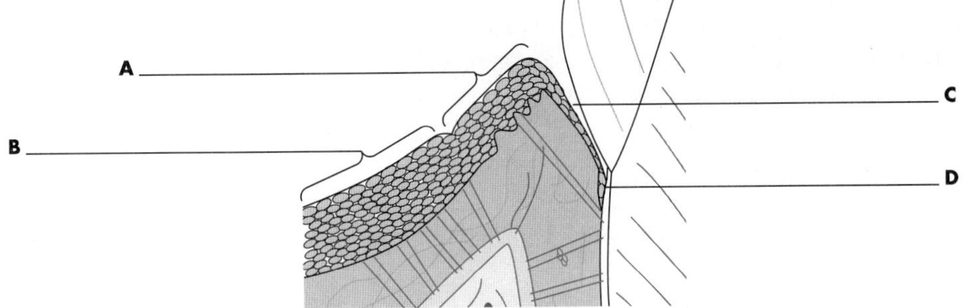

A. free gingiva
B. attached gingiva
C. sulcular epithelium
D. attachment epithelium

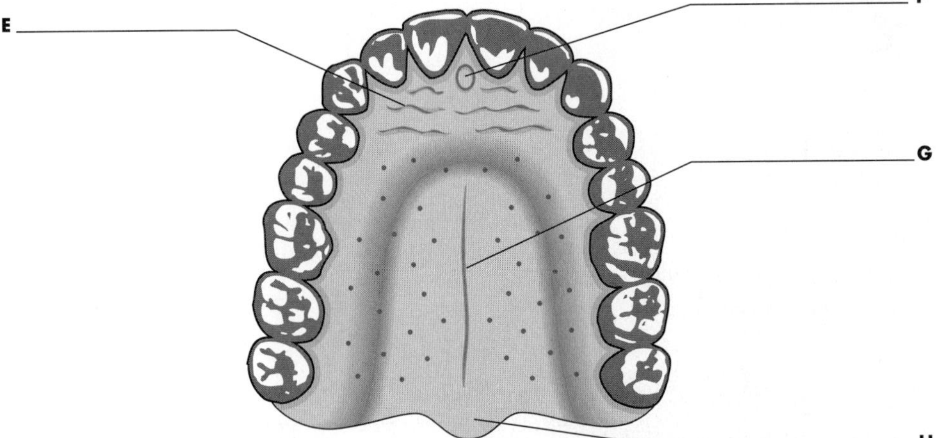

E. rugae
F. incisive papilla
G. midpalatine suture
H. uvula

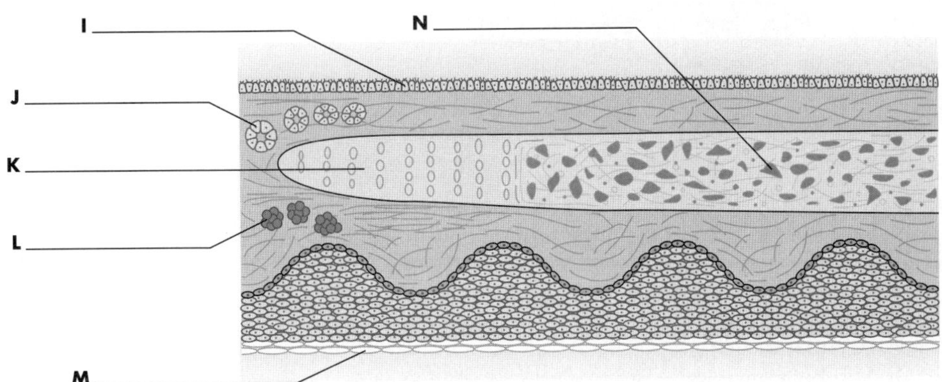

I. nasal mucosa
J. gland
K. cartilage
L. muscle fibers
M. palatal mucosa
N. bone

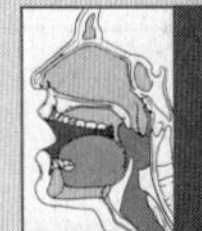

1.2

Lining Mucosa

With the exception of the areas just described covered with masticatory mucosa, the rest of the oral cavity and pharynx (throat) is covered with lining mucosa. In general, **lining mucosa** is a thin and very vascular mucosa, redder than masticatory mucosa. It is fragile and easily damaged, but repairs quickly. It is **nonkeratinized** mucosa.

masticatory mucosa, masticatory mucosa

Compare a section of lining mucosa with one of masticatory mucosa. Which tissue is thicker? Which is keratinized?

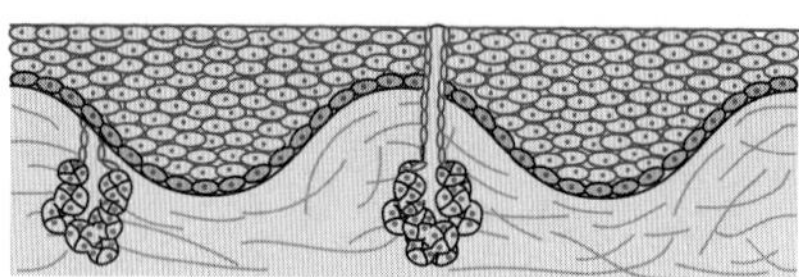

Lining mucosa

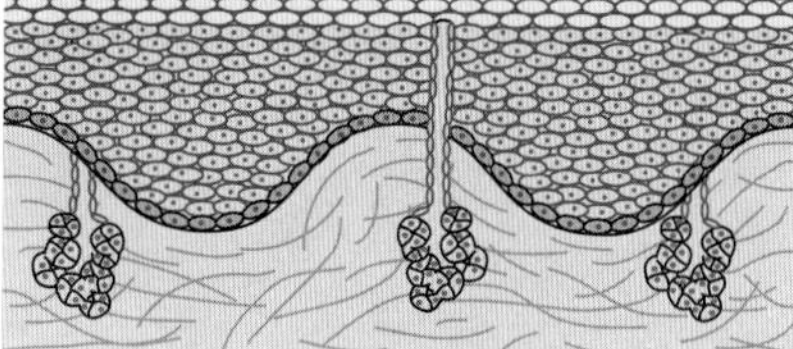

Masticatory mucosa

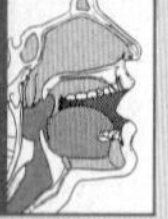

A. mucosa proper
B. lamina propria

Lining mucosa also consists of an upper epithelial layer called the ______________ and a lower connective tissue layer called the ______________. Glands, again, may appear in the lamina propria.

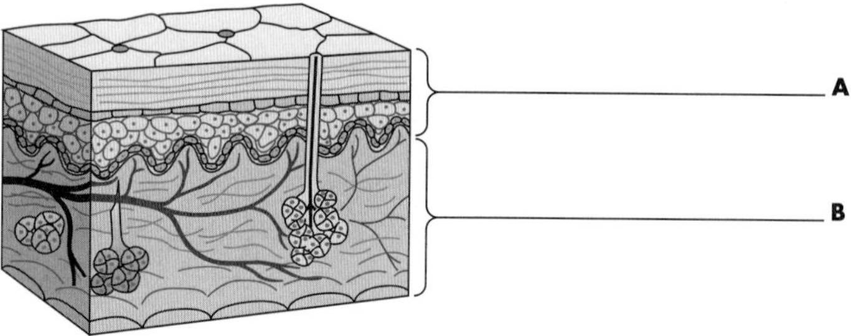

Lining mucosa begins at the end of the masticatory mucosa on top of the alveolar bone, goes down over the end of the jaws, turning upward again to line the cheeks and lips in a continuous sheet of mucosa. Lining mucosa is named for the location in which it is found. Histologically, there is not much difference between the different types:

1. Alveolar mucosa
2. Vestibular mucosa
3. Buccal mucosa
4. Labial mucosa
5. Ventral tongue mucosa
6. Pharyngeal mucosa

ALVEOLAR MUCOSA

As its name implies, **alveolar mucosa** covers the rest of the alveolar ridges. It begins where the gingiva ends, at the **mucogingival junction.** You can see this in your own mouth as a border between the coral pink tissue surrounding the teeth and the red tissue just below it.

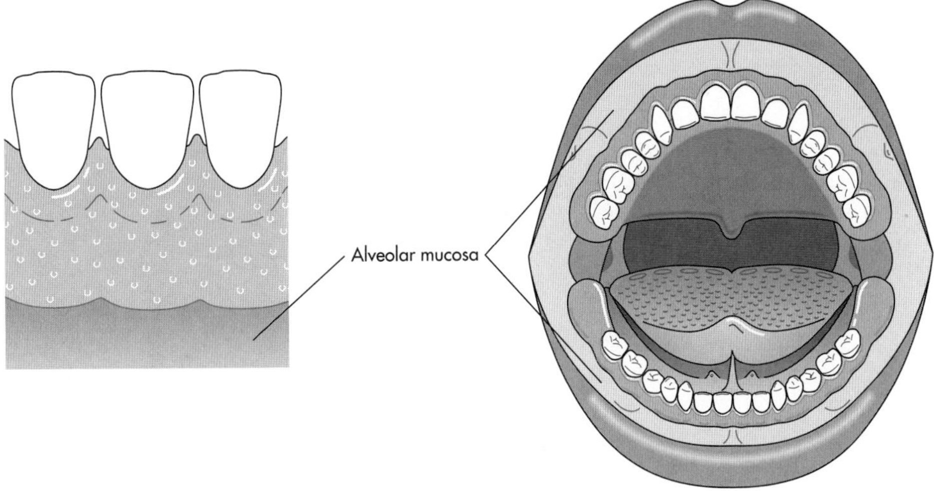

The ______________ junction is a line or border between the gingiva and the alveolar mucosa. What was the line between the free gingiva and the attached gingiva?

mucogingival,
free gingival groove

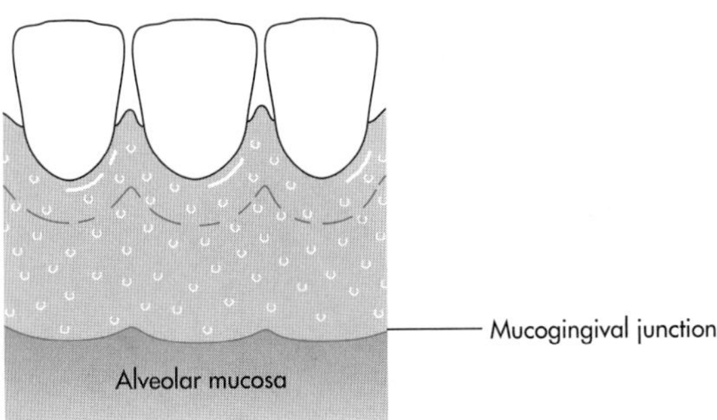

Find the mucogingival junction. What tissue lies above it?

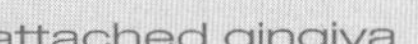

attached gingiva

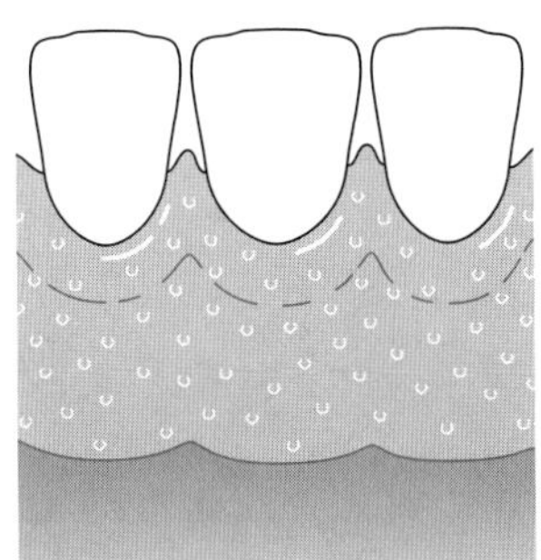

Alveolar mucosa appears much thinner than the gingiva above it and is much more loosely attached to the underlying bone than the gingiva. In fact, you can pull on the alveolar mucosal tissue in some areas, moving the tissue. This is possible because of the lack of strong attachment fibers from lamina propria to underlying bone. Which tissue is strongly attached?

attached gingiva

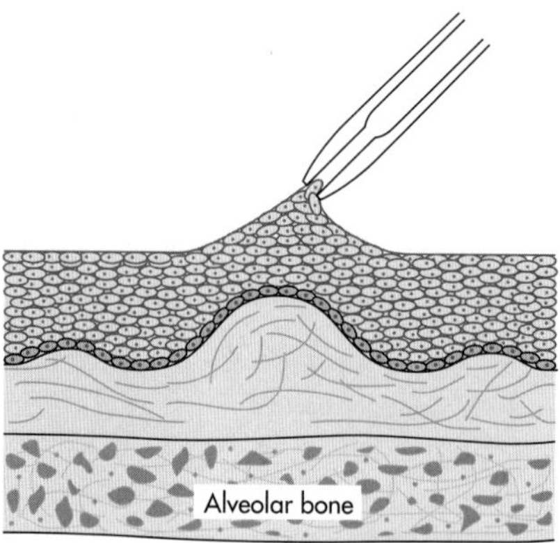

Alveolar mucosa is folded over in several places in the mouth. These folds of mucosa are called **frena** (singular, frenum). Each frenum is named for the location in which it is found. There are usually two **labial frena.**

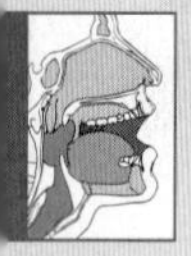

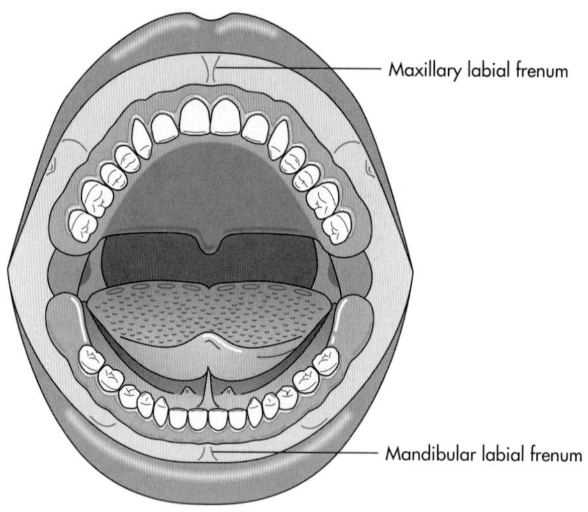

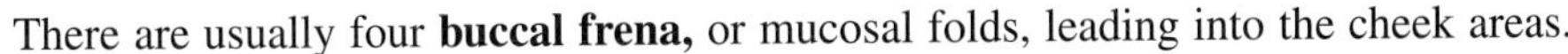

There are usually four **buccal frena,** or mucosal folds, leading into the cheek areas.

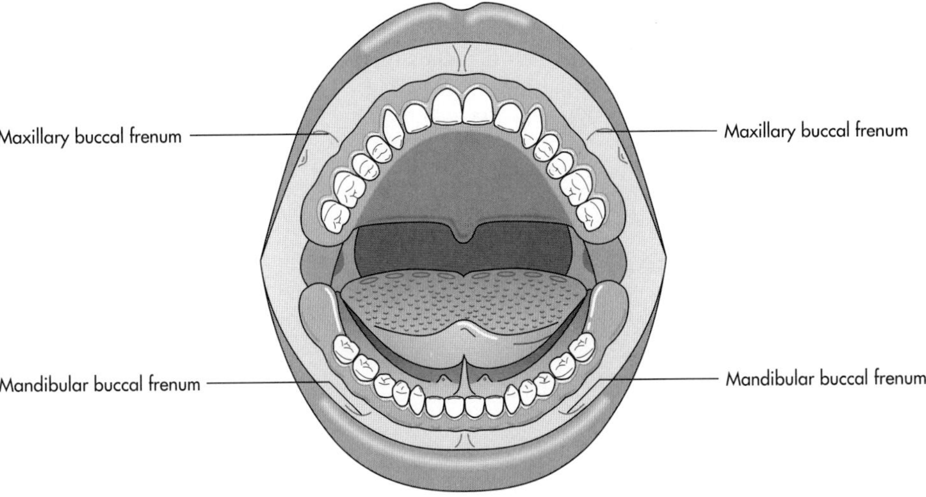

The **lingual frenum** is found under the tongue as a fold of the ventral tongue mucosa.

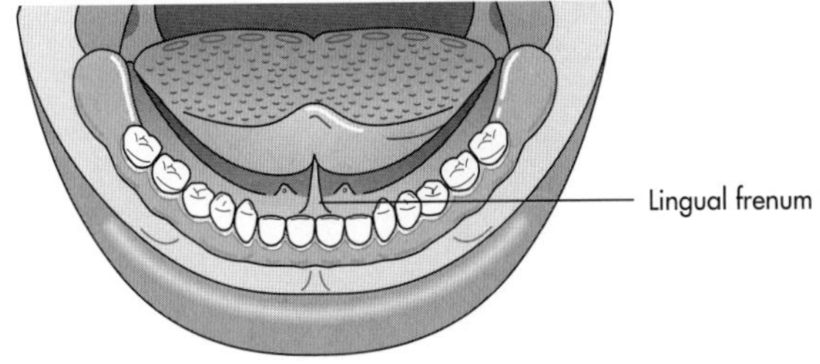

Label the different frena found in the drawing.

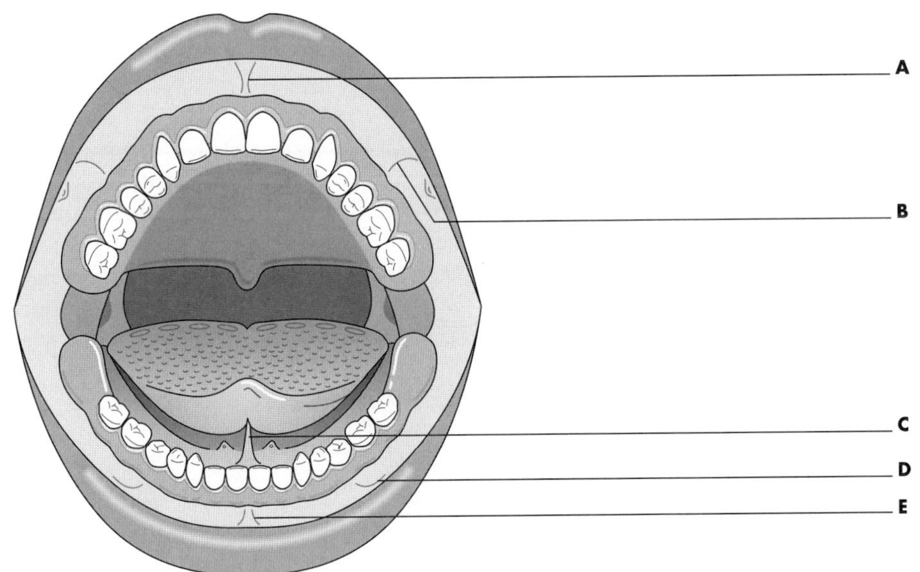

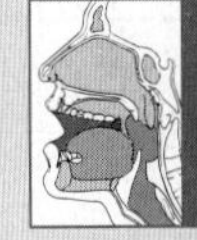

A. maxillary labial frenum
B. maxillary buccal frenum
C. lingual frenum
D. mandibular buccal frenum
E. mandibular labial frenum

VESTIBULAR MUCOSA

Lining mucosa continues off of the mandible and maxilla, turning up to line the cheeks, lips, and tongue. The area created when it makes this turn is a horseshoe-shaped trough called a **vestibule,** and the tissue that lines it is called **vestibular mucosa.**

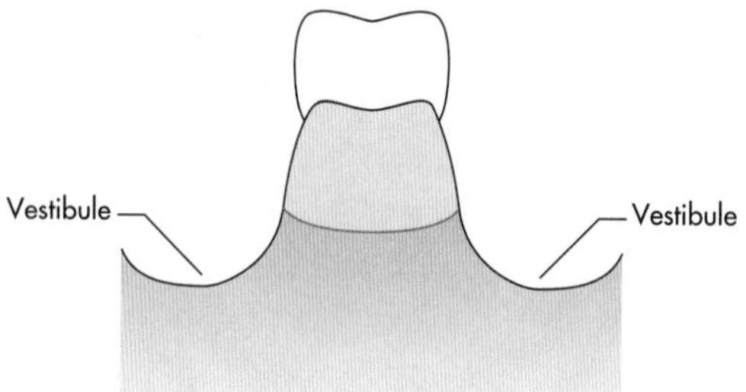

mucosa

Two long vestibules are created at the bottom of each alveolar area. Vestibular mucosa is just a continuation of alveolar ______________. Two horseshoe-shaped troughs are created.

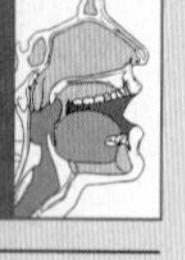

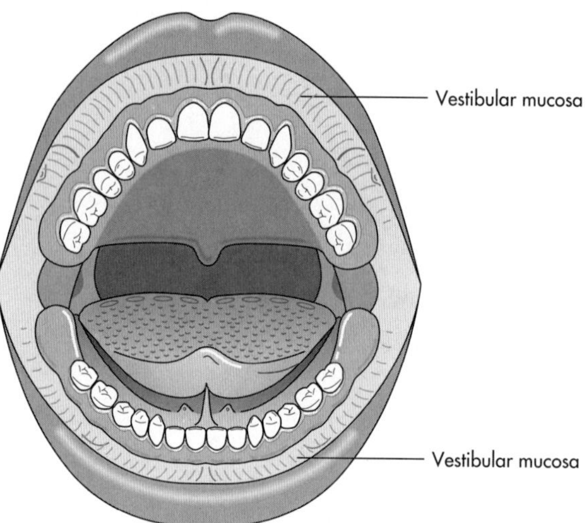

In the lingual area, where mandibular alveolar mucosa ends, a trough-like area of vestibular mucosa forms the **floor of the mouth.** This is a particularly thin area of lining mucosa where you can even see the blood vessels beneath it. Because there is easy access to the bloodstream from this area, several medications may be administered beneath the tongue.

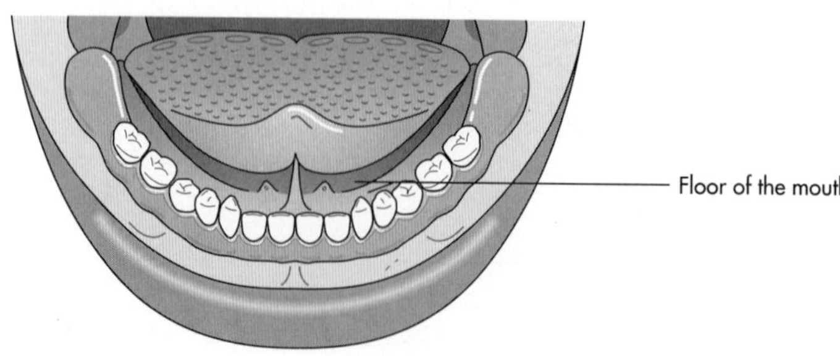

The floor of the mouth also is an area where the ducts of two major salivary glands are found. The **sublingual caruncles** or papillae are where **Wharton's ducts** from the two submandibular salivary glands empty.

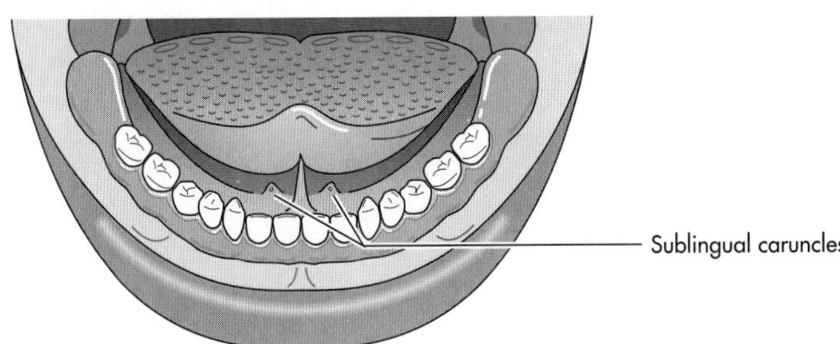

The mucosa of the floor of the mouth rises in two folds on both sides creating the **sublingual plicae.** These folds contain the **ducts of Rivinus,** which are tiny ducts from the sublingual salivary gland.

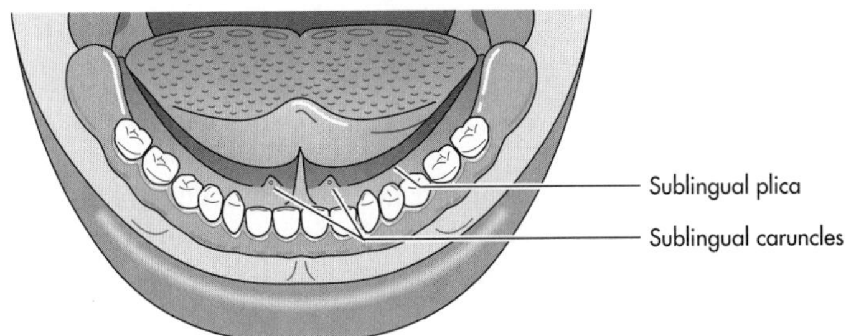

Identify the structures associated with the vestibular mucosa and floor of the mouth.

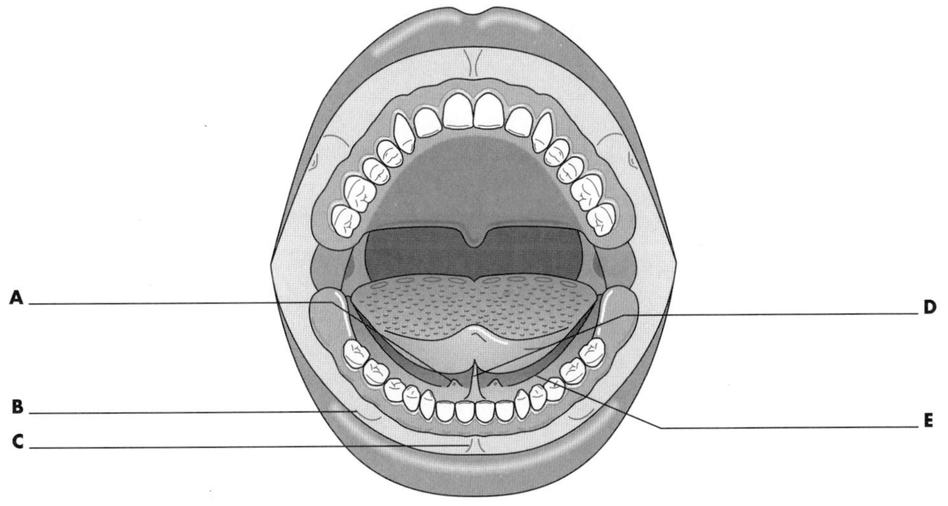

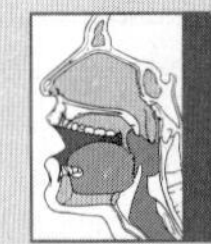

A. sublingual caruncle
B. buccal frenum
C. labial frenum
D. lingual frenum
E. plica

BUCCAL MUCOSA

The lining of the cheeks is called the **buccal mucosa.** It comes from a word meaning "cheek" and covers the chief muscle of the cheek, the **buccinator muscle.**

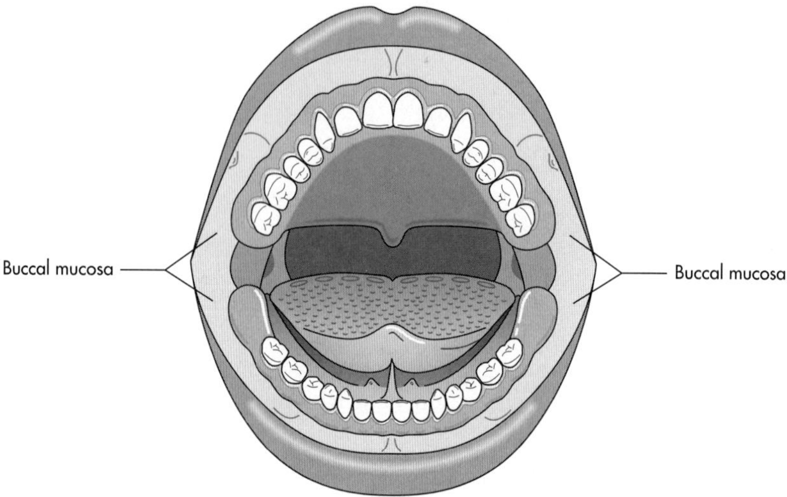

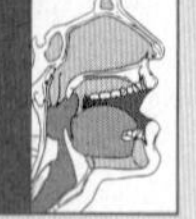

buccinator

At the top and bottom of the buccal mucosa lies the vestibule, which is lined with the same type of lining mucosa. See the diagram of a section through buccal mucosa. It is like any of the preceding lining mucosas, except it lies over muscle tissue, the ______________ muscle in particular.

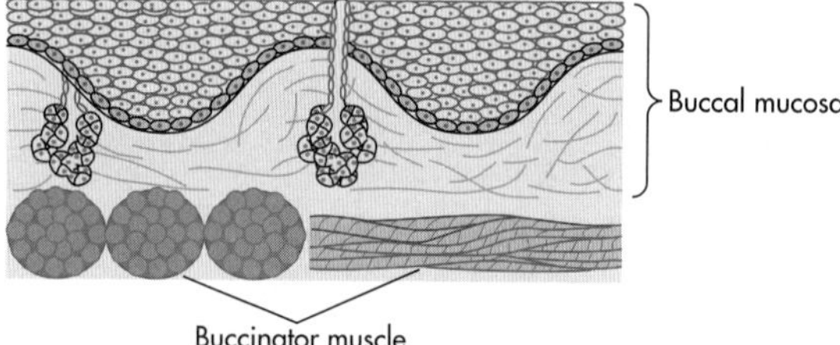

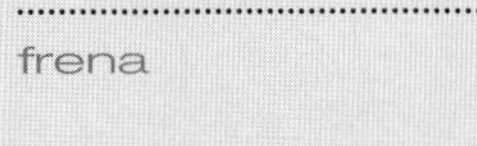

frena

Remember that the buccal mucosa sends folds over the vestibular area and into the alveolar mucosa called ______________. There are usually four buccal frena, one on each side of the mandible and maxilla.

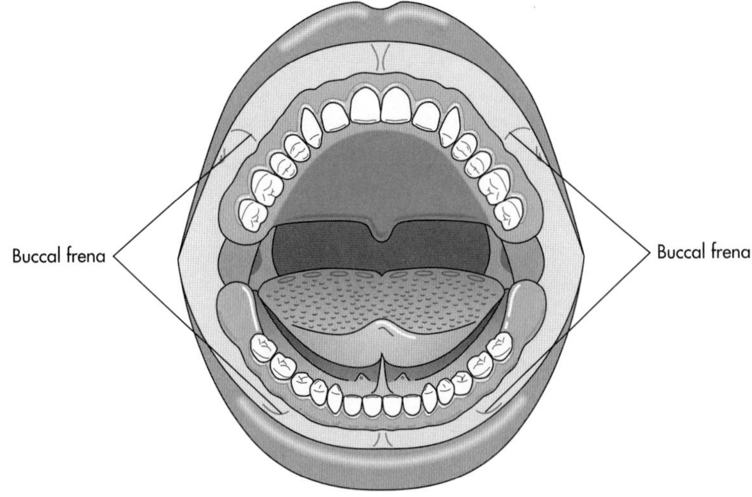

Stensen's, parotid gland

A structure found in the buccal mucosa is the papilla that houses the opening into Stensen's duct. ______________ duct comes from the parotid gland and pierces the buccinator to empty into a papilla directly opposite the maxillary second molar, the **parotid papilla.** From which major salivary gland does Stensen's duct arise?

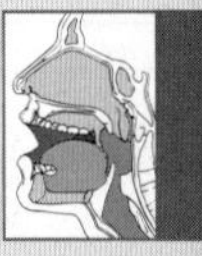

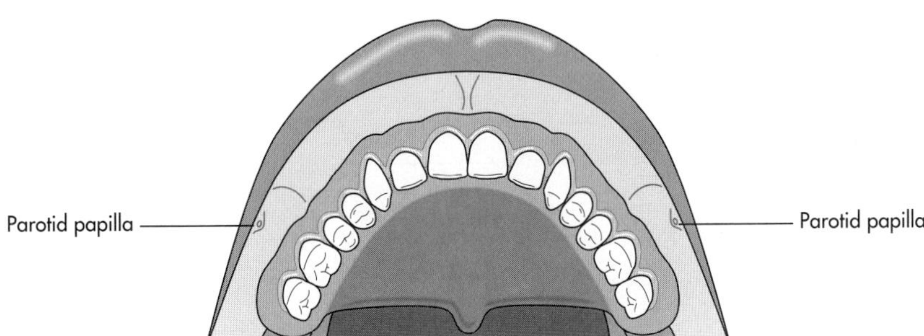

There are a pair of **parotid glands** on the outermost aspect of each cheek, directly below the skin and above the muscle.

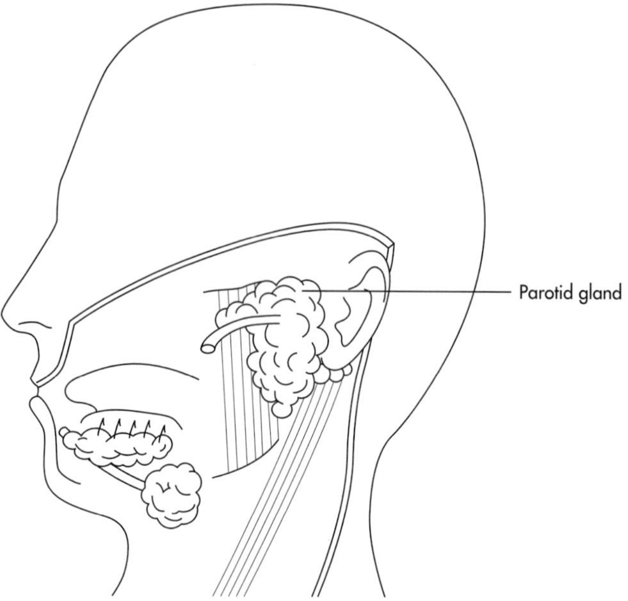

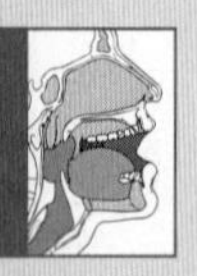

The teeth may occlude with the buccal mucosa between them in some people, creating a rough horizontal fold of tissue in a line along the occlusal plane. This is called a **linea alba** and is normal for some patients.

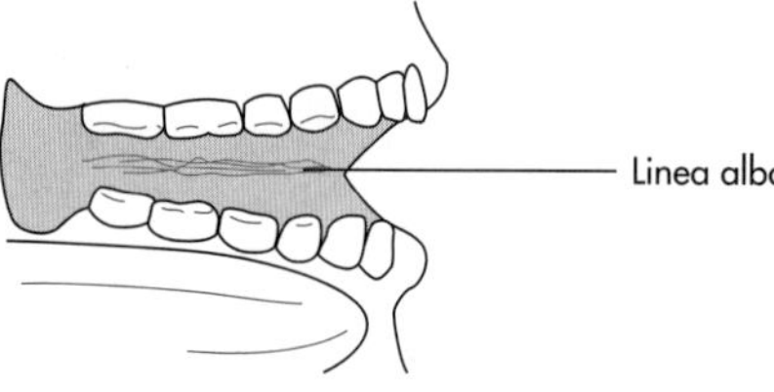

At the end of the oral cavity and buccal mucosa is a vertical line created when the patient is asked to "open wide." It looks like a cord of tissue and shows beneath the mucosa, where the end of the buccinator muscle joins the beginning of the superior constrictor muscle of the pharynx. This "line" is called the **pterygomandibular raphe** or just raphe. It is one of the borders between the oral cavity and the oropharynx.

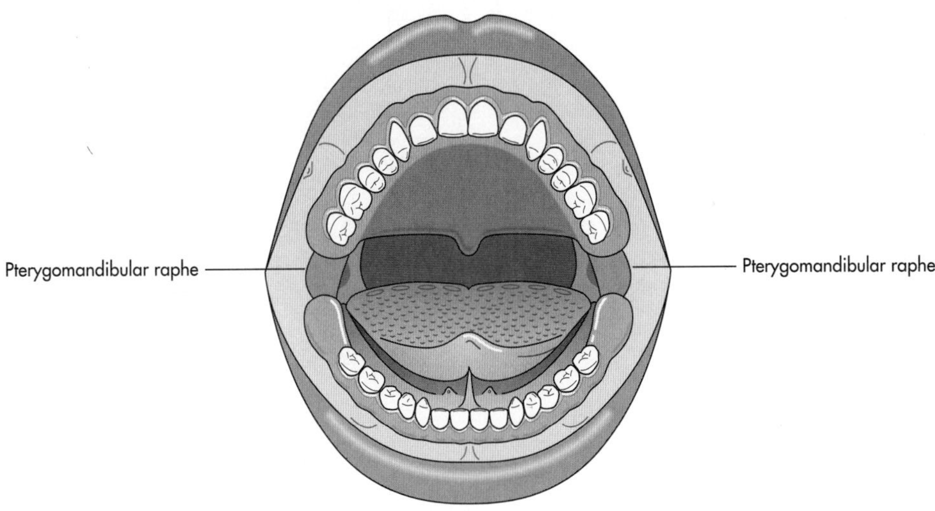

The buccinator and superior constrictor muscles come together to create the _______________ under the mucosa.

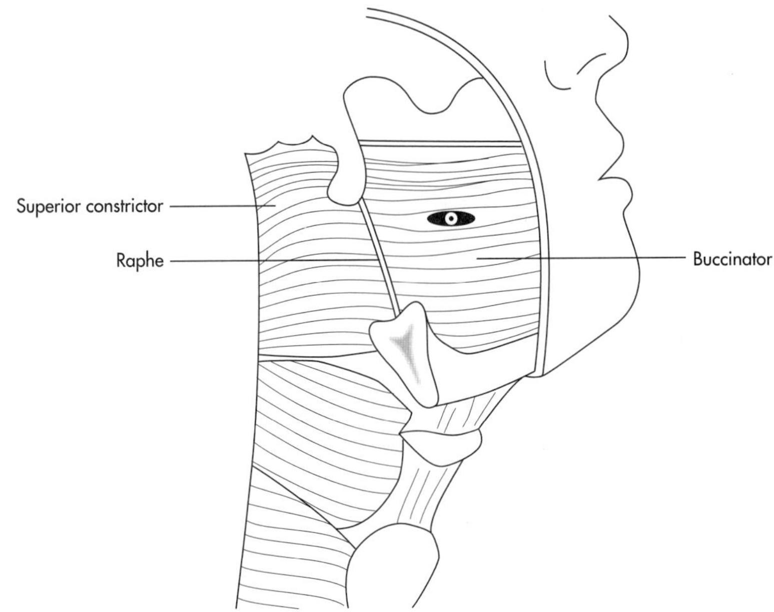

pterygomandibular raphe

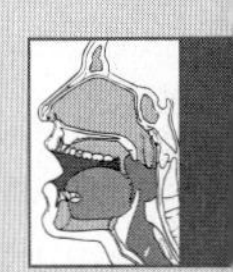

Color the area of the buccal mucosa in the drawing. Label the papilla for Stensen's duct. Find frena. Find the raphe. Refer to the previous text for your answers.

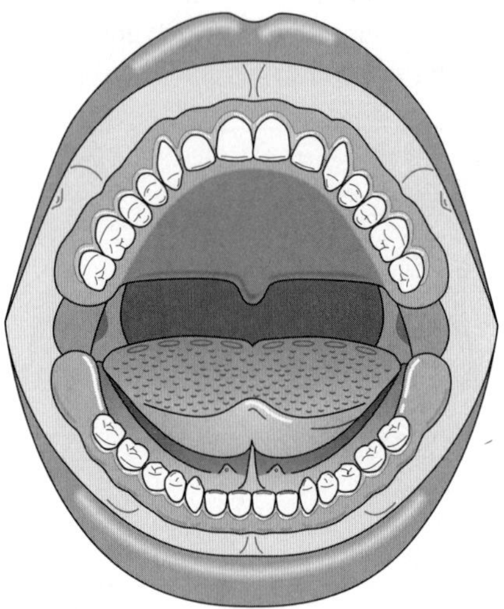

LABIAL MUCOSA

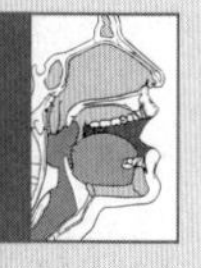

The lining mucosa of the oral cavity continues from the cheeks anteriorly to the lips, where it becomes labial mucosa.

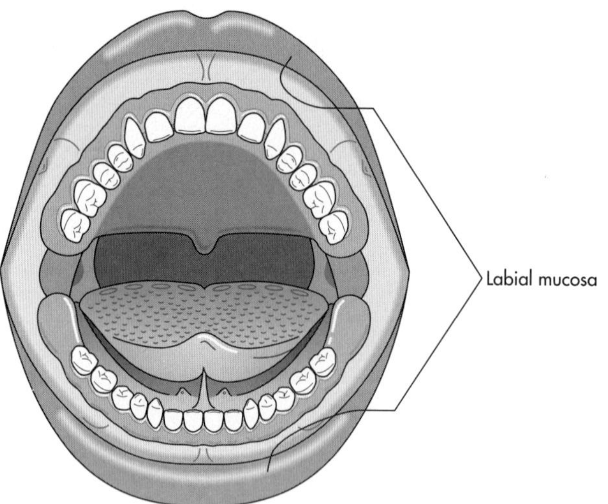

Labial mucosa is the mucosa that lines the ________________. The tissues directly below the labial mucosa are the muscles of the lip and then the outer skin of the lip. A section through a lip is diagrammed.

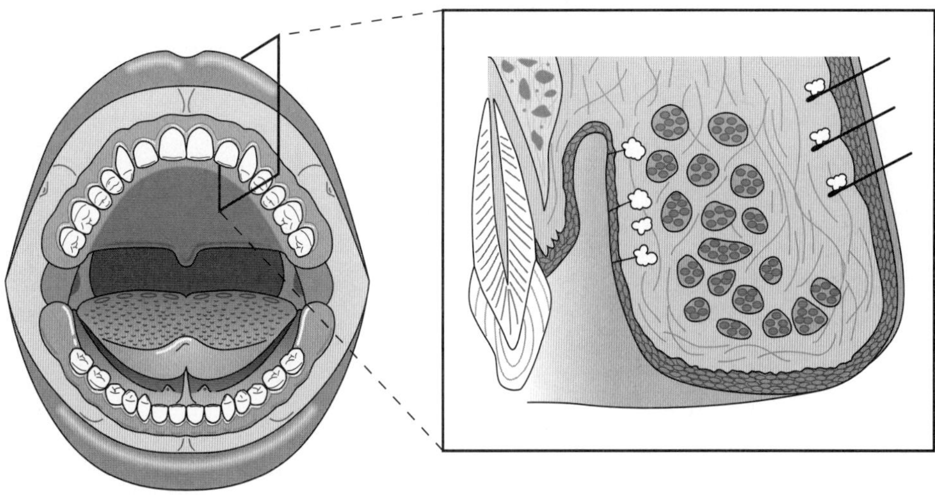

lip

The lip is an unusual area because it demonstrates a transition from skin to oral mucosa. The first difference you can see is the change in thickness. Which is thicker?

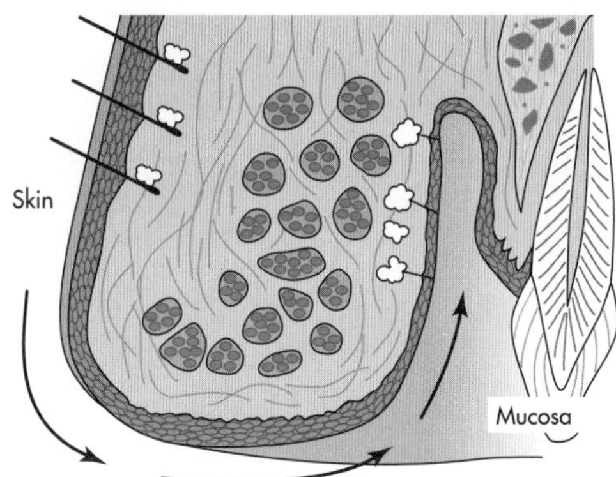

skin

The keratinized, stratified squamous epithelium of the skin is thicker than the stratified squamous epithelium of the mucosa. Also, the skin contains the protein ________________ and several layers of dead cells called the stratum corneum.

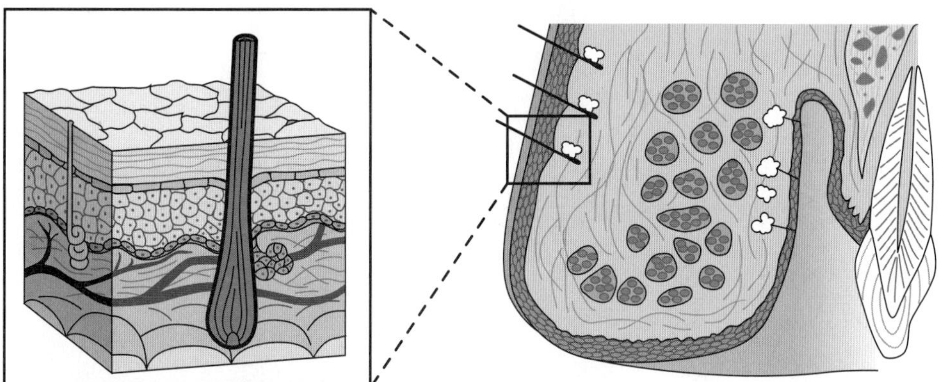

keratin

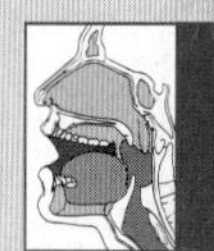

vascular; no—it has sweat and sebaceous glands

Labial mucosa, like the other lining mucosas, has a thin epithelium and a lamina propria with salivary glands. The lamina propria also has many blood vessels, making it very ______________. Does skin have salivary and mucous glands?

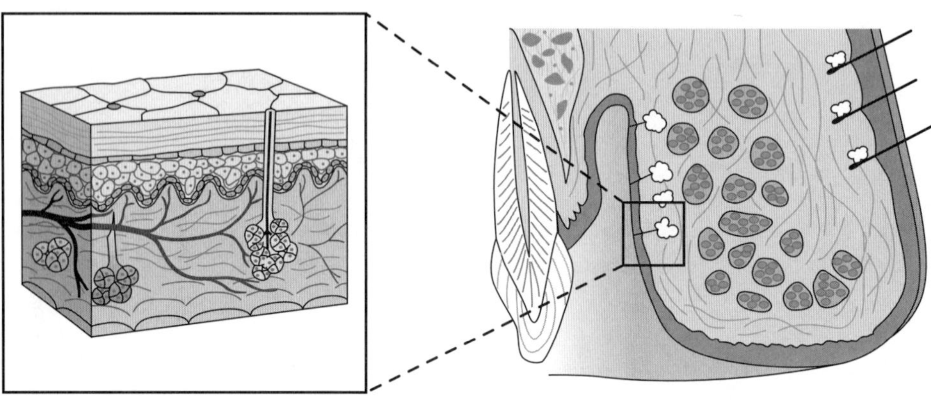

hair follicles

The skin has several "projections" that the mucosa does not have. What are these?

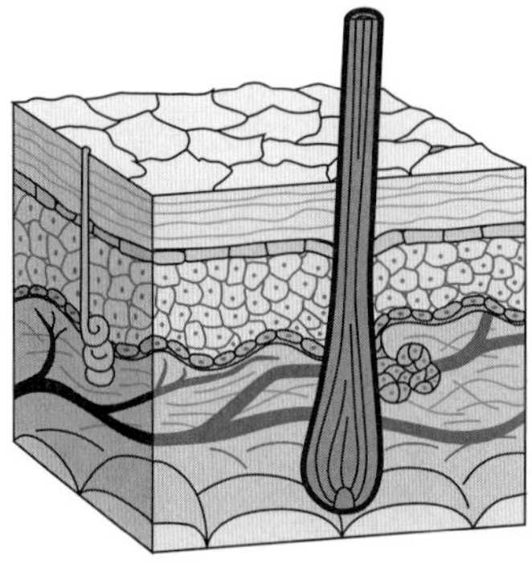

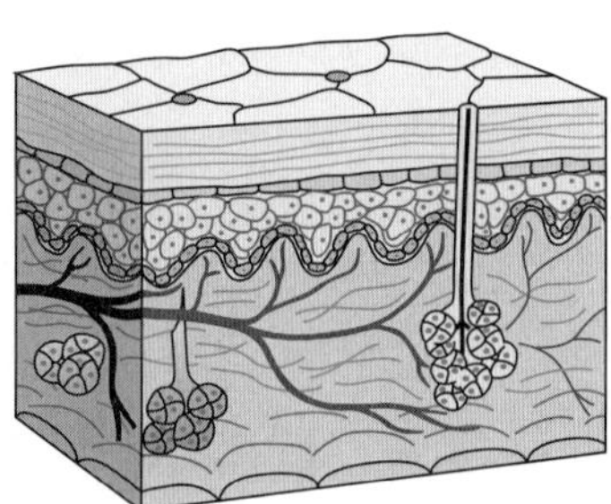

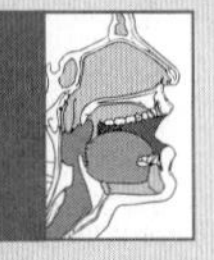

The zone of transition from skin to mucosa occurs in that part of the lip that can be seen just outside the mouth; it is called the **vermillion border** or "red border" for its color. In this zone the epithelium is becoming thinner, gaining glands, losing hair, and starting to look more like mucosa.

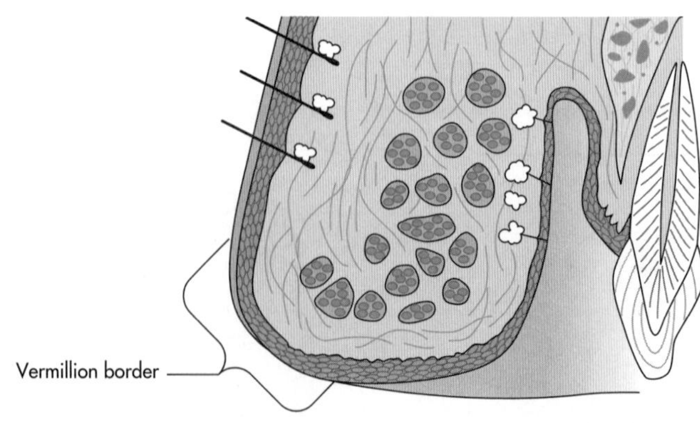

The ______________ border is a zone of transition from skin to mucosa. Remember what slices through these tissues would look like. Which is which?

vermillion

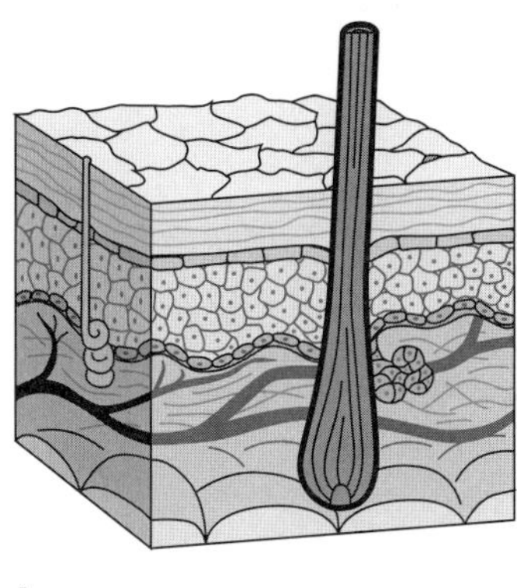

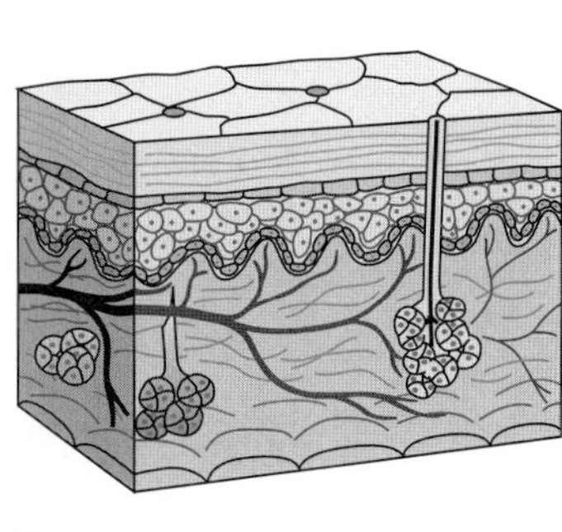

A. skin
B. mucosa

On occasion, sebaceous glands may appear in the vermillion border. What is the vermillion border?

a transition zone

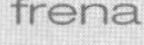

Remember that the labial mucosa contains two ______________ or folds located under the lip in the midline.

frena

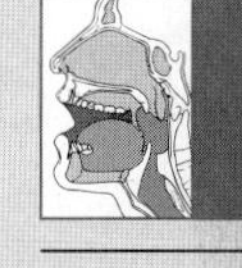

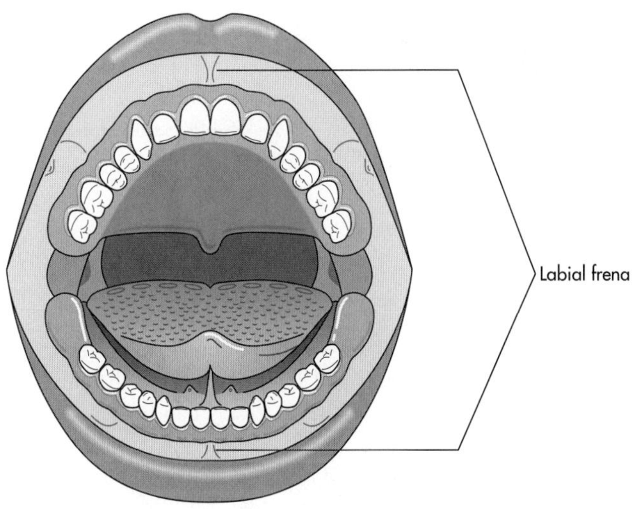

VENTRAL TONGUE (FLOOR OF MOUTH)

Lining mucosa is also found on the underside or **ventrum** of the tongue and in the floor of the mouth.

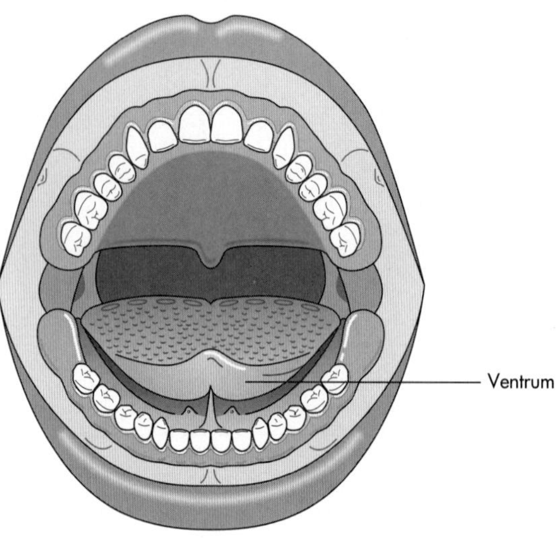

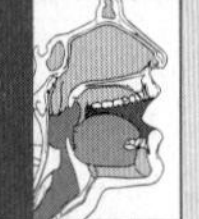

thin and nonkeratinized

Lining mucosa of the ventral tongue is very fragile because it is ________________. It is so thin that the blood vessels running below it, the lingual arteries and veins, can be seen.

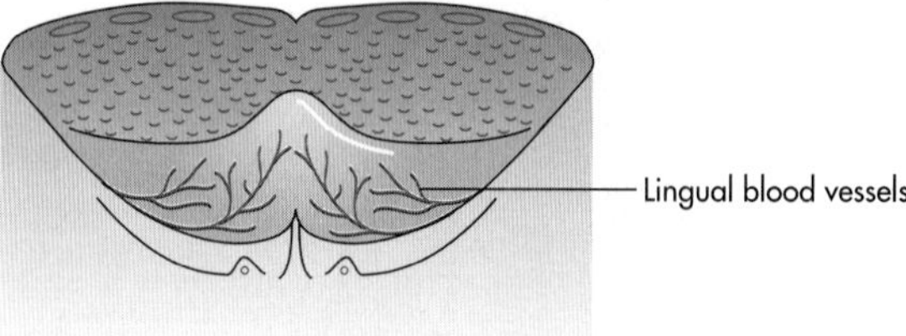

The lining of the **floor of the mouth** is the mucosa directly under the tongue. It runs from the right side of the mandible to the left and is interrupted in the midline by the tongue. This mucosa is also very thin, and major blood vessels can be seen coursing below it.

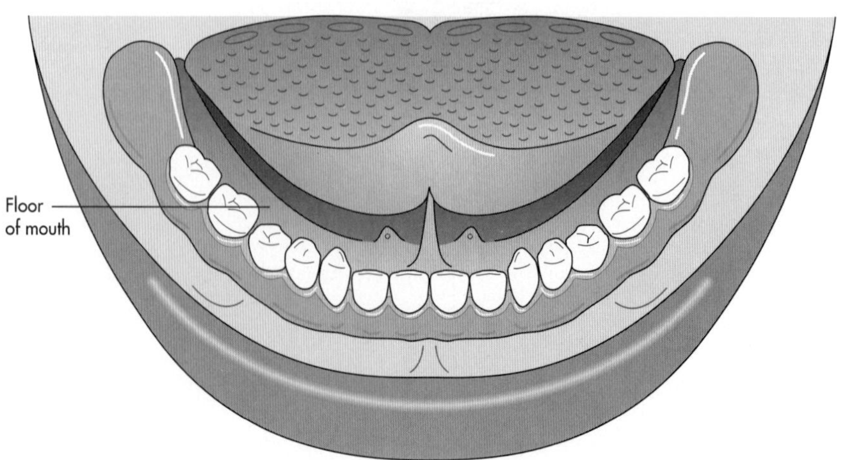

The floor of the mouth has two folds on either side called the **sublingual plicae.** Find them in the drawing.

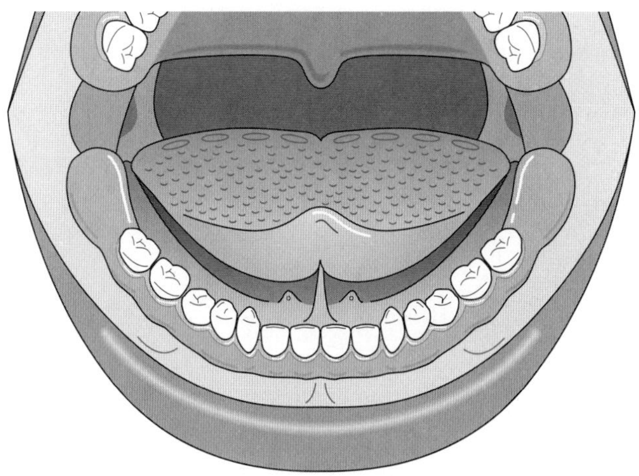

The sublingual ______________ are two folds in the mucosa of the floor of the mouth. They contain the openings of one of the major salivary glands, the sublingual salivary gland.

plicae

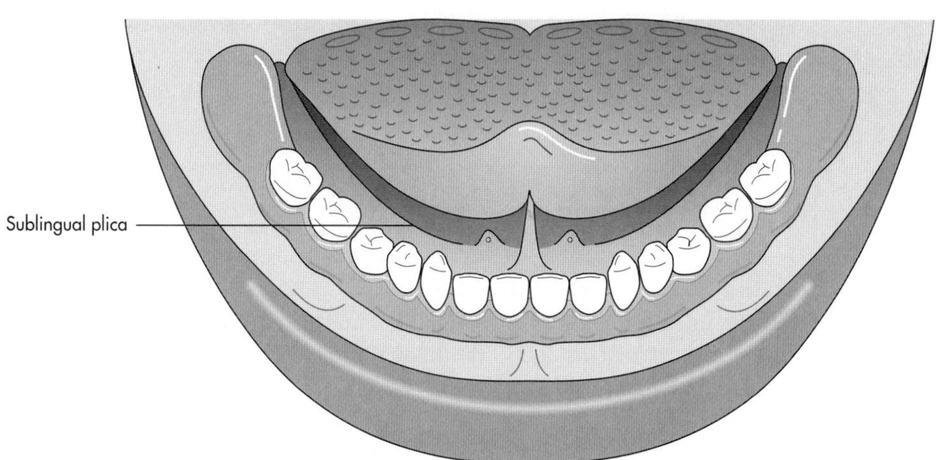

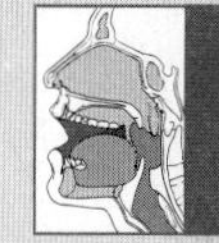

The ______________ salivary glands have multiple ducts called the **ducts of Rivinus** and they empty through the plicae on both sides.

sublingual

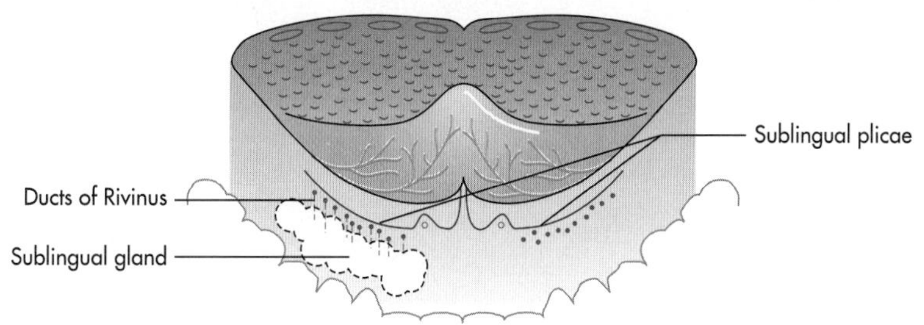

from the ventral tongue to the floor of the mouth

On the anteriormost portion of the tongue is a single frenum, the **lingual frenum.** Where does it run?

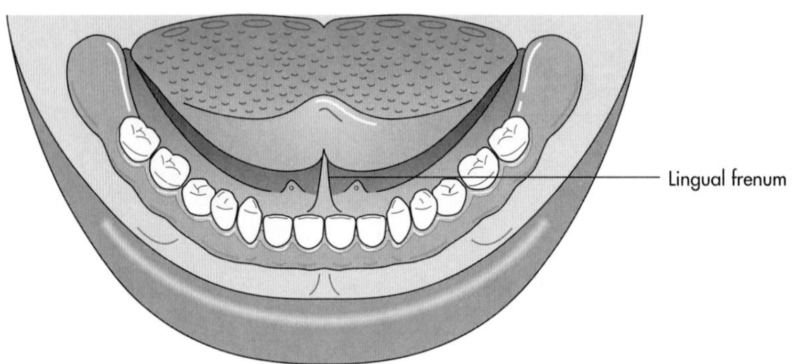

frenum

The lingual ______________ is a midline fold of mucosa dividing the mucosa of the floor of the mouth into right and left halves.

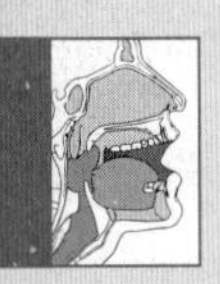

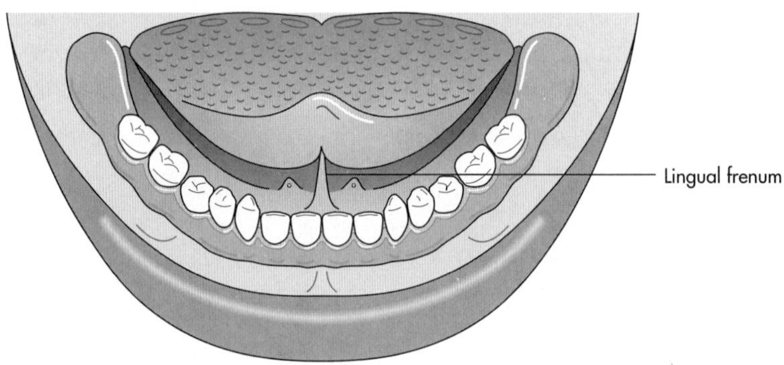

submandibular

On either side of the lingual frenum are two small bumps, the **sublingual caruncles.** The "bumps" house the orifices of two ducts, **Wharton's ducts.** These ducts empty each of the ______________ salivary glands.

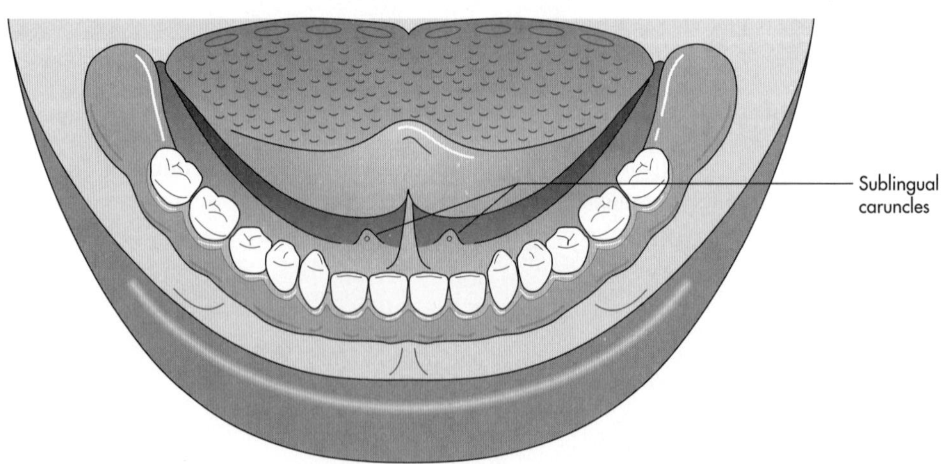

The **submandibular salivary glands** lie under each angle of the mandible, and their ducts travel under the floor of the mouth, parallel to the blood vessels, to empty in the anterior area through the sublingual ________________.

caruncles

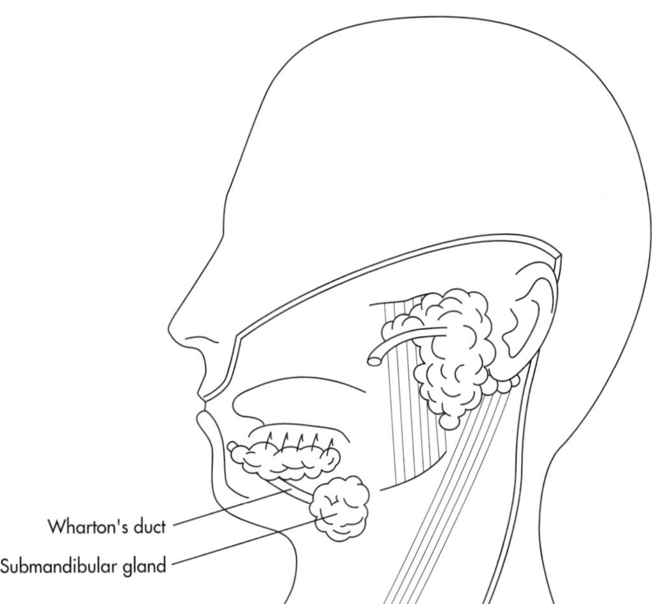

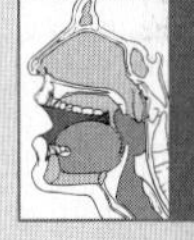

The sublingual area is an area rich in blood vessels that course just below a thin mucosa. It is an ideal area for introducing medications directly into the bloodstream.

Label the structures we have studied on the ventral tongue and floor of the mouth.

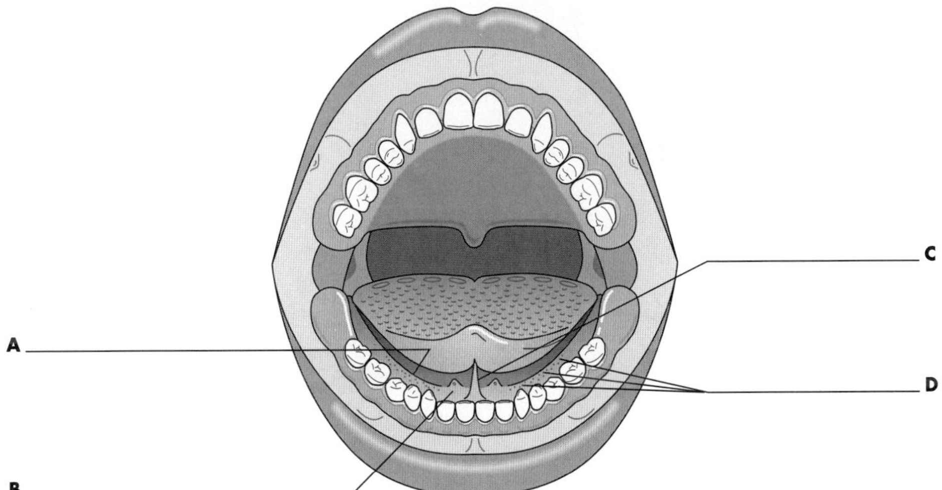

A. plica
B. sublingual caruncle
C. lingual frenum
D. ducts of Rivinus

PHARYNGEAL MUCOSA

Lining mucosa continues beyond the oral cavity back into the area known as the **oropharynx.** The oropharynx is that portion of the pharynx or "food tube" that we can see by looking back through the oral cavity, or the "back of the throat."

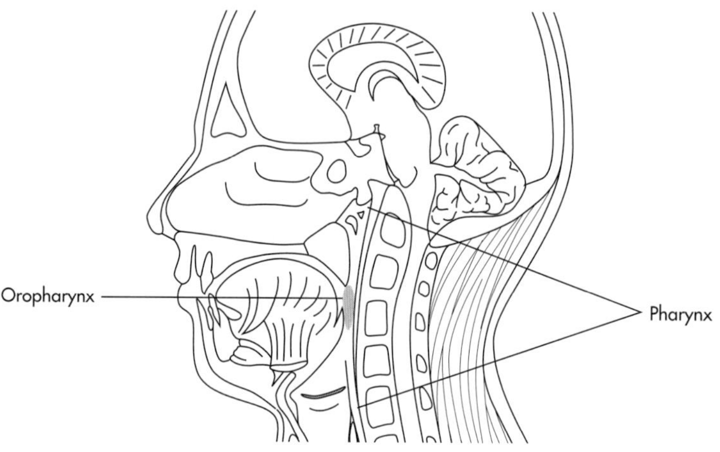

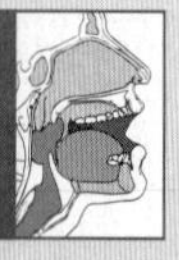

A view of the oropharynx from the oral cavity, is diagrammed here.

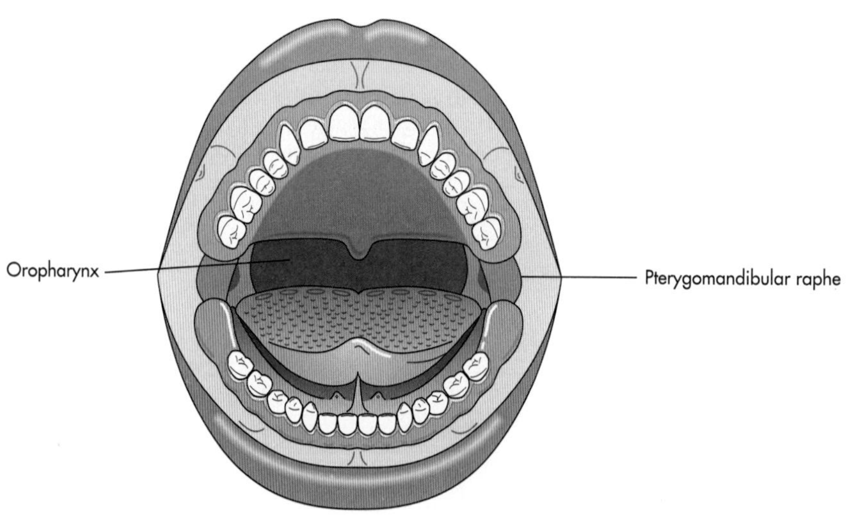

Note the diagram of a section through the head. The shaded area is the oropharynx. Where is the palate?

between oral and nasal cavities

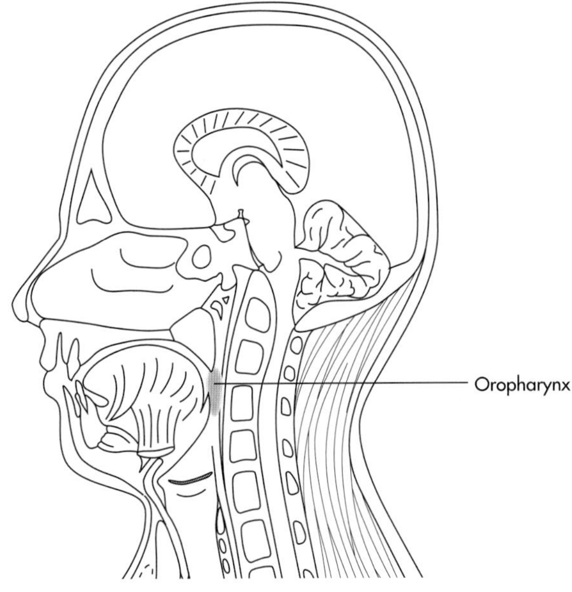

Viewed from the side you can see that the pharynx continues up and down from the oropharynx. The portion that continues up into the nose is called the **nasopharynx;** that part going down past the tongue is called the **pharynx proper.** The pharynx leads into the esophagus.

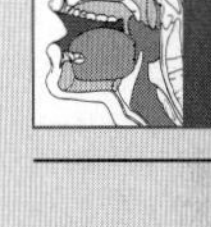

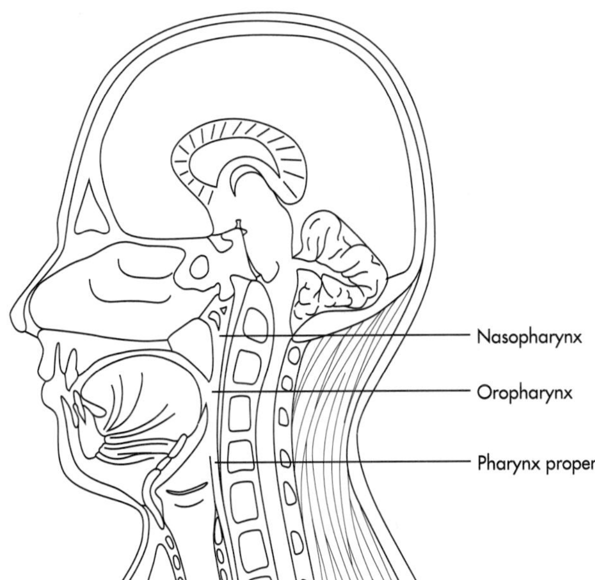

The structure dividing the nasal cavity from the oral cavity is the **palate.** Which portion is the hard palate and which is the soft palate?

hard palate is anterior; soft palate is posterior

The oropharynx is directly across from the soft palate. The soft palate, remember, is a flap of muscular and glandular tissue, covered with palatal mucosa on one side and nasal mucosa on the other. It comes up to touch the pharynx, sealing off the nasopharynx during a swallow.

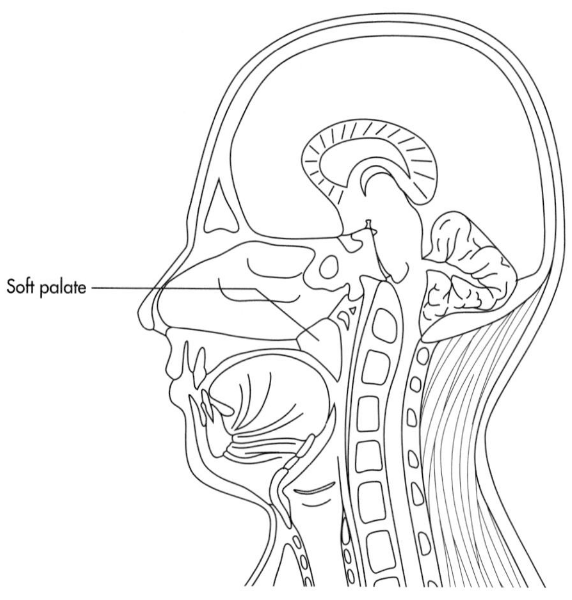

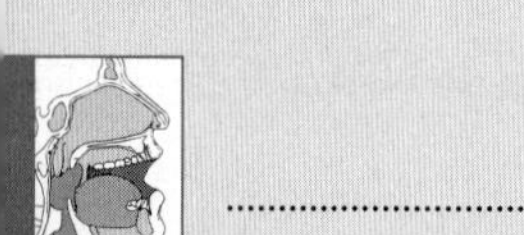

The oropharynx and pharynx proper are lined with lining mucosa. This mucosa rests on top of the muscles of the pharynx, the constrictors. A slice through **pharyngeal mucosa** is diagrammed here.

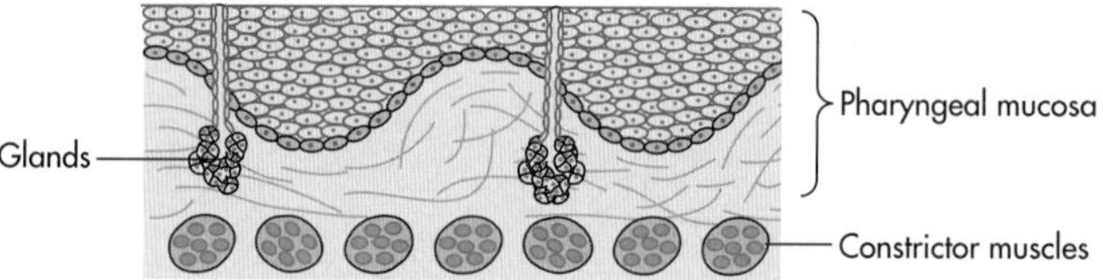

salivary, mucous

Remember that there are ______________ and ______________ glands in the lamina propria.

The mucosa of the nasopharynx is slightly different. It is an area of transition. The nasal cavity is part of the respiratory system and its mucosa is different than that of the digestive system.

Respiratory mucosa consists of a ciliated, pseudostratified epithelium resting on a connective tissue base. Check Chapter One for a definition of this epithelium.

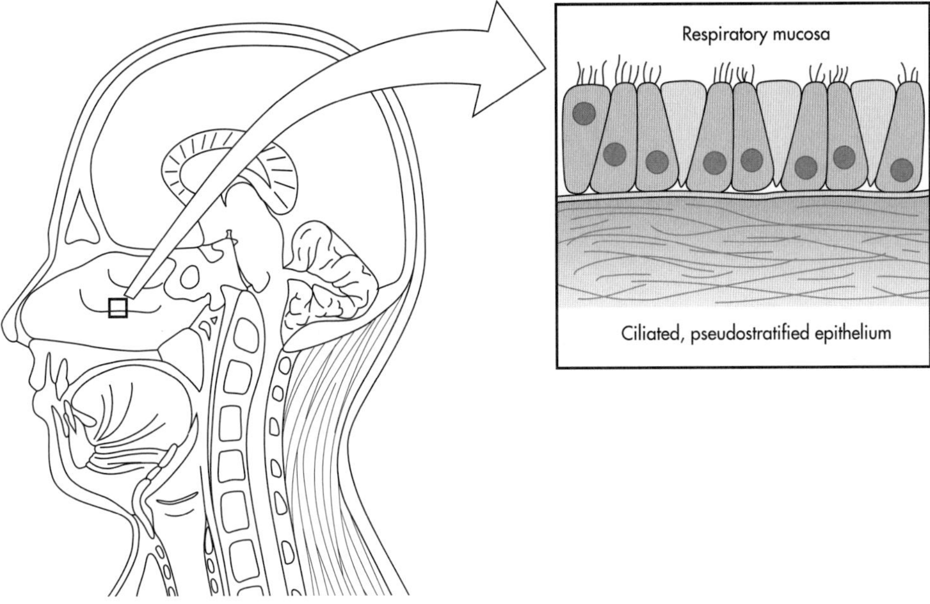

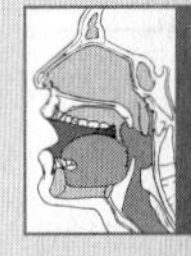

Ciliated, pseudostratified epithelium is an epithelium with only one layer of cells, the nuclei of which are at different levels, so that it appears to have many layers. Ciliated means that the epithelial cells have cilia—hairlike appendages that can move. Within the pseudostratified epithelium of the respiratory tract, are found single mucus-producing cells. These are called **goblet cells** because of their shape. They constantly produce a layer of mucus to cover the epithelium, and the cilia move the mucus along the surface, trapping and eventually ridding the tract of foreign particles at the nasal end.

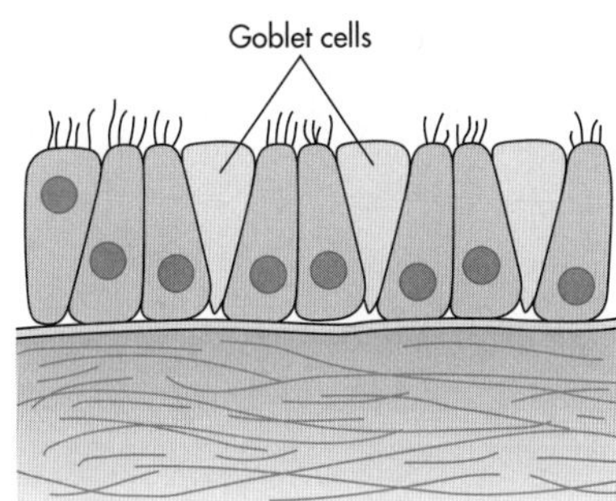

nasopharynx, ciliated pseudostratified, pharyngeal

The oropharynx leads up into the ______________ portion of the pharynx. This is an area of transition from stratified squamous epithelium to ______________ epithelium of the nasal cavity. Which tissue has salivary glands?

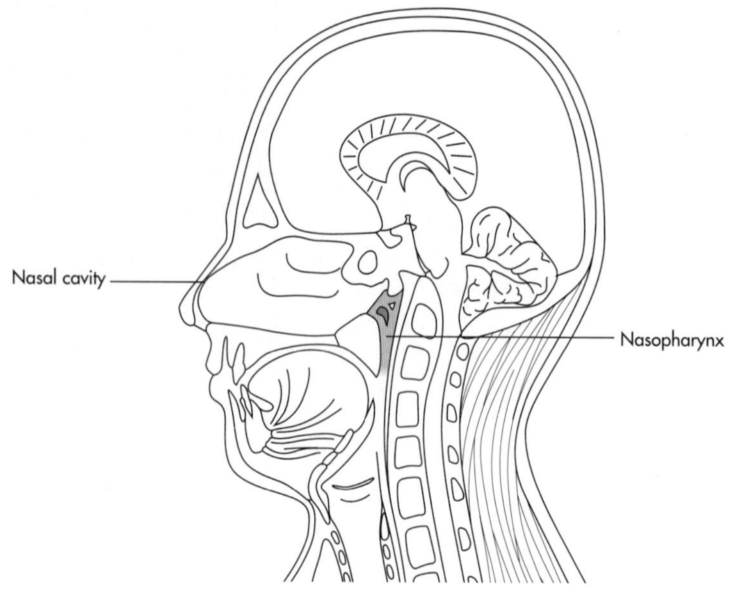

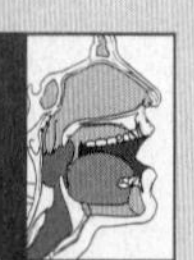

Both tissues produce mucus. In the nasopharynx, on either side of this passageway are the openings of two tubes, the **Eustachian tubes,** which open during most swallows as the soft palate rises.

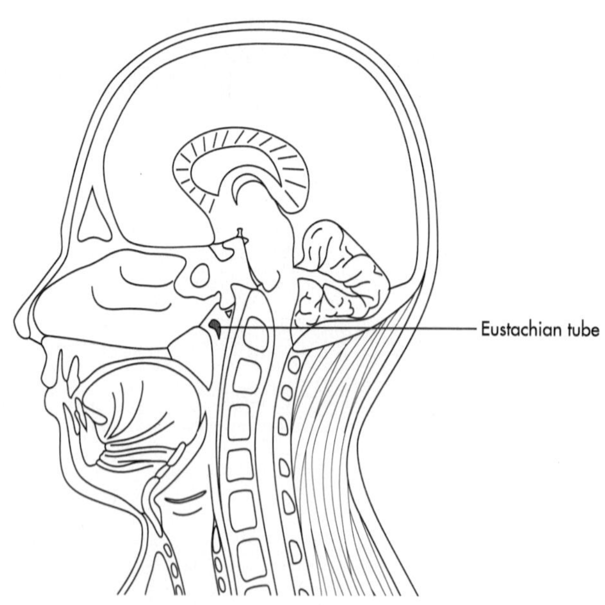

muscle

At the junction of the oropharynx and oral cavity on the sides of the "tube" lie two pairs of "columns" of mucosa-covered tissue. These are called the **pharyngeal pillars** or **fauces.** What do you think lies underneath them?

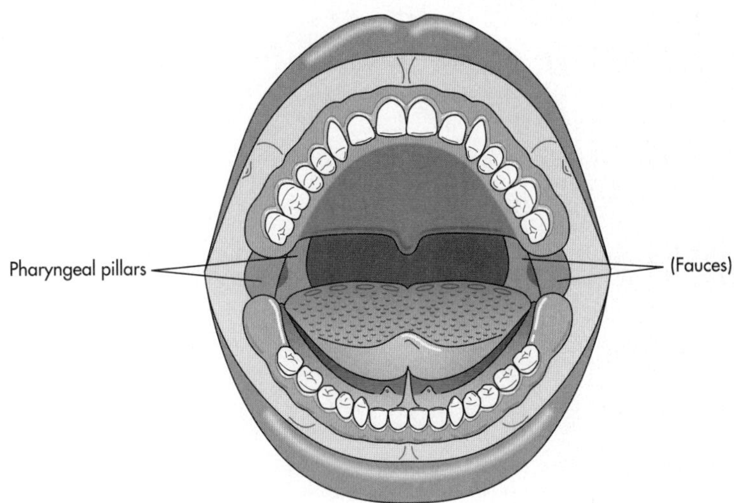

Below the fauces lie two sets of muscles running from the tongue to the pharynx and from the palate to the pharynx (**glossopharyngeus** and **palatopharyngeus**). Both pairs of muscles are covered with pharyngeal mucosa.

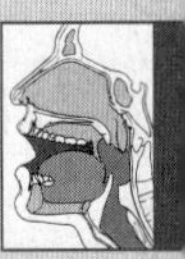

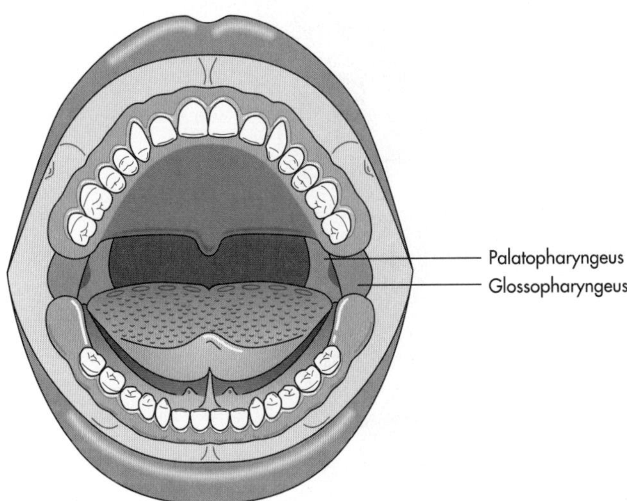

These pairs of muscles form the posterior border of the oral cavity and the beginning of the oropharynx. Tucked between the pillars lie two "glands" also visible on oral inspection—the **palatine tonsils.**

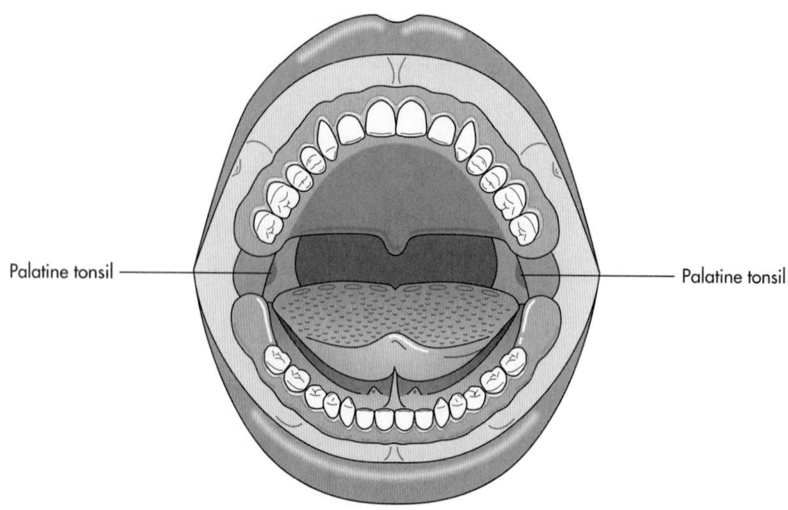

Tonsillar

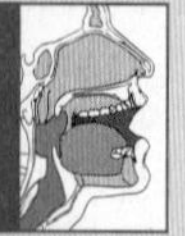

The palatine tonsils are part of a system of tonsils in the pharyngeal area. _______________ tissue is really lymphatic tissue containing lymph cells and their stem cells.

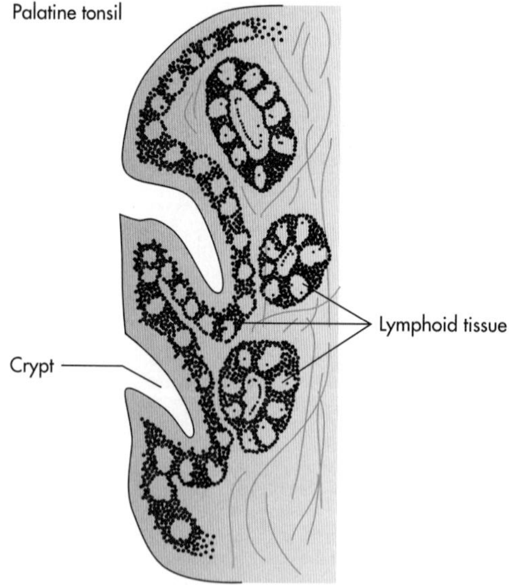

Tonsils are not true glands and do not secrete; however, they do produce white cells called _______________ in case of an infection in the area.

leukocytes (lymphocytes)

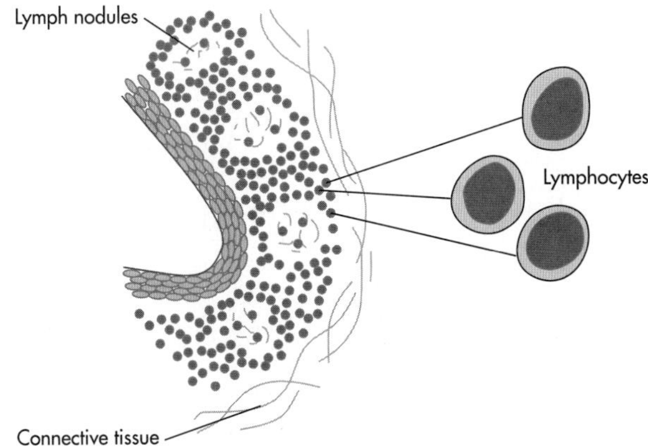

The other tonsillar groups are shown below. The _______________ tonsils lie nestled in the fauces of the oropharynx, and the **pharyngeal tonsils (adenoids)** are a pair of tonsils in the nasopharynx. The **lingual tonsils** are found on the very back or root of the tongue.

palatine

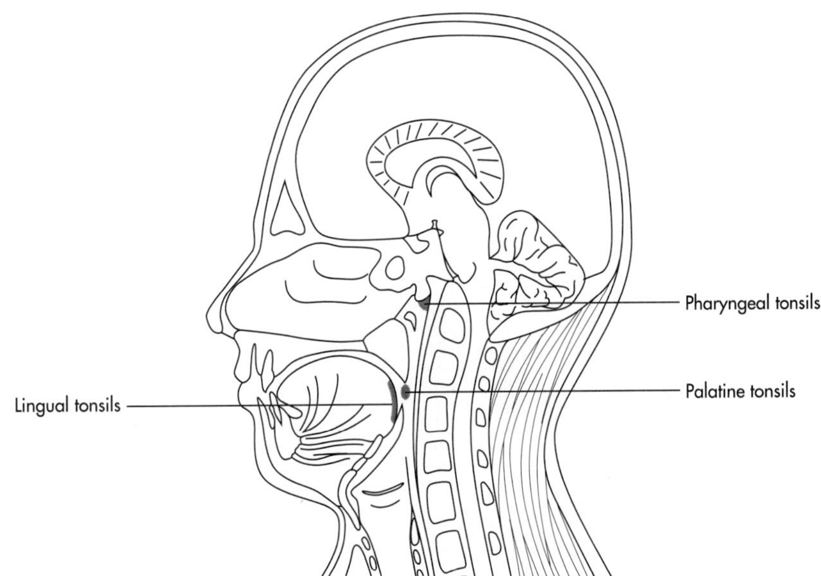

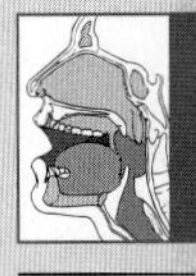

Together all three types of tonsils constitute **Waldeyer's ring;** the tonsils form a protective "ring" around the pharynx.

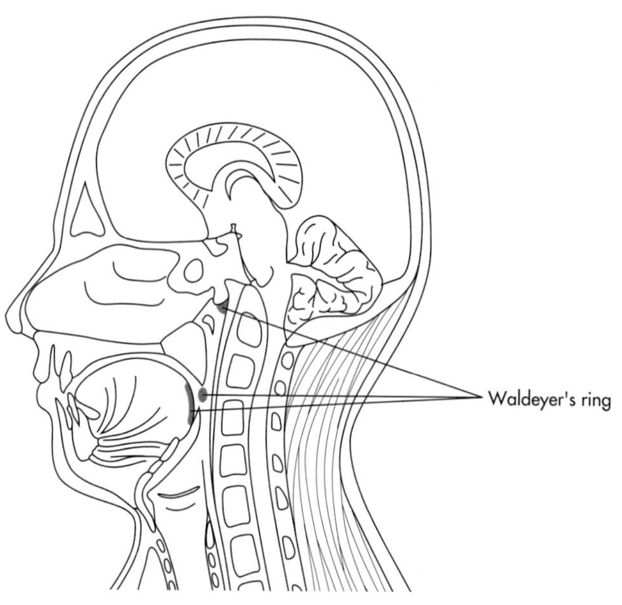

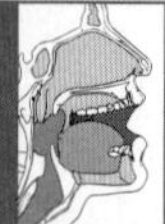

A. fauces
B. palatine tonsil
C. raphe

Review the structures assoicated with pharyngeal mucosa.

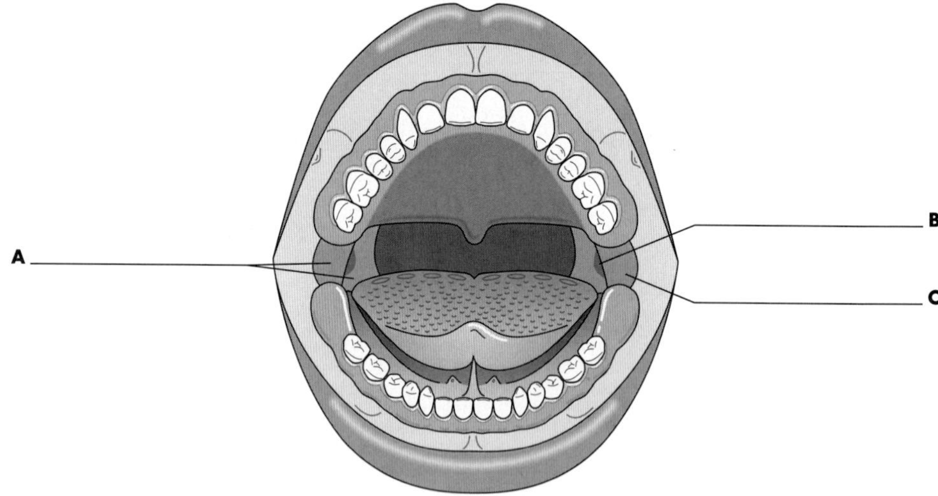

continued

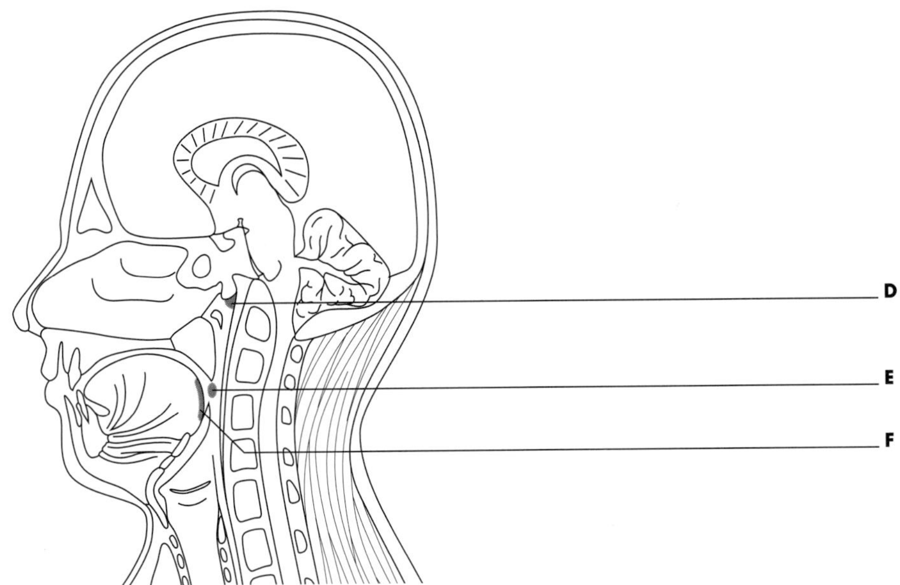

D. pharyngeal tonsil
E. oropharynx
F. lingual tonsil

Specialized Mucosa

1.3

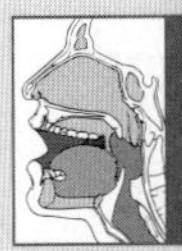

The last type of mucosa is found on the top or dorsum of the tongue. It is called **specialized mucosa** because it has specialized cells and cell structures different from the other types of mucosa. These specialized structures help in the sensory function of the tongue, which is taste.

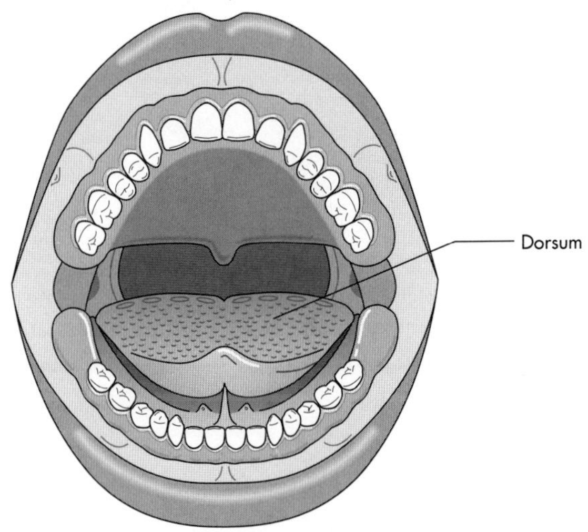

The tongue is, essentially, a "sac of muscles" covered by mucosa. This is a section through the tongue.

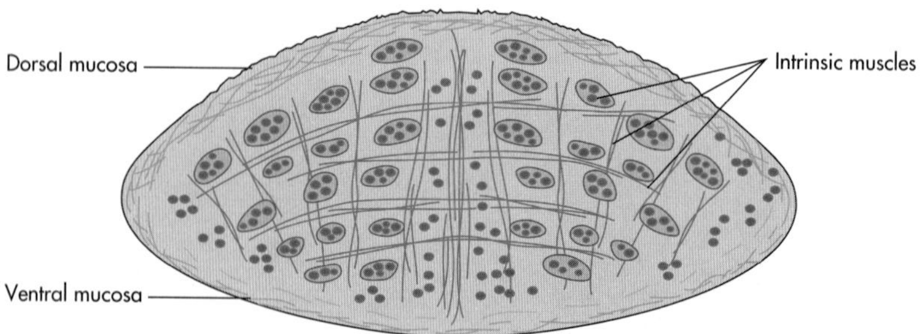

The muscles inside the tongue are called the **intrinsic muscles** and are striated skeletal muscle, the fibers of which run in three major directions. There are other muscles that attach the tongue to the mandible and pharynx.

lining mucosa

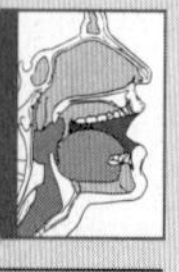

What type of tissue covers the underside or ventrum of the tongue? (Remember that it is the same tissue that covers the floor of the mouth.)

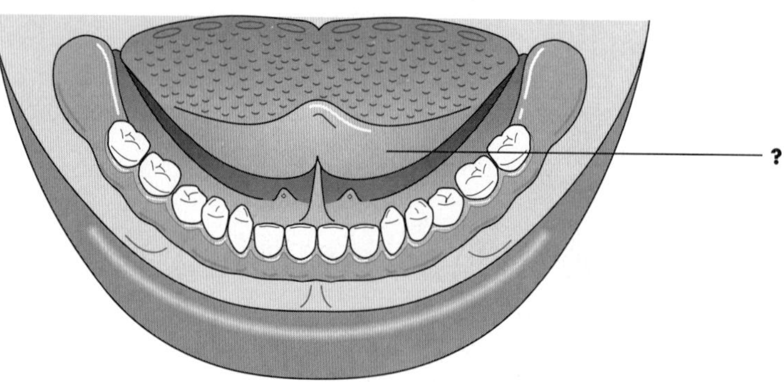

dorsum

If you answered lining mucosa, you are correct. It is a thin, nonkeratinized mucosa similar in structure to the mucosa of the floor of the mouth. Which area of the tongue gets the most wear and tear: dorsum or ventrum?

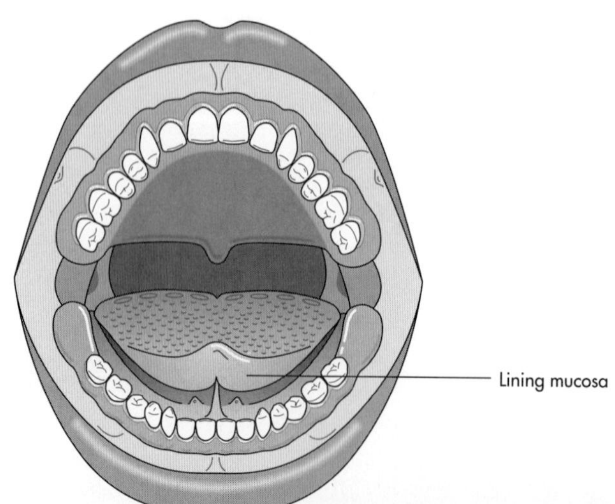

The top or **dorsum** of the tongue receives the most wear and tear and, therefore, is a tougher tissue. The mucosa of the dorsum of the tongue is a very thick, keratinized mucosa, more similar in structure to the mucosa of the palate than to that of the ventrum.

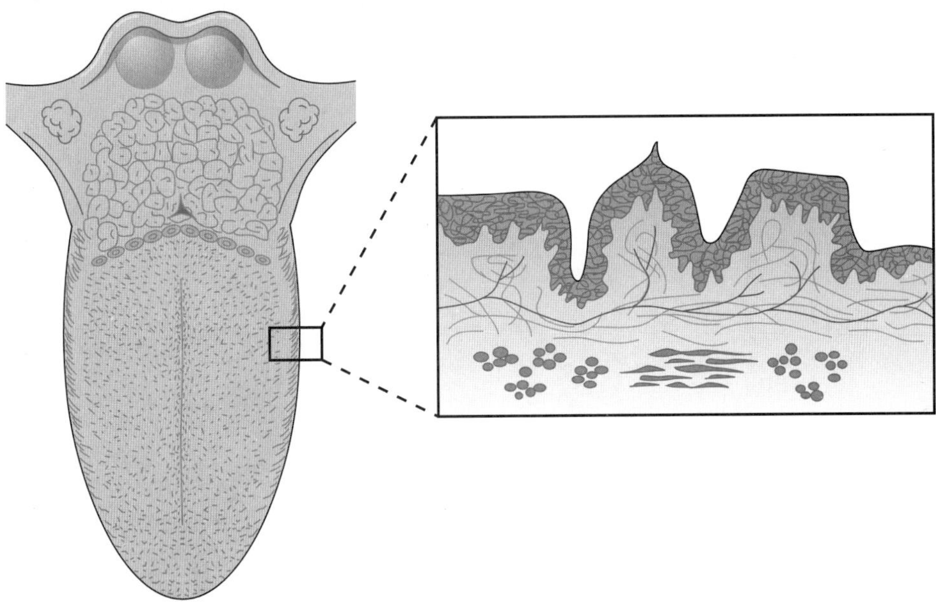

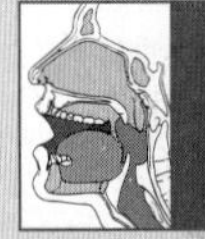

The epithelial layer of the dorsal tongue mucosa forms many peculiarly shaped structures on its surface called **papillae.** (Anything called a papilla is usually a small projecting structure!)

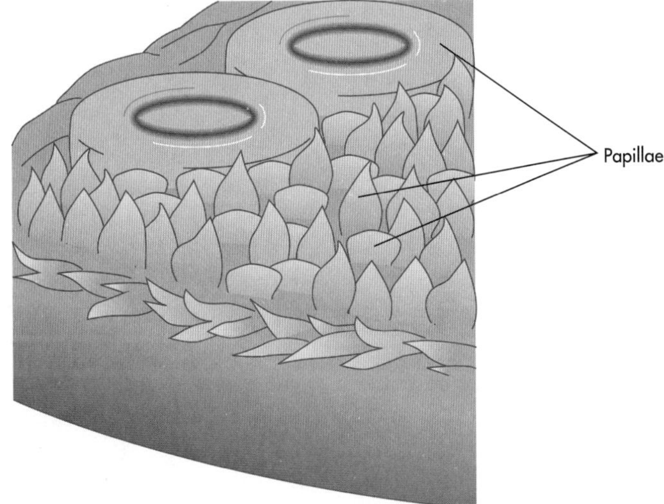

Papillae of the dorsal tongue come in one of four shapes, named for what they resemble:

1. Filiform papillae
2. Fungiform papillae
3. Foliate papillae
4. Circumvallate papillae

Filiform papillae are flame-shaped papillae. They are many and are scattered on the entire surface of the body of the tongue.

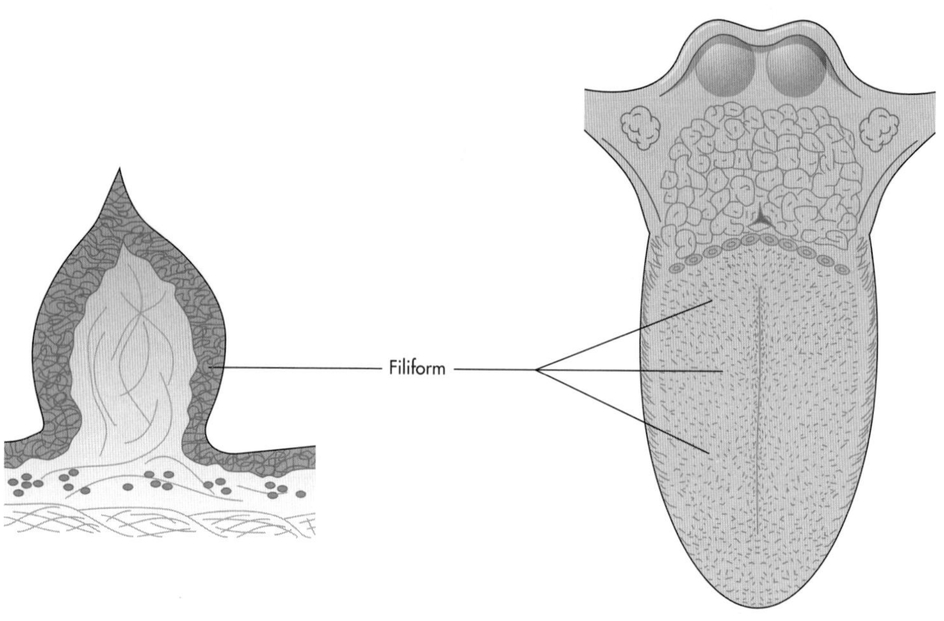

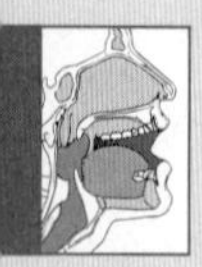

Fungiform papillae are mushroom-shaped papillae that are not as abundant as filiform papillae and are scattered across the dorsal surface also on the body of the tongue.

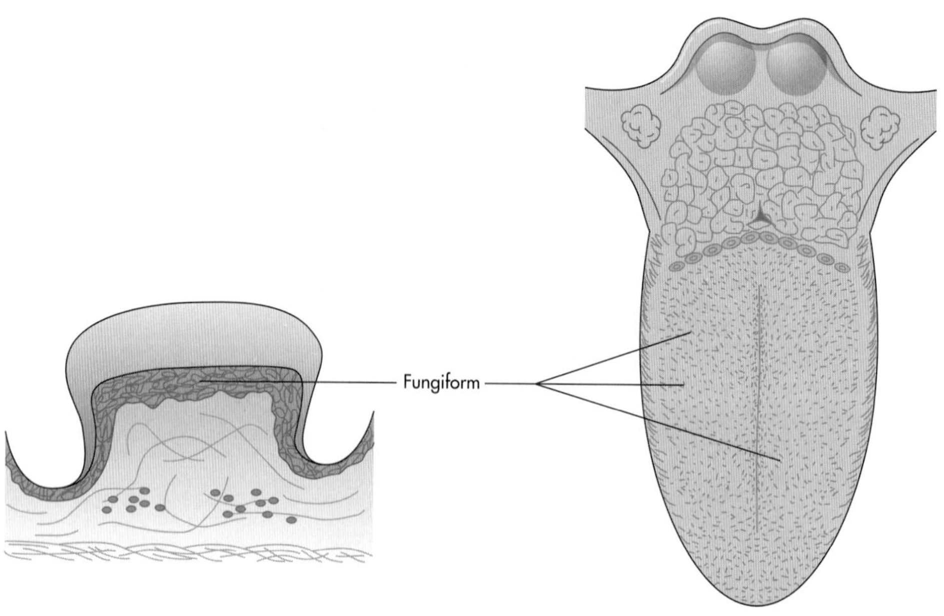

Foliate papillae are like huge filiform papillae. This type is found only on the lateral borders (sides) of the tongue.

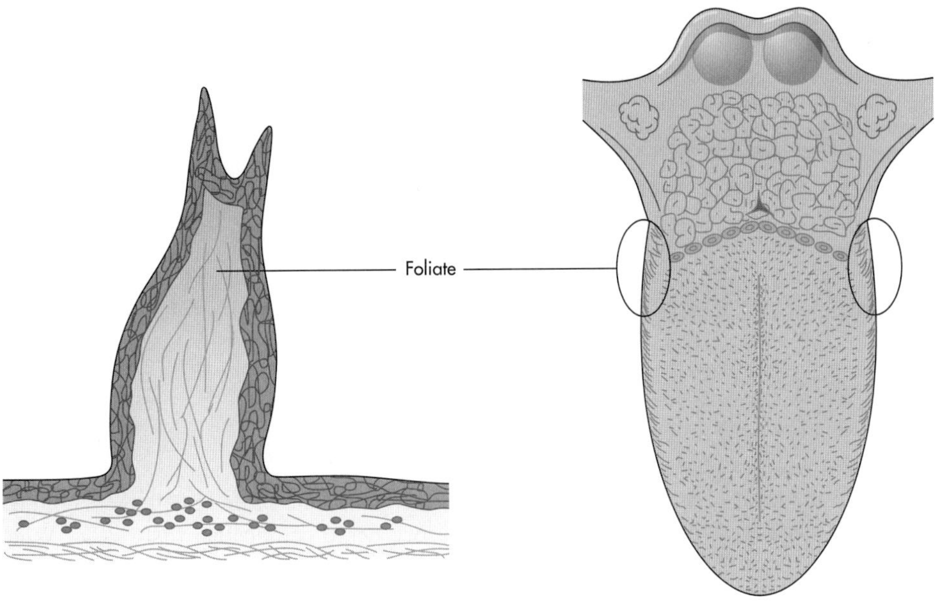

The **circumvallate papillae** are very elaborate. They have a round, mushroom-shaped central portion surrounded by a trough. This trough is then surrounded by a donut-shaped area that encircles the center.

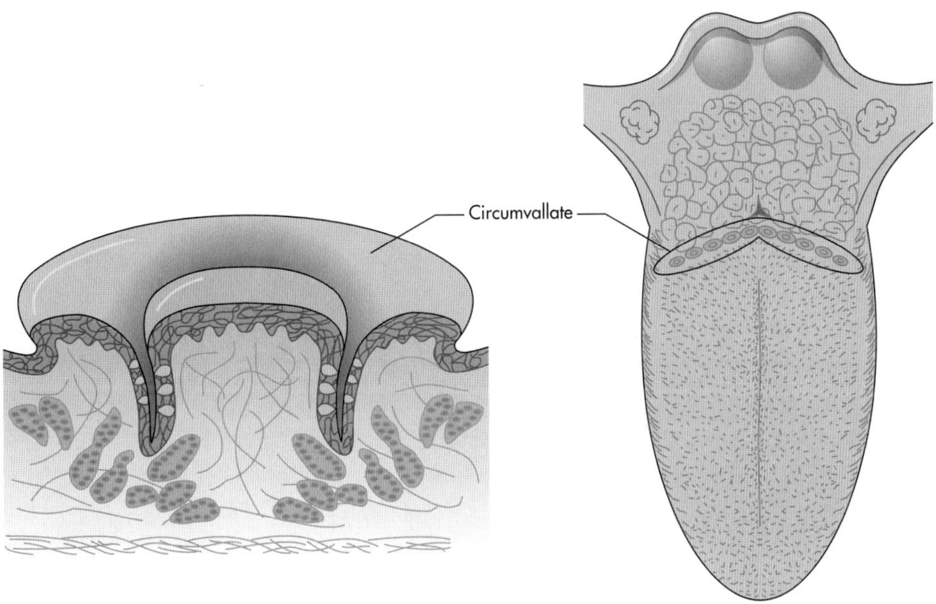

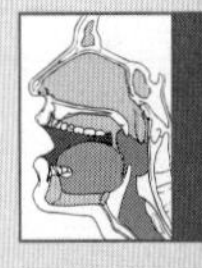

In the diagram of a histologic section through a circumvallate papilla, note that the trough around the center guides fluids around the structure. Some of the fluid comes from serous glands, **Von Ebner's glands,** that empty directly into the trough.

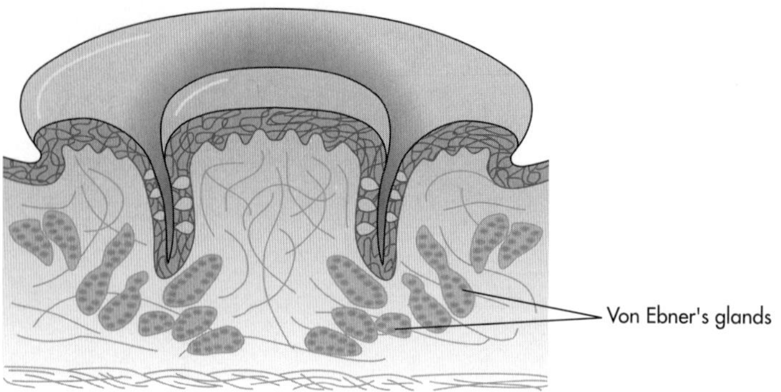

taste

Note also the clear cells lining the trough of the papilla. One of these cells is magnified here. It is actually a group of specialized sensory nerve cells called **taste cells.** What sense is it responsible for conveying?

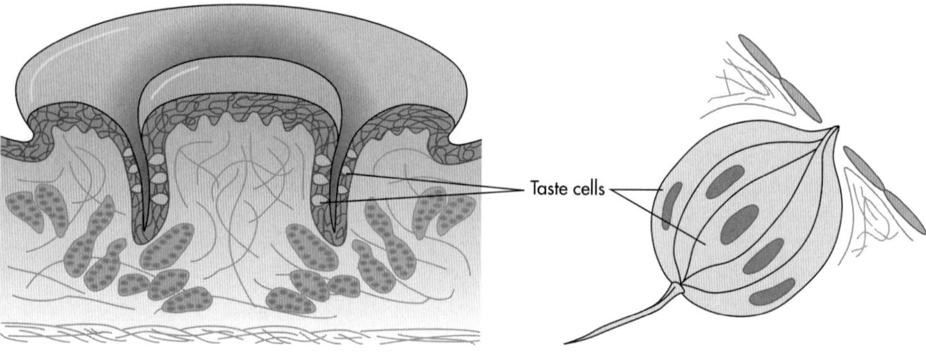

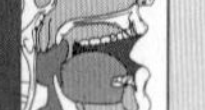

A. foliate,
B. filiform,
C. fungiform

Identify the different types of papillae.

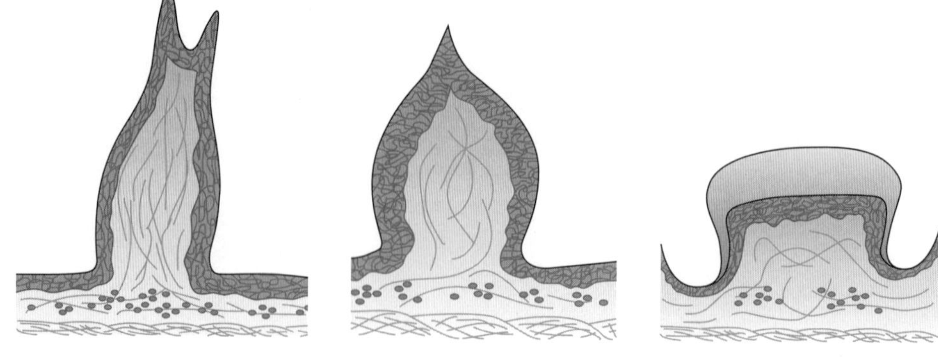

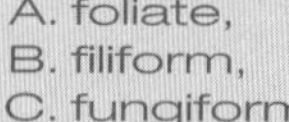

Note that the circumvallate papillae number about 8 to 10 and form a V-shaped border on the tongue between the ______ and ______ portions of the tongue. What embryologic tissues meet here?

anterior two thirds, posterior one third; ectoderm and endoderm

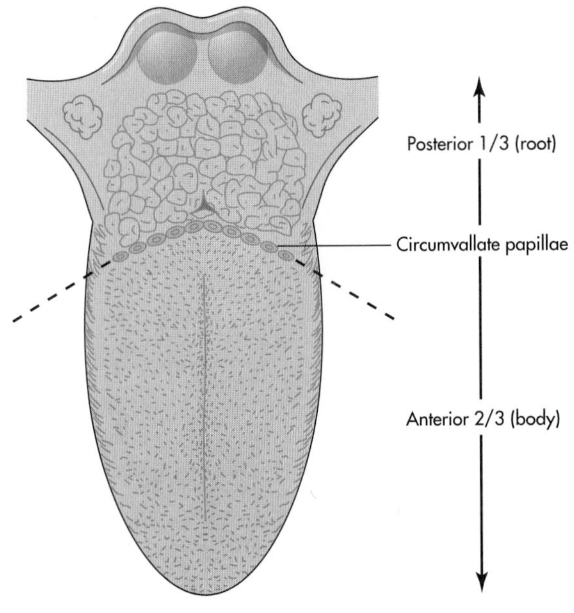

The circumvallate papillae form an important border between the anterior two thirds, or body, of the tongue and the posterior one third, or root, of the tongue. It shows where embryologically the ectoderm of the anterior two thirds and oral cavity meets the endoderm of the posterior one third and pharynx. Between the circumvallate papillae at the point of the "V" is a remnant of thyroid development, the ______.

formen cecum

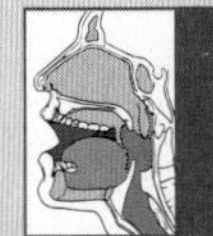

Taste cells are sensory neurons capable of distinguishing between four major tastes: (1) sweet, (2) sour, (3) salty, and (4) bitter. Taste cells are scattered throughout the dorsal tongue mucosa, with some even occurring in other mucosa as the palate. Most taste cells, however, are located on the walls of the circumvallate papillae. Bits of food dissolved in saliva are presented to the ______ cells for recognition.

taste

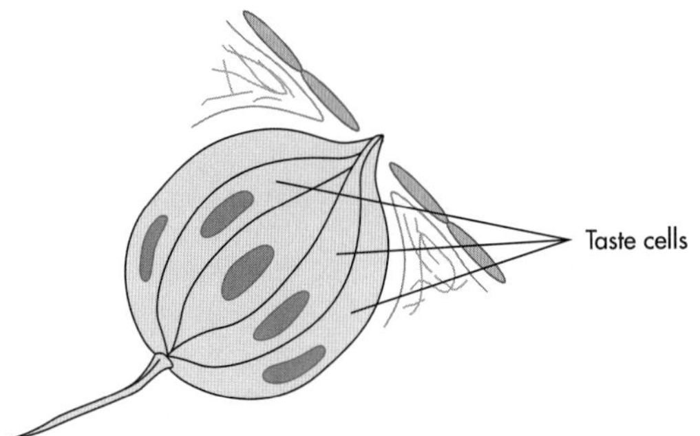

The tongue can be divided into regions where the four basics tastes are more acutely sensed. The wide variety of taste sensations is due to the combination of the sensations of smell and taste.

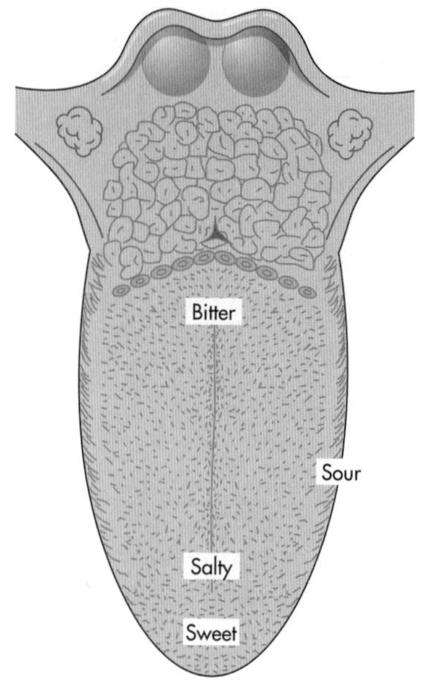

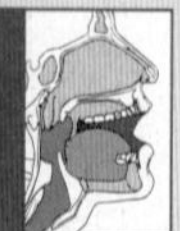

thyroid

The **foramen cecum** appears as a bump or hollowed-out area of tissue at the point of the "V" of the circumvallate papillae; it is a reminder that the ____________ gland began its development there. Behind it begins the root of the tongue, an area covered with very different looking lymphoid tissue or the **lingual tonsils.**

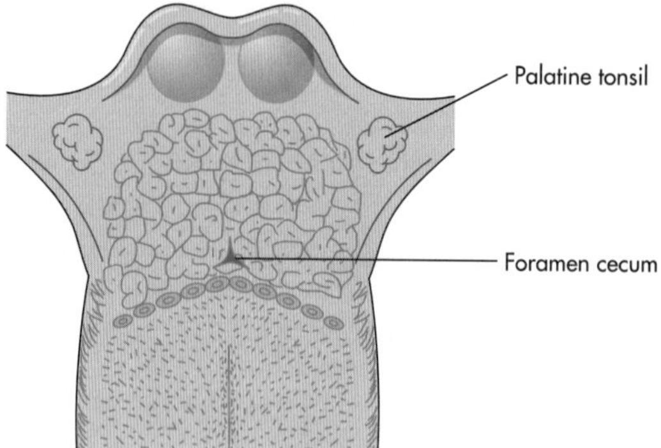

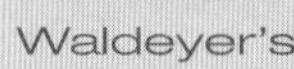
Waldeyer's

As part of ______________ ring, the lingual tonsils constitute part of the body's defense system. Beyond the lingual tonsils, the root of the tongue ends in a flap of mucosa-covered elastic cartilage called the **epiglottis.**

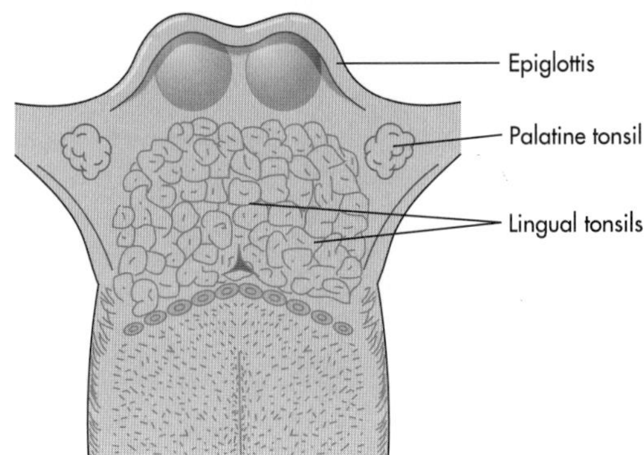

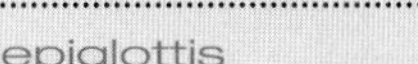
epiglottis

The ______________ is the flap of tissue that covers the windpipe or larynx so that food flows downward into the pharynx instead of into the respiratory system.

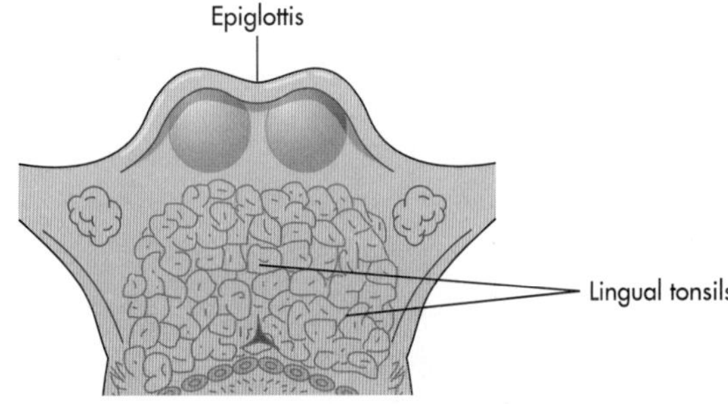

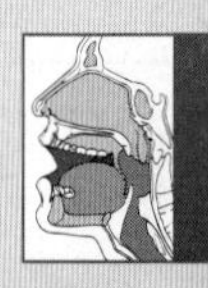

A section through the epiglottis shows a center made of elastic cartilage covered on the dorsal side by keratinized lining mucosa and on the ventral side by respiratory mucosa.

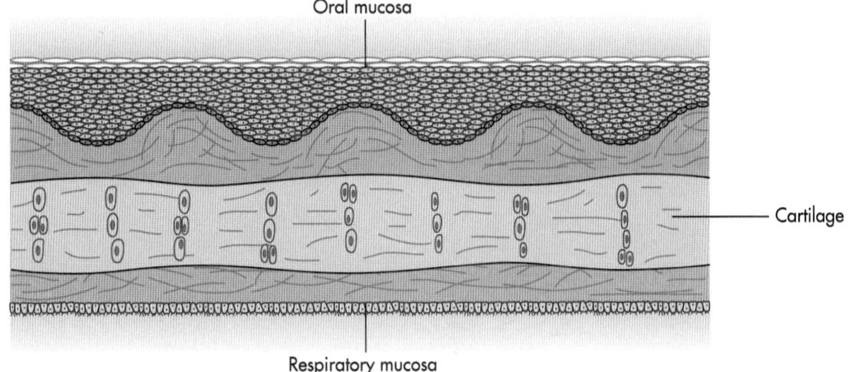

Label the lingual structures shown.

A. circumvallate papilla
B. filiform papilla
C. fungiform papilla
D. folliate papilla

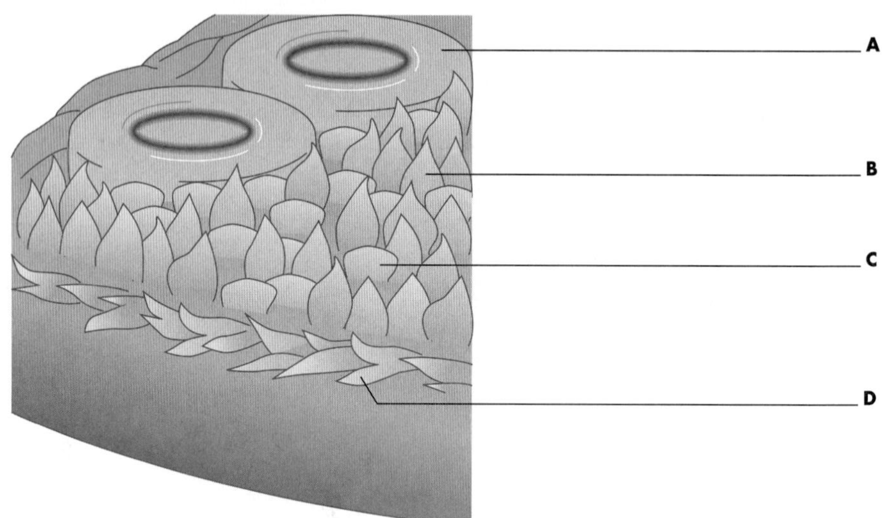

E. lingual frenum

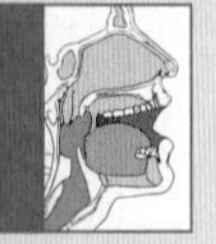

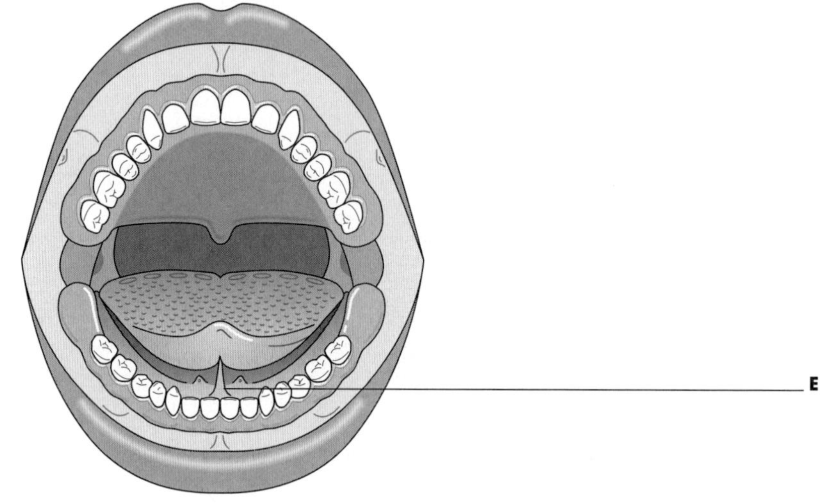

continued

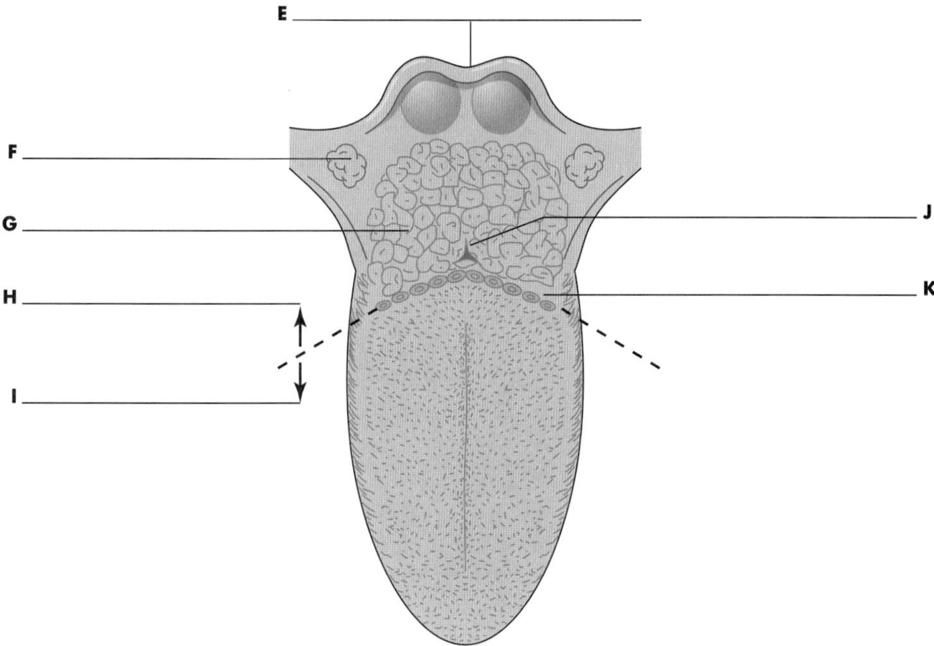

E. epiglottis
F. palatine tonsil
G. lingual tonsil
H. posterior one third (root)
I. anterior two thirds (body)
J. foramen cecum
K. circumvallate papillae

SALIVARY GLANDS 2.0

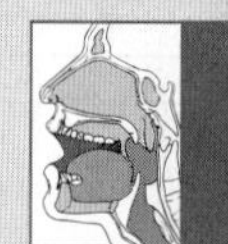

Important to the maintenance of the oral mucosa is the liquid that keeps its surface wet—saliva. **Saliva** consists mainly of water plus some mucus and some dissolved proteins. Saliva is produced by **salivary glands.**

Let's review the structure of a gland from Chapter One. Remember that glands develop from epithelium and are usually composed of two parts: a duct and a secretory unit.

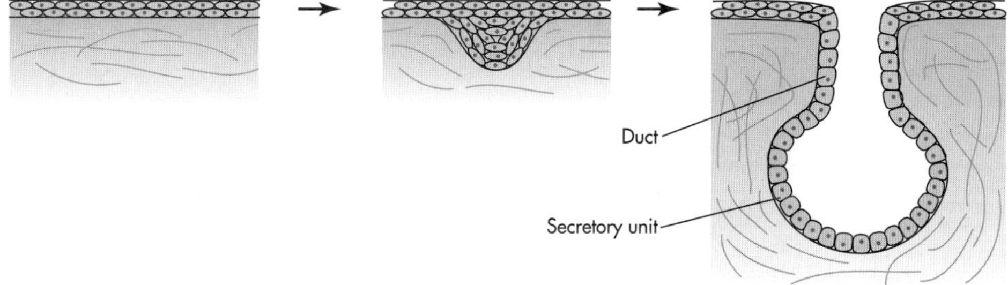

A **secretory unit** is composed of cells that produce a cell product that is expelled into the center or **lumen** of the secretory unit. The product (e.g., saliva) is pushed out of the unit into a tube that leads to the epithelial surface called a **duct.**

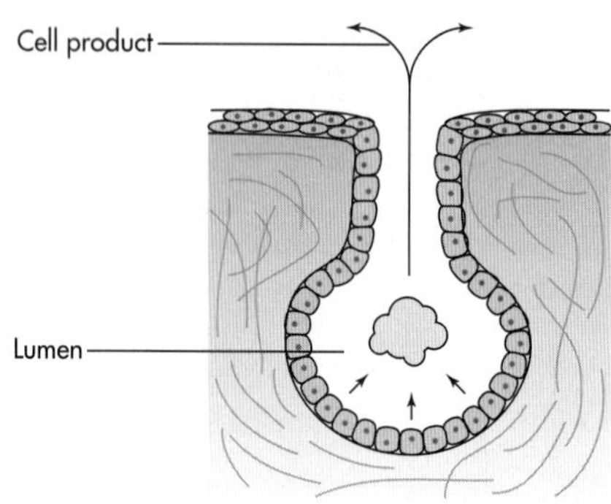

duct, acinar

A _______________ is a tube made of cells that carries the cell product or secretion to a surface. Salivary glands carry their product to the mucosal surface. What type is the gland shown based on the shape of its secretory unit?

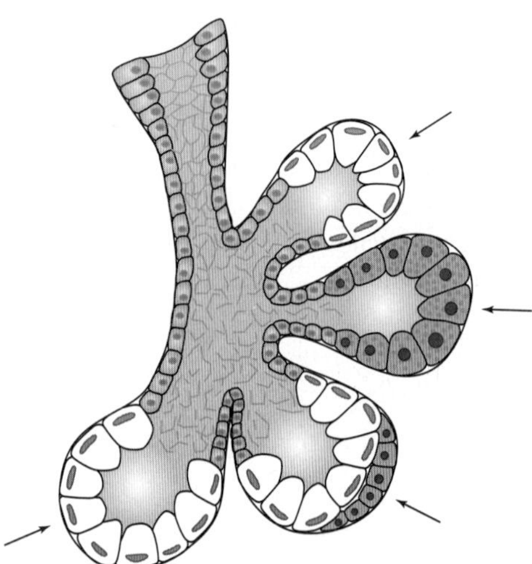

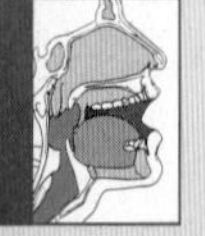

A sphere-shaped secretory unit, as found in salivary glands, is called an acinar-type gland. Are the units in the salivary gland shown multiple or single?

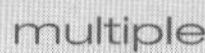
multiple

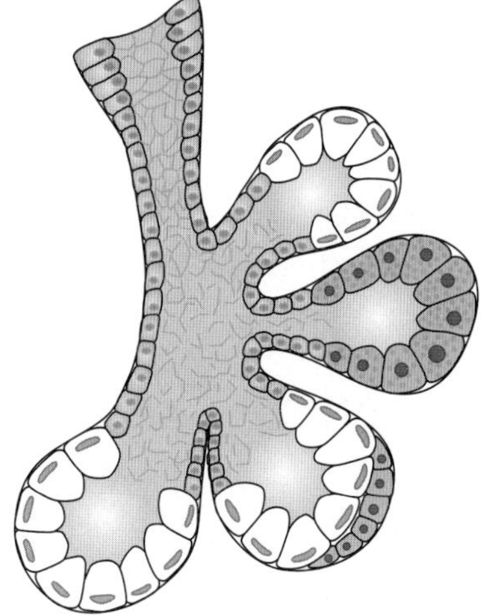

Multiple units make the salivary gland a compound gland. So the salivary gland is a ______________-type gland.

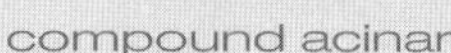
compound acinar

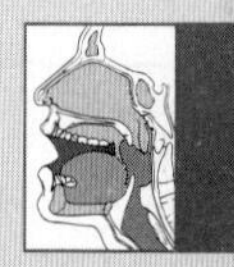

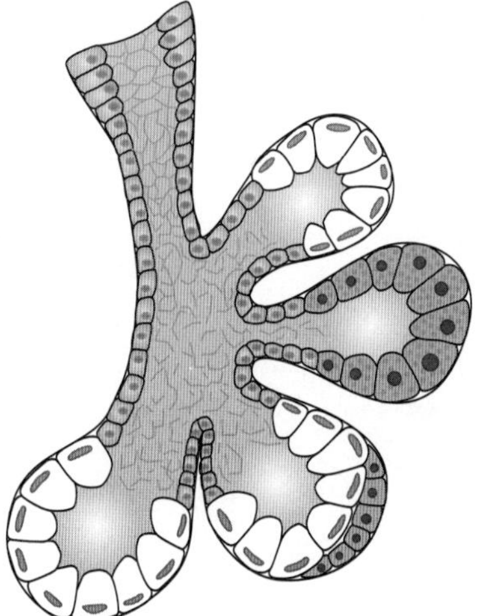

protein

Let's look at the secretory units. Saliva is a watery, mucinous secretion with a protein component. Two different types of secretory units are found within salivary glands: **mucous secreting units** and **serous secreting units.** The word *serous* must mean ______________.

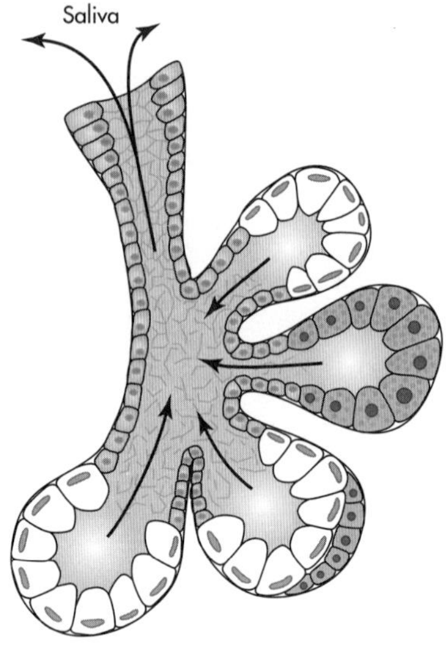

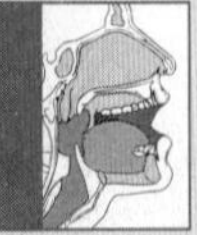

serous unit

The cells of **mucous secreting units** are clear because of the mucus produced within the cells, and the nuclei are squeezed to the side. The other type of unit is a ______________.

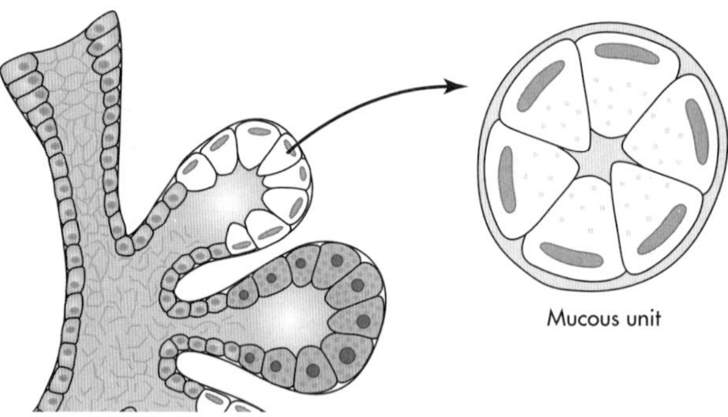

Serous secreting units are composed of cells that have many protein granules in their cytoplasm and stain more darkly. The nuclei remain in the center of the cell.

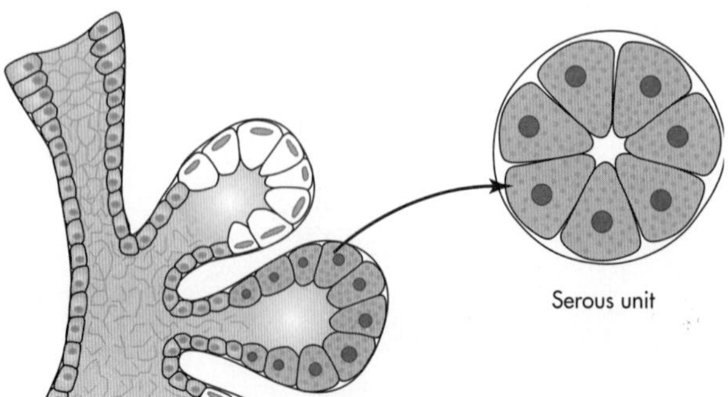

Which type of salivary secreting unit is pictured?

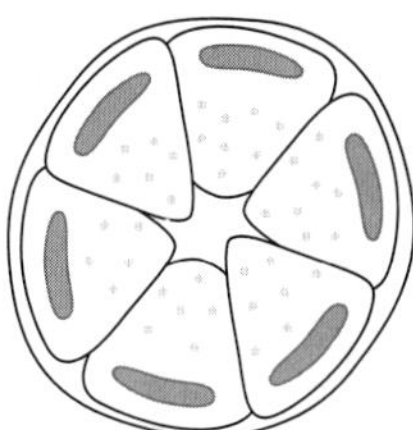

mucous secreting unit

In some instances a combination of units occurs. A group of serous cells caps a unit of mucous cells as a **serous demilume,** so called because of its lunar shape. Both secretions pass into the lumen.

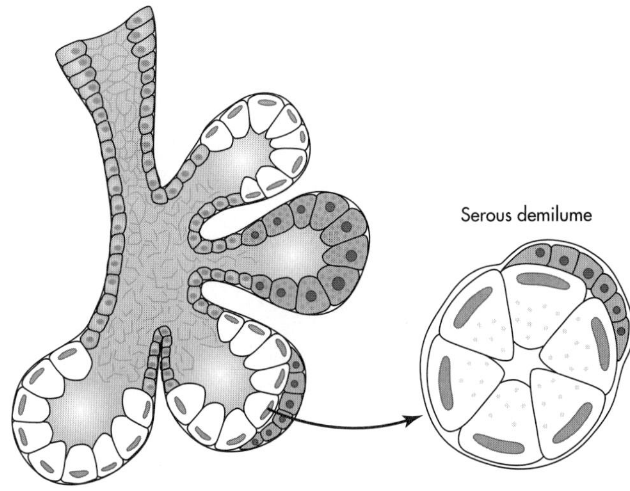

The duct system of salivary glands is very complex, with smaller ducts branching into larger and larger ducts.

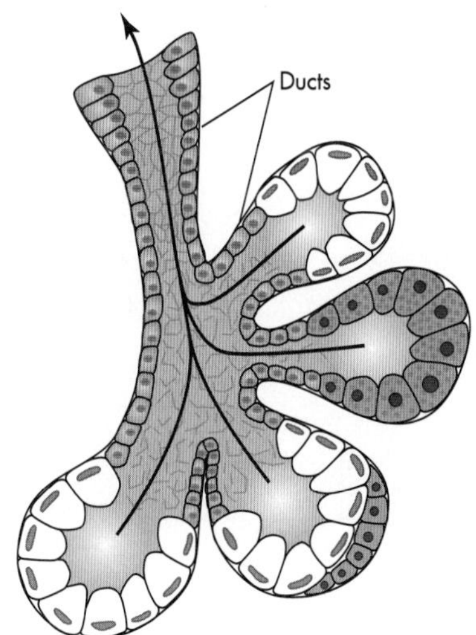

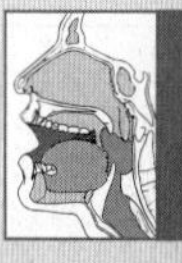

Ducts are composed of simple cuboidal and stratified cuboidal epithelium. A sectioned duct does not look very different from a sectioned secretory unit.

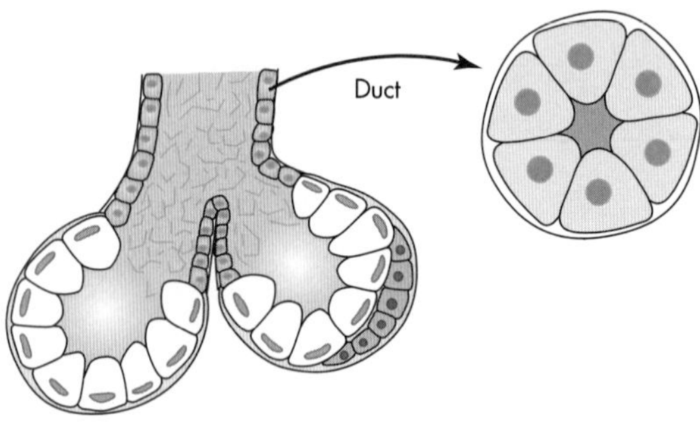

There are two types of salivary glands: small ones, called the **minor salivary glands,** and large ones, called the **major salivary glands.**

Minor salivary glands are found in the lamina propria of many areas of oral mucosa, especially the lining mucosa, although quite a few are found in the palatal mucosa.

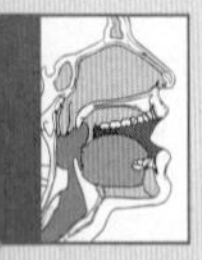

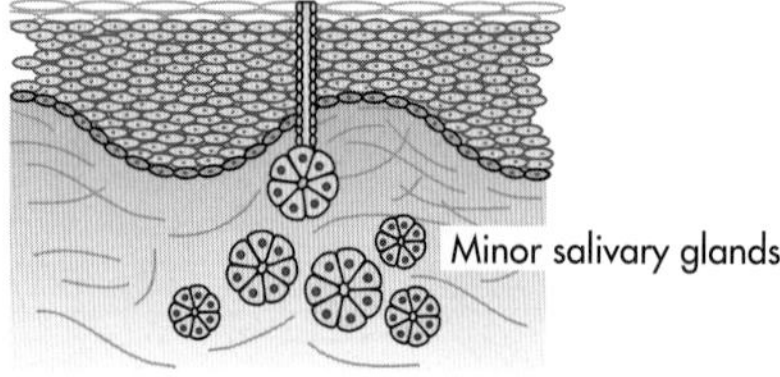

One concentration of minor salivary glands can sometimes be seen by the observer in the palate. Scattered in the mucosa of palate are a series of small dots. These dots are the ducts of the minor salivary glands.

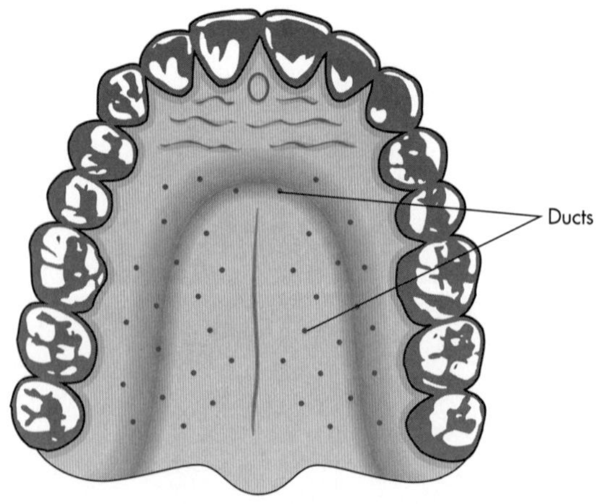

There are three pairs of **major salivary glands:**

1. Parotid glands
2. Submandibular glands
3. Sublingual glands

Each major salivary gland is invested in a connective tissue capsule, and all empty into large major ducts.

PAROTID SALIVARY GLANDS

The **parotid glands** are found directly under the skin of each cheek. They are large, flat glands that spread across a large portion of the midface and may even extend behind the ears and under the ramus of the jaw. Their tissue mingles with subcutaneous fat and the buccal fat pad areas of the cheek.

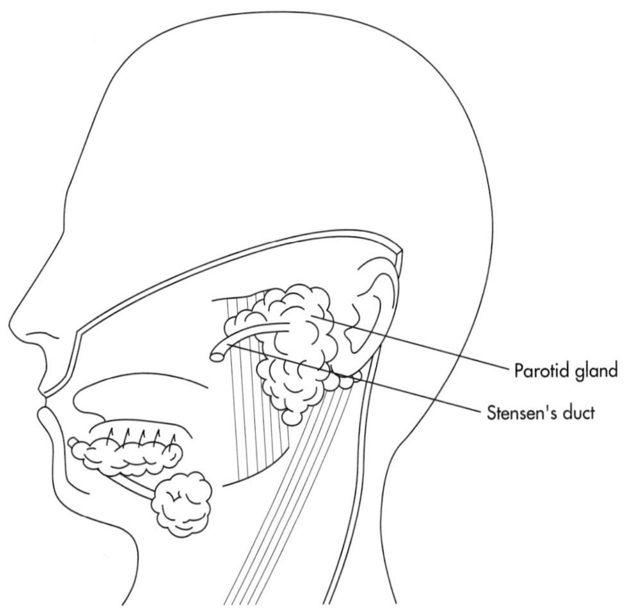

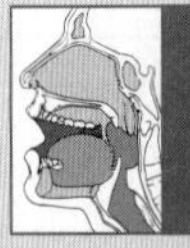

Parotid glands are mostly serous in composition, having mainly serous secretory units. They produce a watery, proteinaceous saliva.

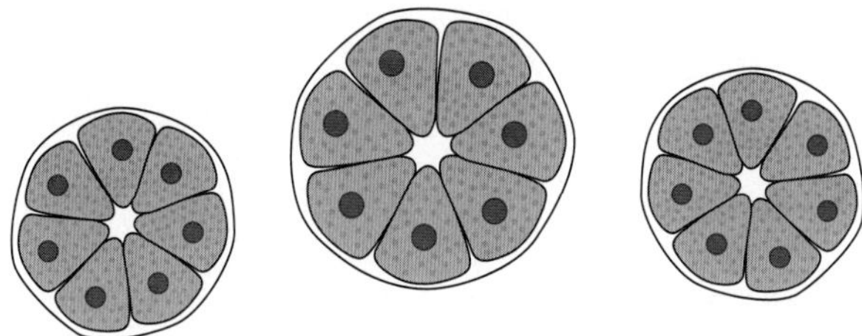

Parotid

_______________ gland ducts collect into one major duct that empties into the oral cavity; this is called **Stensen's duct.** It is shown in the diagram.

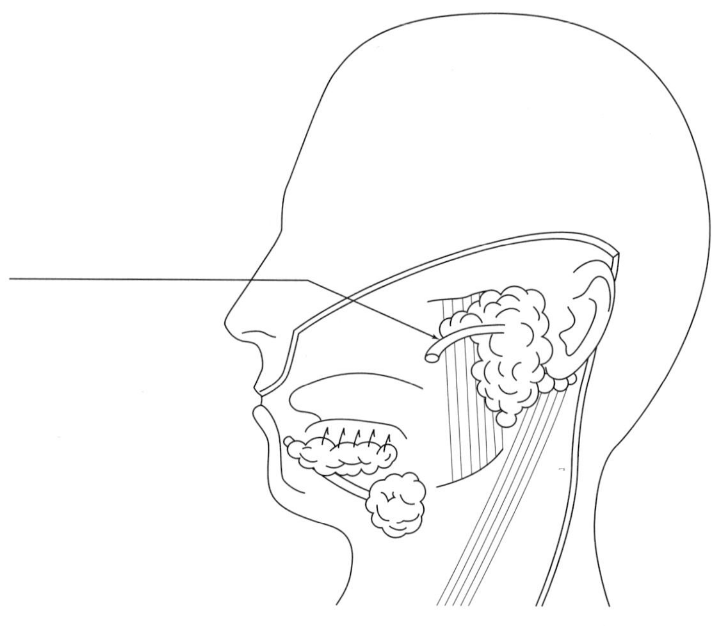

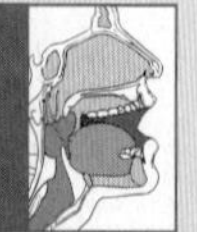

Stensen's

_______________ duct is a large pencil-sized duct exiting from the parotid gland horizontally, piercing the substance of the buccinator muscle to enter the oral cavity.

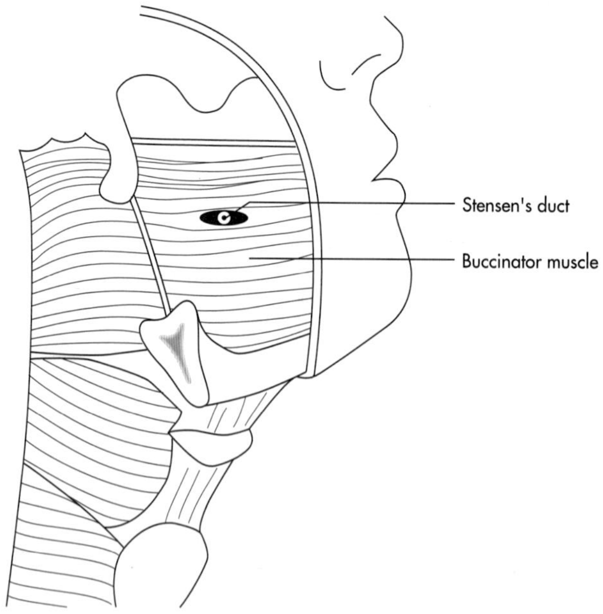

Stensen's duct exits in a papilla of buccal mucosa directly opposite the maxillary second molars and is easily visible in the mouth. Locate this opening in the drawing.

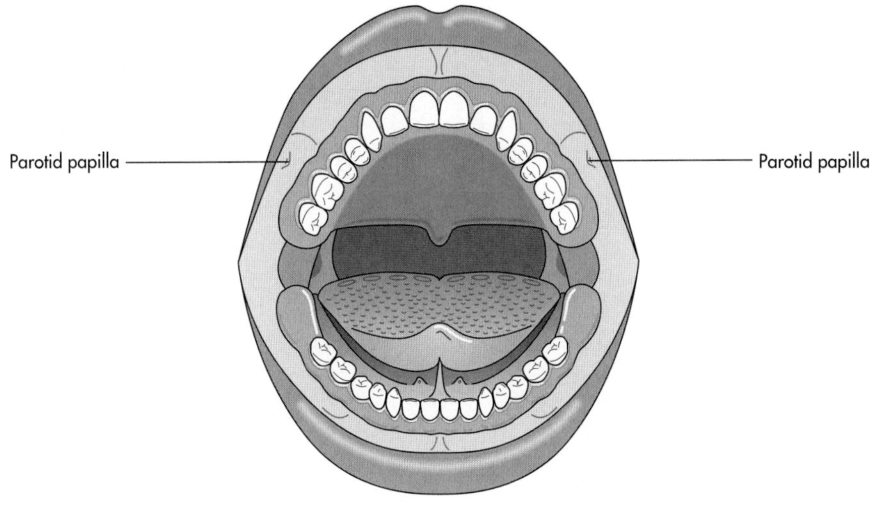

What type of secretion do the parotid glands produce? Why?

watery; serous secretory units predominate

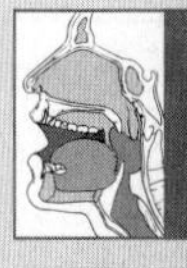

SUBMANDIBULAR SALIVARY GLANDS

The **submandibular salivary glands** are a pair of well-encapsulated glands located on either side below the angles of the mandible, directly below the surface skin and on top of the suprahyoid muscles.

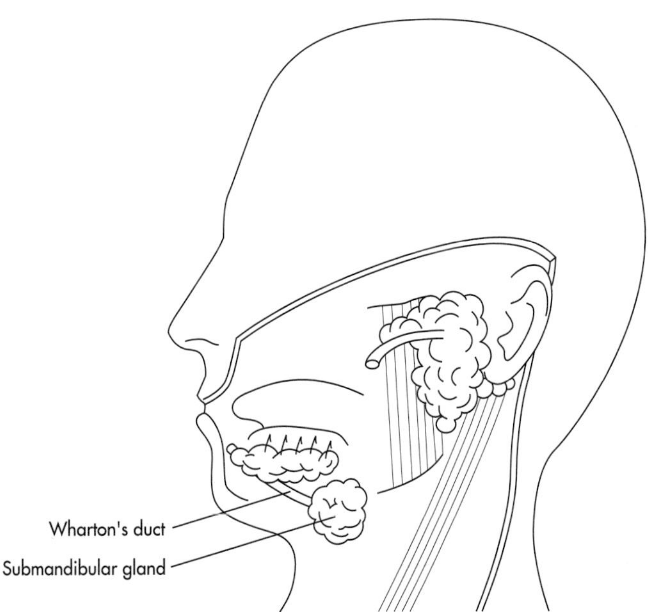

no, the opposite

The submandibular glands are composed mainly of mucous secreting units. Is this similar to the parotids?

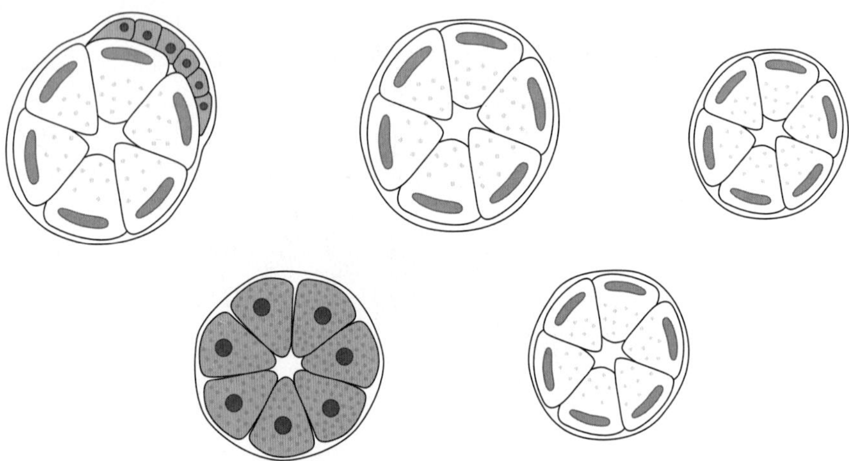

submandibular

From the secretory units, the ______________ gland ducts collect into larger and larger ducts, which empty into the major duct, **Wharton's duct.** This duct is shown in the diagram.

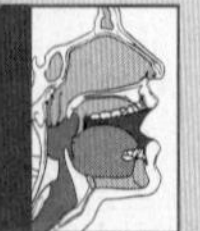

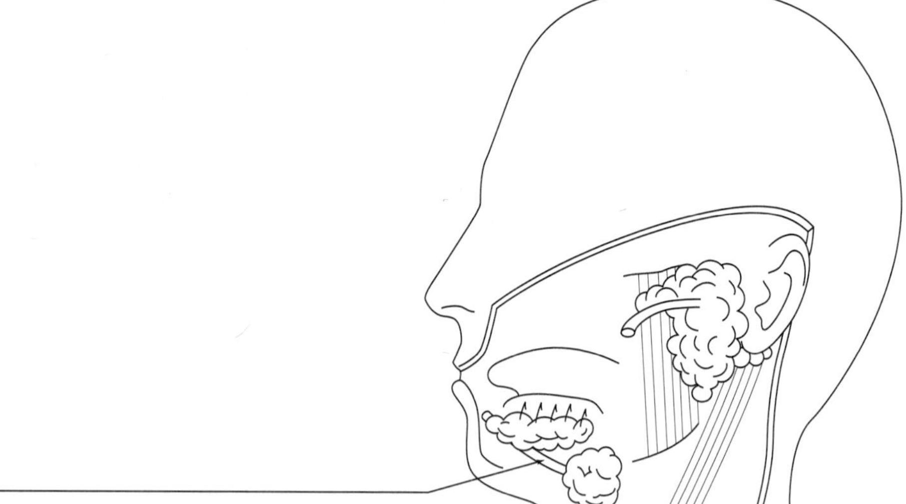

Wharton's ______________ travels a long distance from the gland in the floor of the mouth toward the anterior midline, where it empties through a mucosal papilla, a **sublingual caruncle.** Find these on the drawing.

duct

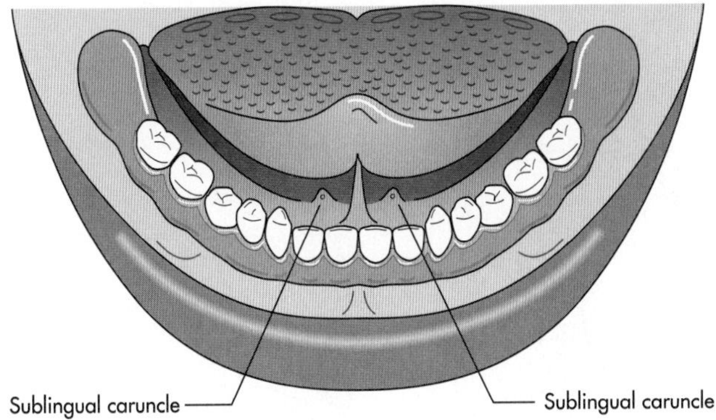

Remember that there is a right and a left submandibular gland, two Wharton's ducts, and, therefore, two sublingual ______________. The caruncles are located on either side of the lingual frenum.

caruncles

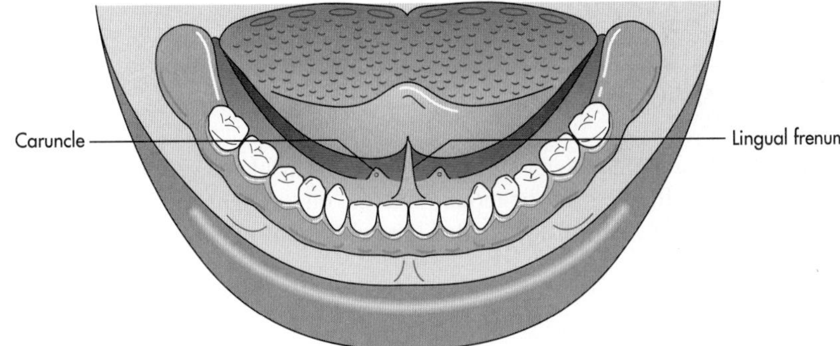

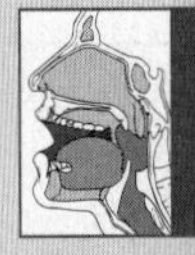

mostly mucus because of the predominance of mucous units

What type of secretion comes from the submandibular glands and why? Label the parts of the gland on the drawing.

A. Wharton's duct
B. submandibular gland

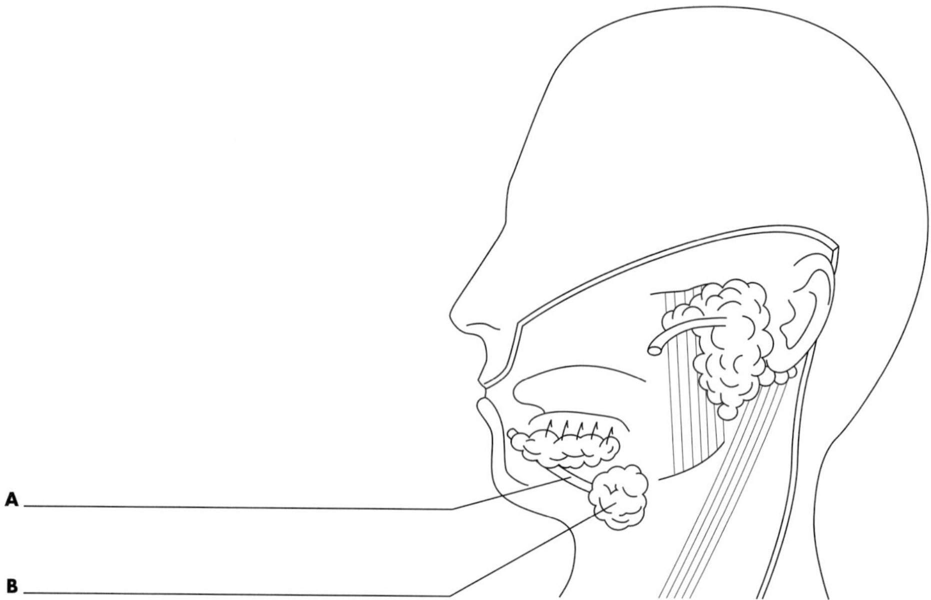

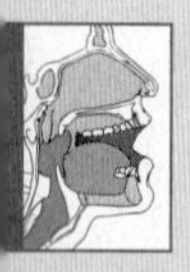

SUBLINGUAL SALIVARY GLANDS

The **sublingual salivary glands** are a pair of poorly encapsulated glands located beneath the tongue, just under the floor of the mouth mucosa, on the right and left sides. They lie beneath the two folds of floor mucosa called the **sublingual plicae.**

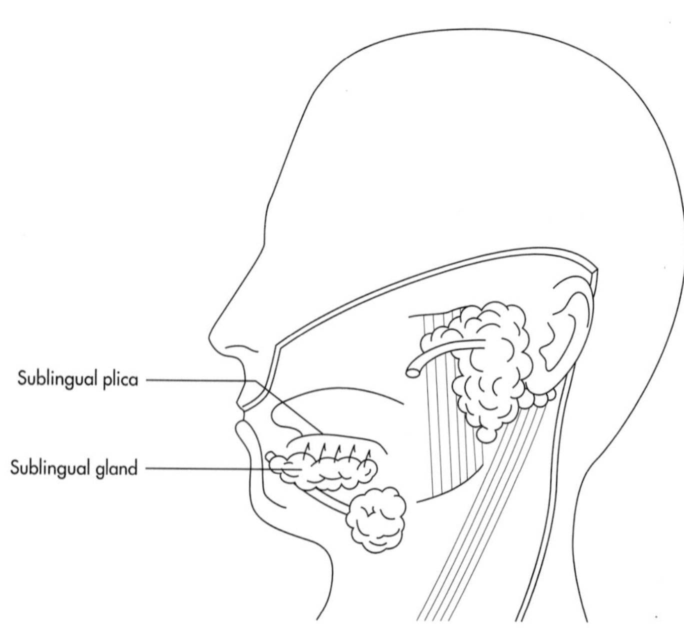

_______________ glands are also composed of mainly mucous units and produce a thick saliva. The ducts from these glands do not collect into a main duct, but rather branch out into multiple small ducts called the **ducts of Rivinus.**

Sublingual

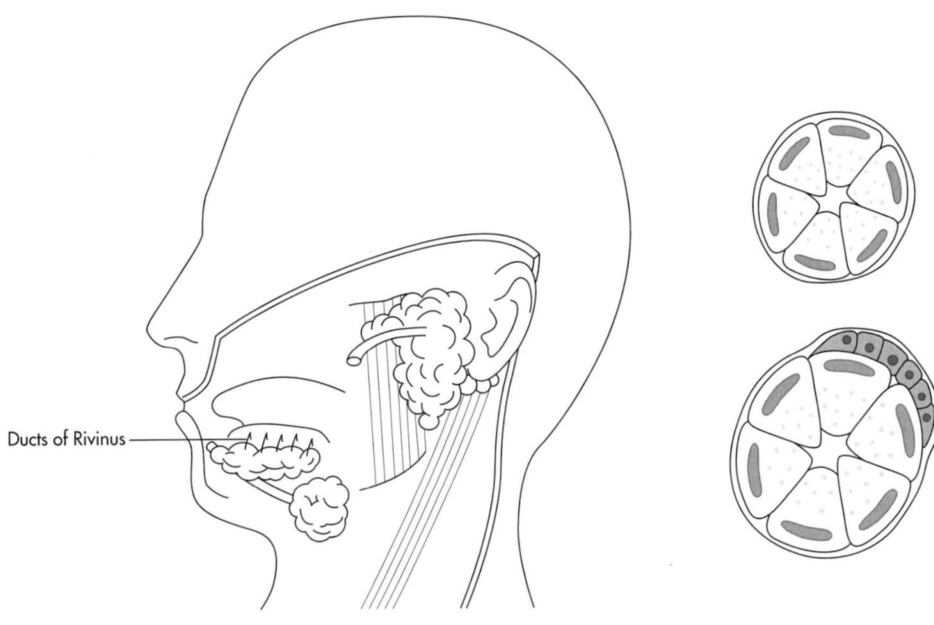

What are the ducts of the parotid and submandibular glands called?

parotid: Stensen's duct; submandibular: Wharton's duct

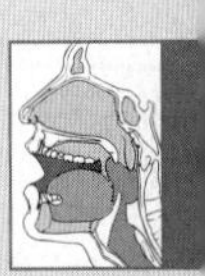

The ducts of Rivinus empty directly through the sublingual plicae. Find them in the diagram. Some of the secretion also makes its way into the duct of the submandibular gland, Wharton's duct.

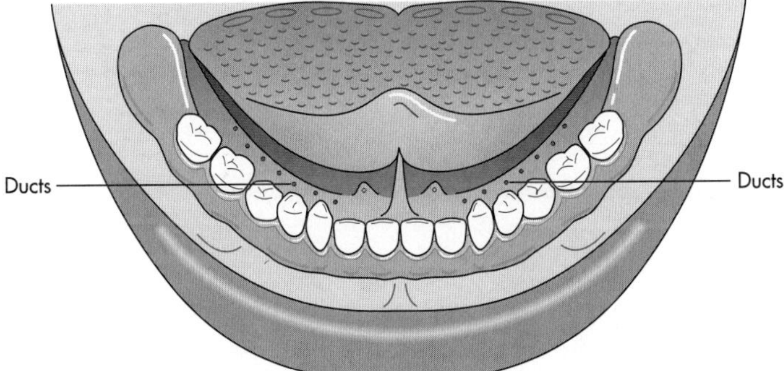

Locate the three major salivary glands and their ducts.

A. parotid gland
B. Stensen's duct
C. ducts of Rivinus
D. sublingual gland
E. Wharton's duct
F. submandibular gland

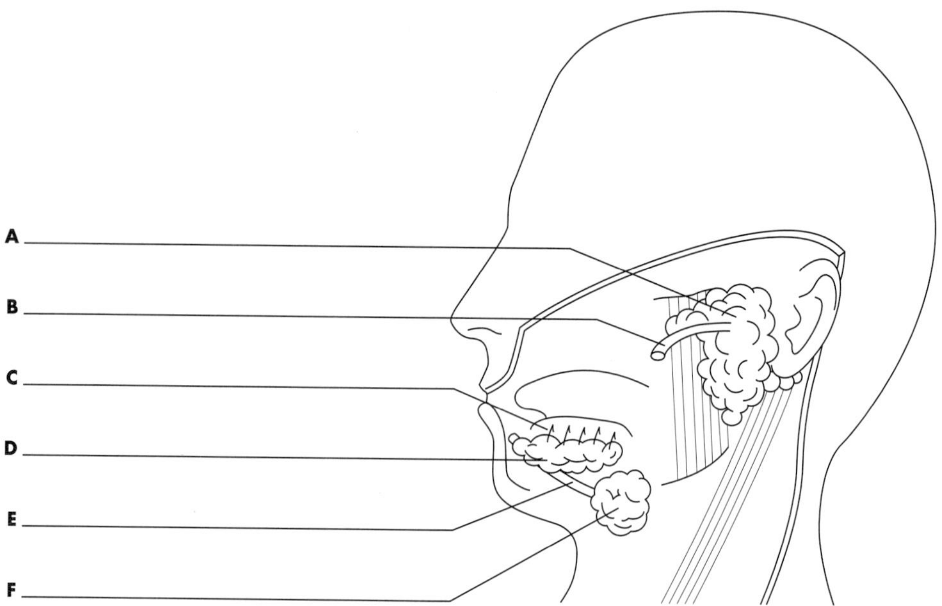

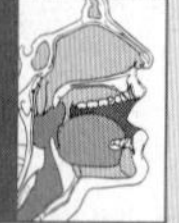

3.0 ORAL LANDMARKS

When looking into a patient's mouth, knowledge of several structures is necessary for orientation and diagnosis. Many of these structures are covered with oral mucosa. The following diagrams show you these **oral landmarks.** We have already studied many of them. Please review them at this time, then look at the unlabeled drawing to test your knowledge.

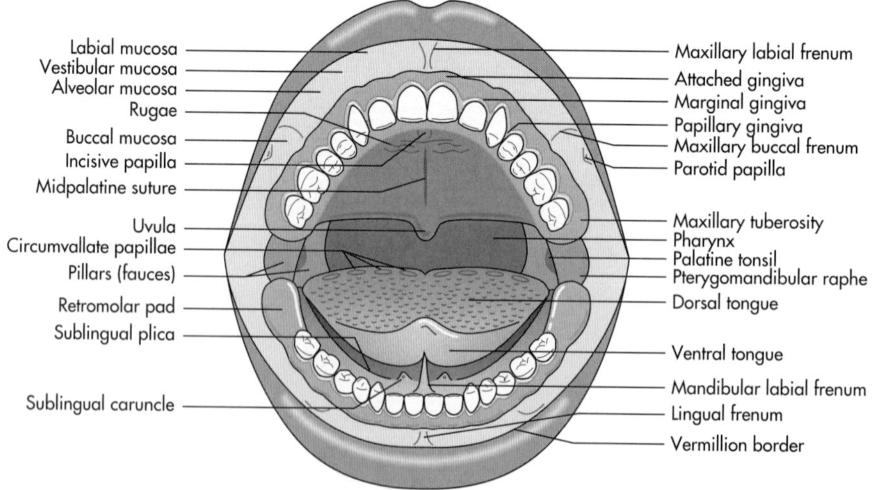

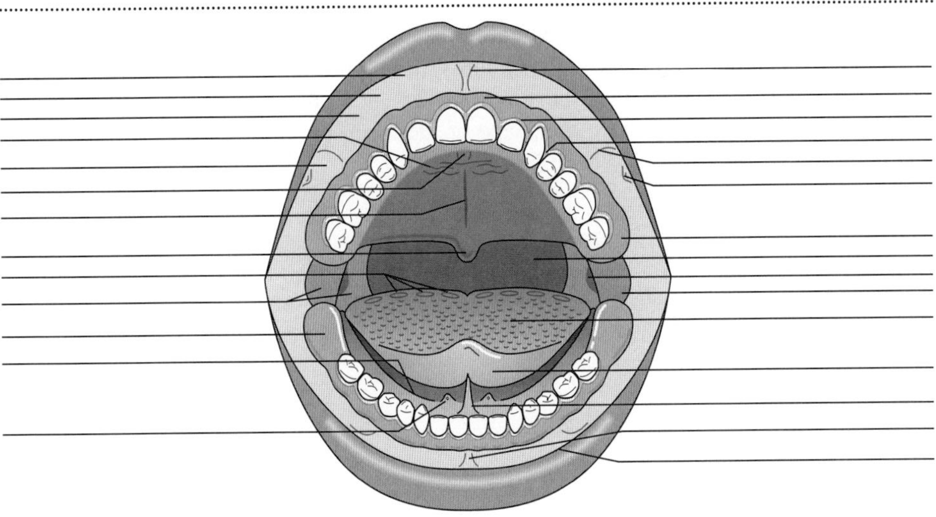

TEMPOROMANDIBULAR JOINT

4.0

We turn now to the tissues of the "jaw joint" or **temporomandibular joint,** where the mandible articulates with the cranium within the temporal bone. Remember that where two bones are joined together by connective tissue, they create a joint.

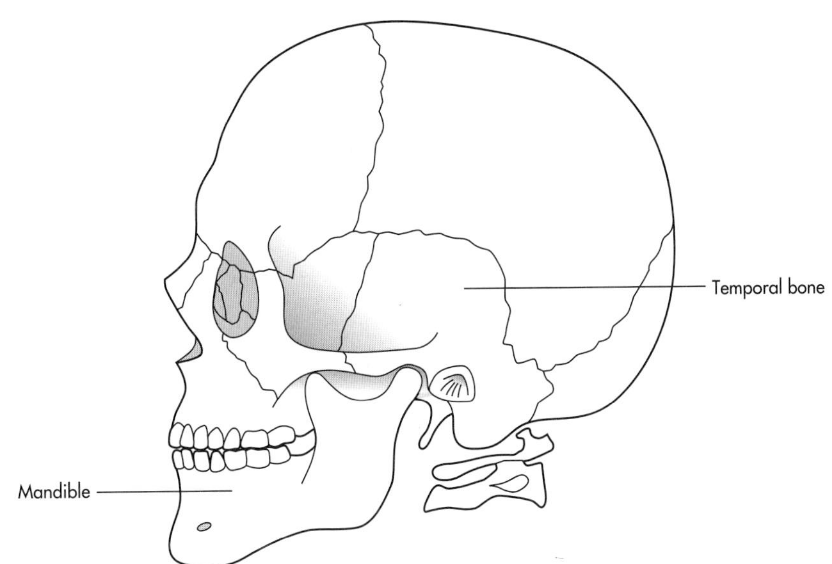

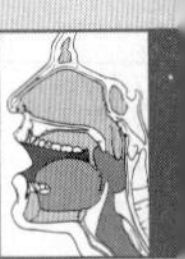

We study the temporomandibular joint (TMJ) because, histologically, it is a unique joint of the body. This joint allows **hinge-type movement, gliding-type movement,** and various combinations of these two movements. This not only allows movement of the mandible that is compatible with the shape of the teeth, but allows a varied diet, as humans are **omnivores** (plant and meat eaters).

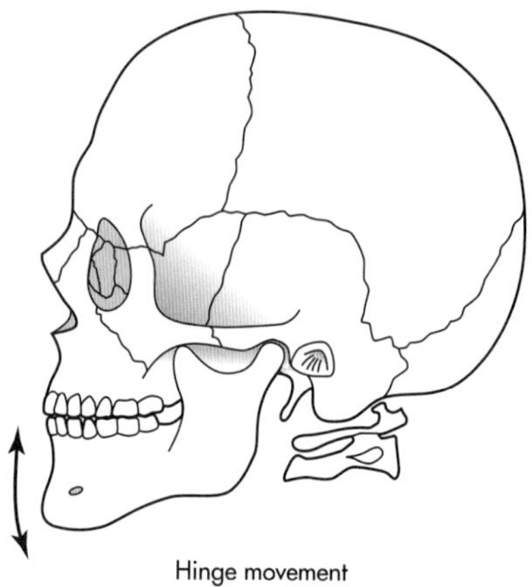

Hinge movement

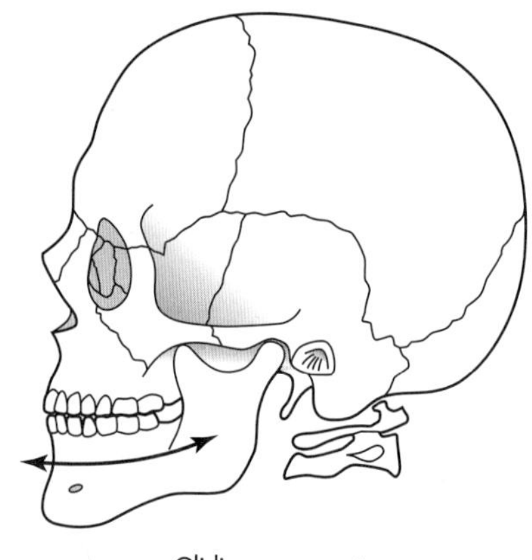

Gliding movement

Let us begin with the two bones that come together: the **condyle** of the mandible and the **mandibular fossa** and the **articular eminence** of the temporal bone. Find them below.

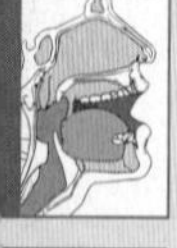

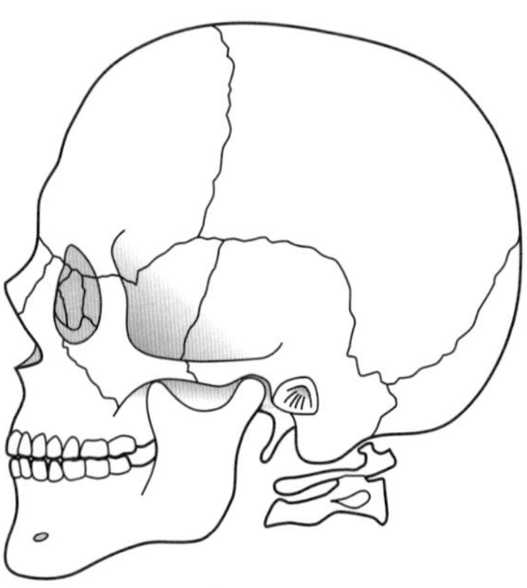

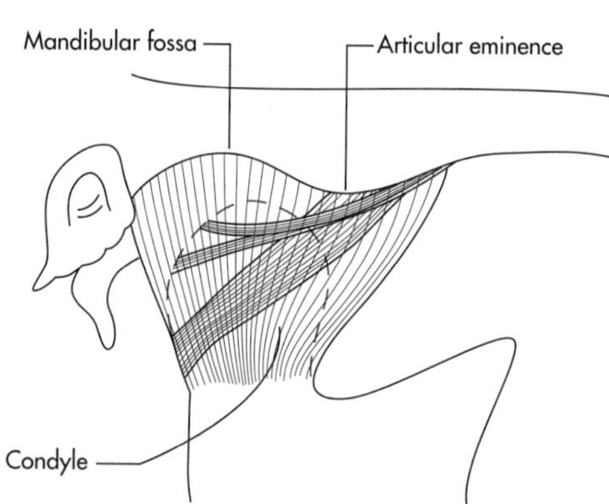

The **condyle** is an egg-shaped bone that seems to fit into the **mandibular fossa;** however, it does not articulate here. It articulates against the **articular eminence.**

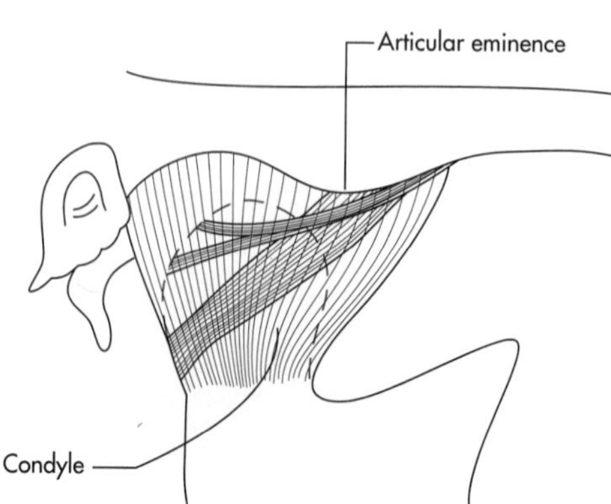

Both the condyle and the eminence are covered by **fibrous connective tissue** with no blood vessels and some cartilage cells. This is different from all other joints, which are usually covered by cartilage. This fibrous covering allows for a great deal of wear and tear, as the TMJ is the most frequently used joint in the body.

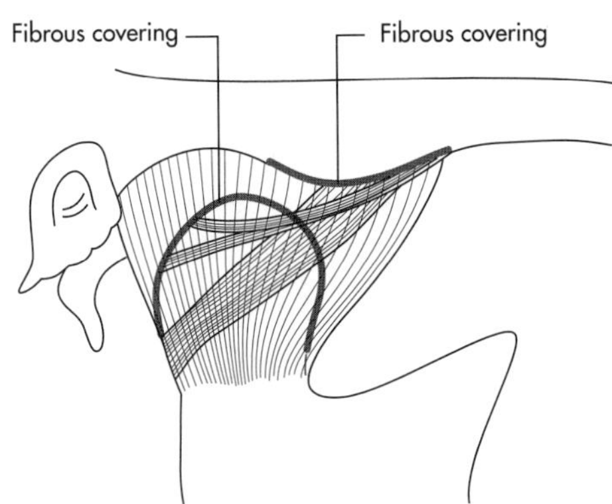

---

fibrous

Besides the ______________ covering of the bones of the TMJ, this joint has a unique **disk** or **meniscus** interposed between the two bones as a cushion. It, too, is composed of fibrous connective tissue with no blood vessels and, with age, a few chondrocytes. It is bi-concave, fitting between the condyle and eminence. Find it on the drawing.

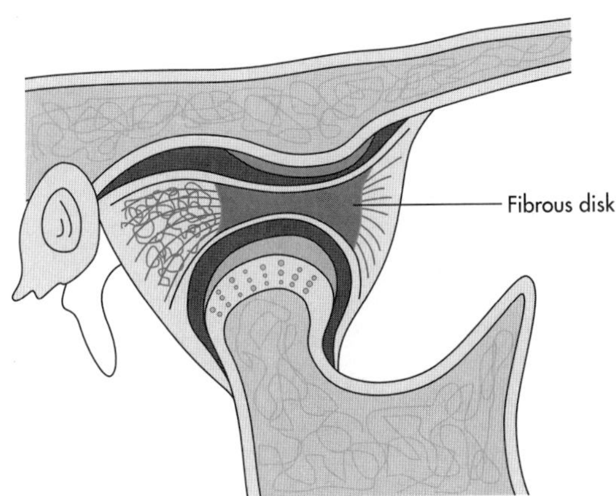

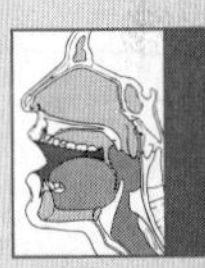

The condyle is attached to the temporal bone by a connective tissue band that encircles the joint. The inner portion of this connective tissue is called the **temporomandibular (TM) capsule** and is thin and avascular. It is barely distinguishable from its outer layer, the **TM ligament,** which is thick.

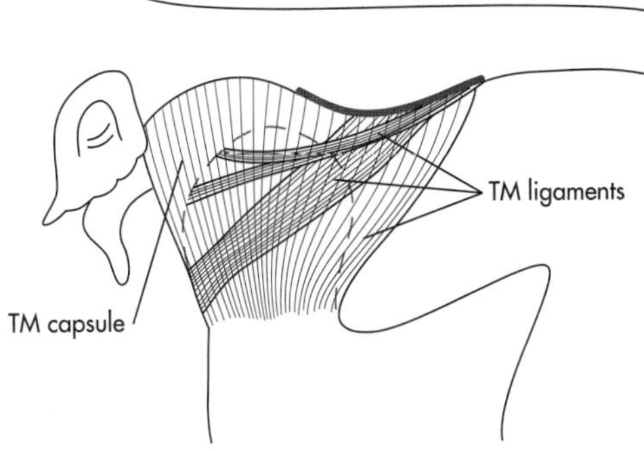

TM capsule

The TM ligament is a thick layer of fibrous connective tissue (dense regular) found on the lateral side of the joint. The fibers of the ligament travel in two directions and are considered, by some, to be two separate ligaments, the **lateral ligaments.** What is the thin inner portion below the ligaments called?

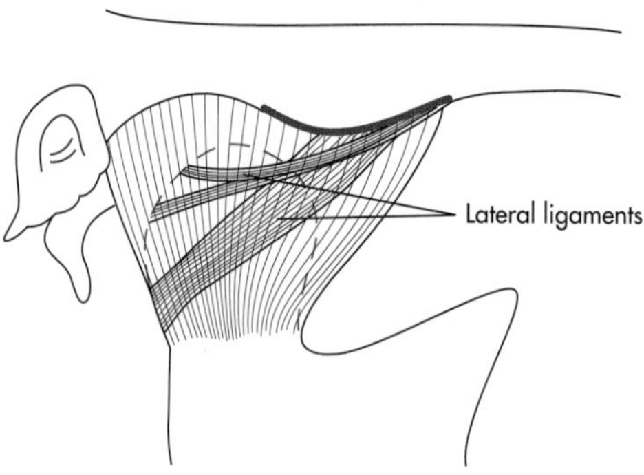

A few other ligaments (accessory ligaments) help attach the mandible to the cranium, but we will look at those in anatomy.

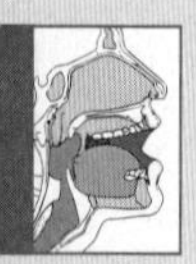

This slice through the joint and its ligaments shows the TM capsule and the TM disk.

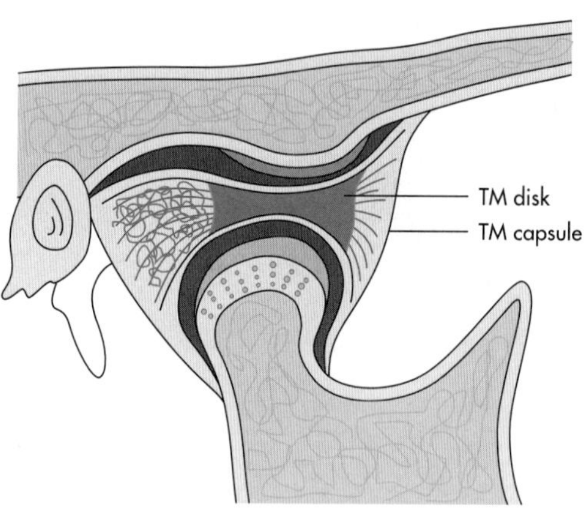

Note that the disk is attached to the capsule by fibrous tissue or ligaments also, as it seems to be suspended in the middle of the capsule. The anterior and medial discal ligaments are collagenous fibrous tissue but the posterior or **retrodiscal tissue** has some elastic fibers. In the medial attachment of the disk are also some of the tendinous fibers of the **lateral pterygoid muscle.**

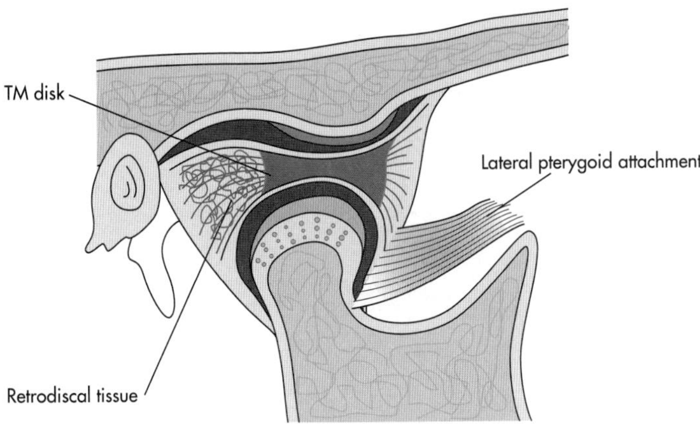

The tissue behind the joint or _______________ tissue is rich in blood vessels and nerve fibers lying in a loose connective tissue. It appears to fall into two layers or a **bilaminar zone,** with the superior layer containing most of the elastic tissue.

retrodiscal

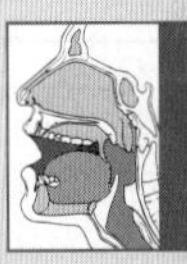

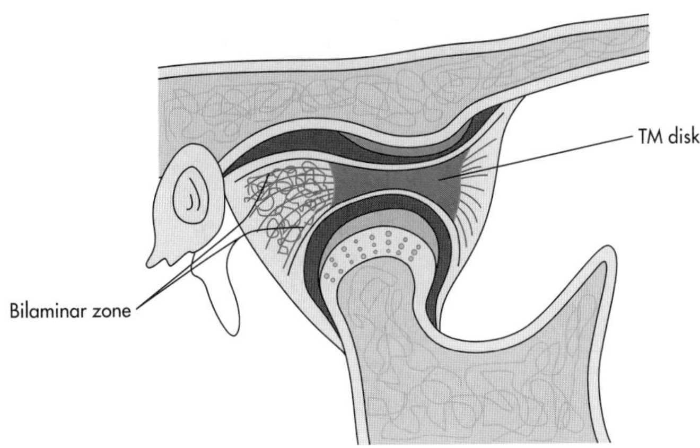

See how the disk separates the joint into two spaces or joint cavities, the **superior** and **inferior joint cavities.**

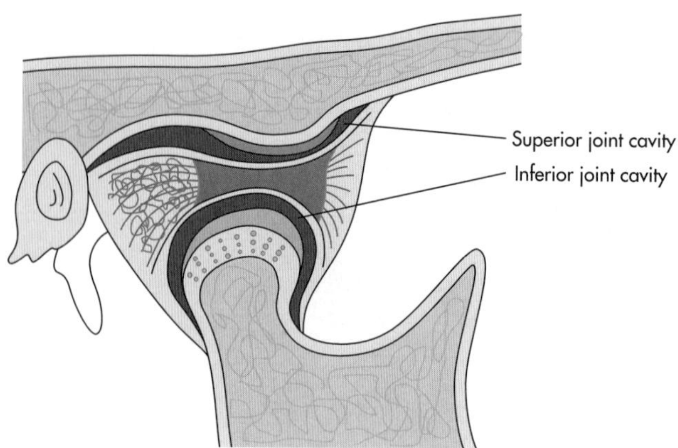

1. fibrous covering on bones
2. disk
3. synovial fluid

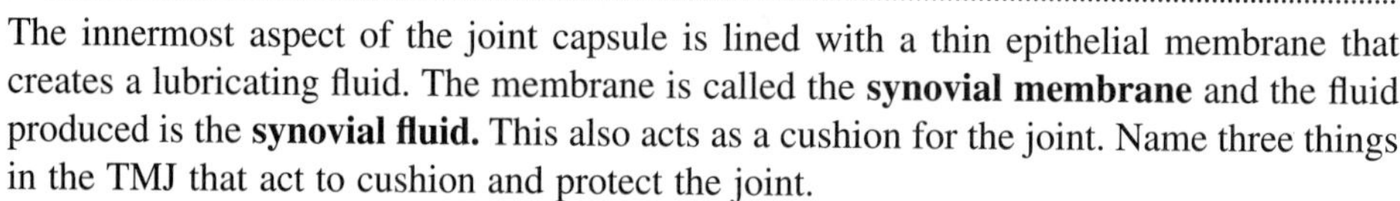

The innermost aspect of the joint capsule is lined with a thin epithelial membrane that creates a lubricating fluid. The membrane is called the **synovial membrane** and the fluid produced is the **synovial fluid.** This also acts as a cushion for the joint. Name three things in the TMJ that act to cushion and protect the joint.

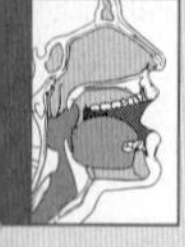

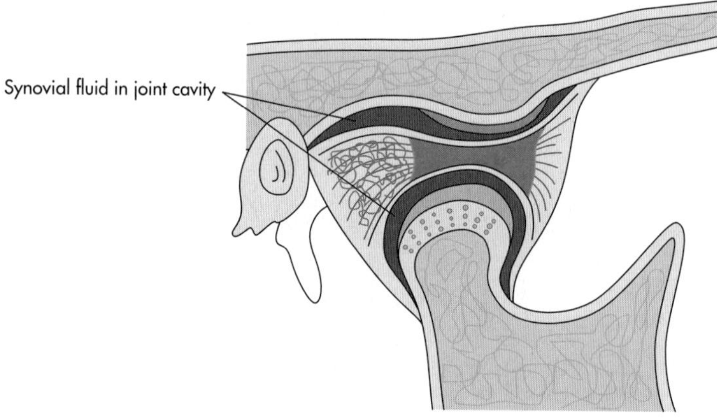

The division of the TMJ into two joint cavities allows its two different types of movement: hinge and gliding. Hinge movement occurs in the inferior joint cavity; gliding movement occurs in the superior joint cavity. Chewing or mastication is achieved by a combination of these basic joint movements.

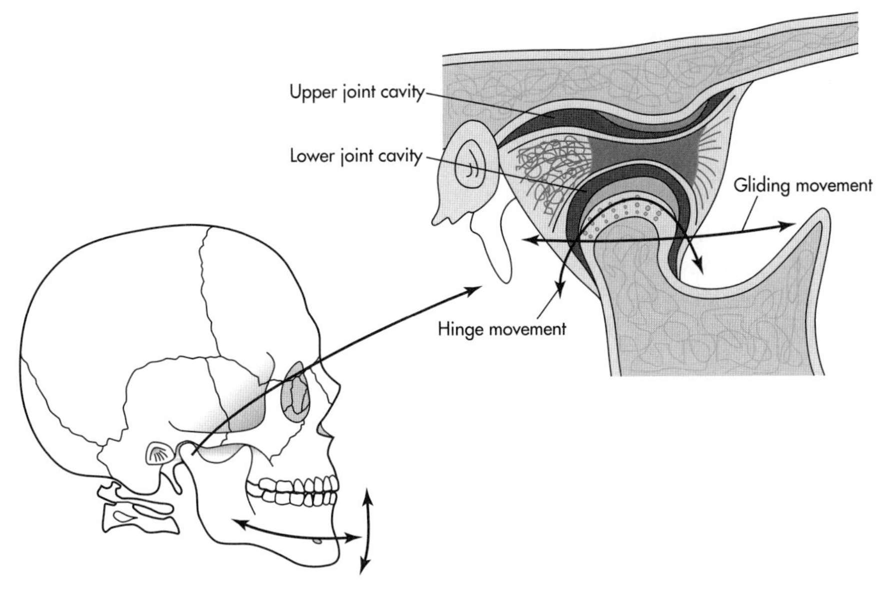

Label the parts of the TMJ.

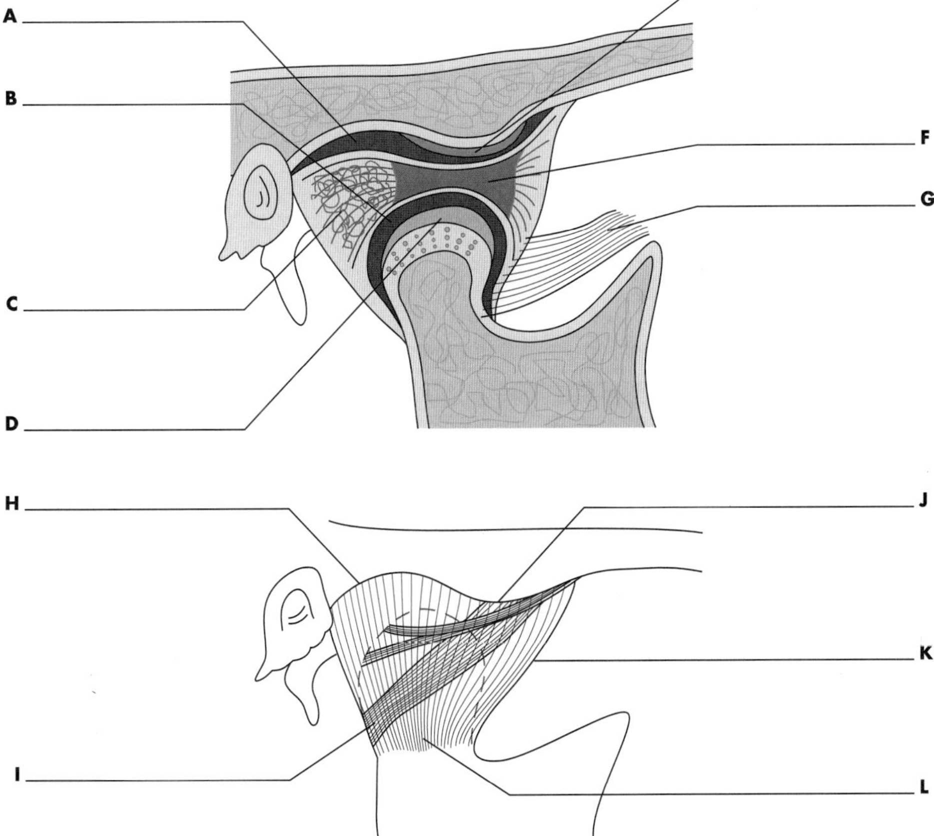

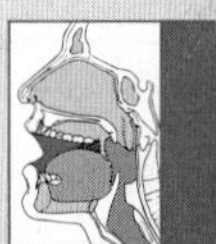

A. superior joint cavity
B. inferior joint cavity
C. retrodiscal tissue
D. fibrous tissue on condyle
E. fibrous tissue on articular eminence
F. fibrous disk
G. lateral pterygoid

H. mandibular fossa
I. lateral ligaments
J. articular eminence
K. TM capsule and ligament
L. condyle

REVIEW TEST 6.1

SELECT THE CORRECT ANSWER.

1. Mucosa is a lining tissue that consists of an upper epithelial layer called the ______________, a middle layer of connective tissue called the ______________, and sometimes a third muscular layer.
   a. epidermis, dermis
   b. mucosa proper, lamina propria

2. The upper layer of oral mucosa is what type of epithelium?
   a. stratified cuboidal
   b. simple squamous
   c. simple cuboidal
   d. stratified squamous

3. Oral mucosa has all of the following characteristics except
   a. great vascularity
   b. hair follicles
   c. thin epithelium
   d. salivary glands

4. Gingiva is a firm, coral pink nonkeratinized tissue that surrounds the teeth. True or false?

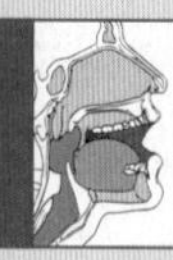

5. Indentations in healthy masticatory mucosa are called
   a. sulci
   b. pockets
   c. stipples
   d. minor salivary glands

6. Gingiva that is attached to the alveolar bone by collagen fibers is called
   a. free gingiva
   b. papillary gingiva
   c. attached gingiva
   d. marginal gingiva

7. The dividing line between the attached gingiva and alveolar mucosa is called the
   a. mucogingival junction
   b. free gingival groove
   c. CEJ
   d. DEJ

REVIEW TEST 6.2

SELECT THE CORRECT ANSWER.

1. The border between epithelium and connective tissue of the gingiva is highly scalloped because of the presence of
   a. keratin
   b. free gingival groove
   c. rete pegs

2. Palatal mucosa is of which type?
   a. lining mucosa
   b. masticatory mucosa
   c. specialized mucosa
3. A bump in the palatal mucosa directly posterior to the central incisors is called
   a. incisive papilla
   b. papillary gingiva
   c. rugae
   d. midpalatine suture
4. Tissue of the hard palate consists of palatal mucosa, a middle layer of bone, and then another layer of palatal mucosa. True or false?
5. Bone in the hard palate is replaced in the soft palate by
   a. muscle
   b. tendon
   c. cartilage
   d. glands
   e. all of the above
6. Which is thicker and contains keratin, lining or masticatory mucosa?
7. Alveolar mucosa is firmly attached to the bone below it. True or false?
8. Folds of lining mucosa found throughout the mouth are called
   a. mucogingival junction
   b. vestibules
   c. frena

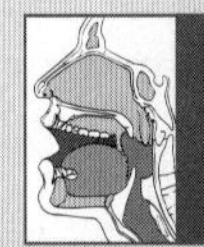

9. The thin nature of the mucosa of the floor of the mouth and ventral tongue makes it a good site for vascular access for some medications. True or false?
10. The two long folds of lining mucosa in the floor of the mouth, under the tongue, are called
    a. sublingual caruncles
    b. sublingual plicae
    c. lingual frena

REVIEW TEST 6.3

SELECT OR FILL IN THE CORRECT ANSWER.

1. Lining mucosa of the cheeks is called ______________ mucosa.
   a. buccal
   b. labial
   c. vestibular
   d. alveolar
2. The "bump" in the buccal mucosa directly opposite the maxillary second molar is called the ______________.
3. The salivary gland duct that leaves the parotid gland, pierces the buccinator muscle, and enters the oral cavity is the ______________ duct.

4. The rough horizontal fold of buccal mucosa that occurs in some people as a result of constant occlusion is called the _______________.

5. Buccinator and superior constrictor muscles meet in the back of the oral cavity and create a mucosa-covered "cord" called the _______________.

6. The area of the lip that becomes a transition zone from skin to mucosa is called the _______________ border.

7. The ventral tongue mucosa is thin enough to see blood vessels beneath it. True or false?

8. The ducts that empty into the sublingual plica from the sublingual salivary glands are called the _______________.

9. The ducts that empty into the sublingual caruncles are _______________ ducts from the submandibular salivary glands.

10. That portion of the pharynx that can be seen by looking into the oral cavity is the _______________.

REVIEW TEST 6.4

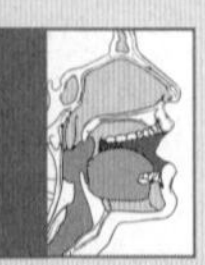

FILL IN THE CORRECT ANSWER.

1. The epithelium of the nasal mucosa (and the rest of the respiratory tract) is ciliated _______________ epithelium.

2. The nasopharynx houses both a tube to the middle ear called the _______________ tube and the _______________ tonsils.

3. Cells responsible for producing mucus in the nasal epithelium are called _______________ cells.

4. Mucosa covers two pairs of muscles in the pharynx and the palatine tonsil rests between them. These are called the _______________.

5. Tissues of the tonsils are not glands, but rather _______________ tissue.

6. The lingual tonsils, palatine tonsils, and pharyngeal tonsils are called _______________.

7. Which side of the tongue is covered by thick, keratinized, specialized mucosa?

8. A smaller, flame-shaped papilla of the dorsal tongue is called a _______________ papilla.

9. Most of the taste cells of the tongue are concentrated in the walls of which type of papilla?

10. The _______________ papillae are large and form a "V" at the posterior/anterior border of the tongue.

REVIEW TEST 6.5

FILL IN THE CORRECT ANSWER.

1. The ______________ lies on the root of the tongue at the tip of the "V" of circumvallate papillae. It is a remnant of the developing thyroid gland.

2. The epiglottis is a cartilaginous structure at the base of the root of the tongue. It has pharyngeal mucosa covering one side and ______________ mucosa covering the other side.

3. The salivary glands are a compound, acinar-type gland composed of two types of secreting units, ______________ and ______________. A third combination unit is the ______________ demilume.

4. Parotid glands are composed mainly of ______________ secreting units.

5. Wharton's duct empties through the pair of ______________ found in the floor of the mouth.

6. Stensen's duct empties through the ______________ in the buccal mucosa.

7. The temporomandibular joint is unique in that it has a ______________ disk and ______________ tissue coverings of the articular surface.

8. The TMJ is a dual-cavity synovial joint with a biconcave disk that allows both ______________ - and ______________-type movements.

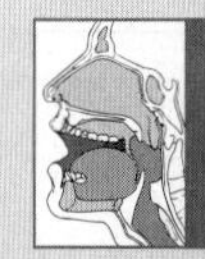

REVIEW TEST 6.6

MATCH THE SALIVARY GLAND WITH ITS DUCT.

1. parotid ______________ a. Wharton's duct
2. sublingual ______________ b. ducts of Rivinus
3. submandibular ______________ c. Stensen's duct

REVIEW TEST 6.7

LABEL THE DRAWINGS.

1.

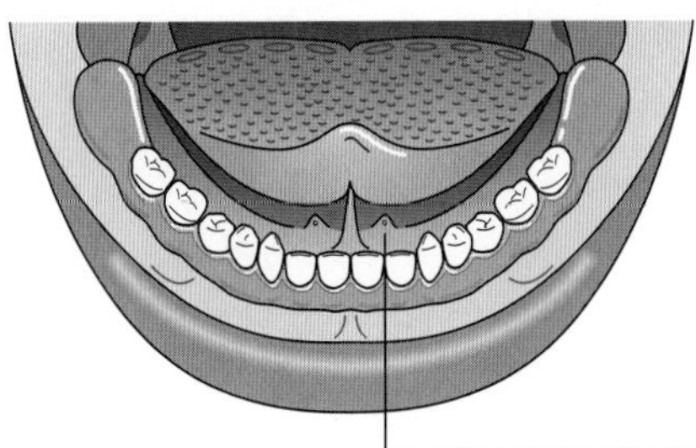
____

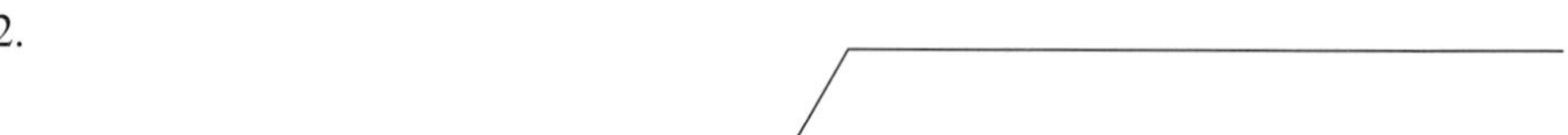

2.

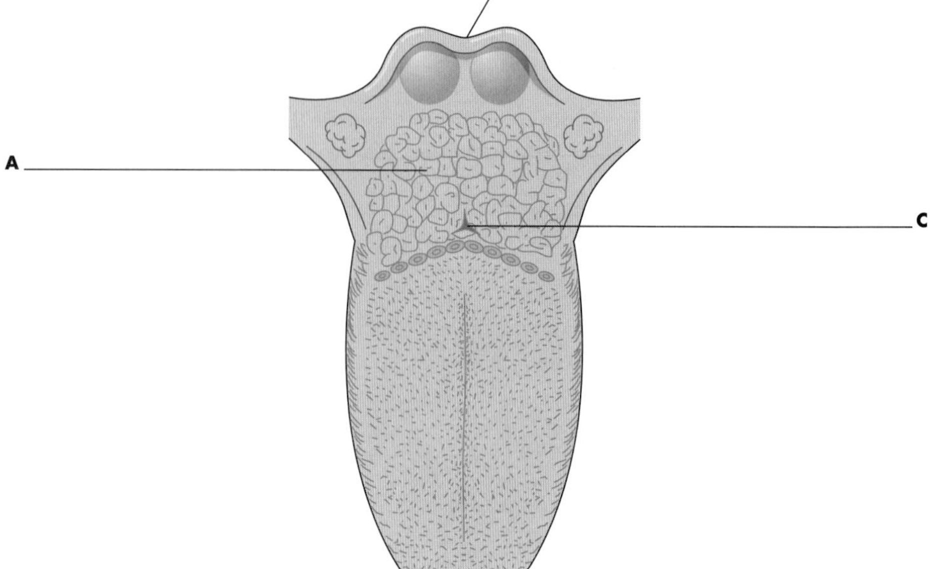

3.

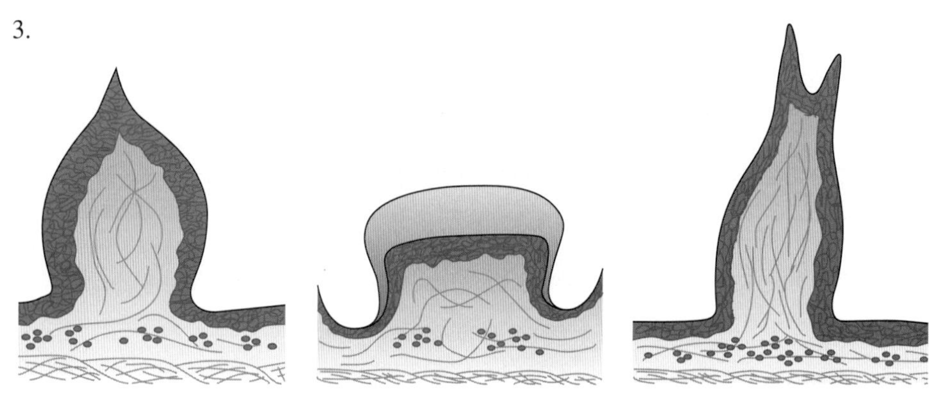

4.

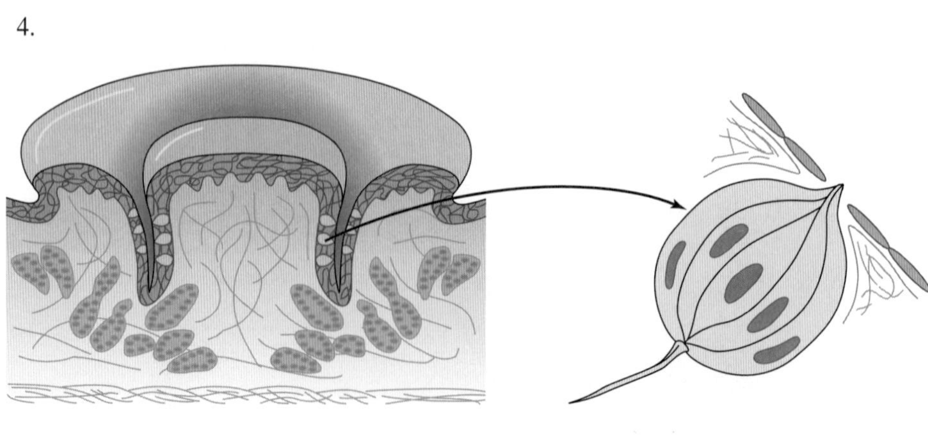

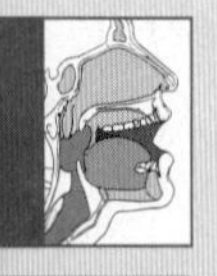

5.

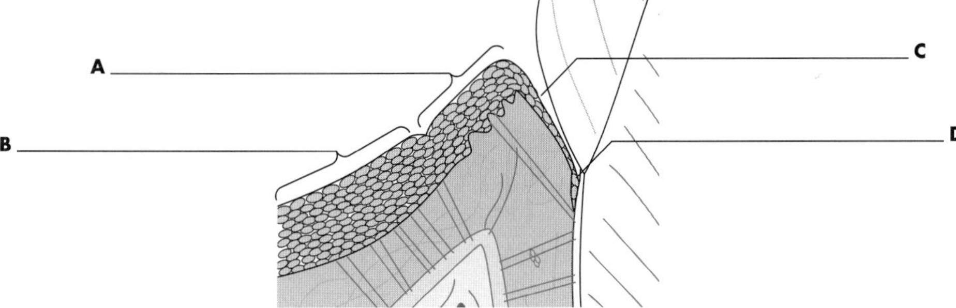

6.

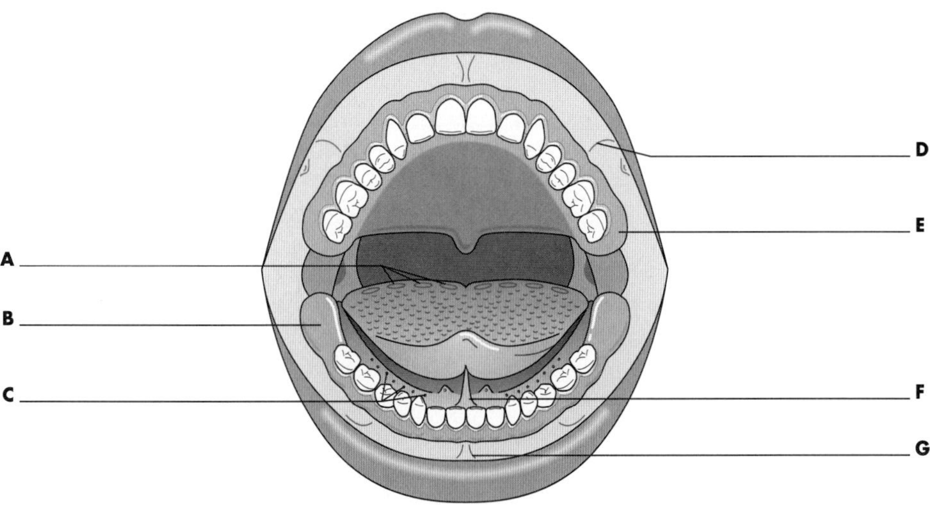

7.

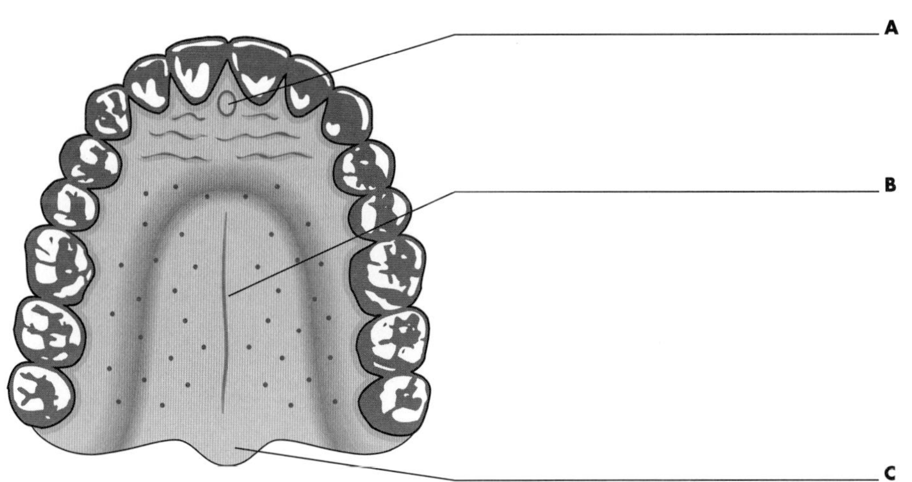

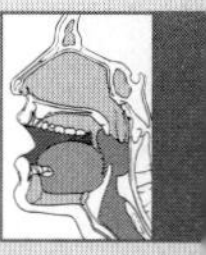

8.

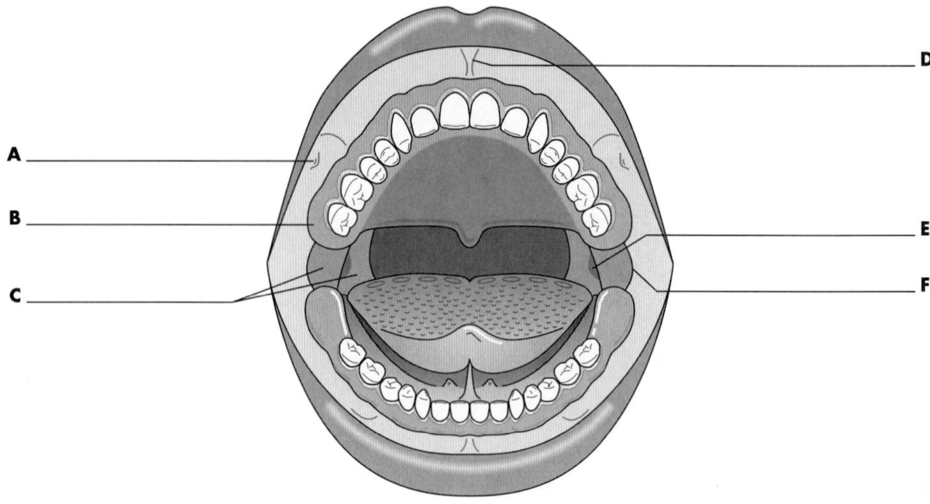

9.

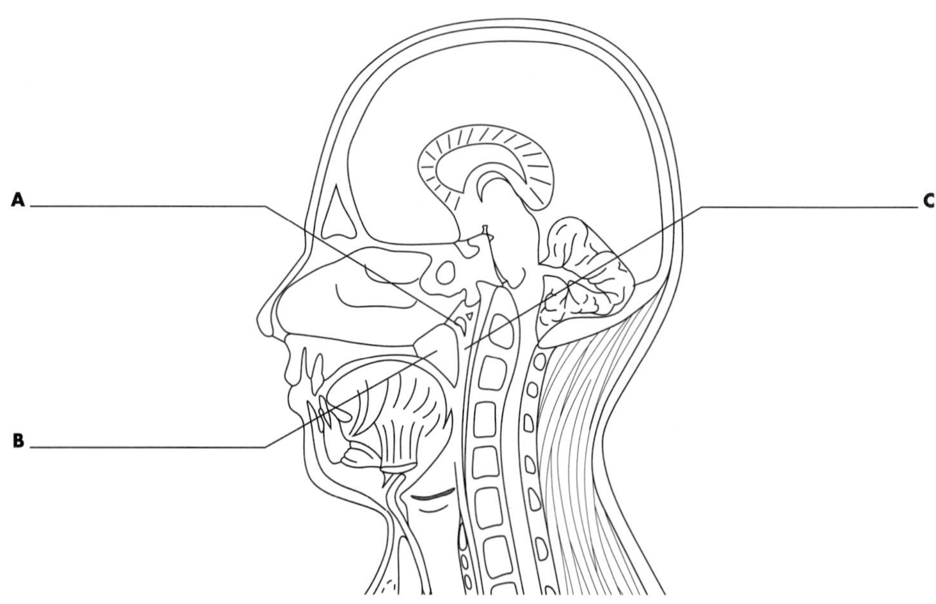

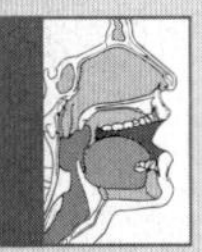

10.

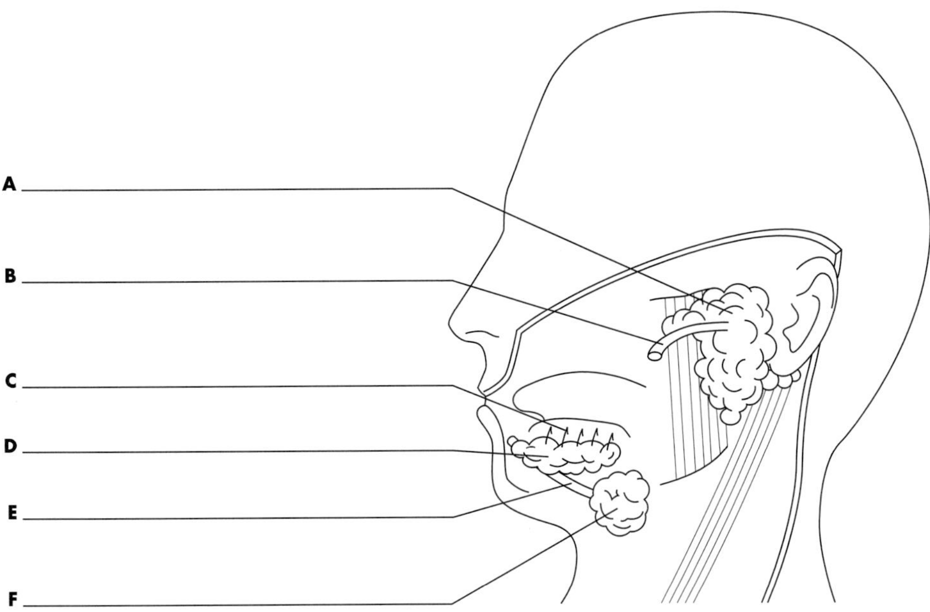

11.

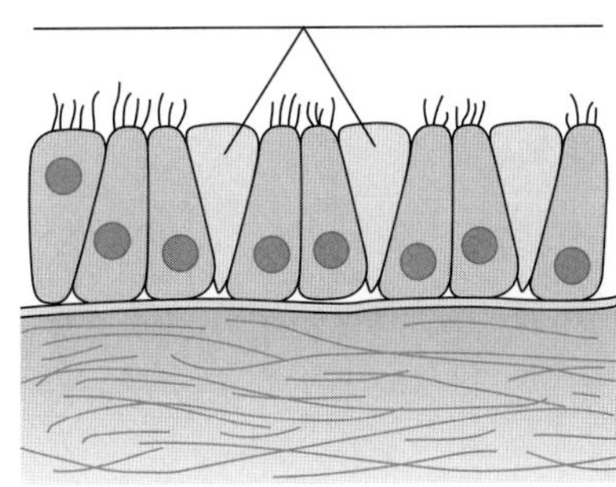

12.

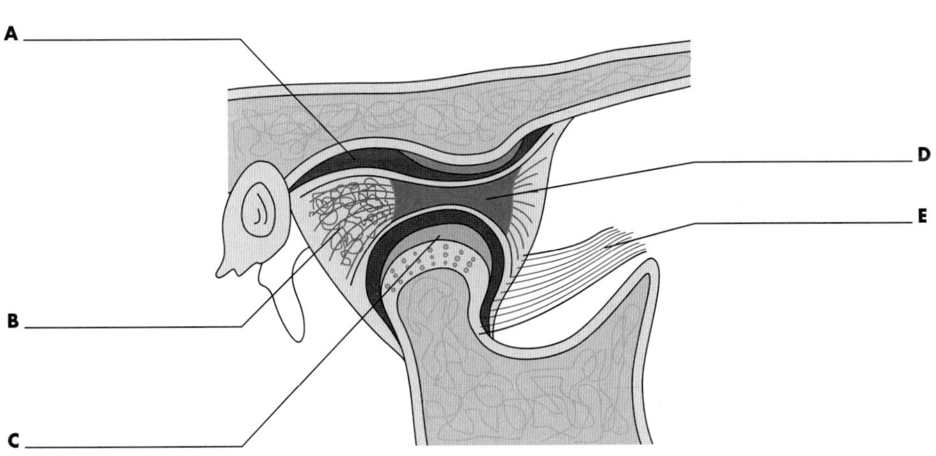

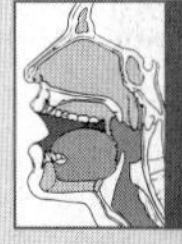

13.

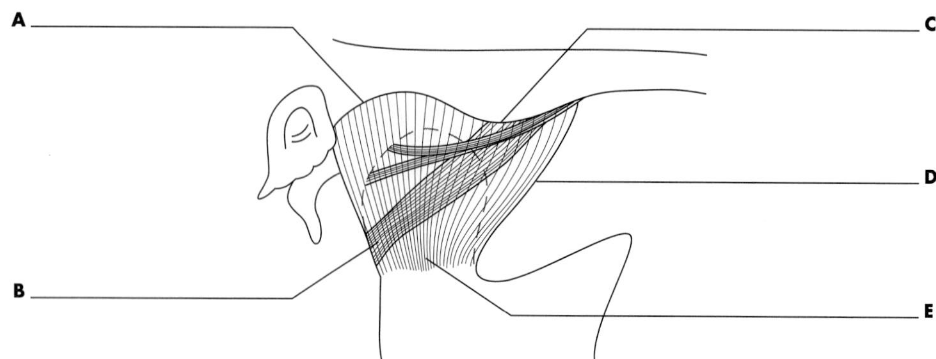

14.

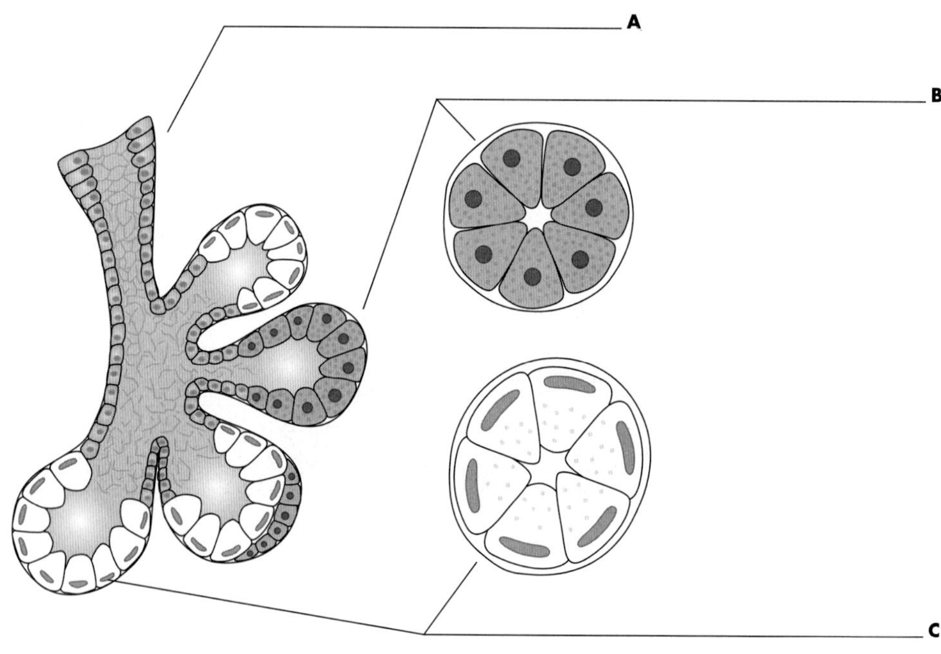

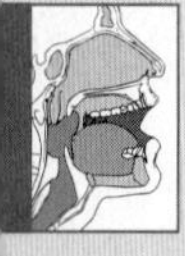

7

Skeletal System

ANATOMIC TERMINOLOGY

1.0

In the first half of the book we explored the head and neck region under the microscope, on the level of cells and tissues. **Histology** is the study of the structure of tissues. We now look at the result of these building blocks, and we can see structure with the naked eye alone. The study of the structure of living things is **anatomy.** In the histology section we studied the microanatomy of the head and neck regions. Now we approach the region from a macroanatomy viewpoint.

Continue your self-study method by reading the text with the attached answer mask, to quiz yourself before you see the answers in the text. You may also find it valuable to color in areas studied with colored pencil for identification and to label structures as you are asked to.

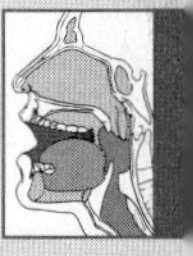

organs

We began with the building blocks of life, the cells; created tissues from them; and went on to build **organs** by combining different tissues. For example, skin was made from epithelial, connective, muscle, and nervous tissues and thus it is an "organ." Organs group together to perform similar functions and are called **systems.** The systems work together to create the **organism,** or whole body. The following schematic shows you this building plan. What is missing?

- Cells
- Tissues
- ______________
- Systems
- Organism (body)

digestive and respiratory

The systems of the human body are well represented in that small region we know as the head and neck. Remember that each system has a job or function. The systems represented in the head and neck region, along with their functions, are as follows:

- Skeletal system: support and protection
- Muscular system: movement
- Nervous system: regulation (electrochemical)
- Circulatory system: provision of nutrients/oxygen, waste/carbon dioxide removal, defense
- Digestive system: food intake, initiation of digestion
- Respiratory system: oxygen intake/carbon dioxide output
- Endocrine system: regulation (chemical)

Some systems such as the reproductive and excretory systems have no portion in the head and neck. In which systems would you place the oral cavity?

Before we begin our systemic look at the head and neck, we need to review some directional terminology. When describing the location of an anatomic structure, we need a specific language. Some of these words will be familiar from histology and from dental morphology.

Humans are delineated by the presence of a backbone. This side of the body is called its **dorsal side.** The "belly side" is called the **ventral side.**

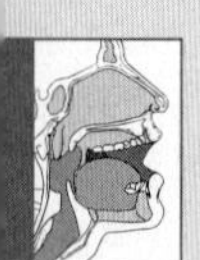

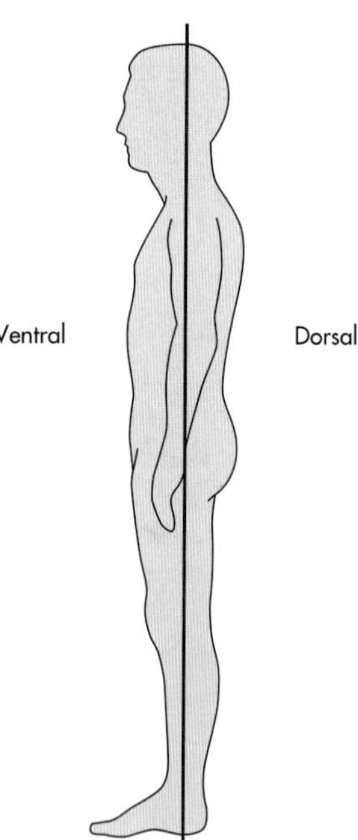

Another way to describe the front of a body or a structure is to call it the **anterior** portion, and the back side, the **posterior** portion.

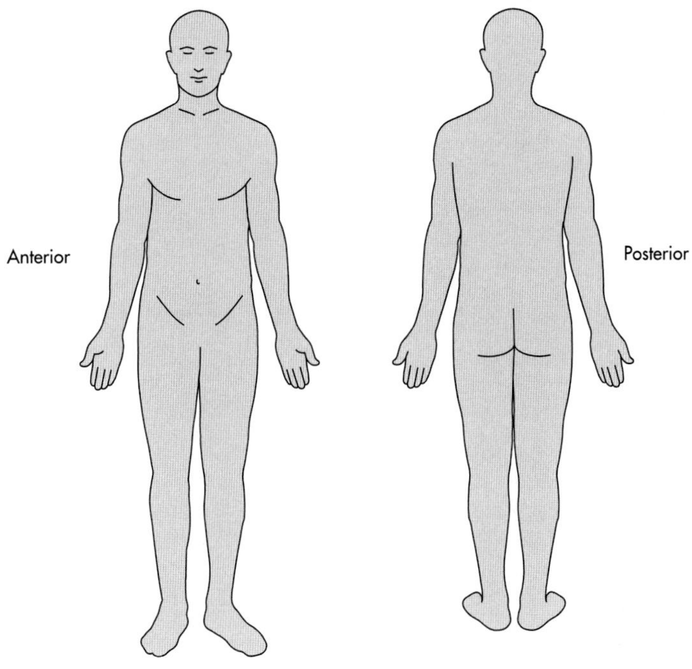

To describe something that is on top or above we say that it is **superior,** and conversely, if it is below or underneath, **inferior.**

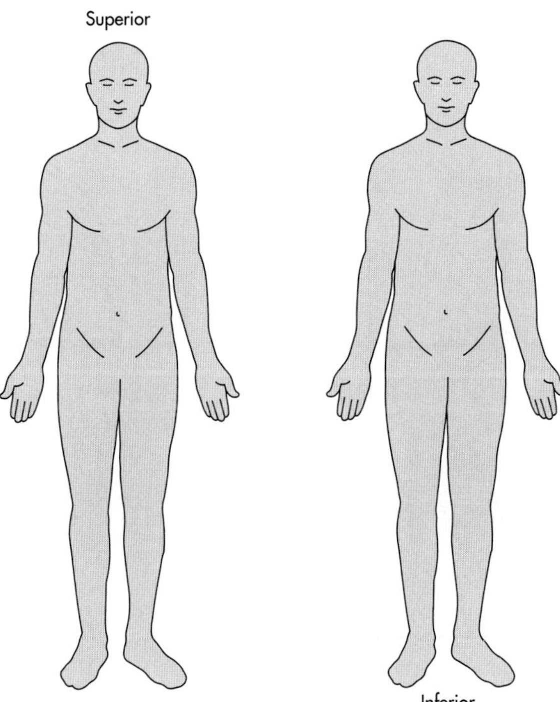

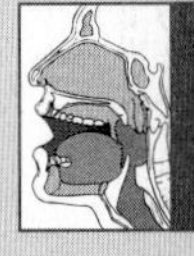

If we run a vertical dividing line down the center of a body, it will give us a **midline.** **Lateral** means away from that midline or to the side of the body, and **medial** means toward the midline.

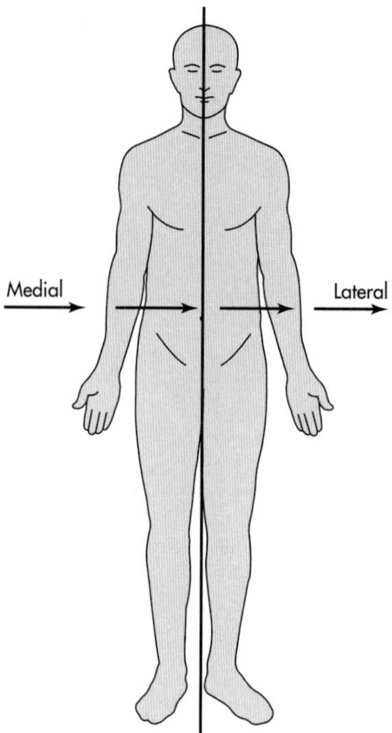

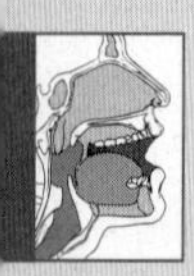

We often look at sections of the head and neck. This means viewing the structures as if they were "sliced" through or as a plane passes through them. Three planes of section are common. A **frontal** section slices through the frontal view of the head and neck.

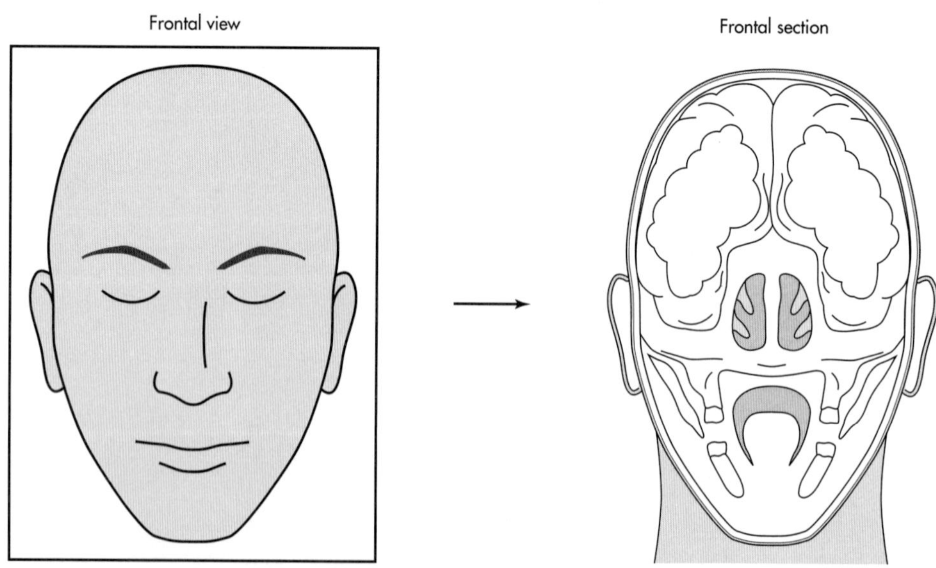

The **sagittal** section slices through the sagittal view of the head and neck.

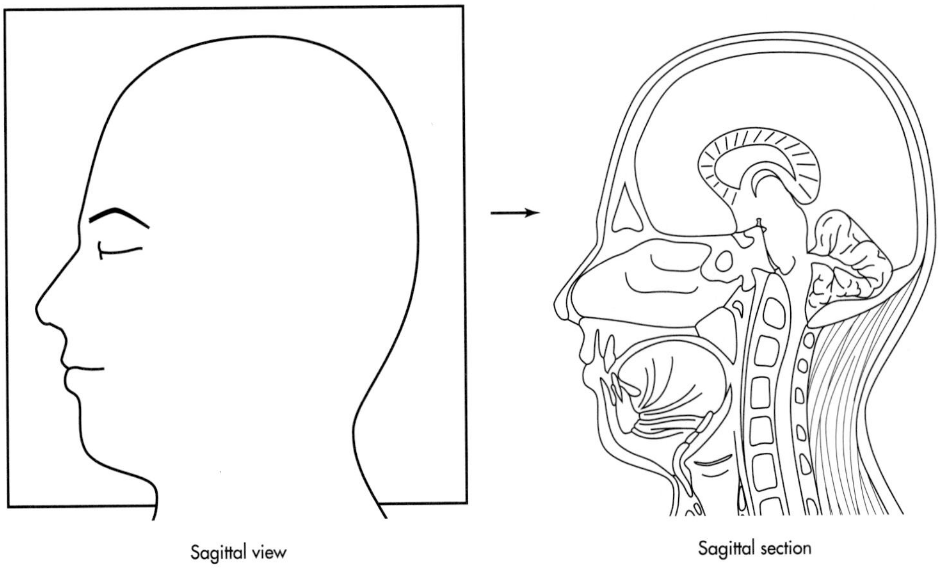

Sagittal view

Sagittal section

The third plane of section is a **transverse** or **cross section** through the head.

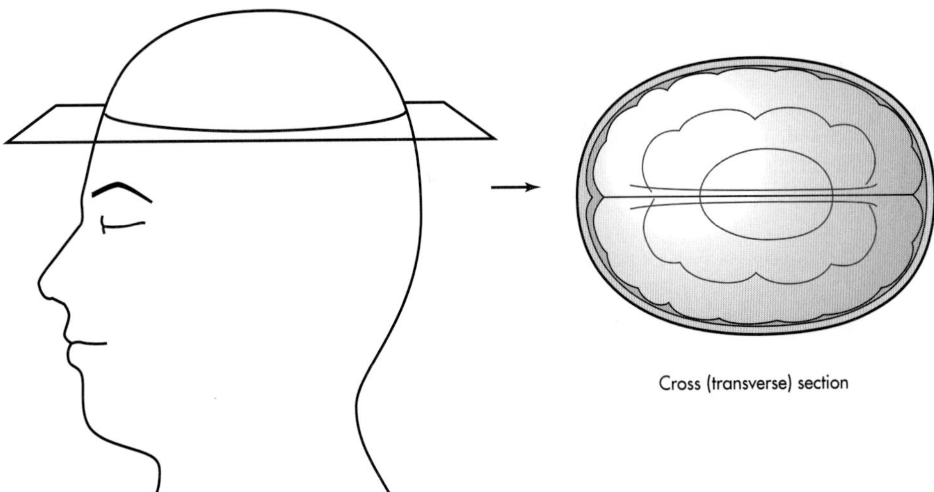

Cross (transverse) section

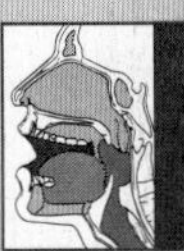

Cranial means "pertaining to the head"; **cervical** means "pertaining to the neck."

A few other terms refer to the surface of the body: **Superficial** means the topmost layer, and **deep,** below it. **Internal** means inside, and **external,** outside.

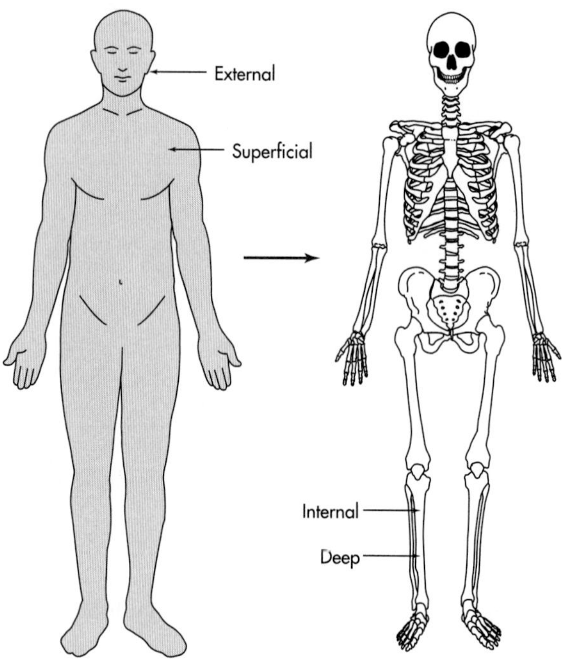

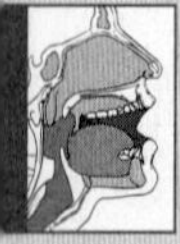

Remember our dental/oral directions: mesial, distal, lingual (palatal), facial (buccal), and incisal (occlusal).

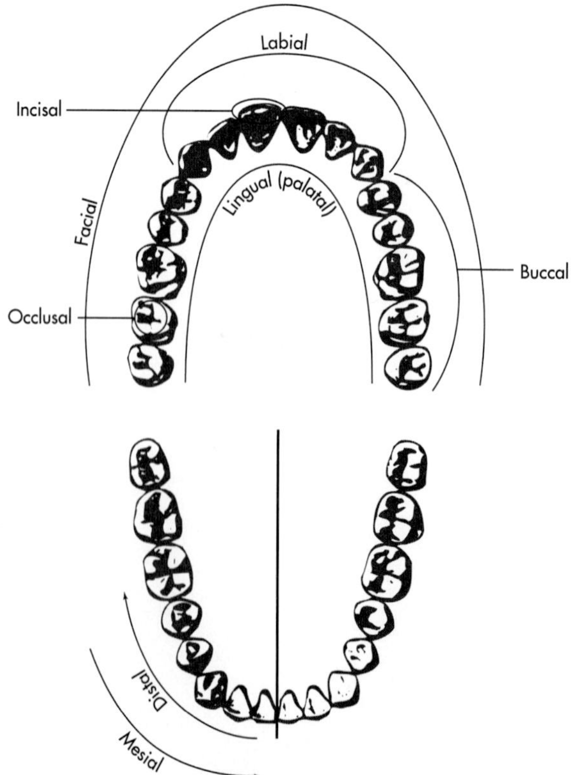

Test yourself on these anatomic words.

Cervical ______________
Posterior ______________
Sagittal ______________
Ventral ______________
Inferior ______________
Superficial ______________
Lingual ______________

Cervical: the neck
Posterior: toward the back side
Sagittal: a view or section showing a "side" view
Ventral: the "belly side"
Inferior: below
Superficial: toward or on the surface
Lingual: toward the tongue (teeth)

SKELETAL SYSTEM

2.0

That portion of the skeletal system within the head and neck region is composed of the cranium, mandible, hyoid bone, and seven cervical vertebrae. What function does the skeletal system serve in the head and neck?

supports and protects the organs of the head and neck

Review the structure of bone tissue in Chapter One at this time. In general, each bone of the body consists of one type of loose bone tissue covered by another type of denser bone. What are these two types of bone?

trabecular bone covered by compact bone

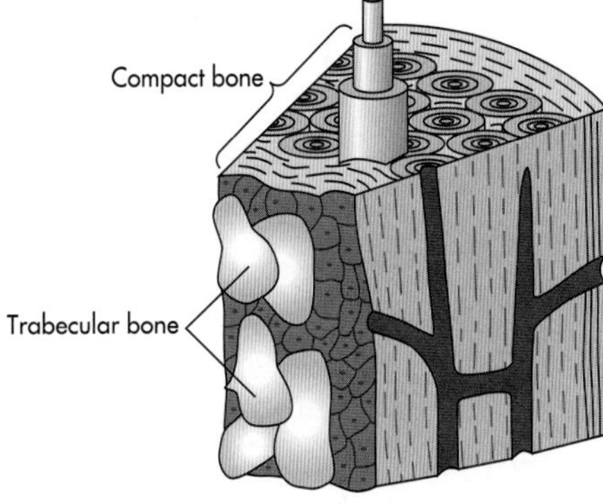

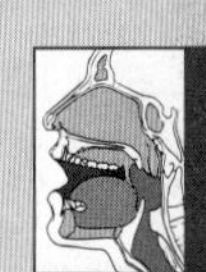

All bones of the head and neck consist of an inner layer of trabecular or cancellous bone covered by a thin, hard outer layer of compact bone. Within the spaces of the trabecular bone lie blood-making cells, blood cells, and fat tissue collectively called marrow.

The joining of two bones is called a **joint.** They are usually joined by strong connective tissue called **ligaments.** Ligaments hold ______________ together.

bones

Joints are classified by the type of movement they allow between the two bones. There are two types of joints in the head. Joints between the cranial bones allow no movement and merely unite the bones. These joints are called **sutures** and appear on the skull as "cracks." They are **immobile** joints.

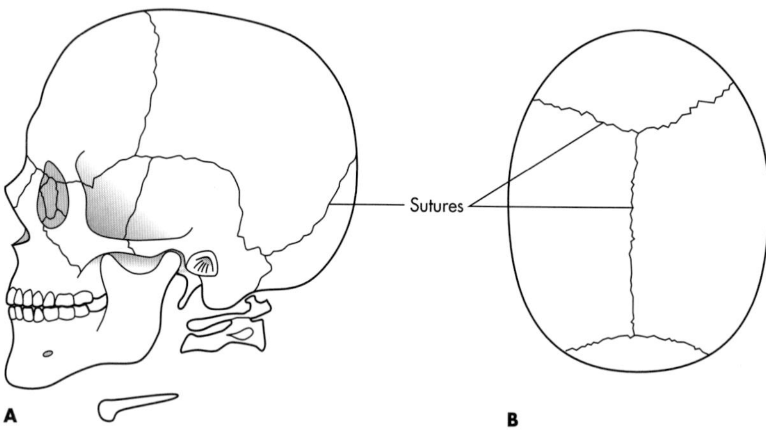

Remember that in development the sutures of the fetus and infant are not totally closed, creating two **fontanels** or membranous areas.

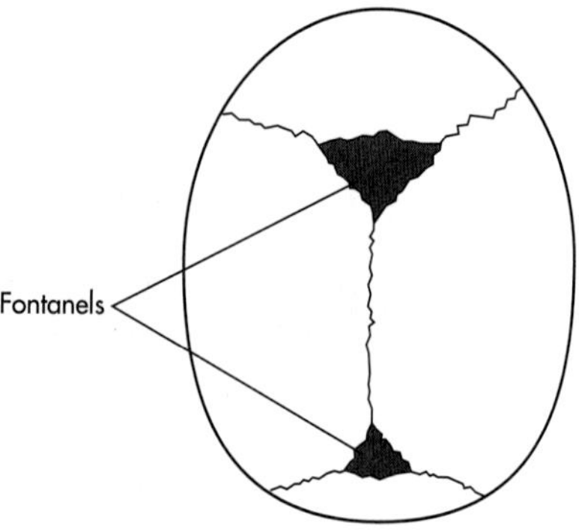

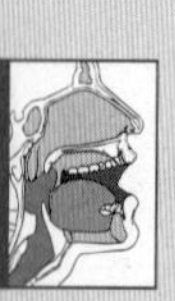

temporomandibular (TMJ)

The other joint involving the cranium is its joint with the mandible. Remember from Chapter Six, that this is called the ______________ joint.

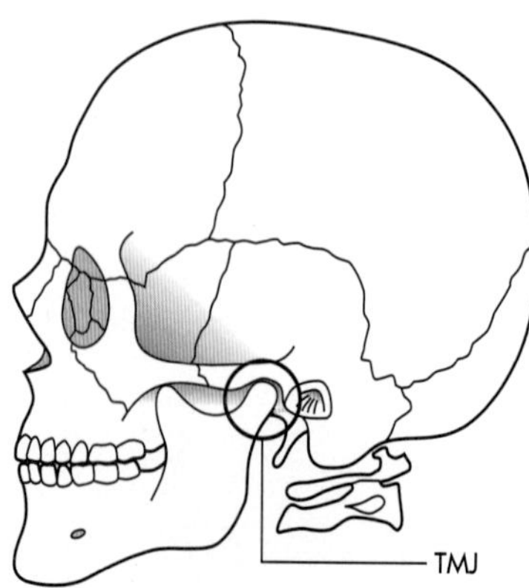

The TMJ is a unique joint with a wide variety of movement. Temporomandibular movement can be classified into a combination of two types of joint movement: **hinge** and **gliding.** The terms are self-descriptive.

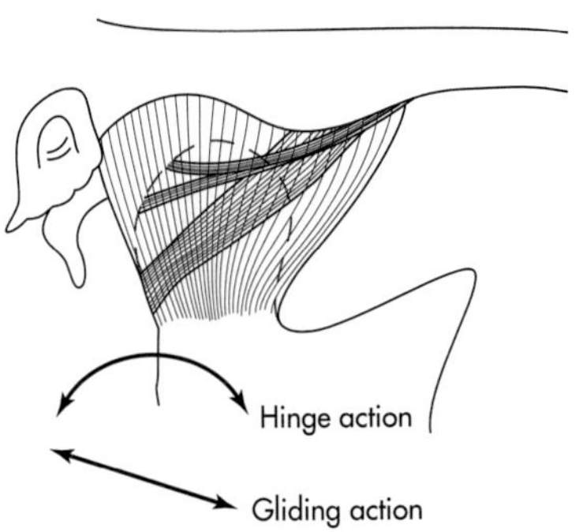

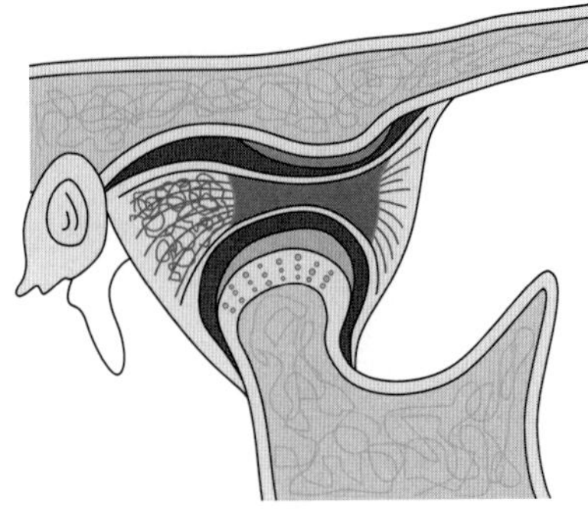

Gliding joints are also found between the cervical vertebrae, and between the first and second vertebrae there is a **rotating joint.**

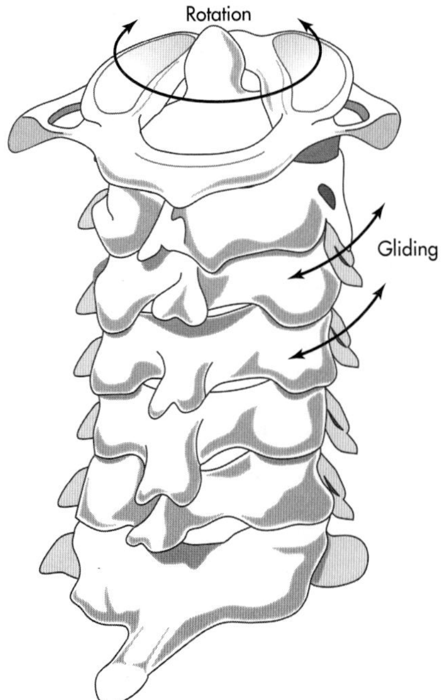

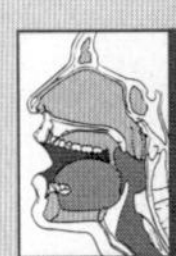

Let us look at each bone found in the head and neck, beginning with the bones of the neck.

2.1 Bones of the Neck

CERVICAL VERTEBRAE

The bones of the neck are built to provide strong, but light support for the head. They also form a protective "tunnel" or passageway for some important nerves and blood vessels. There are seven **cervical vertebrae.**

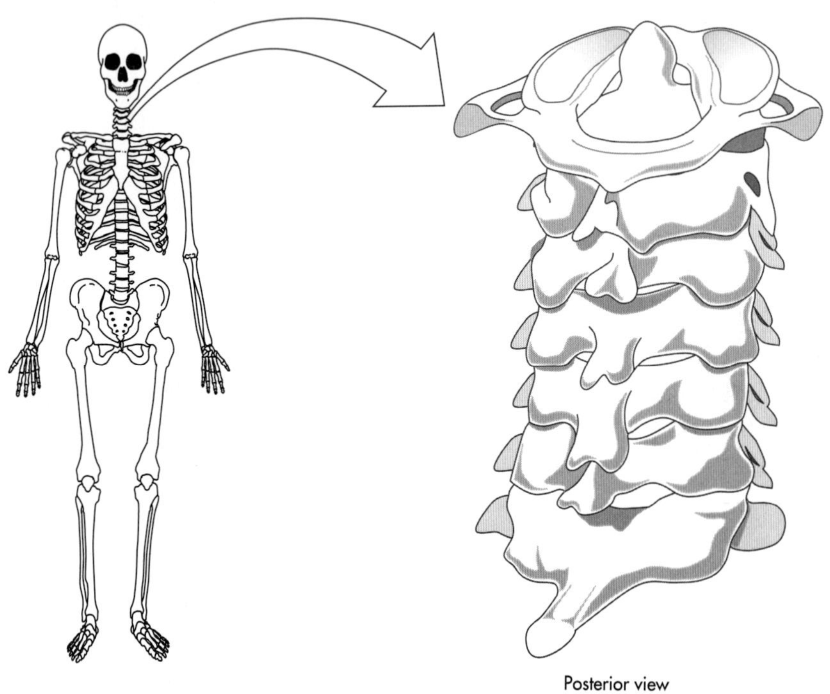

Posterior view

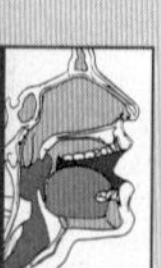

A single cervical vertebrae is diagrammed here. The cervical vertebrae look similar, though each differs slightly.

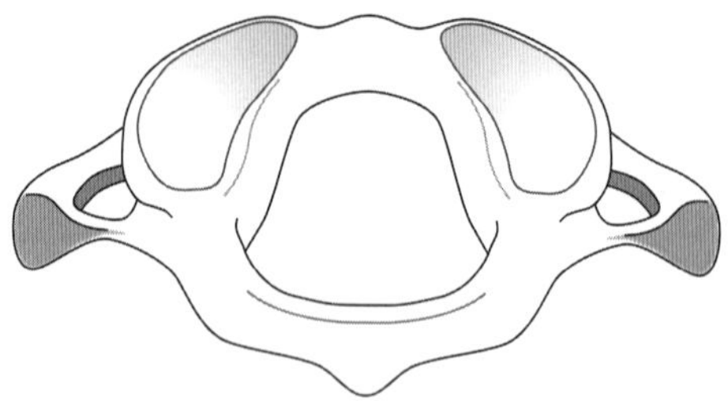

A passageway for the spinal cord, a major grouping of nervous tissue, is provided by the vertebrae—a tunnel created by stacking the vertebral "holes" on top of each other. How many cervical vertebrae are there?

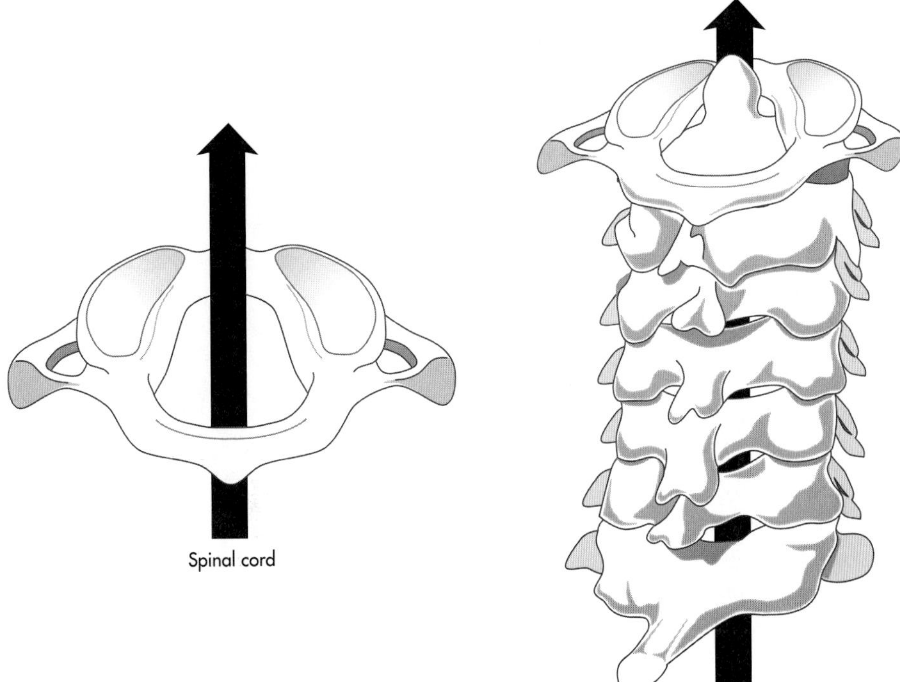

Major blood vessels pass through these holes to and from the brain.

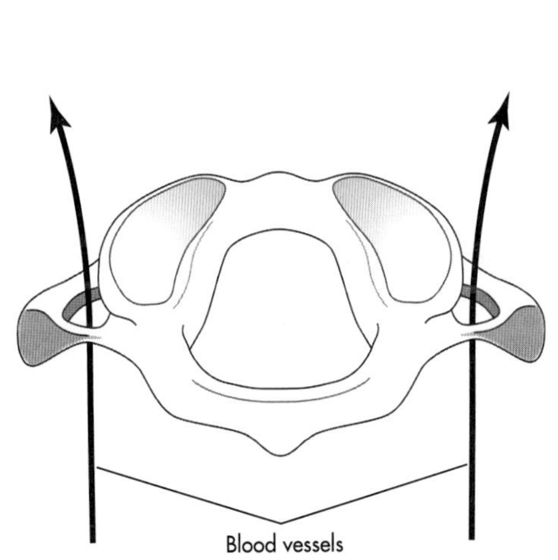

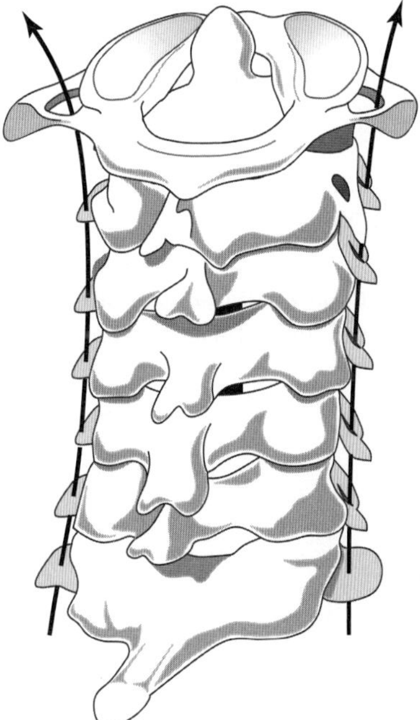

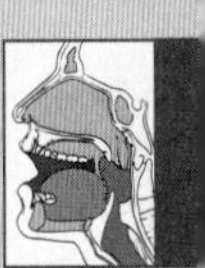

The cervical vertebrae are named by number: C-1, C-2, C-3, C-4, C-5, C-6, and C-7. C-1 and C-2 have special names because of their unique shapes and functions. C-1 is called the **atlas,** as it "holds up" the cranium. C-2 is called the **axis** because of a medial protuberance that allows rotation around it. This joint allows a wide range of bending and twisting movements between the head and neck.

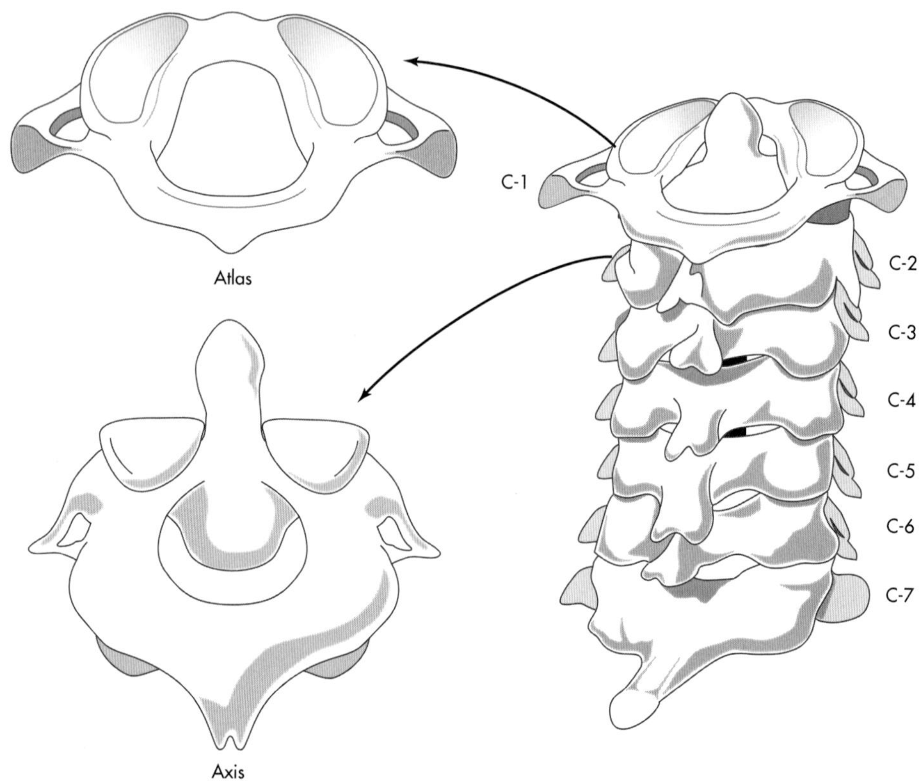

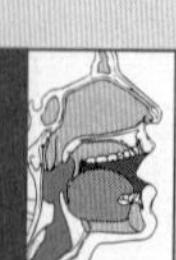

axis

Which vertebrae allows rotations?

HYOID BONE

An unusual bone found in the neck, attached to several muscles but to no other bone, is the **hyoid bone.** It is a derivative of arch cartilage and has a unique shape.

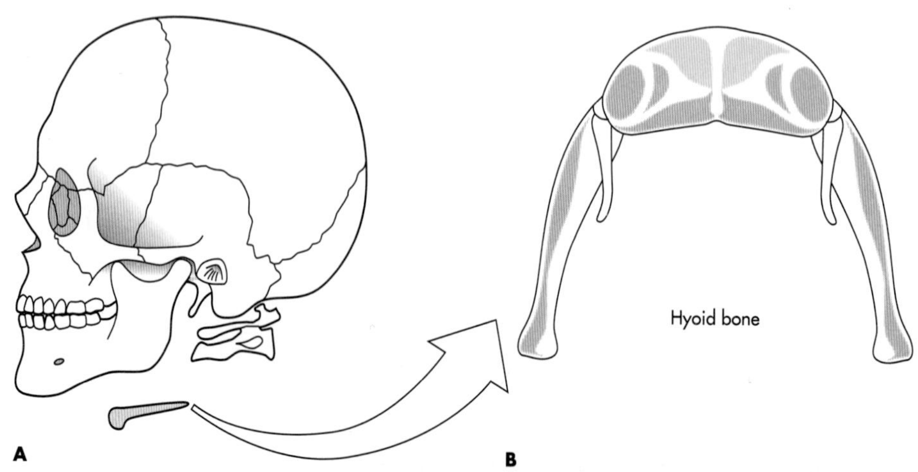

In the diagram of the hyoid bone surrounded by its attaching muscles, note how it seems to be "buried" within the substance of the neck.

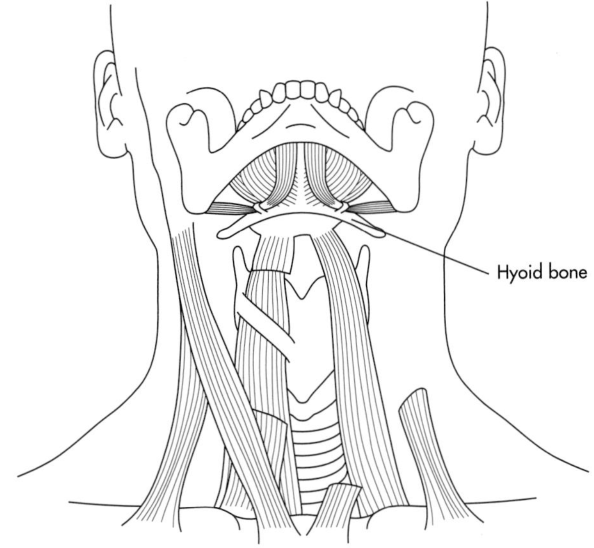

Label the cervical bones.

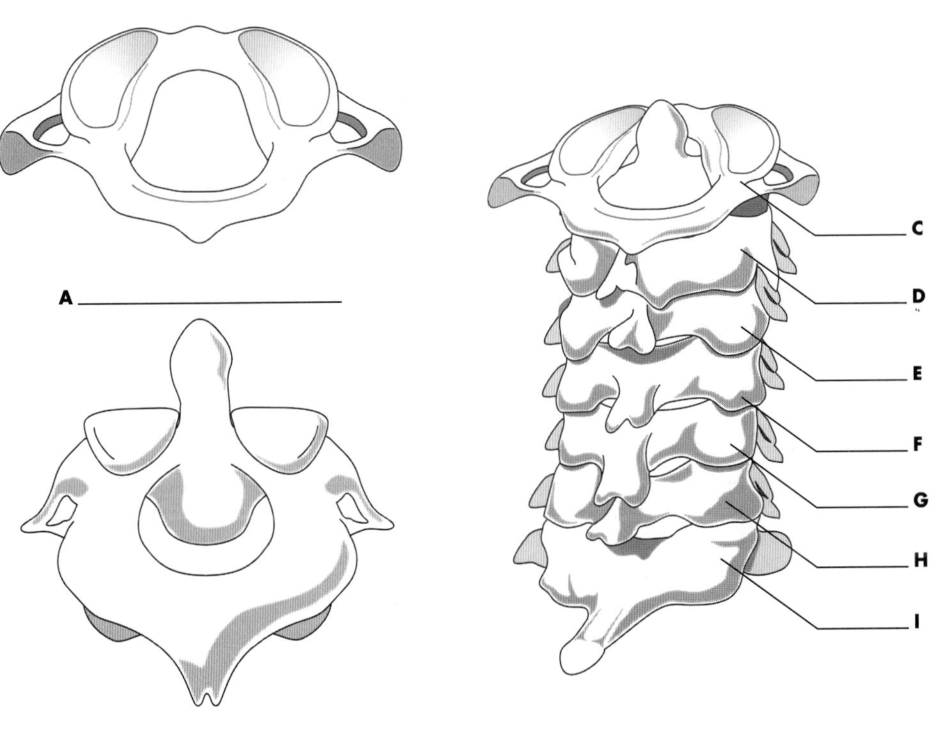

A. atlas
B. axis
C. C-1
D. C-2
E. C-3
F. C-4
G. C-5
H. C-6
I. C-7

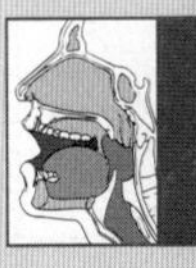

2.2

Bones of the Cranium

There are 12 **cranial bones**—some are paired and others are single—all joined by fibrous sutures so that it appears that the cranium is a single bone. Note that the cranium does not include the mandible.

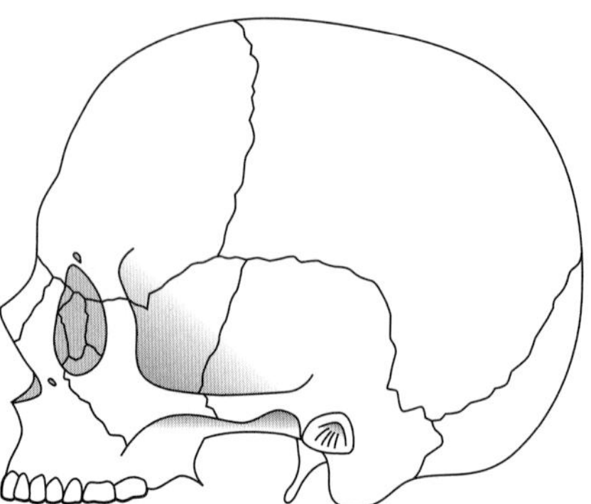

foramina

The cranium has a number of "holes," called **foramina** (singular, foramen). Foramina are passageways for nerves and blood vessels, allowing them to go from one side of the cranium to the other. For example, a number of nerves exit the brain through the cranial foramina. Major blood vessels supply the brain with blood through ______________ into the cranium.

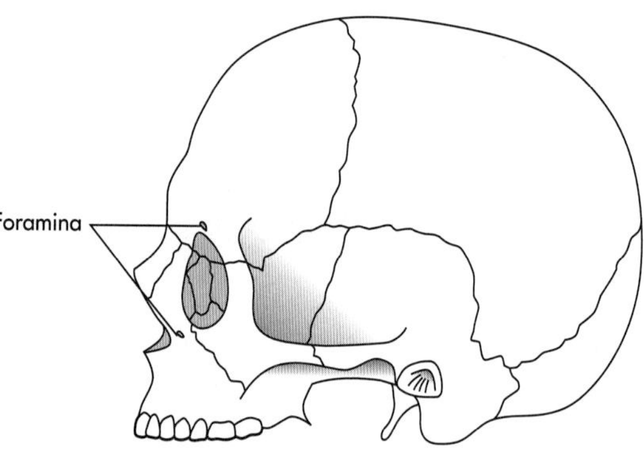

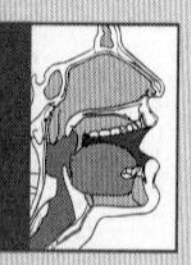

foramina

The cranium also has a number of shallow, concave areas, called **fossae** (singular, fossa). Convex or protruding areas are called **processes.** Holes in bone are called ______________.

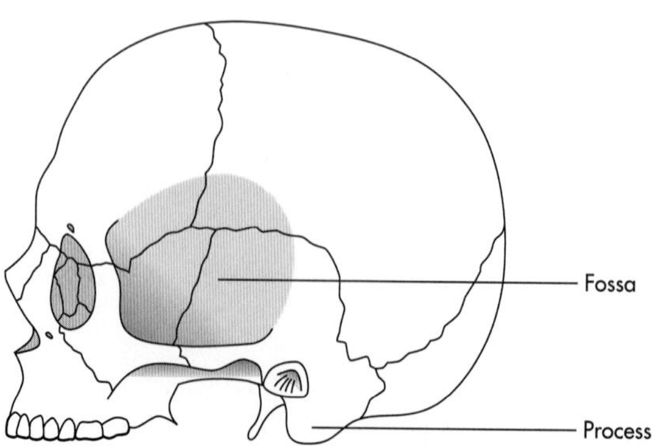

As we locate each of the cranial bones, you may color it in a particular identifying color. We will examine the foramina, fossae, and processes associated with each bone.

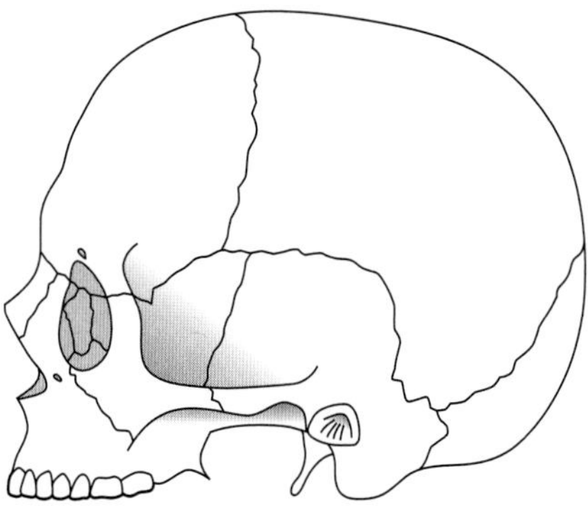

FRONTAL BONE

Two embryonic frontal processes unite to create a single membranous bone, the **frontal bone.** The borders of its sutures are highlighted. You may color in the area in the frontal view of the cranium.

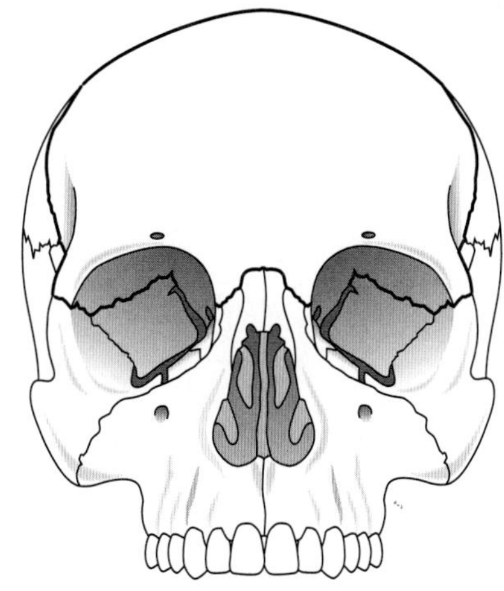

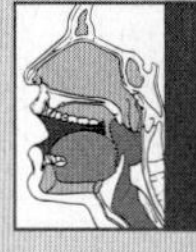

In the sagittal view, find the frontal bone and color it in.

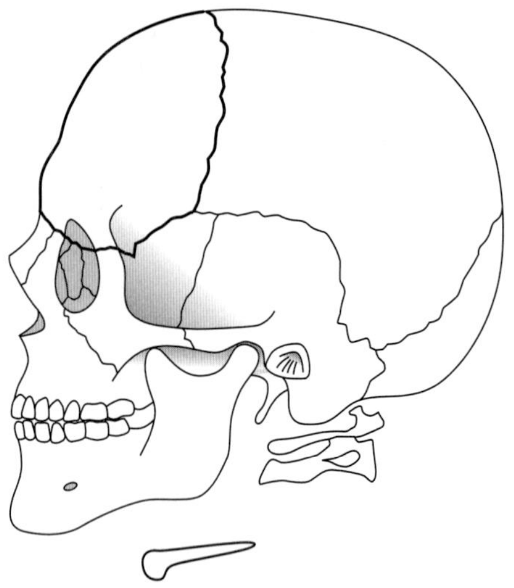

frontal

The _____________ bone comprises the forehead and eyebrow area of the face. It extends into the eye sockets or **orbits.** Looking at the brow ridge, you can see one foramina on each. These are called the supraorbital foramina.

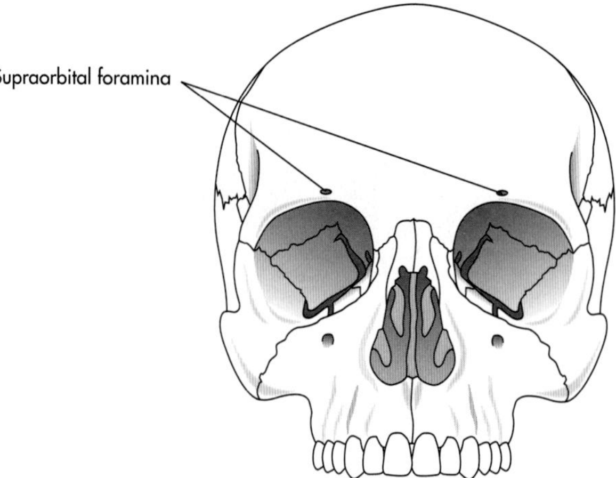

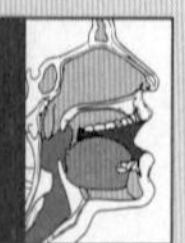

Looking down on the top of the cranium, you can see the extent of the frontal bone. Find its sutures. Which are the anterior and posterior sides of the drawing?

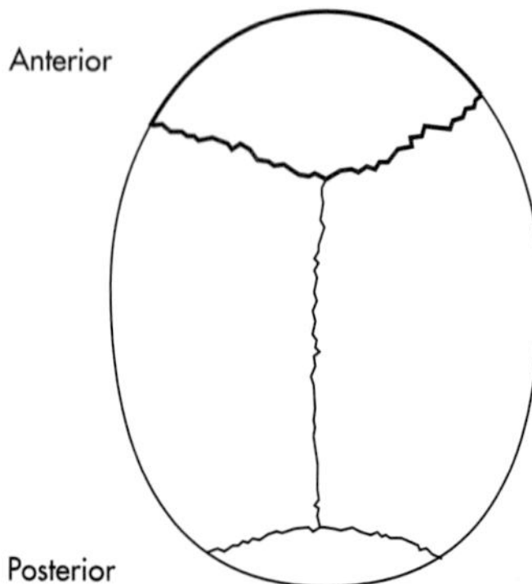

If you were to saw the top of the cranium open, you would obtain a view of the interior of the cranium. Follow again the sutures to find the extent of the frontal bone.

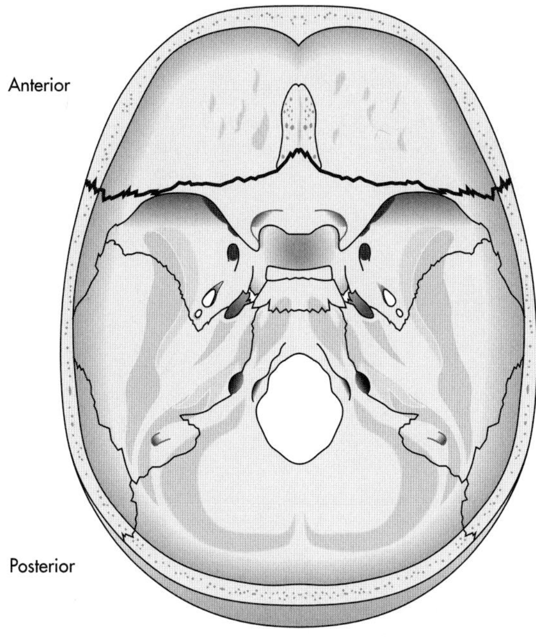

Lying in the middle of the ______________ bone is another cranial bone, which looks a bit like a walnut. It comes together with another bone, the sphenoid, that helps to form a sort of "shelf" here. This area of the frontal bone is concave because this is where the anterior portion of the cerebrum rests. This is called the **anterior cranial fossa.**

frontal

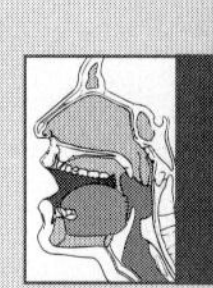

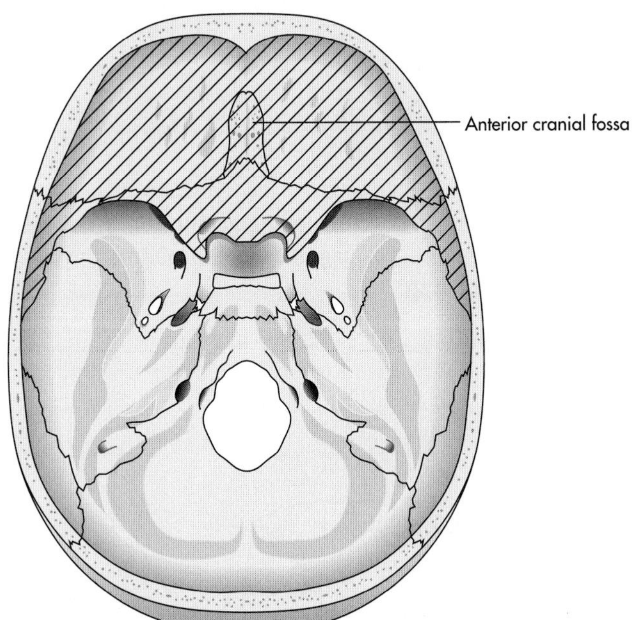

Find the frontal bone and its formina and fossae on the drawings.

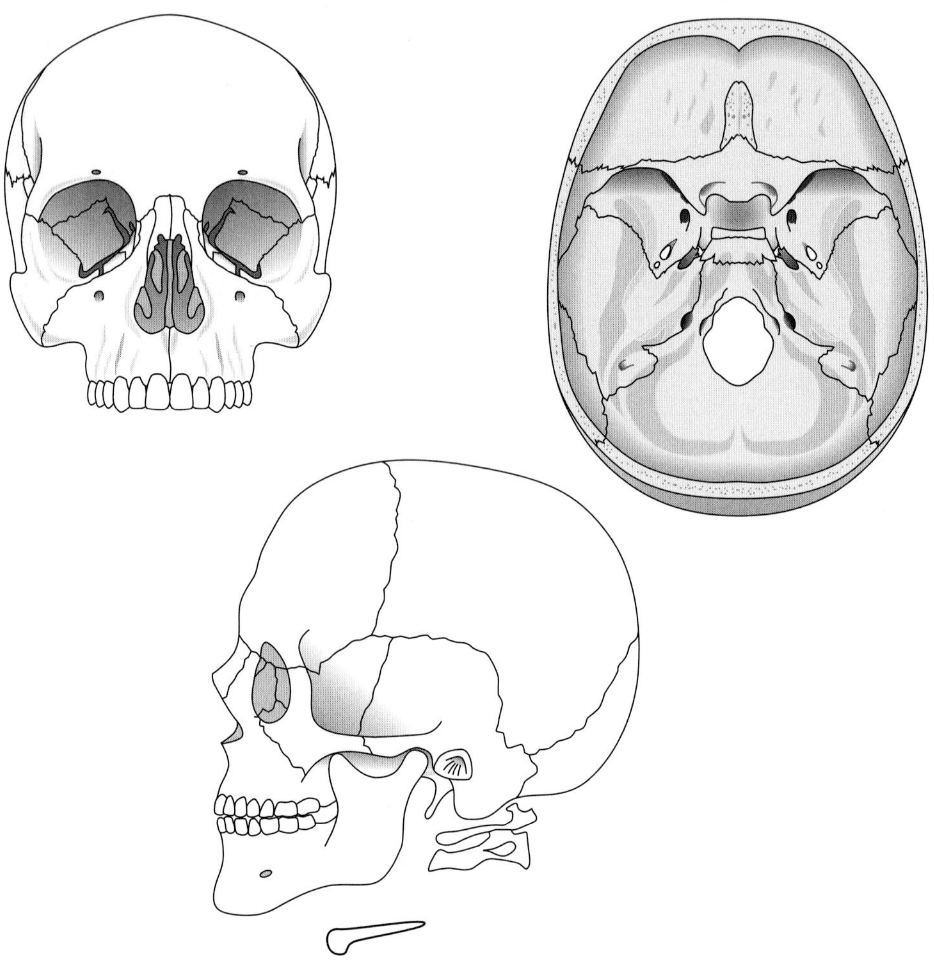

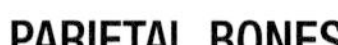

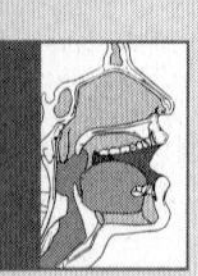

PARIETAL BONES

This pair of bones, membranous in development, constitutes most of the top and sides of the cranium. Follow the sutures on this sagittal view to outline the extent of one of the **parietal bones.** You may color it in.

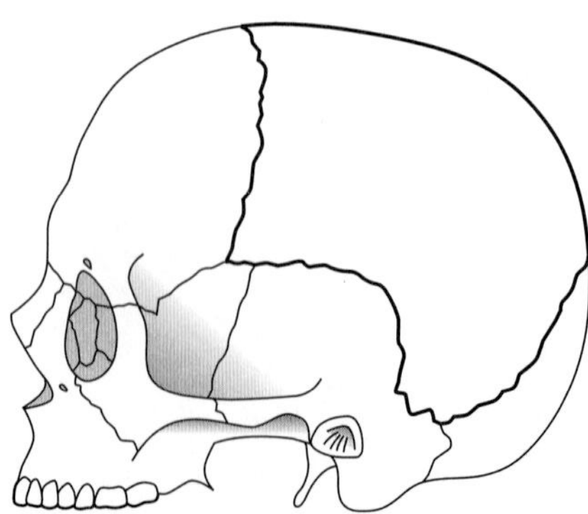

Looking at the top, find both parietal bones. The anterior direction is marked. Where is the frontal bone? See the earlier diagrams under Frontal Bone.

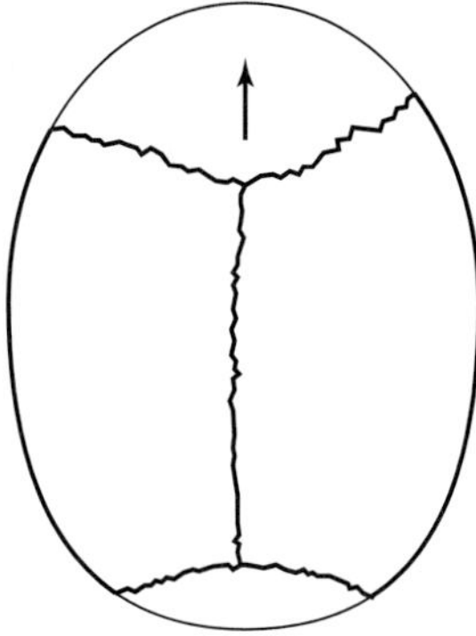

The _______________ bones extend down the sides so that they may be seen in a frontal view.

parietal

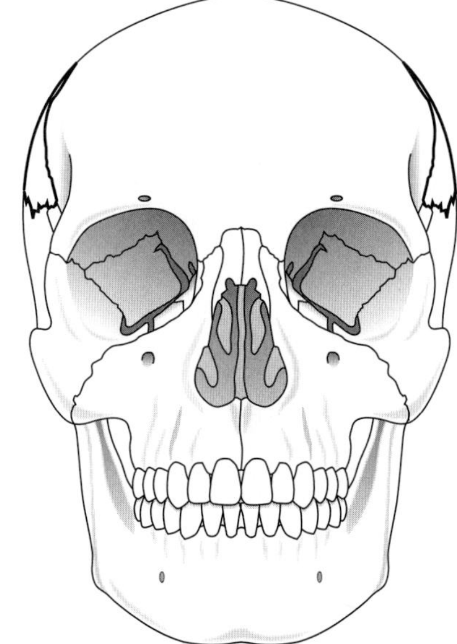

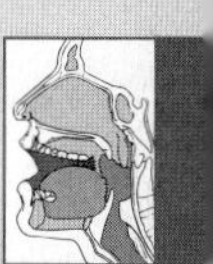

no

In this view inside the cranium, do you see any foramina in the parietal bones?

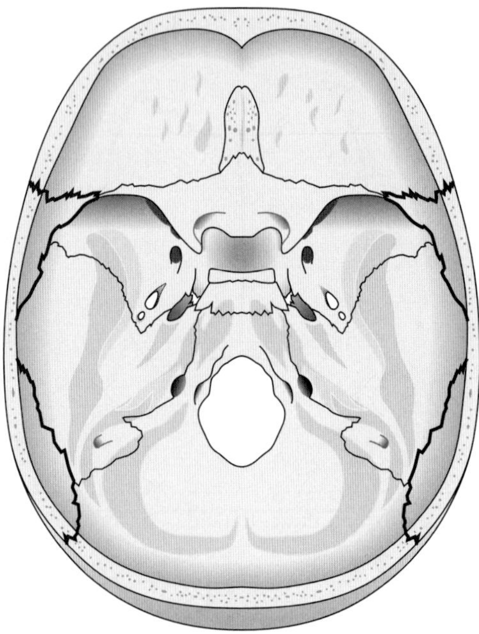

The inner aspect of the parietal and frontal bones shows the concave impressions of the lobes of the cerebrum, the division between their two halves, and a sulcus between them for a major vein, the superior sagittal sinus.

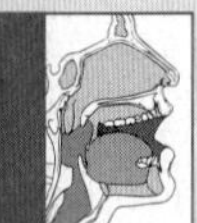

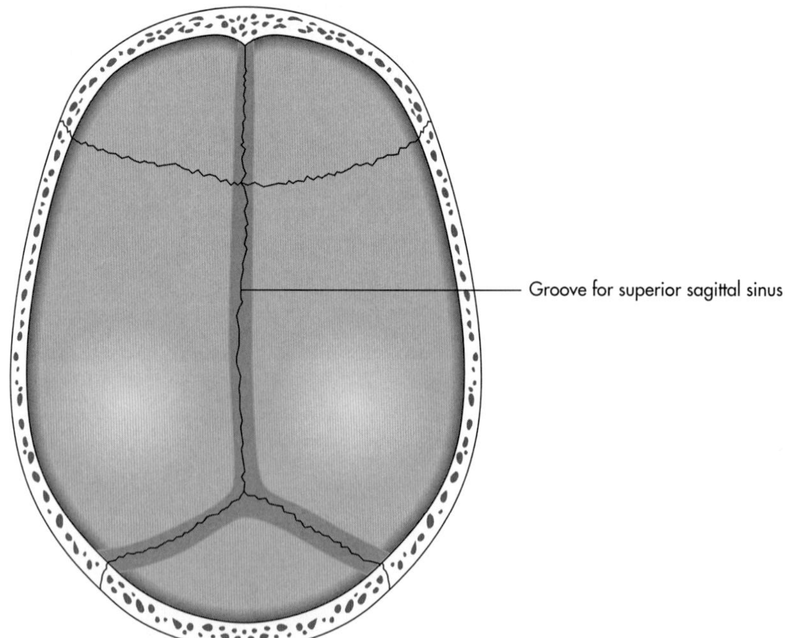

Locate the parietal bones in the drawings.

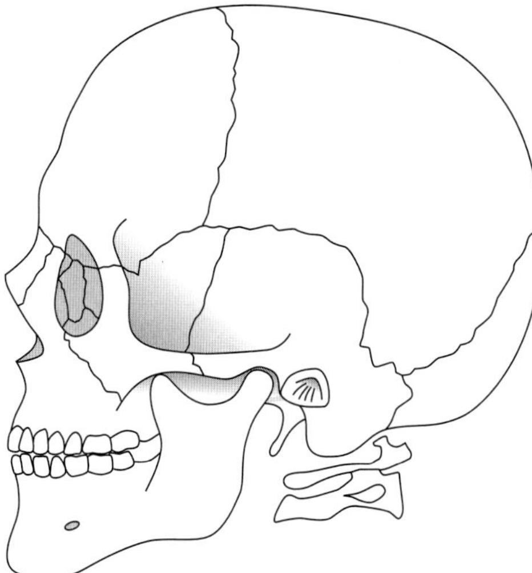

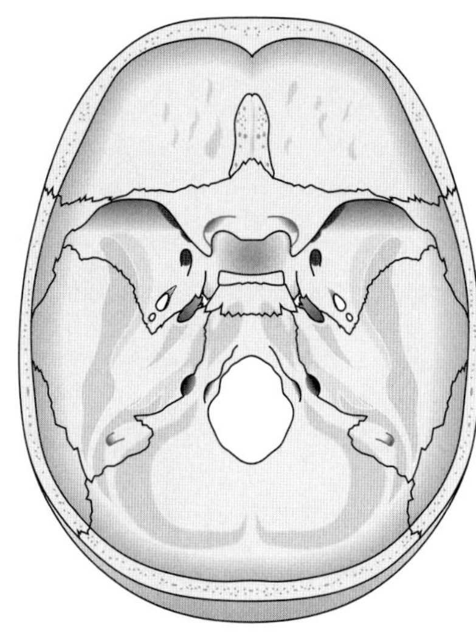

OCCIPITAL BONE

The next cranial bone is singular, formed by both types of bone formation and containing a singularly large foramen. Locate the extent of the **occipital bone** on the inferior view.

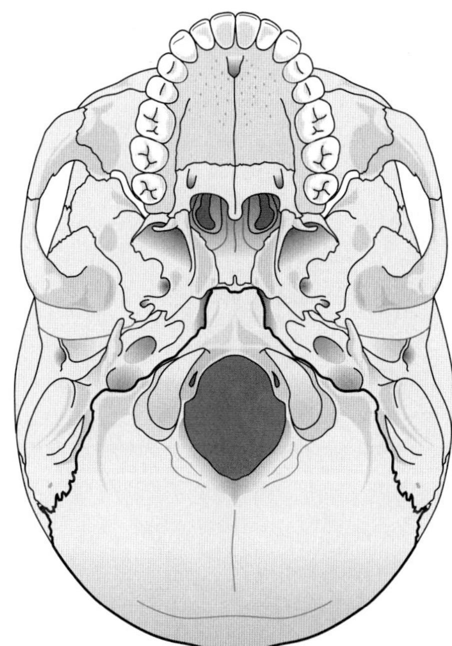

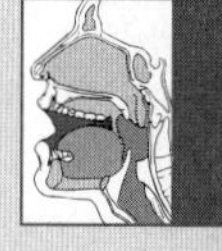

Locate the occipital bone in the sagittal view. You may color it in.

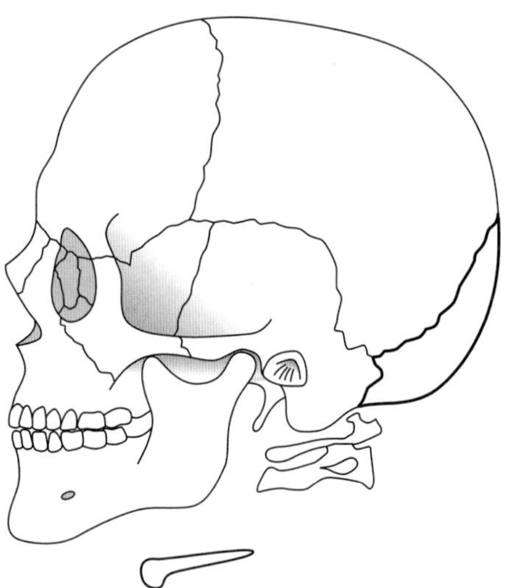

occipital

From the interior view of the cranium, you may appreciate the large foramen that passes through the ______________ bone. This provides passage for the large spinal cord as it exits the brain. Other smaller nerves and blood vessels use this **foramen magnum** to enter and exit the brain.

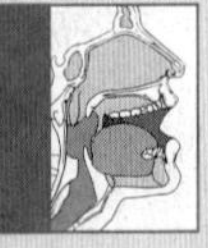

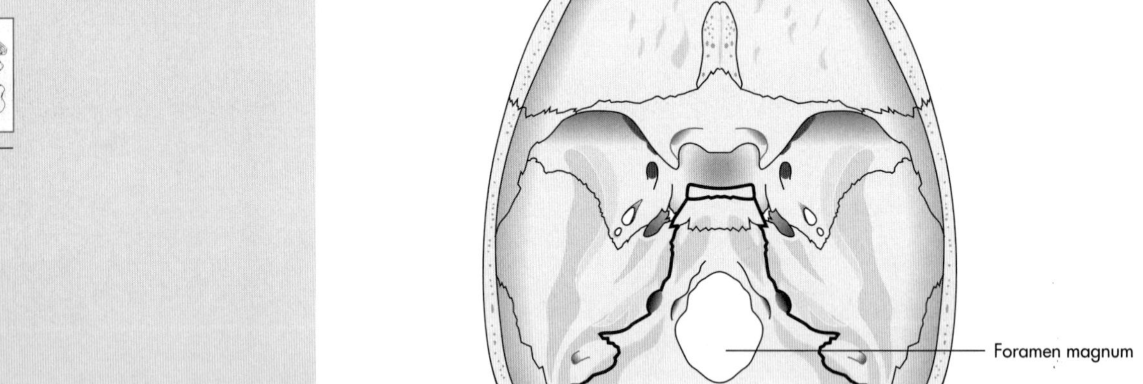

On either side of the foramen ____________ are two lesser foramina that allow passage of the hypoglossal nerve. These are called the **hypoglossal foramina.** Find them.

magnum

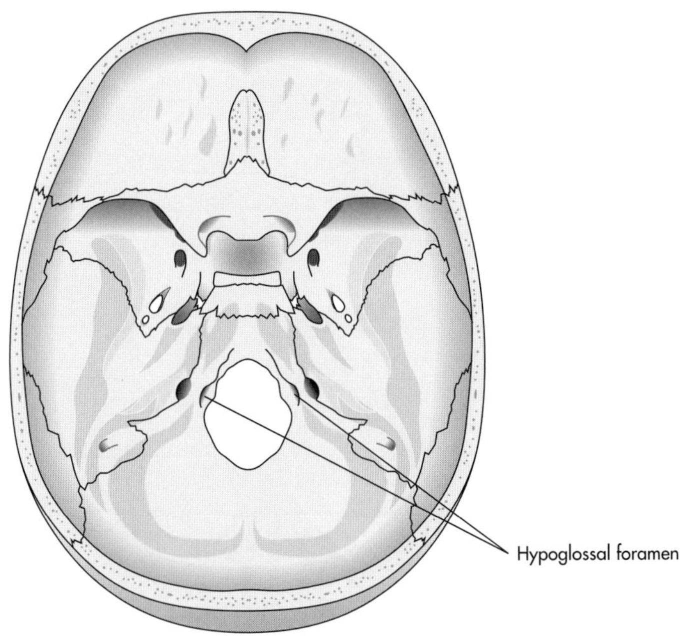

From this view you can appreciate the concavity of the occipital bone that supports the posterior portion of the brain or cerebellum. This concavity is called the **posterior cranial fossa.**

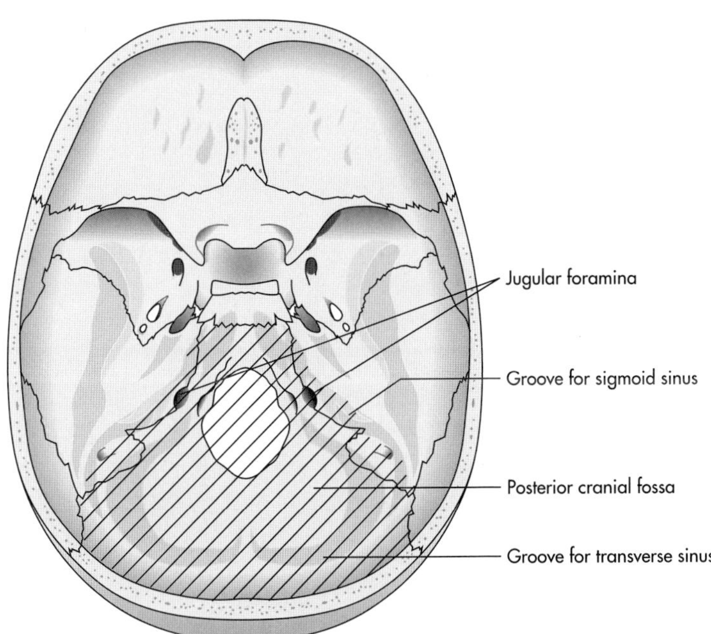

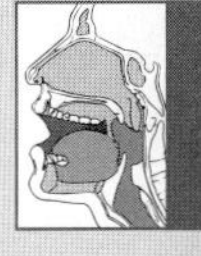

Within the fossa two S-shaped sulci join into a single vertical sulcus. These are the locations of the large veins of the brain, the sigmoid and transverse sinuses. At the end of each sulcus is a large, jagged foramen through which the veins exit—the **jugular foramina.** Find them.

atlas

Looking beneath the cranium again, find the occipital bone and the foramen magnum from the opposite aspect. Find the hypoglossal foramina. Look for two flat processes on either side of the foramen magnum. These are the places where C-1 or the _______________ articulates with the cranium.

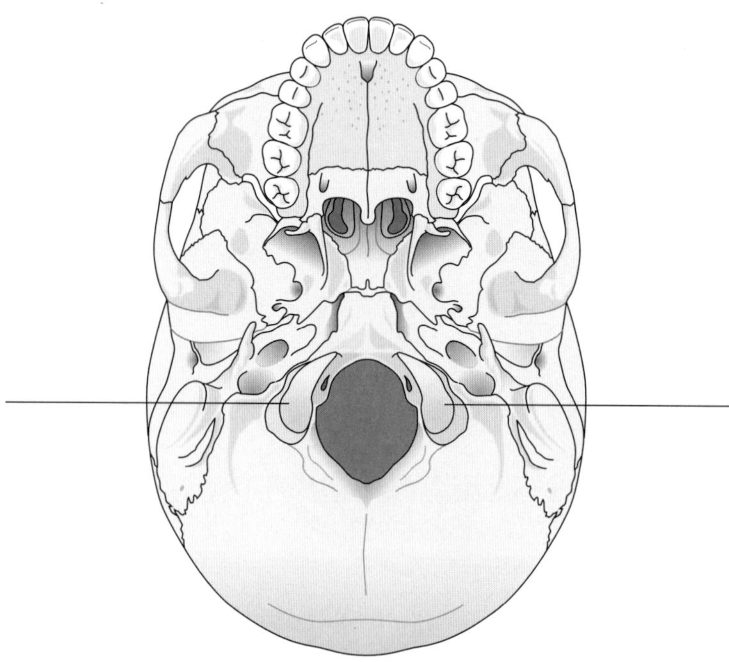

Find the occipital bone and its fossae and foramina.

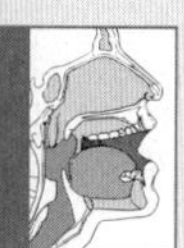

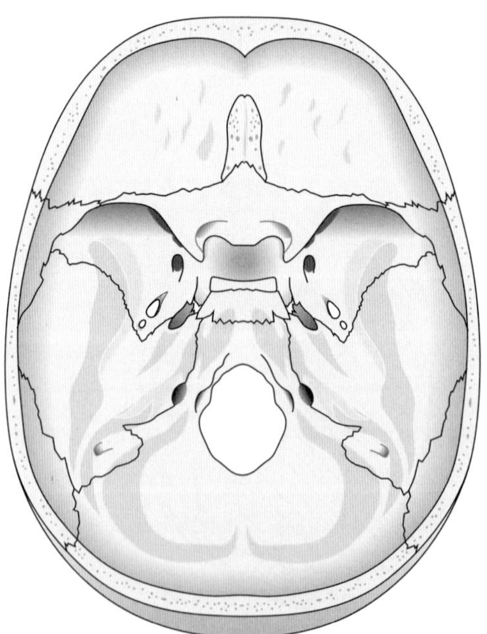

TEMPORAL BONE

Formed by both processes, the pair of **temporal bones** are among the most elaborate of the cranial bones. The word *temple* is derived from the name of this bone. Find its suture outline on the sagittal view. Color it in.

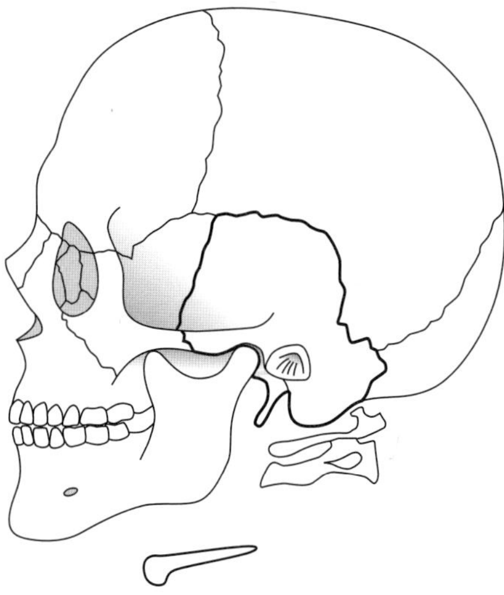

From the underside of the cranium, the extent of the temporal bone can also be appreciated. Find it.

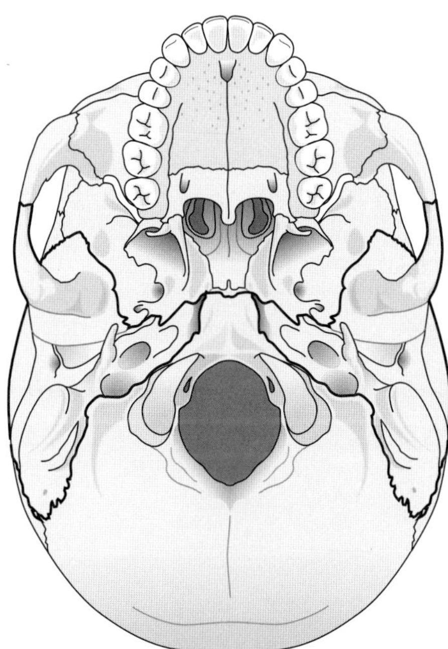

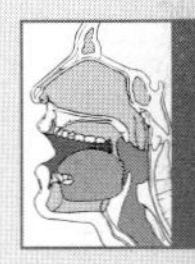

external meatus, ear

Note the large foramen through the temporal bone shown. What is this opening for and where does it go?

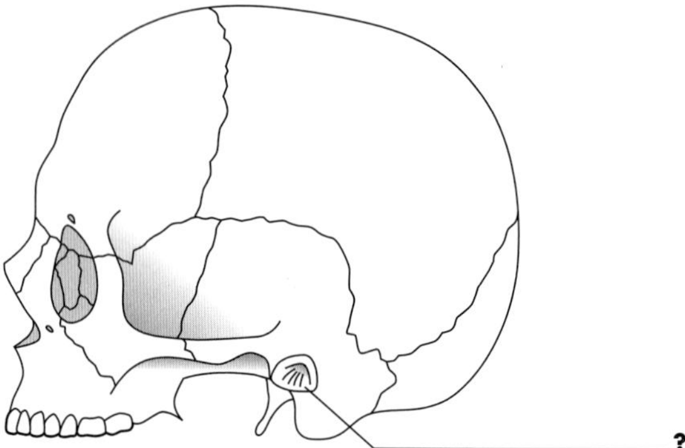

This opening is not a foramen, but rather a bony canal called the **external auditory meatus.** It is the canal that leads the outer ear into the middle ear and then the inner ear. The temporal bone houses the structures of the ear.

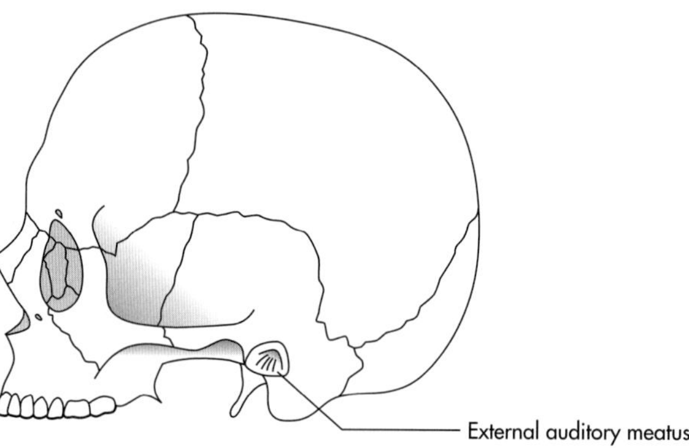

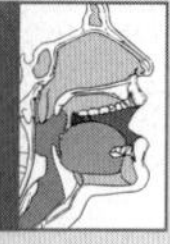

If we look at the interior of the cranium, we can see where the ear is housed. Look for a pyramidal or tent-shaped bony process on either side within the temporal bones. Look at the extent of the temporal bones.

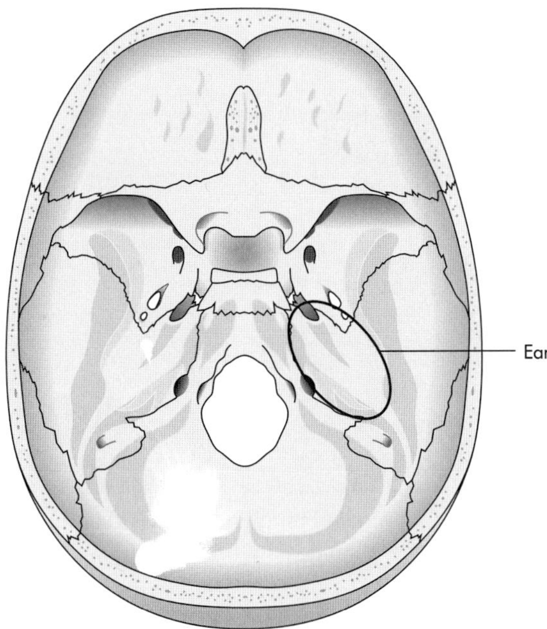

If we were to slice into each of these areas we would find the middle ear and inner ear. They are well protected in their bony houses. Other foramina, including the Eustachian tube (tympanic tube) and internal meatus, exit here.

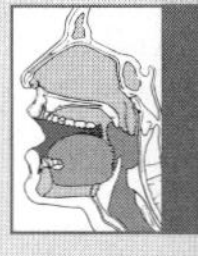

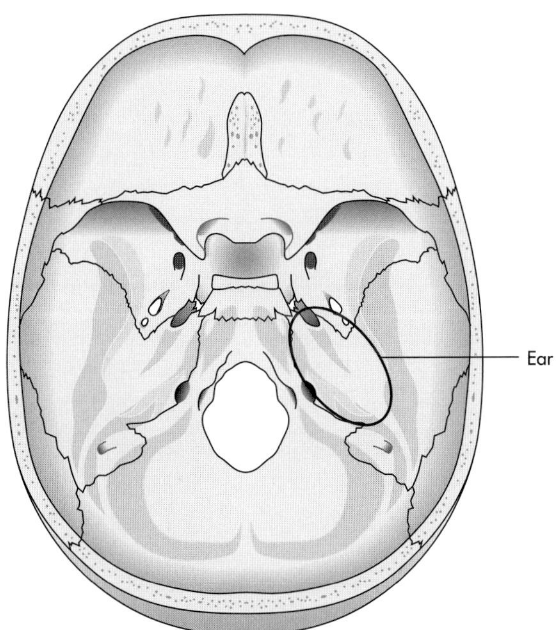

From a sagittal view, the temporal bone is seen to have three interesting processes and two fossae. First find the pencil-shaped process just inferior and medial to the ear. This is called the **styloid process,** and it is the site of muscle and ligament attachment.

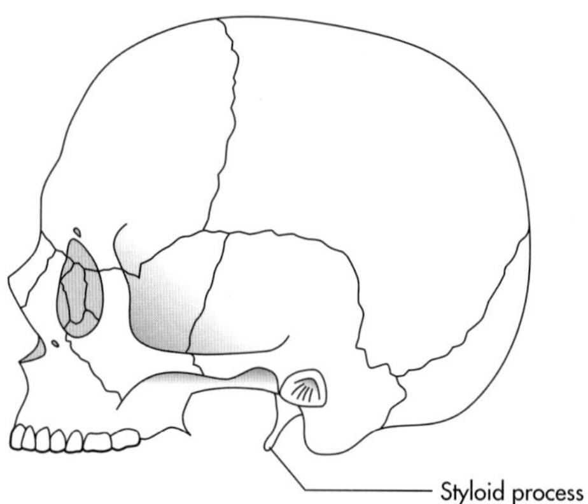

Directly posterior to the ear is a large "bump" or process that also provides muscle attachment. It is the **mastoid process.** Find it on the drawing.

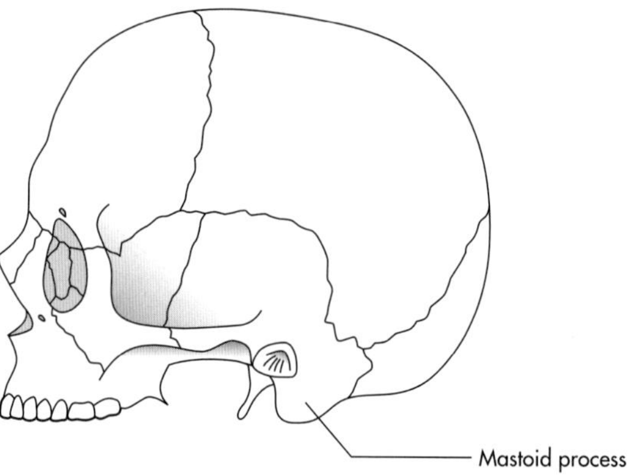

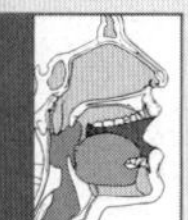

zygomatic

A slender process begins on the temporal bone, connecting with another two bones to create what we commonly call the cheek bone. It is part of the **zygomatic process.** Three bones make up the ______________ process.

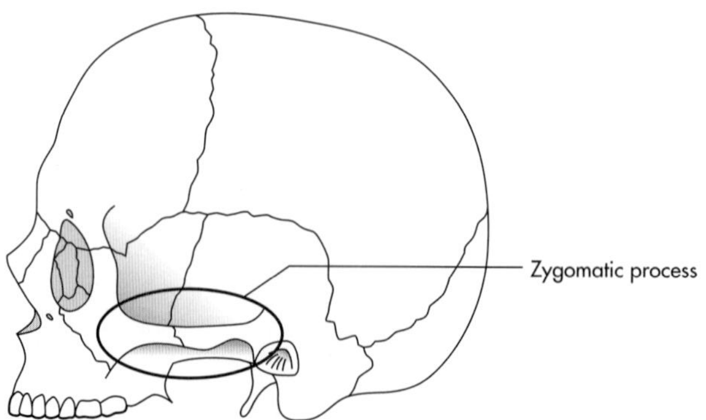

Note that the jaw or mandible articulates with the temporal bone, creating the _______________ joint or **TMJ.**

temporomandibular

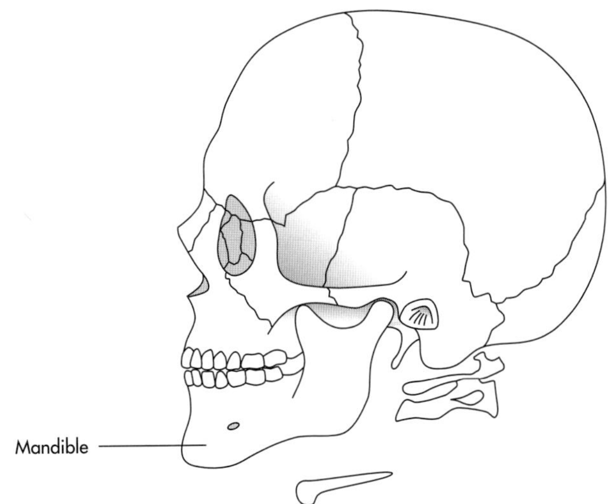

The condyle of the mandible fits into a fossa on the temporal bone. Find it. This is called the **mandibular fossa.** It is not the true site of articulation; rather, the "bump" on the zygomatic process in front of it is—the **articular eminence.**

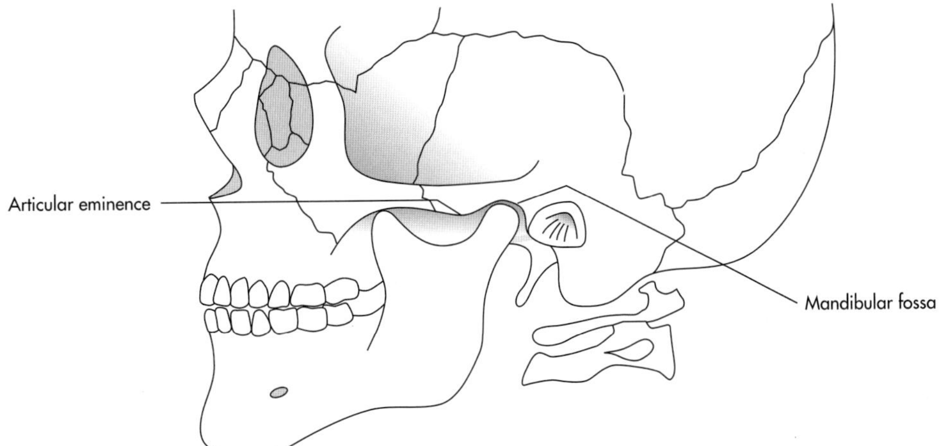

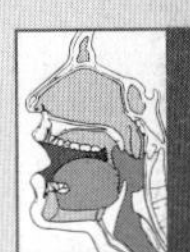

the condyle

In the view of the mandibular fossa, articular eminence, and zygomatic process, what fits into the fossa?

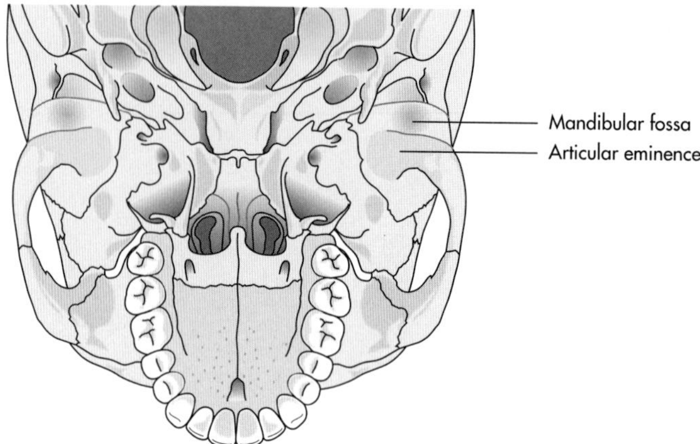

It is difficult to appreciate the next concavity in a drawing. It is a shallow fossa that contains the bulk of the temporalis muscle—the **temporal fossa.** This fossa is continuous and leads into a deeper fossa behind the zygomatic process called the **infratemporal fossa.** Besides the tendon of the temporalis muscle and the coronoid process of the mandible, a number of important nerves and blood vessels pass through this area.

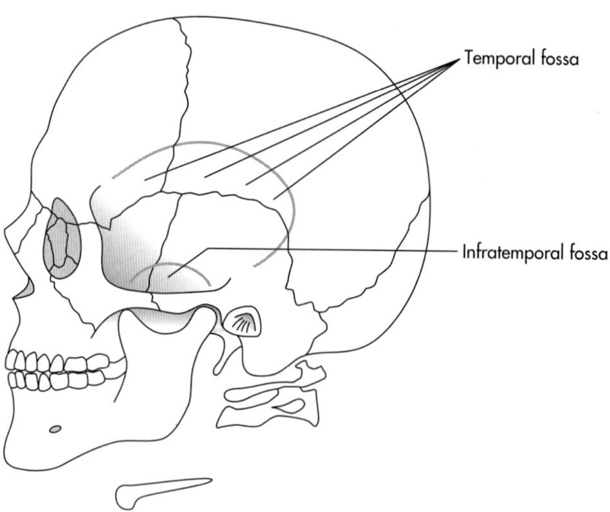

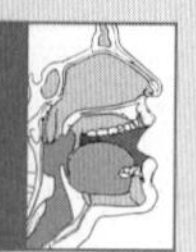

Find the temporal bone and its processes, fossa, and foramina.

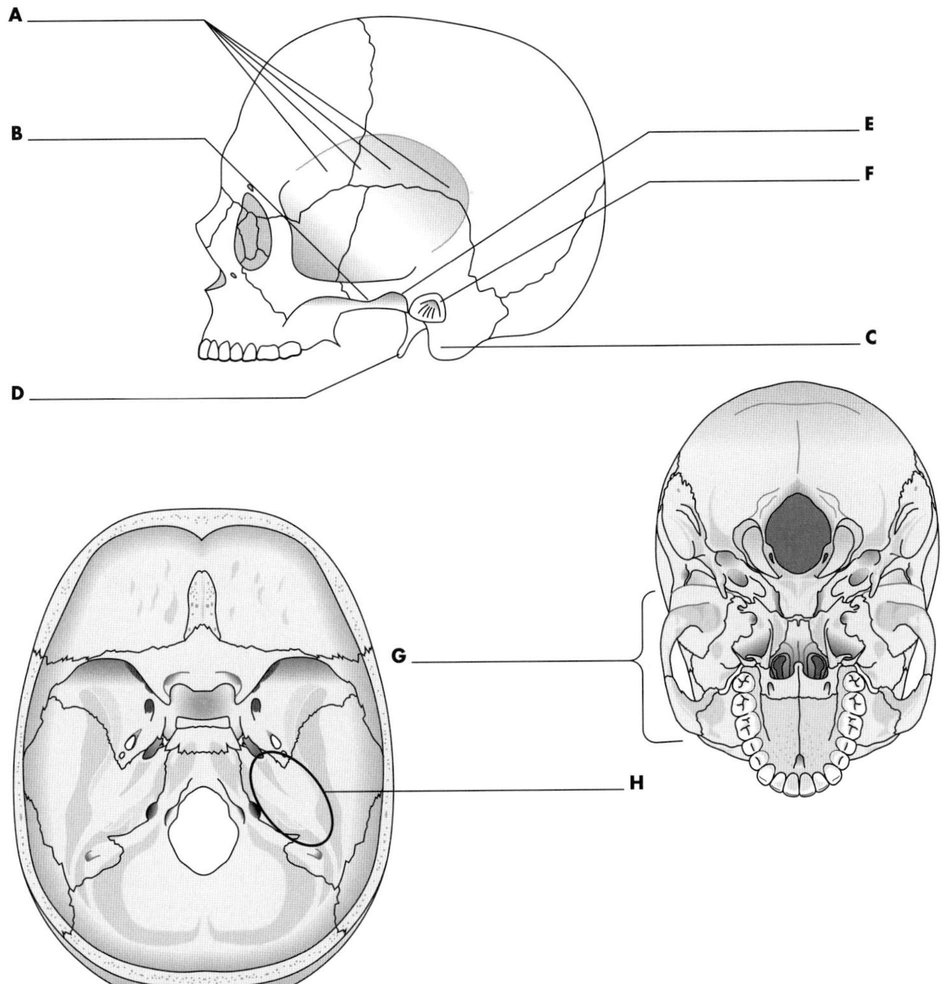

A. temporal fossa
B. articular eminence
C. mastoid process
D. styloid process
E. mandibular fossa
F. external auditory meatus

G. zygomatic process
H. ear

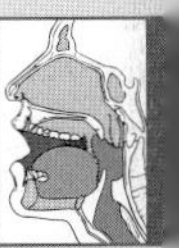

SPHENOID BONE

This single butterfly-shaped cranial bone supports the base of the brain and is the site of several foramina through which major nerves exit the brain. The best view in which to find it is the interior view of the cranium. Find it and color it in.

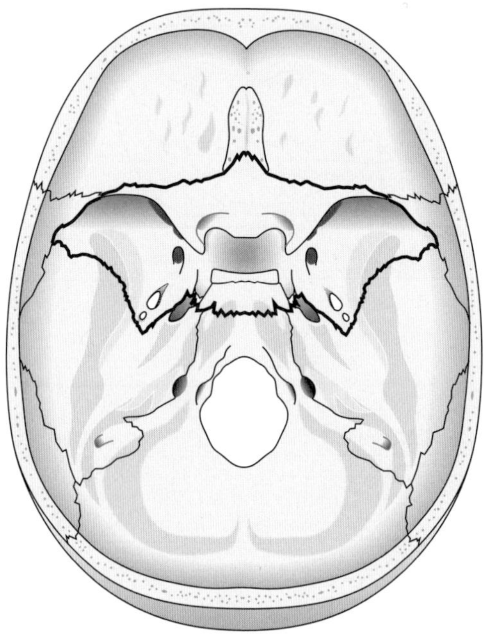

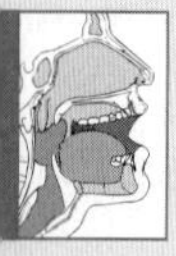

In the middle of the **sphenoid bone** is an unusually shaped area. It is a depression, the **pituitary fossa,** with anterior and posterior processes that make the whole area look like a "turkish saddle" or **sella turcica.** The pendular pituitary gland rests in the fossa, attached to the base of the brain.

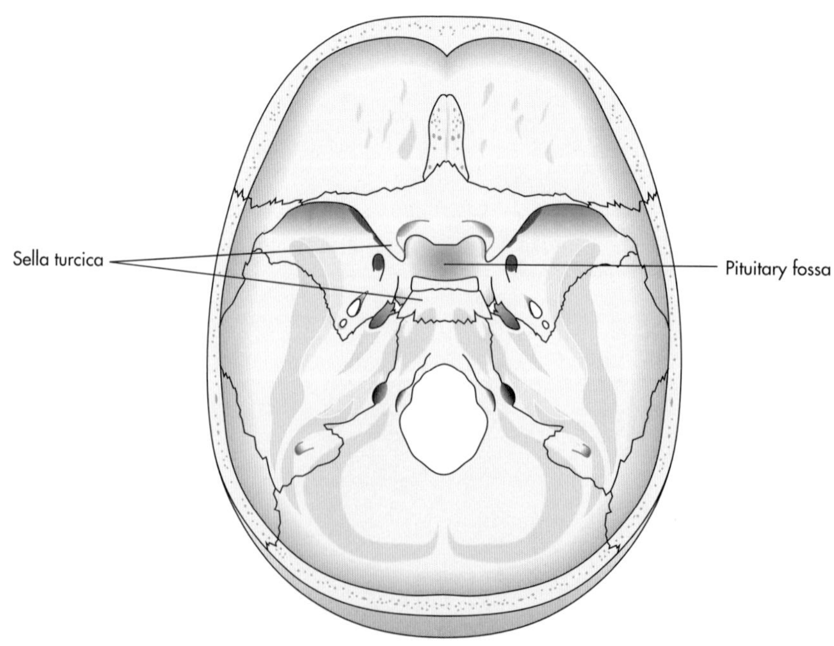

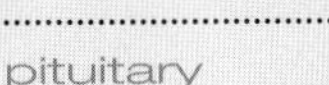

On either side of the ______________ fossa lie two bony canals. In life they carry the major supply of blood into the brain. They are called the **carotid canals** and they carry the internal carotid arteries.

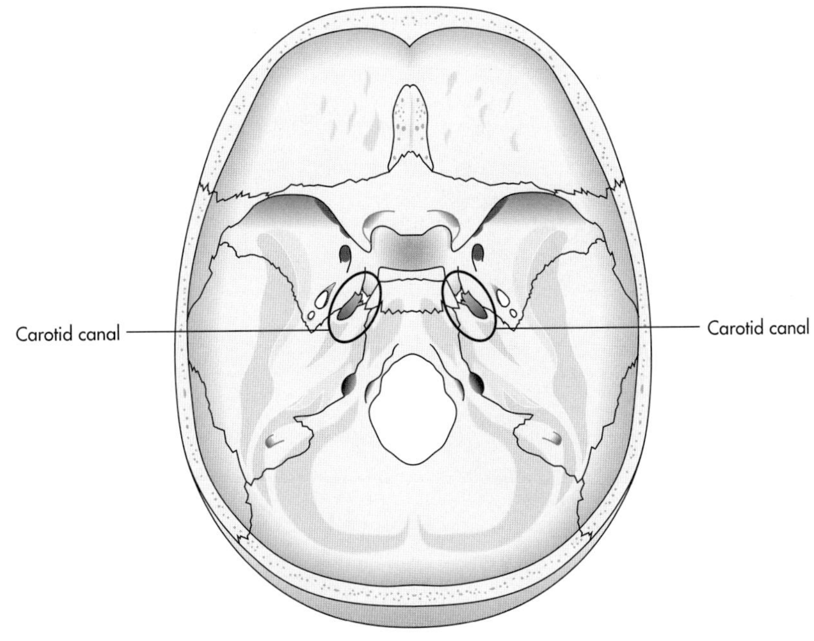

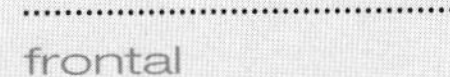

You will note that the sphenoid bone shares a suture with the ______________ bone, up in the anterior cranial fossa, creating a small ledge. Just under this ledge, the **middle cranial fossa** begins and two pair of foramina can be seen.

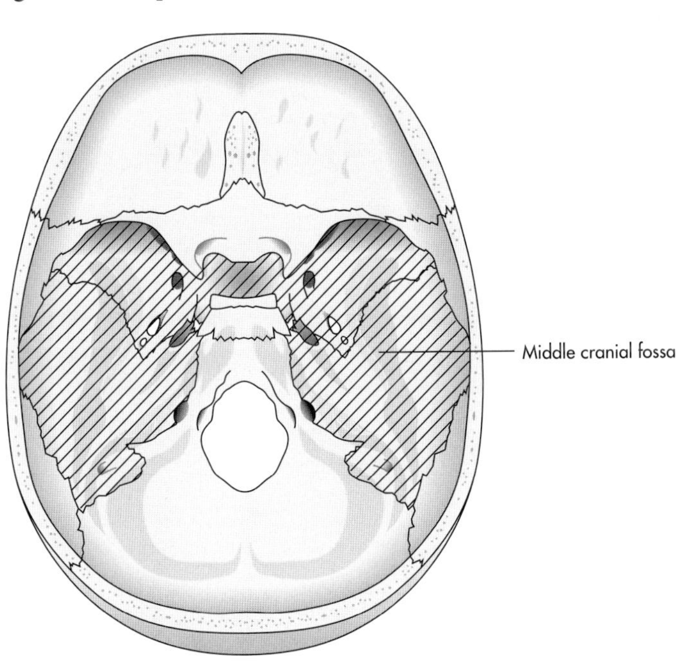

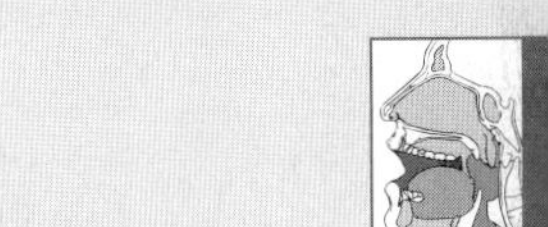

The first pair of foramina exit close to each other in the area of the sella turcica. If you were to take a wire and pass it through one of these foramina, it would exit as shown through this foramen in the orbit. This foramen is called the **optic foramen** and it houses the optic nerve from the eye.

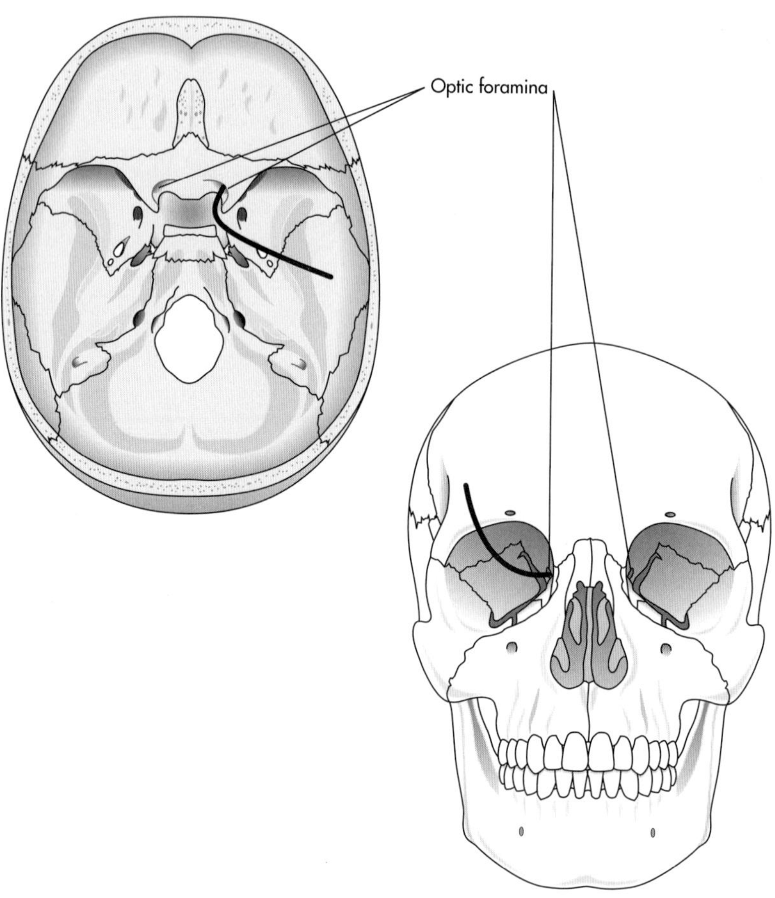

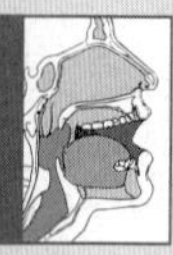

The second pair of "holes" under the sphenoid "shelf" are large fissures, rather than foramina. So, these are called the **superior orbital fissures.** Watch as we pass a wire through one of the fissures, where it will exit in the orbit. This is just next to the _______________ foramen.

optic

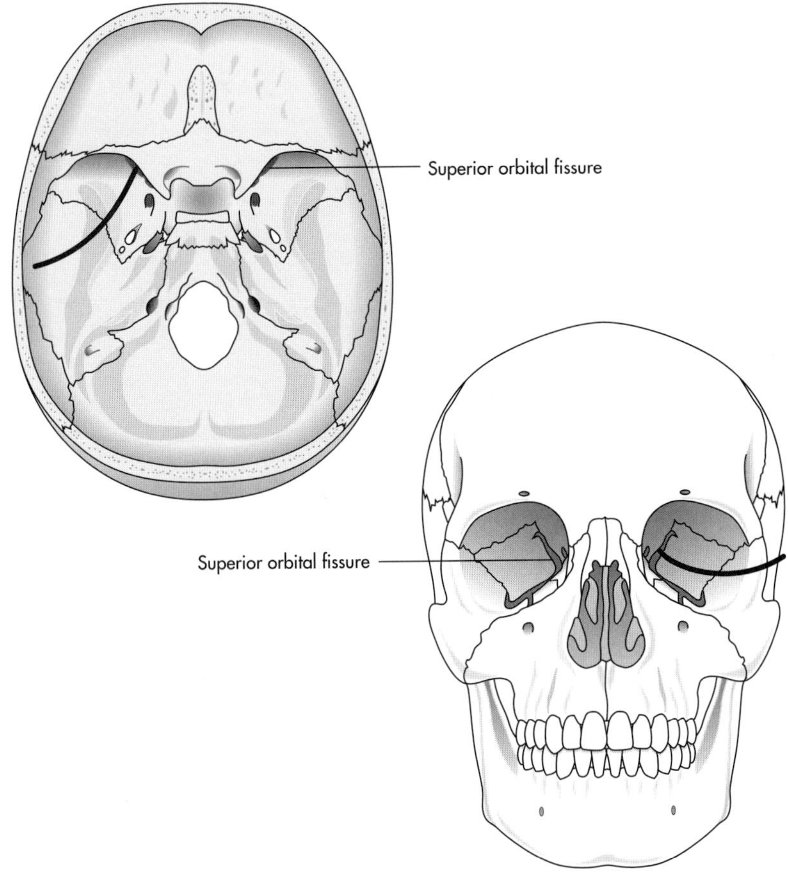

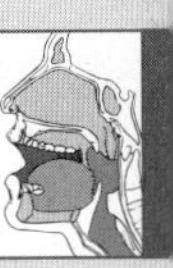

Directly posterior and medial to the superior orbital fissures are two round foramina. Each is called a **foramen rotundum.** If you pass a wire through this foramen, it soon runs into the posterior wall of the maxilla, a bone we will soon study.

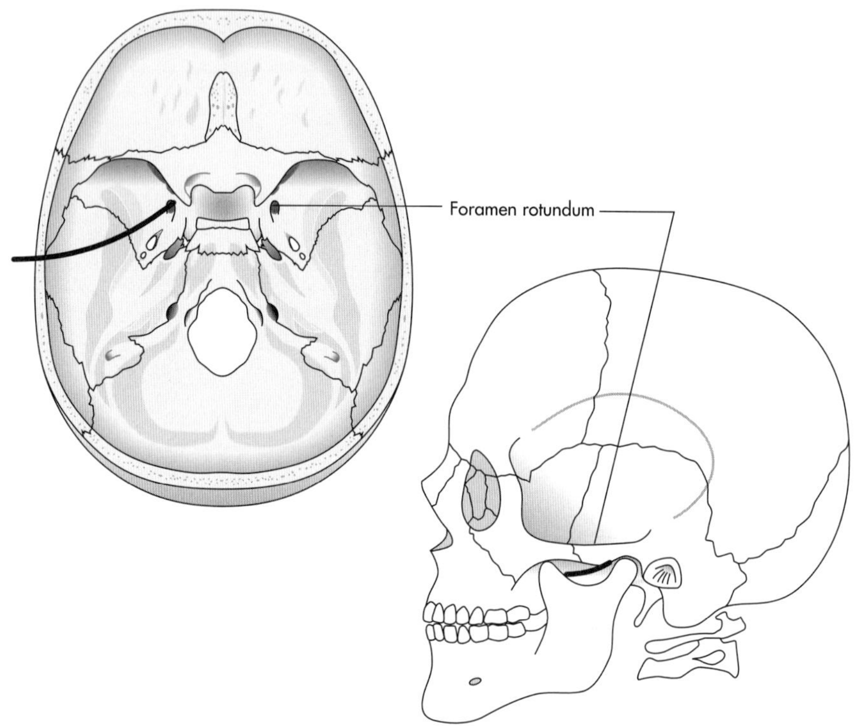

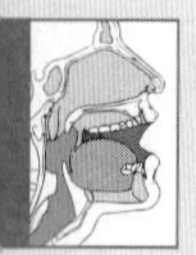

Posterior and lateral to the two foramina rotundi are two larger, oval foramina—the **foramina ovales.** Passing a wire through these reveals a path down toward the mandible or jaw.

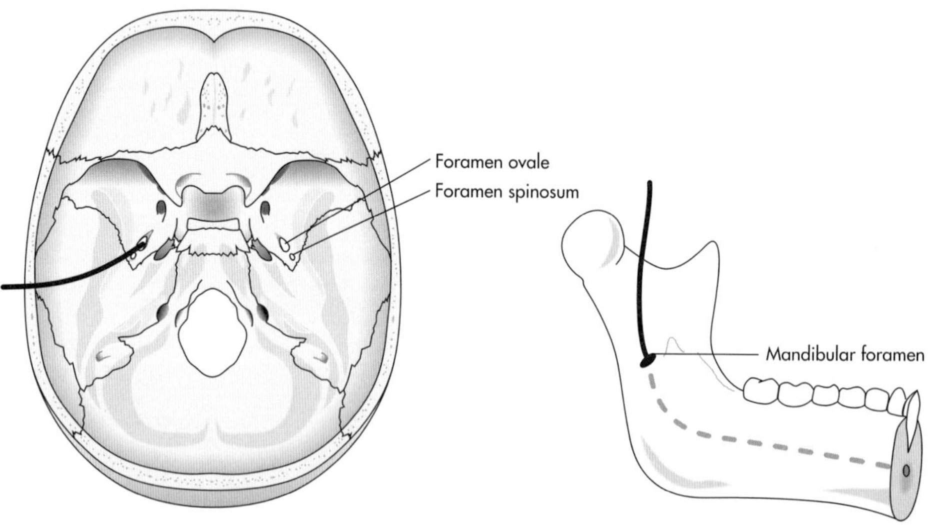

A very small pair of foramina lie just posterior and lateral to the foramina ovales. These are the **foramina spinosa,** so named for the tiny spine of bone next to them.

These three sphenoidal foramina—superior orbital fissure, foramen rotundum, and foramen ovale—are the exit points for three very important divisions of the trigeminal nerve or cranial nerve V. The first division or V1 (ophthalmic) nerve exits the brain through superior orbital fissure and we saw that it travels to the ______________.

eye

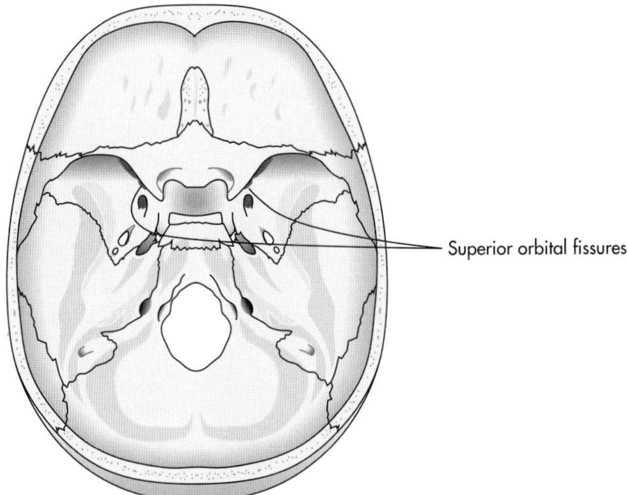

A branch of V1 exits the **supraorbital foramen** on the ______________ bone.

frontal

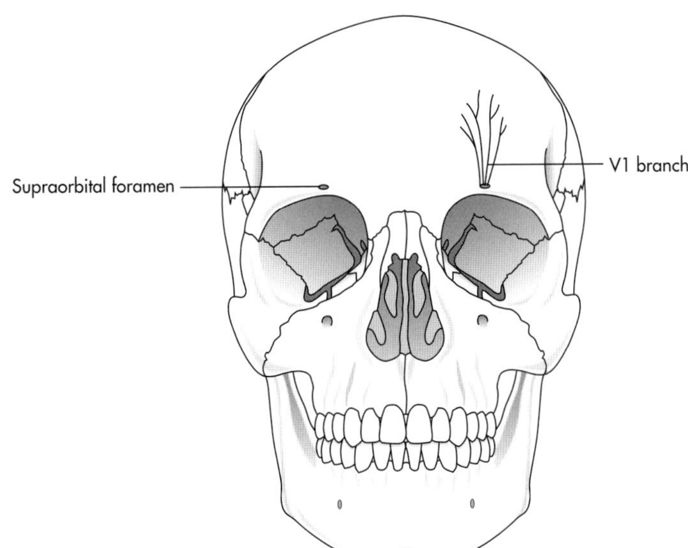

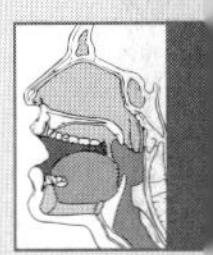

maxillary

The second branch of the trigeminal nerve or V2 (maxillary) nerve exits the brain through the foramen rotundum and butts up against the ______________ bone. A small branch of V2 passes through a foramen under the orbit, the **infraorbital foramen.**

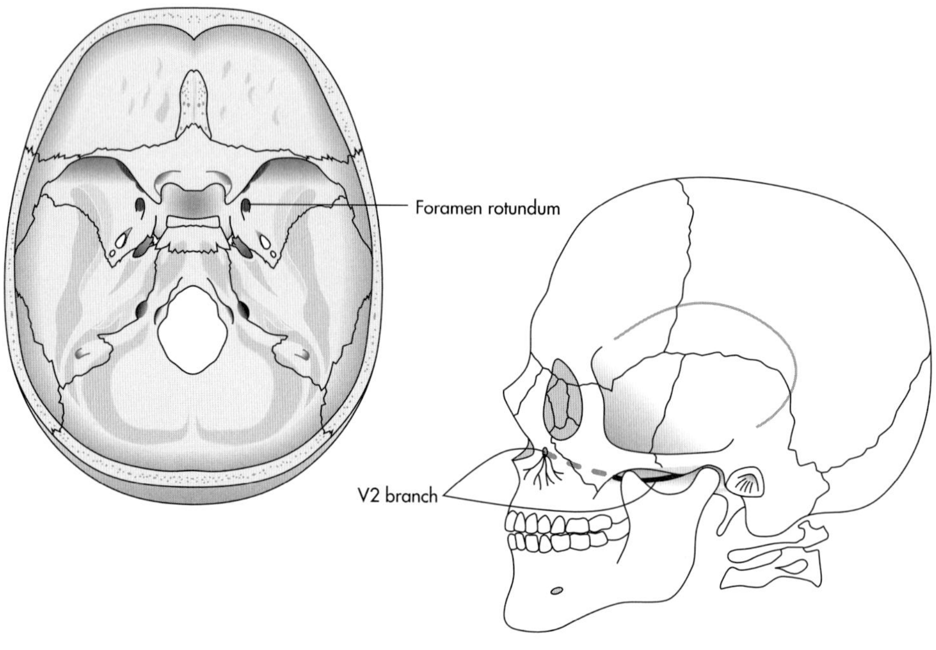

mandible

The third division of trigeminal V3 (mandibular) nerve passes out through foramen ovale and downward to the ______________ or jaw.

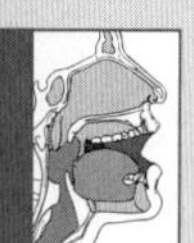

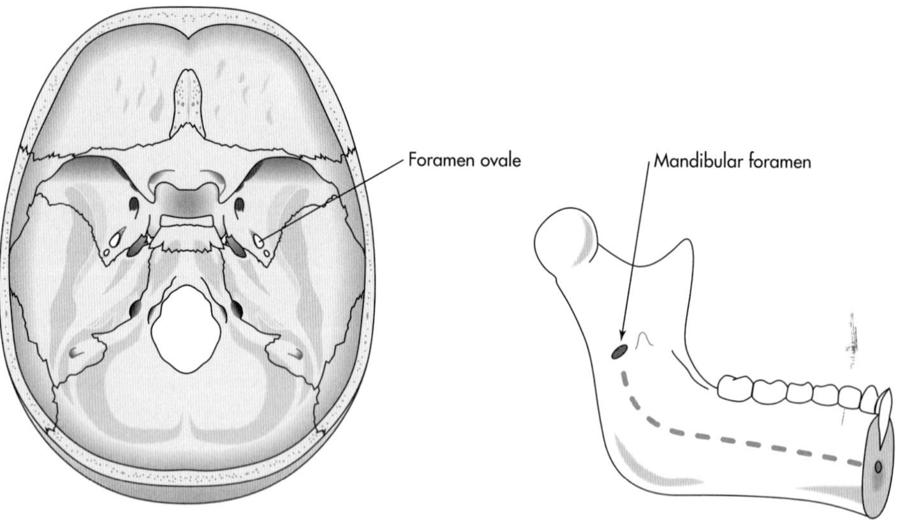

A small branch of V3 exits a foramen in the chin called the **mental foramen.**

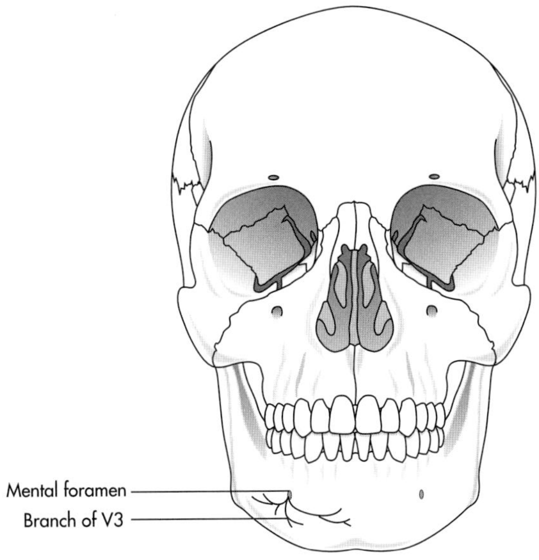

Look, in the interior cranium and on the face, at the pattern of foramina of the divisions of cranial nerve V. We return to these in subsequent chapters.

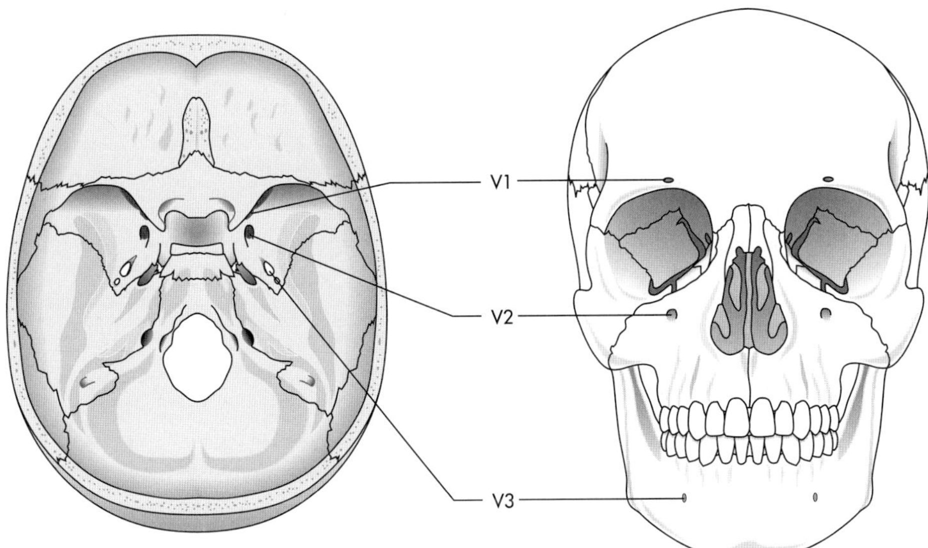

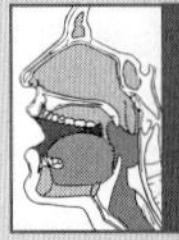

Can you see the small outer aspect of the sphenoid bone from the sagittal view? (Clue: It is next to the temporal bone.)

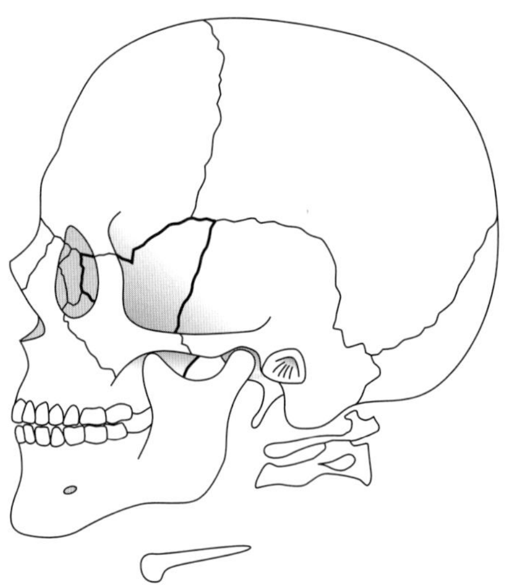

A. carotid canal
B. foramen spinosum
C. foramen ovale

From the underside of the cranium, again, more of the sphenoid is visible. Can you see and identify the foramina from this side? Find the foramen ovale, foramen spinosum, and carotid canals.

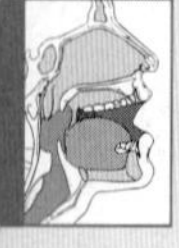

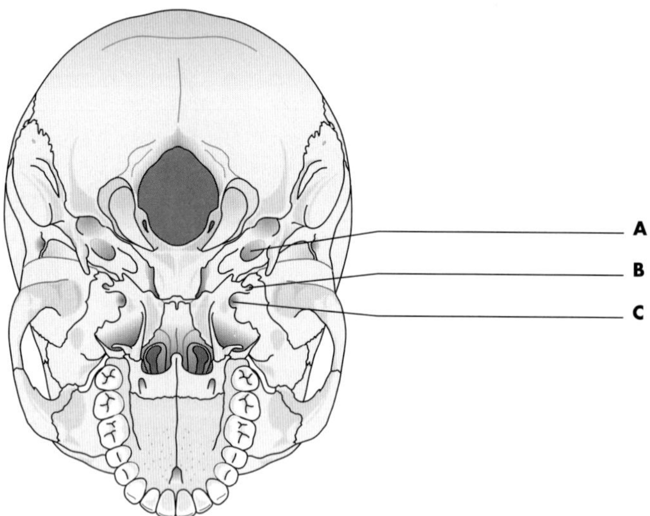

From this aspect, some unusually shaped processes of the sphenoid are seen—the **pterygoid plates.** These four thin "wings" of bone are found directly inferior and lateral to the palate. They provide attachment sites for muscles.

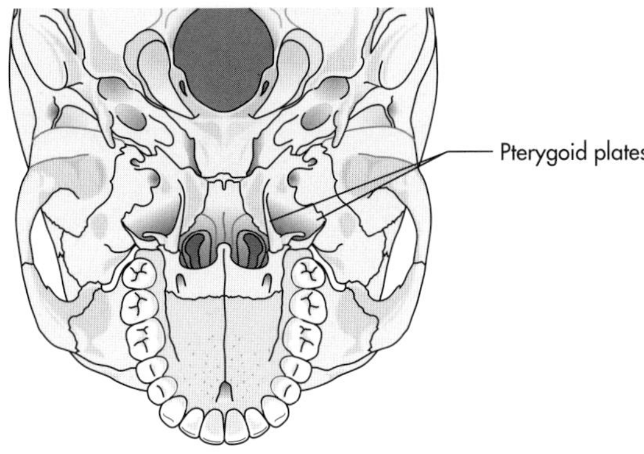

These "wings" of bone of the sphenoid are called the ______________ plates. At their junction with the palate are two tiny hooks. These also are important to muscles that pass around them. They are called the **hamuli** (singular, hamulus).

pterygoid

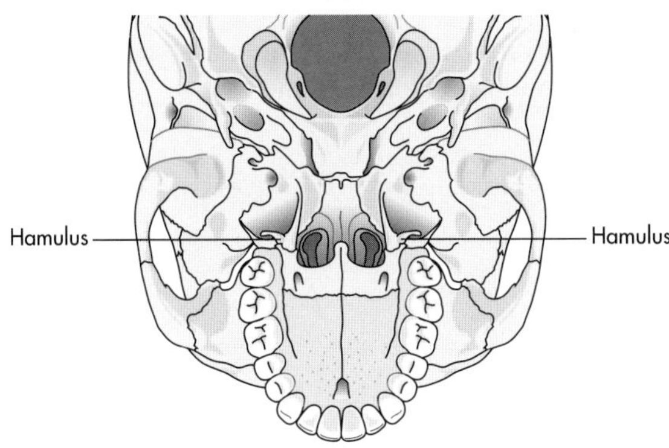

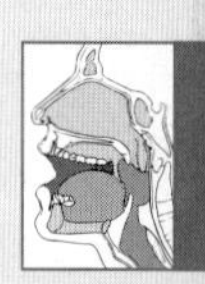

Find the hooks of the hamuli and the pterygoid plates on the drawing.

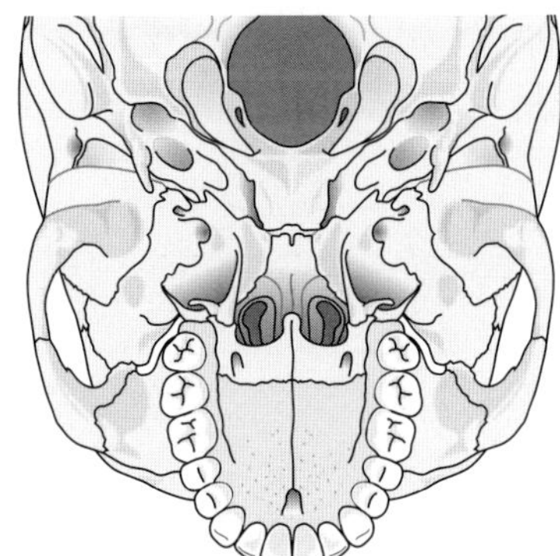

A. foramen rotundum
B. foramen spinosum
C. superior orbital fissure
D. carotid canal

Find the sphenoid bone and its foramina.

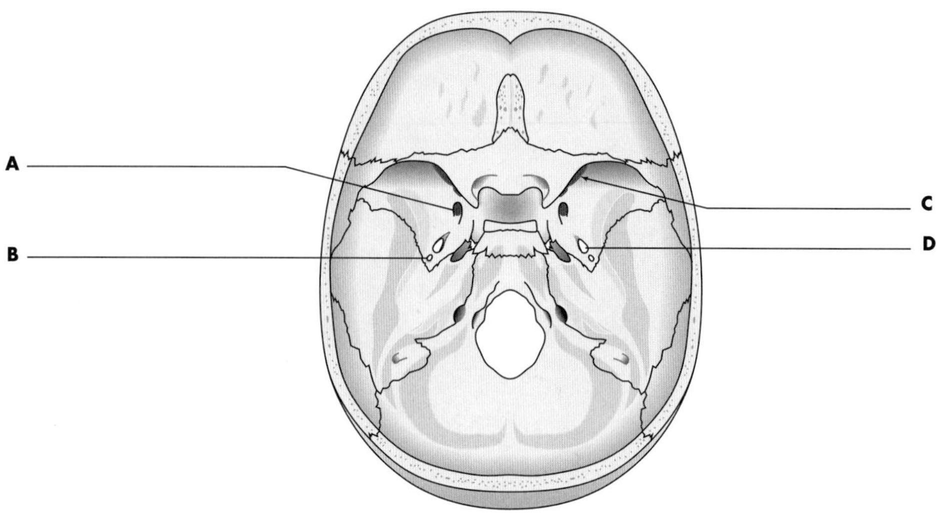

ZYGOMA BONES

At the corners of the "cheekbones" lie the two **zygoma** bones. Find them outlined on the frontal and sagittal views. You may color them in.

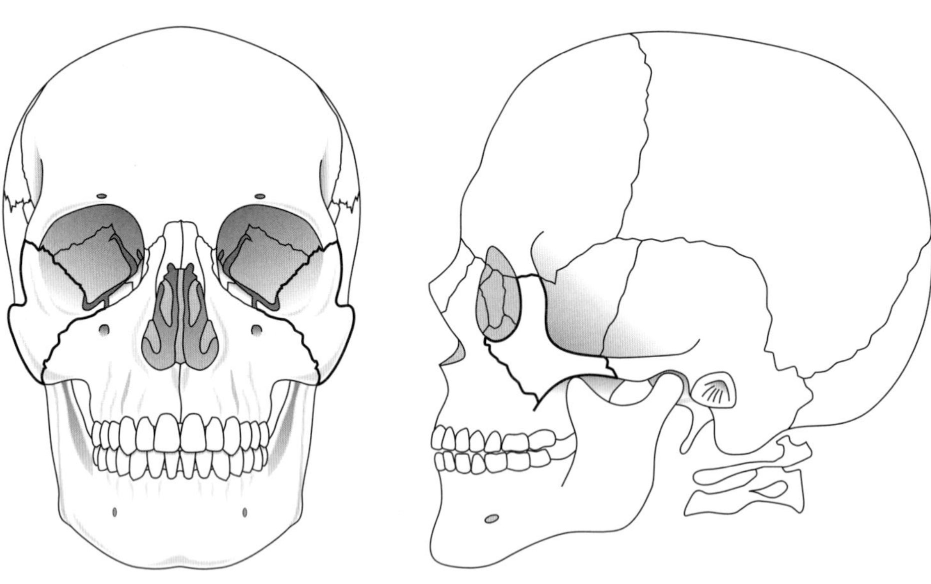

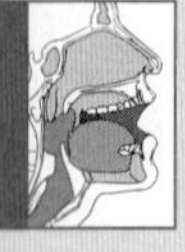

The zygoma is only a portion of the entire "cheekbone," the scientific name of which is **zygomatic process.** The ______________ process is composed of portions of the temporal bone, the zygoma bone, and the maxillary bone. Older texts may call the zygomatic process the **malar bone.**

zygomatic

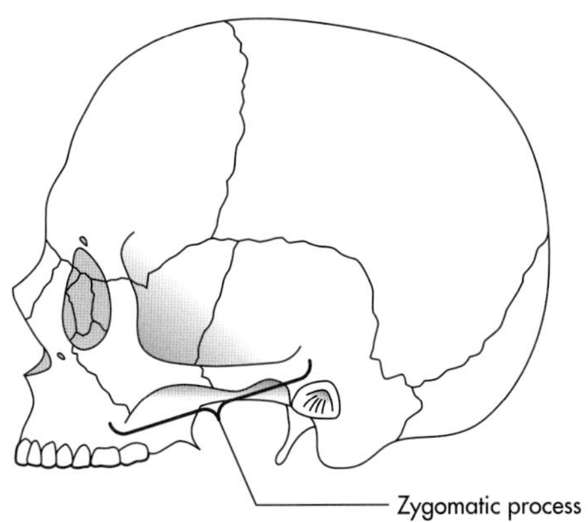

Remember that the infratemporal fossa is the space that lies behind the zygomatic process. The coronoid process of the mandible rests within that space.

MAXILLARY BONES

The large area occupied by the right and left **maxillary bones** can be appreciated in a frontal view of the skull. Not only does the maxillary bone house the maxillary arch of teeth, but it also constitutes the middle third of the face. Find and color them on the drawing.

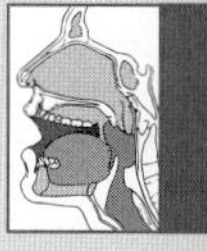

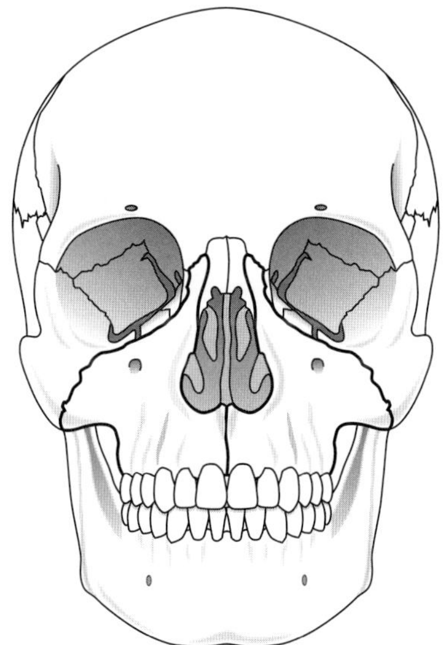

zygomatic process, V2

Find the maxillae on the sagittal view. What process in this view does the maxilla form part of? Note a foramen directly beneath the orbit. This is the **infraorbital foramen** and it provides an exit for a nerve branch of V that innervates the skin of the middle face. Which branch?

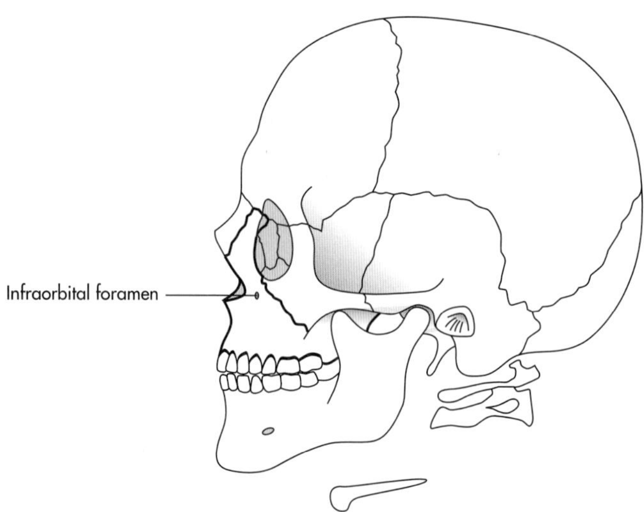

Find the infraorbital foramina on the drawing. Refer to the above sagittal view.

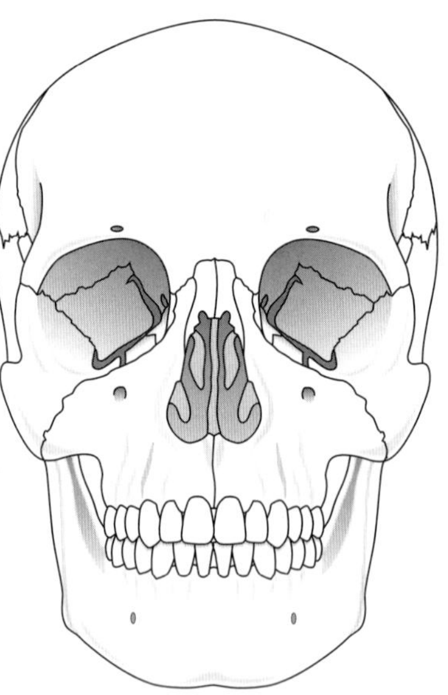

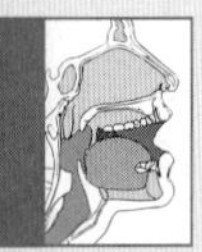

You can see how the maxillary teeth are placed within the alveolar bone of the maxillae. The prominence for each root is visible, especially over the canine roots. These are called the **canine eminences.**

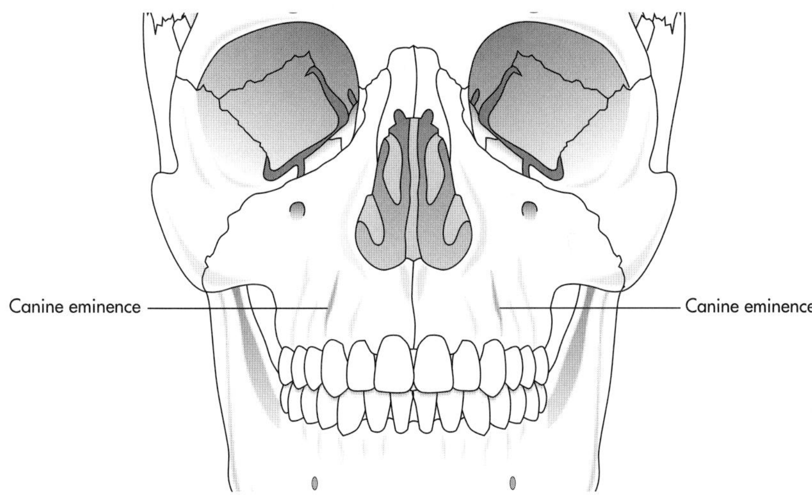

The maxillae also form the bottom portion of the openings for the eyeballs, the _______________.

orbits

If you tip up the cranium to look at the maxillae, you can see the **hard palate.** Find it. The palate was created by the coalescence of three processes. You can often see sutures where they came together. Find them.

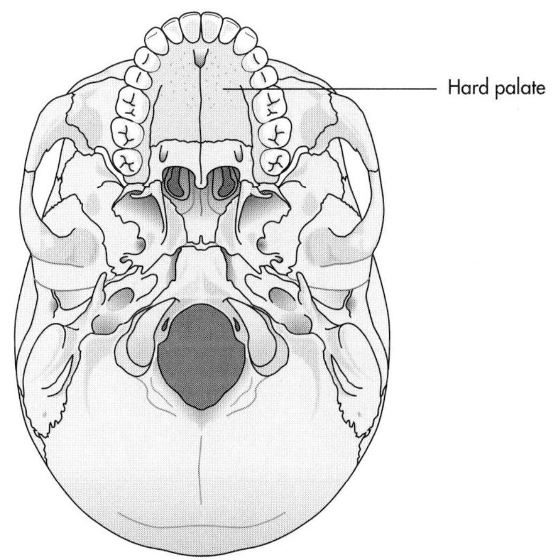

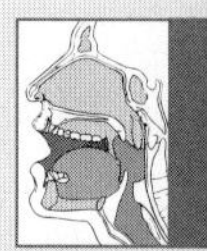

midpalatine

The suture dividing the palate in half is called the **midpalatine suture.** There may be one suture v-shaped just behind the central incisors. This shows the extent of the primary palate, one of the three embryonic processes that formed the palate. The other two are on either side of the ______________ suture. Another perpendicular suture defines a pair of bones separate from the maxillae.

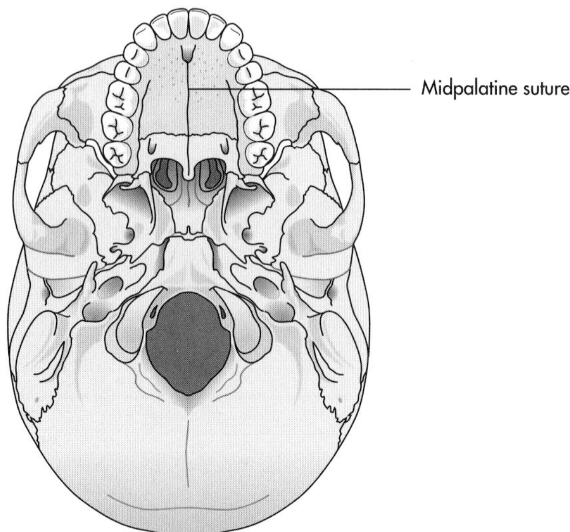

The palate has three foramina. Find them. One is directly behind the central incisors and is called the **incisive foramen.** It carries nerves and blood vessels to the lingual side of the anterior maxillary teeth.

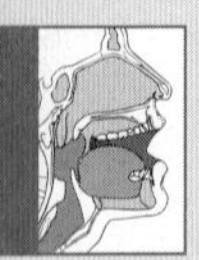

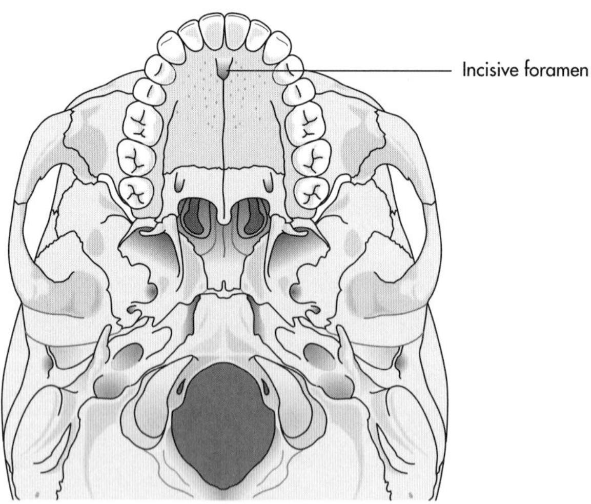

The other two foramina are found on the back of the palate, but are not part of the maxillary bone. They are on either side of the palate, opposite the last molars. These are the **greater palatine foramina.** These carry nerves and blood vessels to the lingual side of the posterior teeth. (There is also a pair of smaller lesser palatine foramina!)

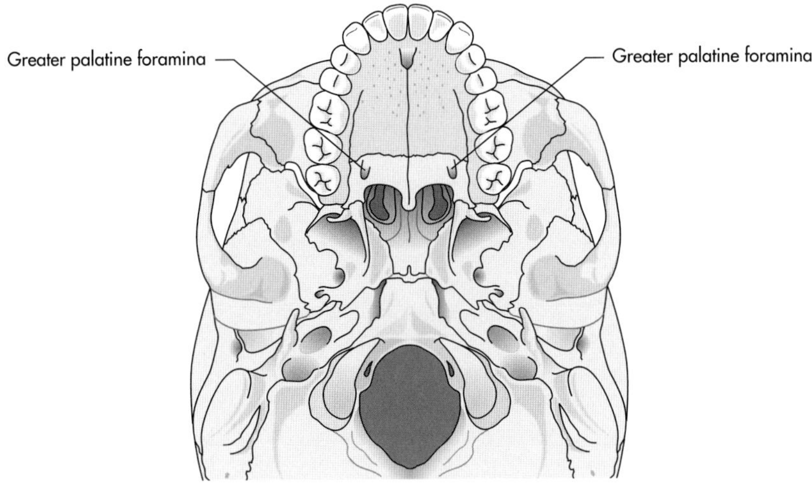

The ______________ foramen carries nerves and vessels to the lingual side of the anterior teeth, and the ______________ foramina, to the lingual side of the posterior teeth.

incisive, greater palatine

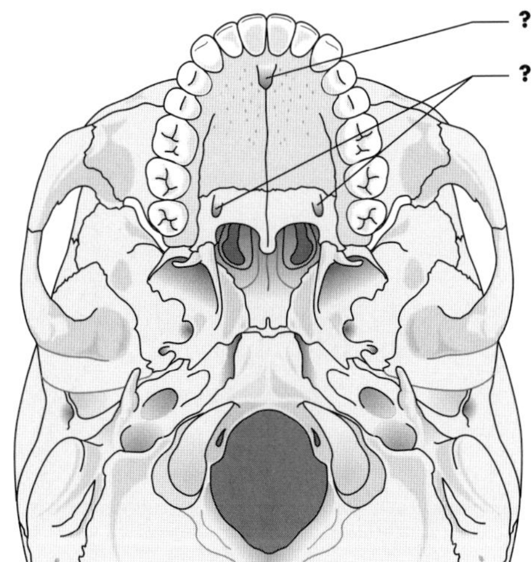

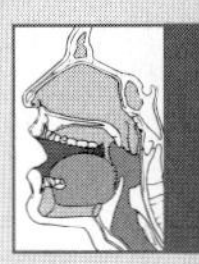

hamulus

That portion of the maxillary bone directly distal to the last molars is called the **maxillary tuberosity.** Distal to it is that hook of bone called the ______________.

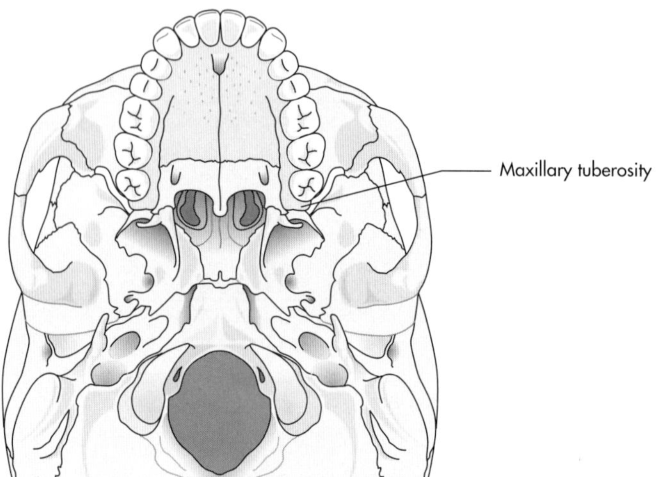

Returning to the frontal view of the cranium, observe that the maxillary bones constitute not only a portion of the orbits but also part of the nasal cavity. You can see a vertical midline structure that divides the nasal cavity into two halves. This is the **nasal septum.** The maxilla forms a small part of it.

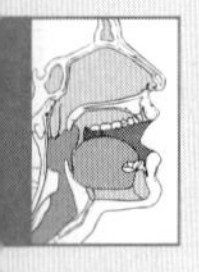

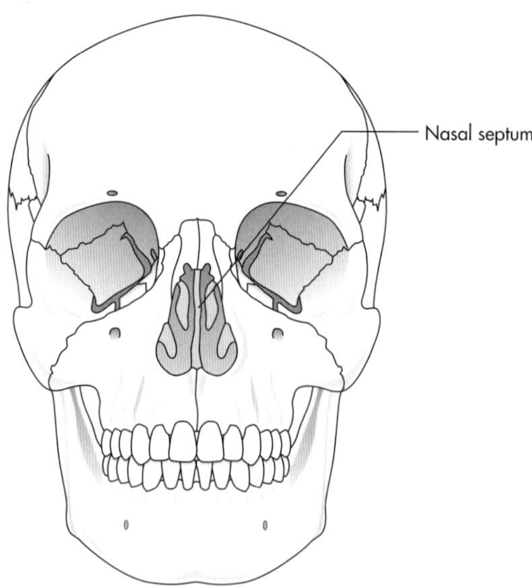

At the beginning of the nasal septum, at its inferior aspect where it joins the outer surface of the orifice, is a small projection of bone called the **nasal spine.** The nasal orifices, nasal spine, or nasal septum may appear in periapical films of maxillary anterior teeth.

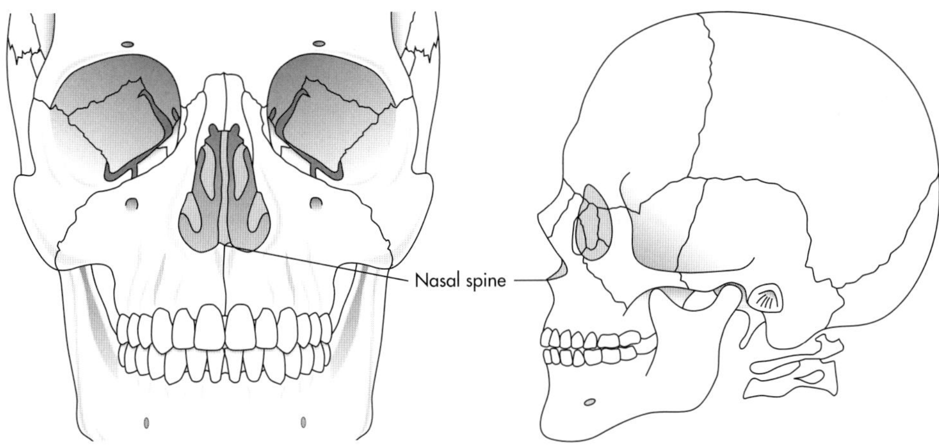

What is not visible when we look at the maxillary bones is the structure within the bones. That is, these bones have a pair of large hollow places within them in the area of the upper "cheeks." These hollow areas are lined with respiratory mucosa and connect by passageways into the nasal cavity. They are called the **maxillary sinuses** and are shown in this "x-ray view."

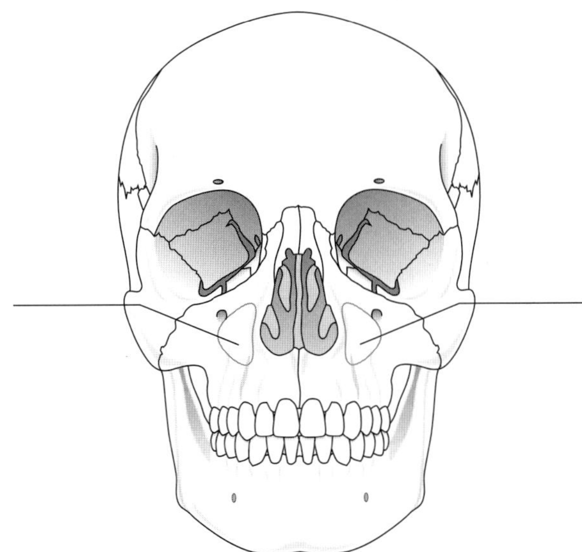

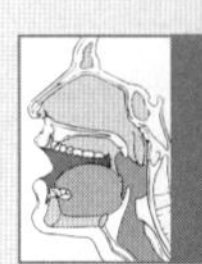

maxillary

The _______________ sinuses are part of the **paranasal sinuses,** a system of hollow areas in several cranial bones that surround the nasal cavity.

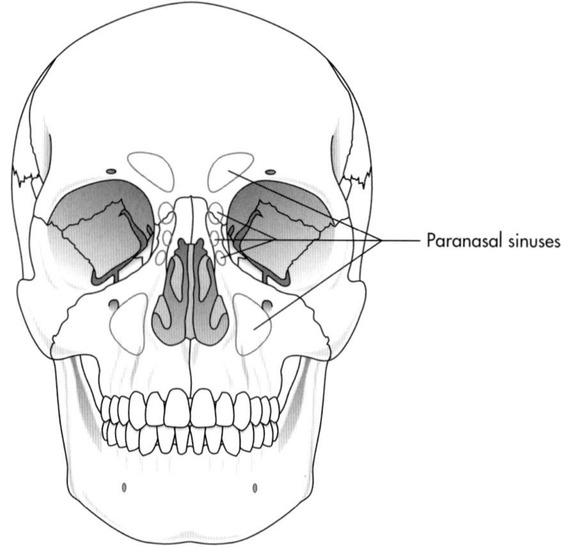

The **maxillary sinuses** are pyramid-shaped spaces that lie in close proximity to the roots of the posterior maxillary teeth. They can also be seen on posterior periapical films.

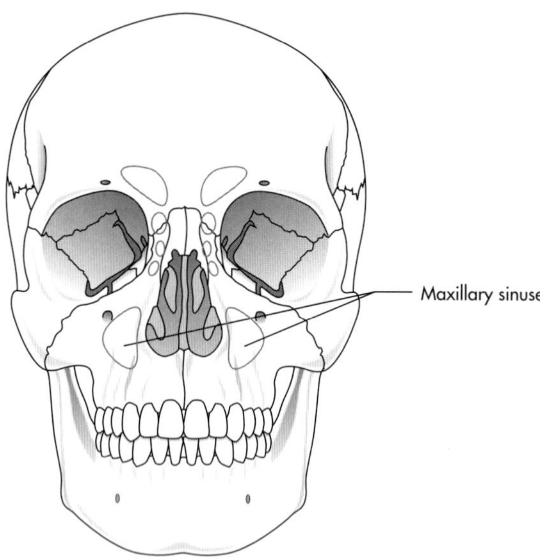

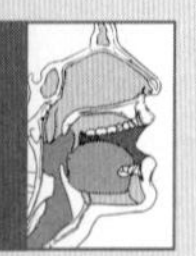

Review the parts of the maxillary bones.

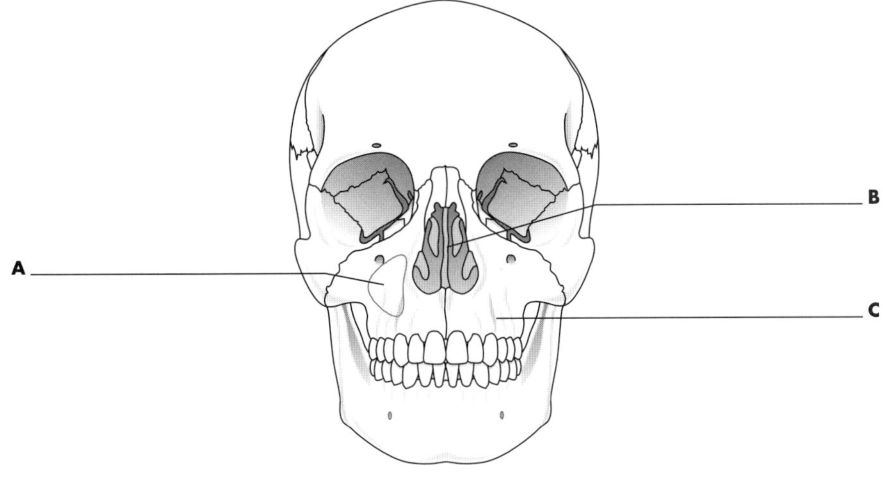

A. maxillary sinus
B. nasal septum
C. canine eminence

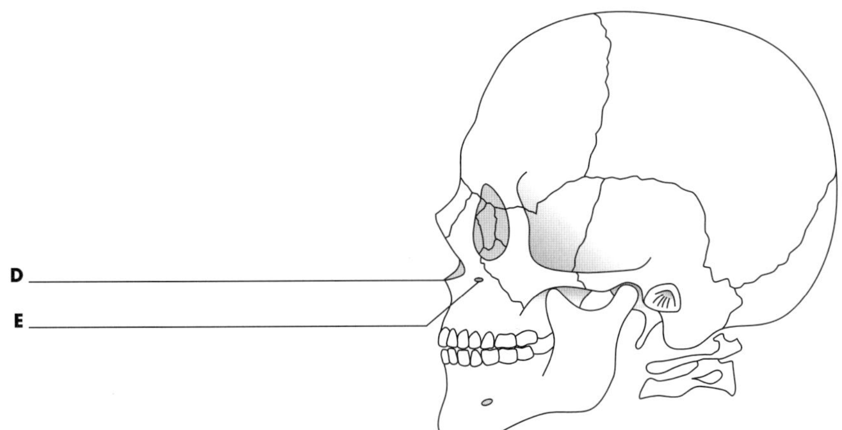

D. nasal spine
E. infraorbital foramen

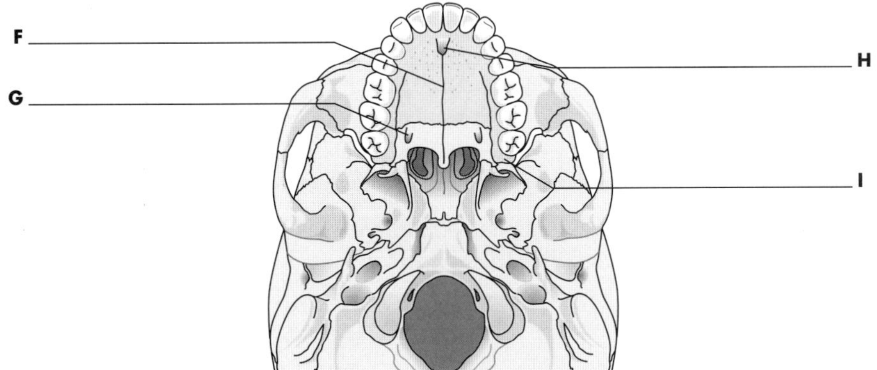

F. midpalatine suture
G. greater palatine foramen
H. incisive foramen
I. maxillary tuberosity

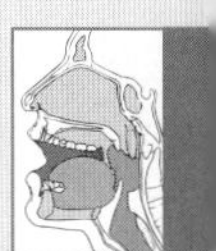

PALATINE BONES

When we looked at the palate, did you notice another suture in the posterior portion? At the most posterior part of the palate is another pair of cranial bones, the **palatine bones.** Find them and color them in on the drawing.

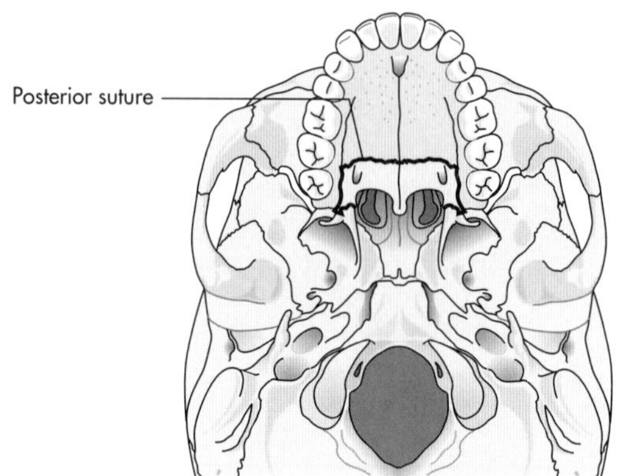

The part that is visible on the hard palate is only part of the palatine bones. Vertical processes from these bones make up part of the posterior nasal septum and some lateral processes not visible on our drawing.

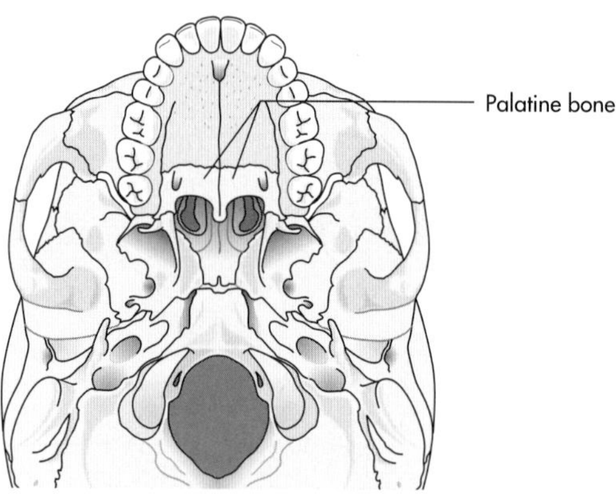

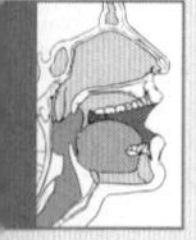

greater palatine, lingual side of the posterior teeth

We have already seen the two foramina of the palatine bones, the ______________ foramina. They carry nerves and blood vessels where?

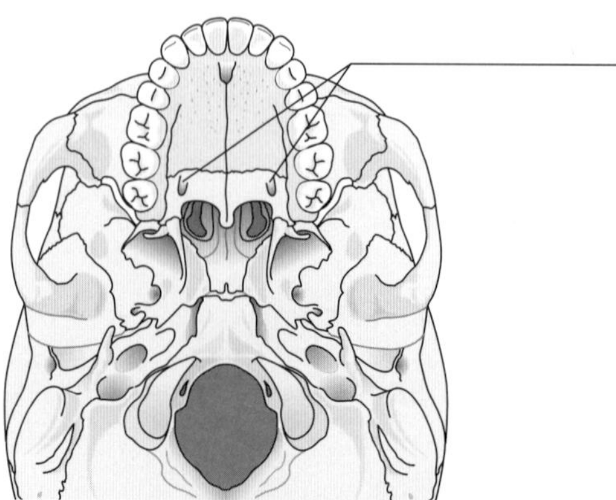

In the view of the palate and nasal cavity, what is the central dividing area of bone called? What lies in the area marked "X"?

nasal septum, oral cavity

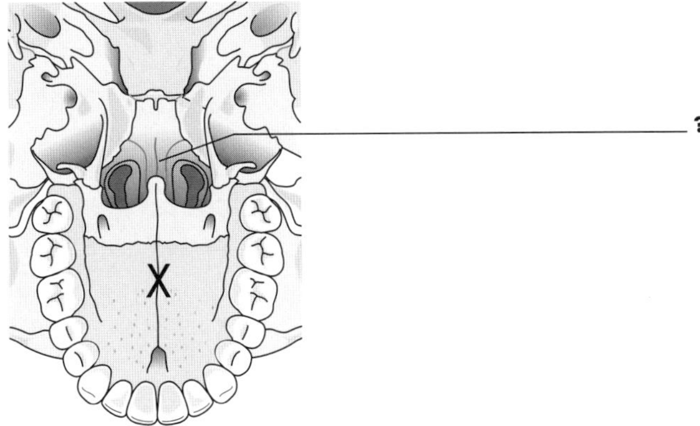

VOMER BONE

Again, in the posterior view of the nasal cavity and palate, look at the bone extending from the base of the skull vertically to the palate. It is shaped like a little plow and thus was named the **vomer.** Find and color it on the drawing.

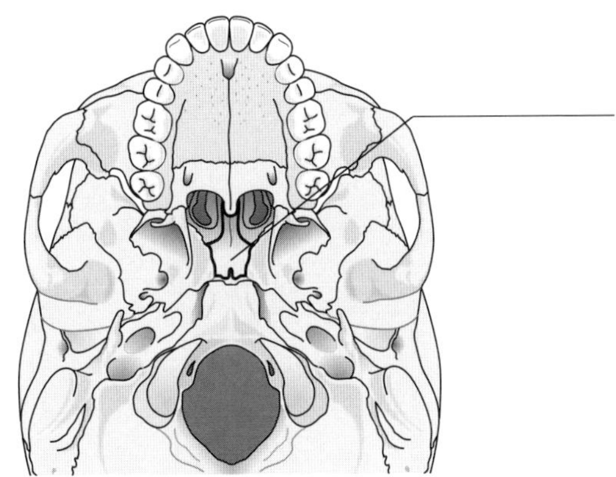

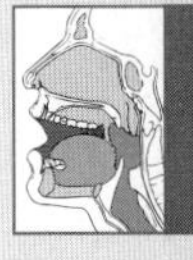

vomer, nasal septum

The _______________ bone forms part of that midline nasal structure, the _______________.

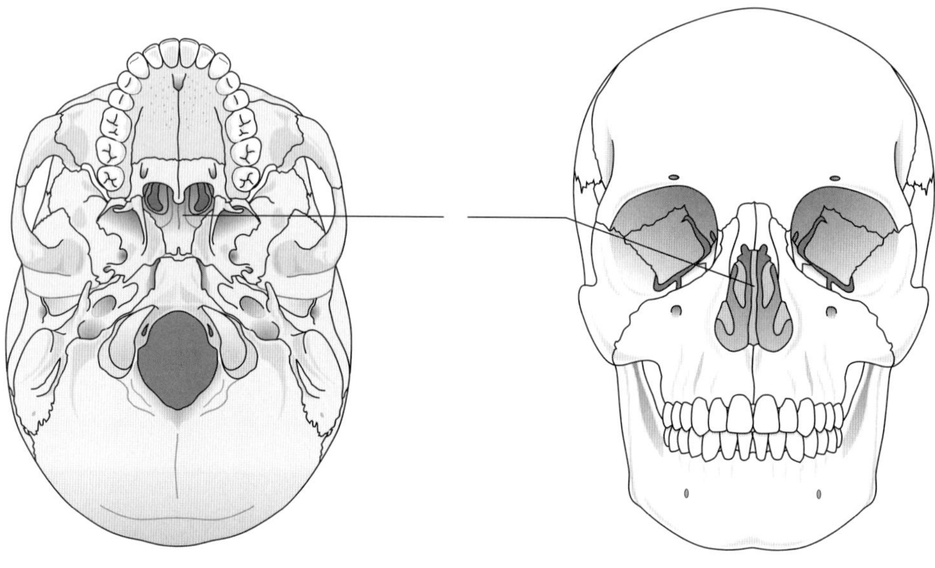

pterygoid plates, hamuli

What other structures of the sphenoid bone can you see in the view of the base of the cranium?

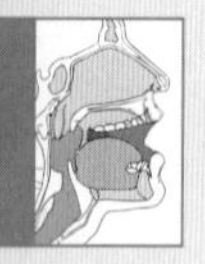

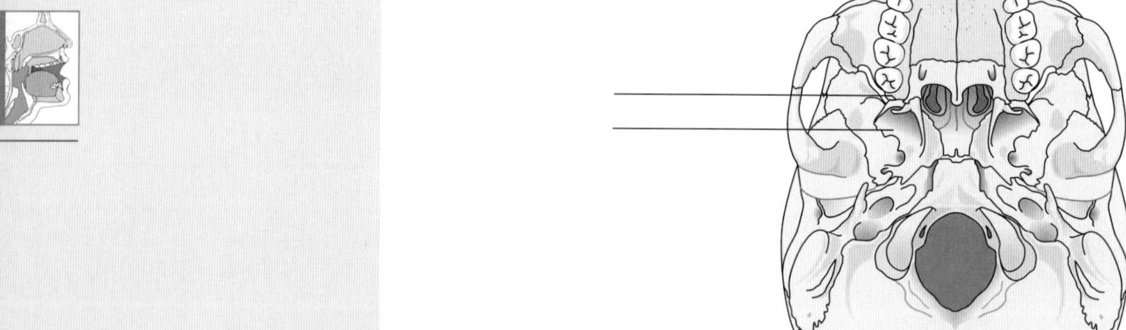

NASAL BONES

Two very small bones are located on the bridge of the nasal orifice in this frontal view. Find them. They are called the **nasal bones.**

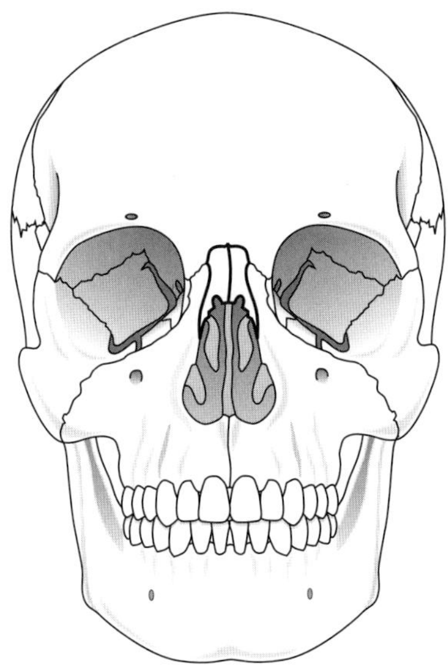

Find the nasal bone in this lateral view. The nasal bones begin the structure that we know as the nose. These bones provide an attachment for the nasal cartilages, which extend out and downward from the bone creating most of the substance of the nose.

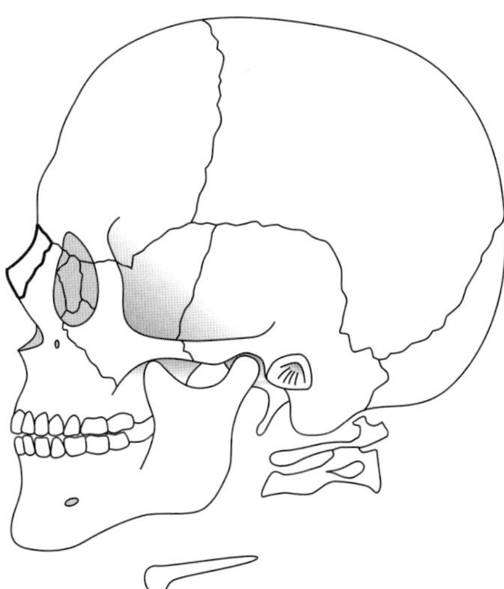

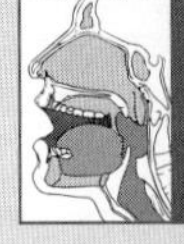

ETHMOID BONE

Return to an interior view of the cranium. Find the frontal bone. A walnut-shaped area of bone is nestled within the frontal bone. It is part of the **ethmoid bone.** Find it and color it in.

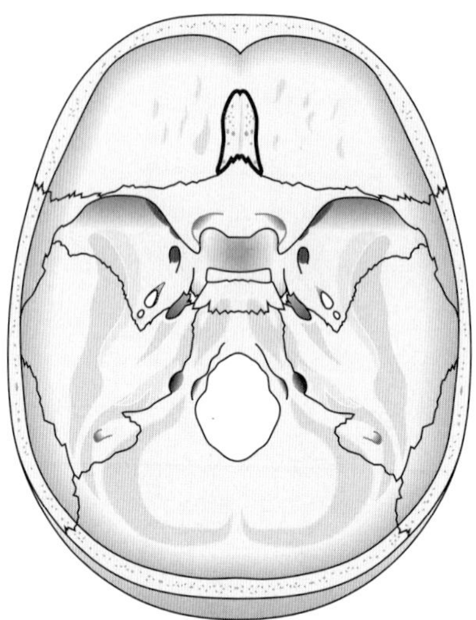

The portion of the ethmoid bone visible to us here is only the "tip of an iceberg." Most of the bone lies below in the nasal cavity, with three vertical processes extending downward.

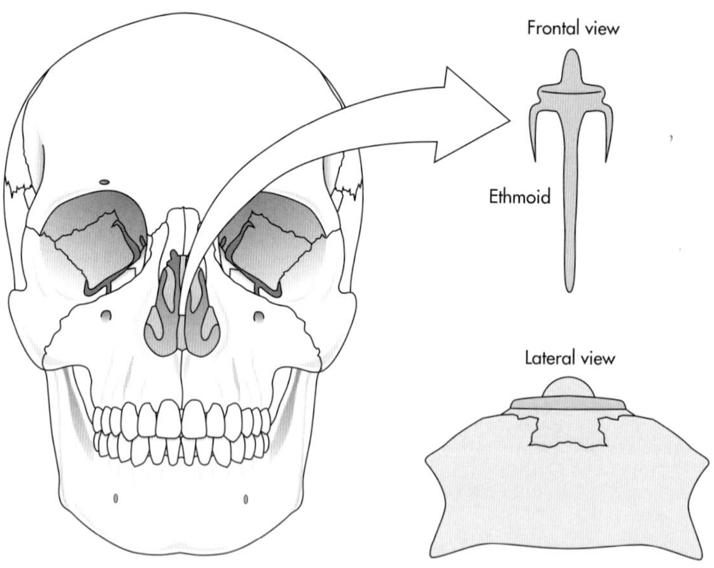

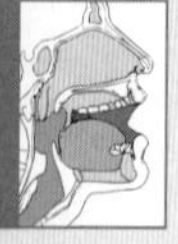

The portion we see in this picture is a single vertical plate or process called the **crista galli** and it is set within a horizontal plate that is perforated with holes called the **cribriform plate.** They are the superior portions of the ______________ bone.

ethmoid

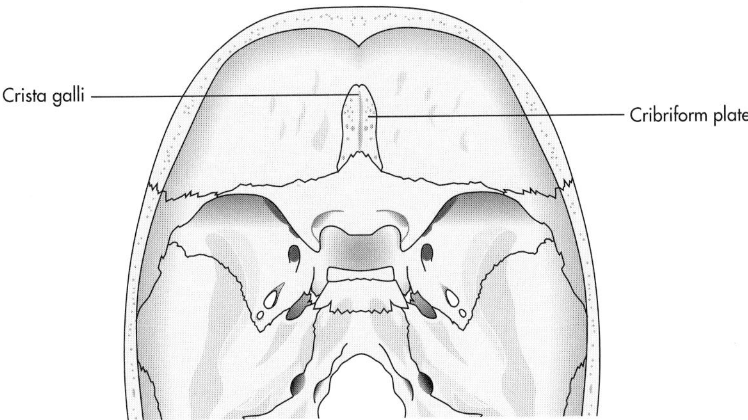

In the frontal view please label the midline structure you can see inside the nasal cavity. Note the lateral bony projections. These are called the **nasal conchae** or **turbinates.** They are three pairs of large vertical processes on the lateral aspects of the nasal cavity, probably functioning to warm air as it enters. They are covered by nasal mucosa. There are superior, middle, and inferior turbinates.

nasal septum

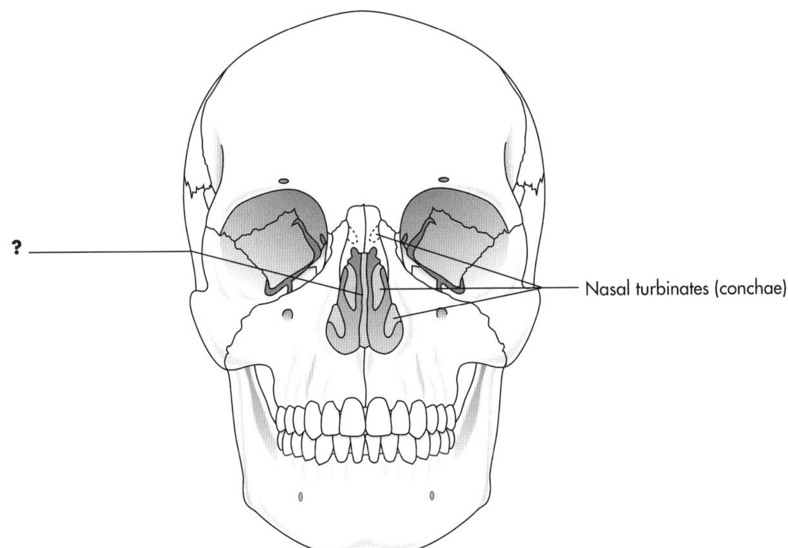

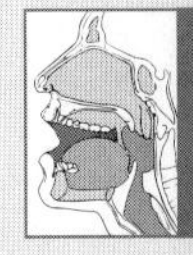

The turbinates are processes from the bones that make up the nasal cavity, the maxillary bones, and the ethmoid bones. The inferior turbinates are sometimes considered separate bones.

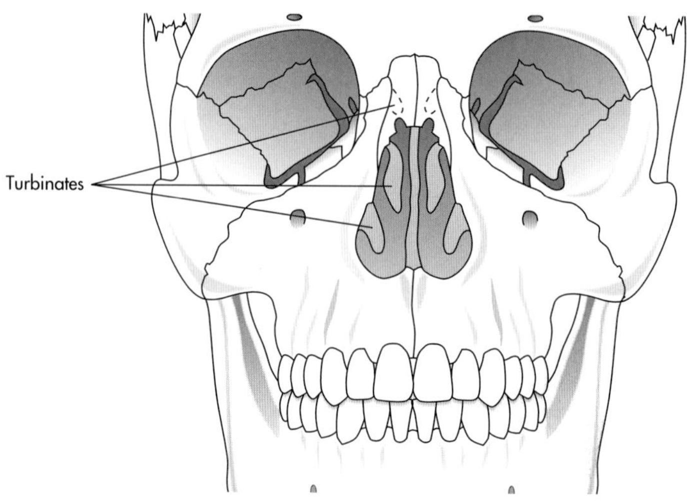

Passageways from the sinuses (frontal, sphenoid, ethmoid, and maxillary) empty beneath the middle turbinate to drain into the nasal cavity. They are called **meatii.**

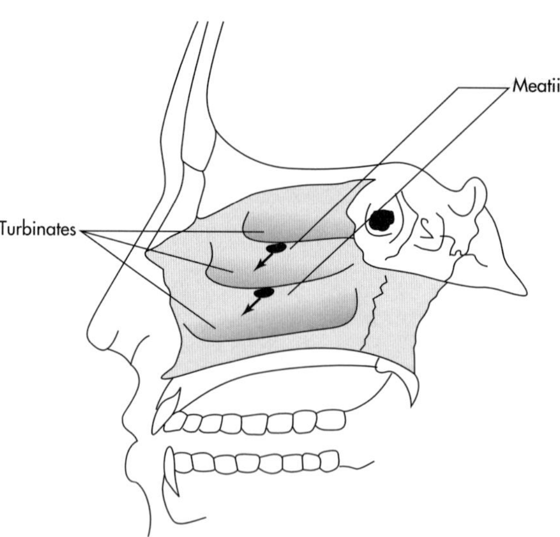

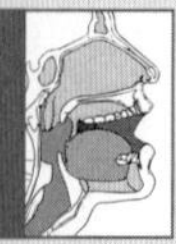

The nasal septum is made of many bones as we have seen. Name them. The end of the septum is made of cartilage.

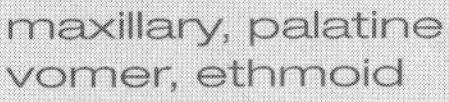

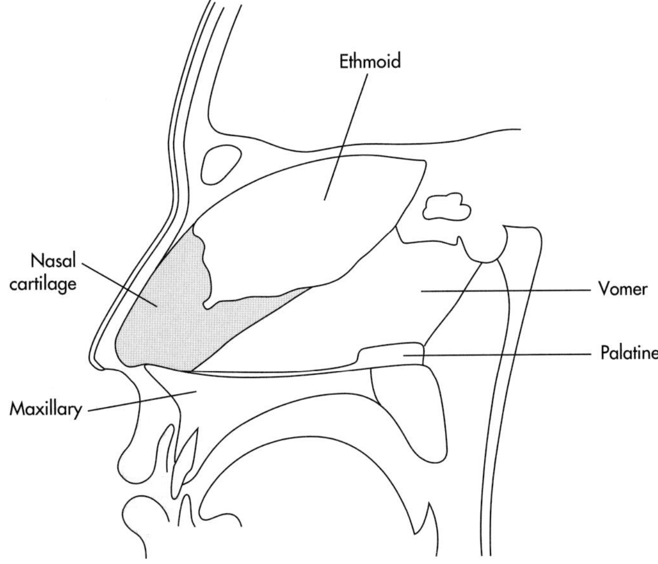

LACRIMAL BONES

The smallest bones of the cranium are the two lacrimal bones. They get their name from a gland, the lacrimal gland that rests on their fossae within the orbit. Find one lacrimal bone on this drawing.

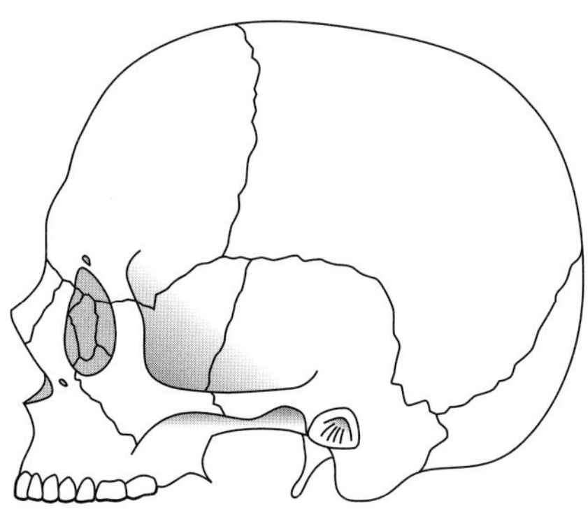

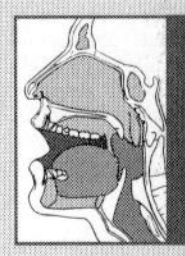

frontal, sphenoid, maxillary, zygoma, ethmoid, lacrimal

Find the **lacrimal bone** in the frontal view. Note how many of the cranial bones make up the orbit. Name them.

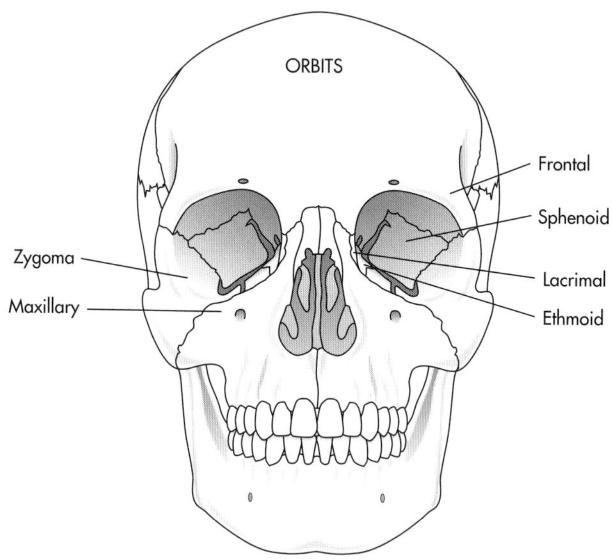

1. frontal
2. parietal
3. occipital
4. temporal
5. sphenoid
6. zygoma
7. maxillary
8. palatine
9. vomer
10. ethmoid
11. nasal
12. lacrimal

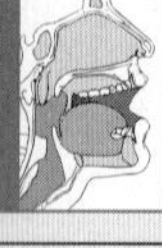

This completes the description of the 12 cranial bones. Can you name them?

1. ____________
2. ____________
3. ____________
4. ____________
5. ____________
6. ____________
7. ____________
8. ____________
9. ____________
10. ____________
11. ____________
12. ____________

Can you find each of the 12 bones in the drawings? If you cannot, check back in the text. Color or outline each.

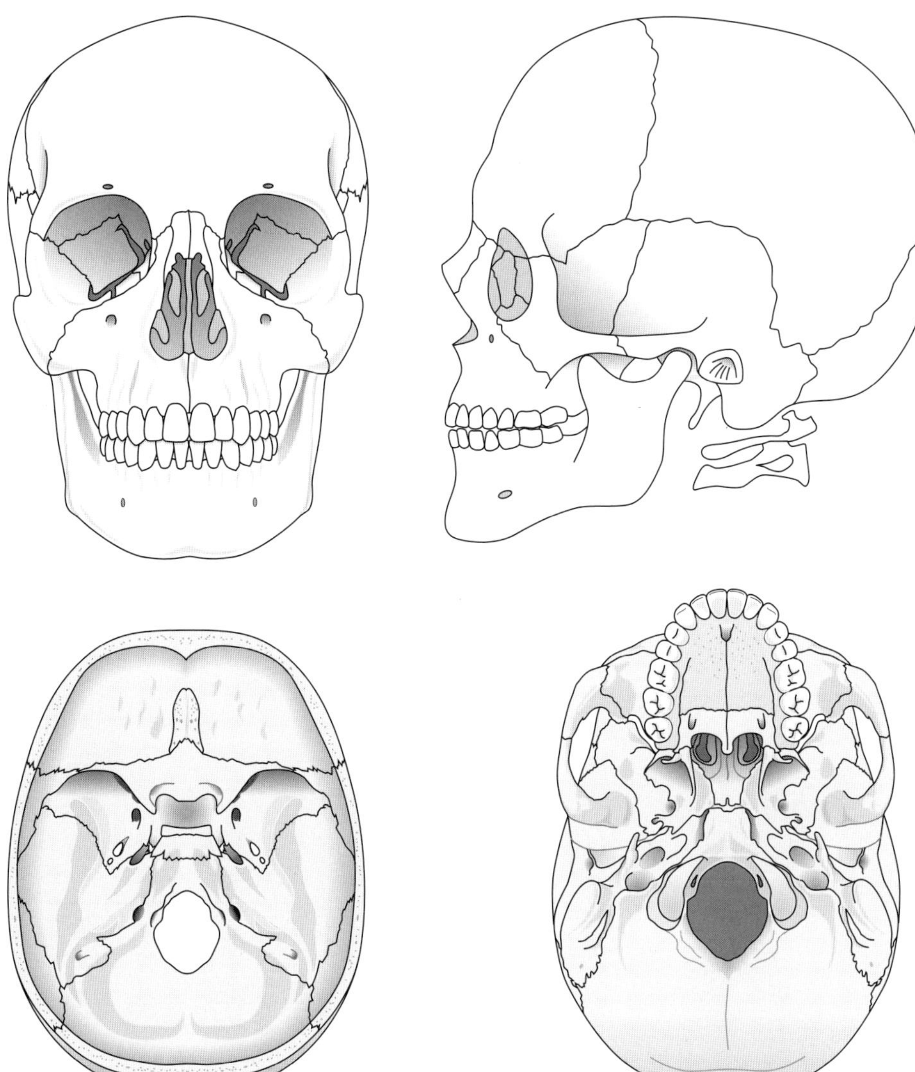

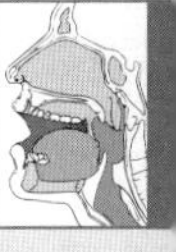

Label the various foramina, fossae, and processes of the cranium.

A. supraorbital foramen
B. nasal septum
C. infraorbital foramen
D. superior orbital fissure
E. nasal turbinate
F. canine eminence
G. mental foramen

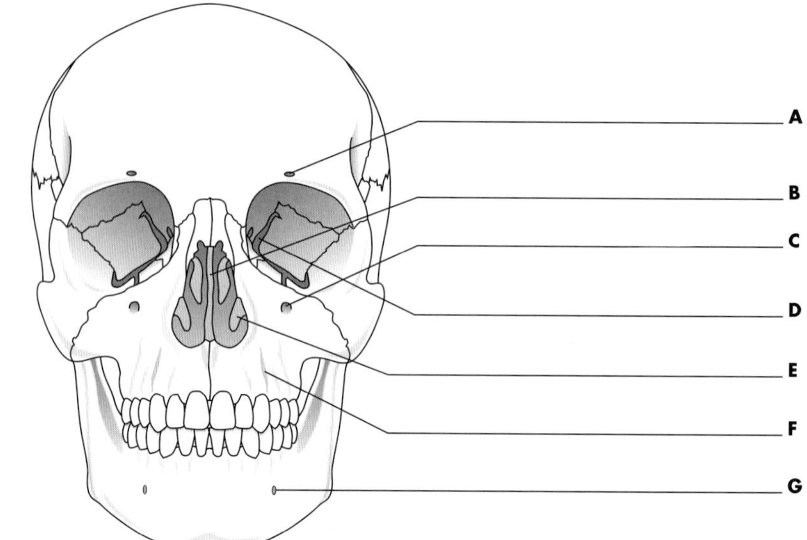

A. mastoid process
B. styloid process
C. nasal spine
D. zygomatic process
E. external auditory meatus
F. articular eminence

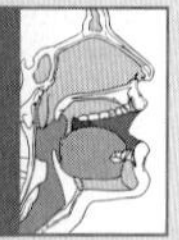

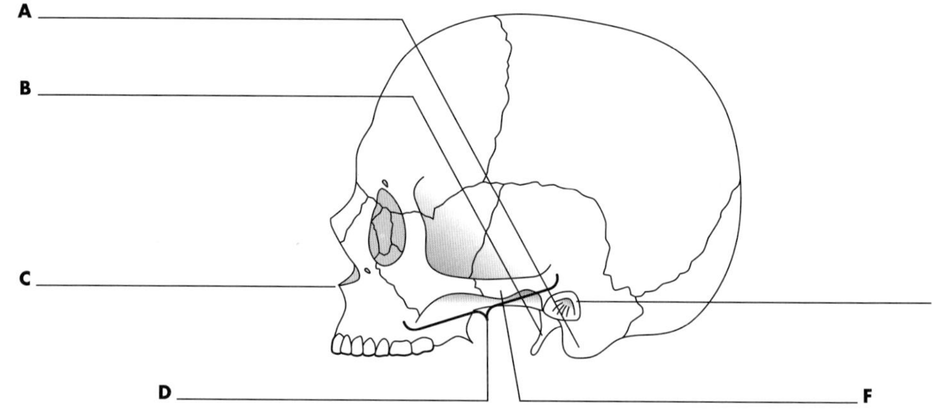

A. foramen rotundum
B. foramen ovale
C. foramen spinosum
D. hypoglossal foramen
E. optic foramen
F. superior orbital fissure
G. carotid canal
H. jugular foramen

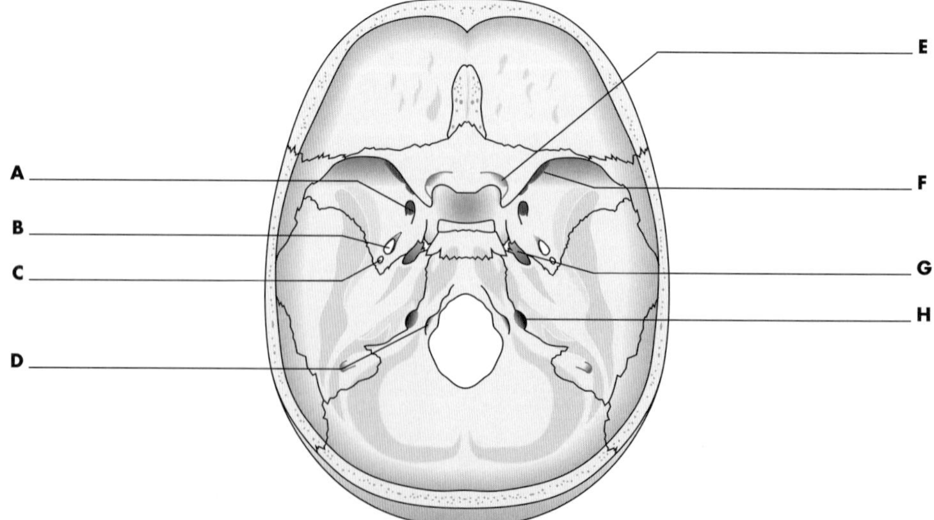

continued

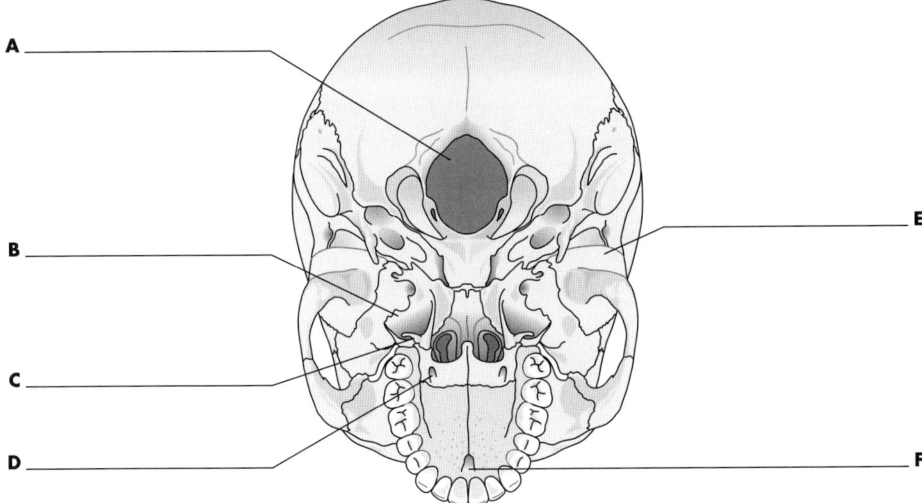

A. foramen magnum
B. pterygoid plates
C. hamulus
D. greater palatine foramen
E. mandibular fossa
F. incisive foramen

The Mandible 2.3

The last separate bone of the head is the **mandible** or jawbone. It developed around that cartilaginous rod, Meckel's cartilage, in the embryo and fetus, from coalescing mandibular processes. It creates two joints with the cranium called the temporomandibular joints. Find the mandible on the drawing. Color it in.

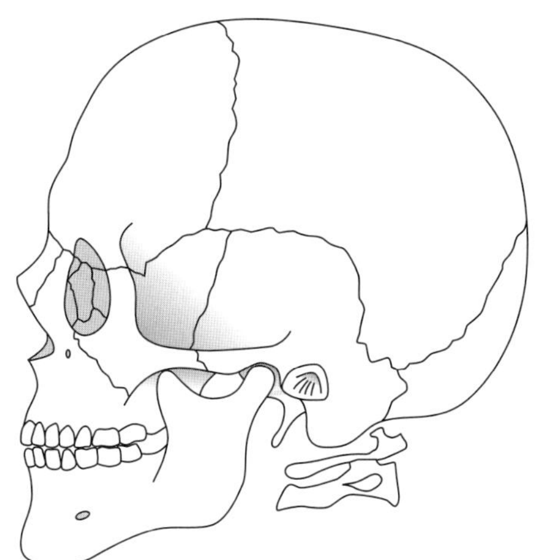

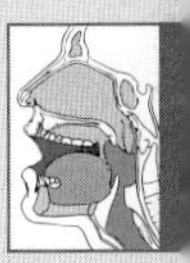

We study the mandible separate from the cranium first.

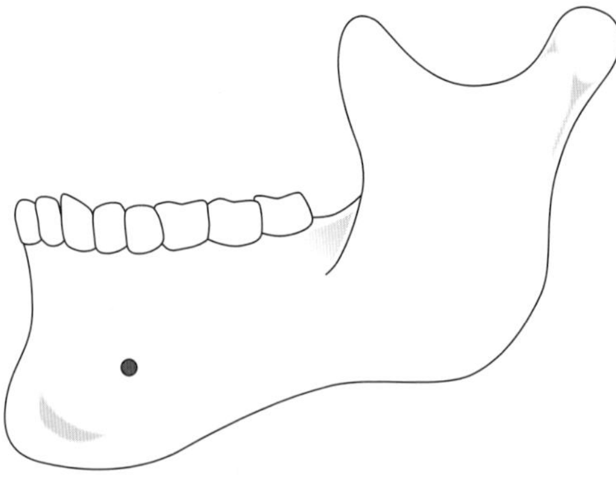

The mandible consists of a horizontal portion bearing the teeth called the **body** of the mandible. On either side, rising vertically are the two **rami** (singular, ramus). The places where they join are called the **angles.**

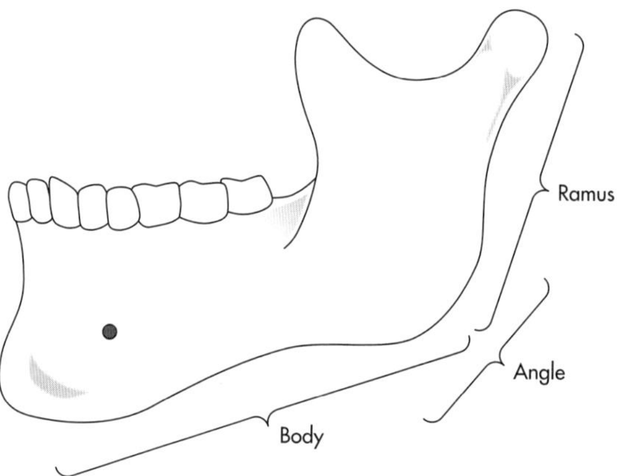

mandibular fossa

Two processes extend from each ramus of the mandible. First is the egg-shaped process that articulates with the temporal bone of the cranium—the **condyle.** Each condyle rests in which fossa?

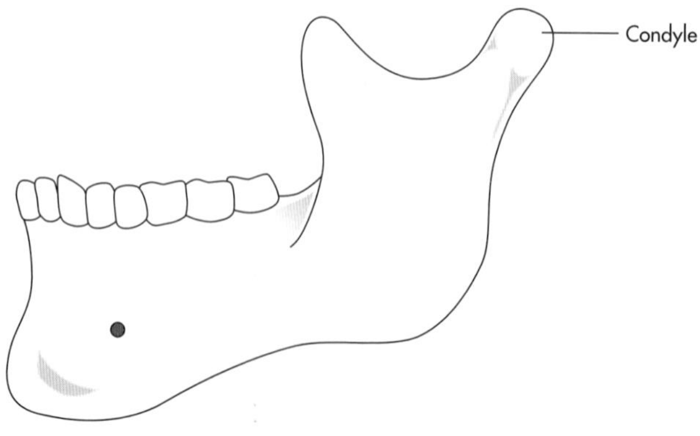

The condyle is part of the temporomandibular joint (TMJ). Return to Chapter Six for a short review of its parts and label the drawings.

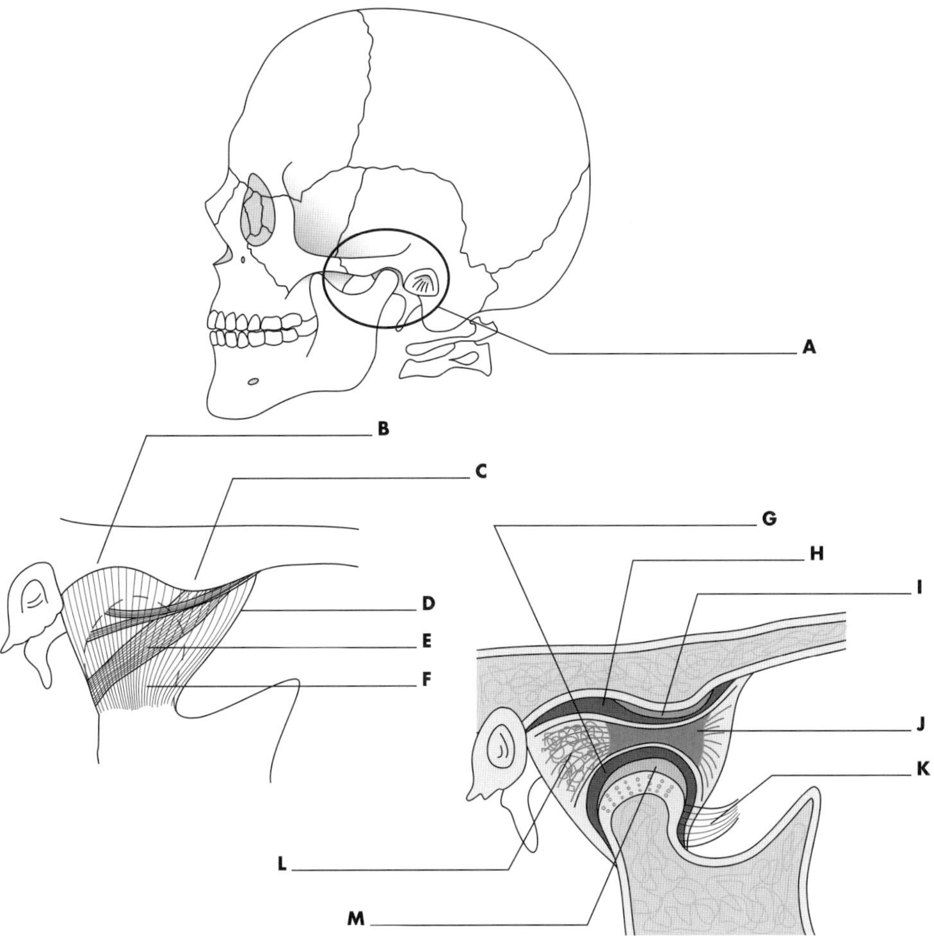

A. TMJ
B. mandibular fossa
C. articular eminence
D. temporo-mandibular capsule
E. lateral ligaments
F. condyle
G. inferior cavity
H. superior cavity
I. fibrous tissue
J. disk
K. lateral pterygoid
L. bilaminar zone (retrodiscal)
M. fibrous tissue

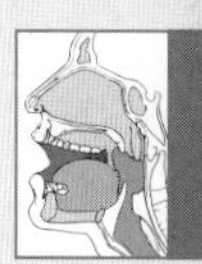

In addition to the **temporomandibular (TM) capsule/ligament,** two other accessory ligaments hold the mandible in place: the **sphenomandibular ligament** and the **stylomandibular ligament.**

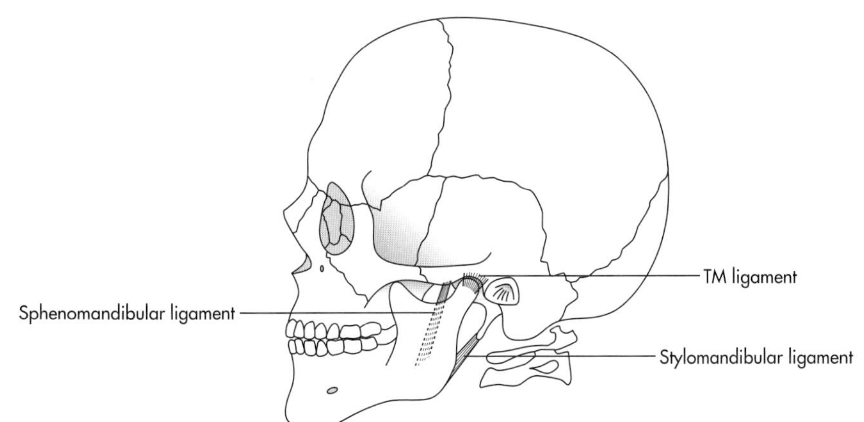

sphenoid

Sphenomandibular ligament runs from the ______________ bone of the cranium to an area just distal to the mandibular foramen.

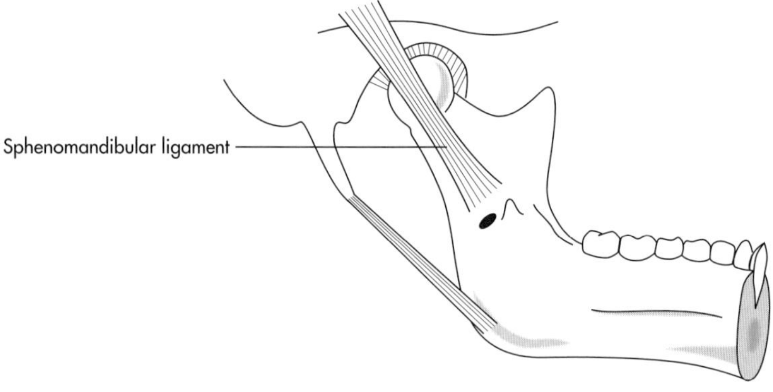

styloid

The **stylomandibular ligament** runs from the ______________ process to the angle of the mandible.

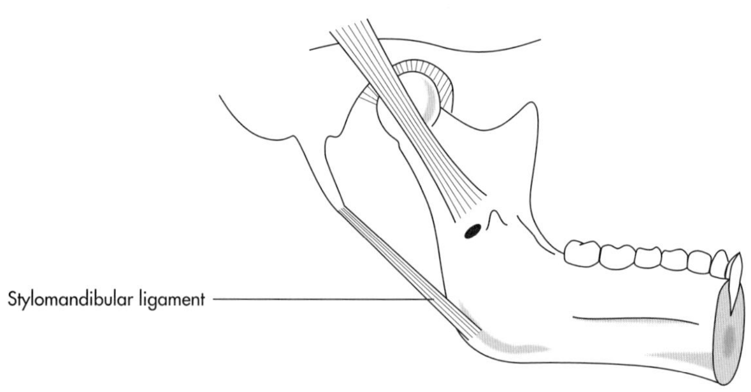

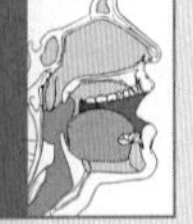

coronoid

The second process is the flat, pointed one below the condyle known as the **coronoid process.** This process provides attachment to the temporalis muscle, which we will study later. When the skull is articulated, the ______________ process lies behind the zygomatic process within the infratemporal fossa.

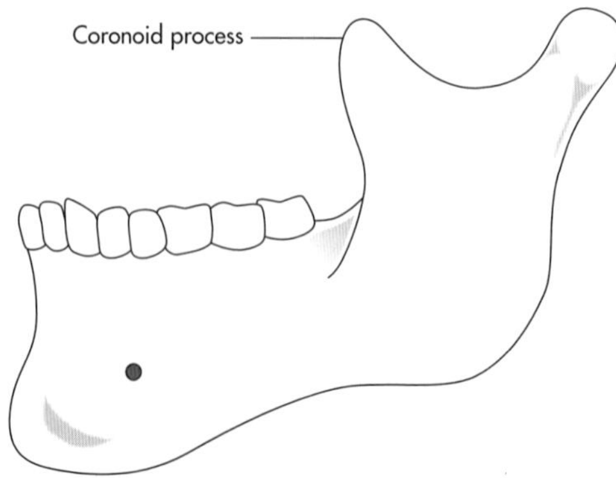

Identify the coronoid process and the condyle. Note that the ramus forms a curved area between the two, known as the **sigmoid notch.**

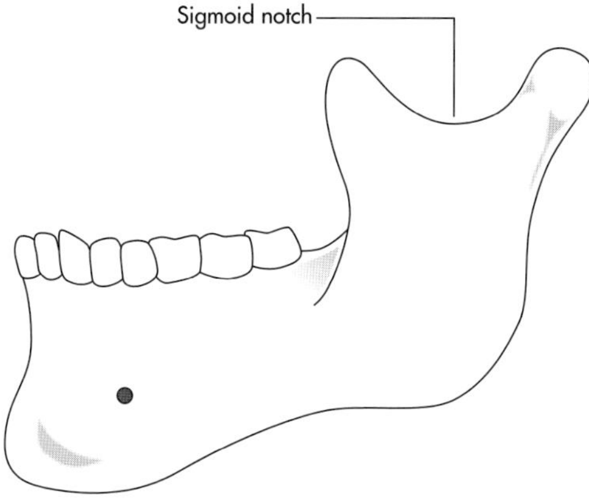

Near the chin or **mentum** of the mandible, a depression and a "hole" can be seen. The depression is the **mental fossa,** an area where the mentalis muscle attaches. The "hole" is the **mental foramen.** Do you remember which branch of the trigeminal nerve exits here?

V3

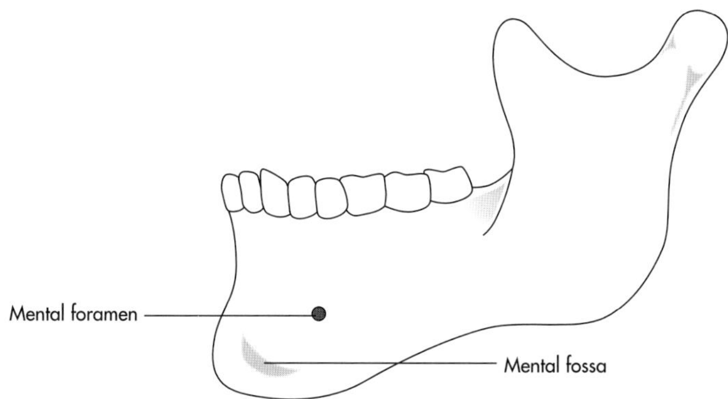

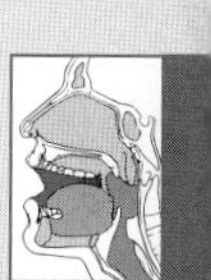

The view below is of the interior side of the mandible, as if it were cut in half and showing the inside portion. Other anatomic structures can be seen.

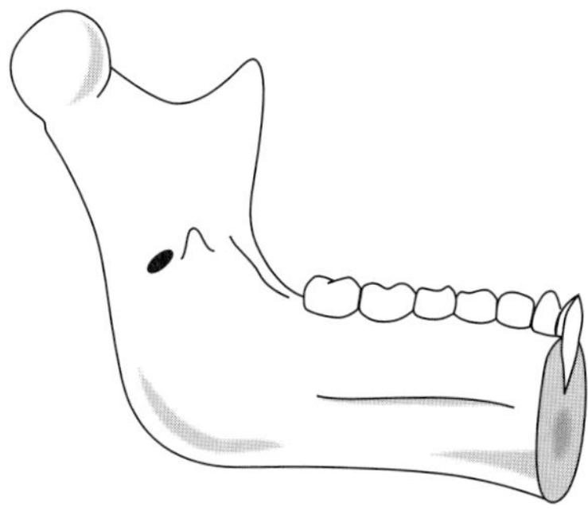

First, another foramen is seen—the **mandibular foramen.** It also carries a branch of V3.

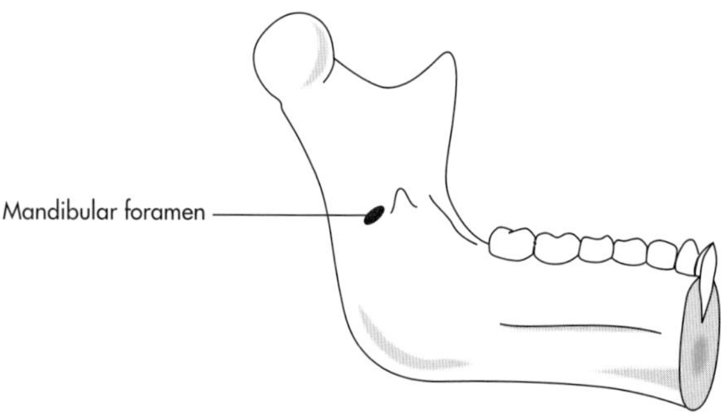

mandibular

Next to the mandibular foramen lies a small projection of bone called the **lingula.** It protects the nerve and vessels entering the ______________ foramen.

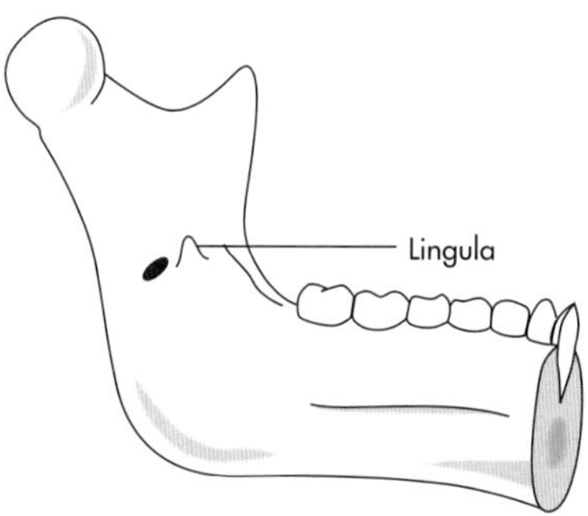

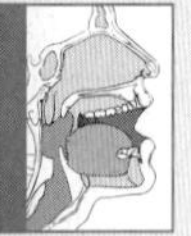

submandibular

A depression or fossa is found right above the angle of the interior mandible. It is the **submandibular fossa** and accommodates the ______________ salivary gland. Another more anterior fossa is the digastric fossa. Digastric muscle attaches here.

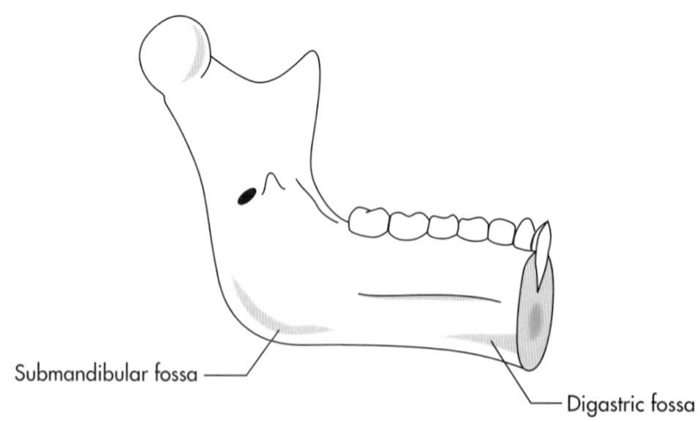

A horizontal ridge or line can be seen on the interior of the body of the mandible. This is the attachment site of a muscle that forms the floor of the mouth—the mylohyoid muscle. The line is called the **mylohyoid line.**

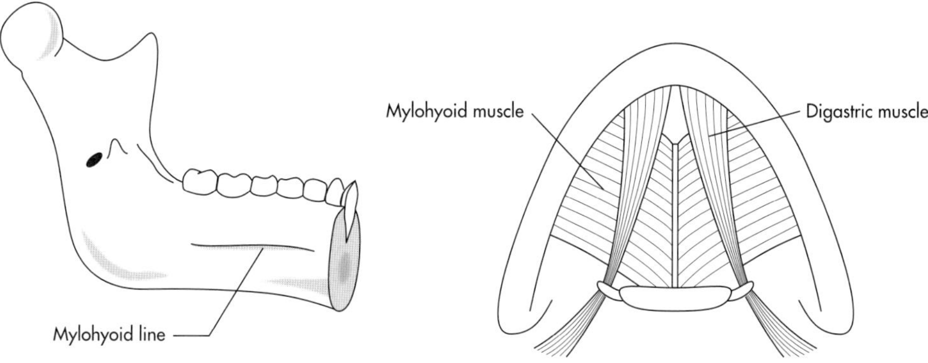

In the midline or interior "chin" area lie a pair of "bumps," which are also muscle attachment sites for the geniohyoid and genioglossus muscles. These processes are called the **genial tubercles.**

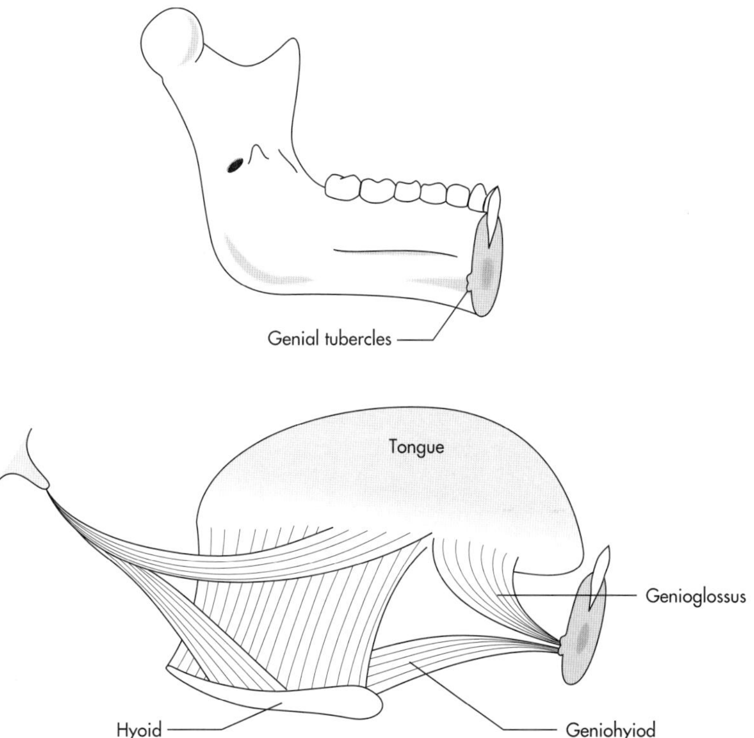

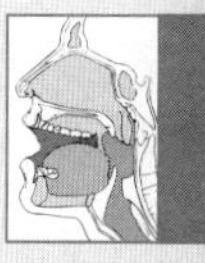

You can also see the attachment sites for the muscle of the cheek, the buccinator, on the mandible. Look at a line running first horizontal, then turning vertical parallel to the ramus. This is the **external oblique line.**

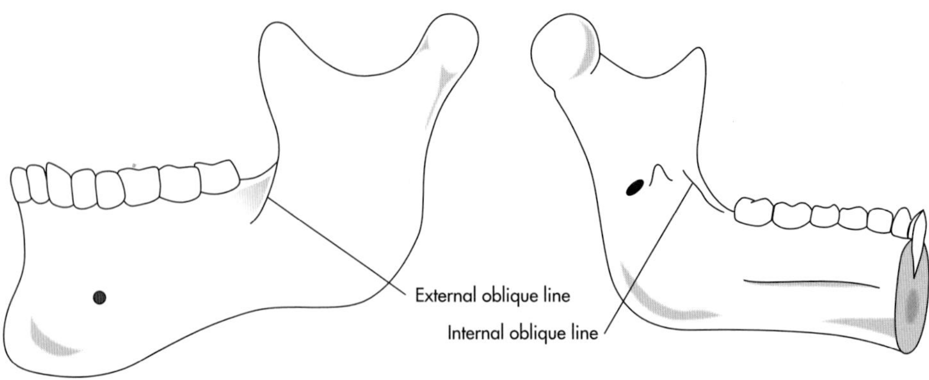

The external oblique line has a companion process on the interior of the mandible, parallel to it, called the **internal oblique line.** It provides attachment for a portion of the constrictor muscle. Both may be visible on x-rays of posterior mandibular teeth.

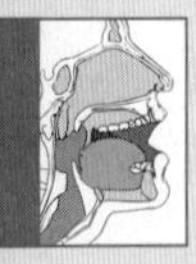

A. condyle
B. sigmoid notch
C. coronoid process
D. exterior oblique line
E. mental foramen
F. mental fossa
G. mandibular foramen
H. lingula
I. internal oblique line
J. mylohyoid line
K. genial tubercles
L. submandibular fossa

Review the structures found on the mandible, exterior and interior. Check back in the text to correct your answers.

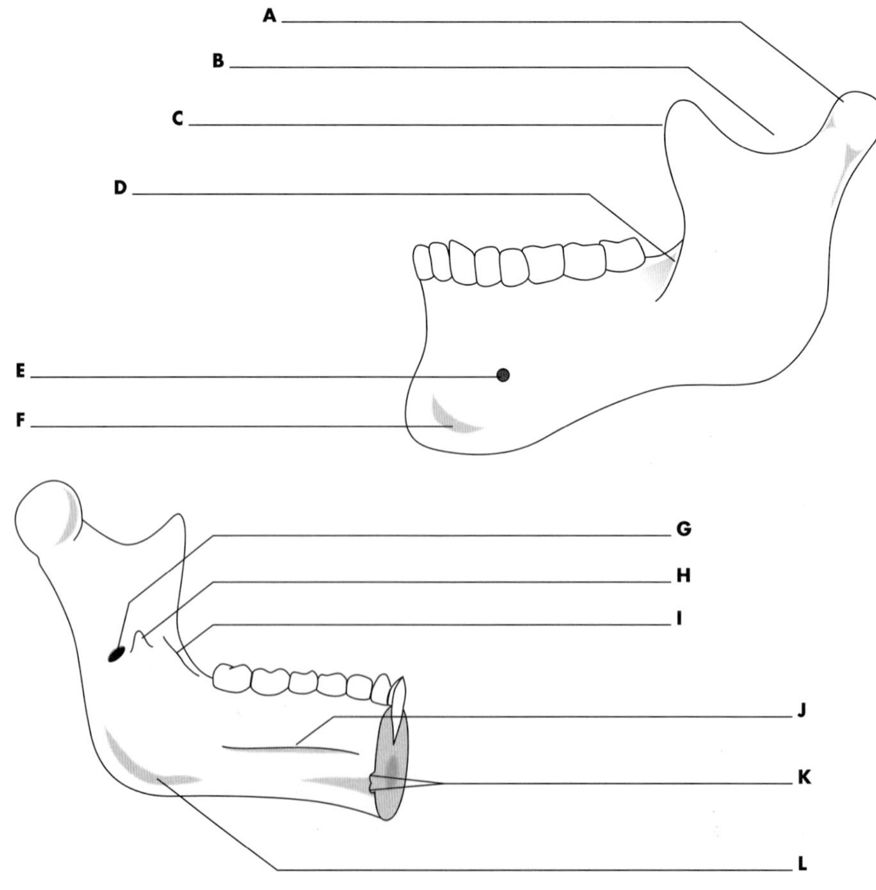

REVIEW TEST 7.1

SELECT OR FILL IN THE CORRECT ANSWER.

1. An anatomic term referring to the "belly side" of a body is
   a. posterior b. interior
   c. dorsal d. ventral
2. An anatomic term referring to the outside surface of a body is
   a. interior b. dorsal
   c. superficial d. ventral
3. The immobile joint between the two parietal joints is called a(n) ______________.
4. In the infant, there are two membranous areas between the cranial bones that will later fill in with bone. They are called ______________.
5. The C-1 vertebra is also called the ______________, and C-2 is called the ______________.
6. How many cervical vertebrae are there in the human neck?
7. The three cranial fossae found in the interior of the cranium are the ______________, the ______________, and the ______________ cranial fossae.
8. The single bone found alone in the anterior neck region is called the ______________ bone.

REVIEW TEST 7.2

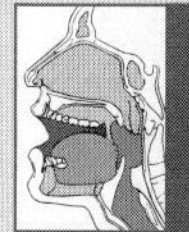

SELECT OR FILL IN THE CORRECT ANSWER.

1. Which pair of foramina are located above the eyesocket or on the "eyebrow" region?
2. The frontal bone in the interior cranial view surrounds another smaller "walnut-shaped" bone called the ______________ bone.
   a. sphenoid b. ethmoid
   c. vomer d. palatine
3. On the interior view of the top of the cranium, the two parietal bones meet in a suture. There is a sulcus or groove for a large vein there called the sigmoid sinus. True or false?
4. Which bone houses the ear?
   a. sphenoid b. parietal
   c. temporal d. occipital
5. What structure passes through the foramen magnum? Which bone contains foramen magnum?
6. The cranial depression that contains the pituitary gland is the ______________ fossa.
7. What pencil-shaped process occurs on the inferior portion of the temporal bone?

8. The TMJ is a joint between the temporal bone and the mandible and is capable of two different types of movement, gliding and hinge. True or false?

REVIEW TEST 7.3

SELECT OR FILL IN THE CORRECT ANSWER.

1. Which three bones constitute the zygomatic process?
2. The condyle of the TMJ doesn't articulate with the articular eminence, but rather with the mandibular fossa. True or false?
3. Nerves pass through the ______________ foramen to the back of the eyeball for vision.
4. What are the "eyesocket" areas of the cranium called?
5. Match the foramina with the branches of cranial nerve V:

a. foramen rotundum	V1
b. foramen ovale	V2
c. supraorbital fissure	V3

6. Of the two foramina found in the orbit, the round one is the optic foramen and the "crack" is the ______________ foramen.
7. Match the foramina with the branches of cranial nerve V:

a. infraorbital foramen	V1
b. supraorbital foramen	V2
c. mental foramen	V3

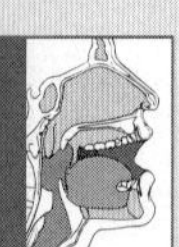

8. The palate is comprised of which two bones?

REVIEW TEST 7.4

SELECT OR FILL IN THE CORRECT ANSWER.

1. Two hook-shaped processes found posterior to the hard palate are called the ______________.
2. Four wing-shaped processes that are inferior and posterior to the palate and are part of the sphenoid bone are called the ______________.
3. The flat processes on the mandible that are the sites of muscle attachment for the temporalis muscle are called the ______________ processes.
4. Major veins exit the brain through the ______________ foramina, and major arteries enter the brain through the ______________ canals.
5. A depression for the ______________ salivary gland is found on the interior of the mandible, in the region of the angle.
6. The ______________ portion of the mandible houses the teeth.

7. Which muscle attaches from one side to the other of the interior mandible?
   a. geniohyoid
   b. mylohyoid
   c. genioglossus
   d. temporalis

8. There are 13 cranial bones. True or false?

REVIEW TEST 7.5

LABEL THE DRAWINGS.

1.

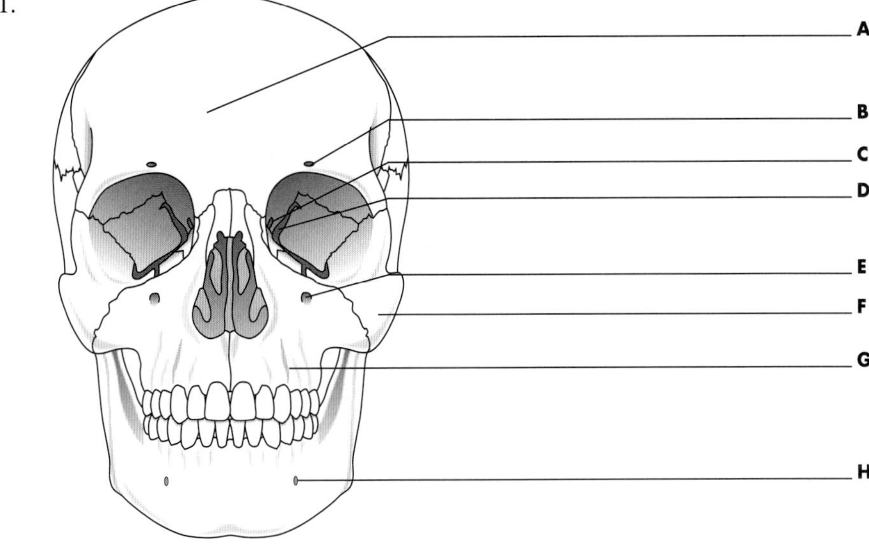

2.

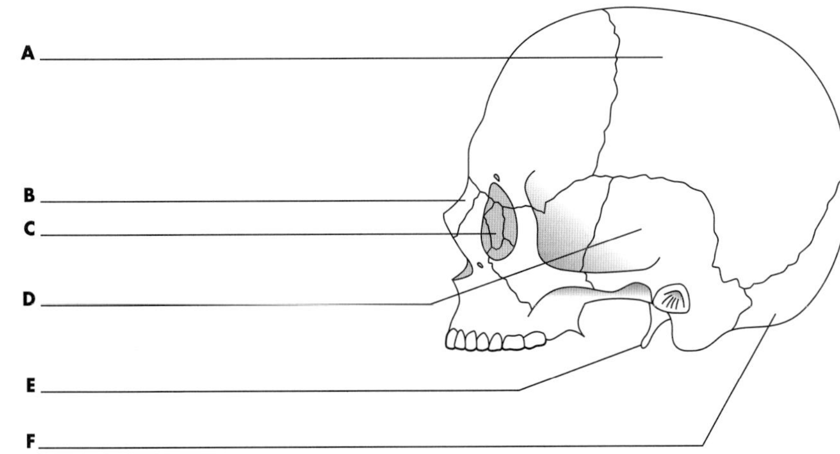

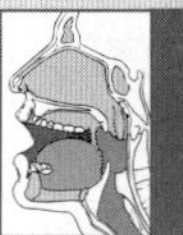

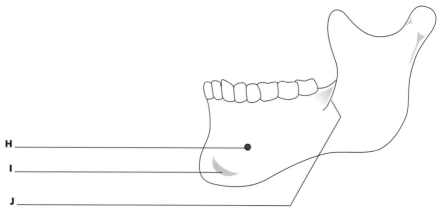

3.

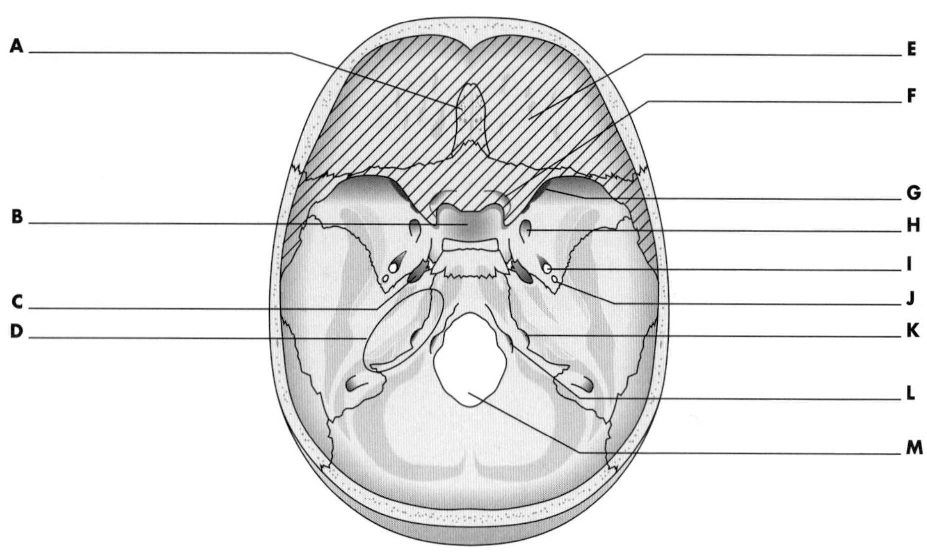

4.

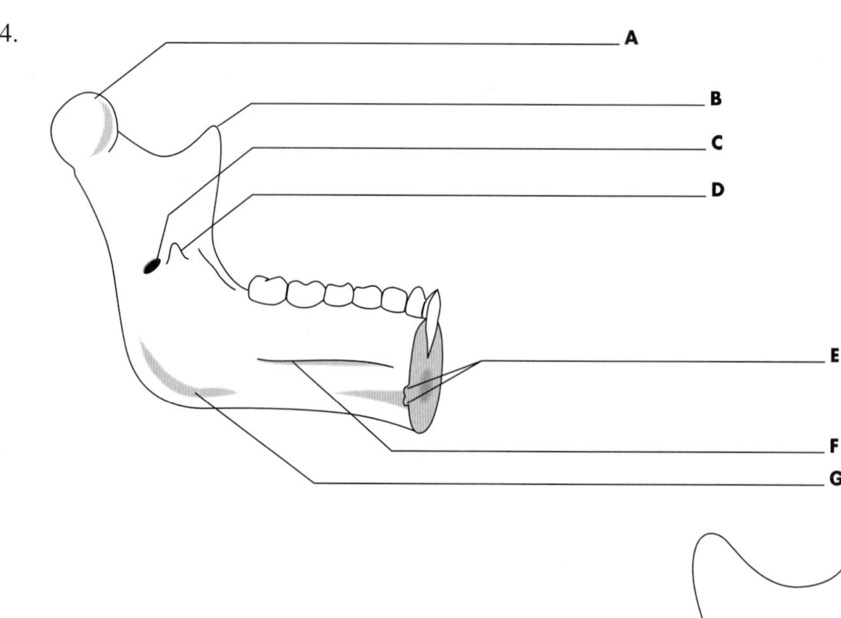

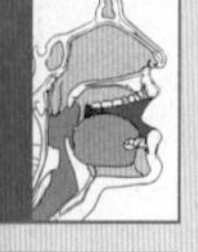

5.

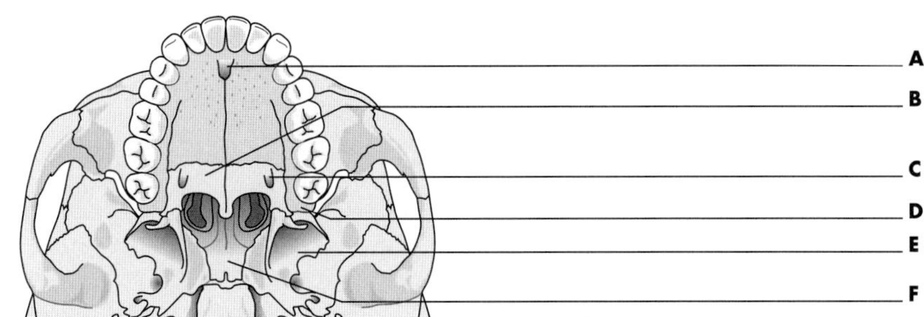

6.

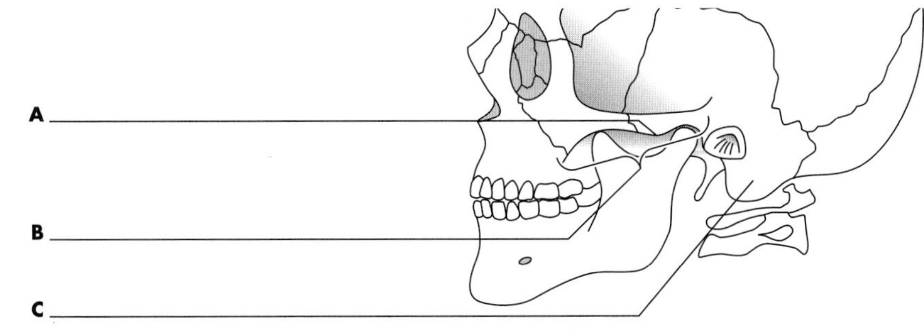

7.

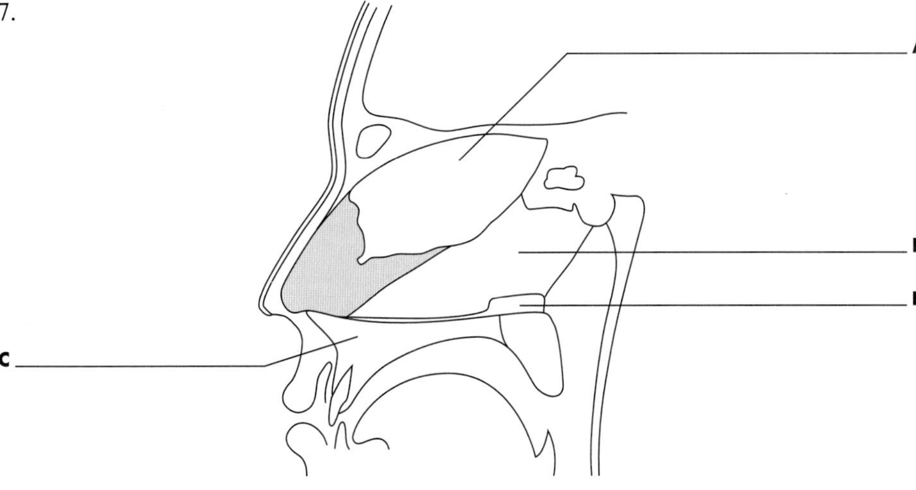

8.

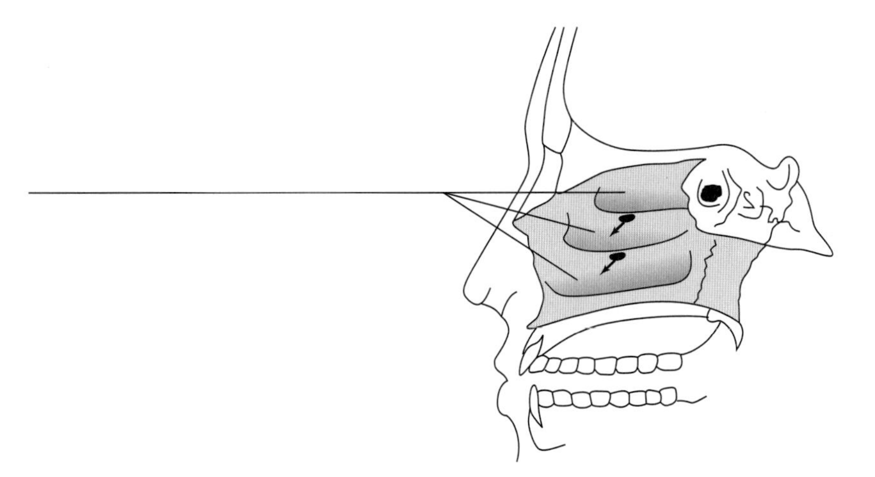

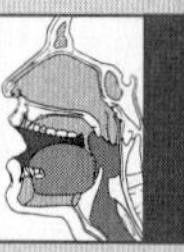

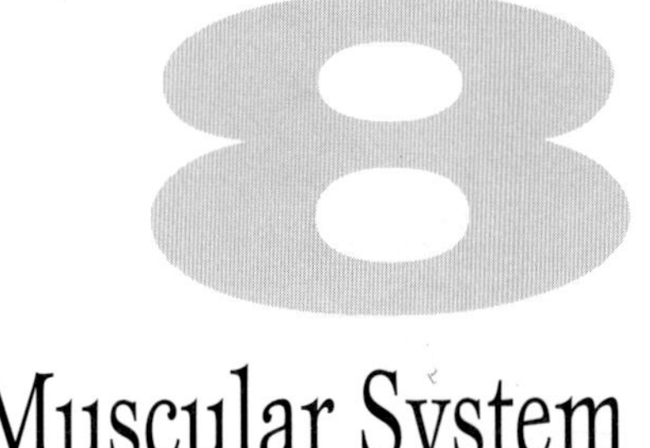

Muscular System

If the primary function of the skeletal system is support, then that of the muscular system is movement. The muscular system consists of the skeletal muscles and their surrounding and attaching tissues.

Muscle, as we saw in Chapter One, is a tissue that produces movement by **contraction.** Contraction makes a muscle grow shorter and produces work, usually, by movement. Contraction occurs when the protein filaments within muscle are caused to slide inward past each other. Contraction is initiated by a neuronal signal.

Contraction makes a muscle grow ______________ (shorter/longer).

shorter

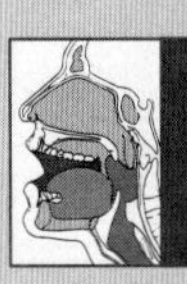

Although there are three types of muscle and they all function in a similar way, we will be speaking only of skeletal muscle. See Chapter One for a picture. Skeletal muscle has long striated fibers, gathered into large bundles running in the same direction. A muscle, as we will describe in the head and neck, is one of these discrete bundles, invested in connective tissue, and having a specific **action.** A single muscle is pictured here.

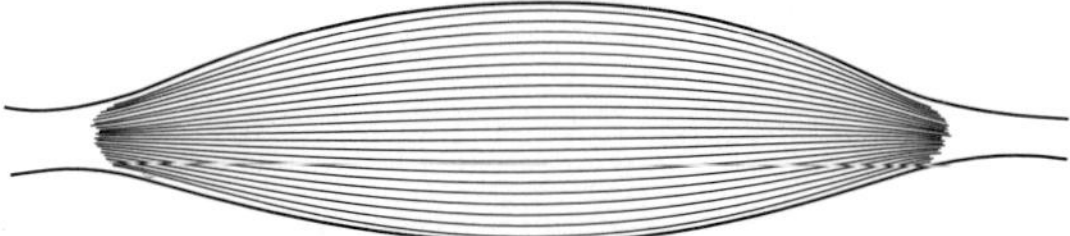

Skeletal muscle works by (1) being attached at two separate points and (2) contracting, thus moving the two points closer together. Which of the muscles has contracted?

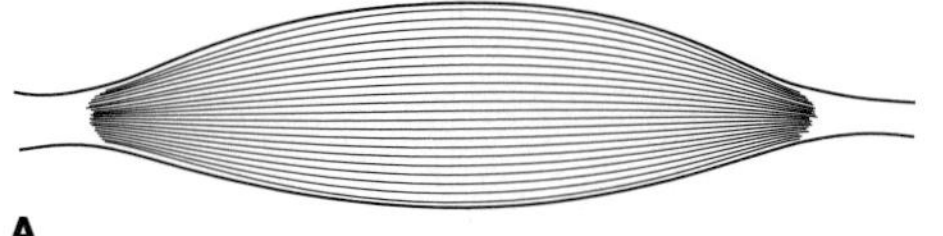

A

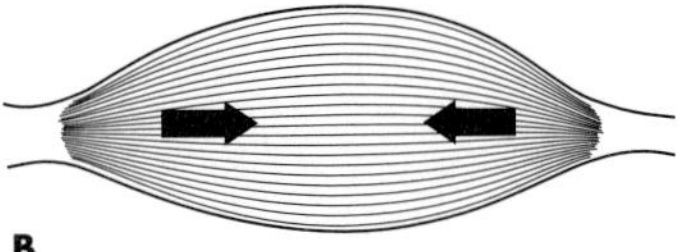

B

B. The bone on the right moved.

If you said B, you are correct. The muscles are attached to bones by connective tissue called **tendons.** Which muscle has contracted? What happens?

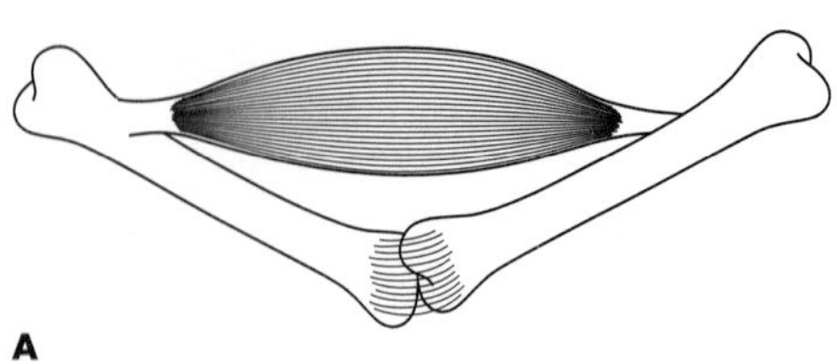

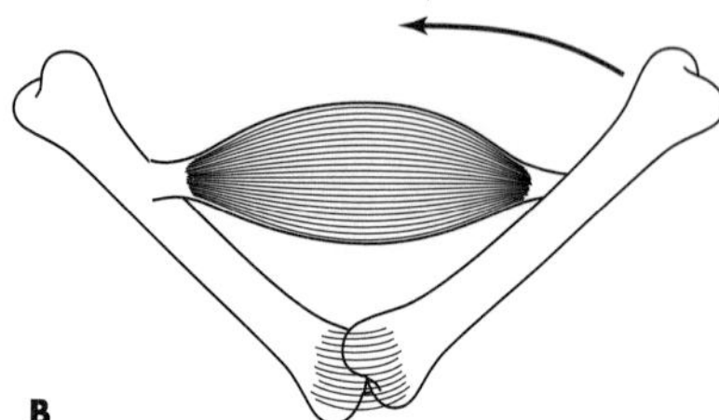

Again, in B, a muscle has contracted and the bone has moved. The attachment site in A, which remained stationary, is called the **origin** of the muscle.

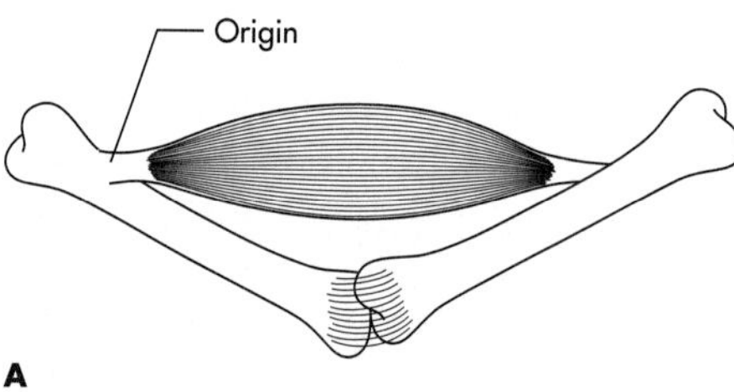

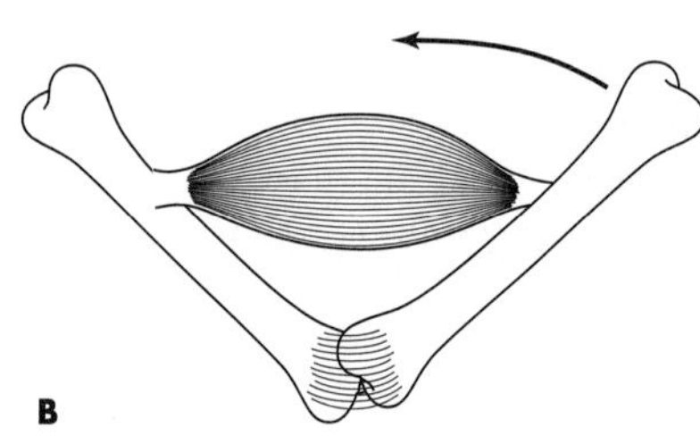

origin

The stationary attachment of the muscle is called the ______________ and the attachment that moves is called the **insertion.**

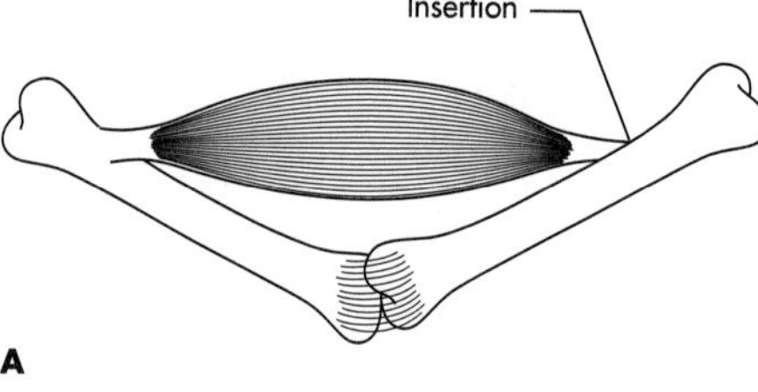

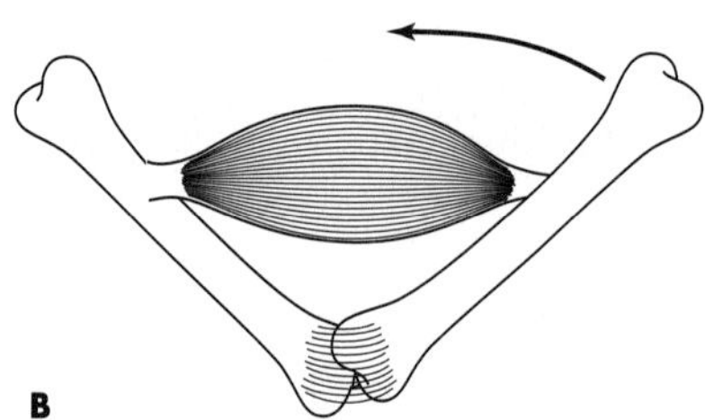

A. insertion
B. origin

Label which end of the muscle is its origin and which is its insertion.

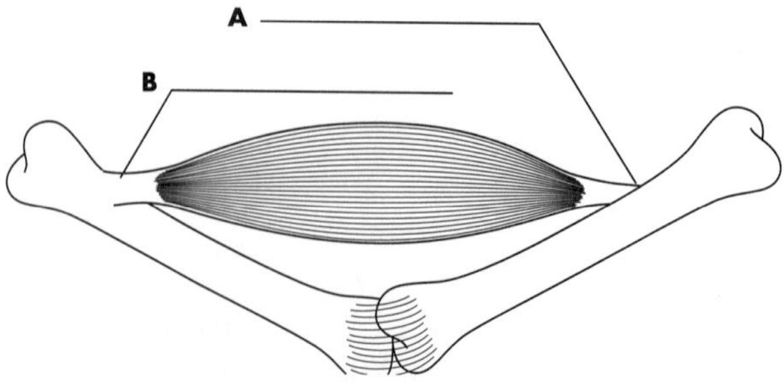

Find on the drawing the dense regular connective tissue that attaches muscle to bone; it is called ________. Also pictured is the dense regular connective tissue that attaches bone to bone; this is called ________. Where two bones come together is called a **joint.**

tendon, ligament

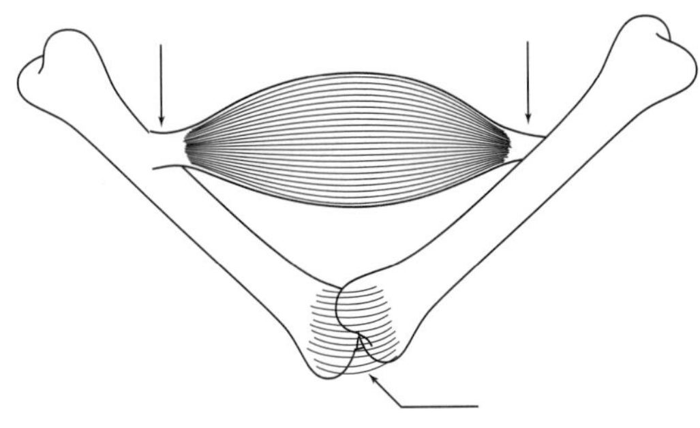

Ligaments are difficult to distinguish from the other connective tissue that surround a joint. This tissue is the **joint capsule** and it is often filled with **synovial fluid.** The bones may have cartilage coverings or pads of tissue between them for protection during motion. What are the four types of joints found in the head and neck? (See Chapter Seven.)

1. suture—cranium
2,3. gliding and hinge—TMJ
2,4. gliding and rotation—cervical vertebrae

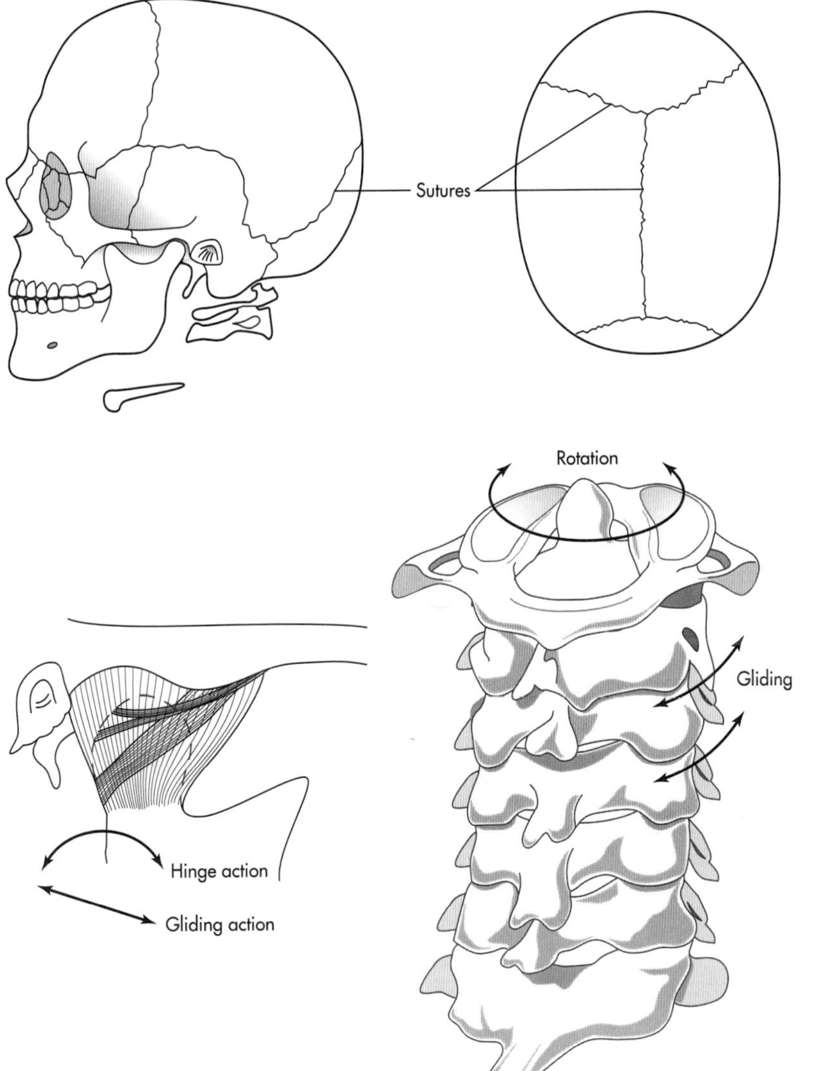

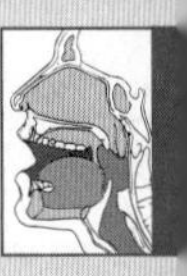

Contracting muscles cause movements or actions about a joint (except for suture joints).

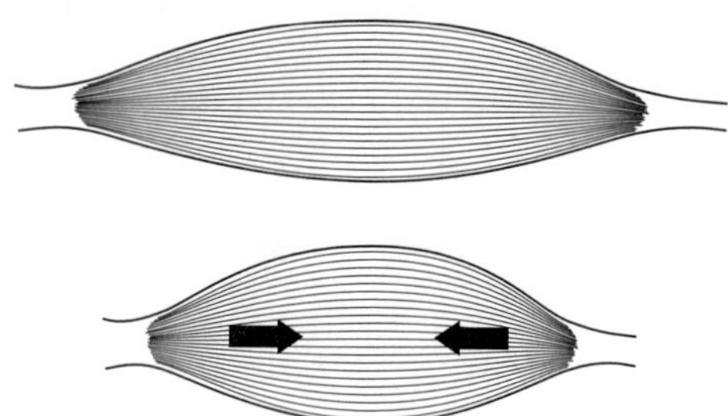

We do have some muscles in the head and neck that attach to skin instead of bone, causing the skin to move.

Particular branches of nerves are associated with particular muscles. We say that such and such nerve innervates such and such muscle. This is a muscle's **innervation.**

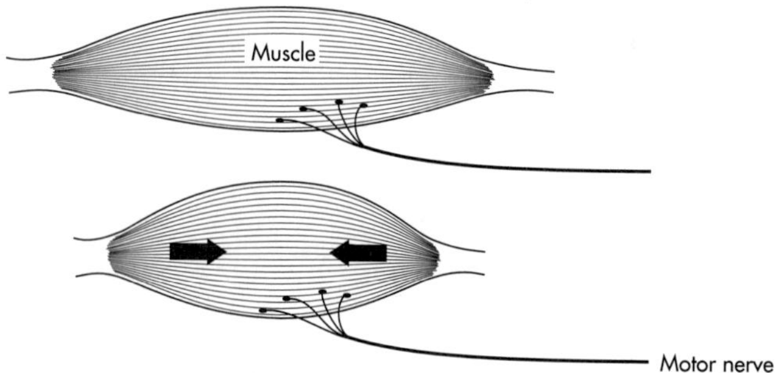

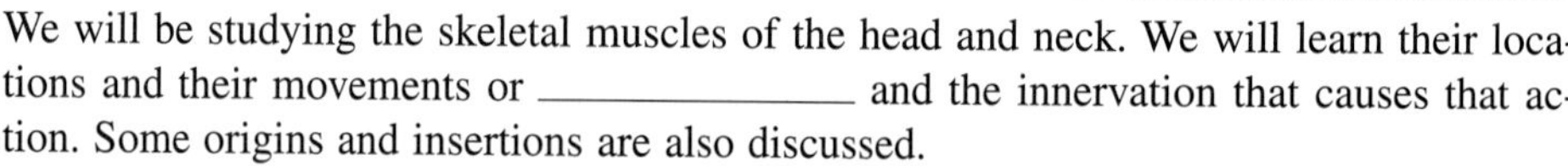

actions

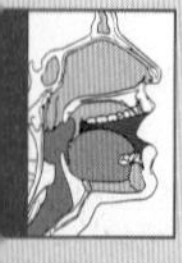

We will be studying the skeletal muscles of the head and neck. We will learn their locations and their movements or ______________ and the innervation that causes that action. Some origins and insertions are also discussed.

Muscles with similar actions are often grouped together. They often have similar innervations. The first group we look at involves the most superficial muscles of the face.

1.0 MUSCLES OF FACIAL EXPRESSION

facial expressions

This group of muscles, as hinted by its name, is responsible for the wide variety of human facial expressions, an important part of communication. They insert for the most part below the skin, causing these actions. The actions of the muscles of facial expression are ______________.

The **muscles of facial expression** are all innervated by cranial nerve (CN) VII (seven), the facial nerve. These are superficial (on the outer surface) muscles of the face and are shown with the facial nerve.

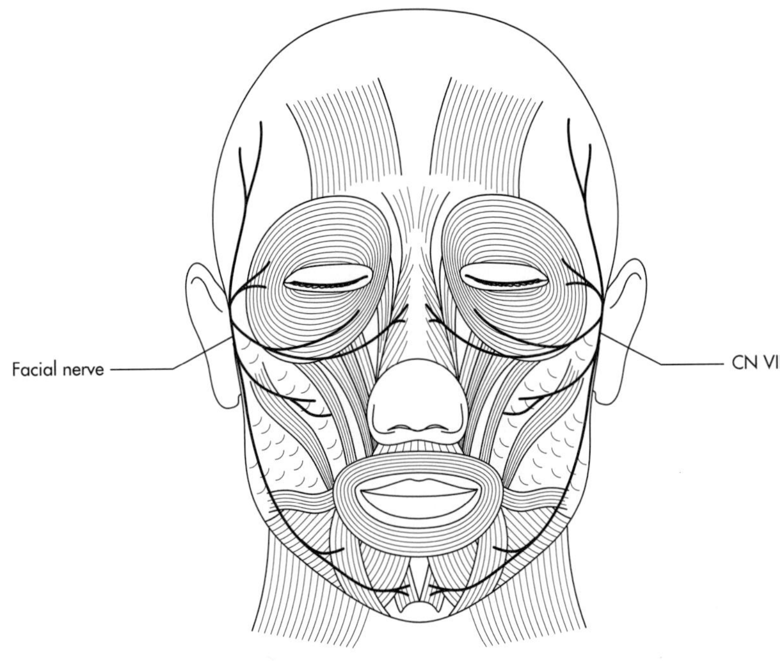

The first pair of muscles of the group are the **frontalis muscles.** They act on the skin of the forehead and eyebrows. (As you locate muscles in the drawings, you may color them in to help you learn their locations.)

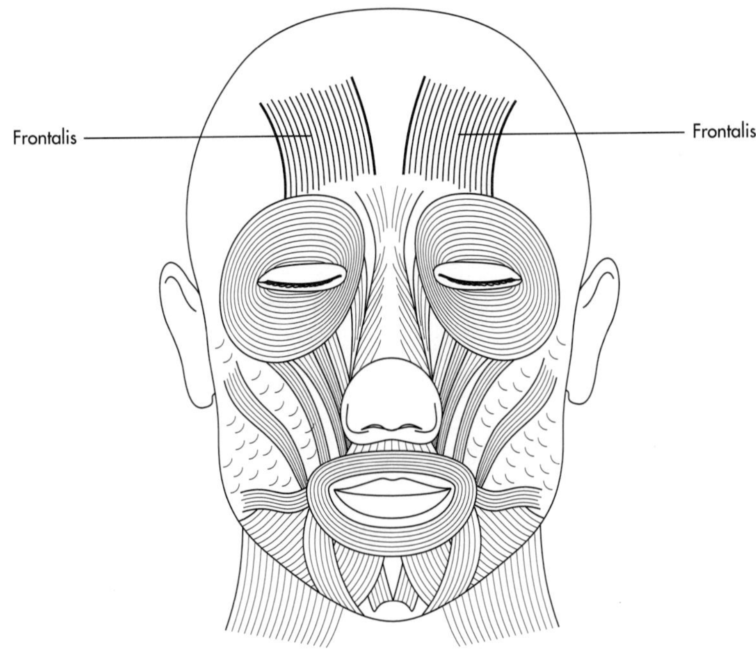

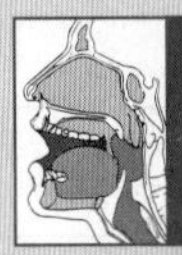

Inferior to frontalis are two circular muscles around the eyes. Each is called **orbicularis oculi** and they aid in closing the eye. Find them in the drawing.

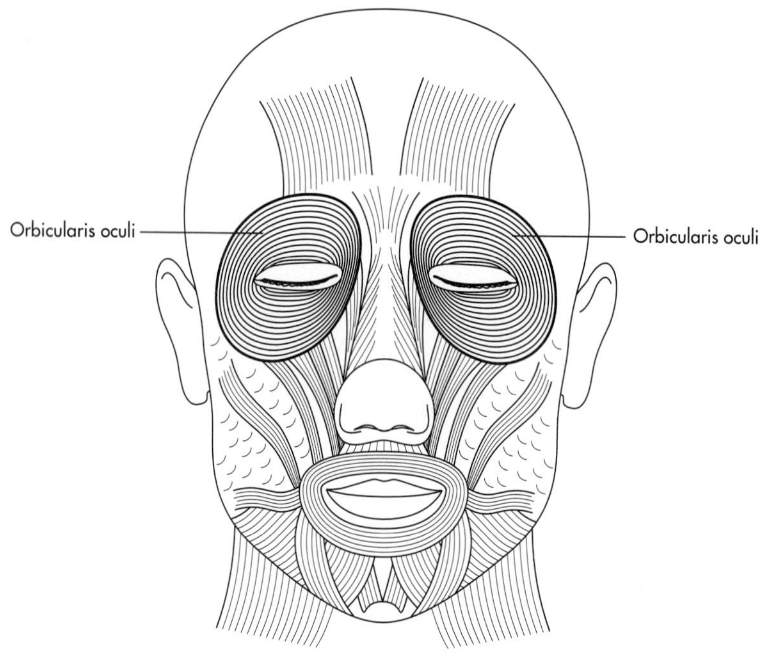

On the midline of the nose and spreading down laterally are the **nasalis muscles,** which wriggle or flare the nose. Find them.

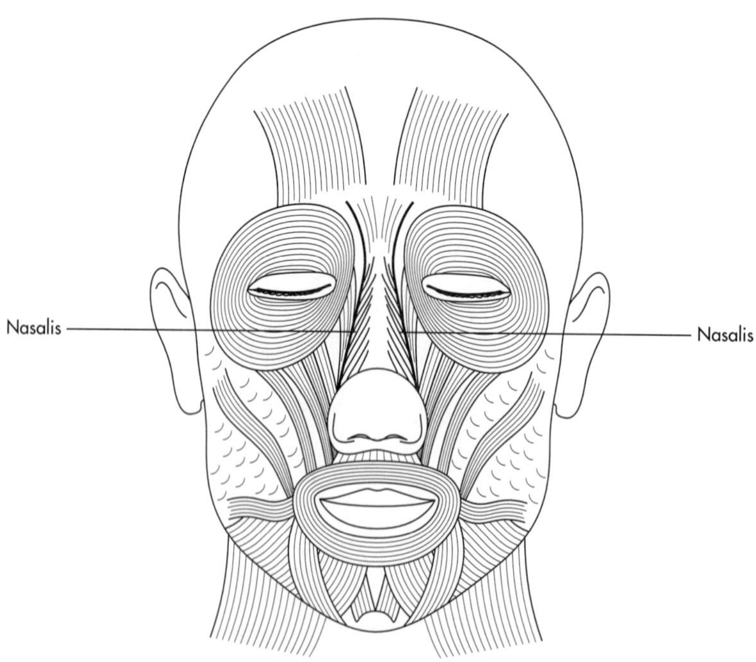

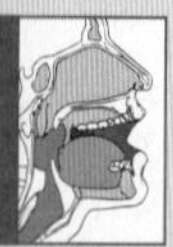

Surrounding the mouth and creating much of the bulk of the lip is the other circular muscle, **orbicularis oris.** When it contracts, the lips purse together. As you can see from the drawing, many different muscles insert into orbicularis oris.

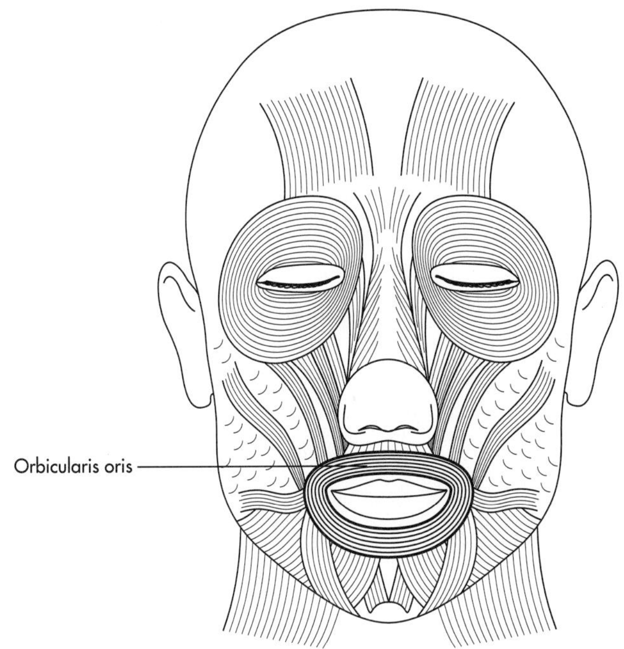

On the drawing, find frontalis, nasalis, orbicularis oculi, and orbicularis oris.

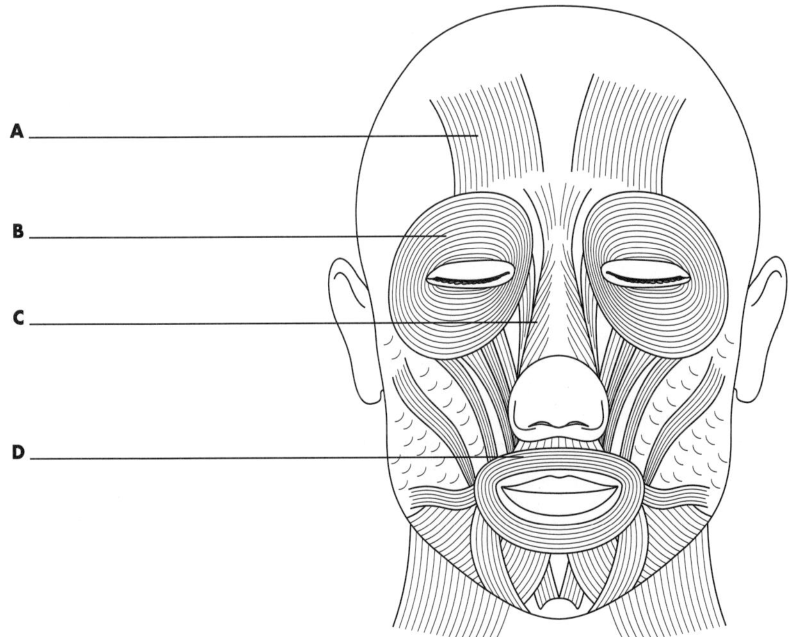

A. frontalis
B. orbicularis oculi
C. nasalis
D. orbicularis oris

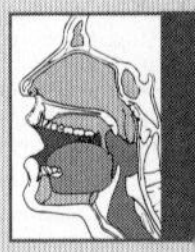

A. frontalis
B. orbicularis oculi
C. nasalis
D. orbicularis oris

Now look at the sagittal section and find the same muscles.

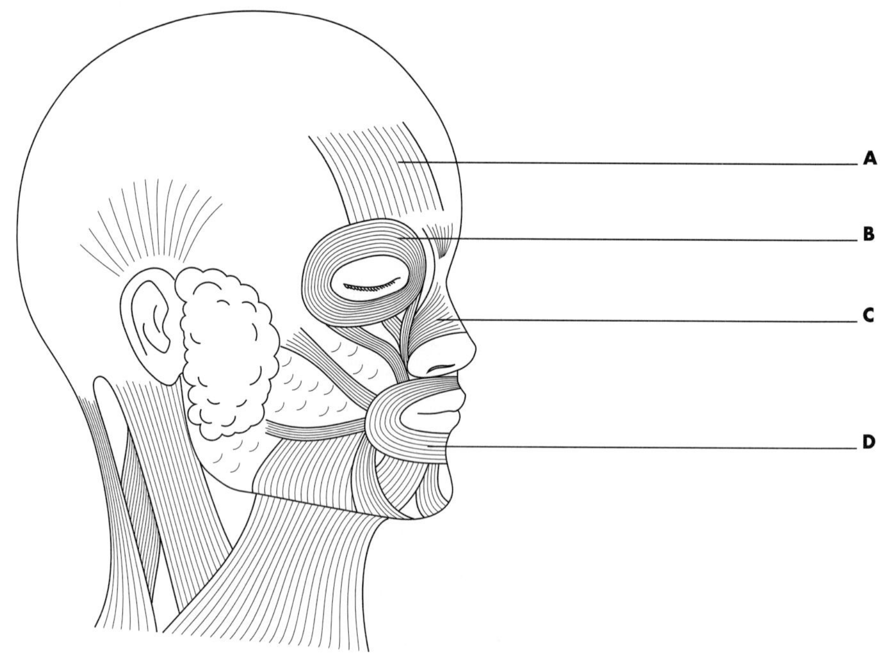

They would raise the lip where attached.

Many muscles insert into orbicularis oris from above and below, and are responsible for the many actions on the lips. Those muscles inserting from a superior aspect belong to a subgroup called the **levators** of the lip. We will not learn each separate muscle. Find them. Imagine that their fibers are drawn shorter. What kind of action would the levators have on the lips?

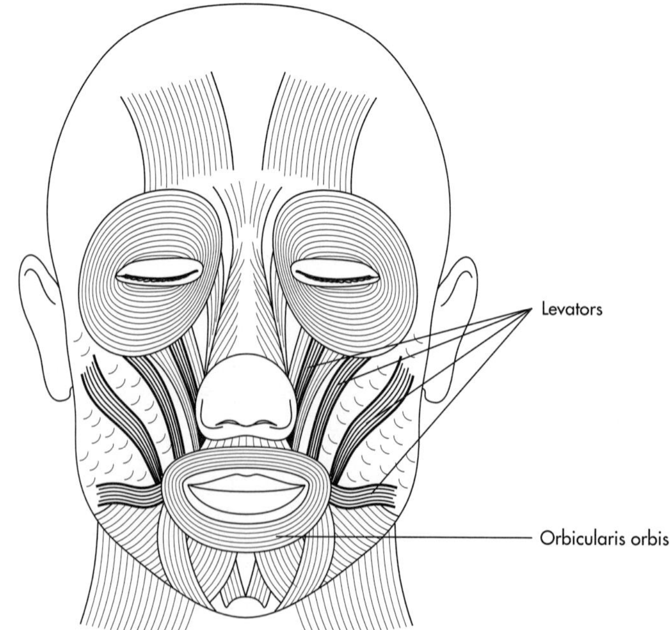

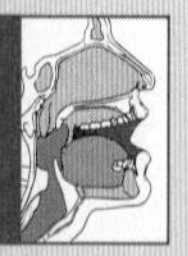

Find the levators from the sagittal view.

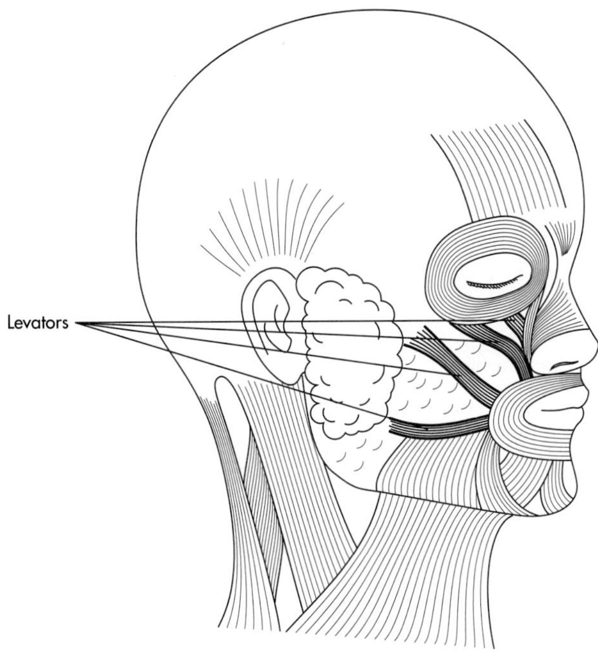

Opposite the levators are the **depressor muscles** of the lip. Find them on the drawing. What would their action be?

to lower or depress the lip where attached

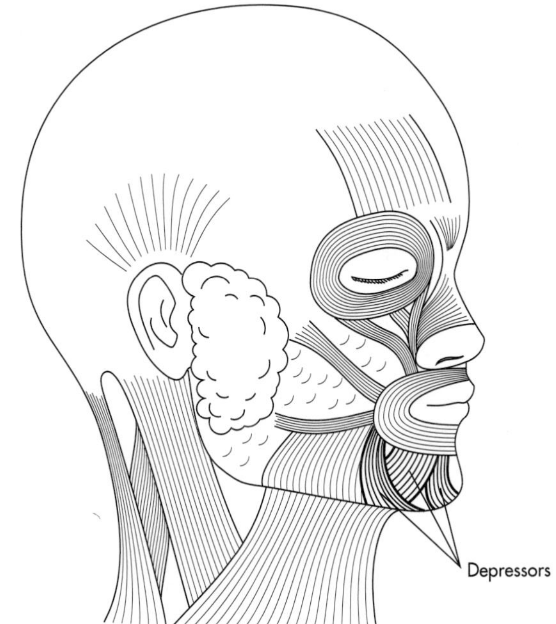

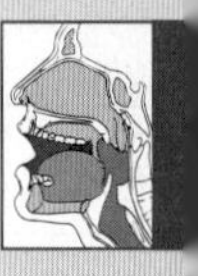

The wide variation of depressor and levator actions helps create facial expressions ranging from frowns to smiles.

The middlemost pair of depressor muscles are called the **mentalis muscles.** Find them on the drawing. These originate in the **mental fossae** and insert into the lower lip. When active they produce a pout. This muscle pair is strong enough in some people to create pressure on the lower anterior teeth. Also find the levators and depressor muscles on the drawing.

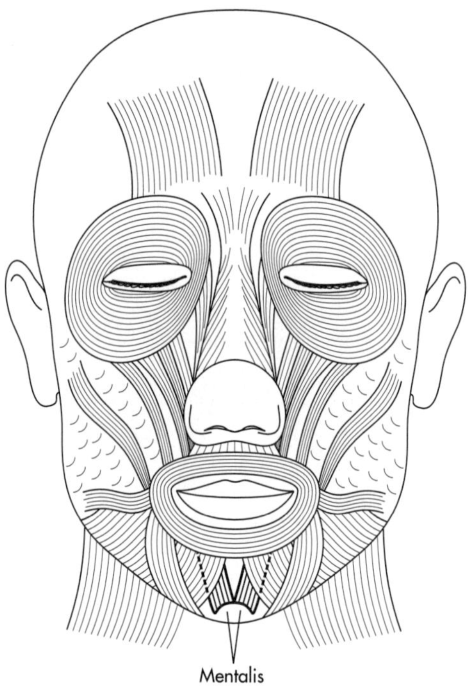

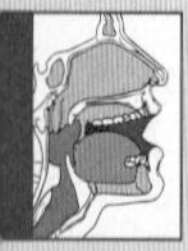

Inferior to the mouth and beginning all about the lower border of the chin (mandible) is **platysma muscle.** This muscle is often absent on anatomic drawings because it is so thin and lies almost entirely in the subcutaneous layer. Thus, it is frequently peeled off during dissections. Find platysma in the drawing.

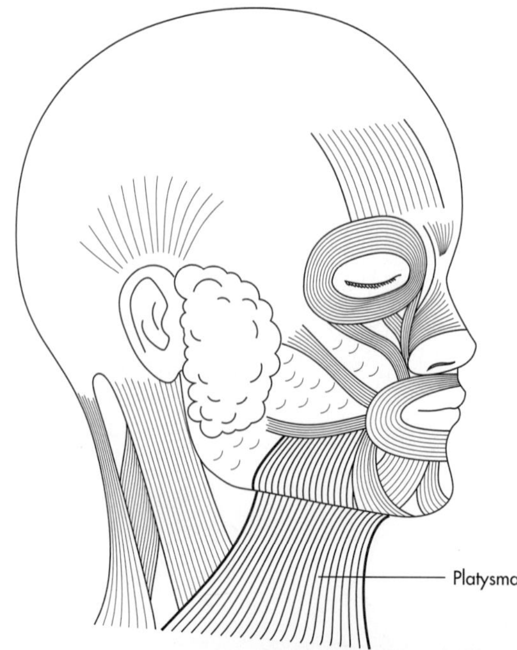

_______________, when contracted, pulls down the corners of the mouth in a grimace.

Platysma

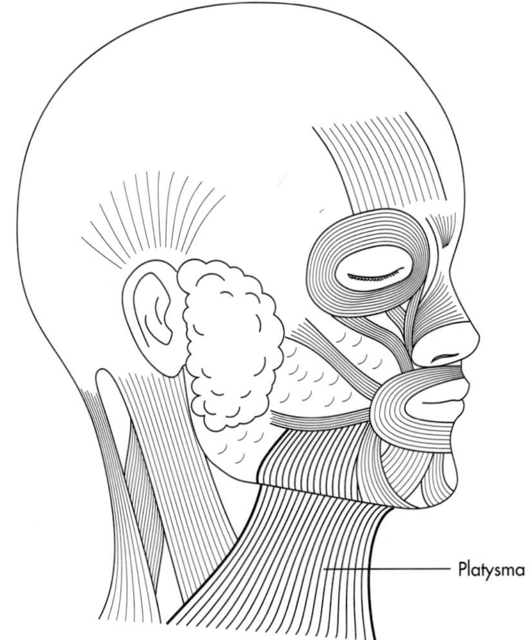

With their insertions into the skin of the face, that is, eyebrows, eyes, nose, and mouth, the muscles of facial expression are aptly named. Communication of emotions such as fear, rage, sadness, and joy were important to our primitive ancestors and primates before the development of language, and they remain so to us. Which nerve activates this muscle group?

CN VII (facial nerve)

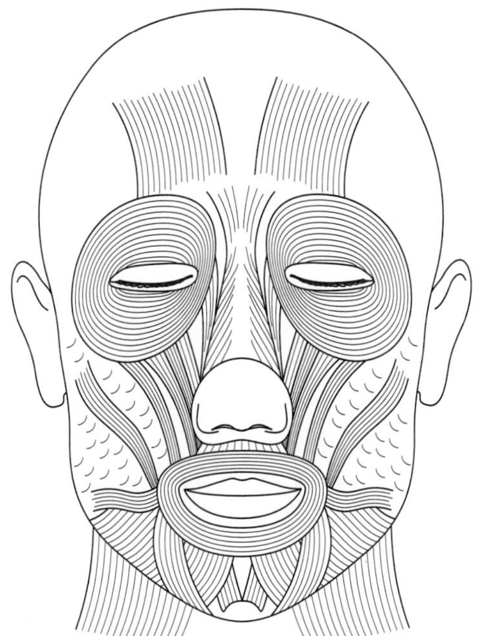

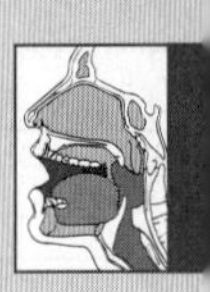

When the skin is removed during dissection, the specimen appears much like the drawing. The drawing after it has fat tissue removed and a few facial expression muscles. The area between the ear and mouth (cheek) has what appears to be fatty tissue. A closer look reveals both fat **(buccal fat pad)** and glandular tissue **(parotid gland).**

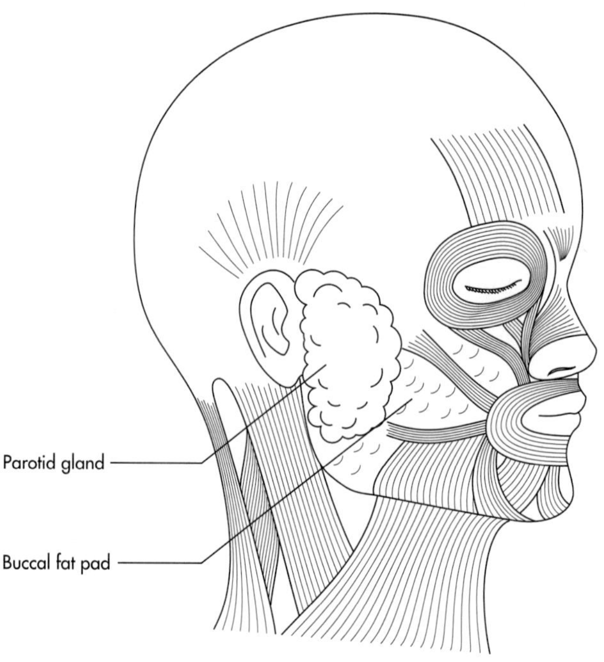

Stensen's duct

In this drawing, the buccal fat pad is removed and only the parotid gland remains. A duct leaves the parotid gland horizontally and appears to pierce the muscle in front of it. What duct is this?

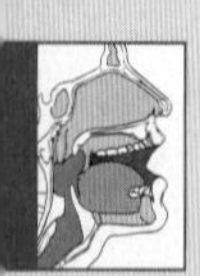

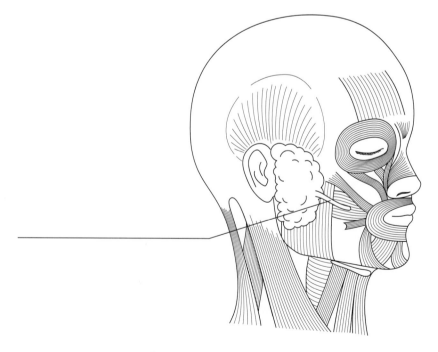

The muscle with horizontal fibers that runs from orbicularis oris back to the ramus of the mandible, below the parotid gland, is called the **buccinator muscle,** and it is the last of the facial expression muscles. Find it on the drawing.

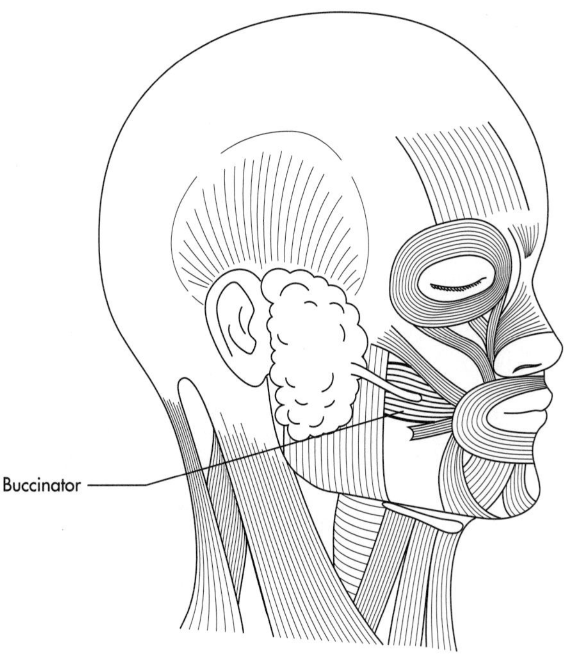

With the parotid gland removed you can better see the buccinator. This is the main muscle of the cheek, and the word *buccal* means "cheek." When this muscle contracts it draws the cheeks inward. This is an important action during chewing and swallowing (mastication and deglutition), centering the food in the mouth. Is this a facial expression-type action?

no

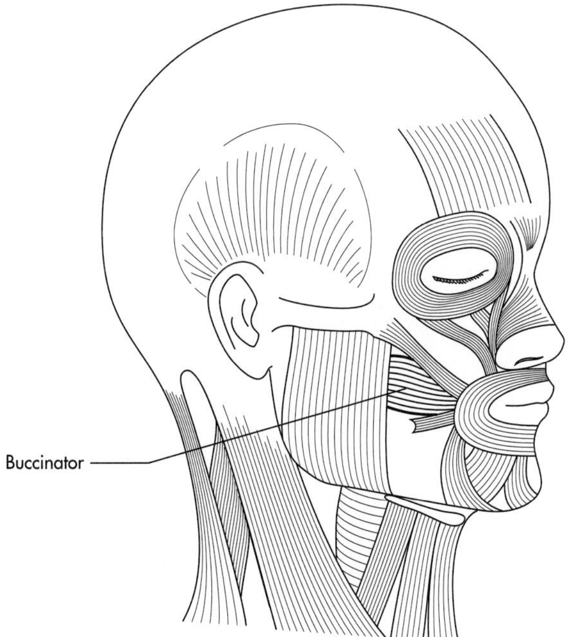

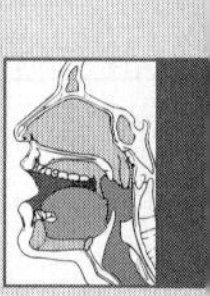

CN VII, facial nerve

The buccinator differs in action from the other facial expression muscles, but it is innervated by the same cranial nerve, which is ______________.

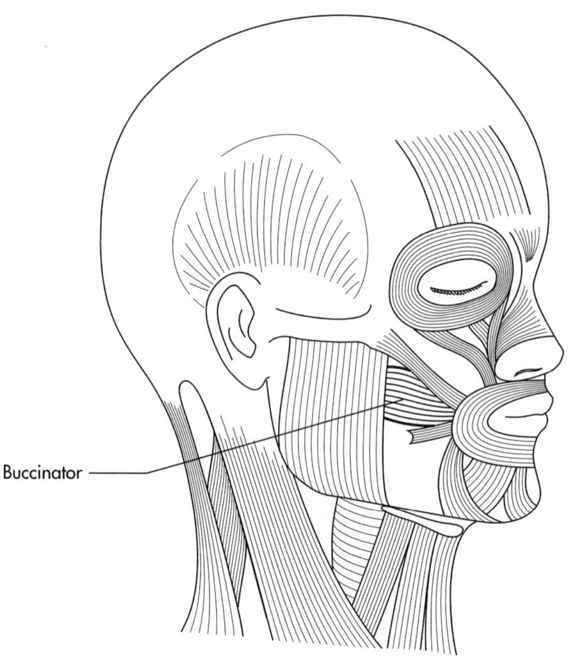

muscles of facial expression

The **facial nerve** (CN VII) is shown in the diagram. It is found directly beneath the skin also, exiting the brain below the ear and then spreading across the face to innervate which muscles?

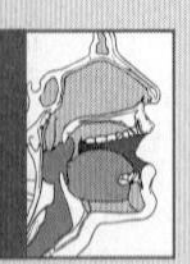

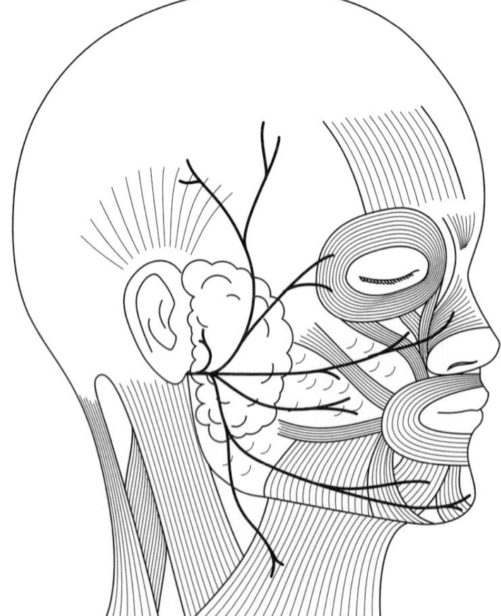

Label the muscles in these diagrams. List the actions they have next to the muscle.

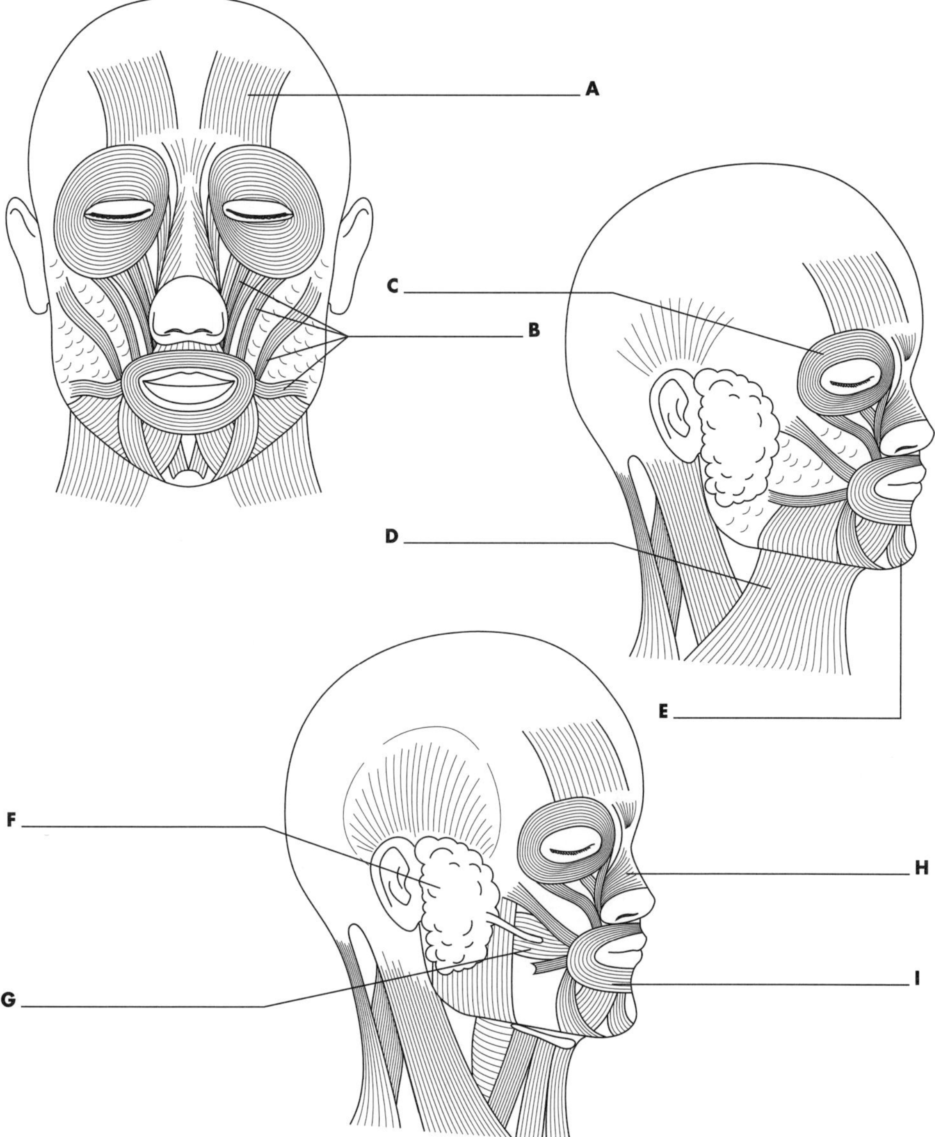

A. frontalis
B. levators
C. orbicularis oculi
D. platysma
E. mentalis
F. parotid
G. buccinator
H. nasalis
I. orbicularis oris

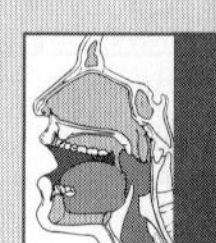

MUSCLES OF MASTICATION 2.0

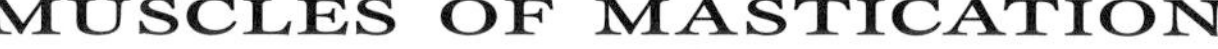

Mastication is the process of breaking food down into smaller and smaller pieces by repetitive occlusion of the maxillary and mandibular teeth. This is accomplished by moving the mandible by way of the muscles attached to it. The mandible, not the maxilla, is the moving bone, and it must be elevated, depressed, and moved laterally (side to side). The **muscles of mastication** are the primary movers of the mandible, with the exception of depression.

The muscles of mastication, then, insert onto the mandible and are located deeper than the facial muscles. In the drawings here, most of the facial expression muscles are removed, to see the muscles of mastication.

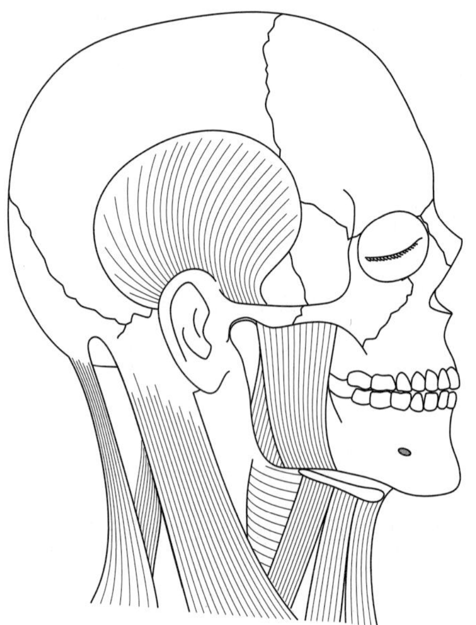

elevation and lateral movement of mandible

The muscles of mastication constitute four pairs and are innervated by CN V, the **trigeminal nerve** (mandibular or third division). What is the major action of the muscles of mastication?

CN V, the trigeminal nerve

There are four pairs of masticatory muscles. We look now at the origin, insertion, and action of each pair of muscles. What is their innervation?

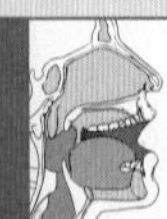

mandible

Remember that the masticatory muscles move the mandible so all four muscles must insert onto the ________________.

The diagram is of the first masticatory muscle, the **temporalis** muscle, from the right side. The origin of temporalis is on the temporal fossa, shown on the skull. Find them.

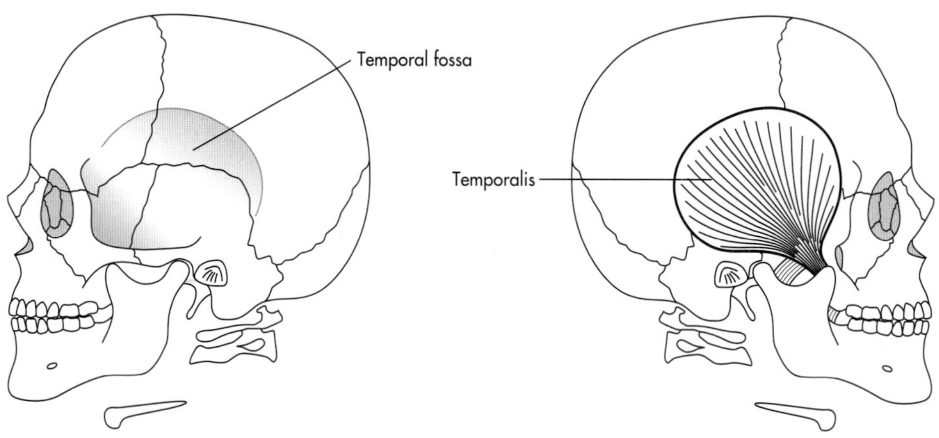

The fibers of temporalis originate on the _______________, come together, and pass inferiorly through the infratemporal fossa directly behind the zygomatic process, which has been cut away.

temporal fossa

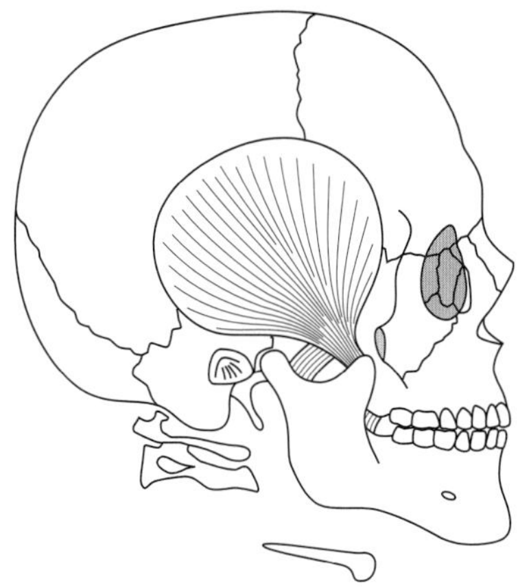

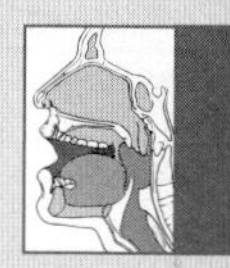

The temporalis muscle then inserts onto the flat process on the ramus of the mandible known as the _______________ process. Find it.

coronoid

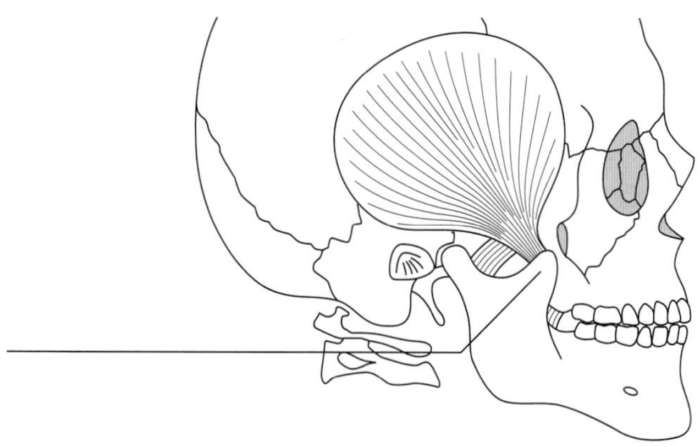

The mandible is elevated.

If you imagine the fibers of the temporalis muscle shorter, you can figure out its action. What happens to the mandible as the fibers grow shorter?

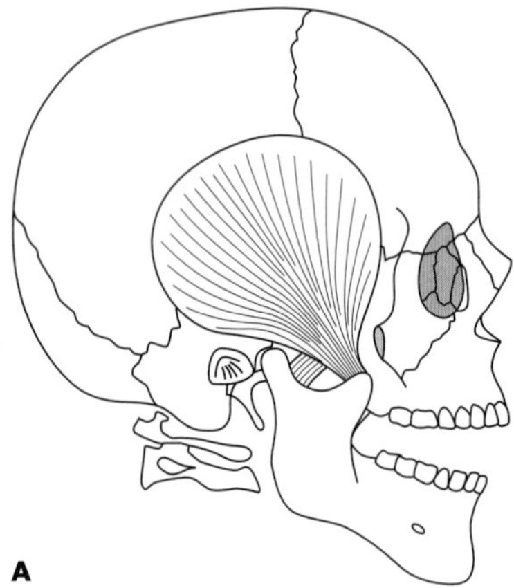

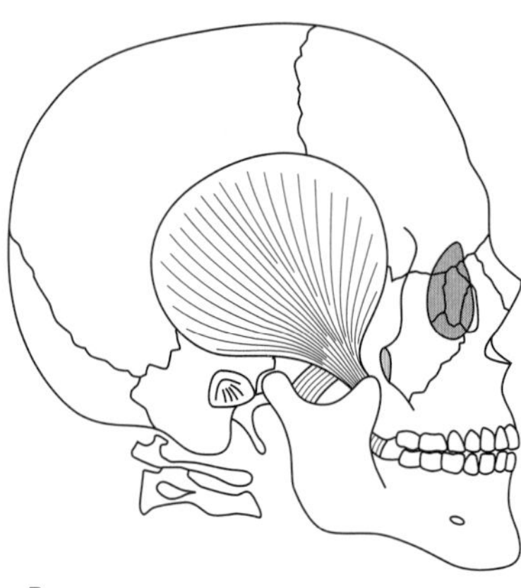

diagram B

The mandible is lifted up or **elevated.** This is also called closing the mandible. In which diagram has the temporalis contracted?

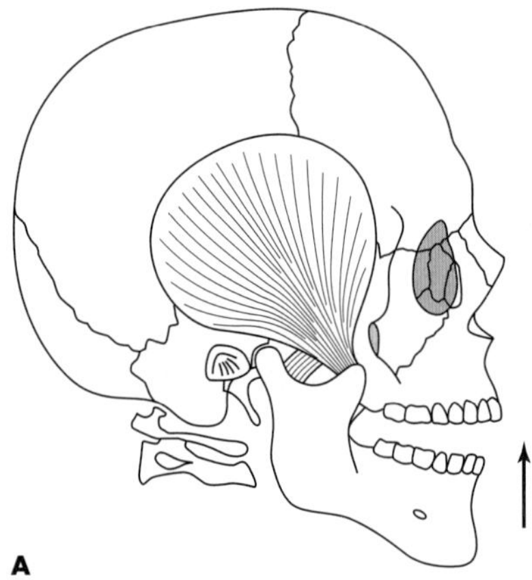

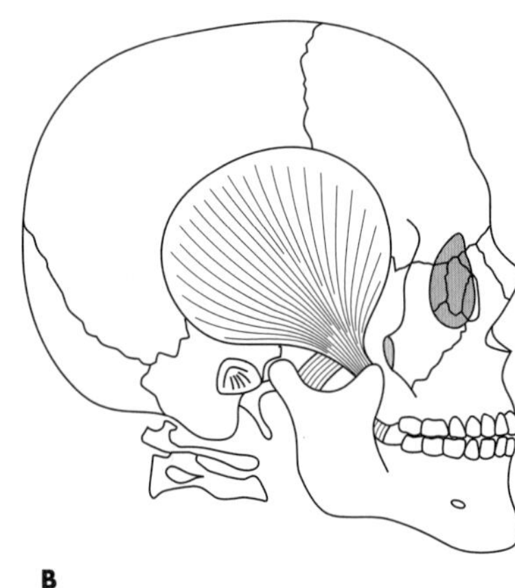

CN V, the trigeminal nerve (third division)

Contraction of temporalis is caused by a branch of which nerve?

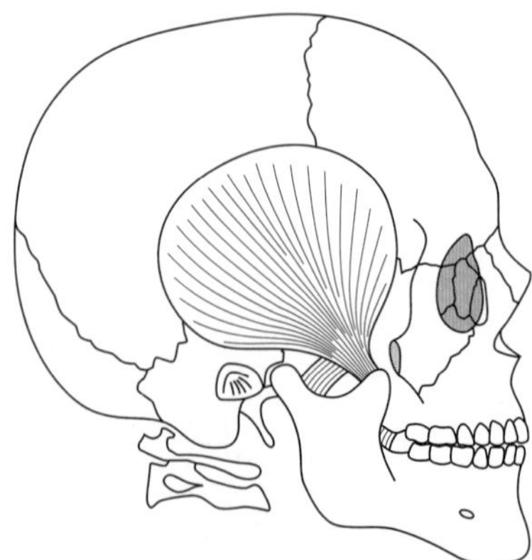

Let's review: The arrow is pointing to which muscle? What is its origin? Insertion? Action? Innervation? Check your answers in the following diagrams, and in the section below.

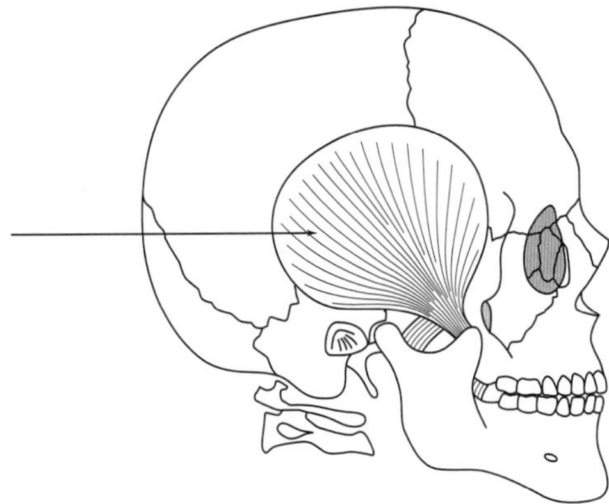

This is the temporalis. Its origin is on the temporal fossa. It inserts into the coronoid process. Its action is elevation of the mandible and it is innervated by the trigeminal nerve, third division.

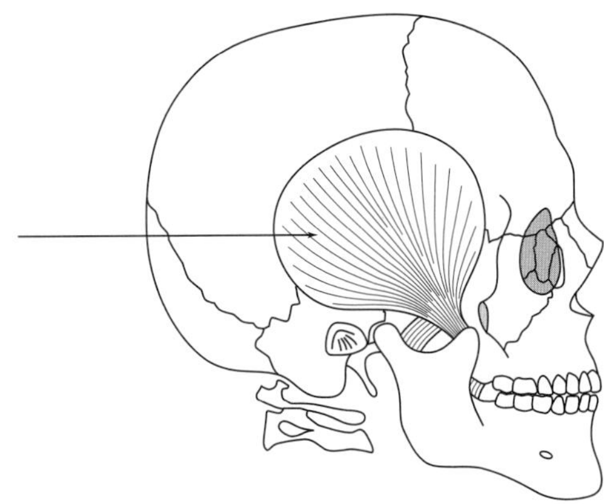

The next masticatory muscle pair is called the masseter. The **masseter** muscle is indicated on the diagram. Find it. You may color it in.

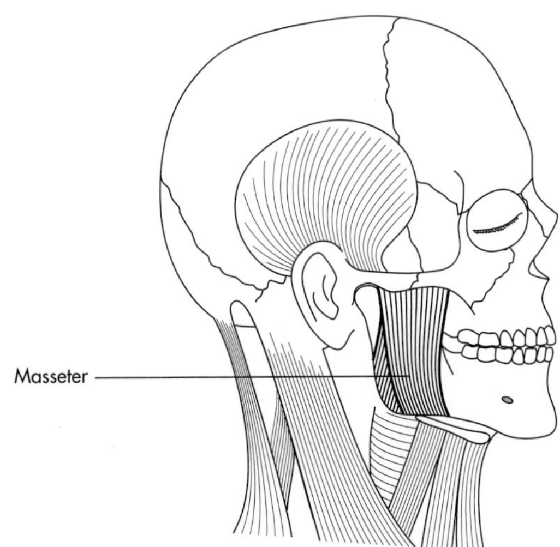

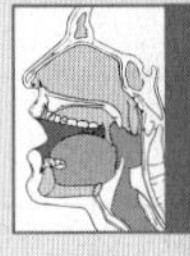

vertically

Masseter muscle originates along the zygomatic process. It has a deep and superficial portion. Find this on diagram B. In which direction does the masseter's fibers run?

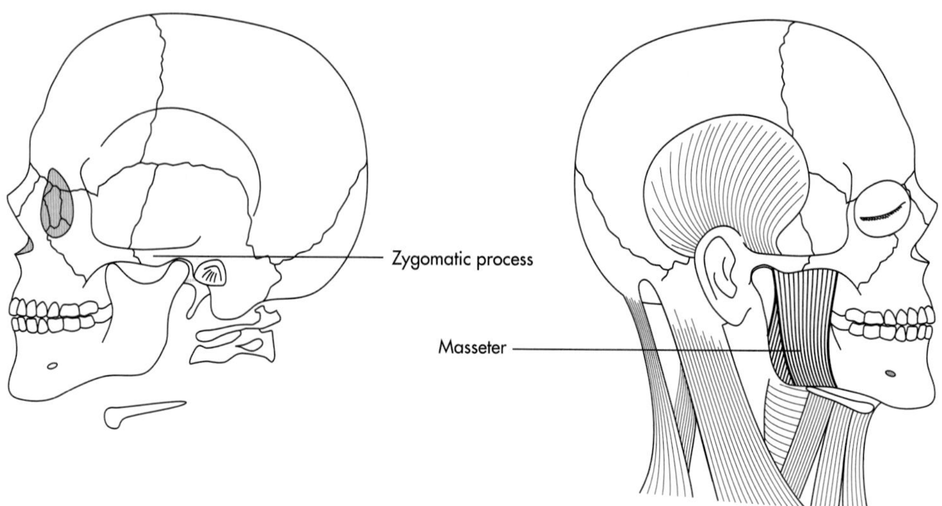

It elevates the mandible.

The masseter runs downward until it inserts on the lower border and angle of the mandible. Imagine the fibers growing shorter. What action does the masseter have on the mandible?

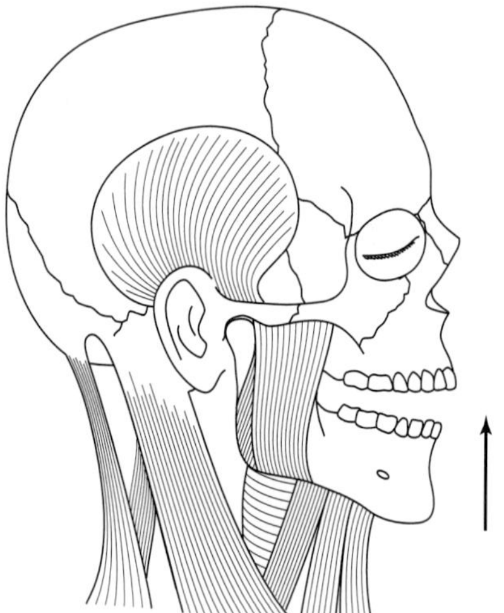

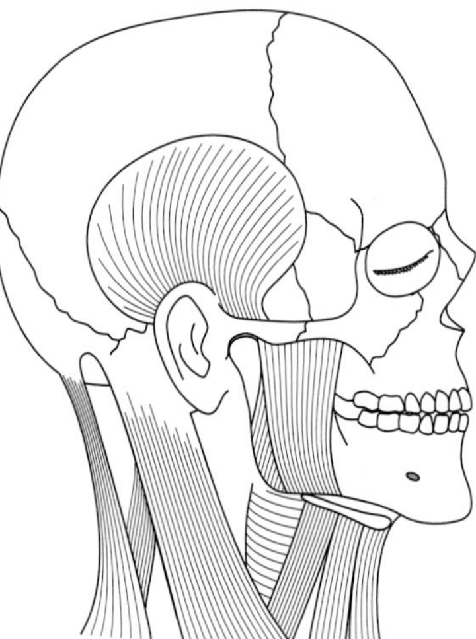

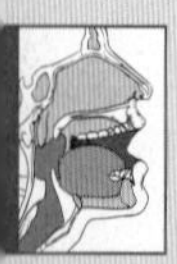

The masseter muscle is also an elevator of the mandible. It is a very strong, thick muscle sometimes called the "clenching muscle." Why?

Strong elevation of mandible causes clenching of the teeth.

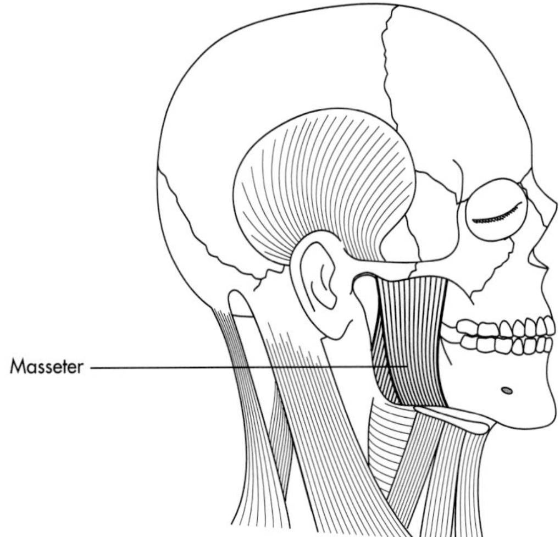

Review. Find the masseter on the drawing. What is its origin? Insertion? Action? Innervation?

origin—zygomatic process; insertion—lower border and angle of mandible; action—elevation of mandible; innervation—CN V, trigeminal nerve, third division

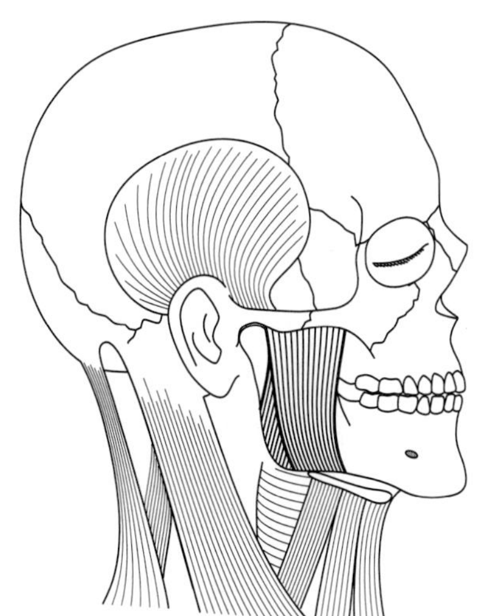

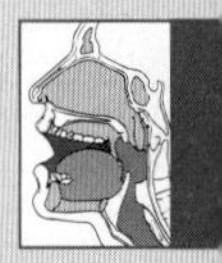

The third and fourth muscles of mastication are "internal muscles"; that is, we need to dissect further to find them. They are both on the "inside" of the mandible. In the drawings, portions of the face have been removed, as has part of the mandible. Temporalis and masseter are more superficial muscles.

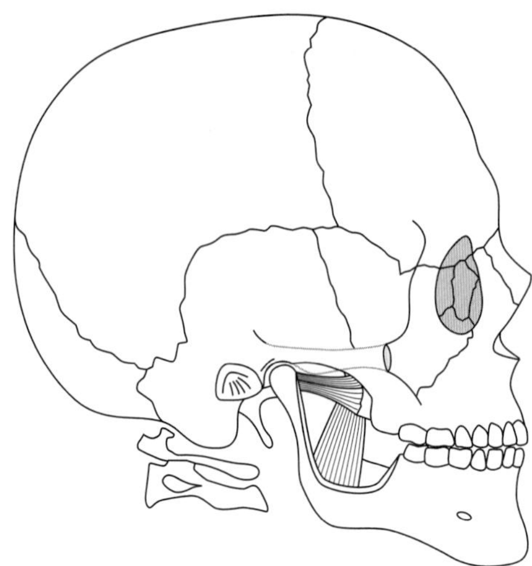

The third muscle of mastication is the **medial pterygoid.** Find and color it in.

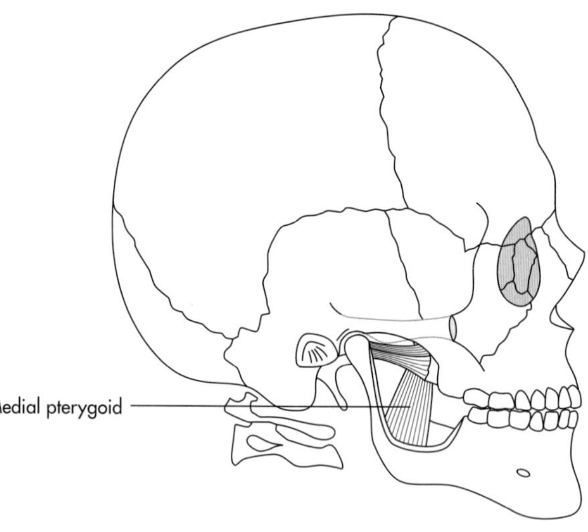

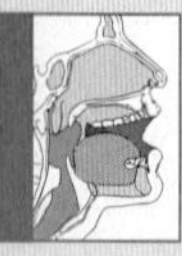

We need to look at the base of the cranium to find the origin of the **medial pterygoid muscle.** The bony "wings" that give origin to the pterygoid muscles are called ______________? Find them.

pterygoid plates

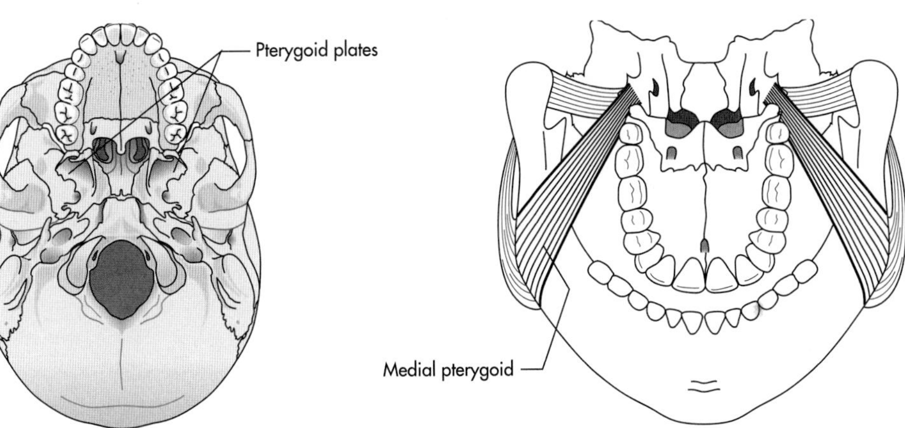

The lateralmost set of pterygoid plates are the origin of both pairs of pterygoid muscles. In which direction do you see the fibers of the medial pterygoid running?

vertically

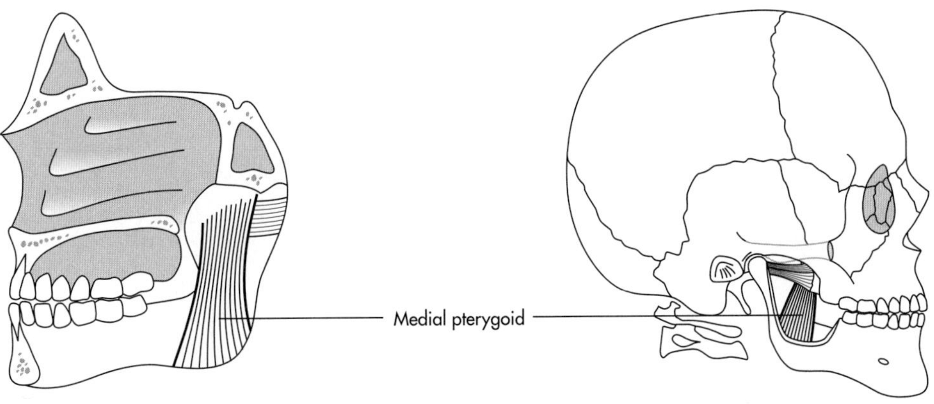

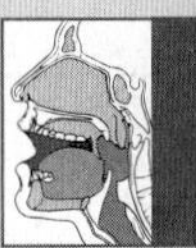

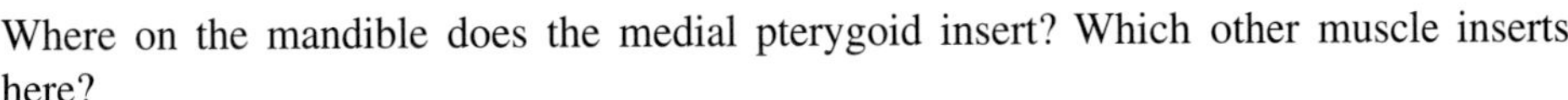

Where on the mandible does the medial pterygoid insert? Which other muscle inserts here?

angle of the mandible, masseter

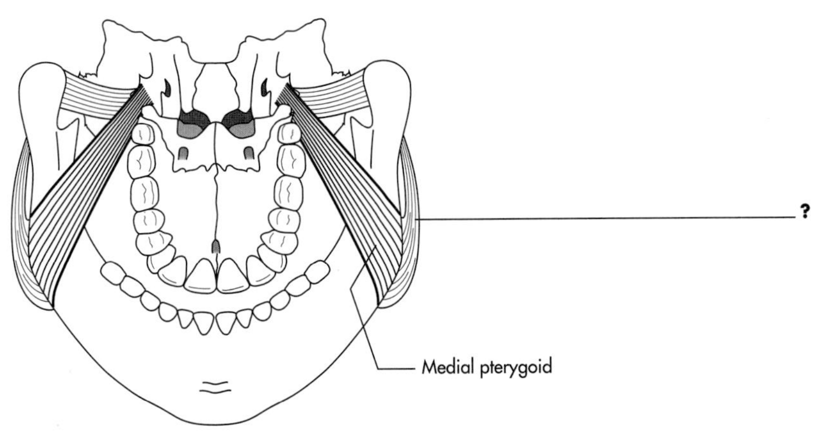

pterygoid plates; it elevates the mandible

The medial pterygoid originates on the ______________ and runs down vertically to insert on the lower border and angle of the mandible. It forms a "sling" with and is parallel to the masseter muscle. What action would it have?

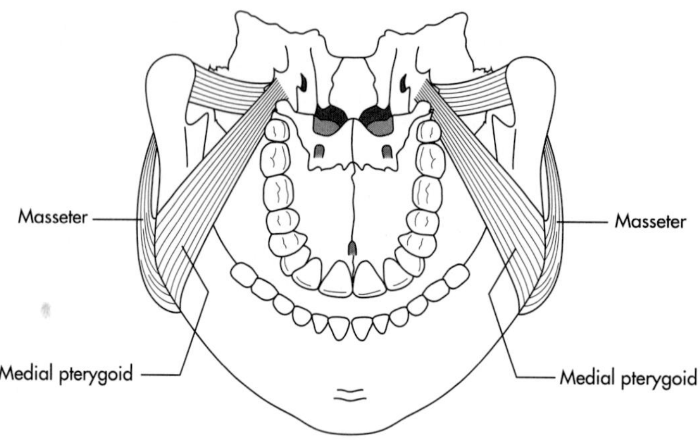

elevate

As the medial pterygoid and masseter run in the same direction, they have similar actions. They both act to ______________ the mandible.

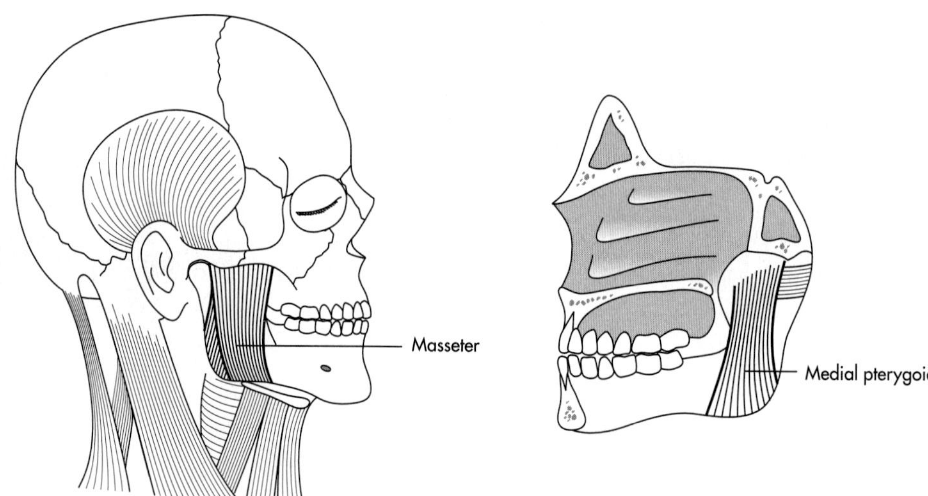

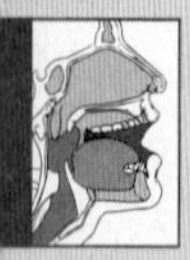

Masseter and medial pterygoid muscles form a "sling" around the mandible, holding it up and elevating it when active. The muscle on the outside of the mandible is the ______________ and the one on the inside is the ______________.

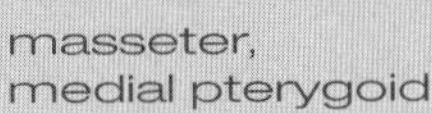

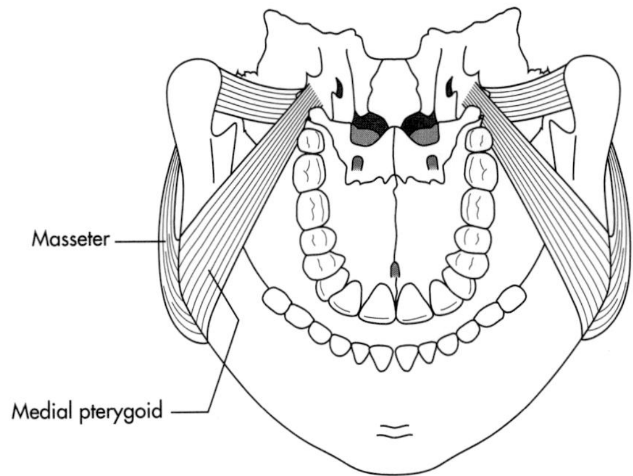

Review. The muscle shown is the ______________. Its origin is ______________; its insertion, ______________; and its action, ______________. It is innervated by ______________.

medial pterygoid, pterygoid plates, angle of the mandible, elevates the mandible, CN V

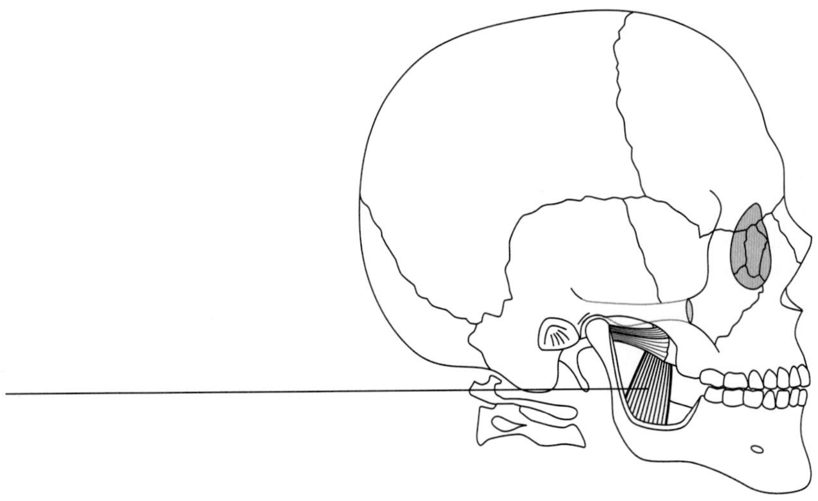

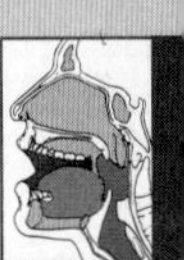

The medial pterygoid originates on the pterygoid plate, inserts on the lower border and angle of the mandible, and is an elevator of the mandible. It is innervated by CN V, the trigeminal nerve, third division.

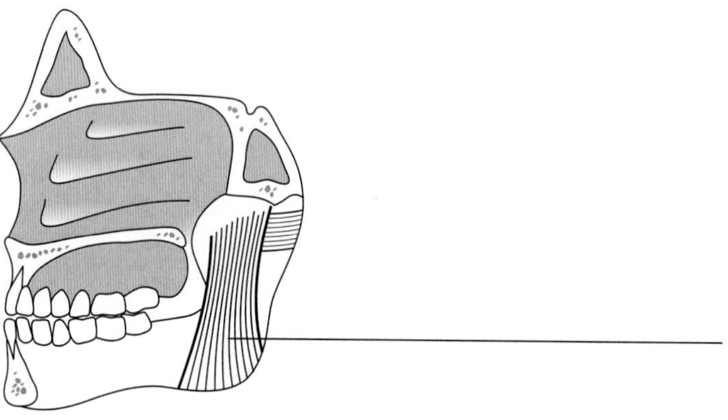

elevation

So far, all three of the masticatory muscles have the same action, which is ______________. Temporalis, masseter, and medial pterygoid are very strong muscles, used every time one swallows or chews. Elevating the mandible is a hard job requiring strong muscles. Depressing the jaw requires only small muscles because gravity aids depression. (Relax your jaw and see what happens!) The muscles that open or depress the jaw belong to a different group. The last muscle of the masticatory group is not primarily an elevator.

The last muscle pair are the **lateral pterygoids.** From their name, you should be able to tell two things: (1) The lateral pterygoid muscle is lateral to the medial pterygoid. (2) The lateral pterygoid has the same origin process as the medial pterygoid. Find the lateral pterygoid muscle and color it in.

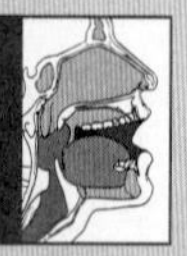

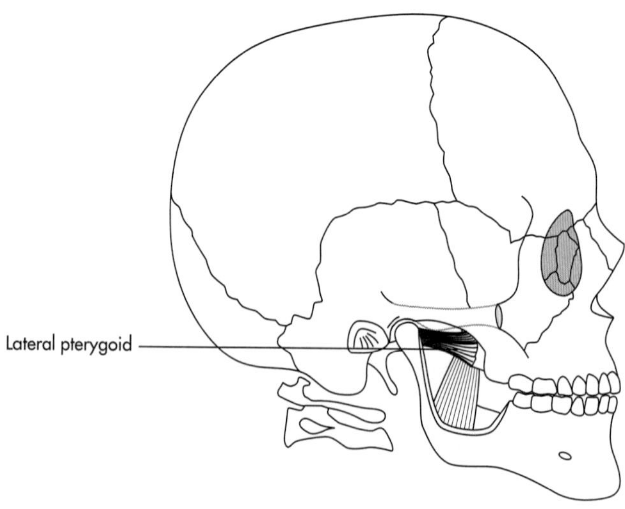

In which direction are the fibers of the lateral pterygoid running? The lateral pterygoid originates on the lateral portion of the lateral pterygoid plate. It can be divided into two portions, a superior portion and an inferior portion.

horizontal

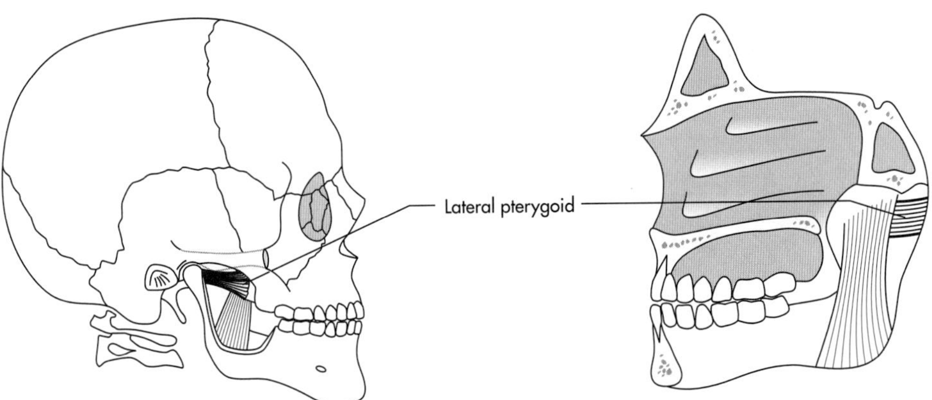

The lateral pterygoid inserts into the neck of the condyle of the mandible and even into the temporomandibular capsule and disk. The lateral pterygoid is the only masticatory muscle that runs horizontally. Do you think it has the same action as the other masticatory muscles?

no

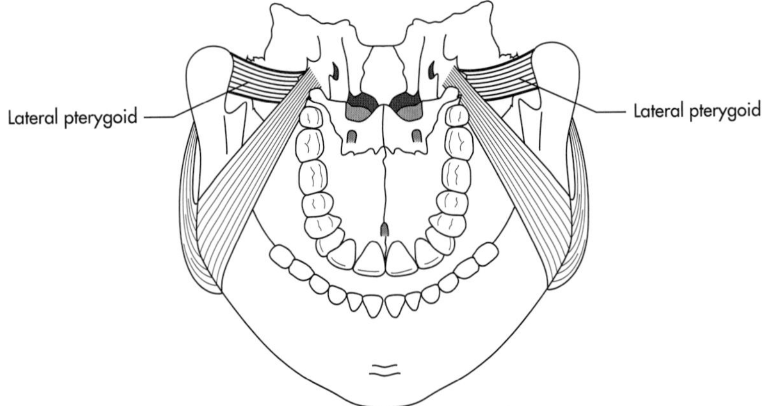

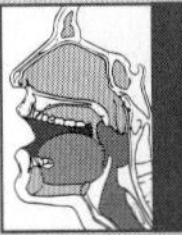

It protrudes.

Imagine the fibers of the lateral pterygoid growing shorter. What happens to the mandible?

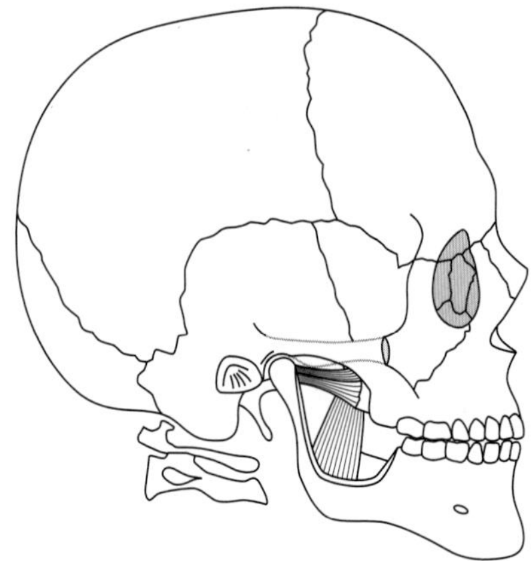

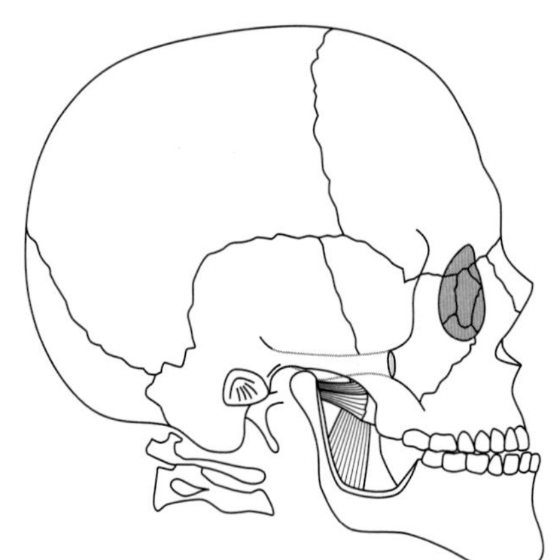

protrusion of the mandible

If both lateral pterygoids contract, the mandible will protrude or come forward. So, one of the actions of the lateral pterygoid is ________________.

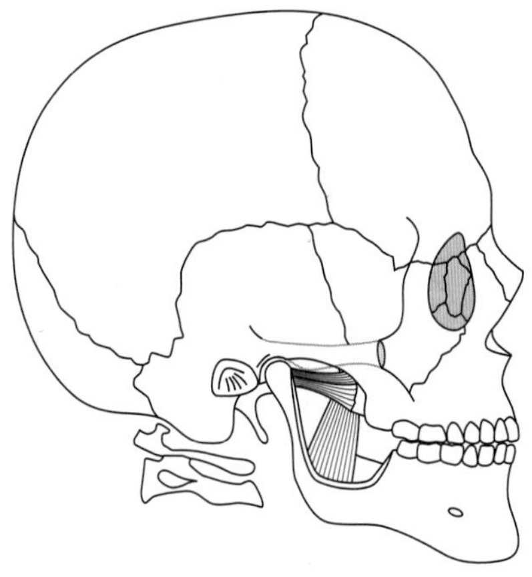

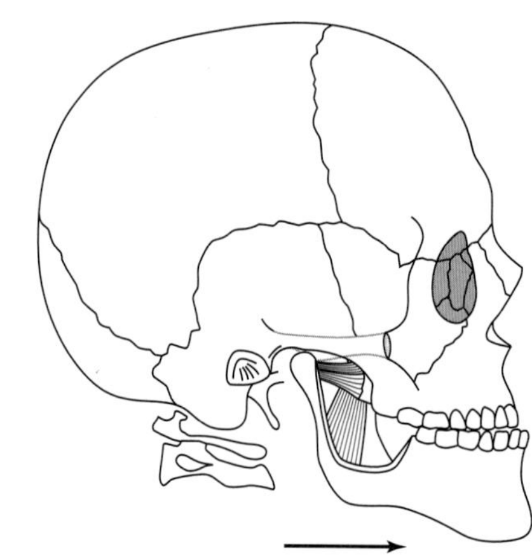

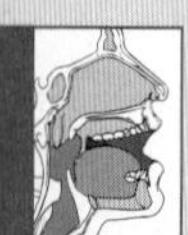

protrusion

A different action occurs if only one side, or one lateral pterygoid, contracts. The mandible moves toward that contracting lateral pterygoid. It gives the mandible lateral movement. What happens if both contract?

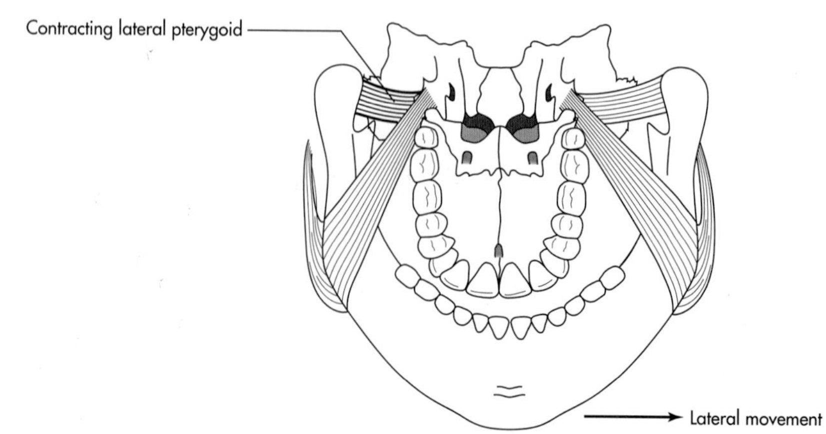

Actually, separate action of the temporalis and medial pterygoid also aids lateral movement of the jaw, but the lateral pterygoid is the primary activator. A last action of the lateral pterygoid muscle is maintenance of tension on the temporomandibular disk during jaw movements or excursions of the mandible. What are the actions of the lateral pterygoids?

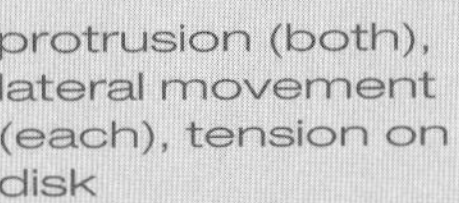
protrusion (both), lateral movement (each), tension on disk

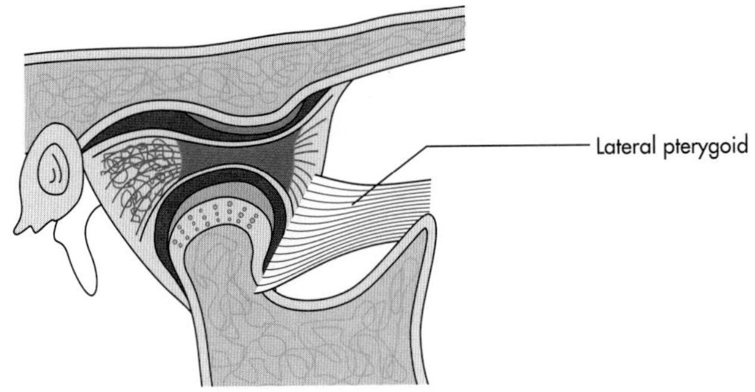

Review. This is the ______________ muscle, innervated by ______________. What is its origin? Insertion? Actions?

lateral pterygoid, CN V

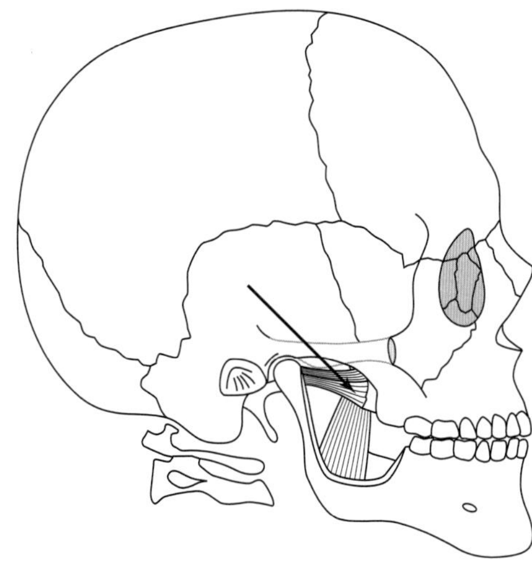

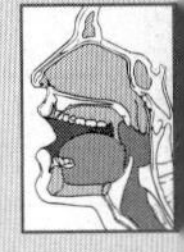

This is the lateral pterygoid muscle, innervated by the trigeminal nerve, third division. It originates on the pterygoid plates and inserts into the neck of the condyle and temporomandibular capsule and disk. If both right and left muscles contract, protrusion of the mandible occurs. If only one contracts at a time, lateral movement is induced. It also maintains tension on the TM disk during mandibular excursions.

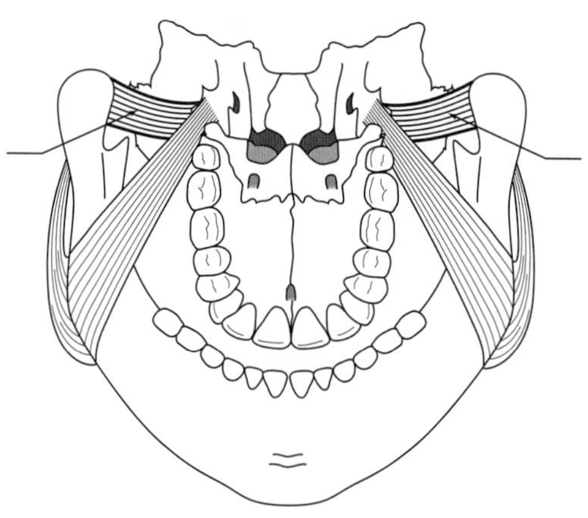

CN V, trigeminal nerve

In summary, list the four muscles of mastication and their origins, insertions, and actions. Check the preceding frames to find your answers. What innervates this group of muscles?

1. ______________
   Origin:
   Insertion:
   Action:
   Innervation:
2. ______________
   Origin:
   Insertion:
   Action:
   Innervation:
3. ______________
   Origin:
   Insertion:
   Action:
   Innervation:
4. ______________
   Origin:
   Insertion:
   Action:
   Innervation

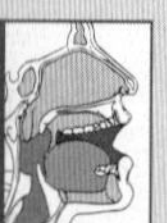

3.0 POSTERIOR NECK MUSCLES

The neck is divided into two areas, the anterior and the posterior, for the study of its muscles. We look first at the **posterior neck muscles.**

The posterior neck is an area of broad, thick muscles running from the occipital bone of the cranium to the shoulders and back. It is an area that contains the cervical vertebrae. So, this region is involved in supporting the head on the neck.

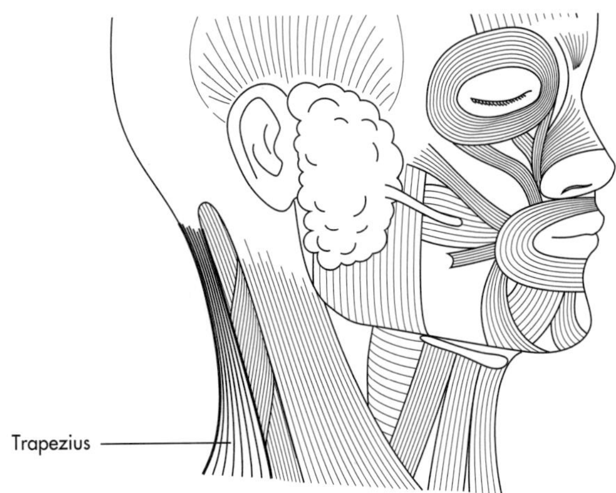

The diagram above and below shows the first layer of these posterior neck muscles and the largest. In fact, the **trapezius** is a large trapezoidal muscle that runs from the head to the shoulders and down the back in a continuous sheet. Find this muscle.

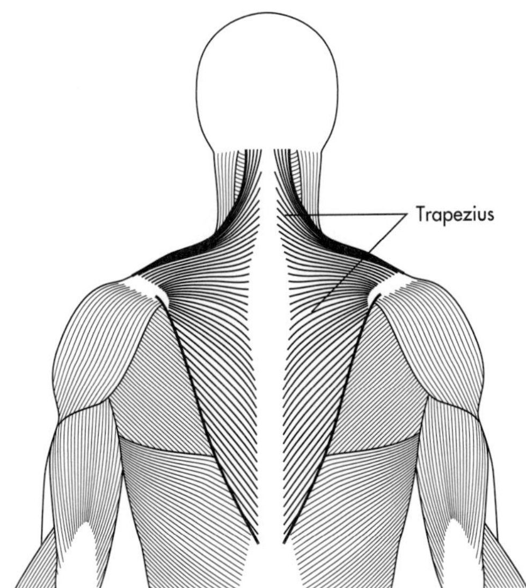

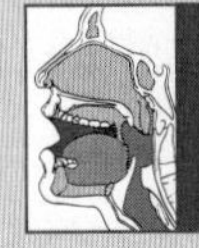

trapezius

The ______________ muscle is important for supporting the head, and it can move the head backward. Trapezius is innervated by CN XI, the spinal accesory nerve.

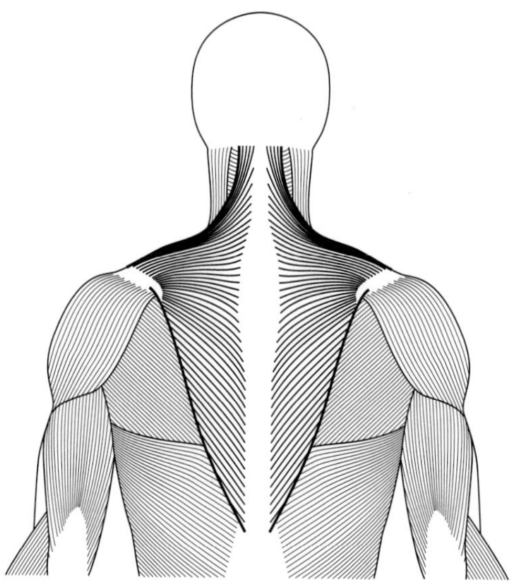

supporting the head, CN XI, seven

What is the trapezius' action? What is its innervation? Below trapezius lie two other large muscle pairs (semispinalis and splenius capitis) and three smaller pairs (oblique and rectus capitii), but we will not study these muscles. Below these muscles lie the cervical vertebrae. How many are there?

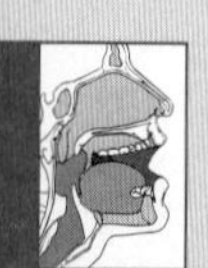

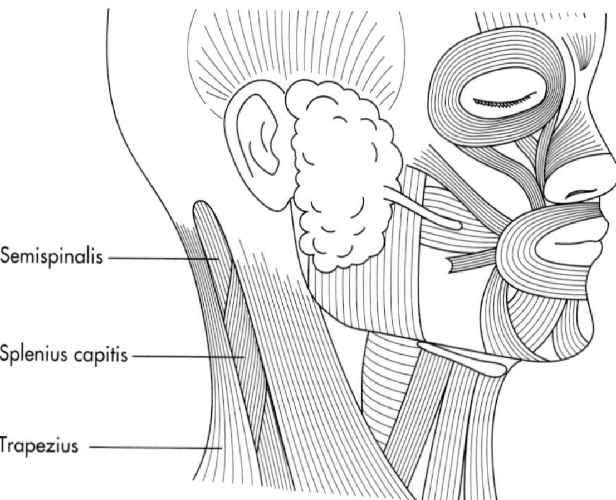

On the sagittal view find the trapezius. Then find a muscle that runs from the mastoid process inferiorly and anteriorly until it inserts on the sternum and clavicle. This three-"headed" muscle is called the **sternocleidomastoid muscle** for its three attachments.

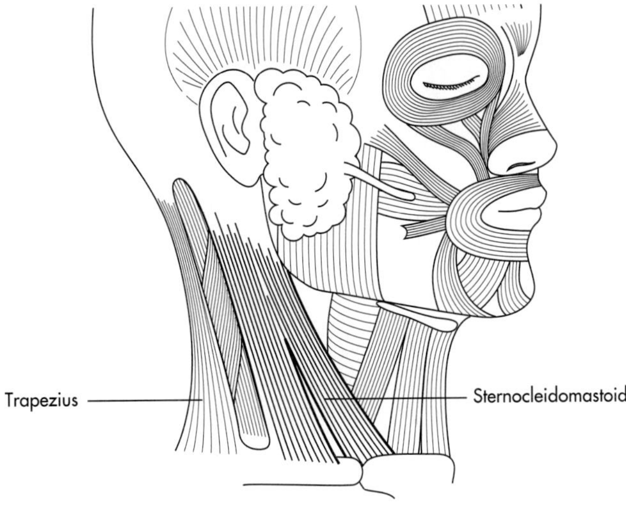

The sternocleidomastoids are a pair of right and left muscles running from the posterior to anterior neck. Abbreviated SCM, this muscle, if imagined shorter, would have what action on the head?

turns head to one side or the other

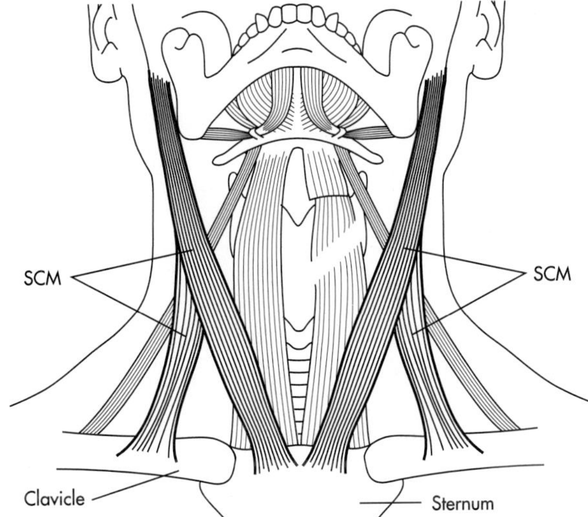

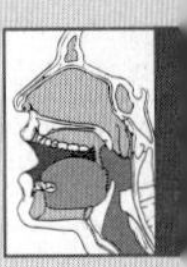

As they contract one at a time, SCM muscles can twist, turn, or flex the head toward the right or left. They are also important, when both are contracting, in supporting the head.

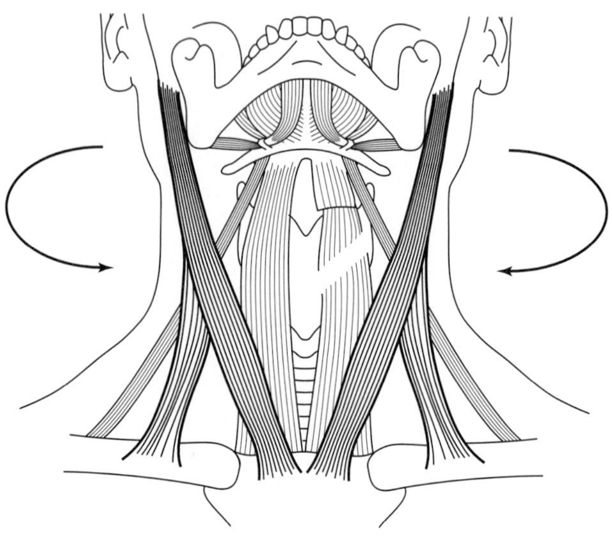

sternocleido-mastoid, turning and supporting head

SCM stands for _______________ muscle. It is also innervated by the spinal accesory nerve, CN XI. What are its actions?

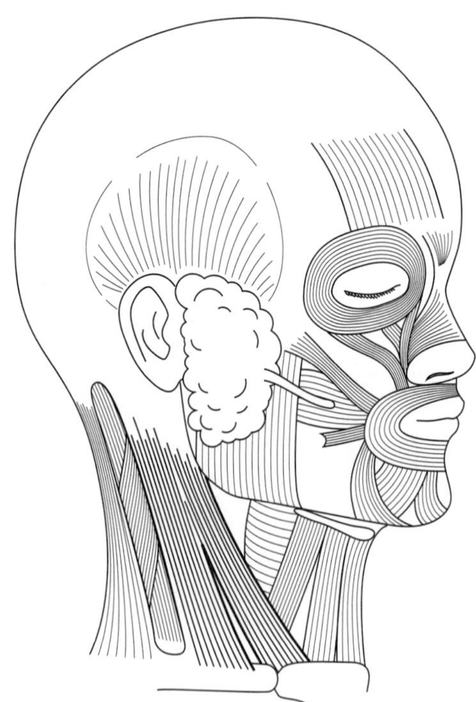

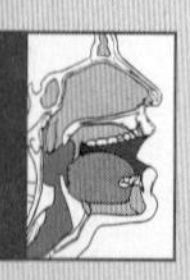

On a sagittal view, the SCM muscle can be used to divide the neck into two triangular areas. These are called the **posterior** and **anterior triangles** of the neck and they are often used by anatomists to describe the location of neck structures.

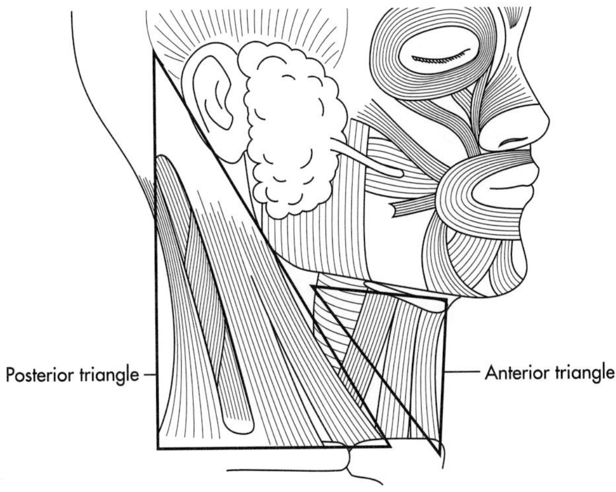

The SCM is known as a landmark muscle, which is an easily found structure that can be used as a reference to find other structures. We will be using SCM as a ____________.

landmark

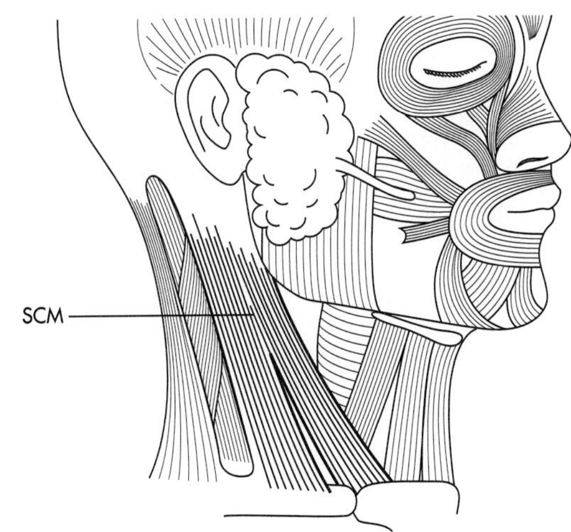

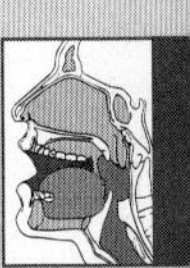

The trapezius and SCM support the head. The SCM turns the head. Both are innervated by CN XI.

Find the sternocleidomastoid and trapezius muscles on the drawing. Describe their actions and innervations. Check the preceding frames for your answers.

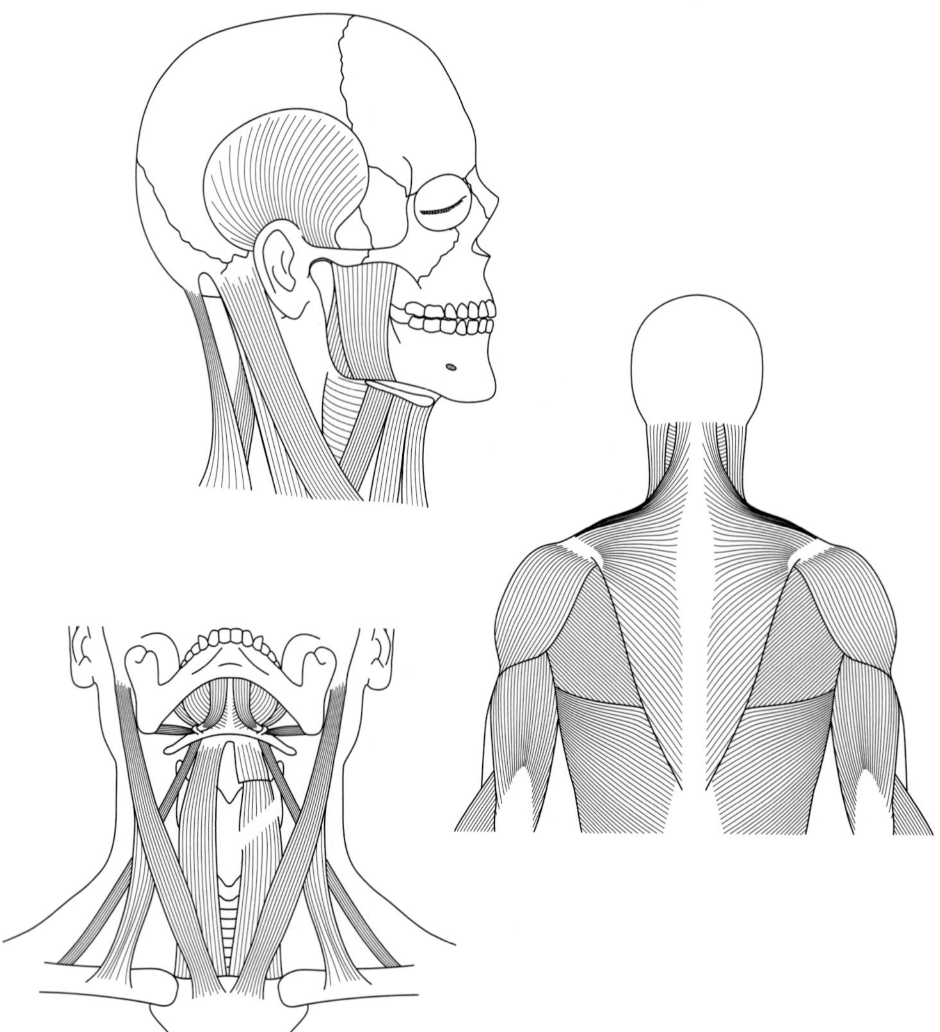

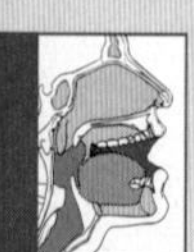

ANTERIOR NECK

4.0

In contrast to the posterior neck, the anterior neck has thin, straplike muscles. Within the anterior neck lie several important structures including the pharynx/esophagus and larynx/trachea. Also, there are many important blood vessels, nerves, and glands.

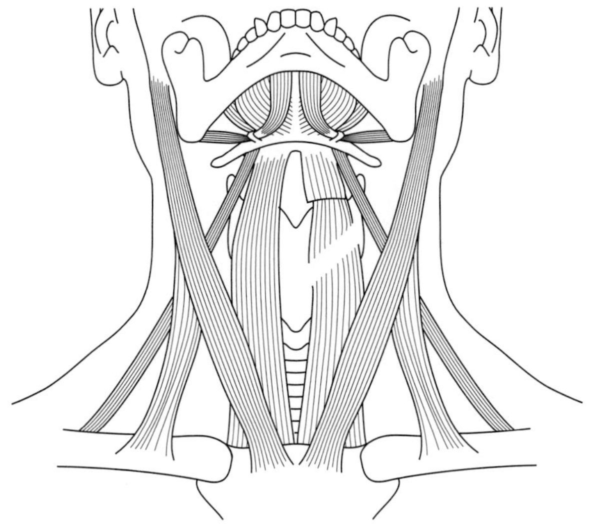

The anterior neck muscles are centered around a separate bone in the neck called the **hyoid bone.** It is found directly beneath the mentum or "chin." Find the hyoid on the drawing.

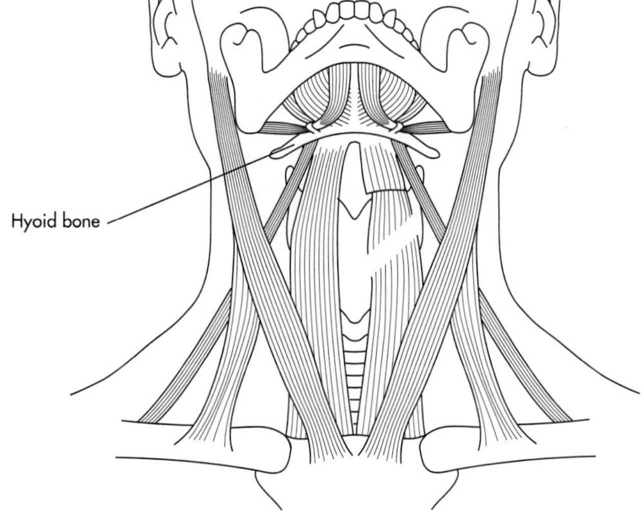

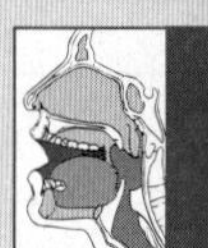

Muscles located above the hyoid bone that belong to the anterior group are called **suprahyoid muscles** and there are four types. Below the hyoid bone are the **infrahyoid muscles.** There are four pairs in this subgroup. Find the suprahyoids and infrahyoids in the diagram and color them in.

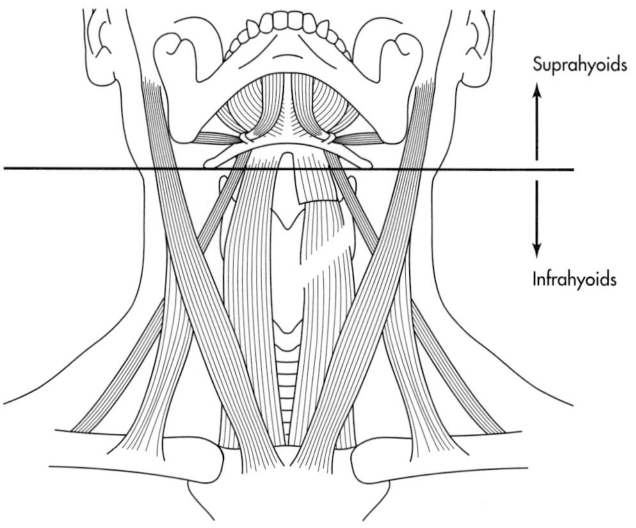

4.1 Suprahyoid Muscles

above, muscles of mastication

This subgroup of anterior muscles is found where in relation to the hyoid bone? In general, this group of muscles acts to open or depress the mandible. This action is opposite that of what muscle group?

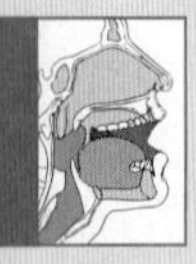

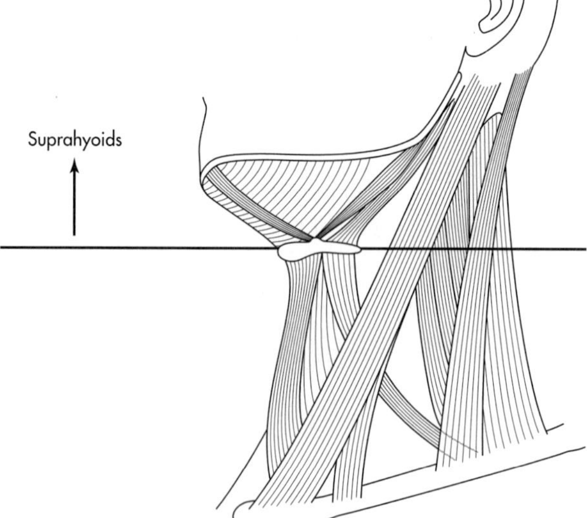

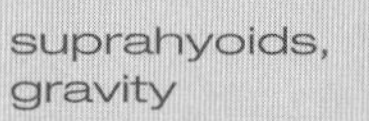

Closing or elevating the mandible requires four pairs of very thick strong muscles, the muscles of mastication, whereas opening or depressing the mandible requires only thin small muscles, called the ______________. Why is this so?

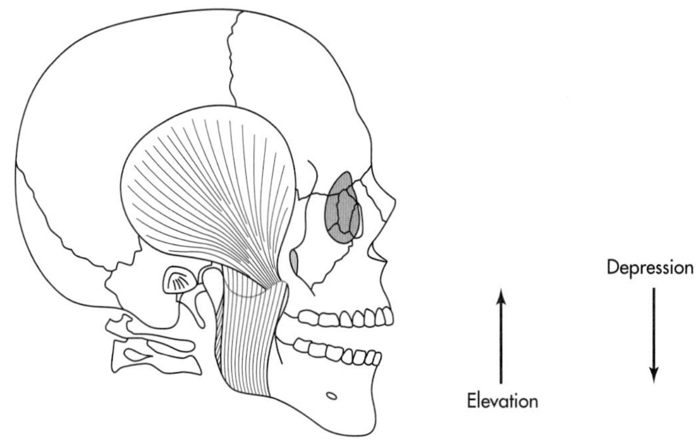

Relax your jaw. What happens? Gravity naturally helps open the mandible and not much further muscular effort is needed to depress the mandible.

The first suprahyoid found is a pair of muscles under the mentum, directly deep to the overlying skin. These **digastric muscles** are unusual in that they have two functioning parts or "bellies" joined together in the middle. Find digastric on the diagram.

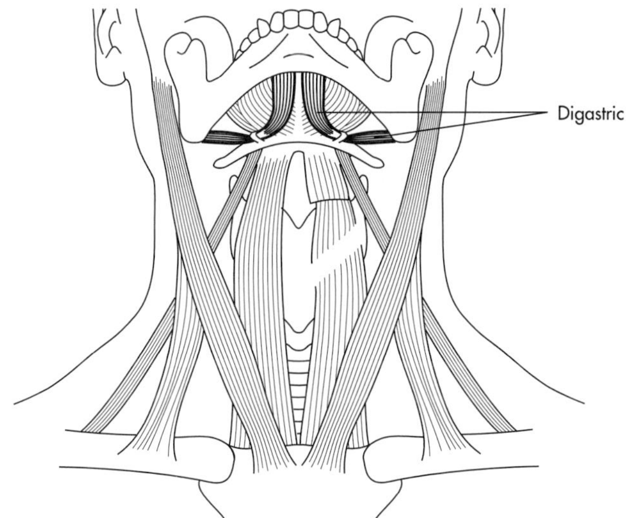

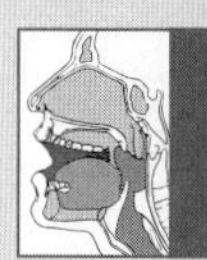

Digastric muscle originates on the mastoid process and passes downward to the hyoid bone, where the first belly ends in a tendon that slips through a loop on the hyoid bone. The second portion passes back up to the mandible, where it inserts on the digastric fossa on the inside of the mentum.

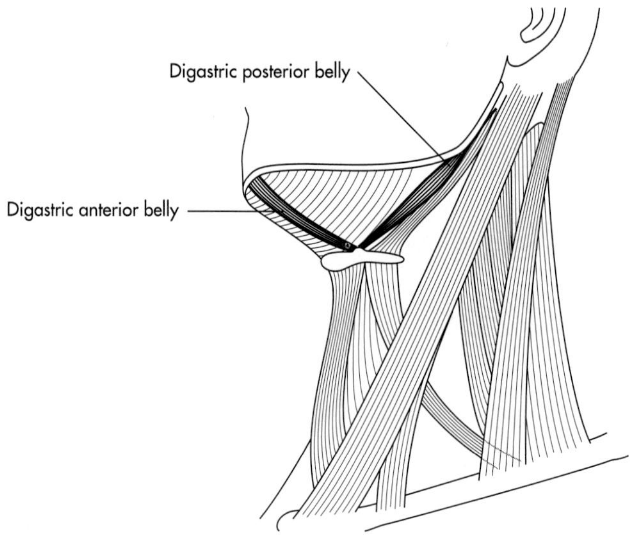

mandible

Digastric muscles act like "pulleys," opening or depressing the ______________ .

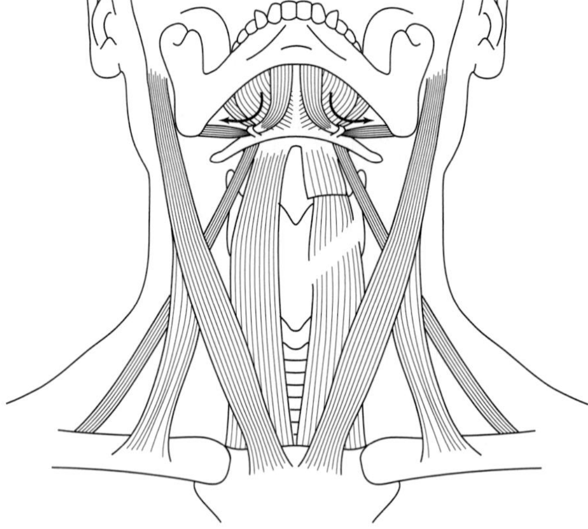

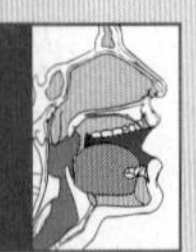

Deep to the digastric muscles is a single broad, flat muscle that runs across the floor of the mouth from side to side. It is the **mylohyoid muscle.** Find it and color it in.

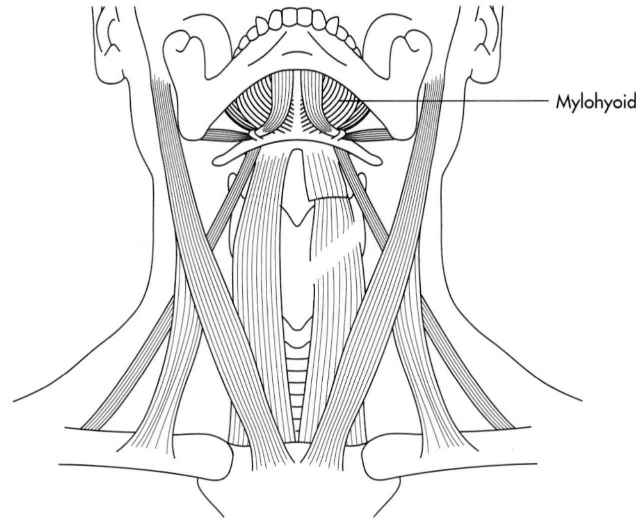

Mylohyoid muscle originates from both mylohyoid lines on the mandible, its fibers merging to insert on the hyoid bone. This is the major muscle of the floor of the mouth. Besides providing a firm base for the tongue, it helps to ______________ the mandible. It is innervated by CN V, the trigeminal nerve.

depress

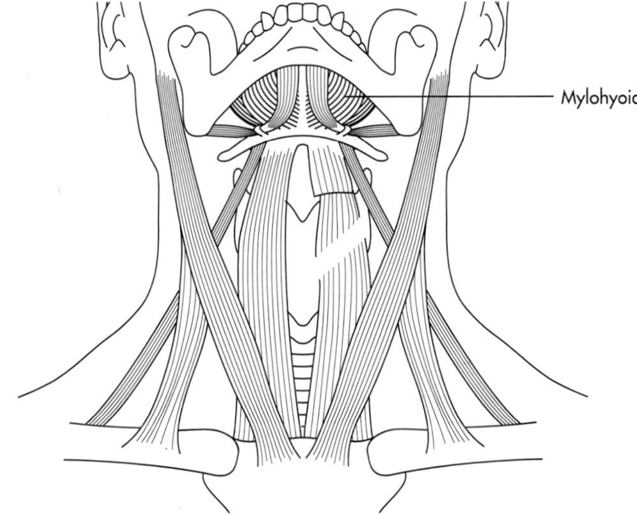

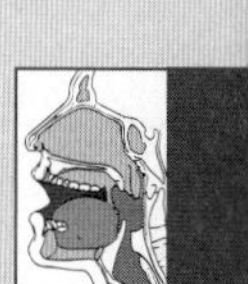

digastric and mylohyoid

Find the digastric fossa and mylohyoid line on the drawing. Which muscles attach to these areas?

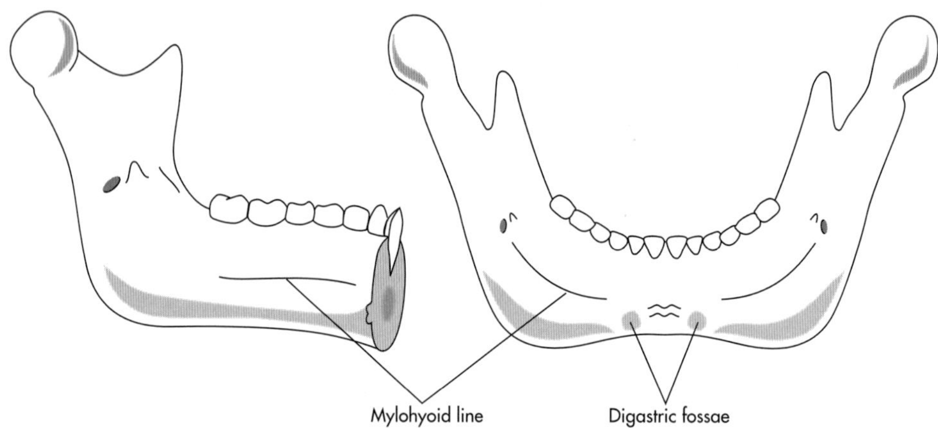

The next suprahyoid pair must be seen on a sagittal view. Find that thin pointed process at the base of the cranium called the styloid process in the diagram.

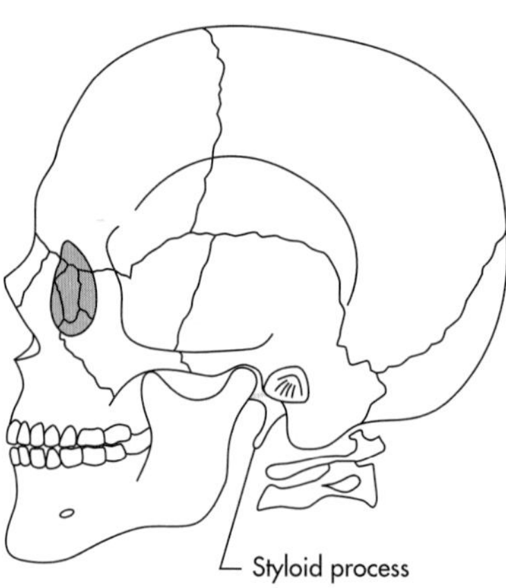

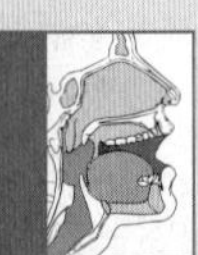

On the sagittal view find the **stylohyoid muscle.** As its name indicates, it originates on the styloid process and inserts on the hyoid bone. You will also note a separate **stylohyoid ligament** next to this muscle.

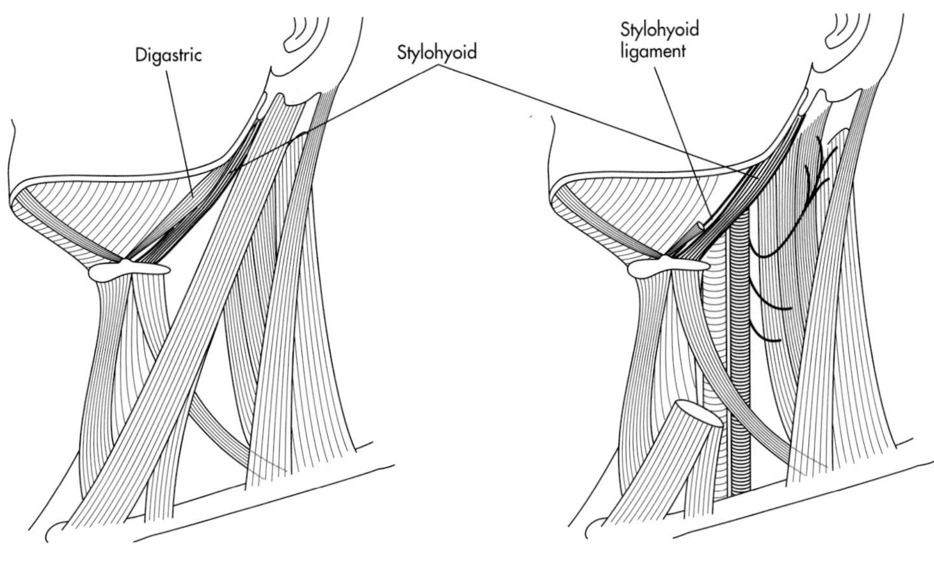

The ______________ muscle helps tighten or stabilize the hyoid bone during the actions of other muscles.

stylohoid

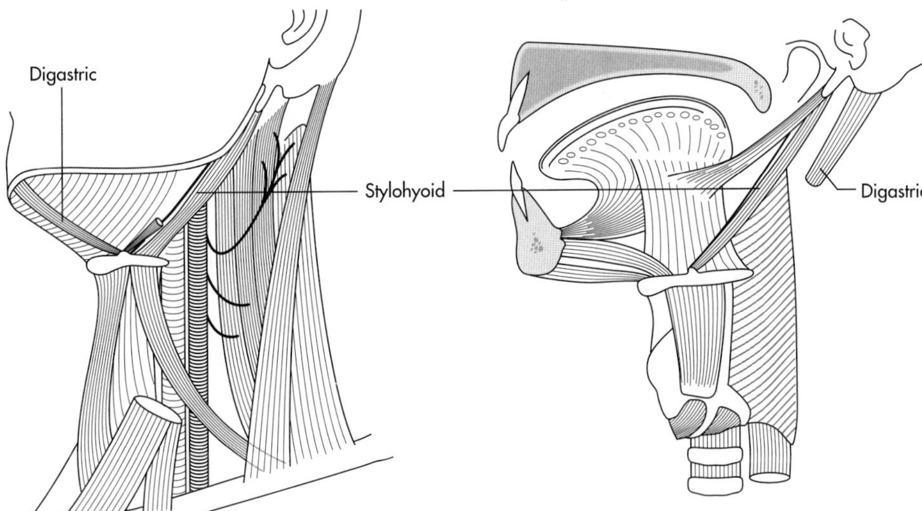

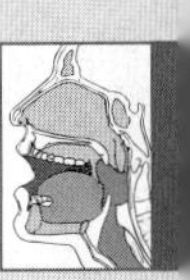

genial tubercles

The last suprahyoid muscle pair originates on processes that we have seen on the interior mandible. What are these processes called?

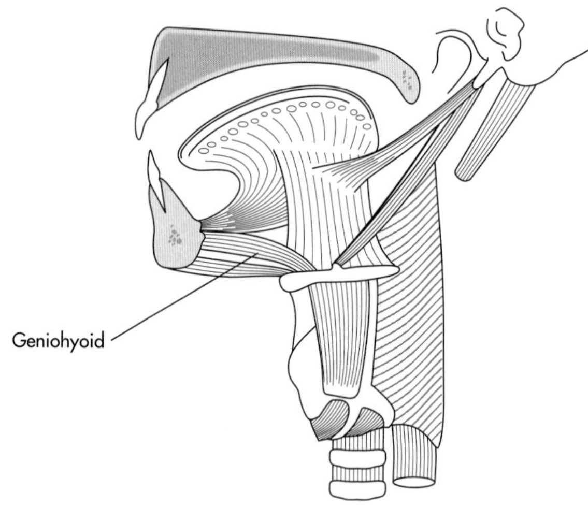

Geniohyoid muscle originates on the genial tubercles and runs down to insert on the hyoid bone. It also is a stabilizing muscle.

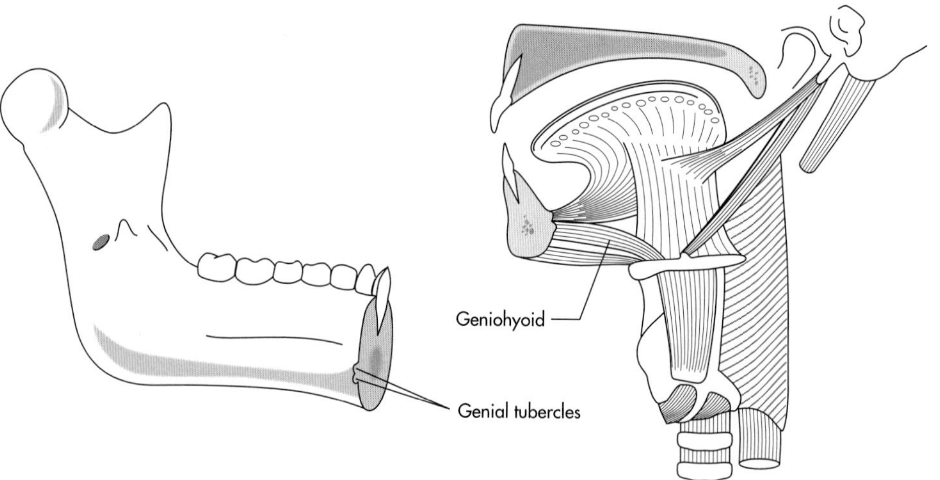

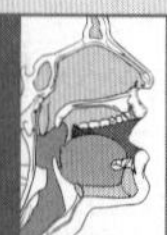

Have you noticed a pattern in the naming of the neck muscles? Usually the name is derived from both the origin and the insertion; the digastric muscle is an exception.

Find the digastric, mylohyoid, stylohyoid, and geniohyoid muscles on the drawing. What muscle group is this? What actions do these muscles have? Innervation is in part by CN V and other nerves. What are some of the origins and insertions of these muscles? Check your answers in the preceding frames.

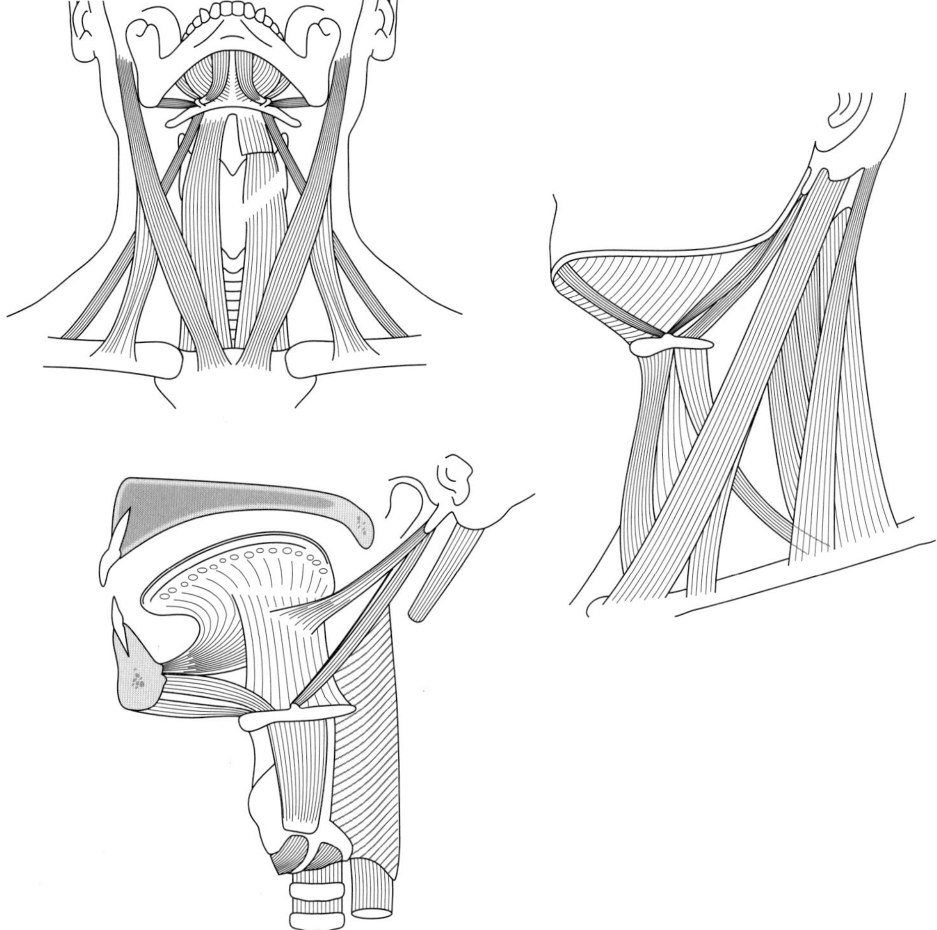

anterior neck suprahyoids, depression of mandible

Digastric
O: mastoid
I: digastric fossa
A: depression of mandible

Mylohyoid
O: mylohyoid lines
I: hyoid
A: depression of mandible, stabilizes floor of mouth

Stylohoid
O: stylohoid process
I: hyoid
A: stabilizes hyoid

Geniohyoid
O: genial tubercles
I: hyoid
A: stabilizes hyoid

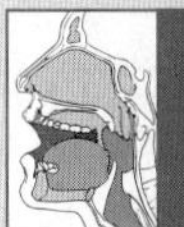

Infrahyoid Muscles

4.2

The anterior neck muscles located below the hyoid bone are the ______________ muscles. There are four pairs. They are also thin, straplike muscles and they act to stabilize the hyoid bone to provide a base against which the suprahyoids, glossal, or laryngeal muscles can act. They help in depression of the mandible, swallowing (base for tongue), and closing of the epiglottis (raising the larynx).

infrahyoid

insertions

The infrahyoid muscles are also named by their origins and ______________, giving us a clue where to locate them.

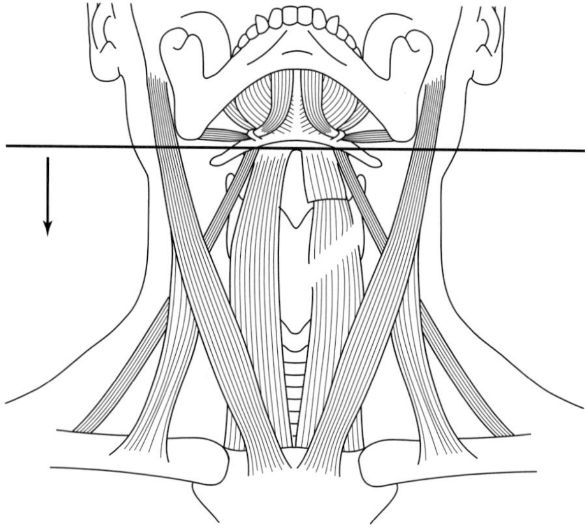

The first infrahyoid is the **sternohyoid muscle.** The sternum is the single large "breast-bone" joining the ribs in the anterior chest. Locate this muscle and color it in.

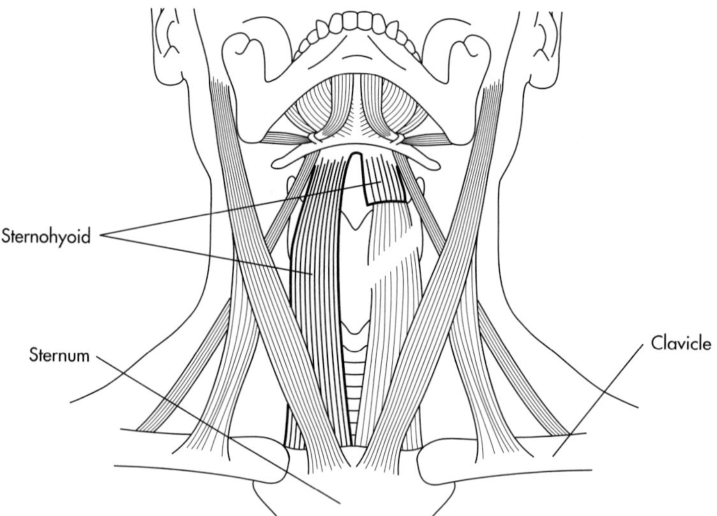

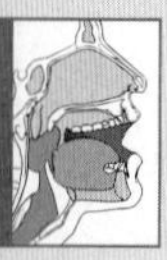

The origin and insertion of the sternohyoid are the _______________ and _______________. There are a right and left sternohyoid, but in the drawing the muscle on one side has been "cut" or removed. Which side?

sternum, hyoid, right

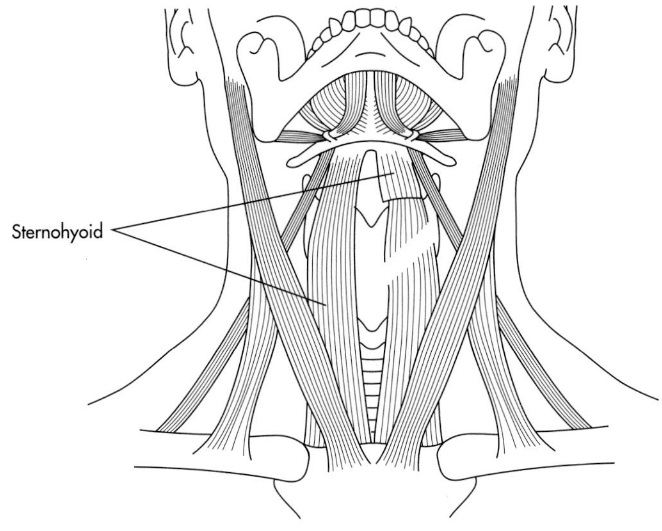

The anterior neck contains the **larynx** and **trachea,** important parts of the respiratory system. The **thyroid cartilage** is a large, shieldlike cartilage plate that covers and protects the larynx. Find the thyroid cartilage and trachea.

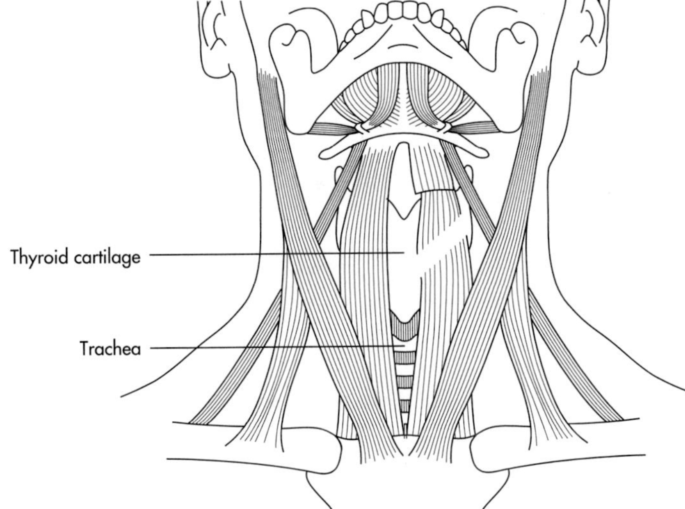

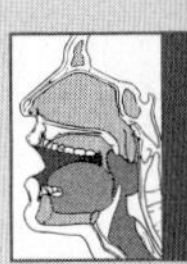

sternum

The next two infrahyoids are found below the sternohyoid muscle, so look to the right side of the drawing where this muscle is removed. The **sternothyroid** originates on the thyroid cartilage and inserts onto the ______________. Find it.

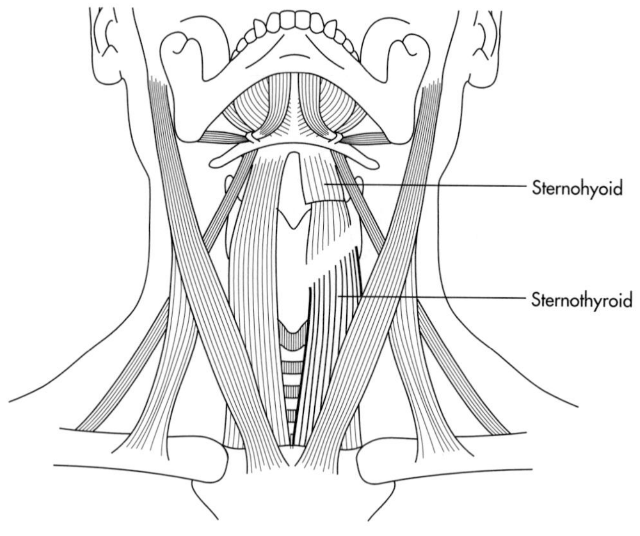

hyoid

The **thyrohyoid muscle** originates on the thyroid cartilage and inserts onto the ______________ bone. Find it.

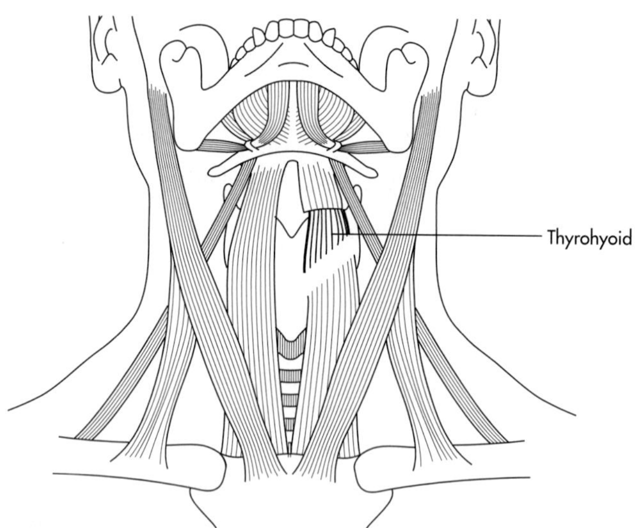

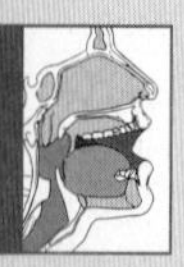

The last infrahyoid muscle needs to be viewed sagittally. It also is a "two-belly" muscle, like the digastric. It is a called the **omohyoid** muscle. The omohyoid originates on the clavicle ("omo") and passes laterally, forming the first belly. Find it.

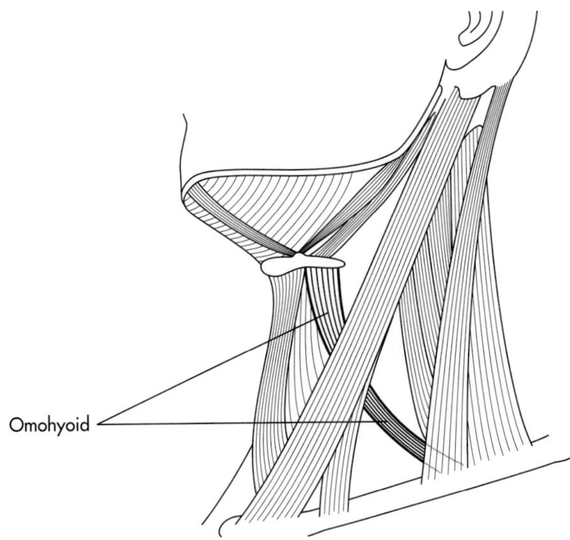

_______________ then becomes tendinous near the jugular vein and forms the second belly, which passes up to insert on the hyoid bone. Find it on the drawing.

Omohyoid

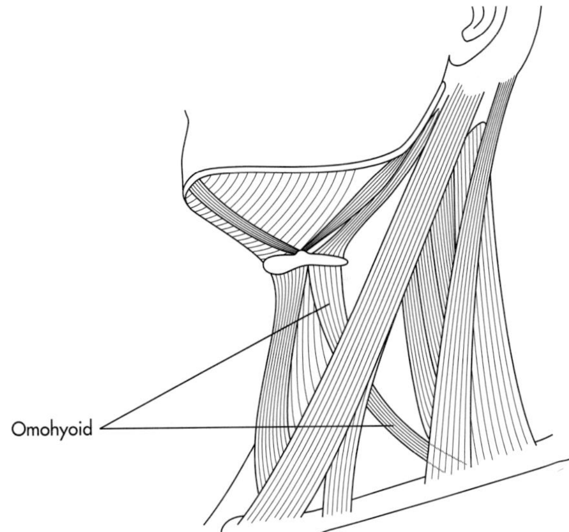

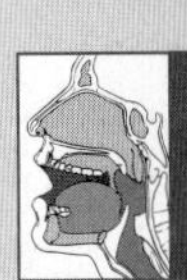

1. sternohyoid
2. thyrohyoid
3. sternothyroid
4. omohyoid

Name the four infrahyoid muscle pairs:

1. ______________
2. ______________
3. ______________
4. ______________

Find them in the diagrams. Refer to the previous text.

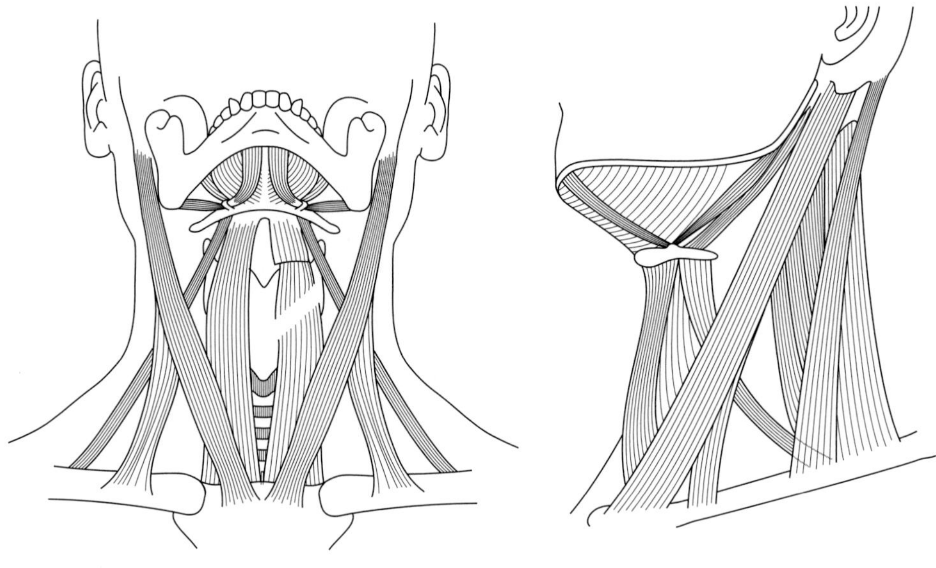

They stabilize the hyoid for depression of the mandible and act as a base for tongue and laryngeal muscles.

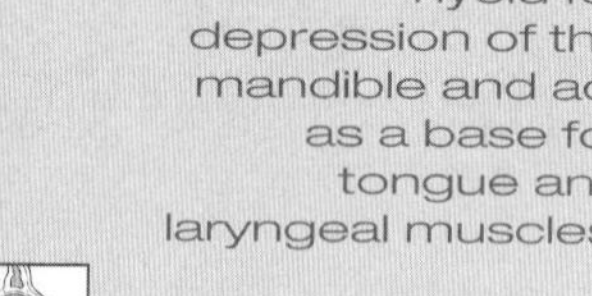

The infrahyoids have what actions? They are innervated by cervical nerves.

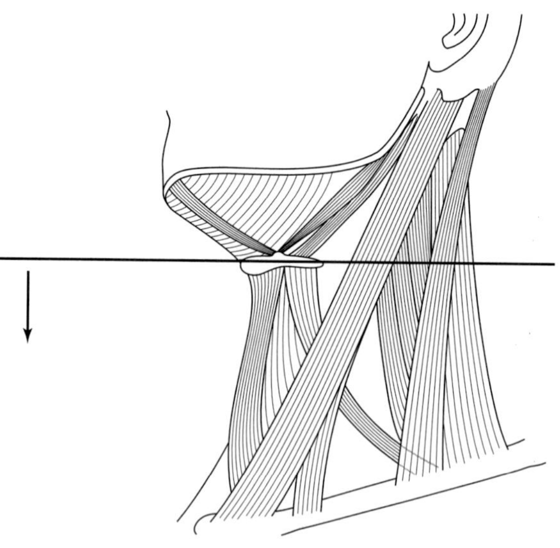

MUSCLES OF THE TONGUE

5.0

The tongue is a very complex structure. It is, in fact, a sac of muscles. Beneath the lingual mucosa are three intermixed layers of muscle fibers in small bundles. These are called the **intrinsic muscles of the tongue.** They are pictured here.

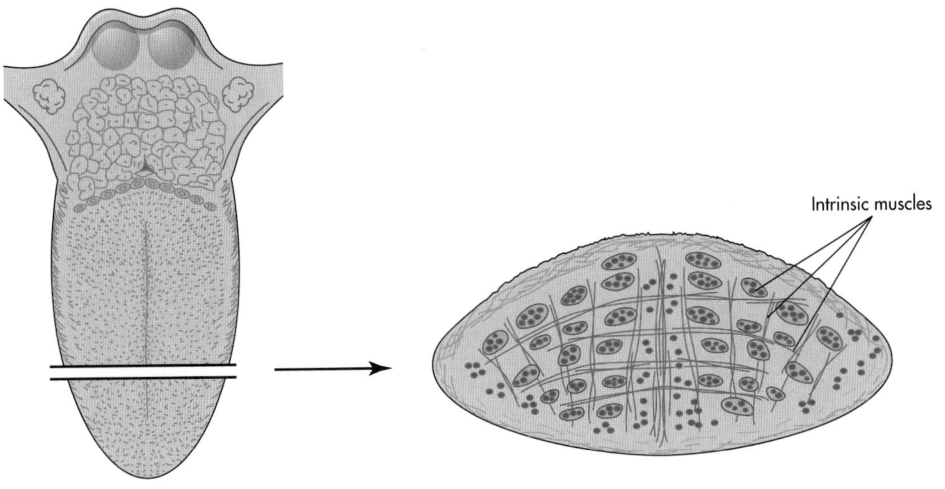

intrinsic

The intrinsic muscles of the tongue are **horizontal, transverse,** and **vertical** in the direction of their fibers. The ______________ muscles of the tongue are capable of many intricate movements associated with swallowing and speech.

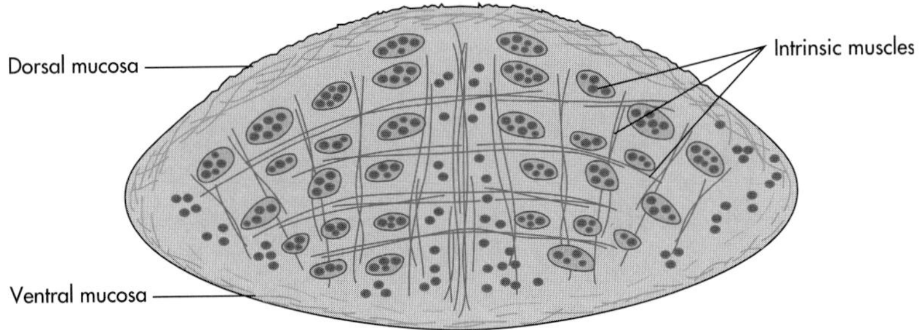

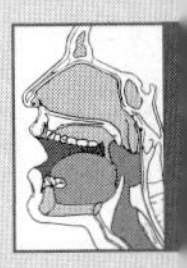

The other muscles of the tongue originate outside of the tongue and then insert into it. These are the **extrinsic muscles of the tongue.** They occur in pairs.

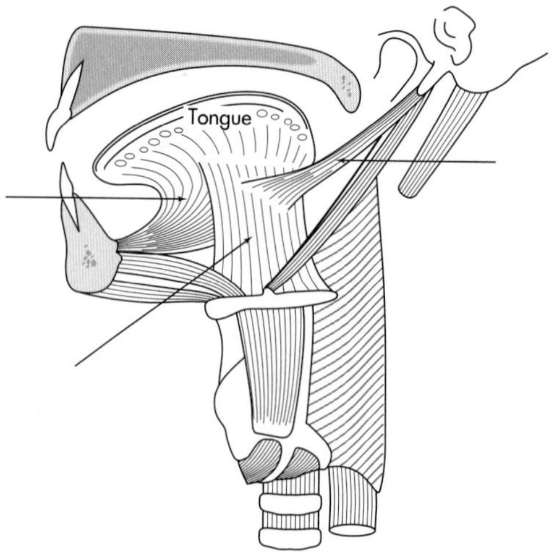

extrinsic, *lingua*

The ______________ muscles of the tongue originate outside of the tongue. They will have the small word *glossus* in their names. What other word means "tongue"?

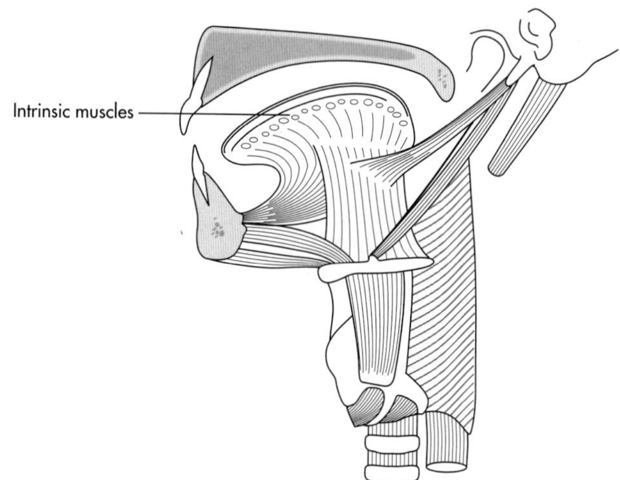

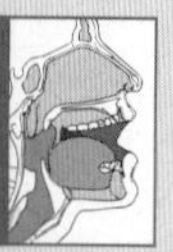

The first intrinsic muscle pair of the tongue is large and strong, forming a strong base below the tongue. It originates on the hyoid bone, inserts into the base of the tongue, and is thus called the **hyoglossus.** Find it and color it in.

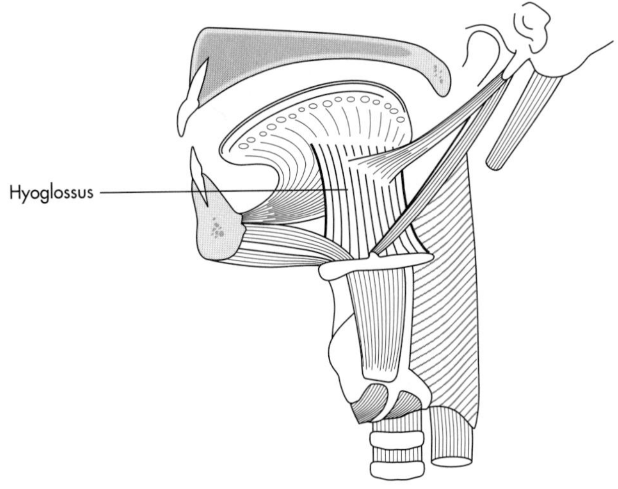

genioglossus

The second extrinsic muscle originates on the genial tubercles and inserts into the tongue. What would you name it?

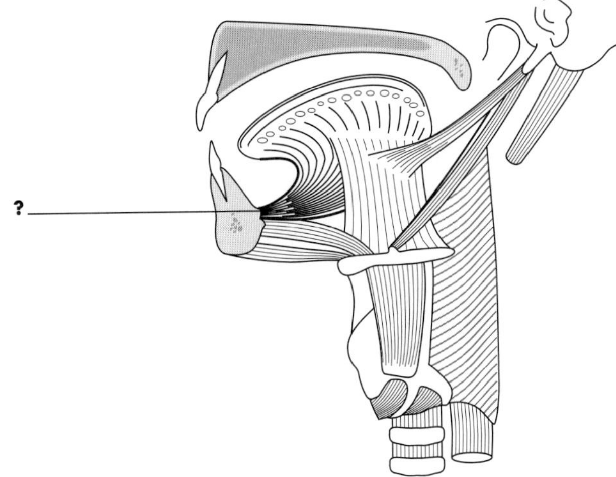

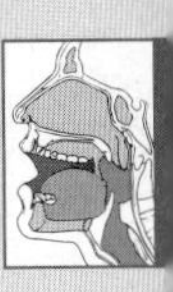

geniohyoid

Color in the **genioglossus muscle.** Which other muscle originates on the genial tubercles?

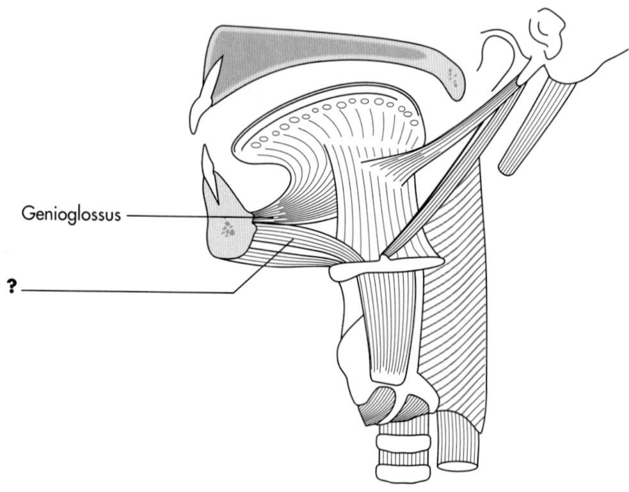

styloglossus

What would you name a muscle that originates on the styloid process and passes down to insert on the posterior and lateral tongue?

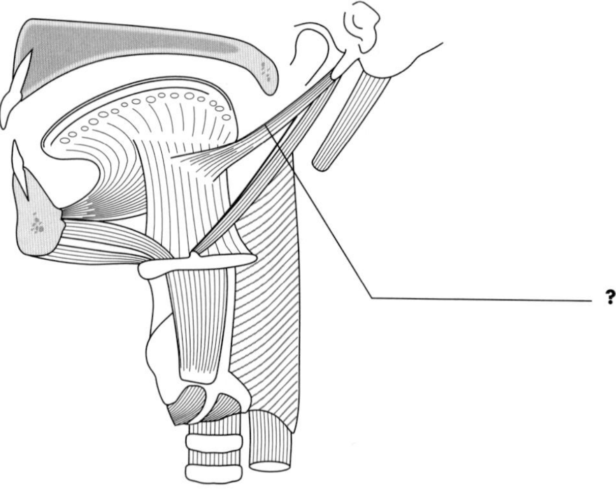

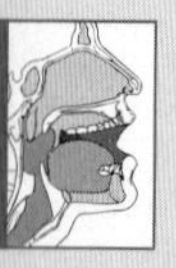

The **styloglossus** shares the styloid process with what other muscle and what ligament?

stylohyoid muscle, stylohyoid ligament

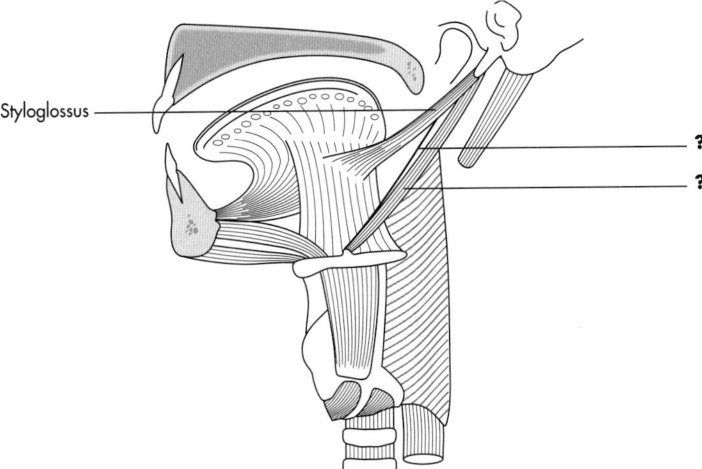

Lastly, there is a muscle that originates on the palate (soft) and passes down to insert on the posterior lateral tongue on either side. It is called the palato________. Find it.

glossus

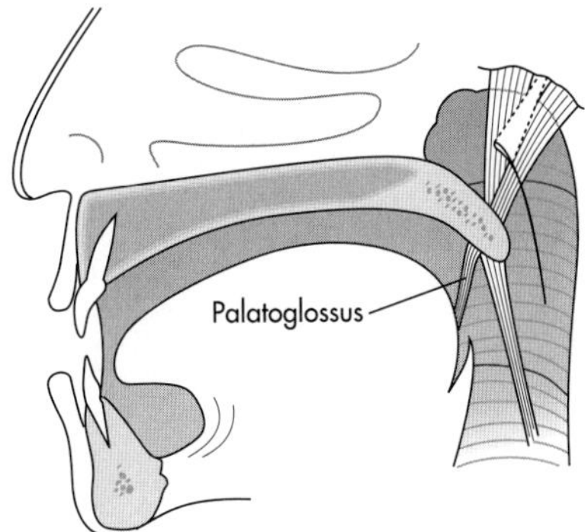

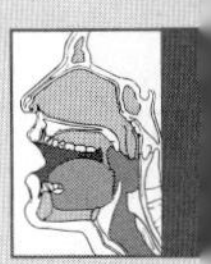

anterior tonsillar pillar

The **palatoglossus** forms the anterior portion of a mucosa-covered landmark in the oral cavity. There are two of these and the palatine tonsil rests between them. It is called the ________________. (Check Chapter Five.)

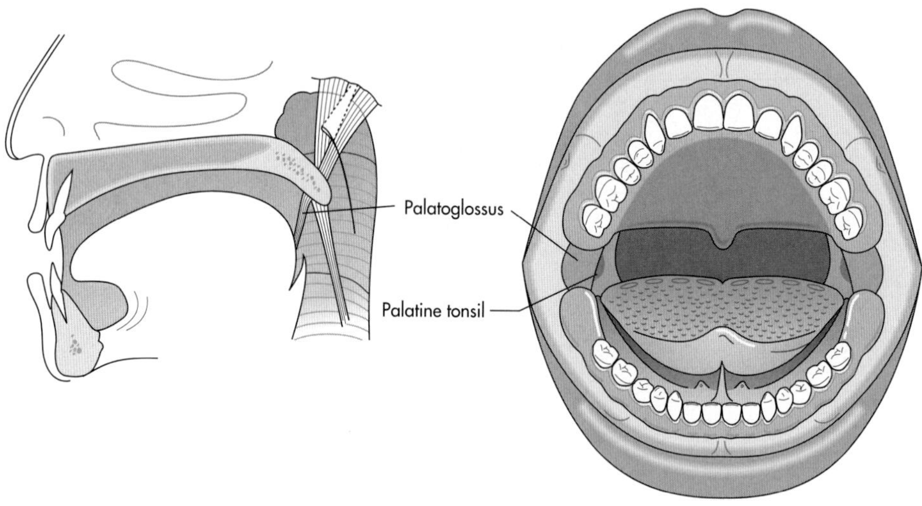

The palatoglossus is beneath the anterior **tonsillar pillar (fauce).** Another muscle of the throat or pharynx forms the posterior pillar.

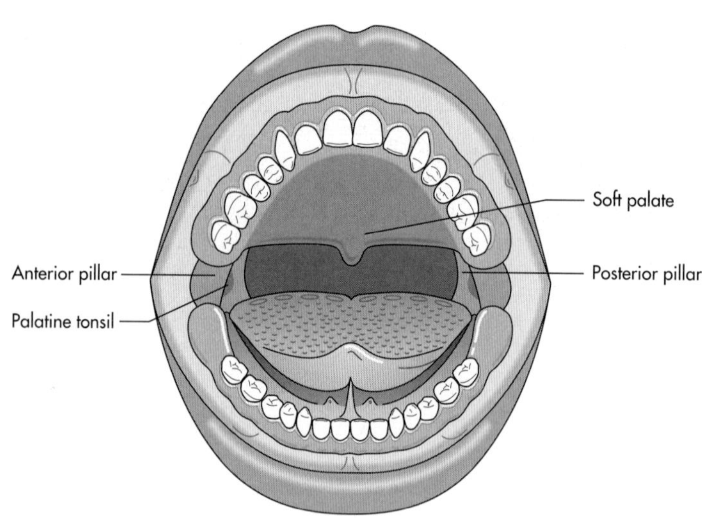

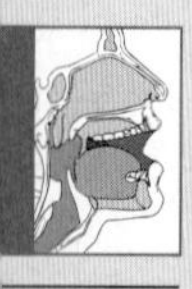

The extrinsic muscles of the tongue act to move the tongue in any direction needed for swallowing and speech. The muscles of the tongue are all innervated by the hypoglossal nerve, CN XII.

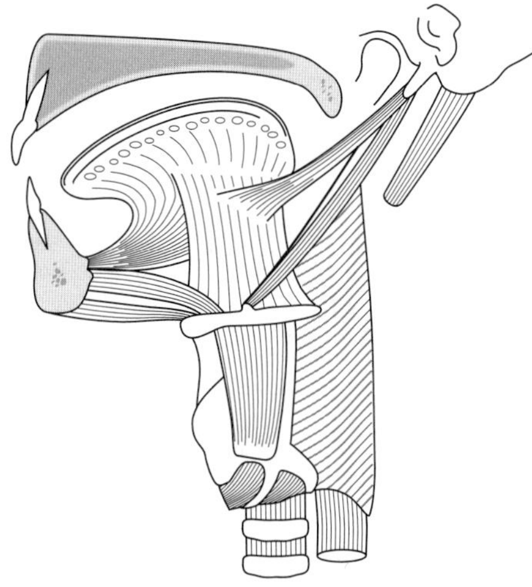

Review the muscles of the tongue. Find each on the drawing. What are their origins and insertions? Actions? Innervation? Check your answers in the preceding text.

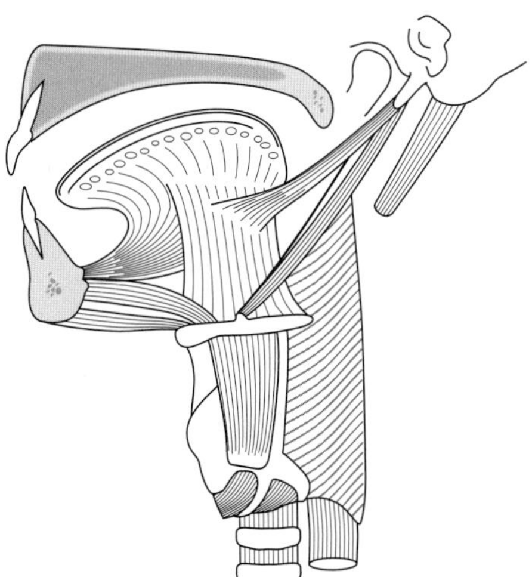

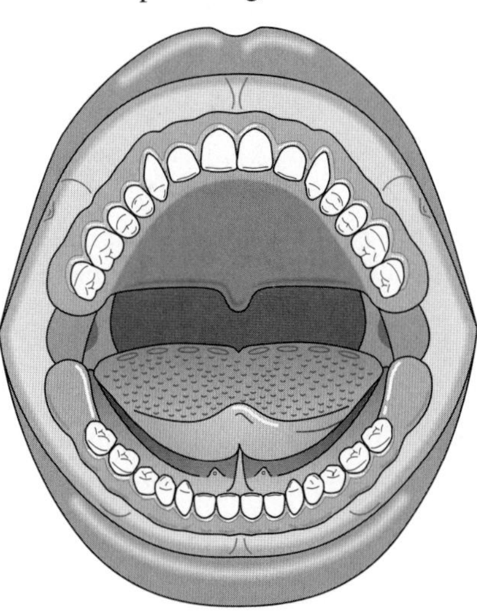

Hyoglossus
O: hyoid
I: tongue

Genioglossus
O: genial tubercles
I: tongue

Styloglossus
O: styloid process
I: tongue

Palatoglossus
O: soft palate
I: tongue

Action for all is movement of tongue during speech and swallowing.

Innerration for all is CN XII.

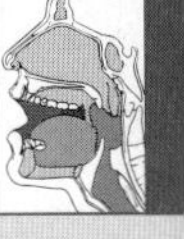

6.0 MUSCLES OF THE PHARYNX

The pharynx, or food tube, begins where the oral cavity ends. Locate the pharynx on the sagittal section of the head. Where are the oral cavity, oropharynx, nasopharynx, and pharynx proper located?

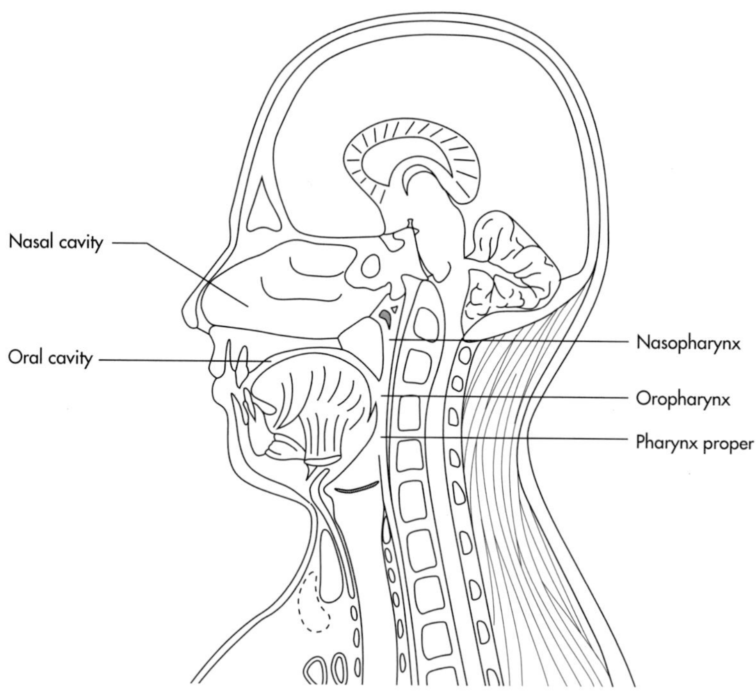

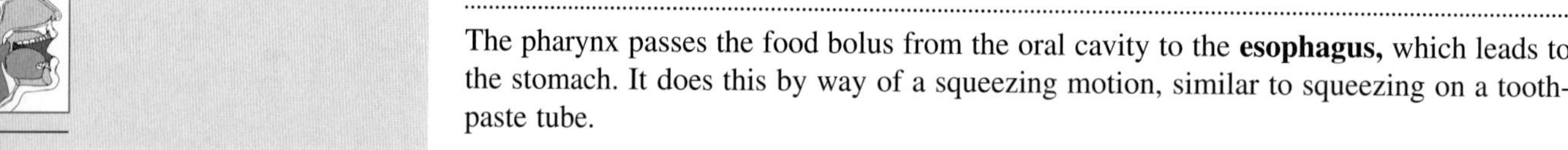

The **pharynx** is a muscular tube. It is lined with mucosa, but the outer portion is wrapped with muscle fibers in almost a circular pattern.

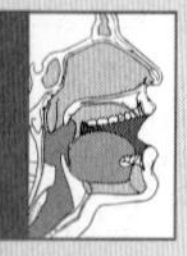

The pharynx passes the food bolus from the oral cavity to the **esophagus,** which leads to the stomach. It does this by way of a squeezing motion, similar to squeezing on a toothpaste tube.

The muscular action of the pharynx is called constriction and is passed downward by the "rings" of muscles called **constrictors.** Find them in the drawing.

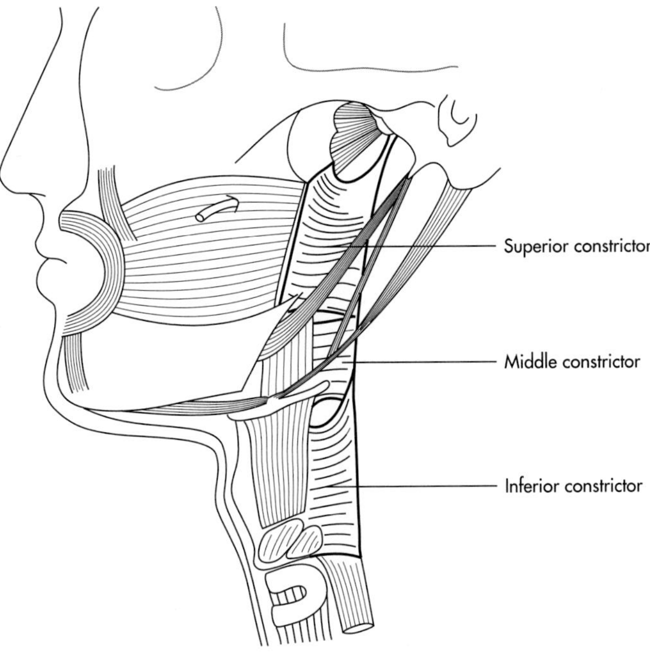

Actions of the pharynx become involuntary at the junction of the oral cavity and pharynx. The constrictors are innervated by CN X, the vagus nerve.

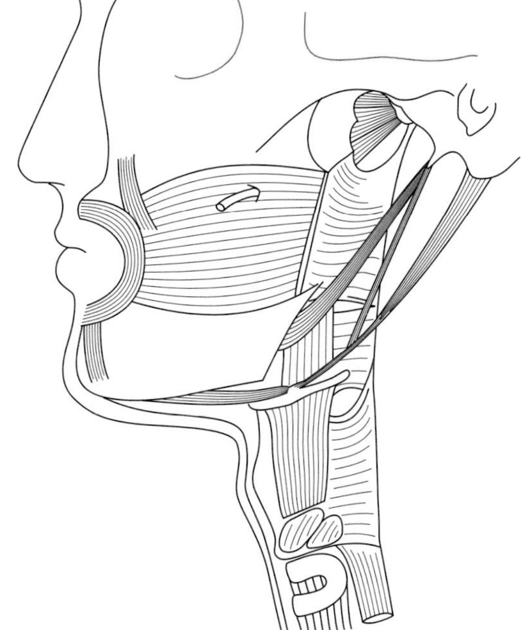

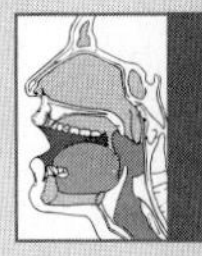

constrictors

There are three sets of ______________, named by location: the **superior, middle,** and **inferior** pharyngeal constrictors. Find and color them in on the drawing.

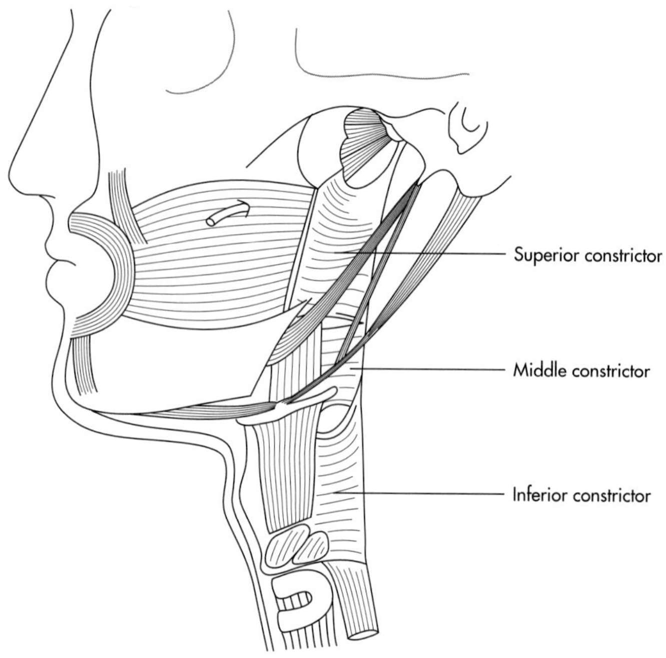

smooth

As the muscular tissue of the pharynx begins, it is composed of striated skeletal muscle, and as it passes from superior to middle to inferior constrictor, it gains smooth muscle and loses skeletal muscle. Which type of muscle is traditionally involuntary in nature?

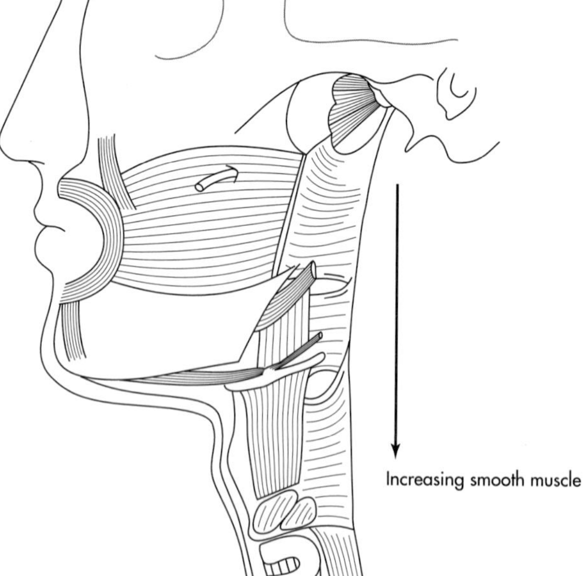

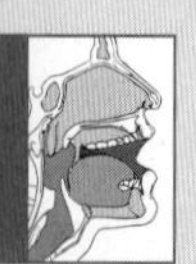

Let's look at the area where the oral cavity and oropharynx meet. Which constrictor lies here? The superior constrictor and buccinator muscle of the cheek meet in a tendinous cord in the back of the mouth here. What is it called?

superior, pterygomandibular raphe

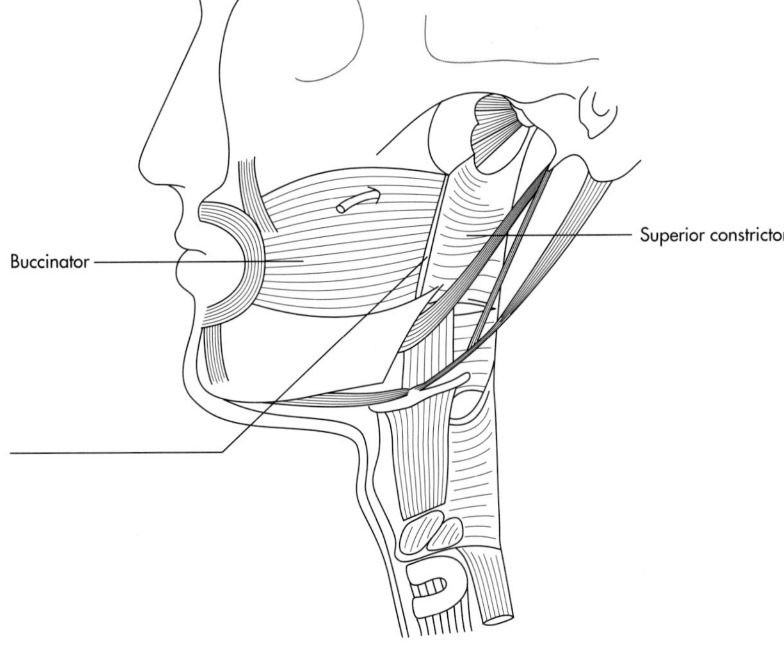

This connection between the ______________ and ______________ muscles runs from the pterygoid plate to the mandible. What other structure do you see piercing the buccinator muscle?

superior constrictor, buccinator, Stensen's duct

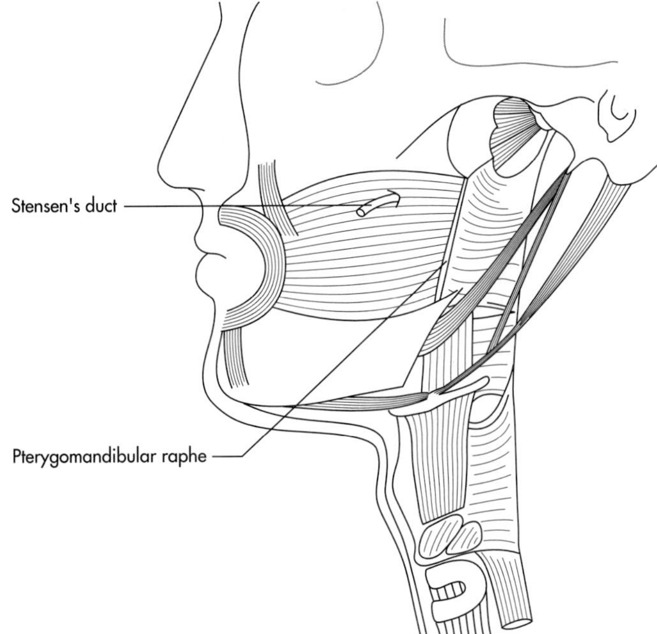

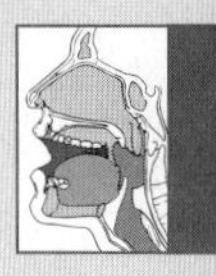

6.1

Palatine Muscles

soft palate

What portion of the palate contains muscle tissue? Find this, as well as the nasopharynx, oropharynx, and oral cavity, on the sagittal section.

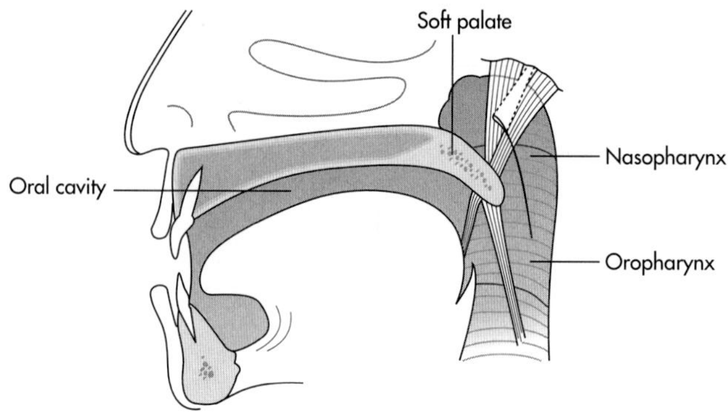

The **soft palate,** which is posterior to the hard palate, forms a wall dividing the oral and nasal cavities. The soft palate is filled with fat, glands, connective tissue, and muscles. It acts as a "flap" that seals the nasopharynx off from the oropharynx during a swallow, so that food does not pass into the nasal cavity. It does this by stretching out and raising up against the pharyngeal wall (the area of the superior constrictor). Diagrams of the soft palate at rest and in contraction are shown.

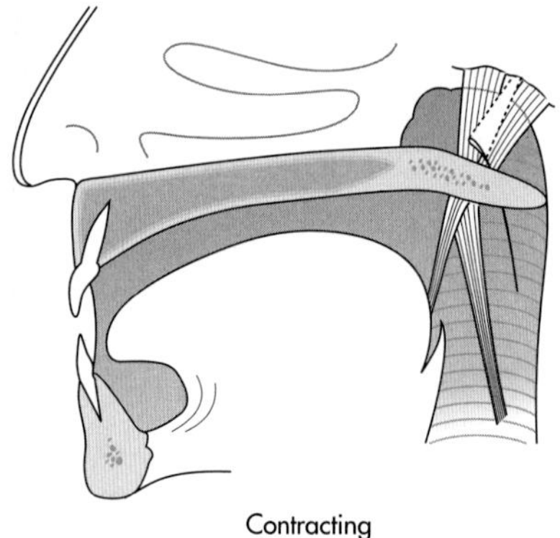

Contracting

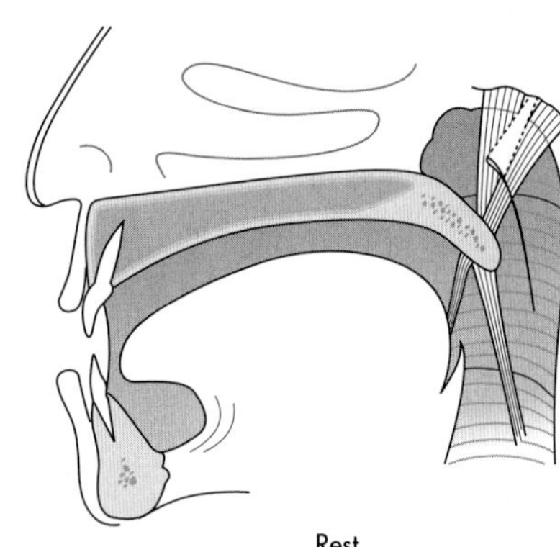

Rest

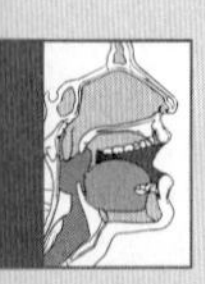

stretching out and raising the palate to seal off the nasopharynx

What is the function (action) of the soft palate muscles?

Two muscles are responsible for stretching and raising the soft palate. We look at them from different views, as they originate from the base of the skull and are difficult to visualize. The first view is of a sagittal section.

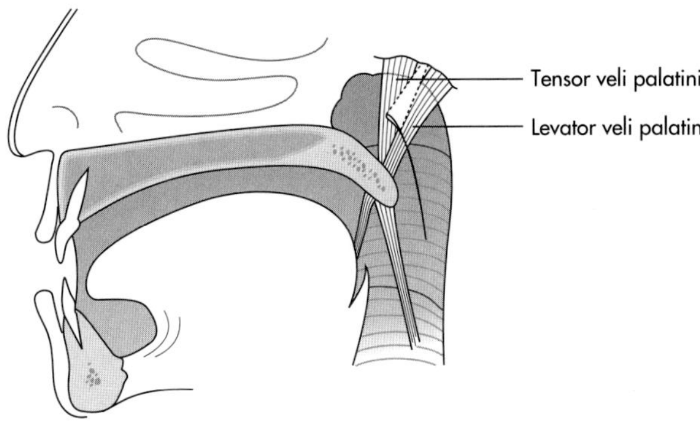

And the second view is of the palate from the rear, as though one were standing on the back of the tongue looking out the oral and nasal cavities.

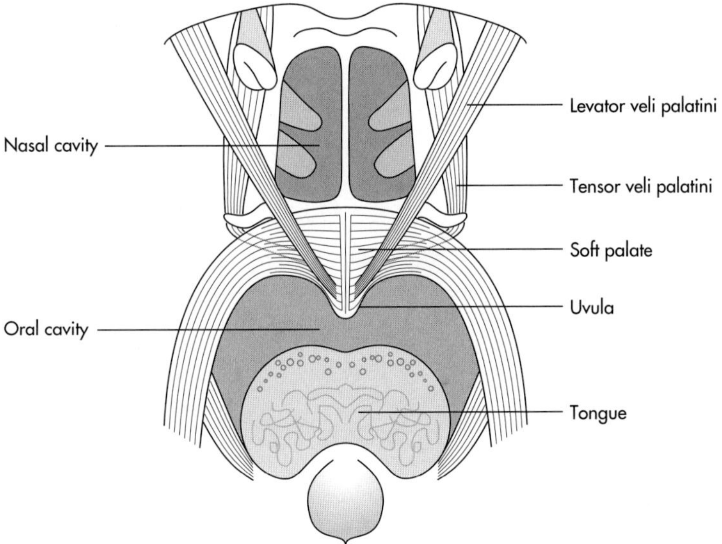

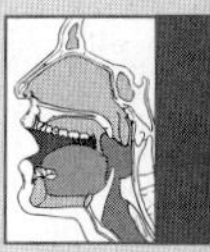

The first palatal muscle is the **levator veli palatini (LVP) muscle.** There are two and each originates on the base of the cranium, passes down toward the soft palate, and inserts on its superior aspect from the right and left sides. Find it below and color in.

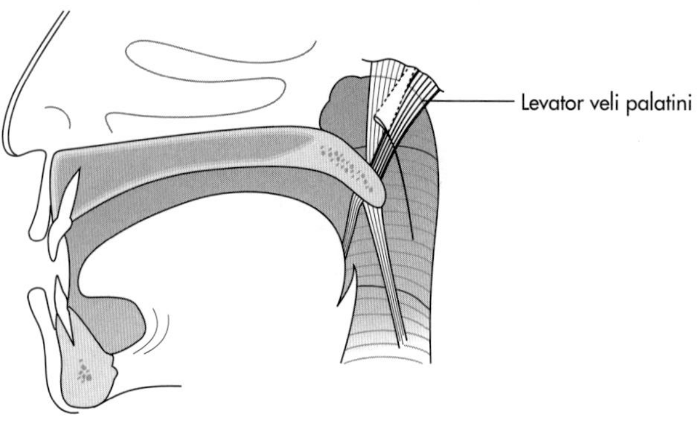

LVP

Find the ______________ on this drawing. It raises the soft palate during swallows and also functions during speech.

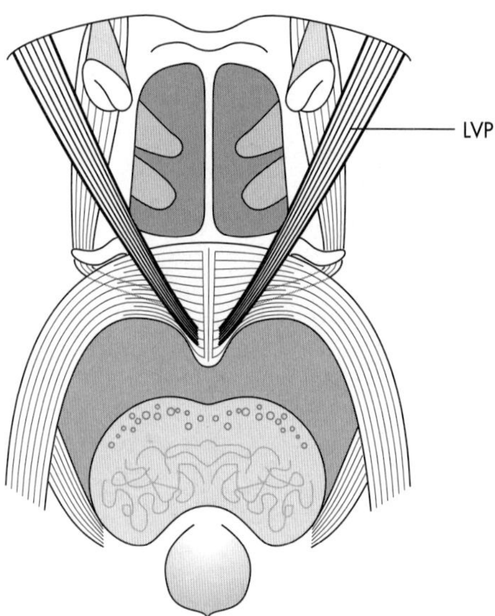

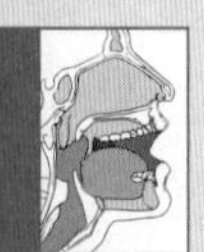

The **tensor veli palatini (TVP)** is the second main palatal muscle and it acts to stretch or tense the soft palate during swallowing and speech. Find it and color it in. Note that it is a "two-belly" muscle.

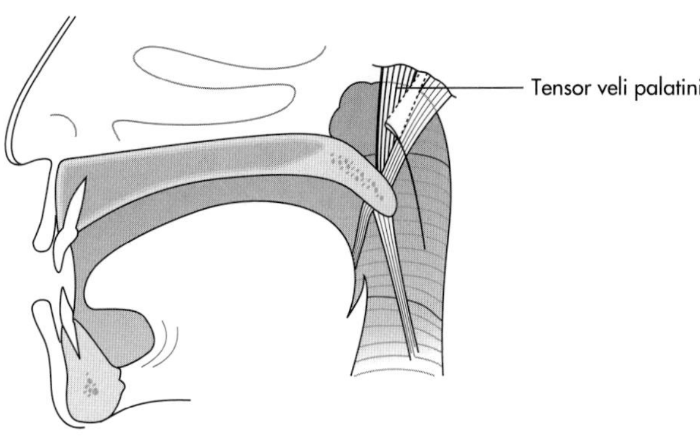

The ________________ is also a paired muscle. It originates from the base of the cranium and passes down to the palatal structures from the right and left, called the hamuli. It is a tendon at this point, hooking around the hamulus.

TVP

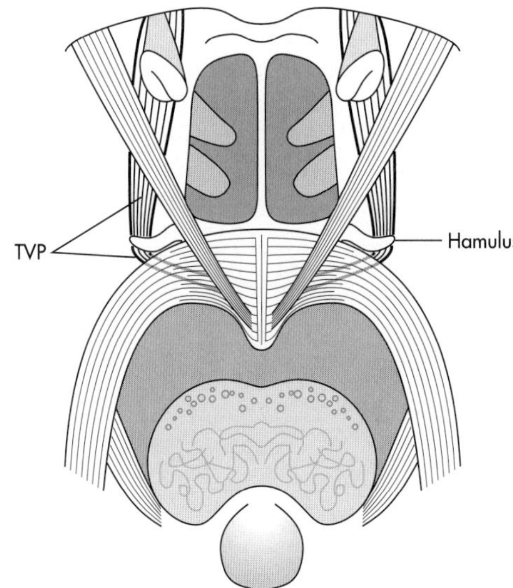

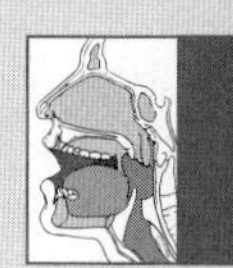

hamulus

The TVP then makes a right angle turn around the _______________ bone, like a pulley, and widens back out in a second belly to insert on either side of the soft palate.

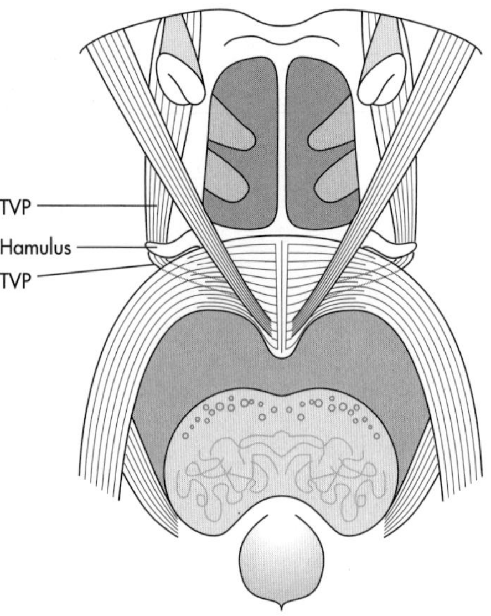

Another portion off of the superior belly of the TVP inserts into the Eustachian or tympanic tube. Not only does the palate tense during a swallow, but also the Eustachian tube is opened. Some anatomists consider this a separate muscle **(dilator tubae).** Find this portion of the TVP on the picture.

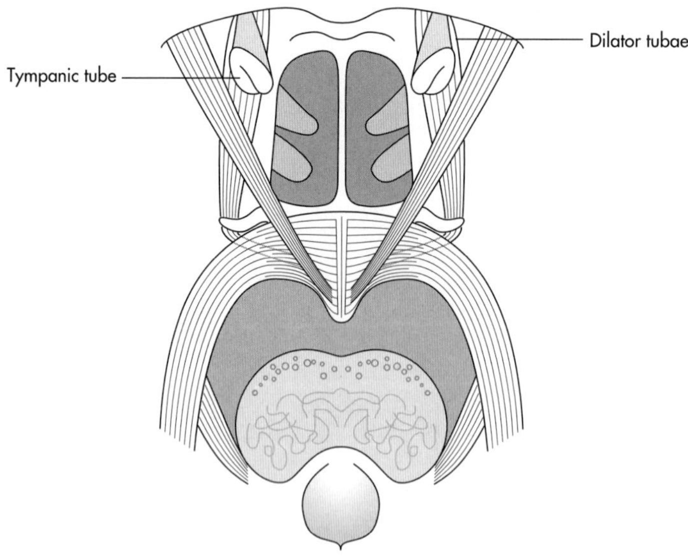

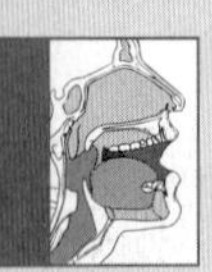

Find the LVP and TVP on the drawings. What are their functions?

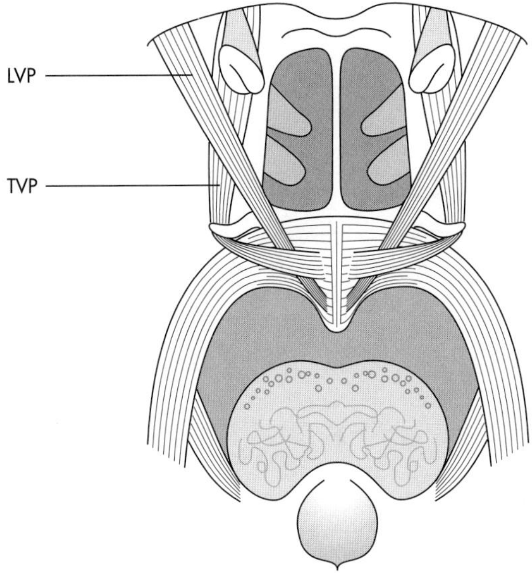

The functions for LVP and TVP are raising and stretching the palate during speech and swallowing. TVP opens the Eustachian tube.

The TVP and LVP tense and raise the soft palate during a swallow. A second action of TVP is to open the tympanic tube during a swallow. The TVP is innervated by CN V and the LVP is innervated by CN VII.

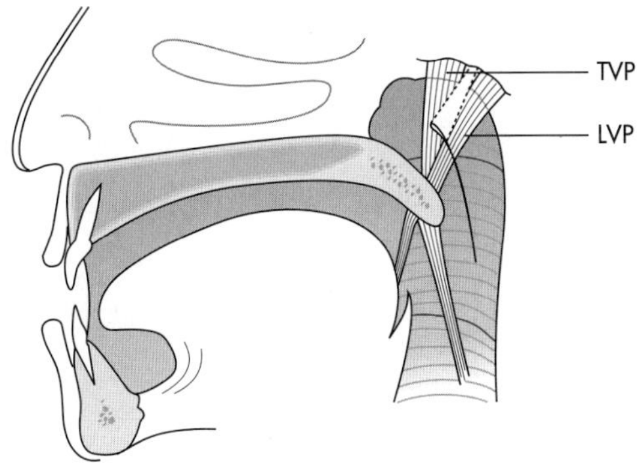

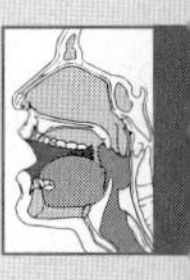

Two accessory palatal muscles are the palatopharyngeus and salpingopharyngeus. The **salpingopharyngeus** is a small muscle originating on the orifice of the tympanic tube and inserting onto the pharyngeal wall. Its function is unclear.

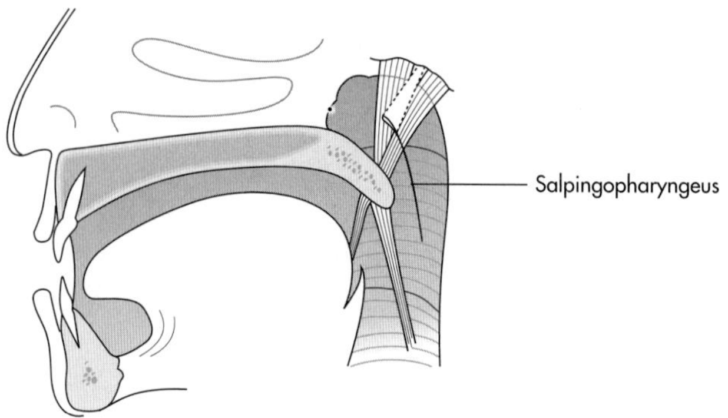

posterior

The **palatopharyngeus** is the ______________ pillar or fauce of the oral cavity. It originates on the soft palate and inserts into the pharyngeal wall. It may be active during swallowing to help the TVP and LVP.

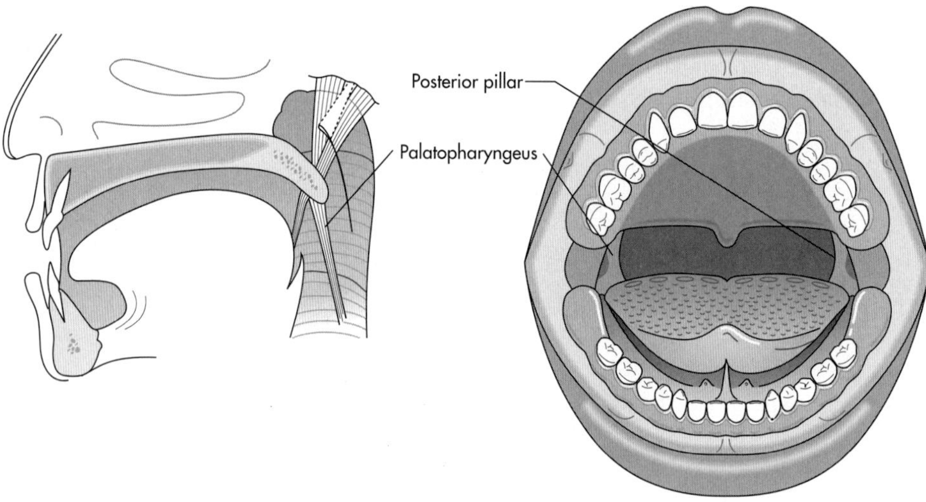

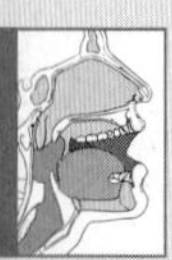

Review the muscles of the pharynx and palate by identifying them in the drawings. What are their origins and insertions? Actions? Check your answers with the preceding text.

LVP
O: base of cranium
I: soft palate
A: raises palate

TVP
O: base of cranium
I: soft palate
A: raises palate

Salpingopharyngeus
O: tympanic tube
I: pharnyx
A: unknown

Palatopharyngeus
O: pharnyx
I: soft palate
A: helps raise and tense palate

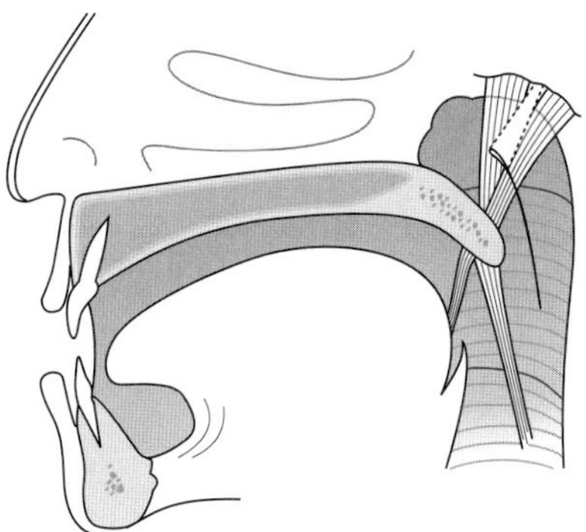

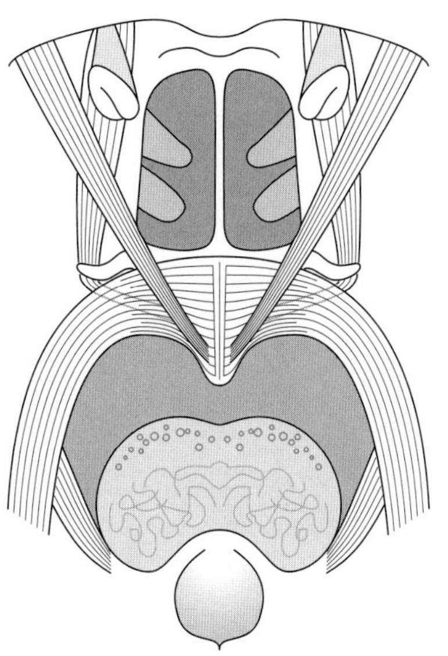

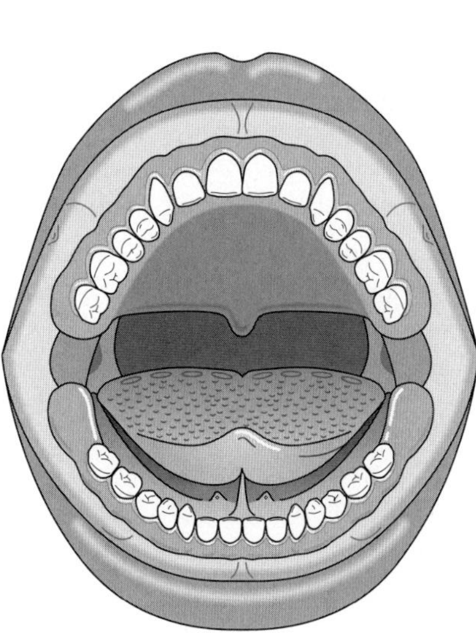

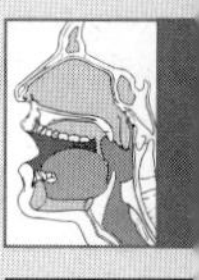

REVIEW TEST 8.1

SELECT OR FILL IN THE CORRECT ANSWER.

1. The stable end of a muscle's attachment is its ______________.
2. Muscles do work by contraction, and the muscle gets longer. True or false?
3. The muscles of facial expression are innervated by the
   a. facial nerve
   b. trigeminal nerve
   c. vagus nerve
   d. hypoglossal nerve
4. Subcutaneous muscles responsible for human and primate nonverbal communication are called
   a. muscles of mastication
   b. posterior neck muscles
   c. anterior neck muscles
   d. muscles of facial expression
5. Closing the eyes is the action of which muscles?
   a. orbicularis oris b. orbicularis occuli
   c. levators d. mentalis
6. The muscles that create a "pout" are called the
   a. orbicularis oris b. orbicularis occuli
   c. levators d. mentalis
7. A muscle that creates a "grimace" is the ______________ muscle.
8. Temporalis originates in the ______________ fossa.
9. Mylohyoid originates along the ______________ lines of the mandible.
10. Digastric muscle inserts on the ______________ fossae of the mandible.

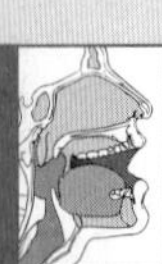

REVIEW TEST 8.2

SELECT OR FILL IN THE CORRECT ANSWER.

1. The nerve that exits the brain under the ear and spreads out across the superficial face to innervate its muscles is the ______________ nerve, or CN ______________.
2. Which structure is not superficial (directly beneath the skin)?
   a. parotid gland b. medial pterygoid muscle
   c. platysma muscle d. CN VII
3. Which muscle of mastication does not have the primary function of elevation?
4. Which two of these muscles have fibers that run parallel to each other and have the same action?
   a. lateral pterygoid c. medial pterygoid
   d. platysma e. masseter

5. Which masticatory muscle maintains tension on the temporomandibular disk?
6. Contraction of one lateral pterygoid results in ______________ movement of the mandible. Contraction of both results in ______________.
7. If one of the sternocleidomastoid muscles contracts, what happens to the head?
8. The SCM is used as a landmark for finding structures of the neck. True or false?
9. What is not a function of the anterior neck muscles?
   a. depression of the jaw
   b. support of hyoid
   c. help with swallowing
   d. elevation of mandible
10. Muscles found above the hyoid bone are ______________ muscles and those found below it are ______________ muscles.

REVIEW TEST 8.3

MATCH THE ACTION WITH THE MUSCLE GROUP.

1. elevation of mandible ______________	a. muscles of facial expression
2. support of the head ______________	b. suprahyoids
3. depression of mandible ______________	c. muscles of pharynx
4. expression ______________	d. muscles of mastication
5. passing food down ______________	e. posterior neck muscles

REVIEW TEST 8.4

MATCH THE ORIGIN WITH THE MUSCLE.

1. genial tubercle ______________	a. medial pterygoid
2. sternum ______________	b. masseter
3. pterygoid plate ______________	c. sternohyoid
4. zygomatic process ______________	d. genioglossus

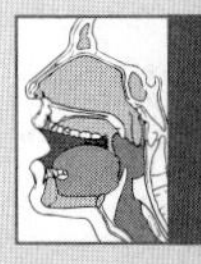

REVIEW TEST 8.5

MATCH THE INSERTION WITH THE MUSCLE.

1. tongue ______________	a. styloglossus
2. condyle ______________	b. masseter
3. angle of mandible ______________	c. lateral pterygoid
4. hyoid bone ______________	d. sternohyoid

REVIEW TEST 8.6

MATCH THE NERVE WITH THE MUSCLE IT INNERVATES.

1. pharynx ______________ a. CN V
2. masseter ______________ b. CN VII
3. trapezius ______________ c. CN X
4. genioglossus ______________ d. CN XI
5. buccinator ______________ e. CN XII

REVIEW TEST 8.7

SELECT OR FILL IN THE CORRECT ANSWER.

1. The floor of the mouth is formed by which muscle?
2. Name three things that originate off of the styloid process.
3. Name two muscles that originate from the genial tubercles.
4. Name two muscles that attach to the mastoid process.
5. Which structure is not found in the anterior neck?
   a. cervical vertebrae b. infrahyoids
   c. trachea d. esophagus
6. Name two two-belly muscles of the anterior neck.
7. The word *glossus* means ______________.
8. Which muscle does not belong to the group?
   a. omohyoid b. sternohyoid
   c. sternothyroid d. stylohyoid

REVIEW TEST 8.8

ANSWER THE FOLLOWING QUESTIONS.

1. Match:
   i. anterior pillar ______________ a. palatoglossus
   ii. posterior pillar ______________ b. palatopharyngeus
2. What tubular structure is found in the nasopharynx and is activated by the TVP?
3. The two main muscles of the soft palate are TVP and LVP. Which one elevates it?
4. The squeezing action of the pharyngeal muscles is done by the constrictors under the involuntary control of CN XI. True or false?

5. Which two muscles meet at the pterygomandibular raphe?
6. What structure pierces the buccinator muscle to enter the oral cavity?
7. What muscle wraps around the hamuli?

REVIEW TEST 8.9

LABEL THE DIAGRAMS.

1.

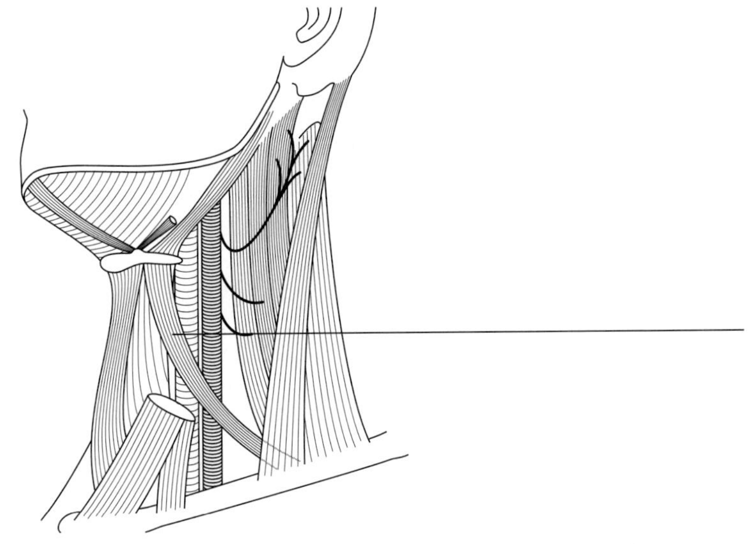

2.

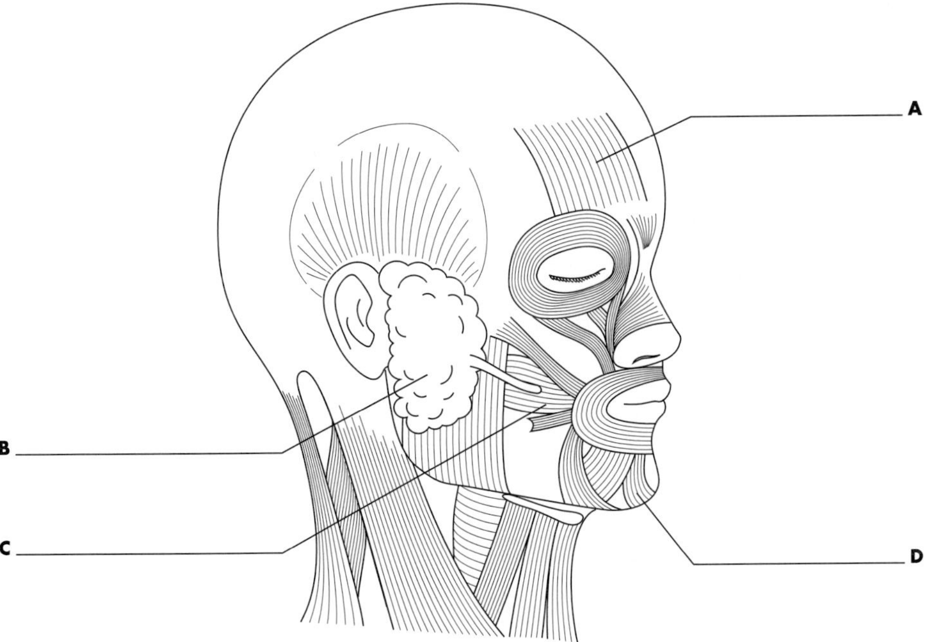

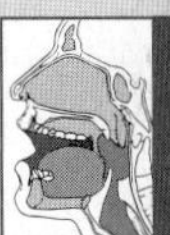

3.

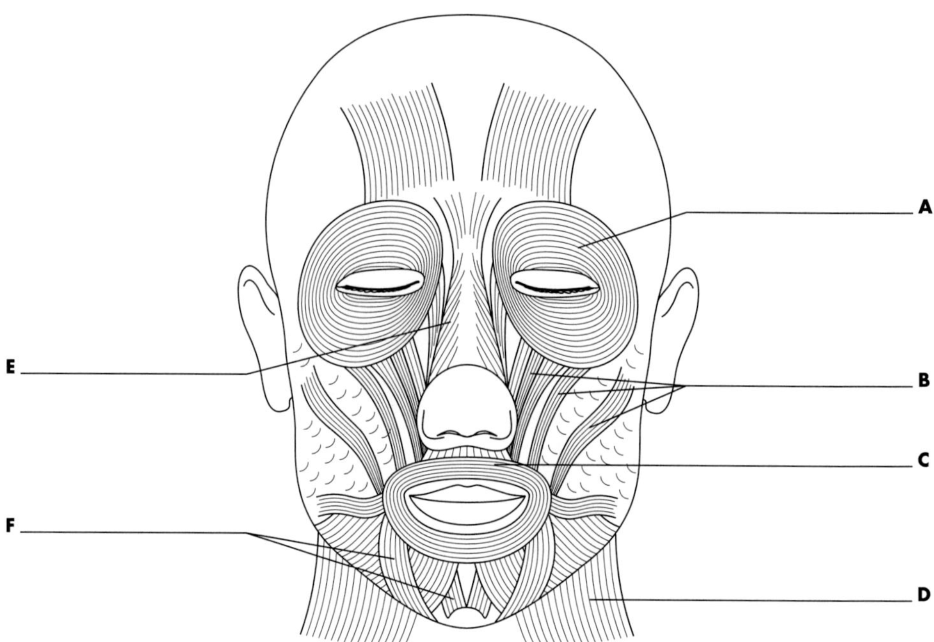

4.

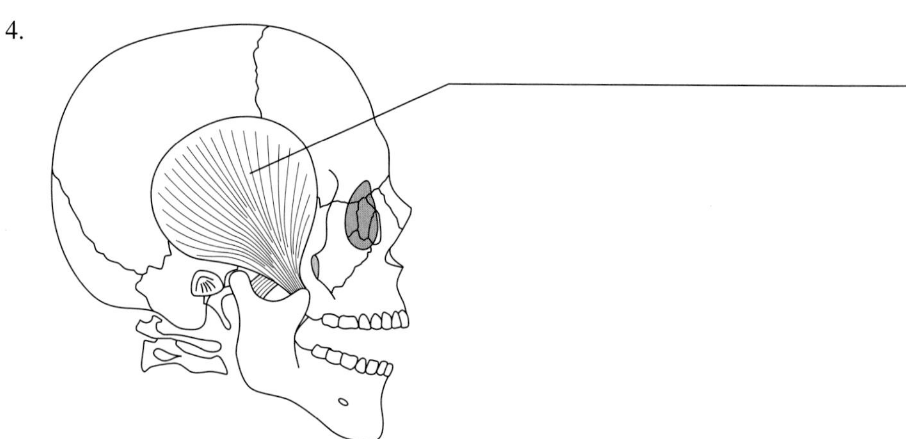

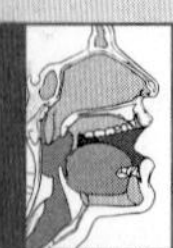

5.

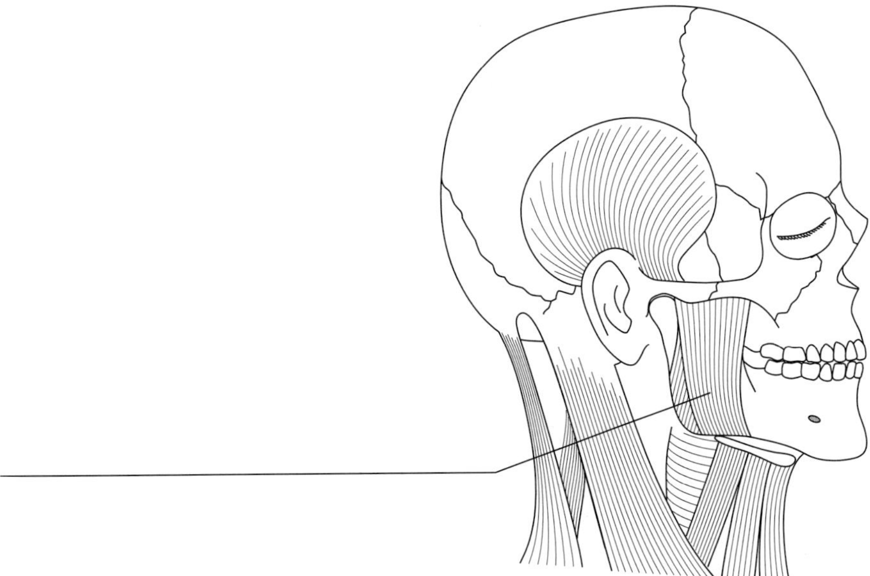

6.

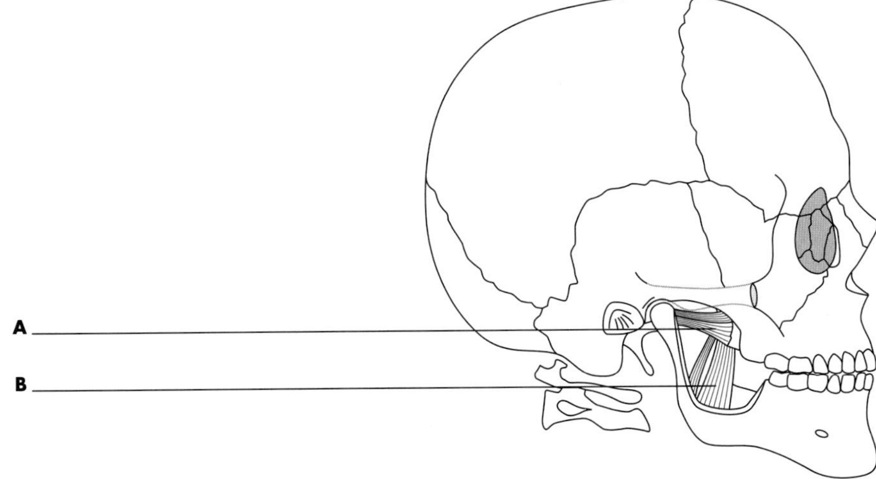

7.

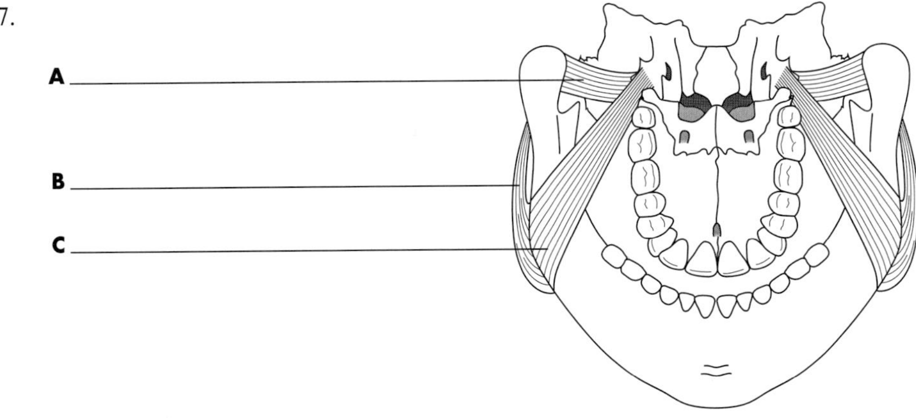

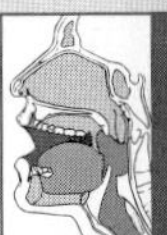

8.

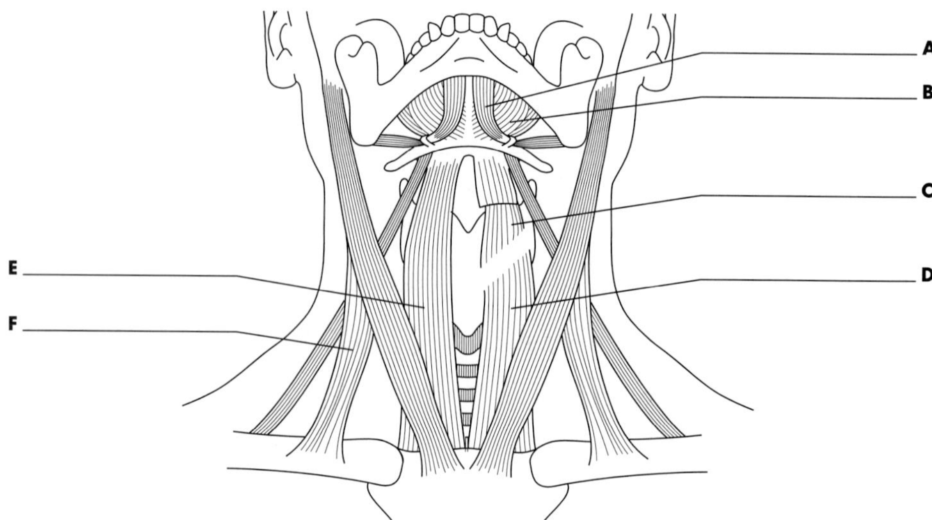

9.

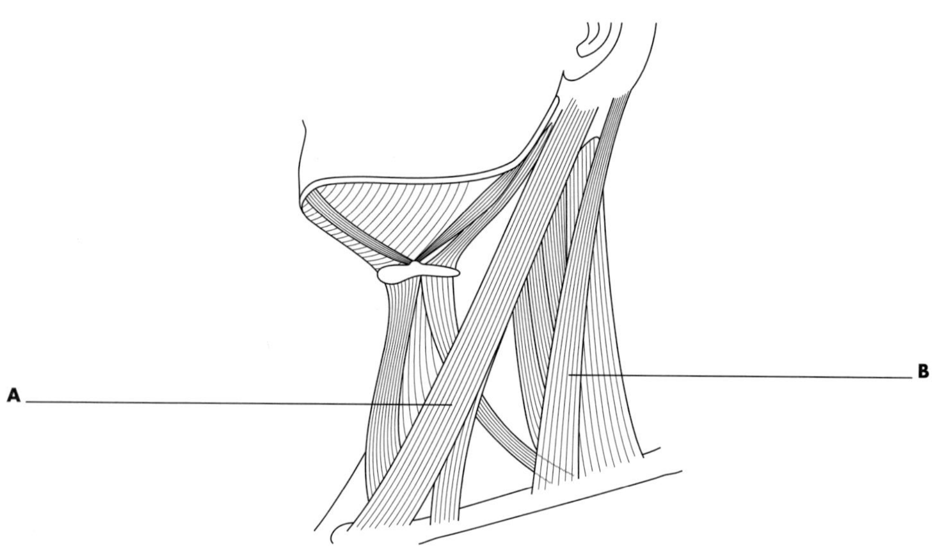

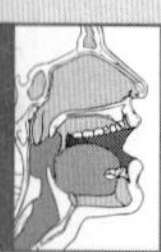

10.

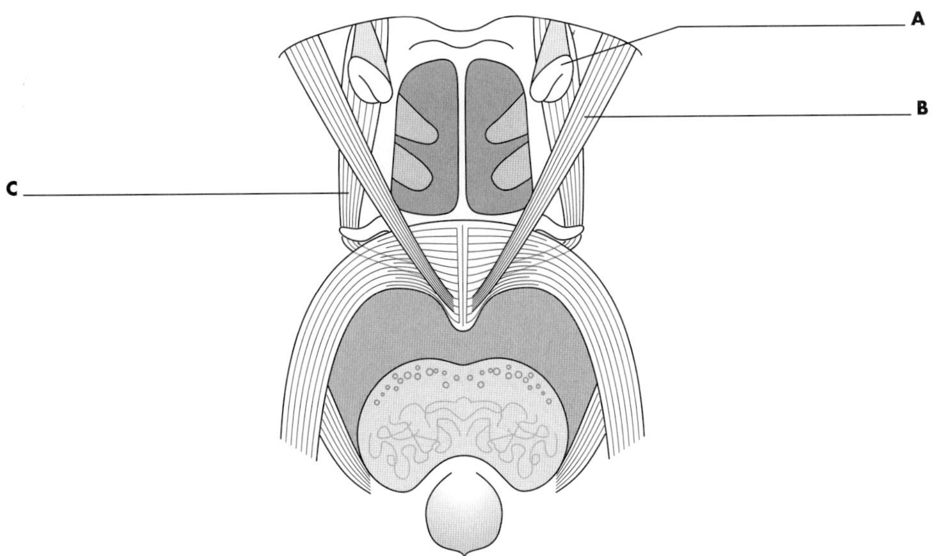

11.

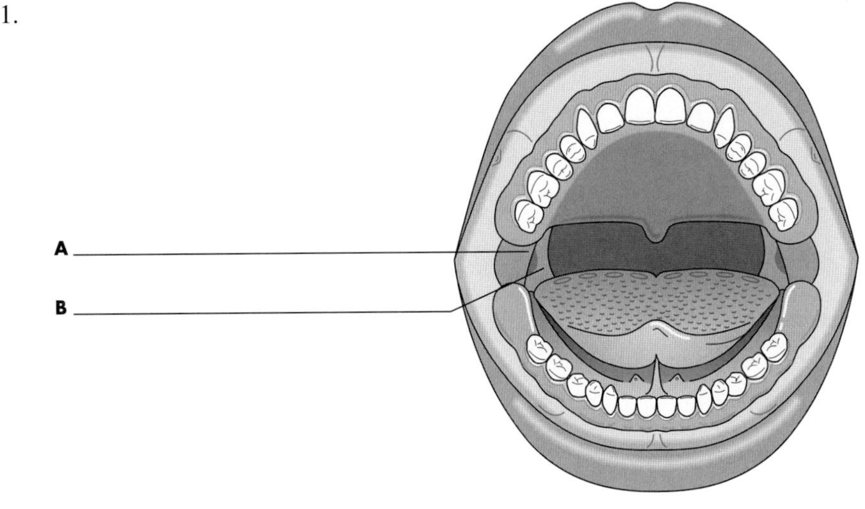

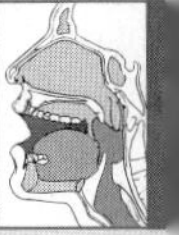

12.

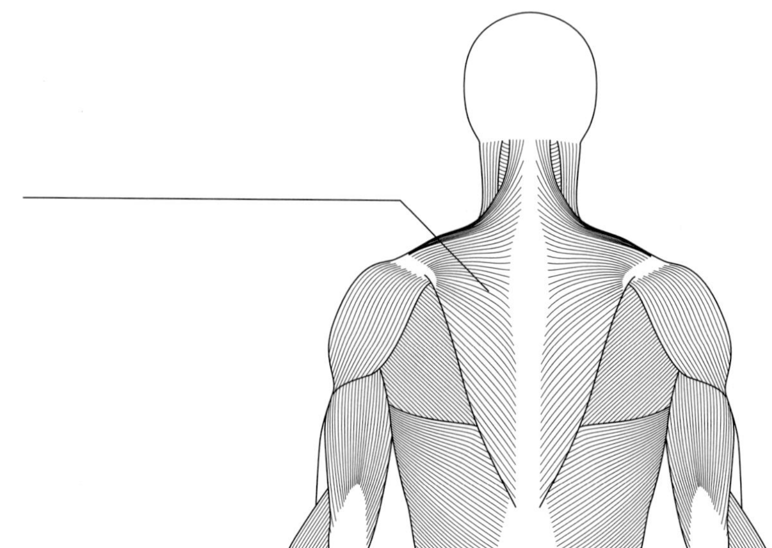

13.

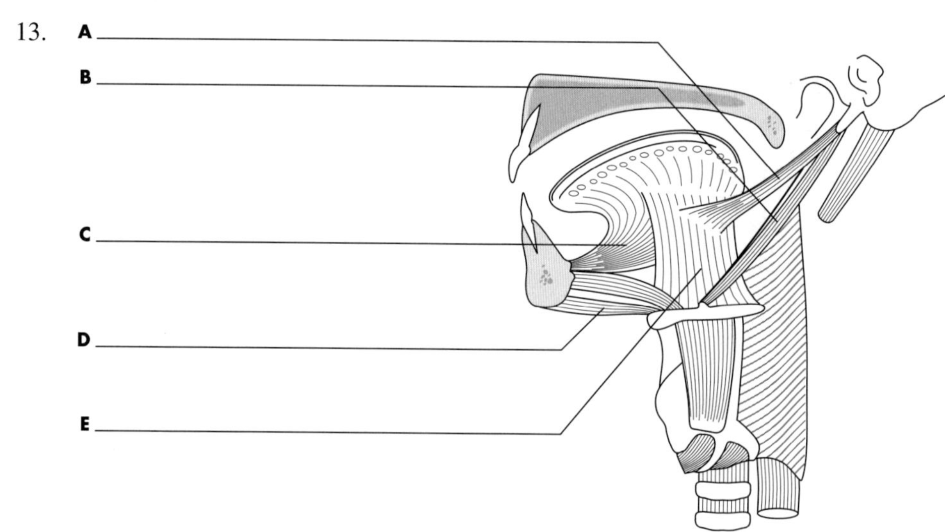

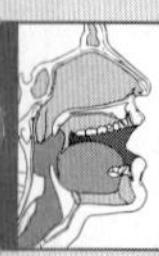

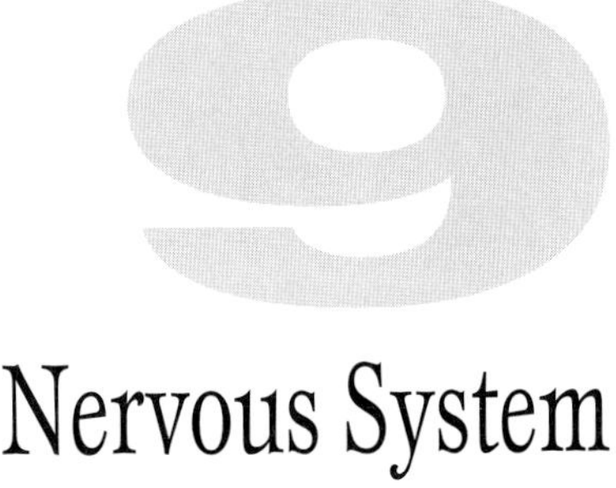

Nervous System

The representation of the nervous system in the head and neck is considerable. The command center of the central and peripheral nervous systems, the **brain,** as well as the **cervical spinal cord and nerves,** is the subject for study. Paired nerves from the brain and brainstem called the **cranial nerves** are also looked at.

First let us review the basic structure of the nervous system as we began in Chapter One. The basic cellular unit of the nervous system is called a ______________. These cells, when strung together in pathways, build that "wiring" of the body together known as the nervous system.

neuron

This drawing represents a **neuron.** In actuality, neurons come in many different shapes and with differing numbers of processes. These cell processes are extensions of the cell that aid in passing a neurochemical signal through the cell and toward another. Processes that receive signals are dendrites and those that send signals away from the cell body are ______________.

axons

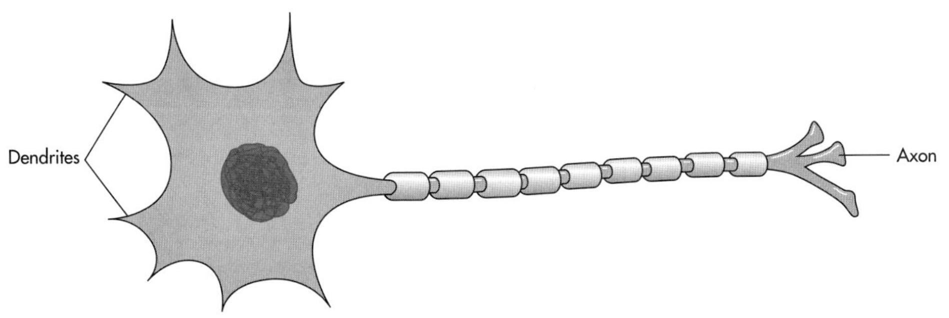

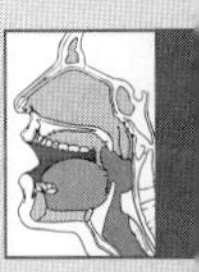

Draw an arrow in the direction that a signal will be passed down this cell.

A neurochemical signal is passed from one cell to another by chemically jumping the gap or **synapse** between them.

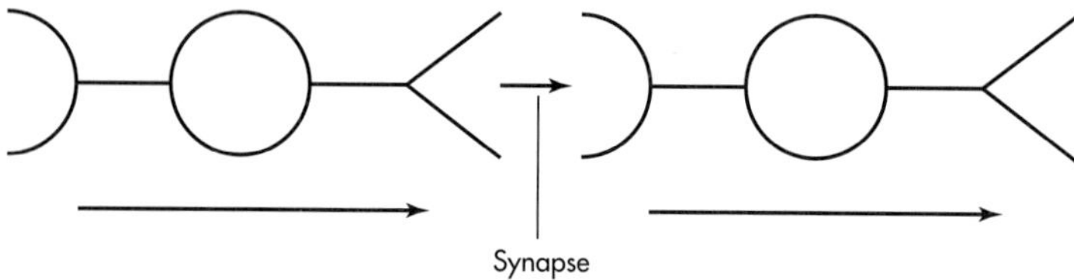

We represent **neuronal pathways** with the symbols that stand for the neuron, axon, and dendrite.

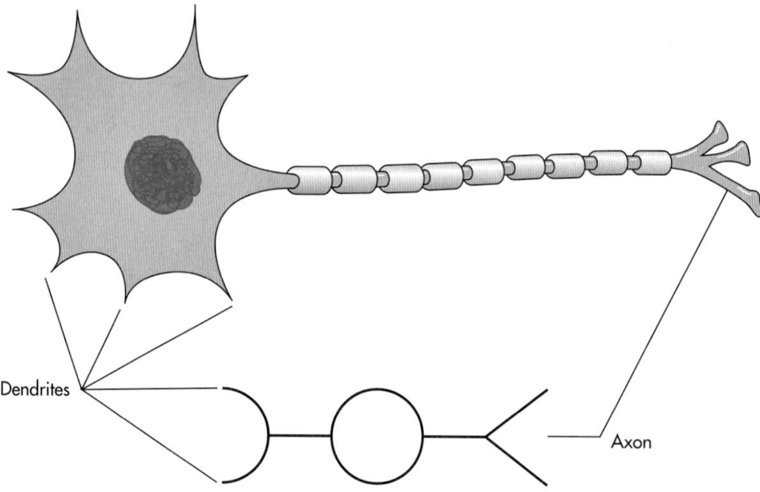

A simple pathway is shown. Remember that each symbol represents several neurons bundled together as a **nerve.**

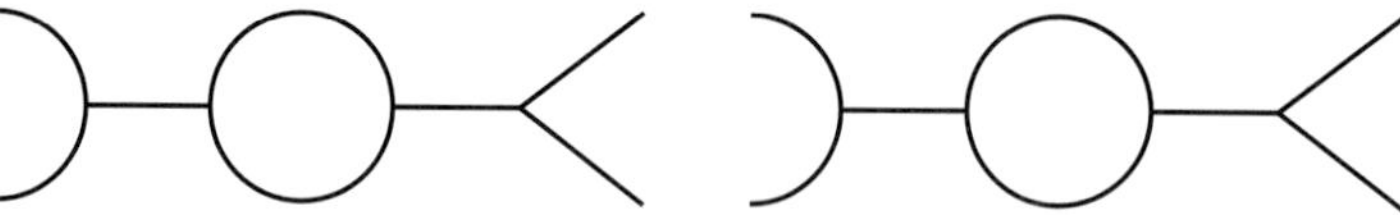

Two-neuron pathway

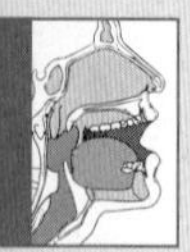

sensory neurons

Neurons are used to sense the environment and to cause a proper response or effect to it. Thus we have two basic neuron types: **sensory neurons (affector)** and **motor neurons (effector).** Which type would tell the body what is going on around it?

Sensation is reception of stimuli from either the outside or inner environment of the body. **Sensory neurons** come in many varied forms to accomplish this job, from the simplest pain receptors to the highly developed rod and cone cells of the eye for vision. Sensation includes:

1. Pain, touch (simple and fine), pressure, thermal, chemical, proprioception
2. Smell
3. Taste
4. Vision
5. Hearing and balance

Sensory pathways begin with **reception** of information. So which end of this sensory neuron is receiving?

dendrite end

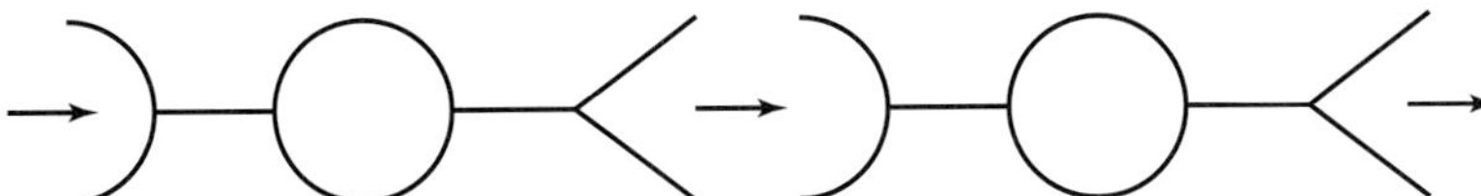

As sensation is gathered by the nervous system it must use this information to respond. The response is handled by **motor neurons.** Motor neurons cause an effect by one of two actions: (1) causing a muscle to contract or (2) causing a gland to secrete. This motor neuron is causing an effect by passing a signal to a muscle. This causes the muscle to ______________.

contract

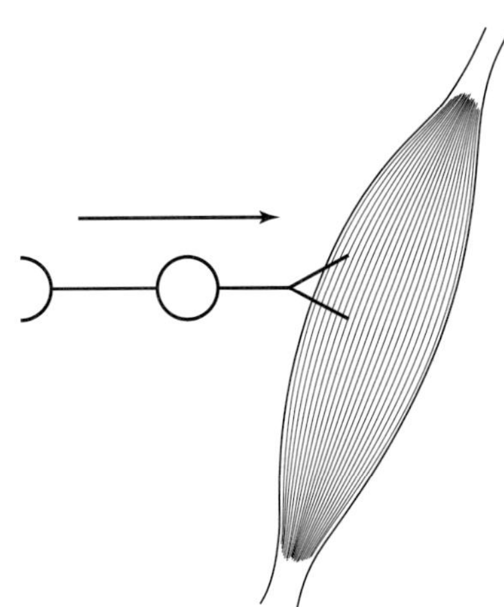

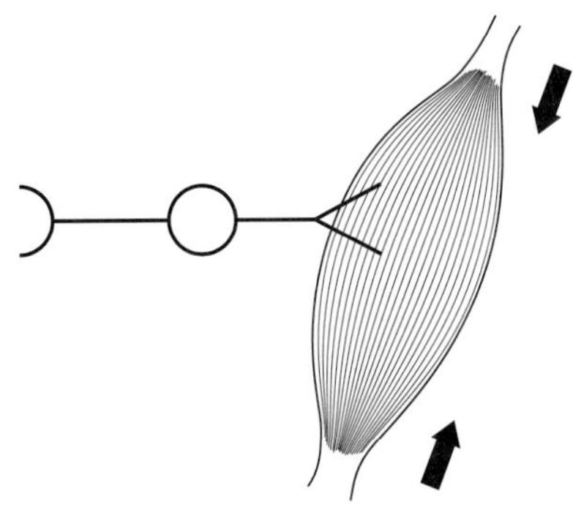

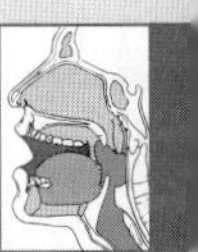

Shown here is a simple effect/response or **sensory/motor pathway.** The receptor of the sensory neuron is located on the surface of the skin. It is receiving a pain signal from the environment and passing it into the body. That signal then synapses to a motor neuron within the spinal cord and passes back out to the same body region, causing muscle contraction that pulls the body away from the pain source.

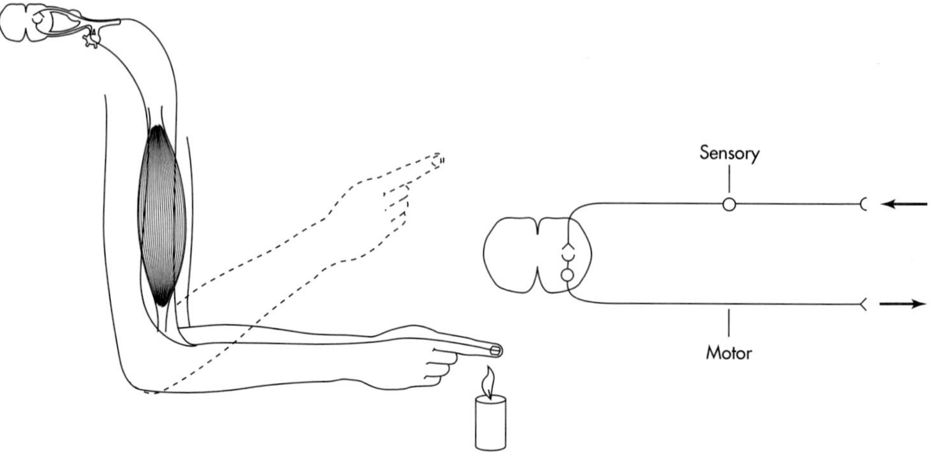

This simple two-neuron pathway is known as a **simple reflex.** Remember again that this represents several neurons bundled together in nerves.

Let's show where this neuronal pathway is in the body. The large oval shape to the right represents a section through the **spinal cord.** The spinal cord is a large tubular structure housed within the spinal column (don't confuse the two!). It contains many neuronal pathways and connections and, thus, neuron processes and cell bodies.

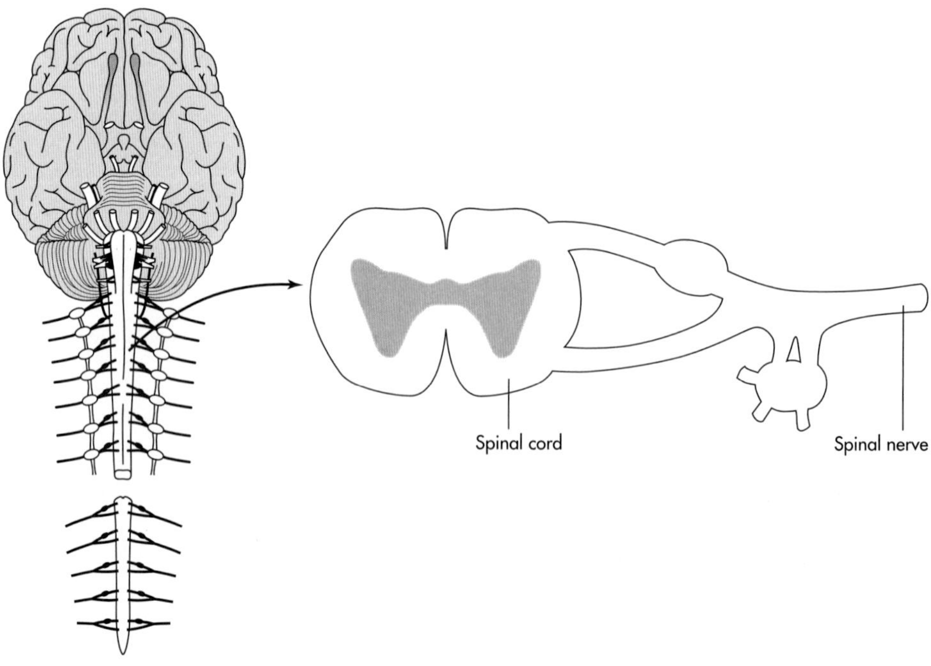

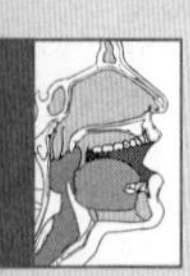

In this drawing we place the preceding simple reflex pathway in the spinal cord section. Note where the sensory neuron's processes and cell body lie.

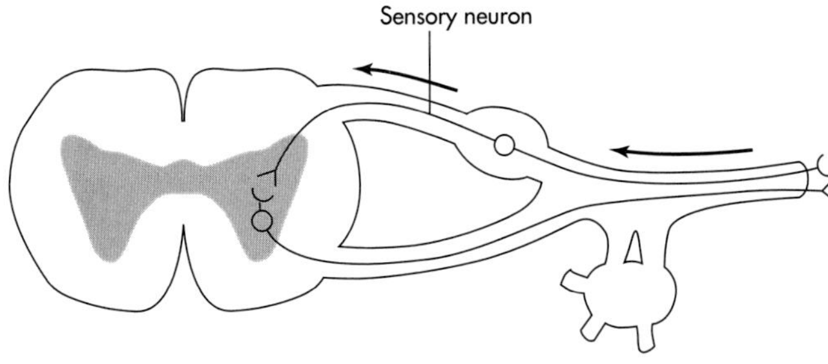

Now look for the motor neuron and its processes and cell body.

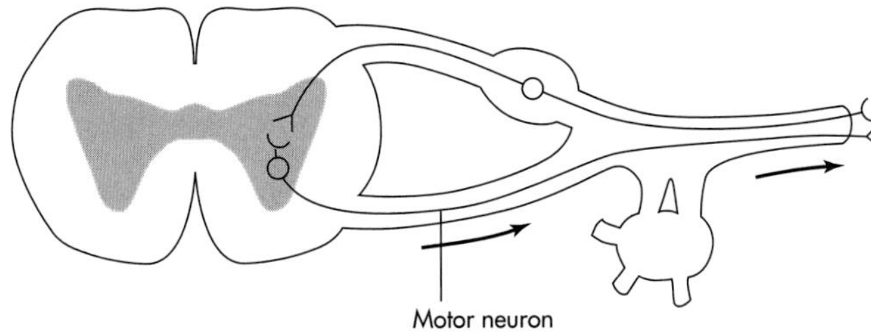

Sensory neuron cell bodies lie outside of the spinal cord. Motor neuron cell bodies lie within the spinal cord. A group of cell bodies (as shown below) is called a **ganglion** if it lies outside the central nervous system (CNS) (spinal cord and brain) and a **nucleus** if it lies within the CNS.

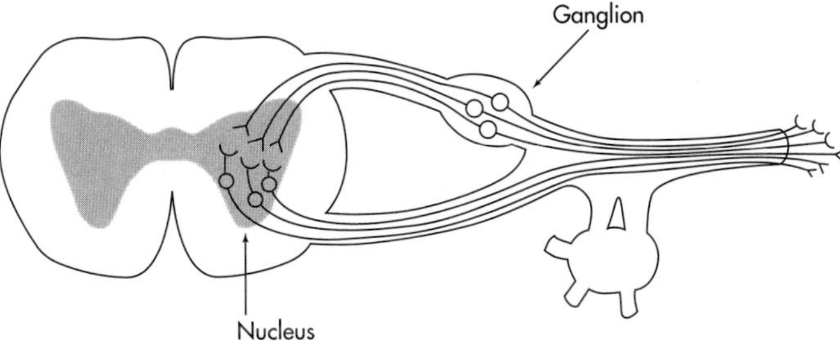

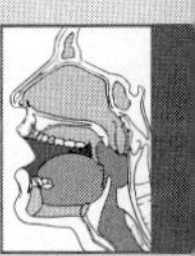

CNS

The sensory neuron may connect to the motor neuron by way of a third neuron called an **interneuron.** A three-neuron pathway is thus created. More complicated pathways are created by interposing more neurons between the sensory and motor neurons. One area for creating a more complex pathway is the spinal cord; another is the brain. Both constitute the ________________.

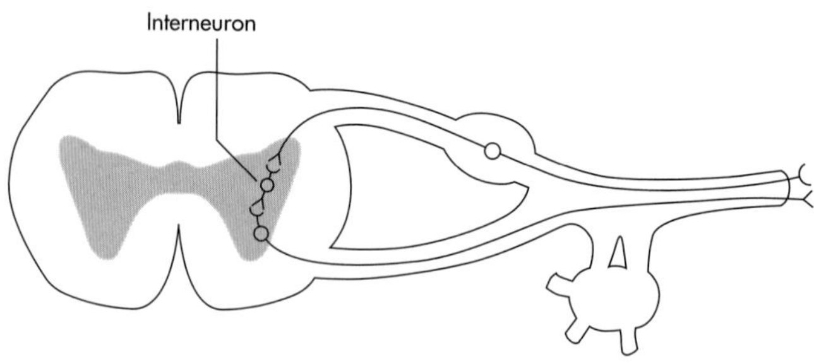

nerve

Remember that we have been symbolizing neuronal pathways by single cells when they are, in effect, multiple cells and processes. A bundle of cell processes, as shown, is called a ________________.

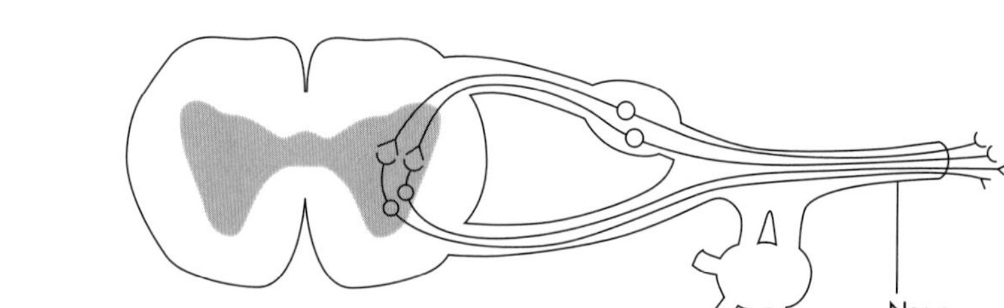

motor nerve

Because it contains only sensory neurons, this bundle of processes is called a **sensory nerve.** The other bundle contains only motor neurons and is called a ________________.

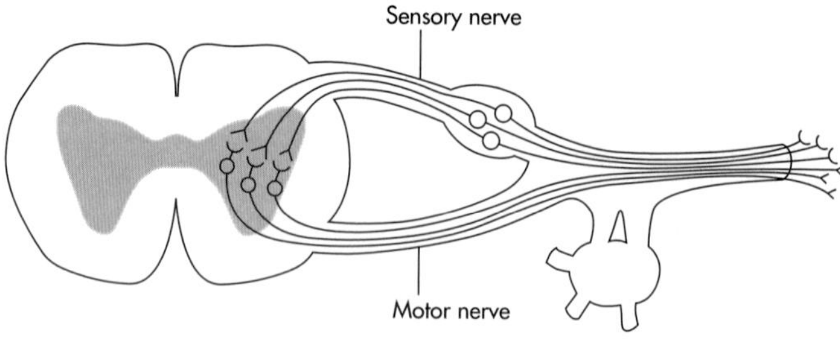

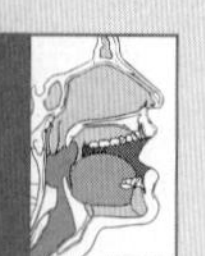

Sensory nerves and motor nerves may travel in the same "bundle" and are then called **mixed nerves.**

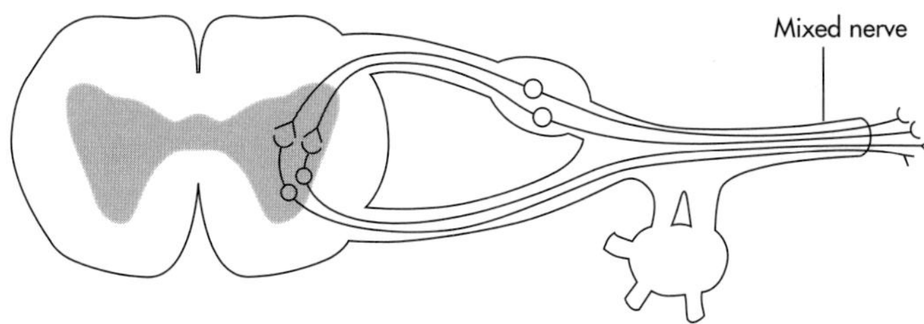

Nerves, then, come in three types: (1) ______________, (2) ______________, and (3) ______________.

1. sensory
2. motor
3. mixed

This is a ______________ nerve. Indicate the direction of signal flow with an arrow. Its cell body is located in a(n) ______________.

sensory, toward CNS, ganglion

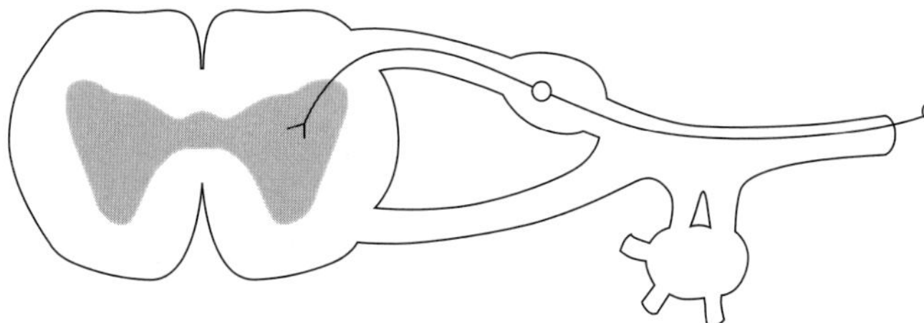

This is a ______________ nerve. Draw an arrow in the direction of signal flow. Its cell body lies in a(n) ______________.

motor, away from CNS, nucleus

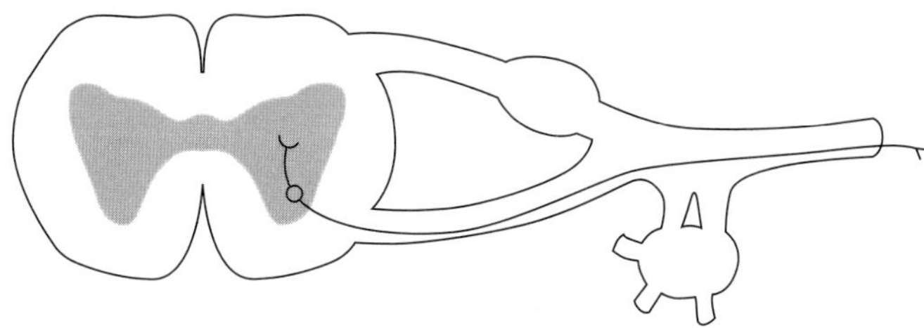

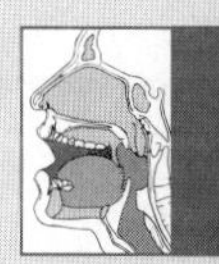

ganglion

The group of cell bodies pointed to in the drawing is called a ______________.

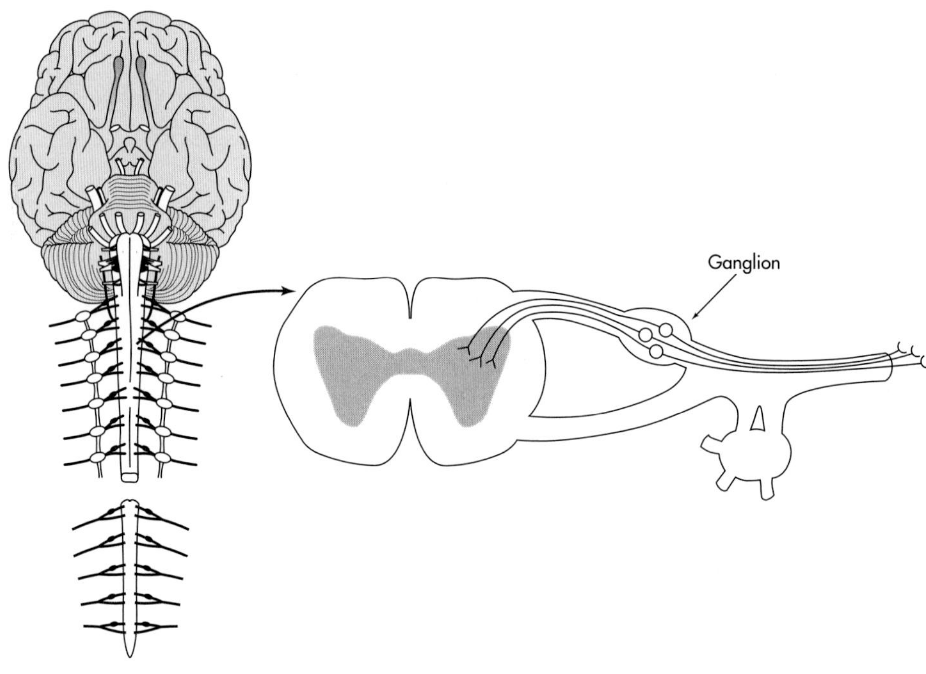

nucleus

And the cell bodies grouped together in the cord are called a ______________.

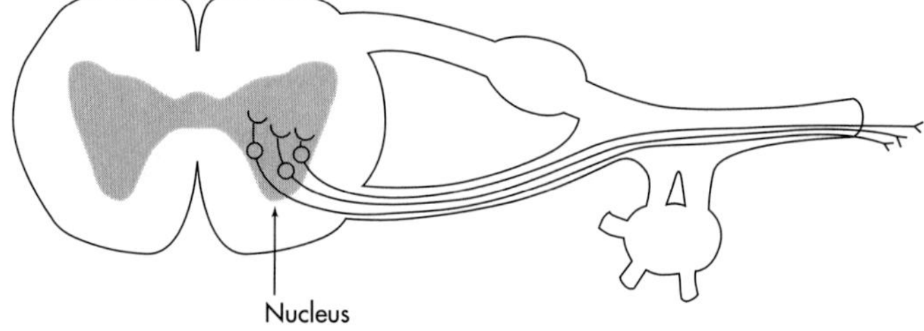

Trace the direction in which a signal is received and passed along.

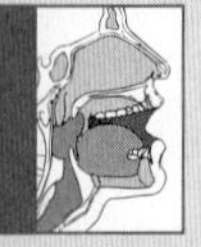

CENTRAL NERVOUS SYSTEM

1.0

With this basic overview of the nervous system, let us look at its major components. We have seen that the cells and processes of the system group themselves by their pathways and functions into nerves, spinal cord, and brain. Find those in the drawing. Remember that each is composed of neurons and also supporting cells called **neuroglia.**

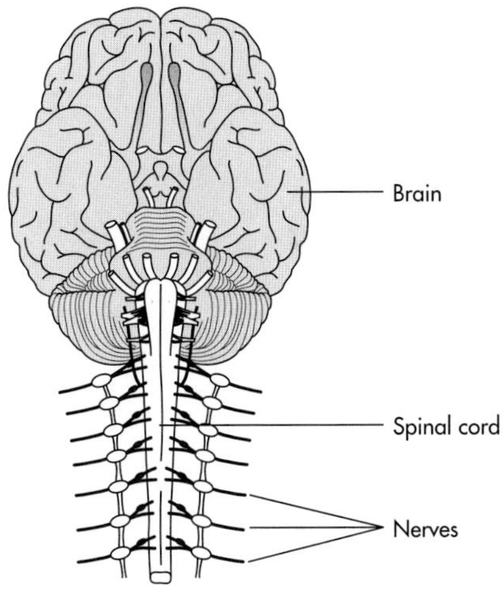

central nervous system (CNS)

The brain and spinal cord portions of the nervous system constitute the ______________. The remaining nerves exiting and entering the CNS are called the **peripheral nervous system** (PNS).

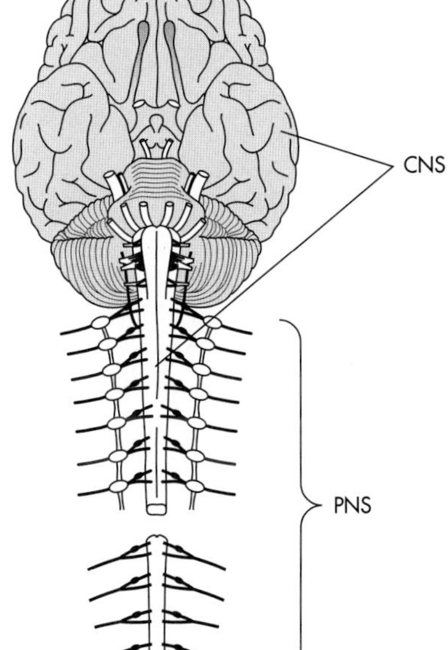

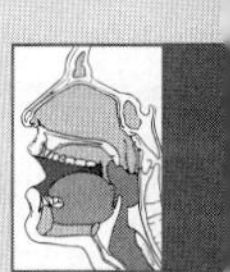

CNS = brain and spinal cord; PNS = nerves and outside CNS

Label the CNS and the PNS. The line and arrow represent the area of the nervous system found in the head and neck.

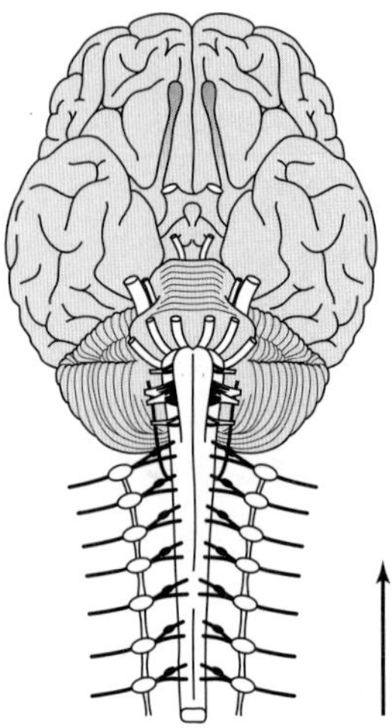

Nerves entering and exiting the spinal cord do so in pairs. These paired nerves are called **spinal nerves.**

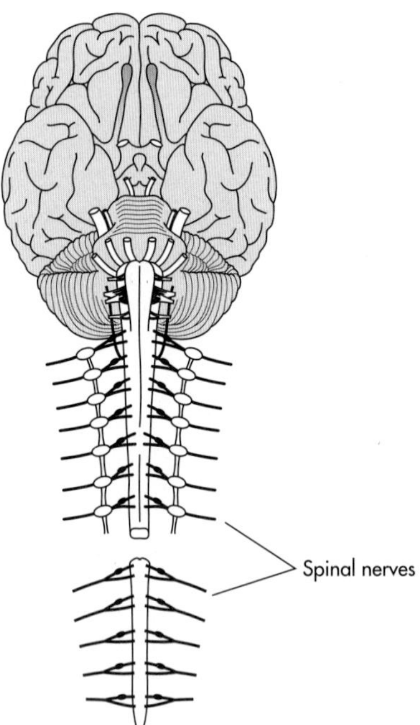

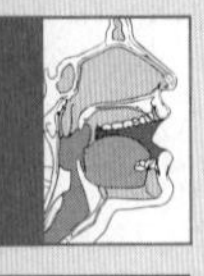

There are 7 pairs of spinal nerves in the neck region, and they are called the **cervical nerves.** They are named C-1, C-2, C-3, etc.

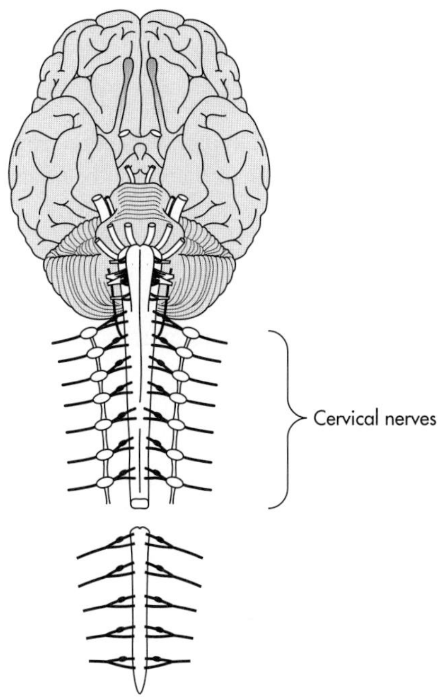

Pairing continues into the brain. The 12 paired nerves of the brain are called the **cranial nerves.**

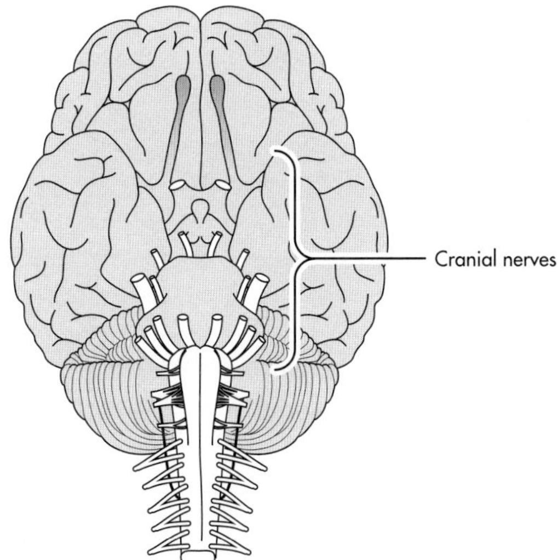

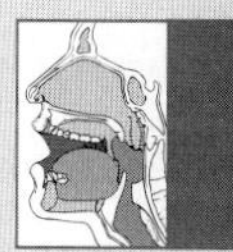

PNS

Anatomically we have divided the nervous system into the CNS and ______________. Functionally (and somewhat anatomically) it can be divided into two other systems: the somatic system and the autonomic system.

The **somatic nervous system** includes all pathways that regulate "conscious" bodily functions. The somatic system includes sensory and motor neurons to and from the skeletal muscles of the body.

The **autonomic nervous system** includes all pathways that regulate the "unconscious" bodily functions. The autonomic system includes sensory and motor neurons to and from the viscera of the body. Its pathways include an extra neuron, the cell body of which lies in a ganglion.

somatic, autonomic

Both systems may travel in the same nerve, so it is physically difficult to see the division of the two; however, the ganglia of the autonomic system can be seen. The two functional divisions are called the ______________ and ______________ nervous systems.

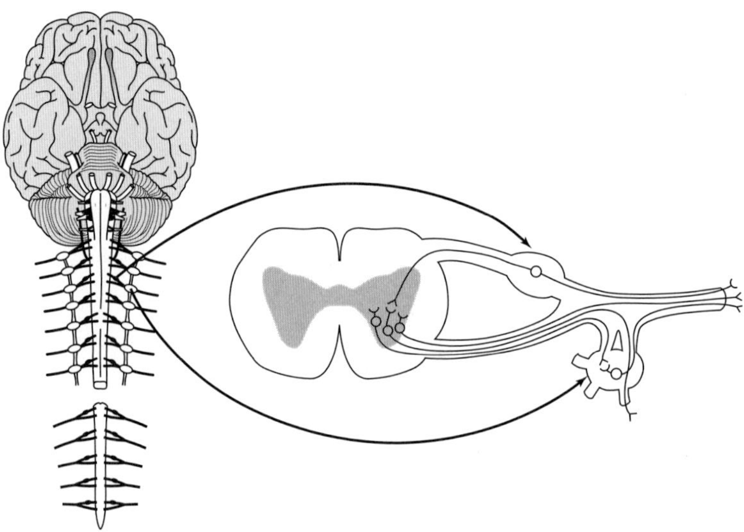

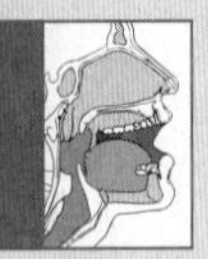

parasympathetic

The autonomic nervous system is further divided into the parasympathetic and sympathetic nervous systems. The **parasympathetic system** comprises those pathways involved with the regulation of everyday life-sustaining functions, such as respiration, heartbeat, and digestion. The ganglia of ______________ neurons are usually located close to and within the substance of the organs that they regulate.

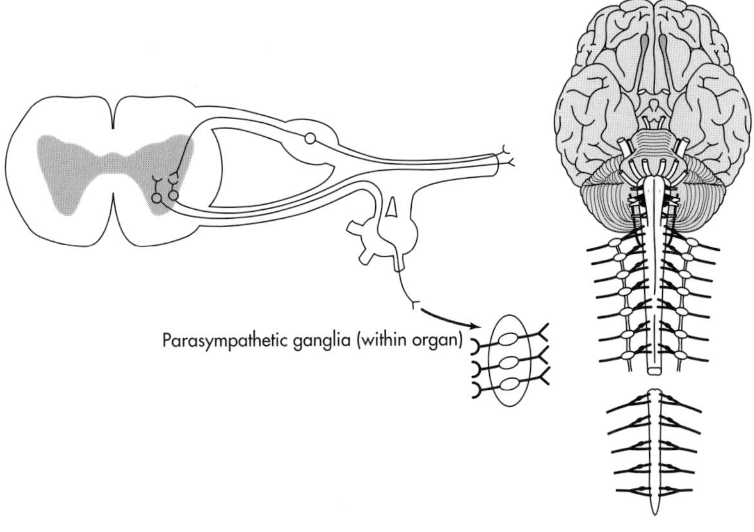

sympathetic

The **sympathetic system** involves neuronal pathways that regulate responses to stress, the "fright or flight" mechanisms that increase heartbeat and respiration and shut down digestion and other secretory responses. The ganglia of ______________ neurons are located in the **sympathetic chain,** a group of ganglia that lies next to the spinal cord and column.

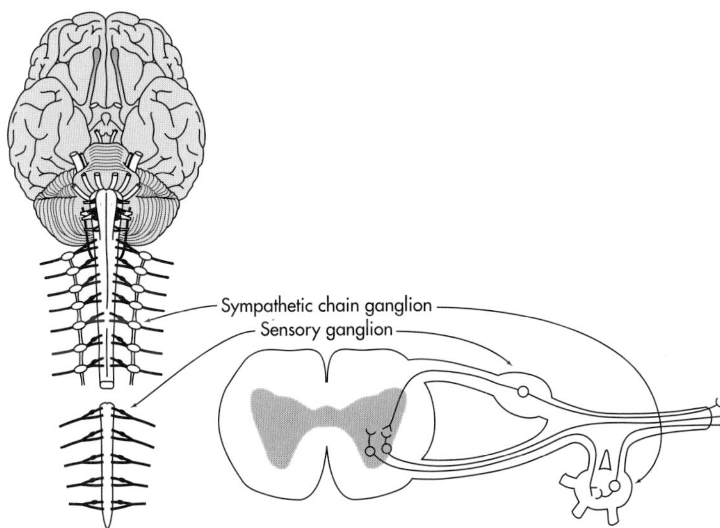

All organs, glands, and blood vessels have dual innervation; that is, they are supplied with parasympathetic and sympathetic nerves to have "speed up" and "slow down" capabilities. For example, the blood vessels have sympathetic innervation to restrict the flow of blood by constriction, and parasympathetic fibers allow flow by dilation of vessels.

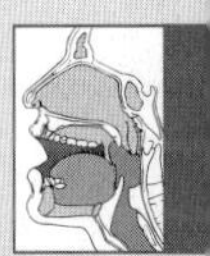

somatic, sympathetic, parasympathetic

Review. Which system is responsible for the innervation of skeletal muscle? Which system regulates emergency situations? Which system regulates daily visceral functions?

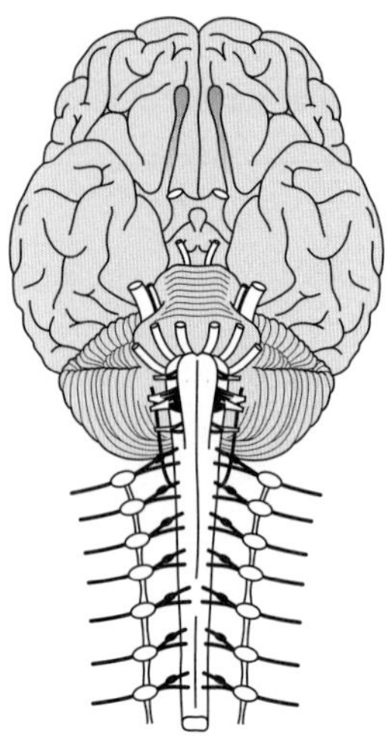

Sensory, motor

Both the somatic and autonomic systems have sensory and motor components in their pathways. ______________ neurons use receptors to sense their environment, and ______________ neurons cause a response to sensation by either contracting a muscle or causing a gland to secrete.

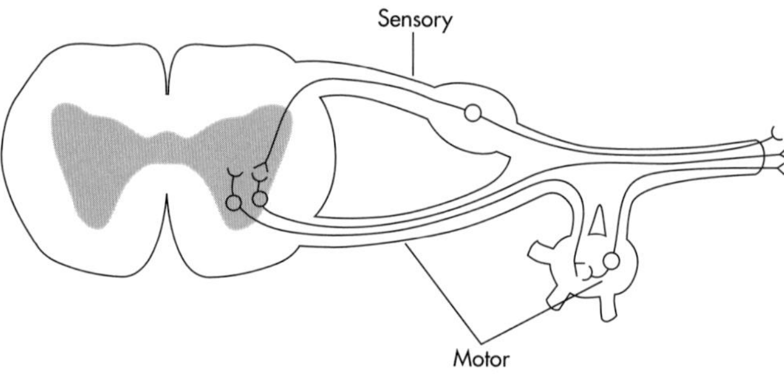

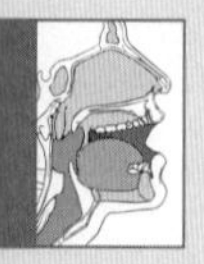

Spinal Cord and Cervical Nerves

1.1

The paired nerves exiting and entering the cervical portion of the spinal cord are called the **cervical nerves.** How many pairs of cervical nerves are present?

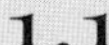
seven

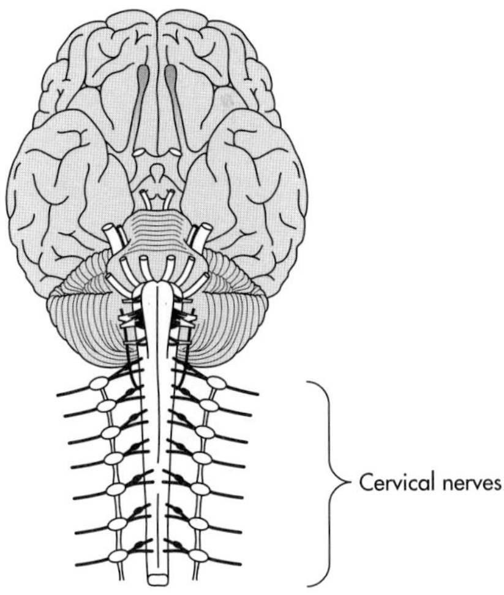

The cervical nerves are named (abbreviated) C-1, C-2, C-3, C-4, C-5, C-6, and C-7. These nerves innervate the muscles and viscera of the neck with sensory and motor neurons.

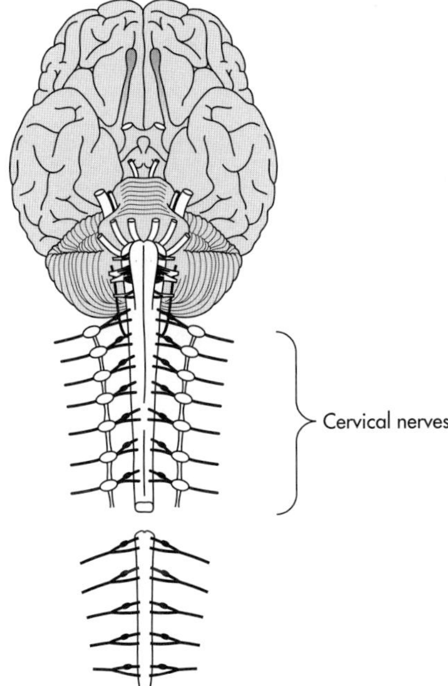

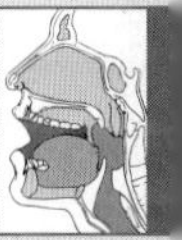

cervical

The ______________ nerves innervate the neck, providing somatic and autonomic regulation of its muscles and glands (and, therefore, organs and blood vessels).

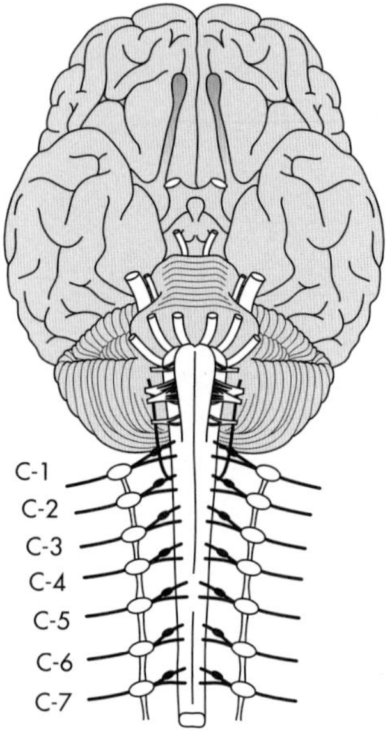

all five

Which of the following are examples of structures that cervical nerves may innervate?

1. Infrahyoid muscles
2. Skin of the neck
3. Posterior neck muscles
4. Blood vessels of the neck
5. Sweat glands of the neck

You may note later on as we study the cranial nerves that there is crossover innervation from head to neck and from neck to head. Some cranial nerves, for example, innervate muscles of the neck and its pharynx, larynx, and carotid vessels.

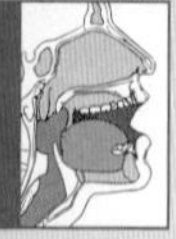

BRAIN 2.0

Cerebrum 2.1

The largest portion of the brain is called the cerebrum. It has a highly folded surface, with **lobes** and **sulci** (folds and fissures). The cerebrum is organized into two halves or **hemispheres,** which are connected by the **corpus callosum.** Find them.

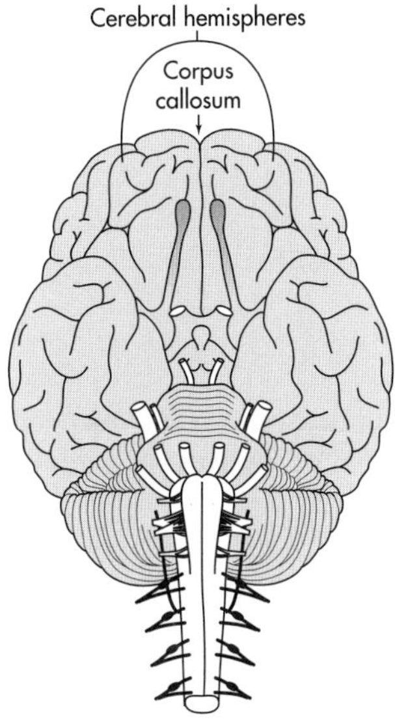

Separating the two hemispheres reveals the deeper structures of the cerebrum, the **diencephalon** and the **telencephalon**. Corpus callosum is now visible. Also seen are the cerebellum and the brainstem, which are not part of the cerebrum.

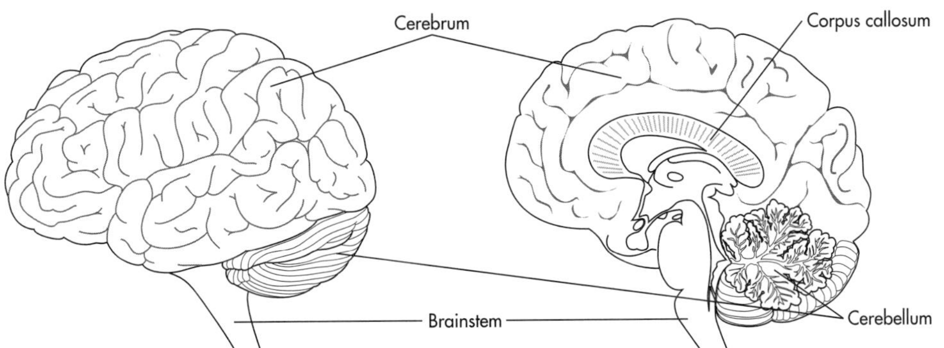

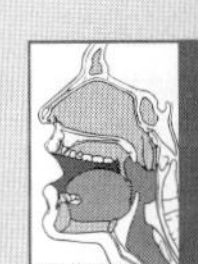

The **cerebrum** is responsible for the so-called higher functions of the brain or its conscious activity. This is the end of many sensory neuronal pathways and the beginning of consciously activated motor pathways. The cerebrum is divided into the ______________ and the ______________.

diencephalon, telencephalon

The **telencephalon** is the largest area of the brain, consisting of the highly convoluted surface area known as the **cortex** plus an inner area of "gray matter" known as the **corpus striatum** or **basal ganglia.**

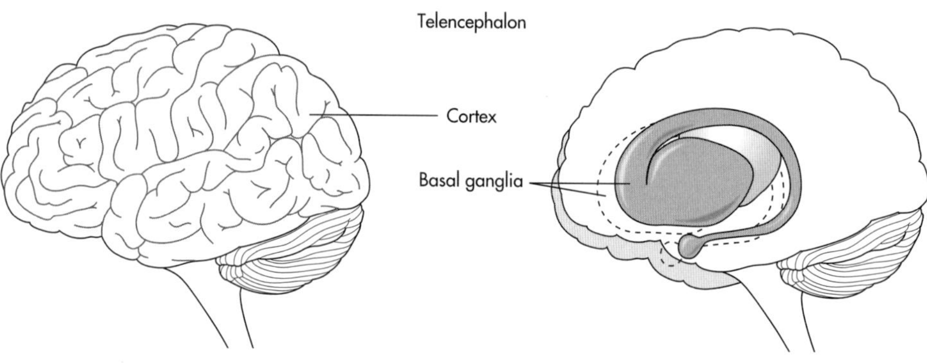

Many functional areas of the cortex have been "mapped out" by their **sulci** and **lobes**. Lobes are convex folds and sulci, the grooves between them.

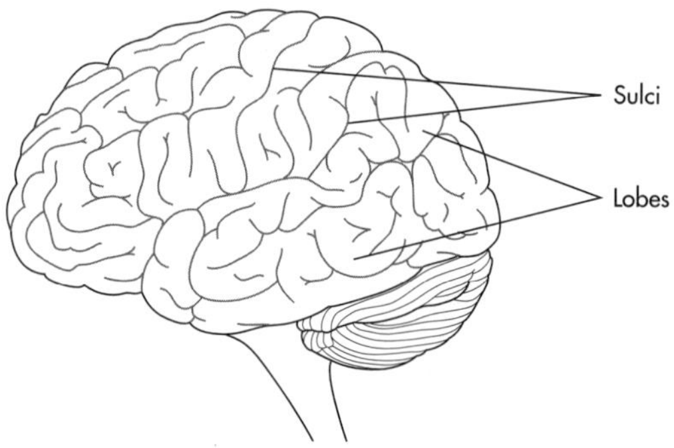

The cerebral cortex is divided into four anatomic "lobes" or areas:

1. Frontal lobe
2. Parietal lobe
3. Temporal lobe
4. Occipital lobe

corpus callosum

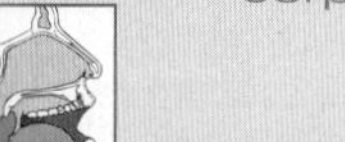

The hemispheres are connected together by the ______________.

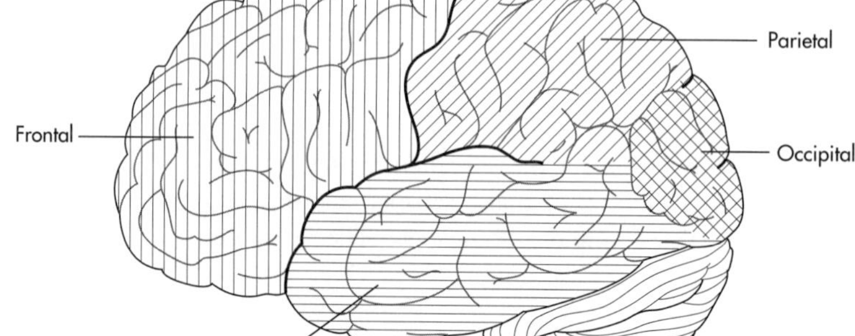

The sulci of the cerebrum are the (1) lateral sulcus, (2) central sulcus, (3) parietooccipital sulcus, and (4) calcarine sulcus.

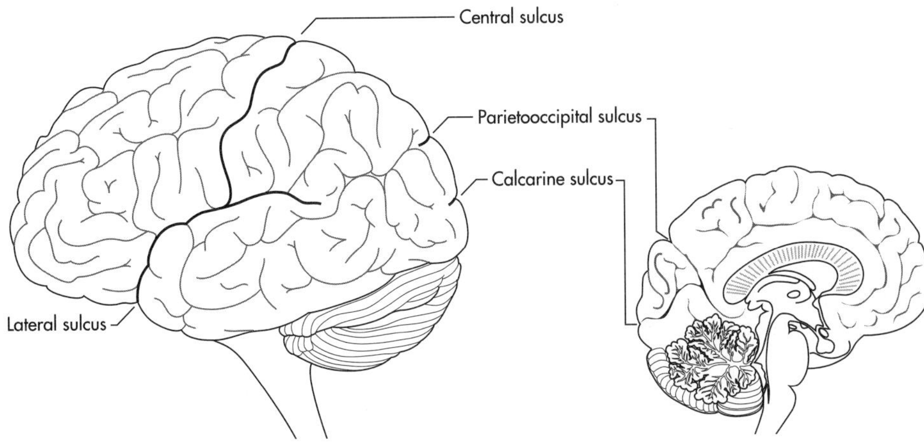

The cerebral cortex has also been mapped by areas of function. For example, the area of the frontal lobe anterior to the **central sulcus** is called the **primary motor cortex,** and that portion anterior to it, the **premotor area.** Both cortical areas are involved with voluntary movement of skeletal muscle.

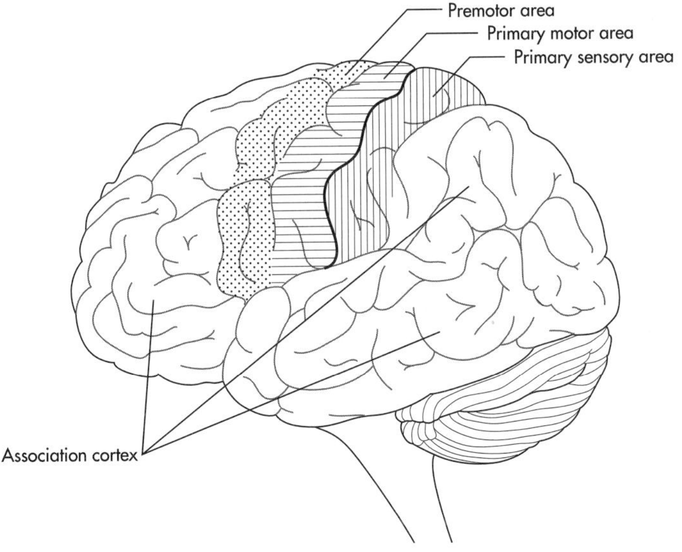

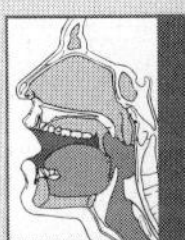

Posterior to the central sulcus in the parietal lobe is the **primary sensory** (or somesthetic) **area.** This region of cortex receives information from sensory neurons and makes us aware of those sensations, such as pain, touch, and temperature.

The remainder of the cortical areas are called **association cortex** and have many functions.

Along the **calcarine sulcus** in the occipital lobe is cortex that is associated with **vision.** Below the **lateral sulcus** in the temporal lobe is an **auditory area.** Find these on the drawing.

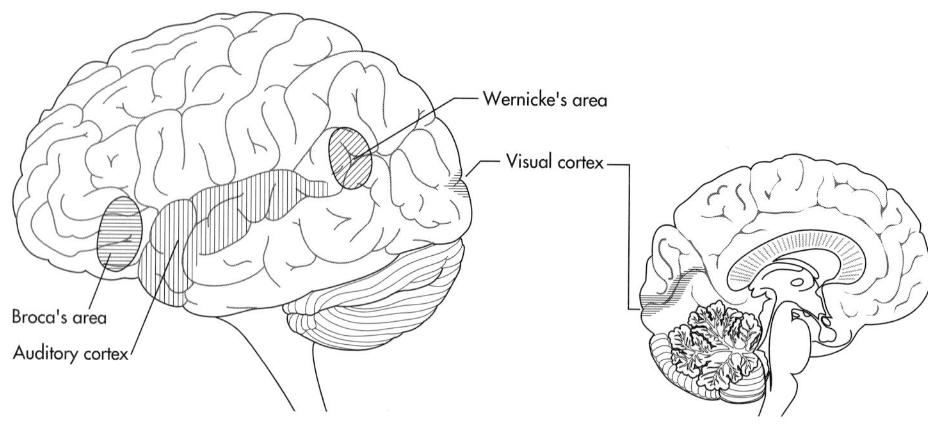

In the frontal cortex lie areas associated with memory and personality. **Broca's area** also lies in the frontal cortex and is associated with speech. Within the occipital lobe is found an area that deals with language comprehension called **Wernicke's area.**

A. frontal lobe
B. temporal lobe
C. central sulcus
D. parietal lobe
E. parietoccipital fissure
F. calcarine fissure
G. occipital lobe

Label all of these anatomic portions of the cerebral cortex. Check the preceding frames for your answers.

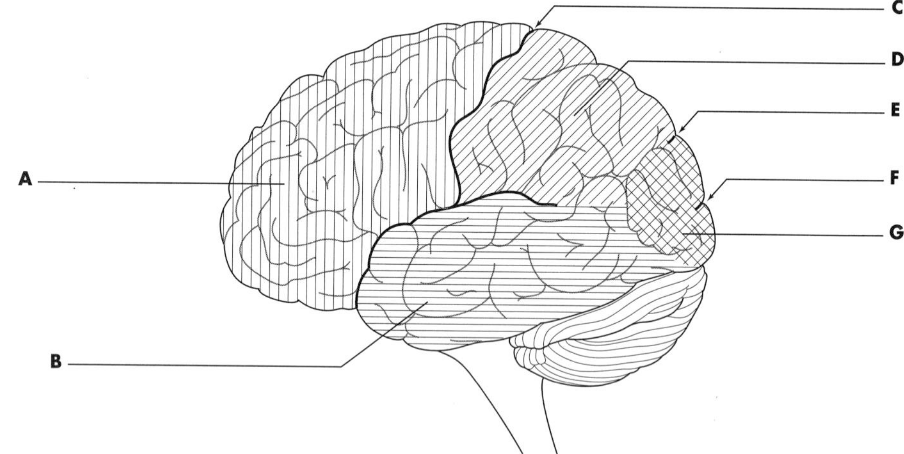

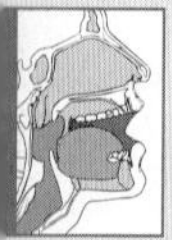

Label these functional areas of the cortex. Write the function beside the name of the area. Check the preceding frames for your answers.

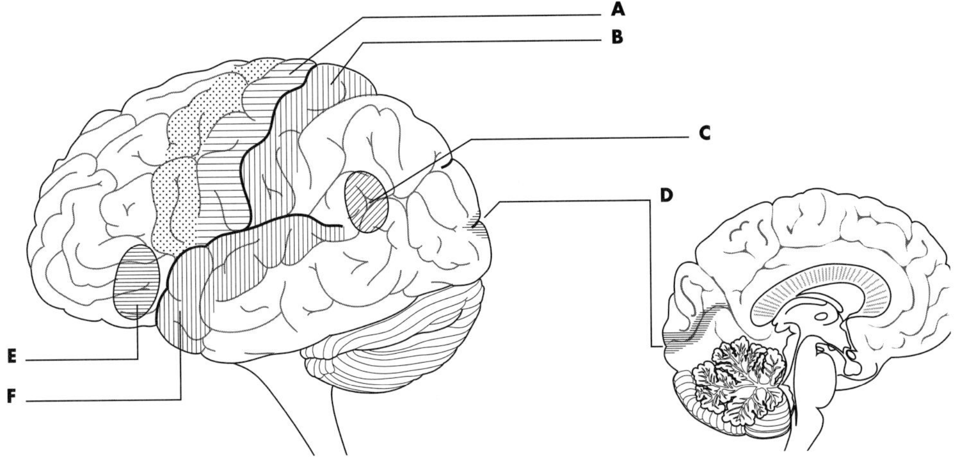

A. primary motor area; muscle function
B. primary sensory area; sensation (touch, etc.)
C. Wernicke's area; language comprehension
D. visual cortex; sight
E. Broca's area; speech
F. auditory cortex; hearing

The second portion of the telencephalon after the cortex is the ______________. This is an inner portion of the cerebrum near the base.

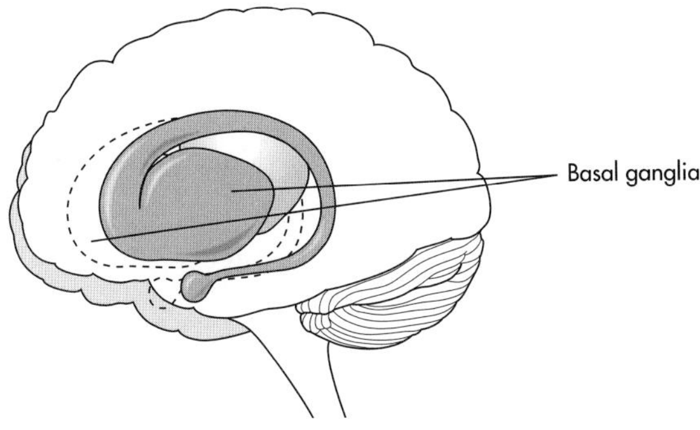

basal ganglia (or corpus striatum)

The **basal ganglia** consist of groups of nuclei associated with muscle or motor movements, making many connections to higher and lower centers of the brain.

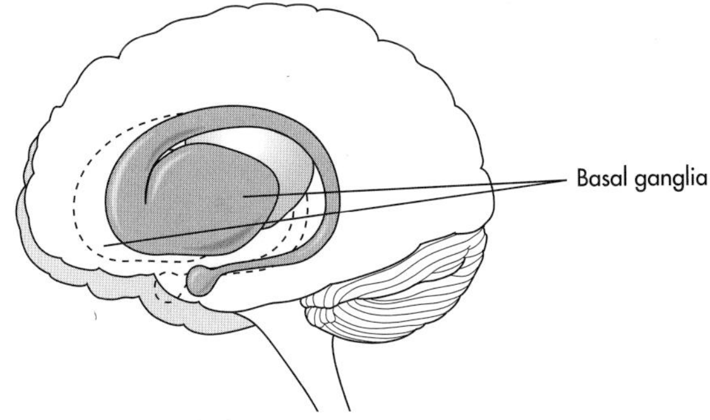

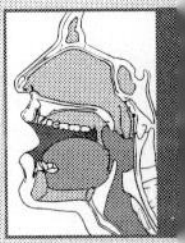

cortex and basal ganglia

Disruptions of the basal ganglia cause **dyskinesias** or involuntary, purposeless movements such as those that occur in Parkinson's disease. What are the two divisions of the telencephalon?

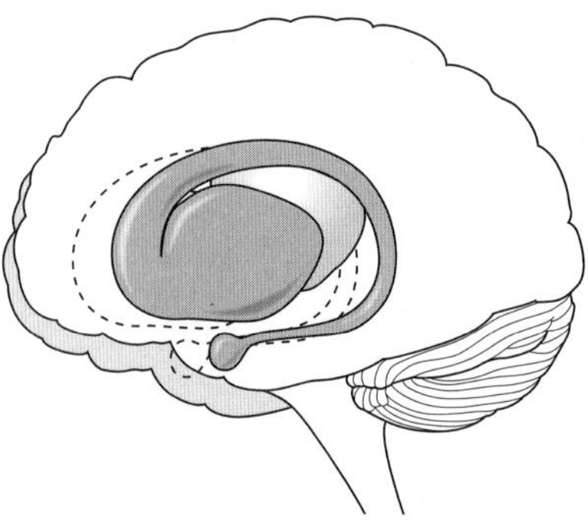

The remaining portion of the cerebrum is called the **diencephalon.** It is tucked within the cerebral hemispheres, medial to the cortex. It is composed of the (1) thalamus, (2) subthalamus, (3) epithalamus, and (4) hypothalamus.

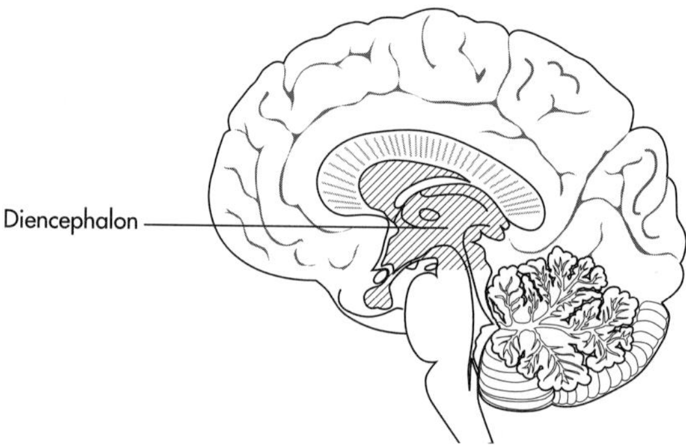

The **thalami** are two egg-shaped areas that act as sensory relay stations for neuronal pathways, deciding which portion of the brain to send these signals. They contain many specific nuclei.

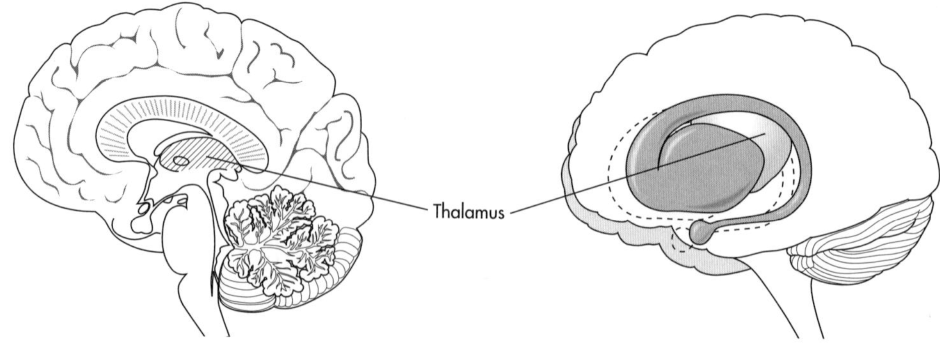

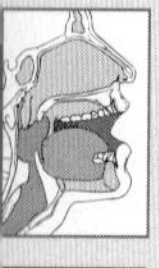

The **subthalami** are areas of nuclei and fiber tracts that relay sensory and motor signals and are found below the thalami.

The **epithalami** are unique areas containing an endocrine gland called the **pineal gland,** which is associated with biorhythmic signals. Find both subthalami and epithalami on the drawing.

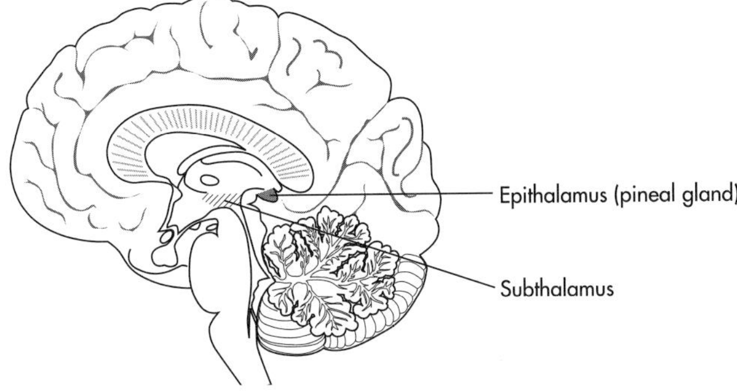

Which area contains the pineal gland?

epithalamus

Find the thalamic, subthalamic, and epithalamic areas. Beneath these areas is the **hypothalamus.** The hypothalamus is the main area for integrating the autonomic nervous system and controlling of some endocrine glands. It is continuous with a portion of the **pituitary gland (hypophysis).** The hypothalamus is integral to the maintenance of the internal environment, involving responses to hunger, thirst, and emotion.

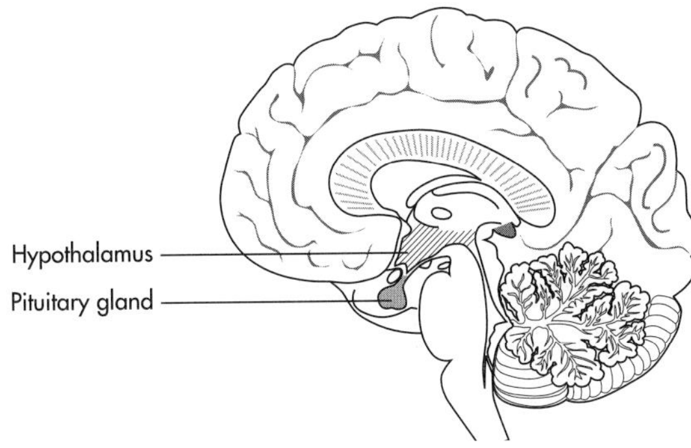

Centers for regulation of hunger and thirst are located in the _______________.

hypothalamus

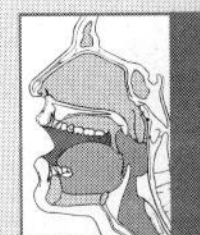

A. cerebrum
B. basal ganglia

The cerebrum is divided into telencephalon and diencephalon. The telencephalon is further divided into the:

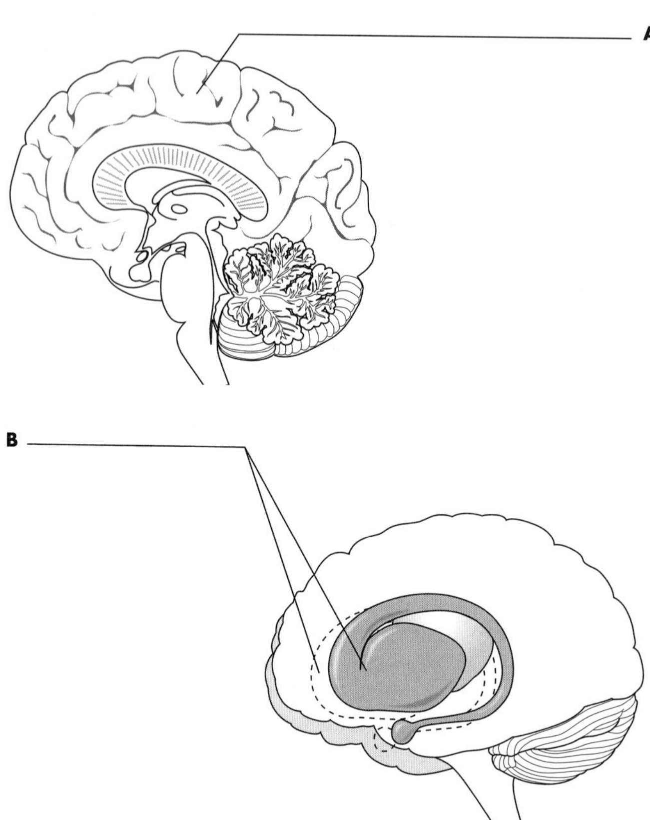

1. thalamus: sensory relay
2. epithalamus: biorhythm control
3. subthalamus: motor/sensory relay
4. hypothalamus: regulation of hunger, thirst, and emotion

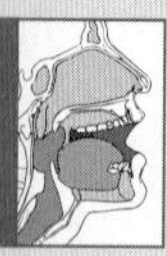

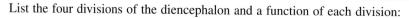

List the four divisions of the diencephalon and a function of each division:

1. ______________________________
2. ______________________________
3. ______________________________
4. ______________________________

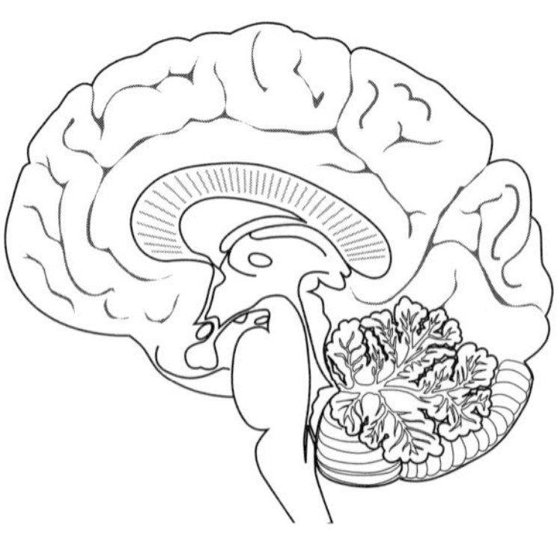

Label on one side the portion of the brain pointed out and also its function.

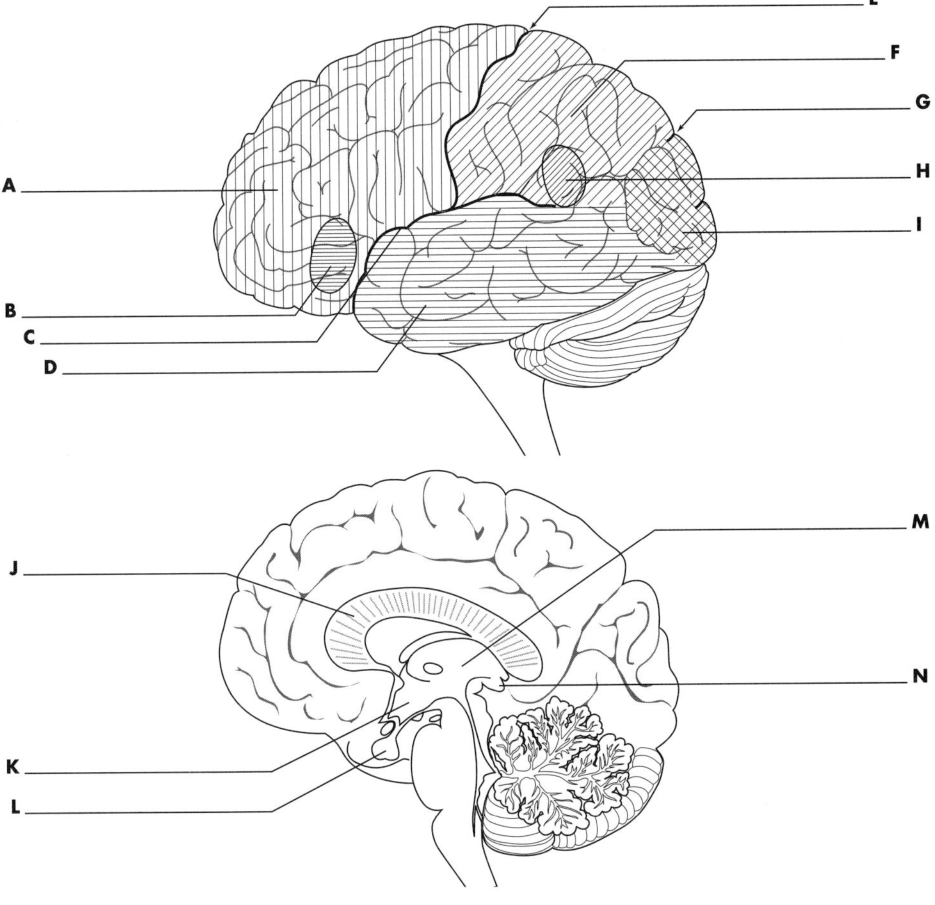

A. frontal lobe
B. Broca's area: speech
C. lateral sulcus: hearing
D. temporal lobe
E. central sulcus: motor—frontal, sensory—parietal
F. parietal lobe
G. parietooccipital sulcus
H. Wernicke's area: language comprehension
I. occipital lobe

J. corpus callosum
K. hypothalamus: hunger, thirst, emotion
L. pituitary
M. thalamus: sensory relay
N. epithalamus: biorhythm control

Cerebellum

2.2

The smaller, more highly folded portion of the brain that is located inferior and posterior to the cerebrum is called the **cerebellum** ("little brain"). The cerebellum has two hemispheres also and is composed of neuron cell bodies and their processes with connections to the cerebrum and brainstem portions.

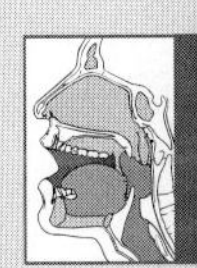

cerebrum

The cerebellum is an important area for the coordination or regulation of skeletal muscle movement (motor movement). Movements of the body such as walking involve several muscle groups, the actions of which need to be coordinated for smooth functioning with minimal conscious activity. Which portion of the brain is concerned with conscious activity?

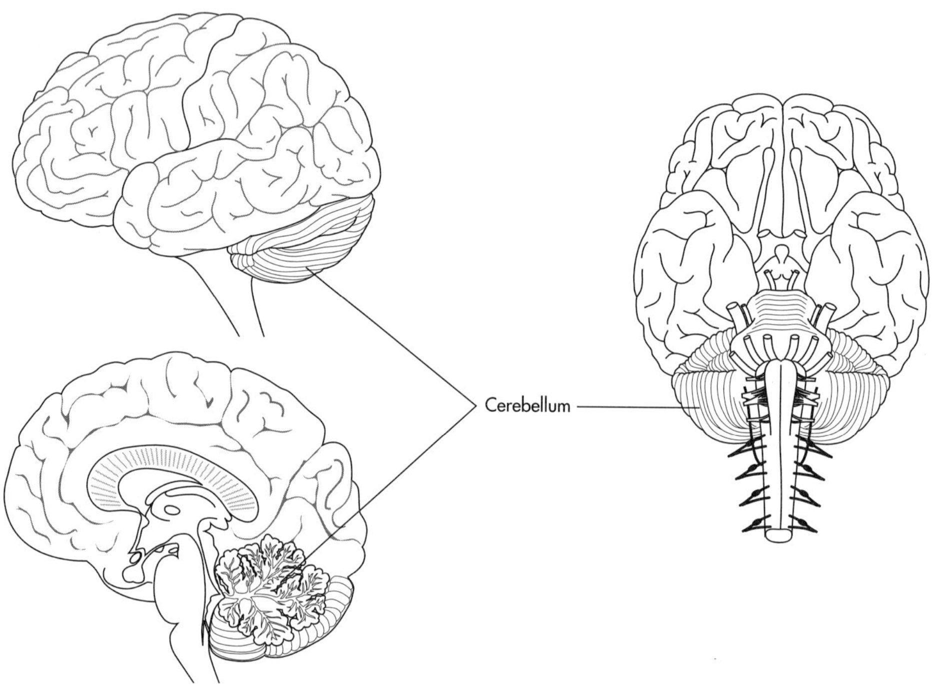

There are three functional areas of the cerebellum.

1. Vestibulocerebellum
2. Spinocerebellum
3. Pontocerebellum

These areas are not shown in the drawings. The first area, or **vestibulocerebellum,** receives information from neuronal pathways from the vestibules of each ear and thus can influence motor neurons with information about the head's position. This is information concerning balance.

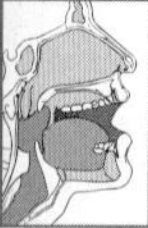

proprioception

The second portion of the cerebellum is the **spinocerebellum** and receives information from touch, pressure, and proprioceptive neurons via the spinal cord. **Proprioception** is the sense of position of the body telling the brain where the various portions of the body are located in space. This sensory information is used to help set muscle tone and to coordinate muscle action by way of cortical and brainstem pathways to motor nuclei that innervate the skeletal muscles. The sense of body position is ______________.

The third portion of the cerebellum is the **pontocerebellum,** so named because it relays information through the pons area of the brainstem into the cerebellum. It relays information about voluntary actions that are about to happen or that have already been initiated so that they can be modified before or during the motor action.

What are the three areas of the cerebellum?

vestibulo-cerebellum, spinocerebellum, and pontocerebellum

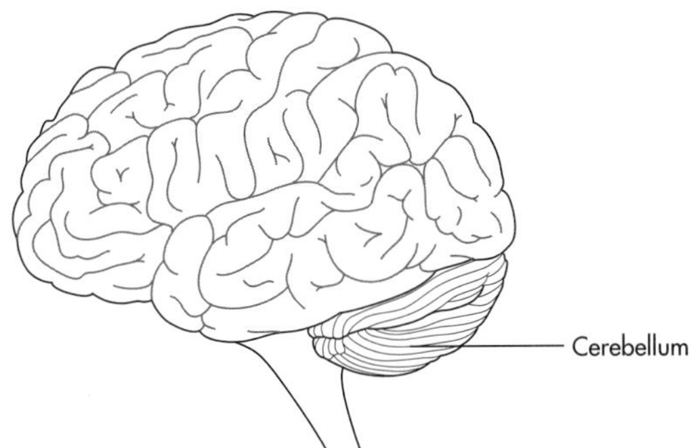

In general, information from visual (sight), auditory (hearing), vestibular (balance), and touch/pressure/proprioceptive neurons converges in the cerebellum to affect muscle activity. Also influencing motor actions is information from higher cortical centers involving learning, emotional input, and memory which is input by pathways into the cerebellum. All of this information is used to coordinate muscle activity and regulate muscle tonus. Output is to the various motor regulation areas of the brain including the basal ganglia, brainstem, and prefrontal cortex.

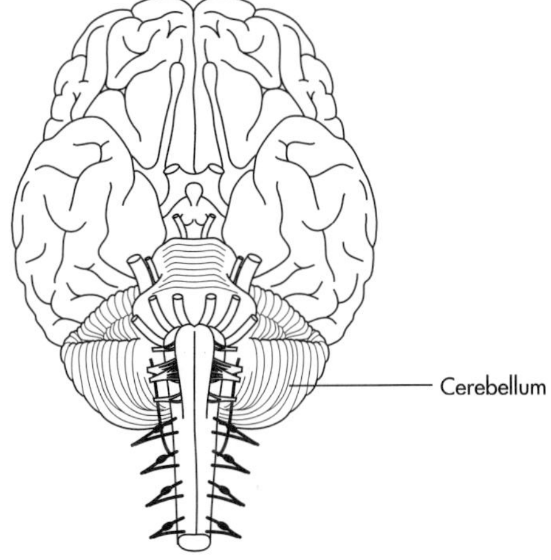

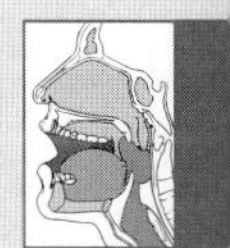

In general, what is the function of the cerebellum?

motor coordination

2.3 Brainstem

The long tubular portion of the brain is the **brainstem.** It continues down from the base of the brain and becomes continuous with the spinal cord, which it resembles in structure. Superiorly it connects with the diencephalon and posteriorly with the cerebellum via three peduncles.

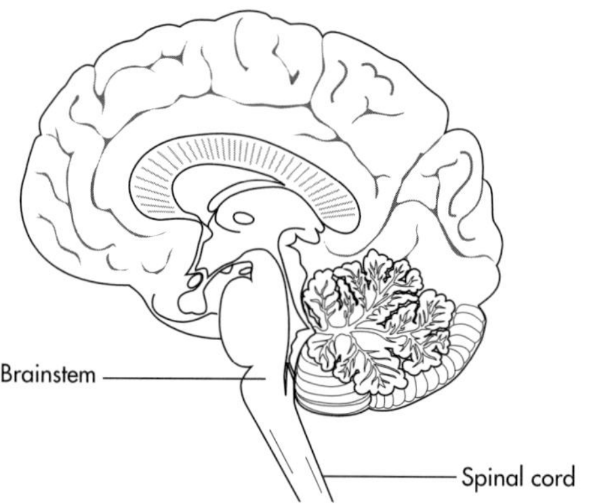

spinal cord

The brainstem is composed of many neuronal processes or pathways that travel up to the cerebrum and cerebellum and down to the ________________. It also contains many regulatory nuclei and 12 pairs of nerves called the **cranial nerves.** Find them.

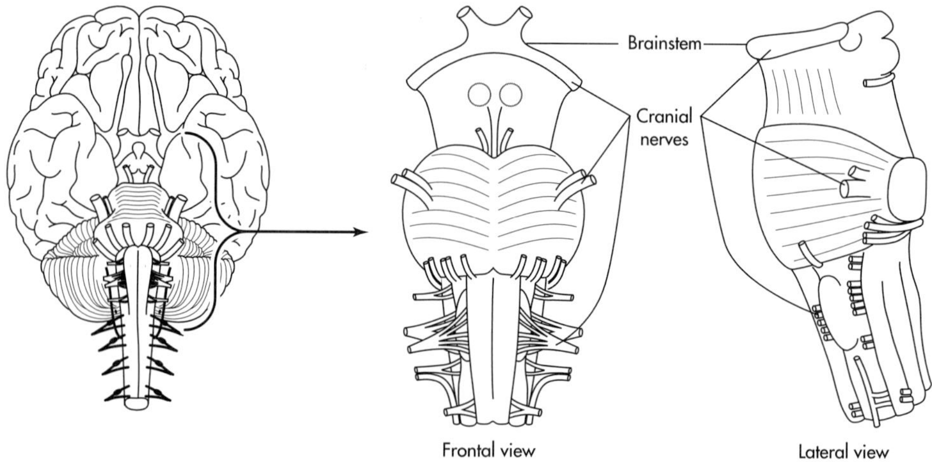

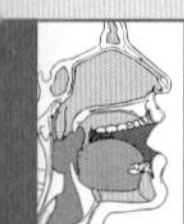

Brainstem functions include the so-called lower or basic functions of the brain, most of which are life-sustaining:

1. Regulation of heartbeat and respiration
2. Regulation of digestion and excretion
3. Mastication and swallowing centers
4. Pain perception and regulation

The brainstem is organized similarly to the spinal cord. It is a solid tubular structure with incoming and outgoing connections via the cranial nerves and with pathways that travel up and down the "tube" in bundles of neuron processes.

Also, cell body groups or ______________ are located in the brainstem, acting as regulatory centers or connecting points for different pathways. Pathways and nuclei for sensory activity tend to be concentrated in the dorsal portion of the brainstem and motor activity in the ventral portion.

nuclei

Compare sections of the brainstem and the spinal cord.

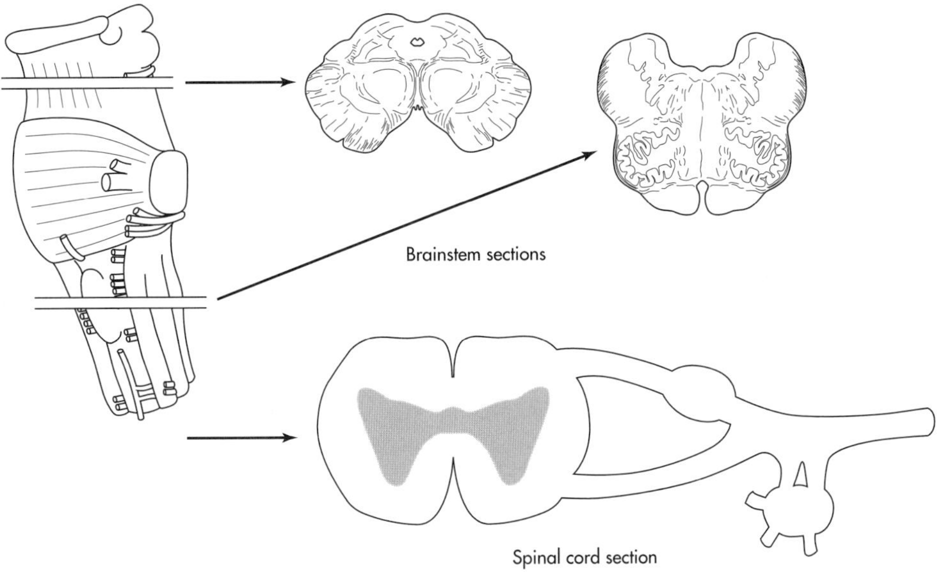

A prominent area of the brainstem on its ventral side is the **pons** or **pontine area.** This is basically an area where several neuronal processes cross over from the right to the left side of the brain. Another area of crossover is called the **decussation of pyramids.** Find them below.

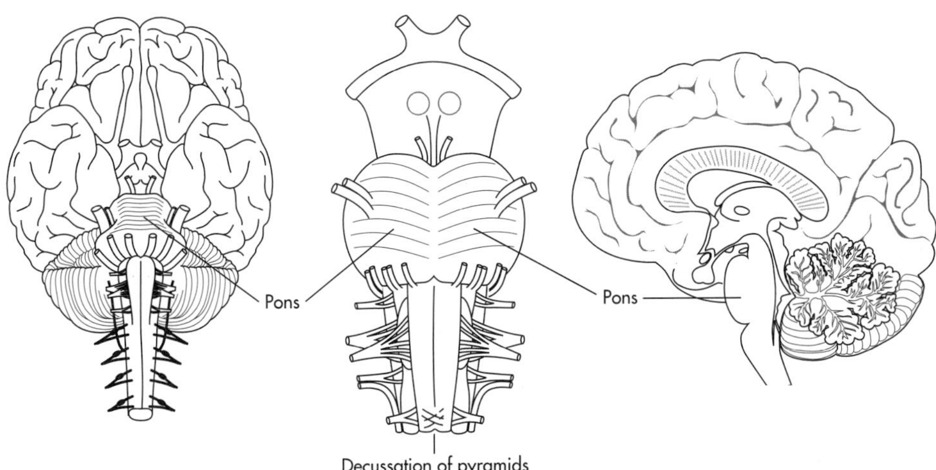

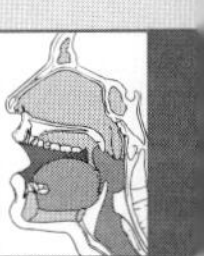

cranial nerves

Twelve pairs of nerves called the ______________ originate from the brainstem area. We will study them in detail later in the chapter. Label these portions of the brainstem. Refer to the preceding frames.

A. pons
B. decussation of pyramids
C. pons

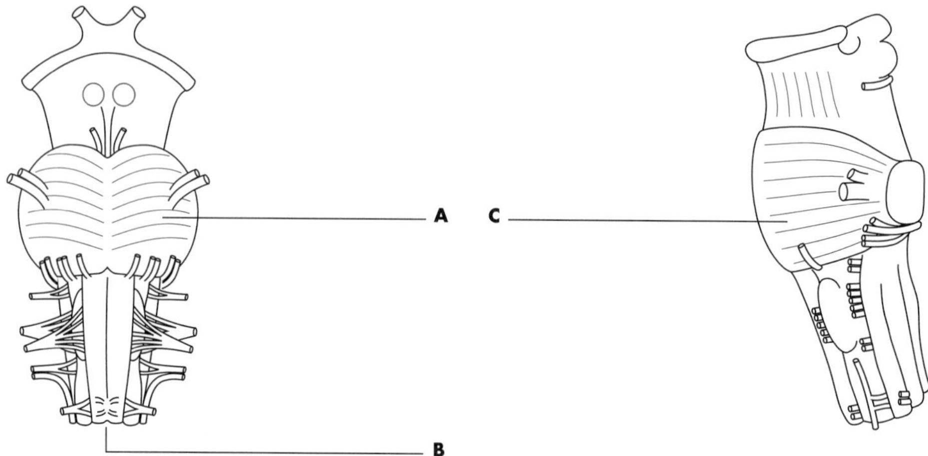

3.0 CRANIAL NERVES

The 12 pairs of **cranial nerves** that exit from the cerebrum and brainstem are similar to the spinal nerve pairs that exit the spinal cord along its length. Cranial nerves carry motor and sensory neurons, somatic and autonomic neurons, although they sometimes tend to carry more of a specific kind. Find the cranial nerves in the diagram.

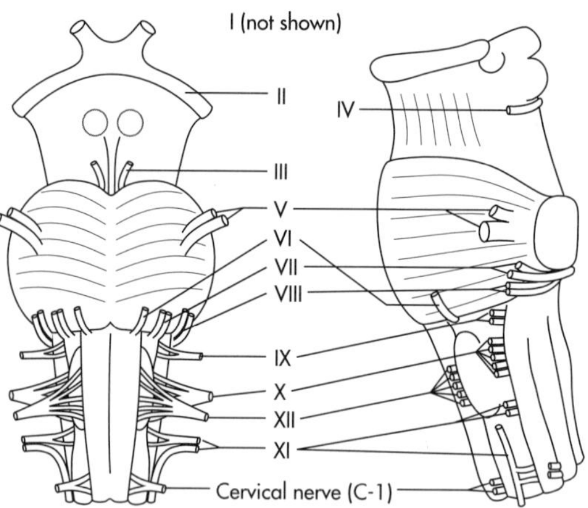

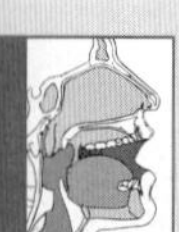

12

How many pairs are there?

ganglia

The neuronal cell bodies of sensory neurons lie outside of the CNS in ______________, as they do in spinal nerves. Ganglia are "lumps" of sensory cell bodies on the cranial nerve roots, just before they enter the brainstem.

Inside the brainstem are the cell bodies of motor neurons in groups called ______________. Nuclei of the cranial nerves are found within the brainstem in very specific locations. Both ganglia and nuclei of the cranial nerves have specific names.

nuclei

How many pairs of cranial nerves are there? We look at each pair of cranial nerves and its location, components, innervation (where it travels to), and function.

12

Each cranial nerve is numbered with a roman numeral (I, II, III, etc.) and each has a name. The names of the cranial nerves are listed here. Take time now to memorize their names and numbers.

I Olfactory nerve
II Optic nerve
III Oculomotor nerve
IV Trochlear nerve
V Trigeminal nerve
VI Abducens nerve
VII Facial nerve
VIII Vestibuloacoustic nerve
IX Glossopharyngeal nerve
X Vagus nerve
XI Spinal accessory nerve
XII Hypoglossal nerve

Each cranial nerve has components, that is, mainly sensory, motor, or mixed nerves. Each cranial nerve innervates a particular structure. Each cranial nerve exits the cranium through a particular foramen.

We will build a chart at the end of this section with information on each cranial nerve number and name, innervation/function, type of nerve, ganglia or nuclei, and foramina.

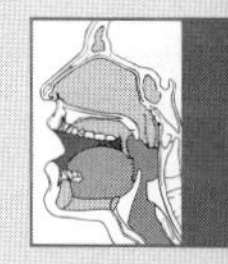

3.1 Cranial Nerve I: Olfactory Nerve

The **olfactory nerve** pair or cranial nerve I is located at the base of the brain (frontal lobes). Find them. They appear as two "antennae" or bulbs, emerging from the base of the cerebrum.

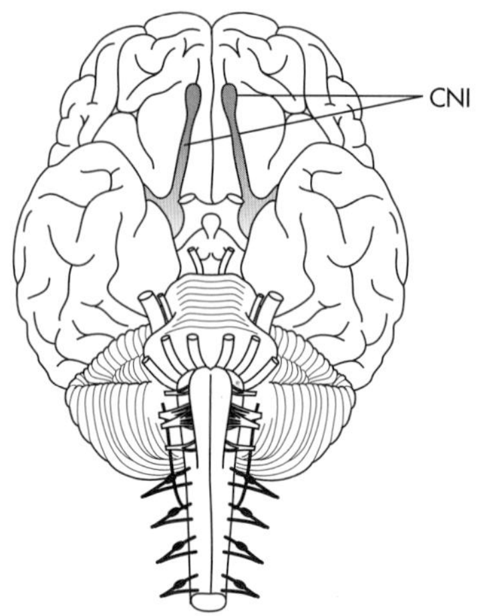

The **olfactory bulbs** are actually clusters of sensory nerve cell bodies associated with the sense of smell. Their receptor neurons originate in the superior nasal mucosa.

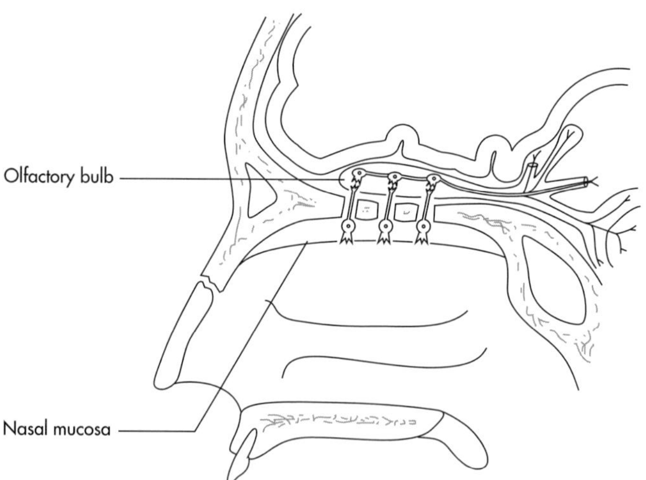

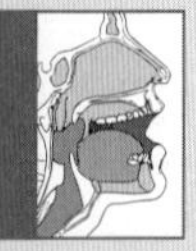

These neurons, as shown, are cranial nerve I or the ______________ nerve. The diagram shows the pathway from the receptor neuron in the nasal mucosa to its synapse in the olfactory bulb and then its connection in the cerebrum.

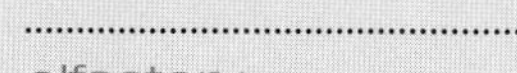

Cerebrum
Olfactory bulb
Receptor neuron
Cribriform plate

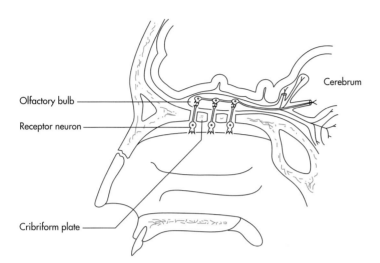

The olfactory nerve fibers pass through perforations in the cranium called the **cribriform plate.** Find them.

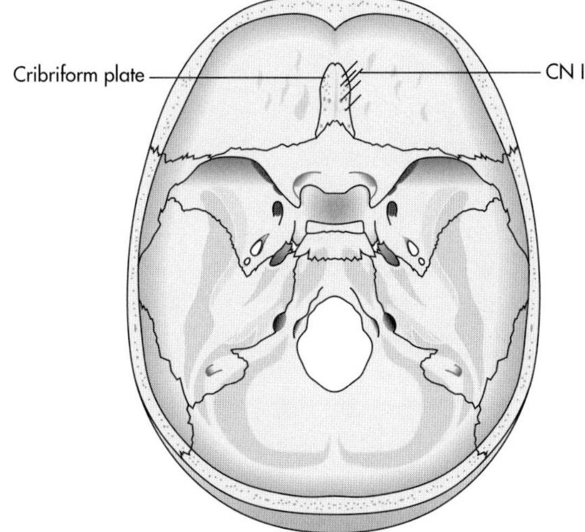

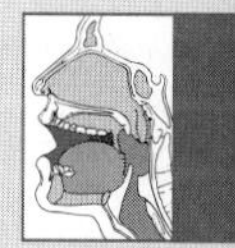

sensory

Look at the diagram of a section of nasal mucosa. Smell receptors are ______________-type neurons and they work through small molecules in the air, attaching to them and causing them to fire and pass a signal to the brain for interpretation. Smell has an especially close connection to that portion of the cerebrum associated with emotion and memory.

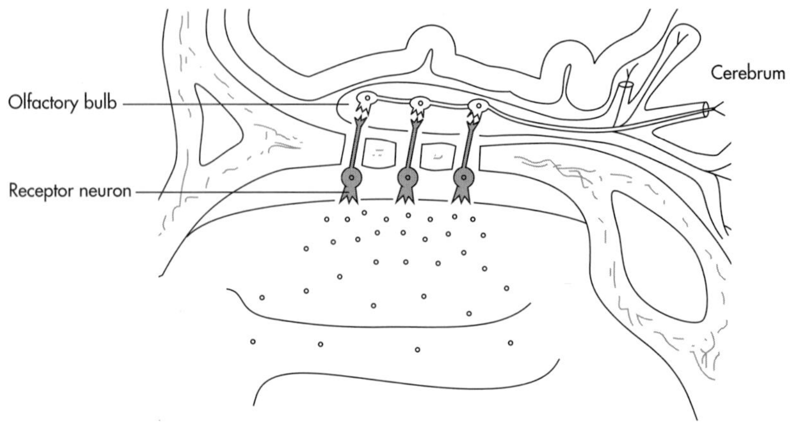

olfactory

Find CN I, the ______________ nerve, in the drawings.

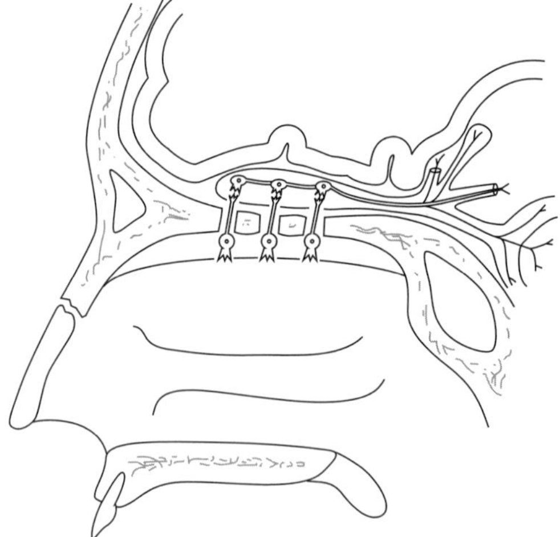

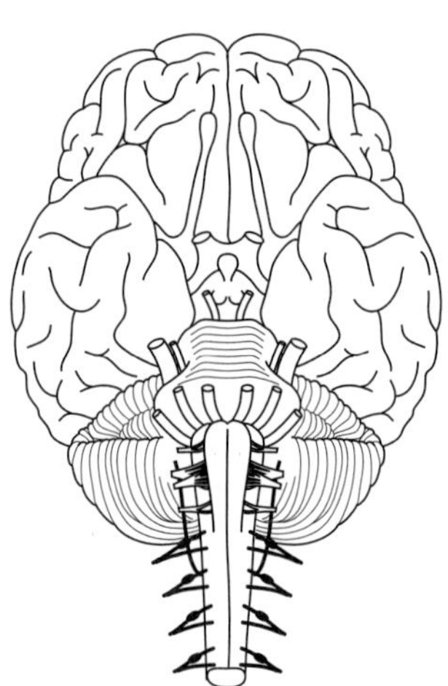

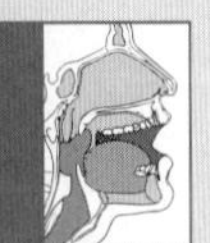

What type of nerve is CN I? Through which foramina does it pass? What does it innervate?

sensory, cribriform plate, nasal mucosa receptors for smell

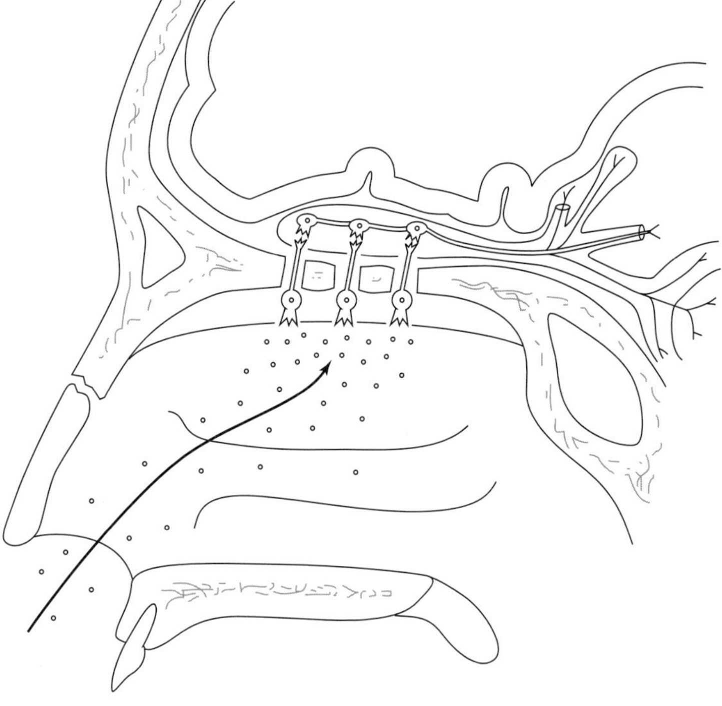

Cranial Nerve II: Optic Nerve

3.2

The **optic nerves** are cranial nerve II. At the beginning of each nerve lies an eyeball. Which special sensation do you think is carried on CN II?

sight

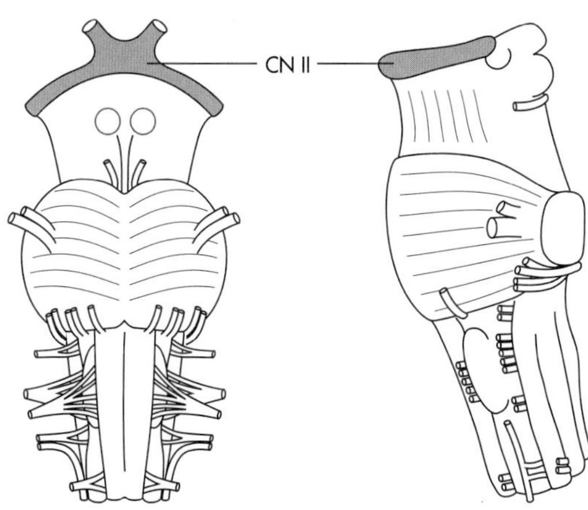

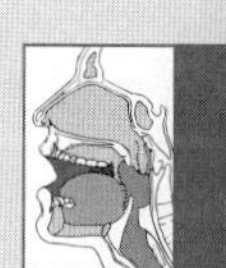

Find the optic nerves on this drawing. Note that they seem to connect to each other. That is because some of the neurons from the right eye cross over to the left side of the brain and vice versa. Information from both eyes is shared by right and left sides of the brain. This area is called the **optic chiasm.**

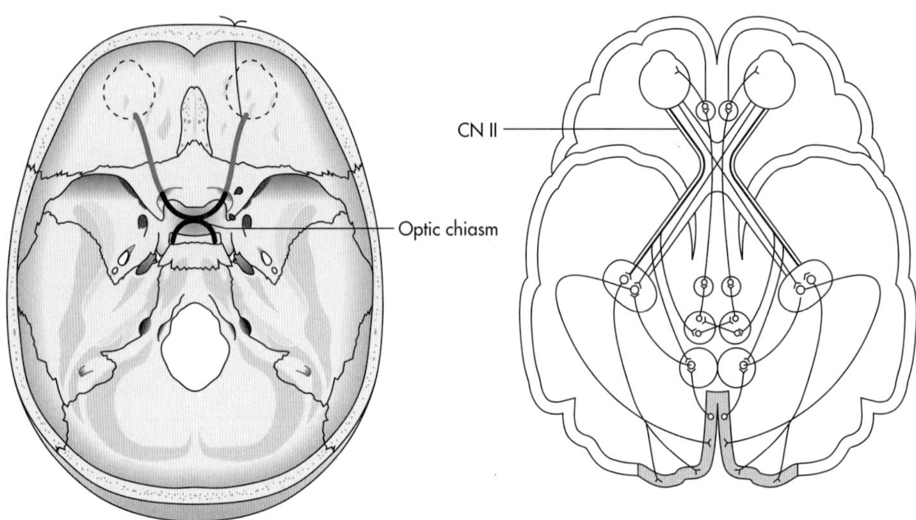

The separate neuronal pathways from the eye to the brain are drawn here. Note that there are different pathways that visual information can take into the brain and that more than one neuron is involved in each pathway.

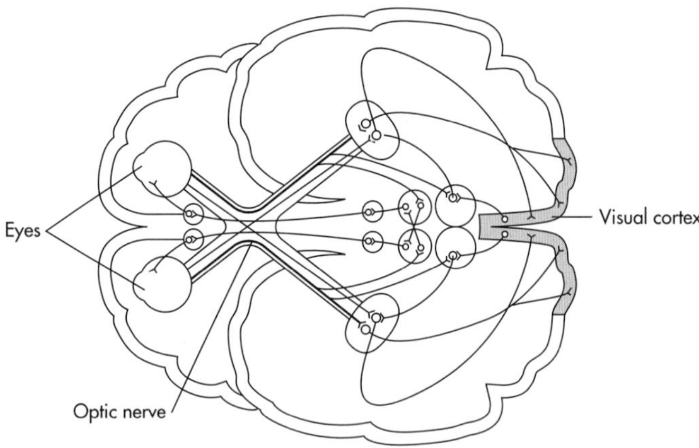

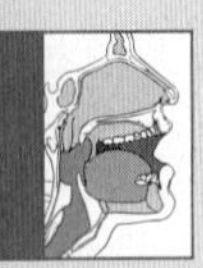

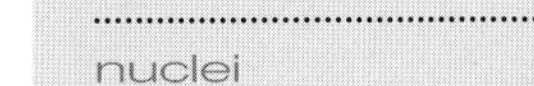
nuclei

Where the cell bodies of the visual neurons lie together, ______________ are created within the brain.

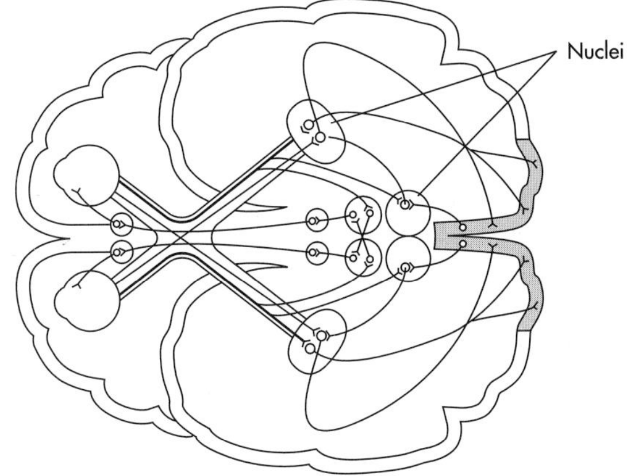

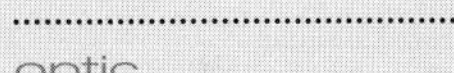
optic

Visual information from CN II (the ______________ nerve) is finally taken to the cortex for interpretation. This area of the cortex is found in the occipital lobe along the **calcarine sulcus.** Find the occipital lobe in both drawings.

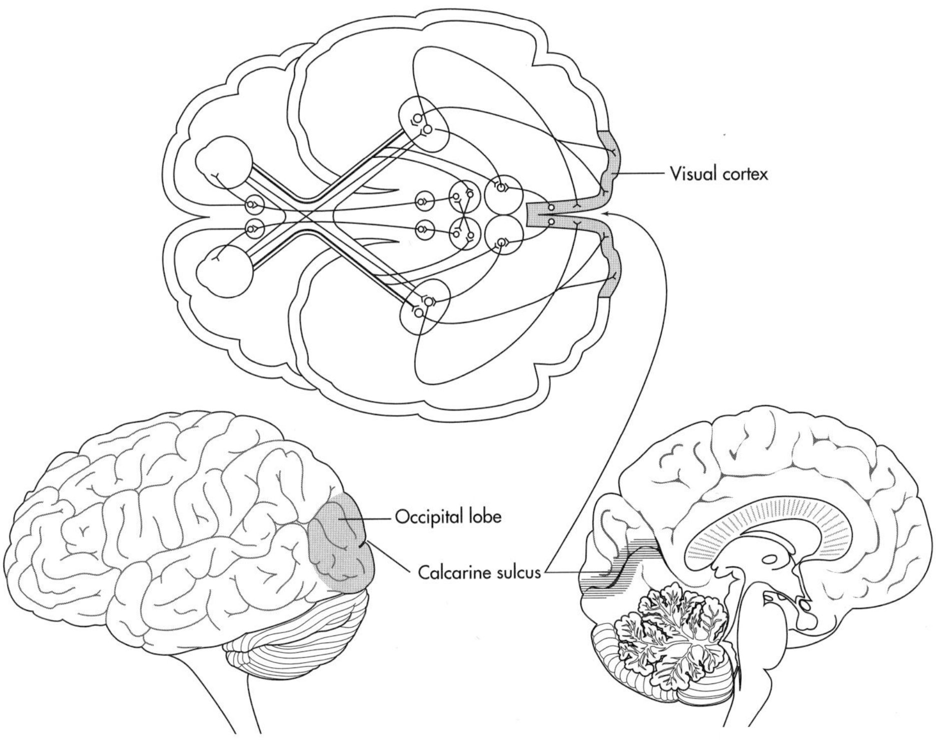

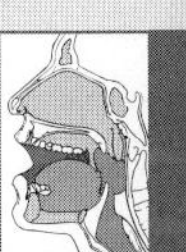

retina

Structurally, the eye is basically a fluid-filled sphere consisting of three layers: the **sclera (cornea),** the **choroid,** and the **retina.** Find these on the drawing. The innermost layer is the ______________.

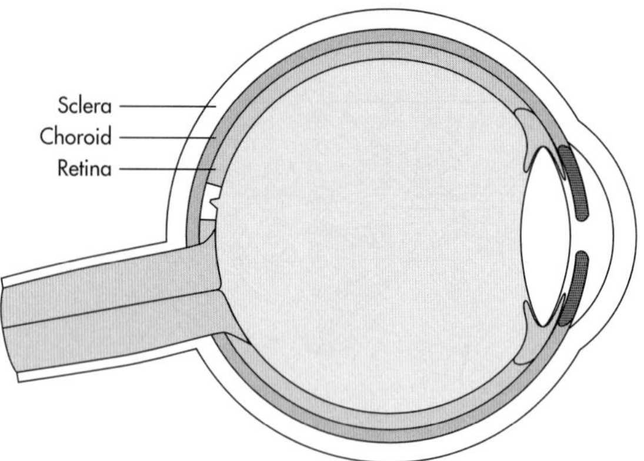

fovea

The **retina** is the layer containing the first group of light-sensing neurons, the **rods and cones.** These receptor neurons are named by their shapes. Rods detect light and dark changes, and cones pick up color sensation. They are concentrated on a small area near the exit of the optic nerve called the __________.

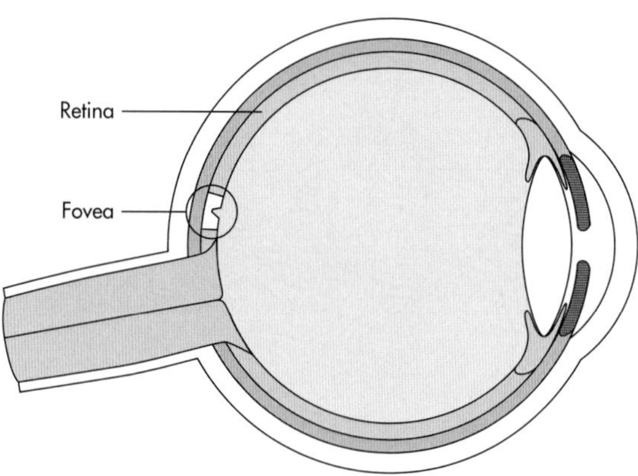

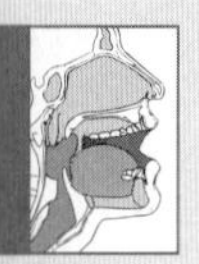

The eye works much as a camera does, focusing light that enters through the **pupil** of the **iris,** passing through a **lens** onto the back of the eye onto the retina. Find these parts of the eye on the drawing.

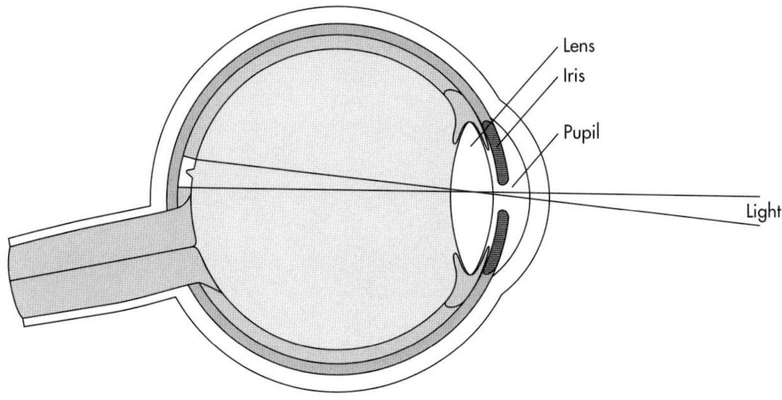

The diagram of an enlarged section of the **retina** shows the neuronal pathways and the nerve cells involved in vision. The first layer comprises the rod and ______________ cells, which are stimulated by light. Three interneurons are used to pass information into the optic nerve.

cone

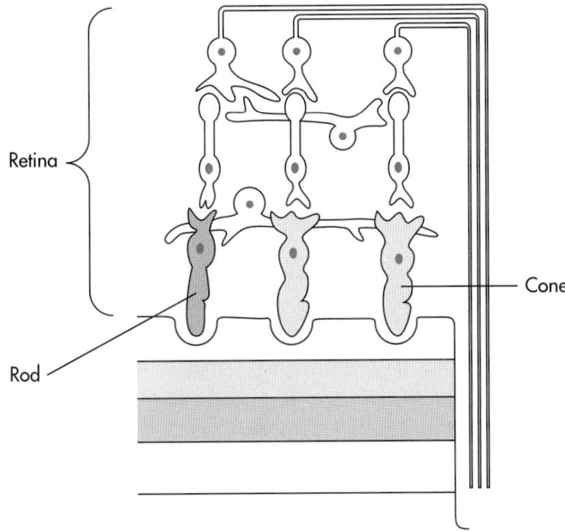

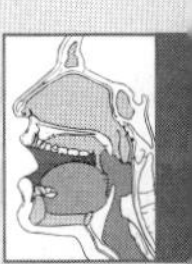

sensory

Cranial nerve II, the optic nerve, is what type of nerve then, because it is responsible for taking visual information to the brain?

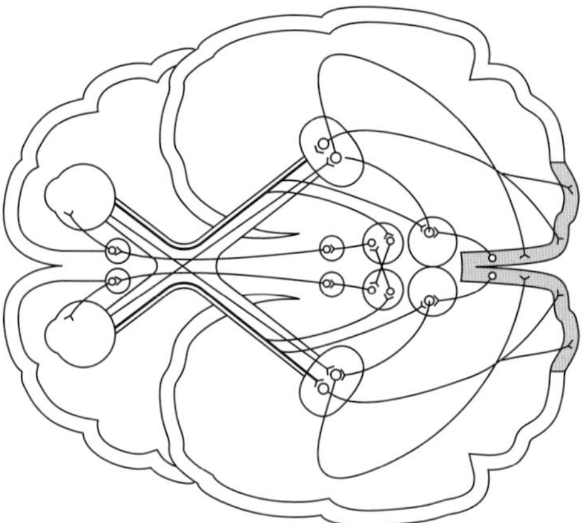

optic

Follow the path of CN II as it passes from the eye, out of the orbit, and into the internal cranium. Through which foramina do you see it pass?

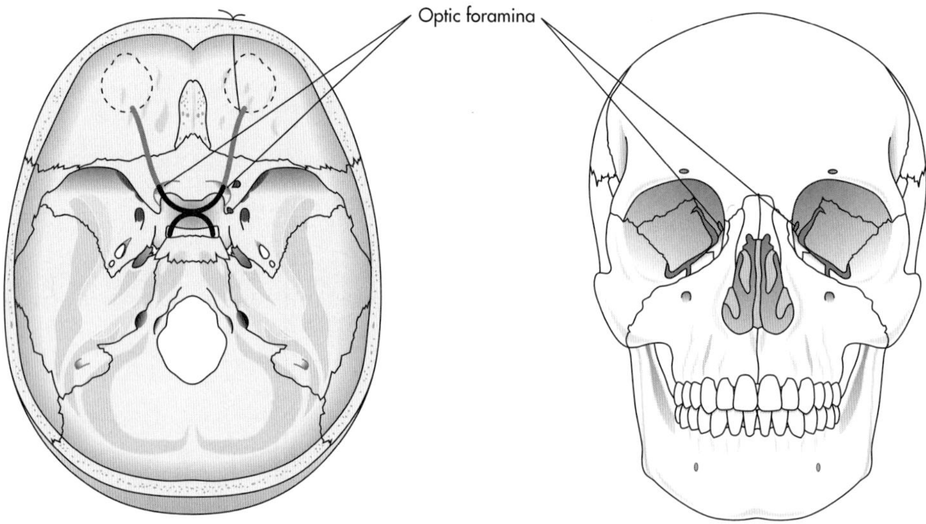

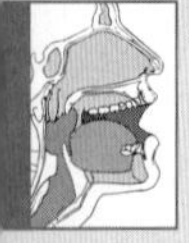

Find the optic foramina in both drawings. Which cranial nerve passes through these?

CN II

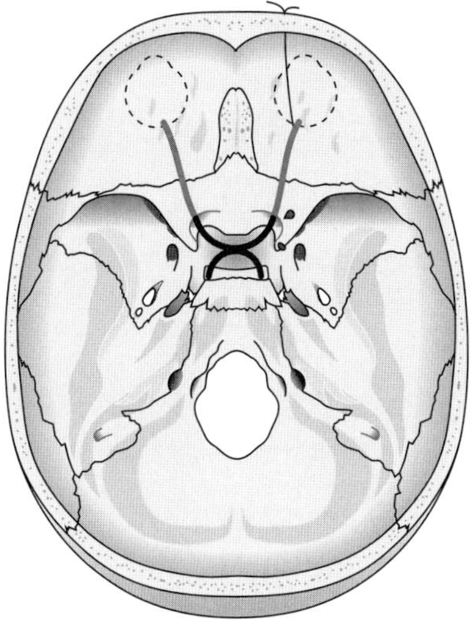

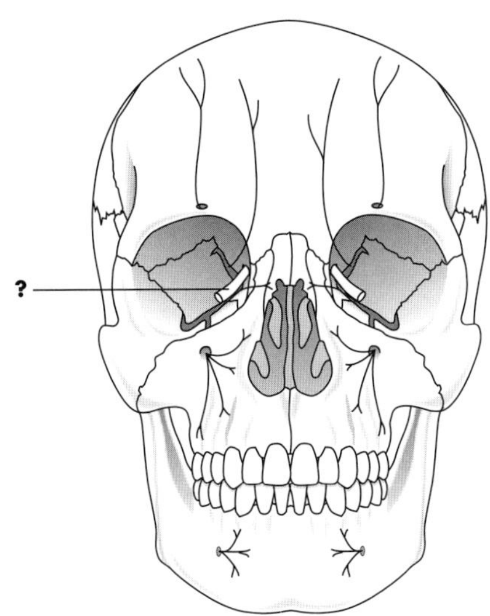

In the diagram of the interior cranium, note how the optic nerves pass out of the optic foramina and join in the area of the pituitary fossa near that gland. They then pass directly into the brain. The area of crossover of the optic nerves is called the ____________. Many important structures are found in this small area.

optic chiasm

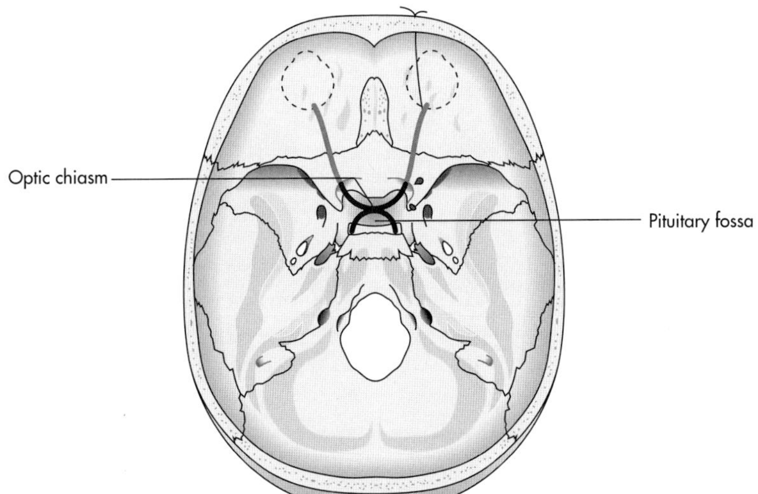

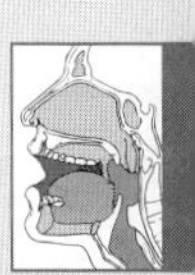

II, eye (vision), sensory, optic, occipital lobe

Review. Find the optic nerve (cranial nerve ______________) on these drawings. What does it innervate? What type of nerve is CN II? Through which foramina does it pass? In what portion of the brain does it end?

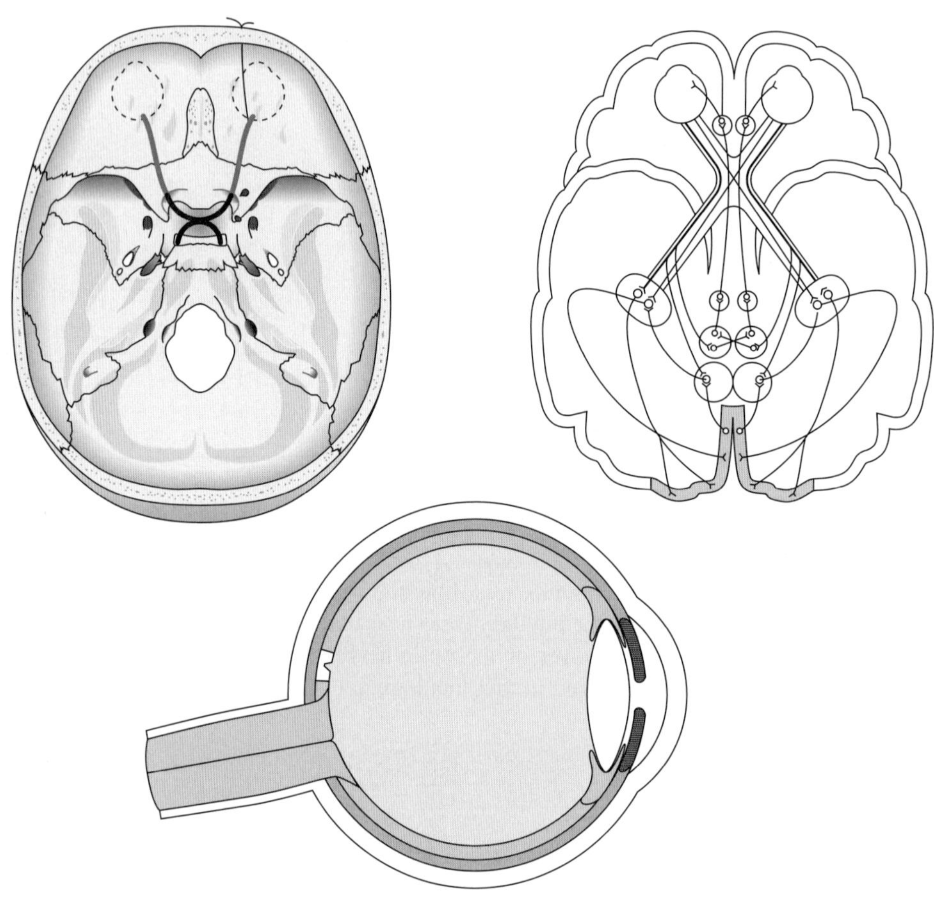

3.3 Cranial Nerves III, IV, and VI: Oculomotor, Trochlear, and Abducens Nerves

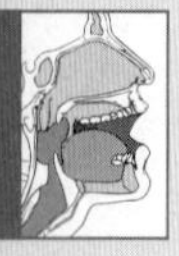

The next three cranial nerves are discussed as a group, as they have very similar functions.

CN III Oculomotor nerve
CN IV Trochlear nerve
CN VI Abducens nerve

The eye is drawn here with its surrounding musculature. These muscles are found within the orbit, originating on the outer layer of the eyeball and passing back to the end of the orbit and sides to insert. They are capable of moving the eye in all directions.

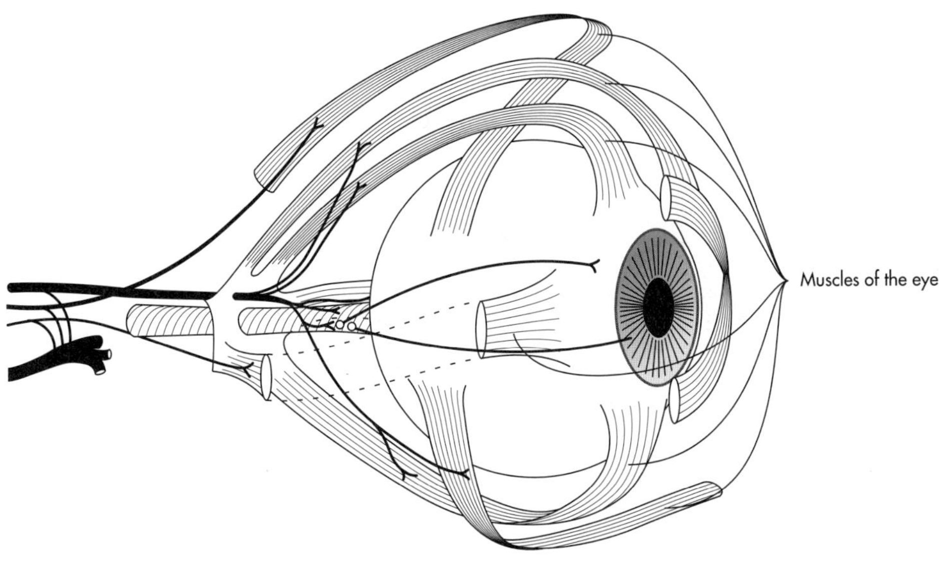

What type of nerve would innervate the muscles of the eye?

motor

Shown with the eye muscles are cranial nerves III, IV, and VI. These nerves innervate the muscles of the eye. **Oculomotor nerve** or CN ______________ also has parasympathetic/sympathetic components that go to muscles of the iris and motor nerves to muscles of the eyelids.

III

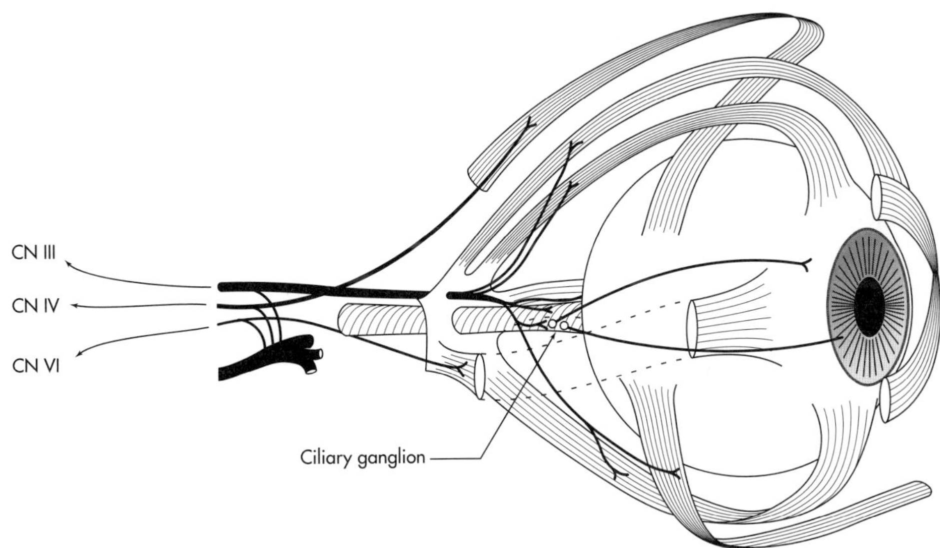

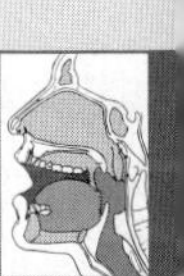

No, CN II passes through the optic foramen.

The interior cranium is shown again with CNs III, IV, and VI as they exit the orbit to enter the cranium, passing through the superior orbital fissure. Is this the same as for CN II?

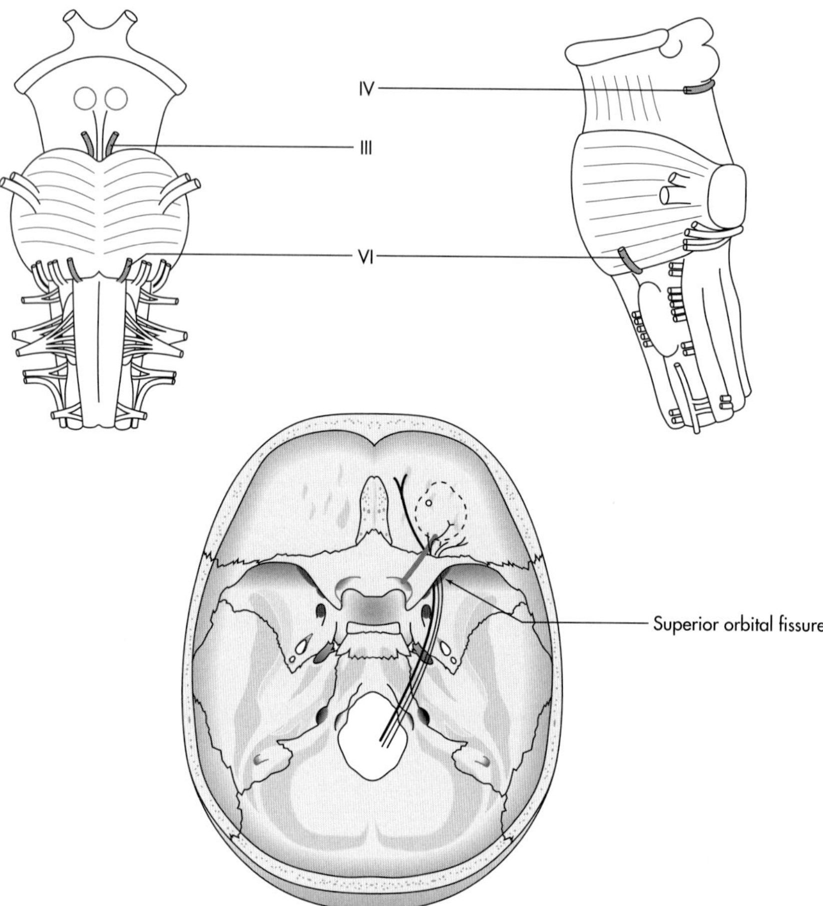

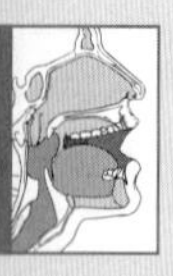

What type of neurons are CN III, IV, and VI? They innervate the muscles of the ______________. As these are motor nerves they begin in the CNS, in the brainstem, going out toward the orbit and passing through the ______________ foramina. Name these cranial nerves.

motor, eye, superior orbital

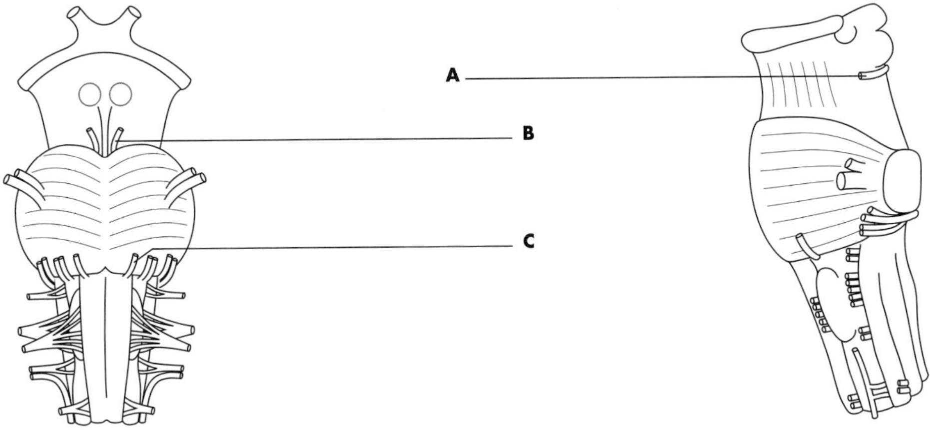

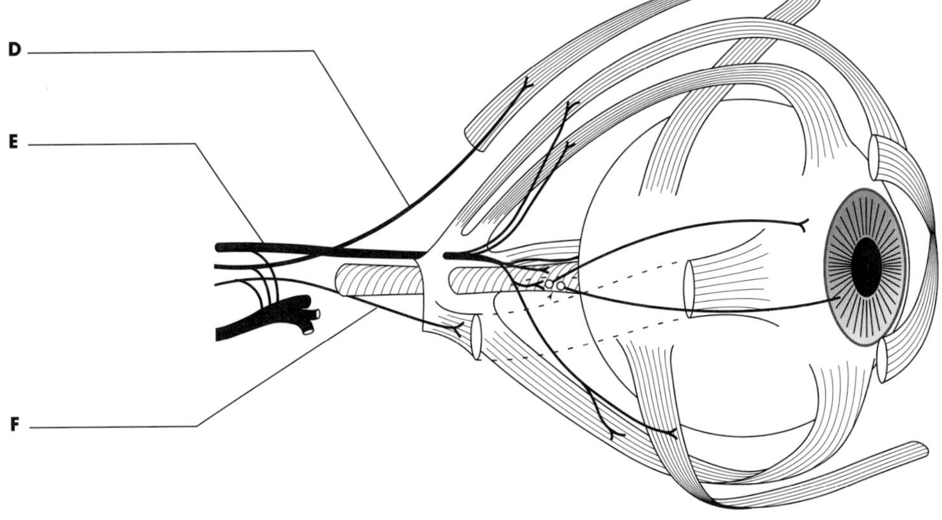

A. CN IV
B. CN III
C. CN VI
D. CN IV
E. CN III
F. CN VI

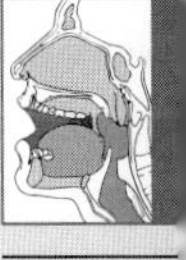

(We return to CN V at the end of the chapter.)

3.4

Cranial Nerve VII: Facial Nerve

The **facial nerve** is so named because of its superficial location on the face. It lies directly below the skin, spreading outward from behind the ear. Find it on the drawings.

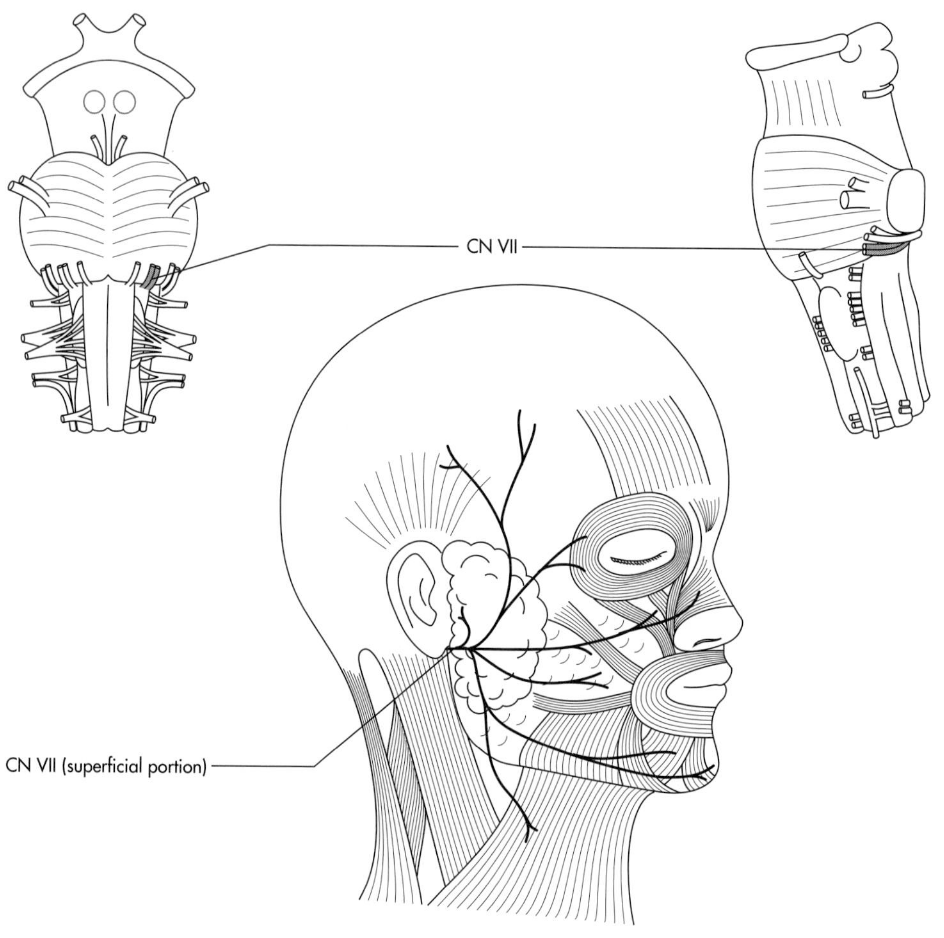

facial

This is the superficial portion of CN VII or the ______________ nerve. There is also a deep component of the facial nerve which we shall see later.

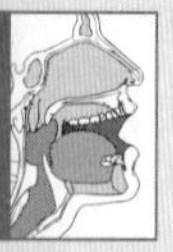

The **superficial portion of the facial nerve** originates in the ventral brainstem in the facial motor nucleus, sending processes out to innervate the muscles of the face. The nerve passes into the **internal auditory meatus,** traveling around the middle ear and extending a branch to the stapedius muscle in the ear. It then exits through the **stylomastoid foramen** behind the ear and spreads across the face.

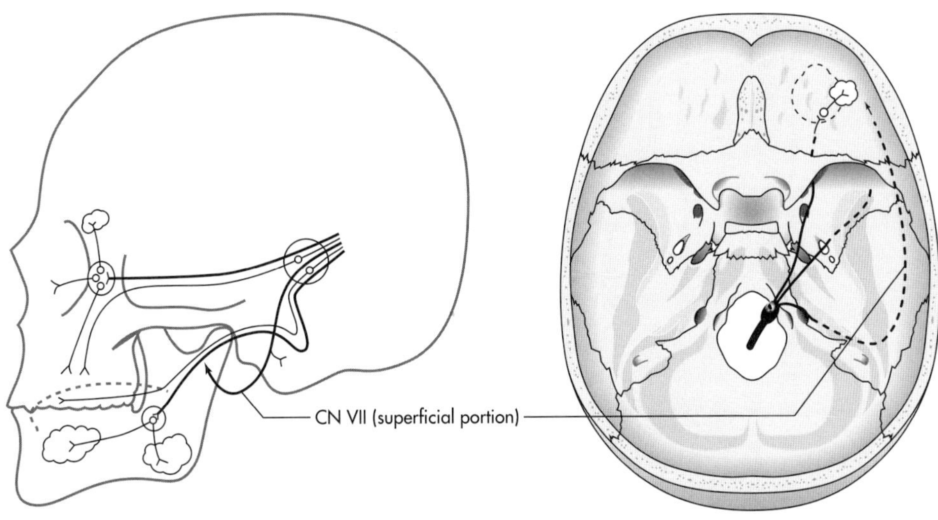

Cranial nerve VII branches across the face, directly below the skin, after passing through the parotid gland, to extend branches to each of the muscles of facial expression.

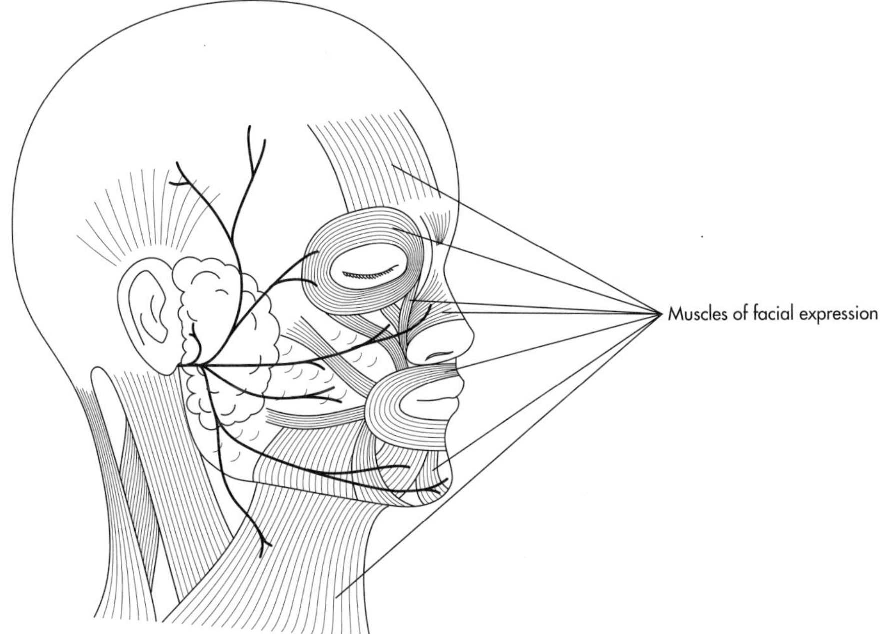

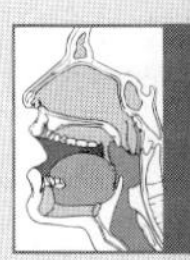

muscles of facial expression, facial expression, motor

What group of muscles does the facial nerve innervate? These thin superficial muscles are responsible for what actions? What type of nerve is this portion of CN VII?

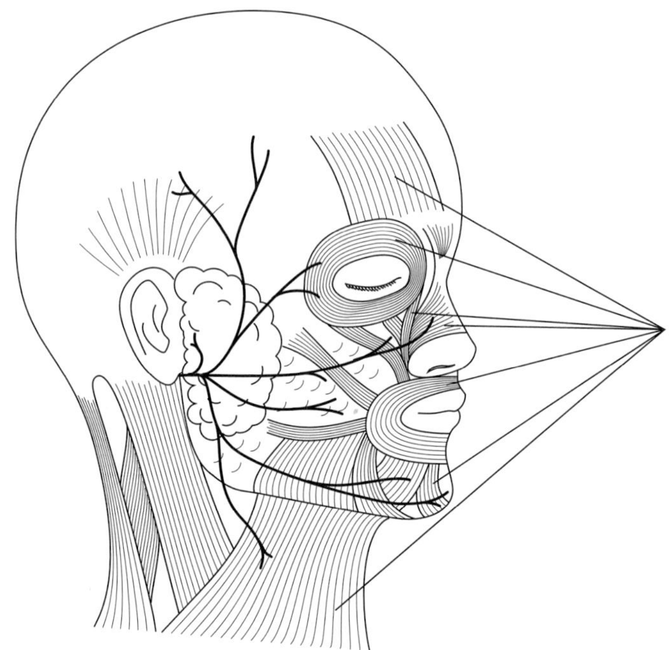

The deeper components of the facial nerve originate in the brainstem and pass out through the **superior orbital fissure** with cranial nerve VI to the nasal mucosa and lacrimal gland, innervating glands (not muscles).

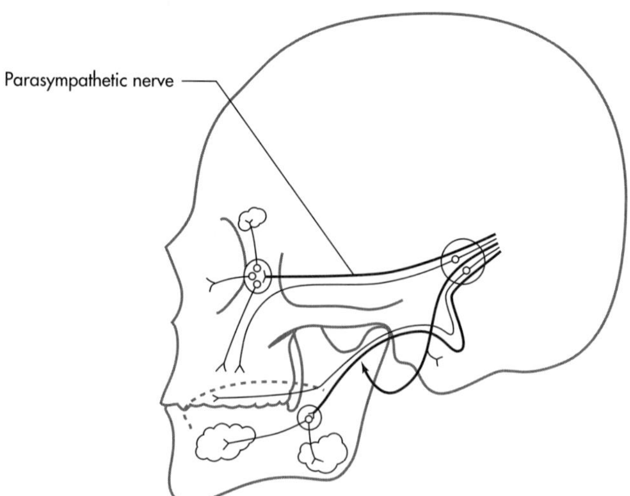

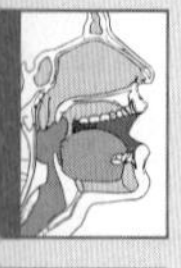

Another branch travels with CN III through the **foramen ovale** to ride on the lingual nerve toward the mandible. It sends a branch to both the submandibular and sublingual salivary glands, innervating these glands. Both of these components are _______________ nerves because they innervate glands. They are also parasympathetic.

motor

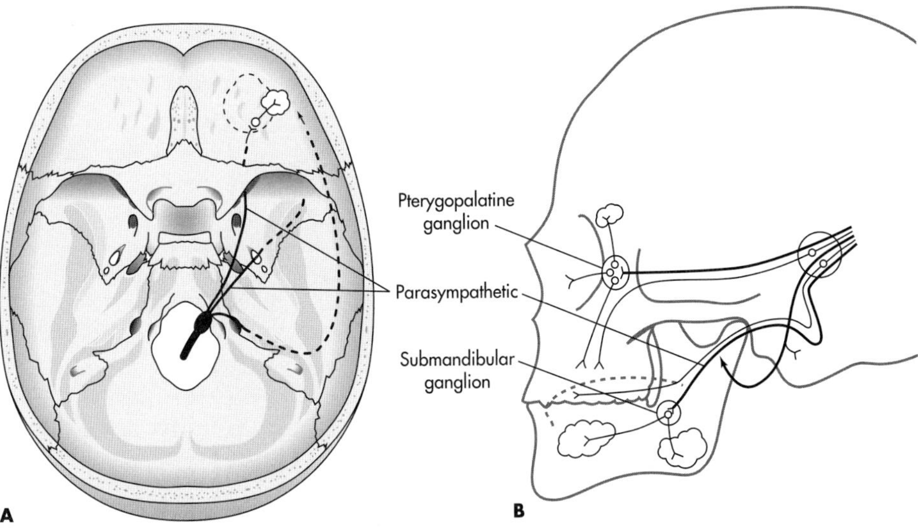

Two ganglia are associated with these portions of CN VII: the **pterygopalatine ganglion** and the **submandibular ganglion.** Find them above.

Lastly, a sensory component of CN VII is shown. It originates on the anterior two thirds of the mucosa of the tongue. These specialized receptor neurons are the **taste cells.**

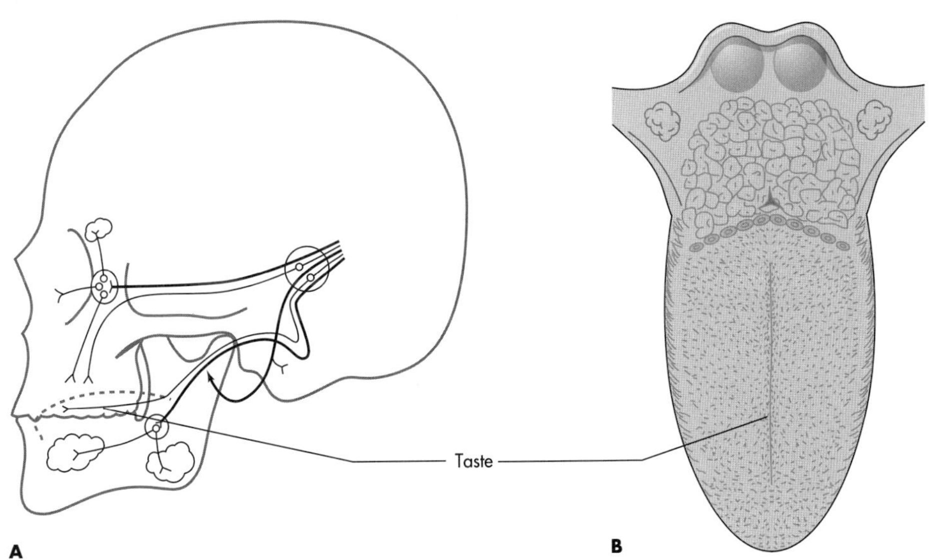

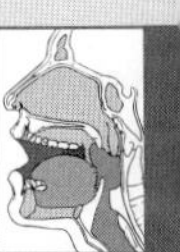

The taste cells of the anterior tongue are responsible for the sense of taste. Taste, as you will remember, is a combination of four major sensations—salty, sweet, sour, and bitter—plus the sense of smell. Locate these four areas of taste on the tongue. See Chapter Five.

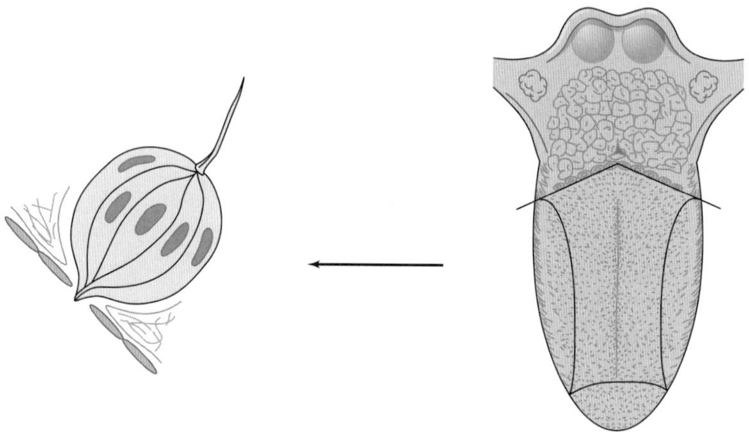

VII

Taste information is gathered and sent on a branch of CN VII that hitches a ride on the lingual nerve (a branch of CN V). This branch of the facial nerve for taste that rides on CN V is called the **chorda tympani.** Facial nerve is CN ______________.

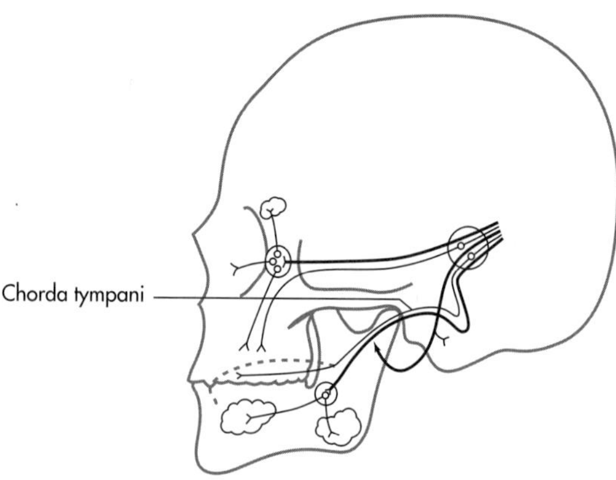

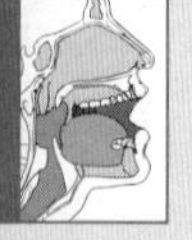

The **chorda tympani** travels up the lingual nerve, branches off, and passes into the middle ear cavity through the **petrotympanic fissure.** It travels over the malleus and joins the rest of the facial nerve to exit the internal auditory meatus and connect with the brainstem after leaving a sensory ganglion, the **geniculate ganglion.** ______________ is the branch of CN VII that carries taste.

Chorda tympani

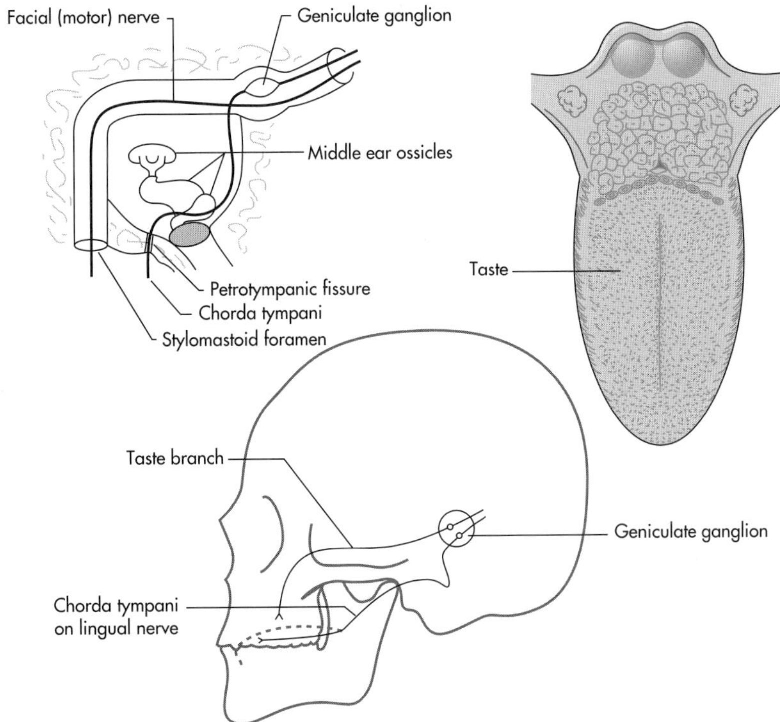

There is also a taste branch to the palate.

As it has both sensory and motor components, the facial nerve is a ______________ type of nerve.

mixed

The motor components of the facial nerve that innervate glands are parasympathetic nerves and you will note that these have two neurons that create separate ganglia. What were these two ganglia?

submandibular ganglion and pterygomandibular ganglion

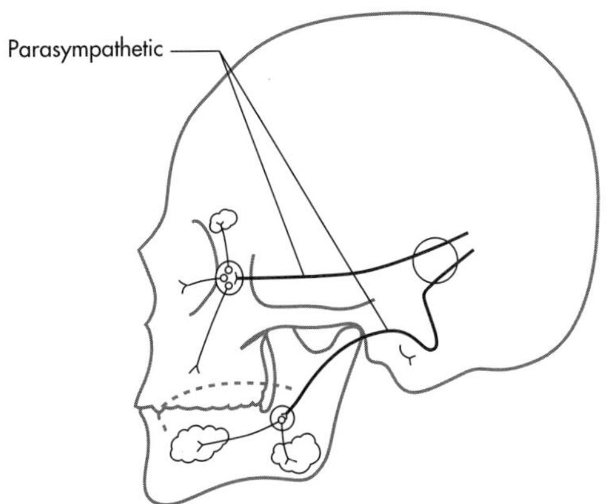

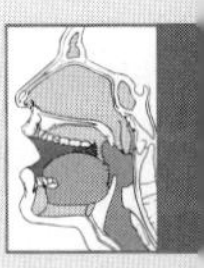

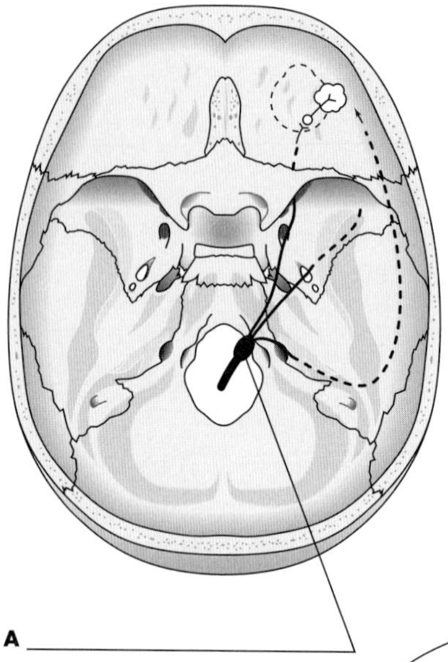

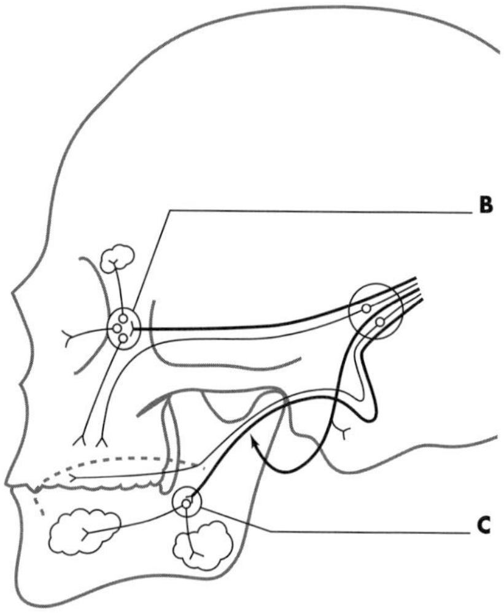

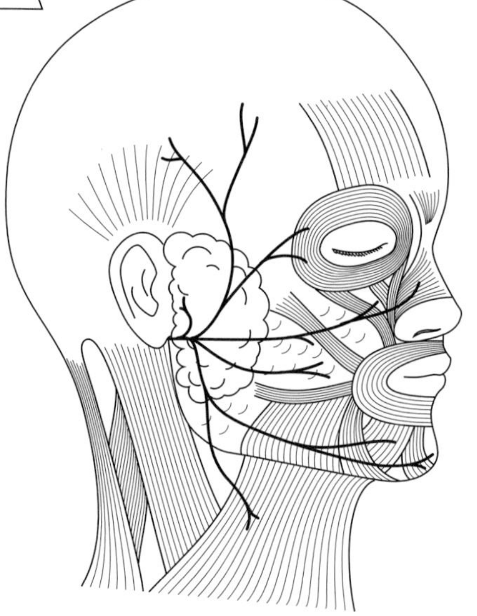

A. geniculate ganglion
B. pterygopalatine ganglion
C. submandibular ganglion

Find the facial nerve ganglia in these drawings. Label the ganglia.

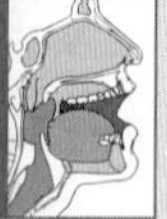

1. muscles of facial expression
2. stapedius muscle
3. lacrimal gland
4. glands of nose
5. submandibular salivary gland
6. sublingual salivary gland
7. taste on anterior two thirds of tongue
8. taste palate

What does the facial nerve innervate? Make a list.

Motor: 1. ______
2. ______
3. ______
4. ______
5. ______
6. ______

Sensory: 7. ______
8. ______

What type of nerve is CN VII? What foramina does it pass through?

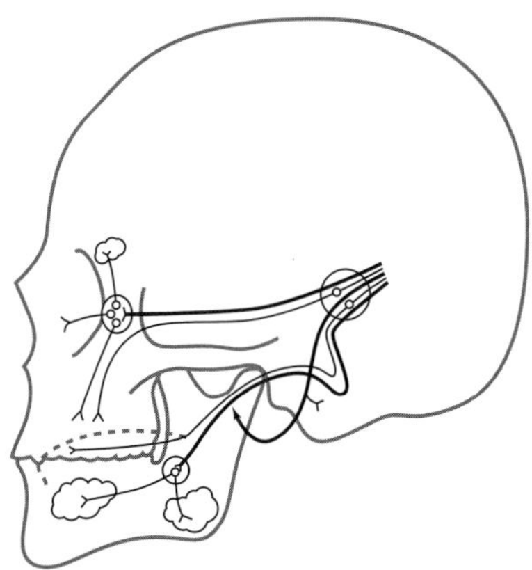

mixed; internal auditory meatus, stylomastoid foramen, superior orbital fissure, foramen ovale, petrotympanic fissure

Cranial Nerve VIII: Vestibulocochlear Nerve

3.5

The eighth cranial nerve has been called a few different names: the auditory nerve, the acoustic nerve, or (more accurately) the **vestibulocochlear nerve.**

Cranial nerve VIII begins with specialized sensory receptor neurons within the inner ear, in both the vestibule and the cochlea. Find those portions of the ear in the diagram.

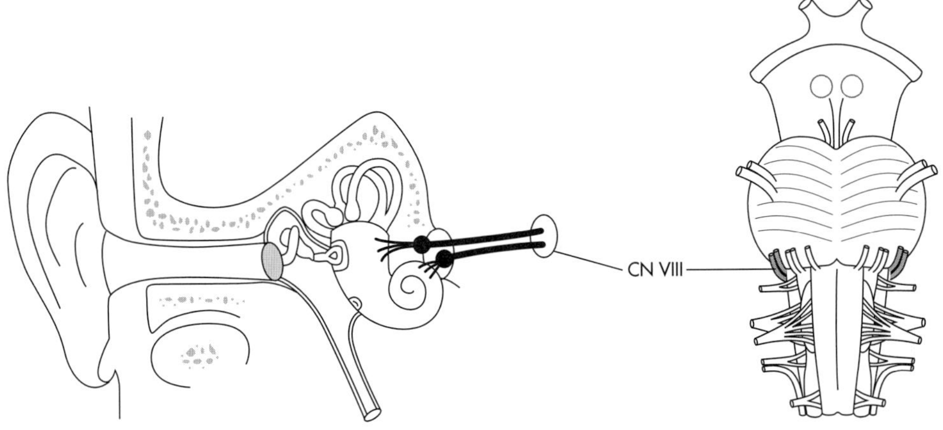

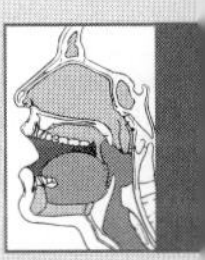

Let us look briefly at the anatomy of the ear. We see that there is an **external, middle,** and **inner ear.**

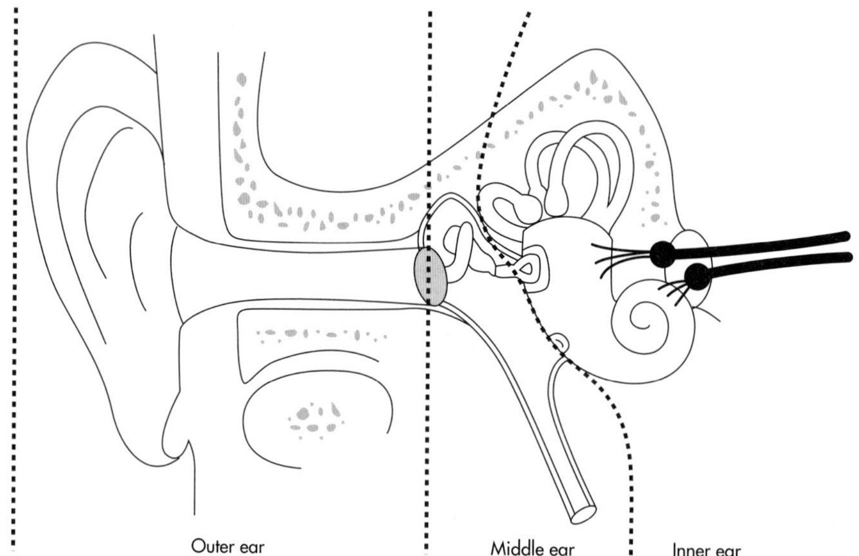

The conversion of sound waves into neuronal signals begins at the outer ear as the **pinna** gathers sound waves and funnels them down the **external auditory meatus.** Sound causes the **tympanic membrane** to vibrate and passes that vibration to the bones of the middle ear.

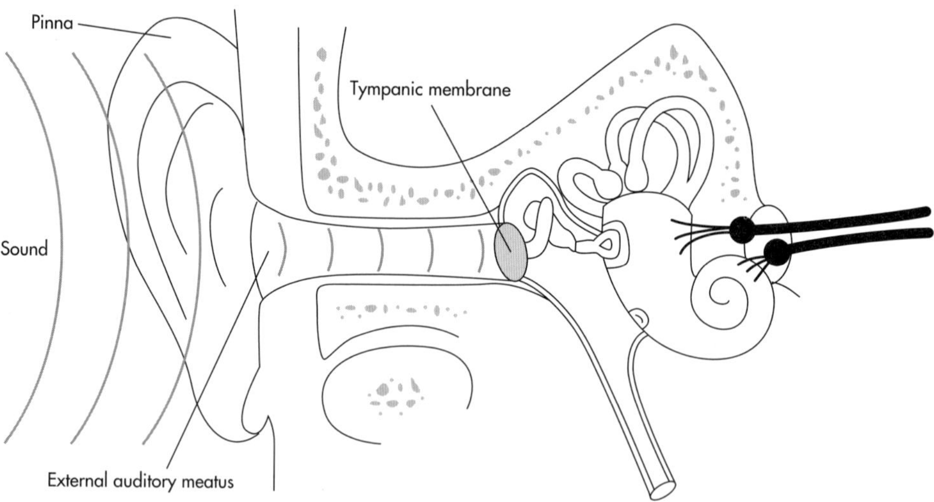

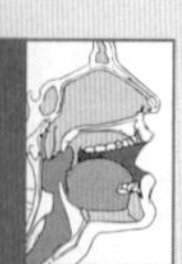

The **middle ear** is a mucosa-lined cavity with three small bones, the ossicles, which are connected and pass vibration mechanically to the inner ear. What are the three **ossicles?**

malleus, incus, stapes

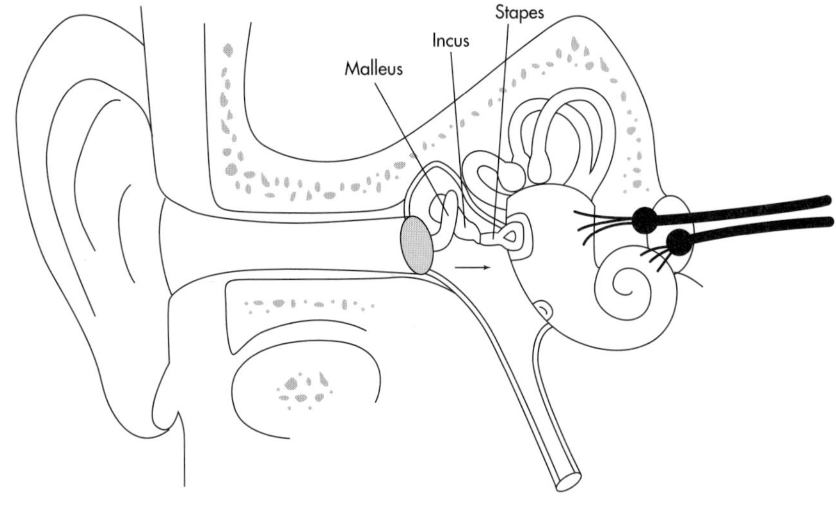

Sound transmission continues as vibration is passed into the inner ear by way of pressure on the fluid-filled sac found there, the **vestibule** and **cochlea,** which are continuous. The **cochlea** is a spiral portion, filled with fluid and lined with a type of hair cell.

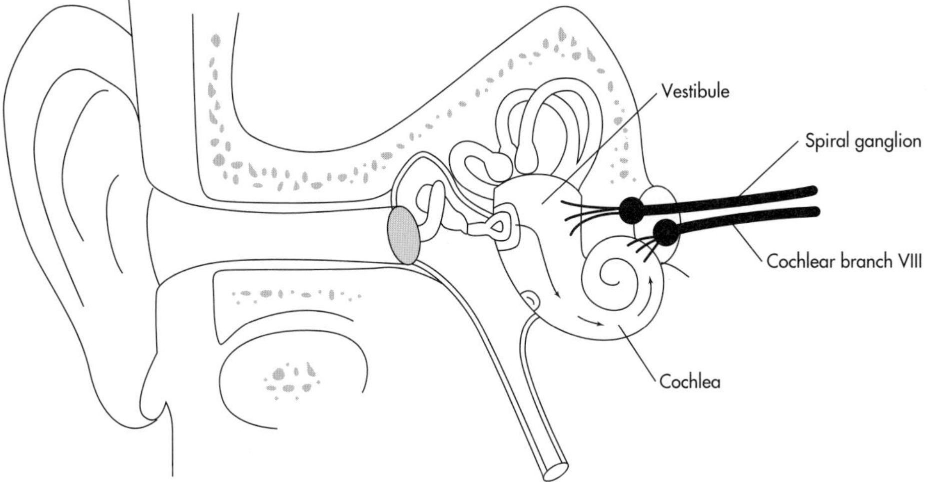

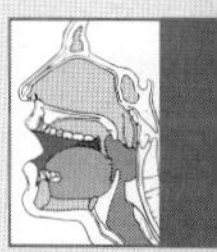

sensory

Fluid movement distorts the **hair cells** of the cochlea and triggers neuronal firing. Thus, the sensation of hearing is produced as it travels down the **cochlear nerve** portion of CN VIII to the brain. What type of nerve is CN VIII?

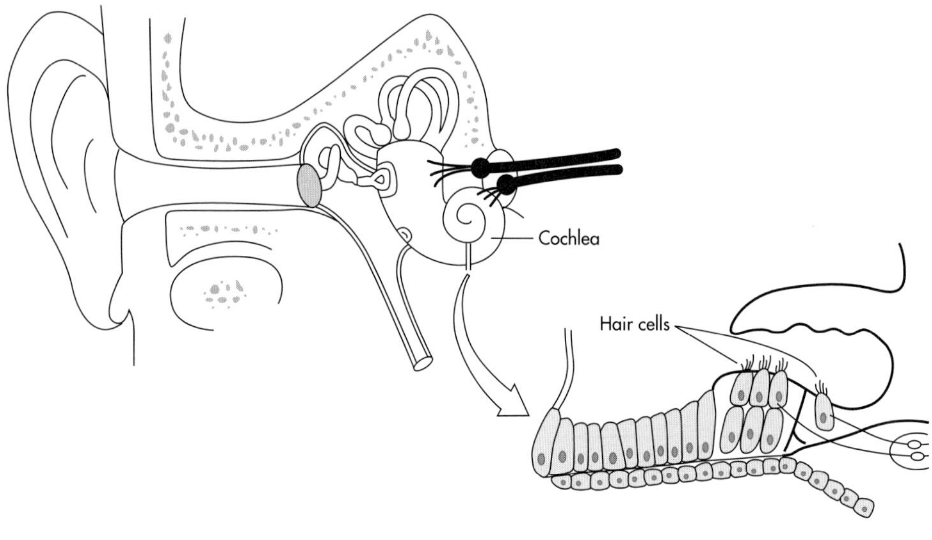

cochlear

The __________ nerve passes out of the inner ear, forming the **spiral ganglion,** and then passes through the **internal auditory meatus** before joining the brainstem. In the brainstem, connections to cochlear nuclei are made.

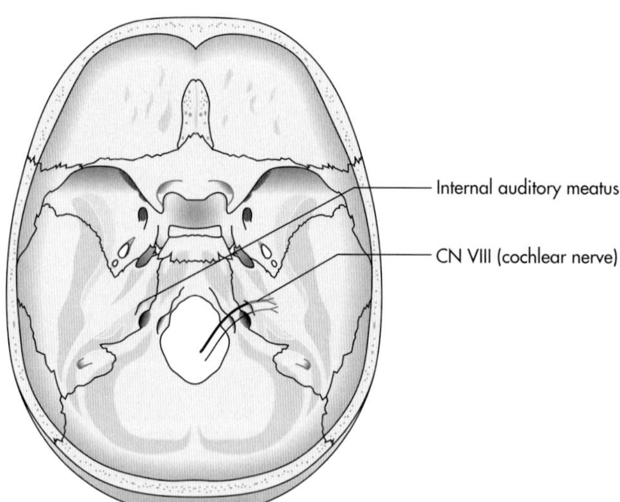

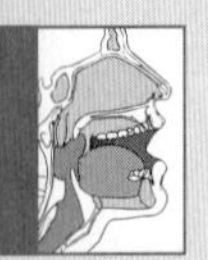

The cochlear nerve then travels to the **geniculate bodies** (nuclei) and the **auditory cortex** in the temporal lobes near the lateral sulcus.

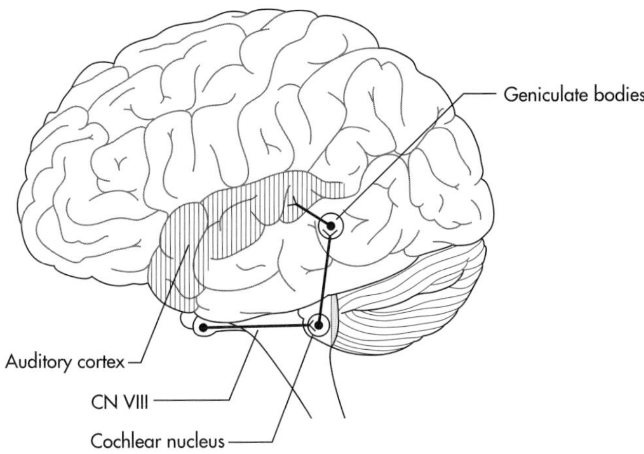

cochlear portion

The **vestibular portion** of CN VIII begins as hair cells within the **vestibule.** These cells are triggered by fluid movements within the vestibule in response to different positions of the head. This acts much as the fluid in a level, giving positional information to the brain, or where the head is located in space. The other portion of CN VIII is the ________ .

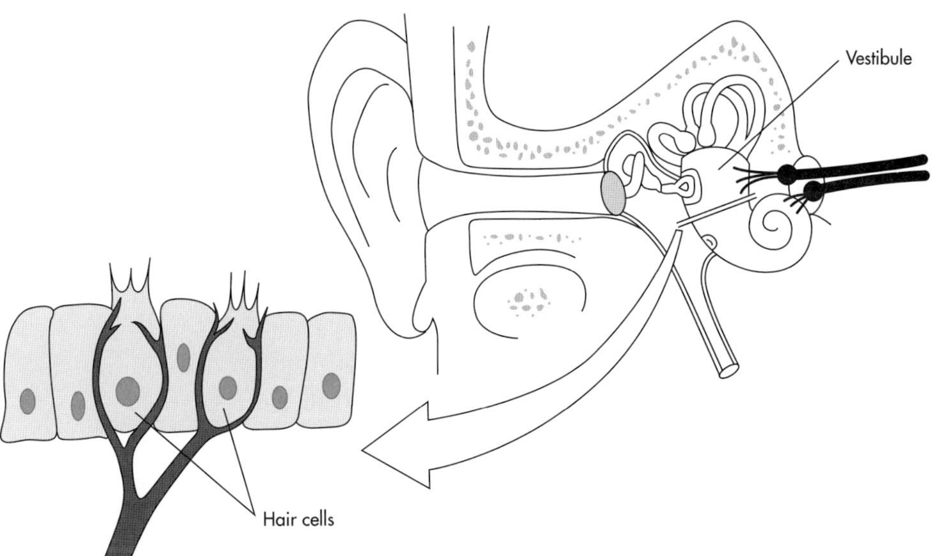

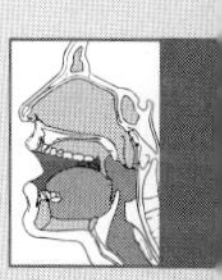

proprioception

Three loops of the vestibule that are sensitive to the three spatial positions are called the **semicircular canals.** Find them on the drawing. Remember that position sense is also called ______________.

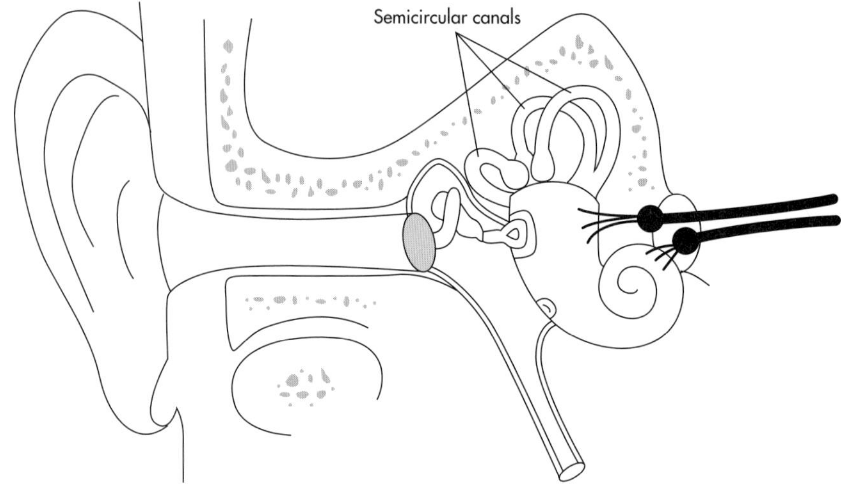

Positional information is passed down the **vestibular nerve** out of the inner ear, forming the **vestibular ganglion.** It then passes with the cochlear nerve out the internal auditory meatus to the brainstem.

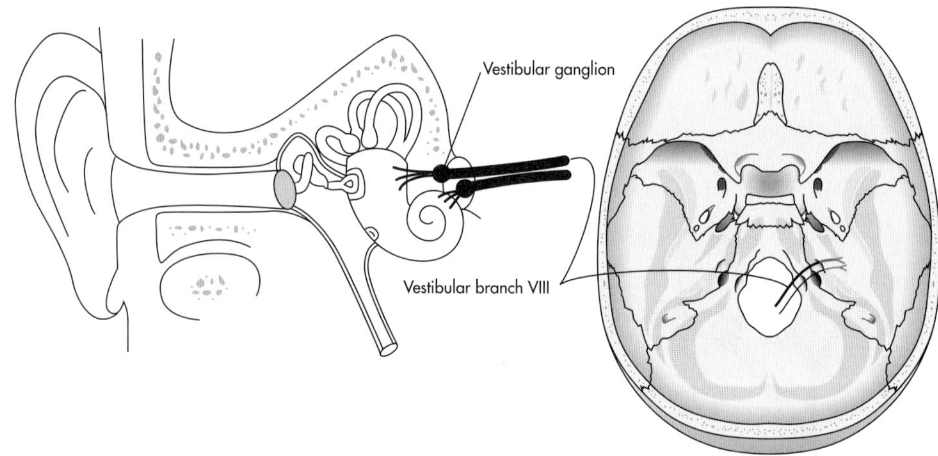

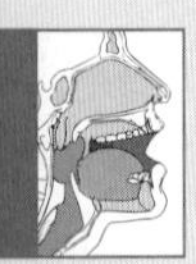

Information from the vestibule passes to the **vestibular nuclei** of the brainstem, making several connections with other nuclei and with the cerebellum, as positional information is important to the function of the body's muscles. Some information connects with the cortex. Find the vestibular nuclei.

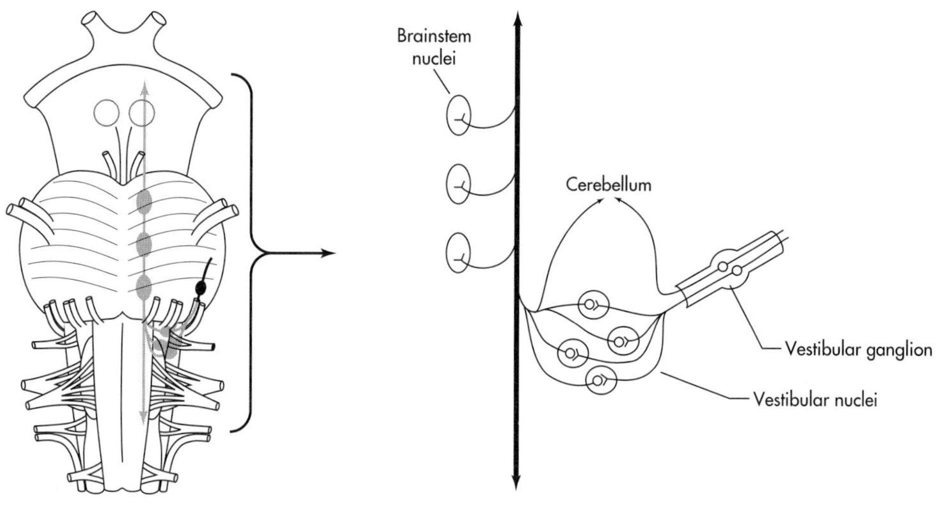

Review. CN VIII, or the ______________ nerve, is a ______________-type nerve, originating in the ______________ and ______________ of the inner ear.

vestibulocochlear, sensory, cochlea, vestibule

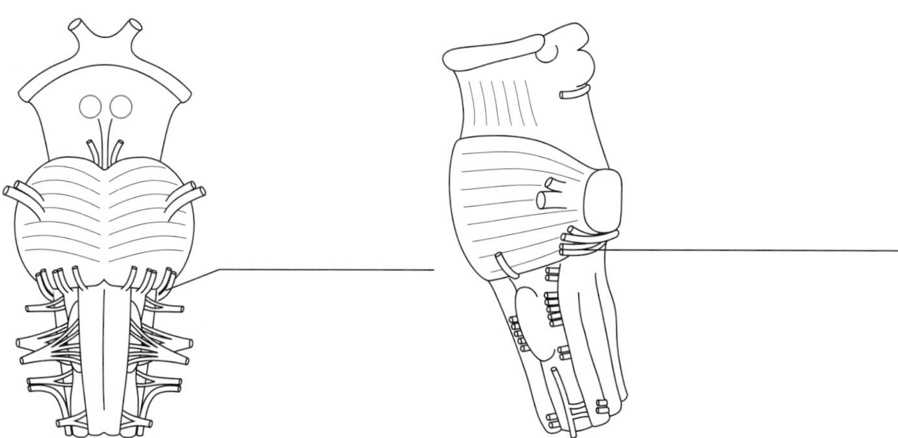

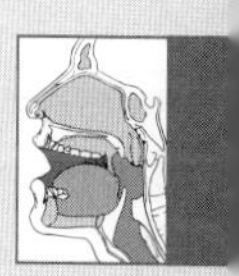

spiral, vestibular, cochlear, vestibular, internal auditory

The sensory ganglia of CN VIII are the ______________ and ______________ ganglia. The ______________ nerve and the ______________ nerve pass together through the ______________ meatus to the brainstem.

geniculate, temporal, hearing

Auditory information passes through the ______________ bodies to the auditory portion of the cortex located on the ______________ lobes. This portion of CN VIII is responsible for the sense of ______________.

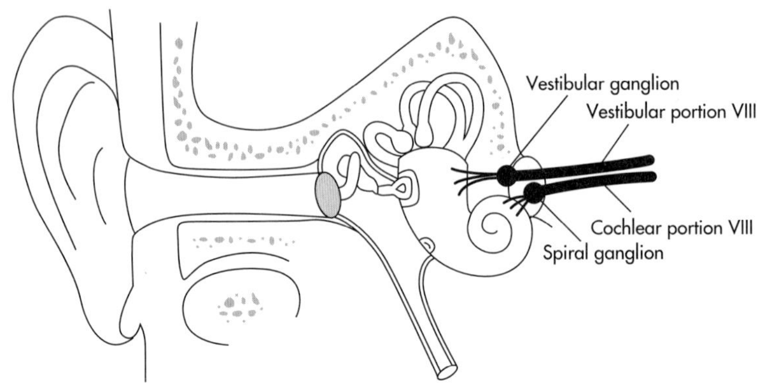

vestibular, vestibule, vestibular, internal, vestibular, position

The other portion of CN VIII is the ______________ nerve, which begins in the ______________. It forms the ______________ ganglia, passing out through the ______________ auditory meatus to the brainstem. The ______________ nuclei connect to several centers of the brainstem, cerebellum, and cerebrum, giving the sense of ______________.

A. external auditory meatus
B. tympanic membrane
C. malleus
D. incus
E. stapes
F. semicircular canals
G. vestibule
H. cochlea

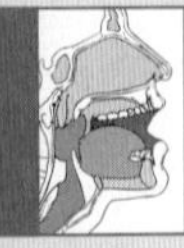

Label these parts of the ear.

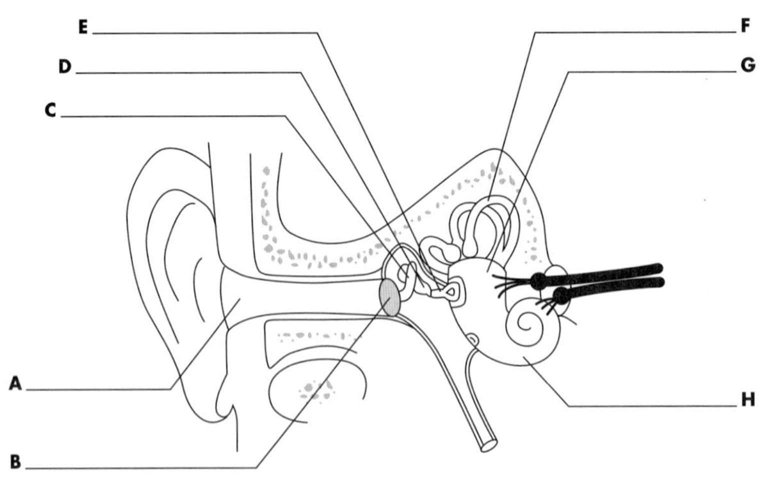

Find these portions of CN VIII on the drawings.

A. CN VIII
B. cochlear branch
C. internal auditory meatus
D. vestibular branch
E. vestibular ganglion
F. vestibular nerve (branch)
G. cochlear nerve (branch)
H. spiral ganglion

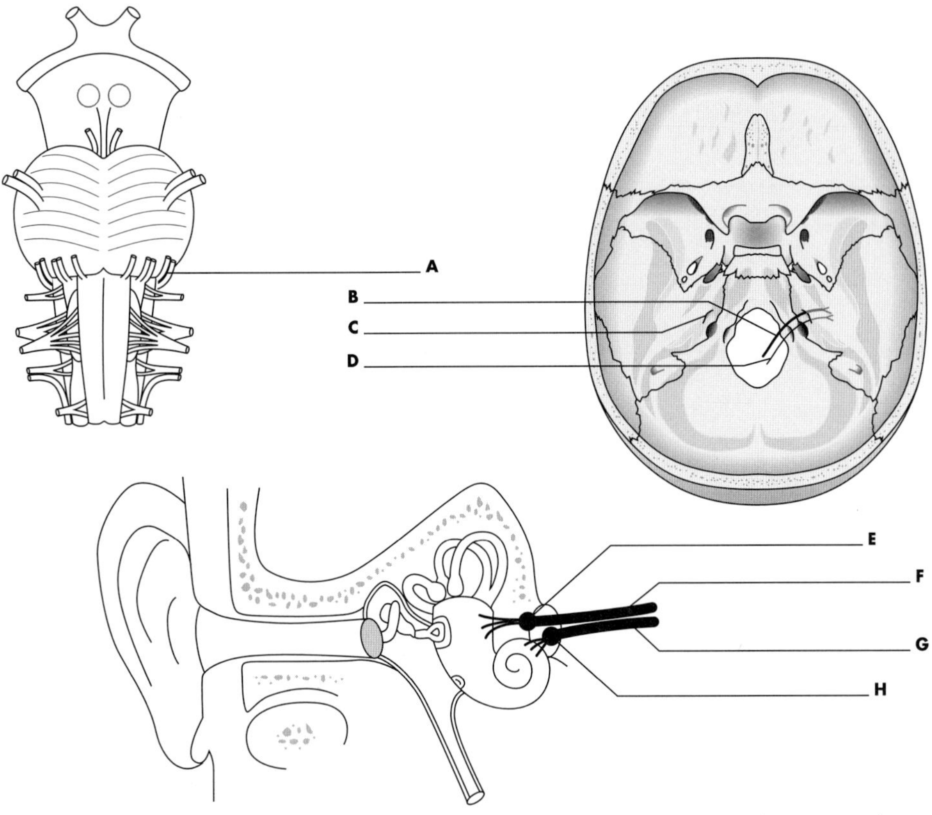

Cranial Nerve IX: Glossopharyngeal Nerve

3.6

The **glossopharyngeal nerve** is cranial nerve IX. The name gives an indication of the destination of this nerve pair: *glosso* means __________, and *pharyngeal,* of the __________. CN IX innervates primarily the tongue and pharynx.

tongue, pharnyx

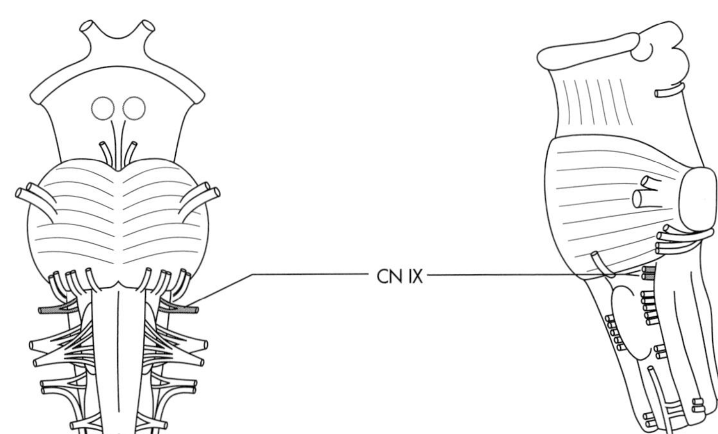

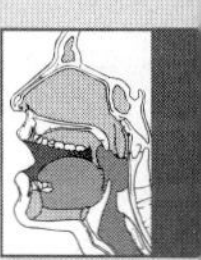

The glossopharyngeal nerve exits the brainstem in this area. It leaves the cranium mostly through the **jugular foramen.**

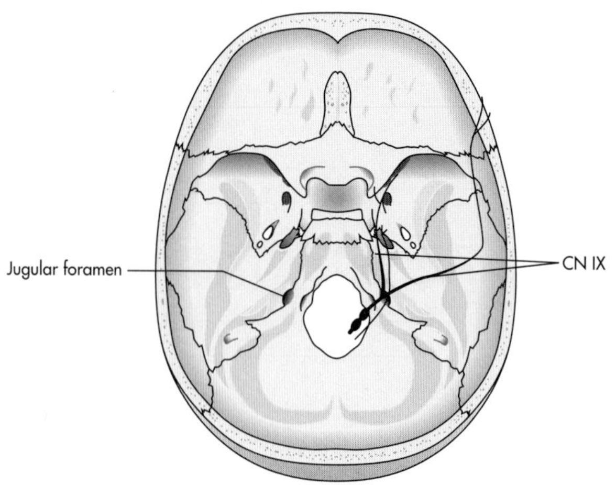

mixed

All of the branches of CN IX run to deep structures in the head and neck. There are sensory and motor branches, so this is a ______________-type nerve.

The first general sensory branches run to the mucosa of the pharynx and posterior tongue. There are also a few to the outer and middle ear and palate. Find these on the diagram.

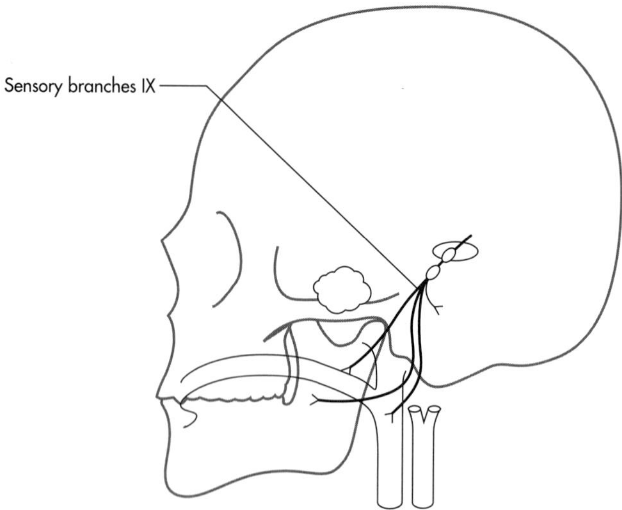

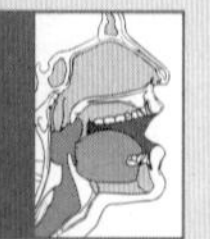

to sense what is about to be swallowed

General sensation is touch, pain, and pressure. Why is it important in this area?

The presence of an object on the posterior tongue and pharynx initiates the swallow reflex. Once initiated, a swallow passes through the pharynx into the esophagus by its muscles, innervated by motor neurons. What type of nerve is CN IX in the pharynx?

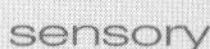

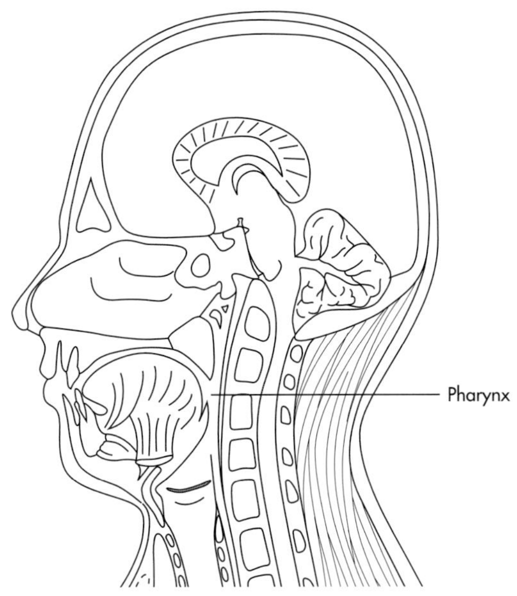

Another sensory branch of CN IX is responsible for a special sense, that of taste. Taste cells innervated by CN IX are located mainly on the posterior third of the tongue. Recall the division of the tongue into thirds based on its embryologic development. What cranial nerve is for taste on the anterior two thirds of the tongue?

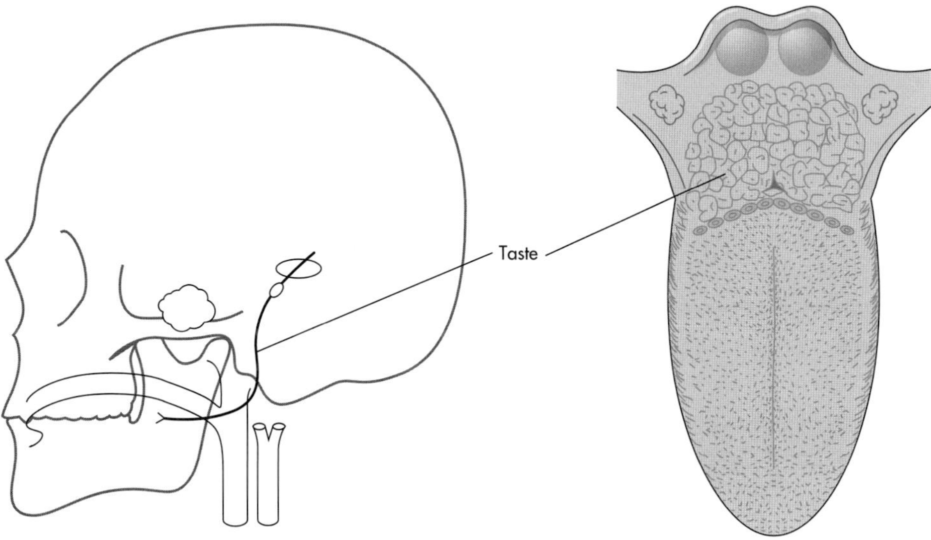

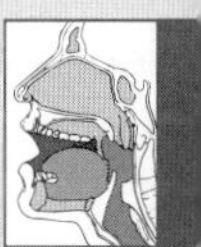

circumvallate papilla

1. CN V
2. CN IX
3. CN VII
4. CN IX

What divides the two areas of the tongue mucosa? Fill in the following information about sensation on the tongue.

1. General sensation to anterior two thirds ______________
2. General sensation to posterior one third ______________
3. Special (taste) sensation to anterior two thirds ______________
4. Special (taste) sensation to posterior one third ______________

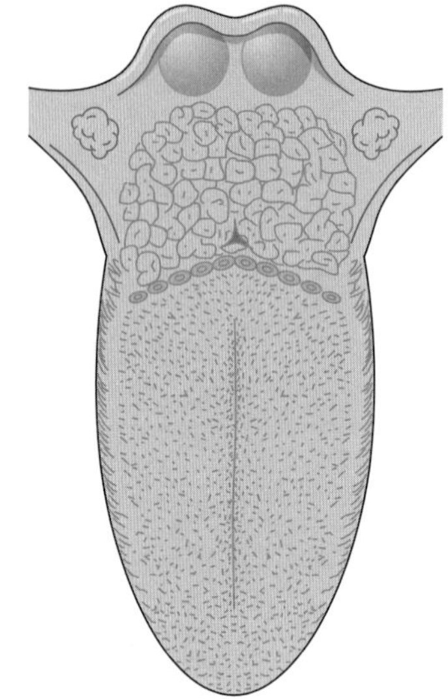

Another type of sensation associated with CN IX occurs in the carotid arteries. Nerve endings in special locations in these arteries sense both changes in blood pressure **(baroreceptors)** and changes in oxygen level **(chemoreceptors).** These are important to the regulation of blood flow to the head.

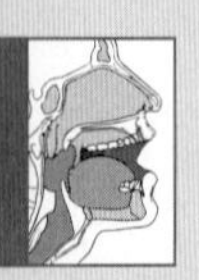

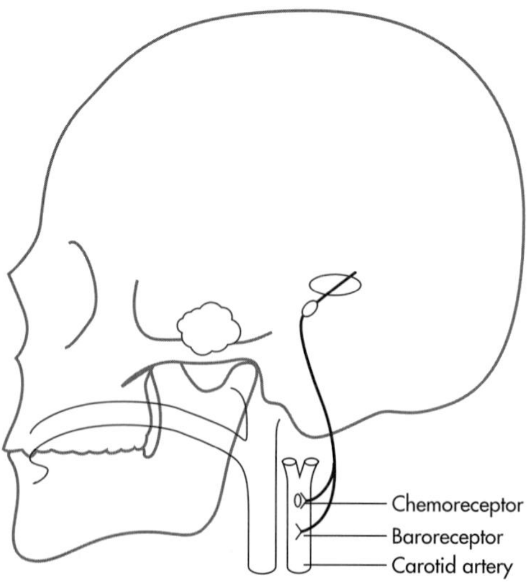

The sensory ganglia associated with CN IX are the **inferior and superior petrosal ganglia.** The nucleus assosiated with the glossopharyngeal nerve in the brainstem is the **nucleus solitarius.**

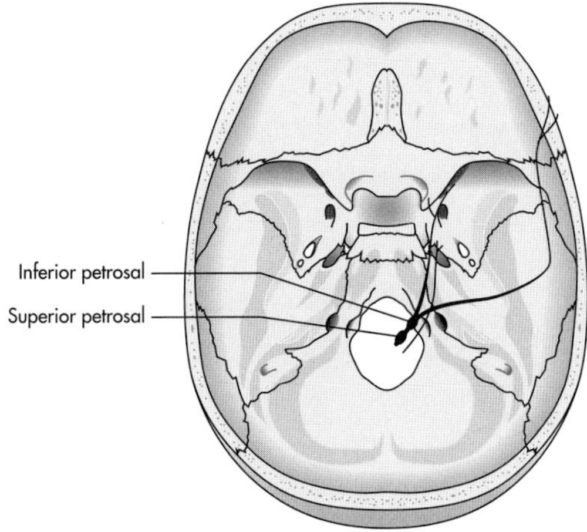

The motor branches of CN IX are of two types. The one shown here operates a gland and is parasympathetic. The gland that is innervated is the ______________ salivary gland.

parotid

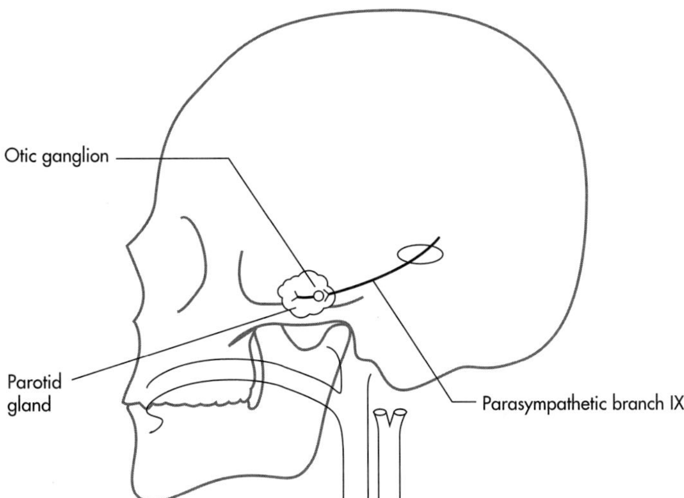

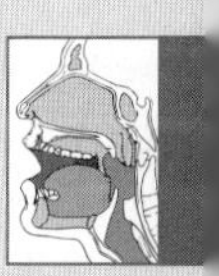

1. CN IX
2. CN VII
3. CN VII

What cranial nerves innervate the (1) parotid salivary glands, (2) sublingual, and (3) submandibular?

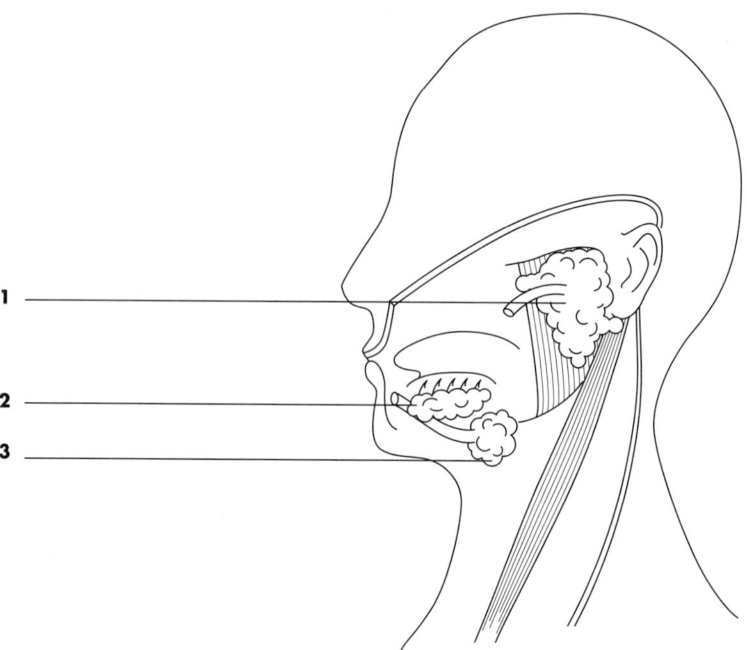

The last motor branch of the glossopharyngeal nerve innervates two small muscles in the pharynx: stylopharyngeus and superior constrictor (a few fibers). Find their pathways.

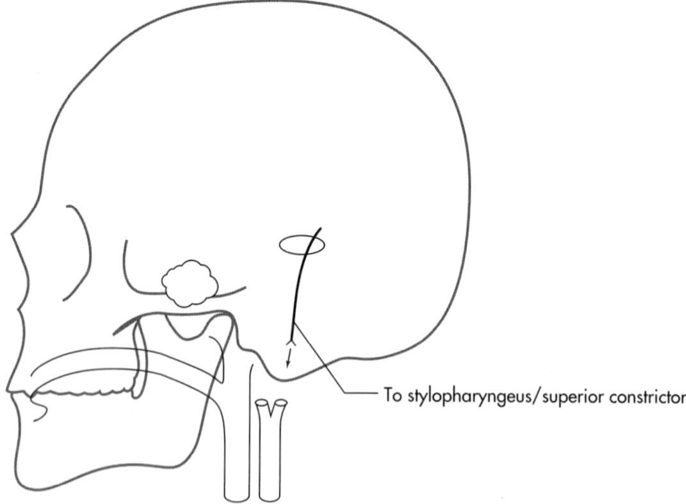

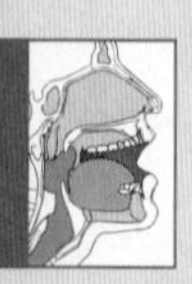

Review. List the structures that CN IX innervates.

Sensory Branches

General sensation to:

1. ______________________
2. ______________________
3. ______________________
4. ______________________

Special sensation (taste) to:

5. ______________________

Baro- and chemoreceptors to:

6. ______________________

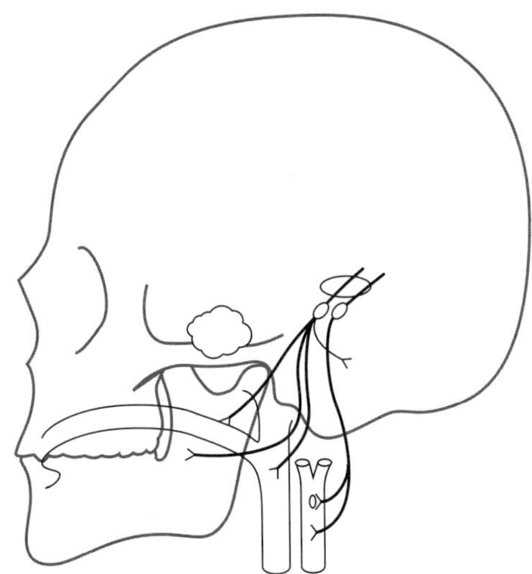

1. pharynx
2. posterior one third of tongue
3. posterior palate
4. outer ear
5. posterior one third of tongue
6. carotid arteries

Motor Branches

Parasympathetic to:

1. ______________________

Muscular to:

2. ______________________
3. ______________________

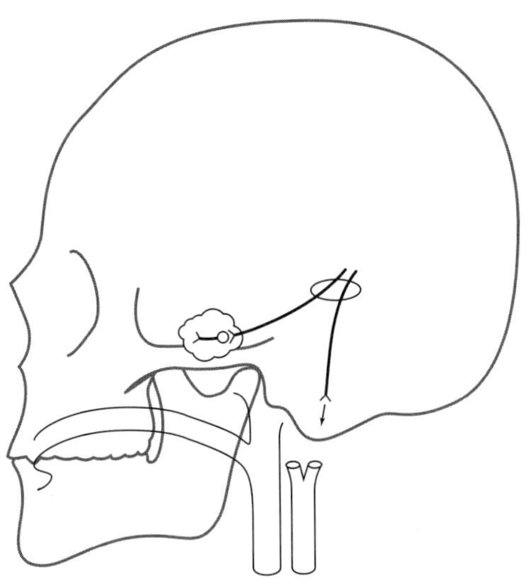

1. parotid gland
2. stylopharyngeus muscle
3. superior constrictor

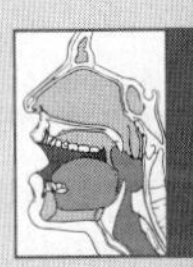

mixed, superior, inferior petrosal, otic nucleus solitarius

CN IX is a ______________ nerve. Its ganglia are the ______________ and ______________ and its nucleus is the ______________.

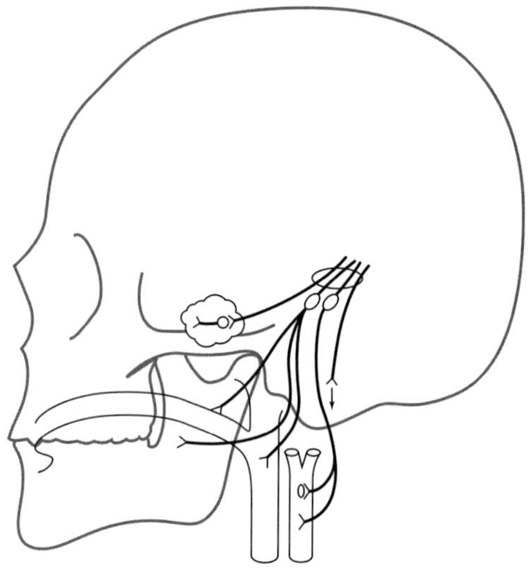

jugular

The glossopharyngeal nerve exits the ______________ foramen to leave the cranium. Find CN IX on the drawing.

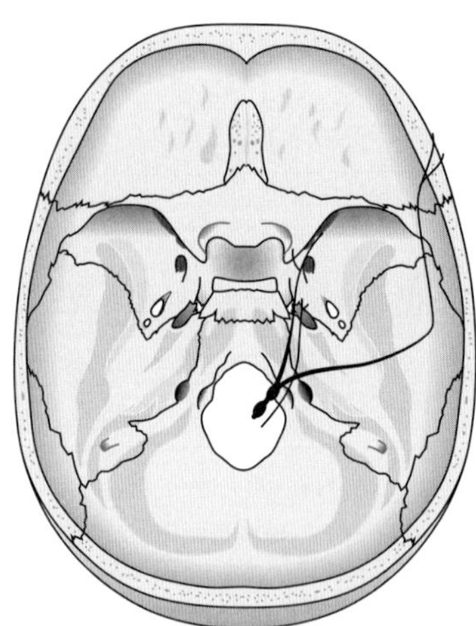

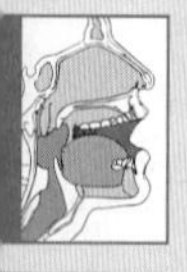

Cranial Nerve X: Vagus Nerve

3.7

mixed

The **vagus nerve** gets its name from a word that means "to wander," and an appropriate name it is, as this cranial nerve travels to most of the organs (viscera) of the body. It is the major parasympathetic nerve supply to the upper and middle body. It carries both sensory and motor nerves, so it is a ____________-type nerve.

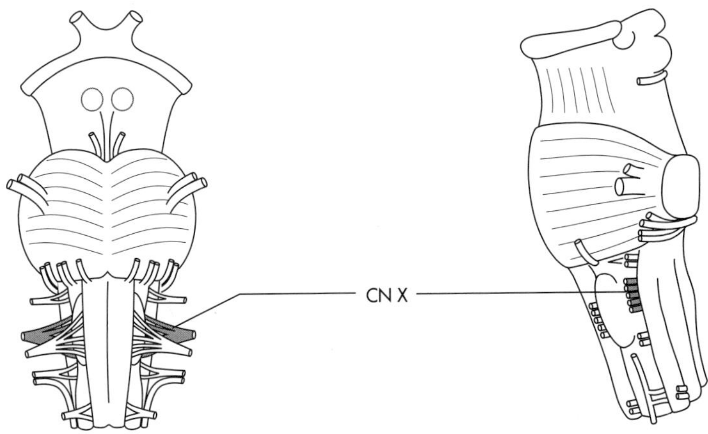

X

The sensory component of the vagus nerve, or CN ____________, is shown here. One small branch gives general sensation to the outer pinna (ear). Many other branches go to the pharynx, larynx, esophagus, stomach, small intestine, part of the large intestine, heart, and lungs for general sensation of visceral sensation. This is a crude sensation that monitors the filling and emptying of organs. Pain sensation travels through other fibers.

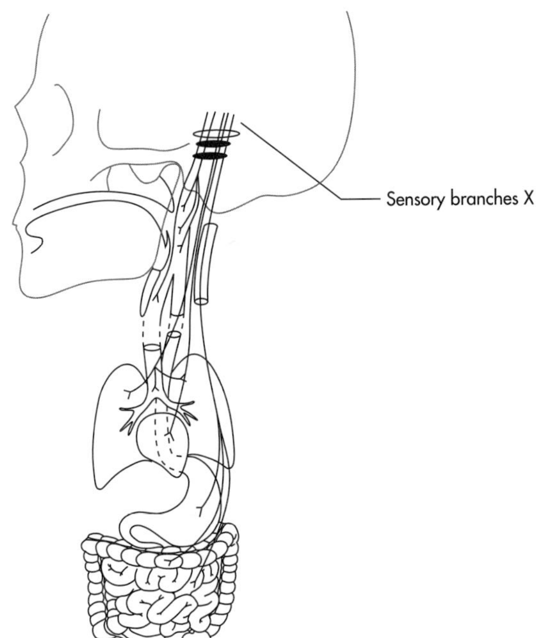

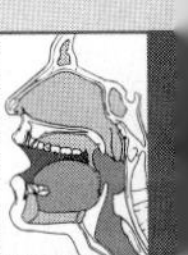

The ganglia associated with the vagus nerve sensory component are the **superior** and **inferior petrosal ganglia,** the same as for CN IX.

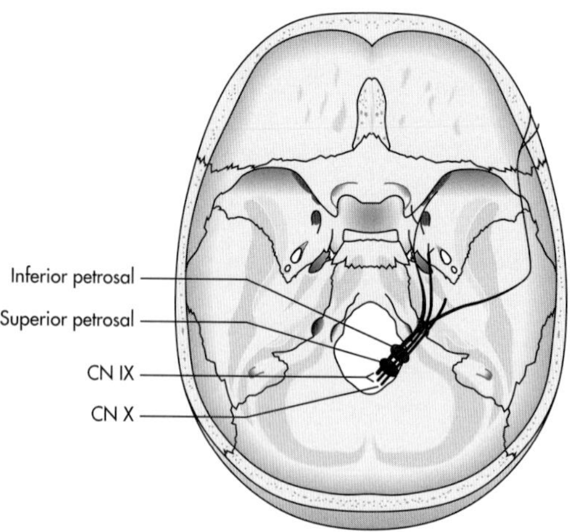

The **motor portion** of CN X contains nerves that cause muscles (smooth and striated) to contract and glands to secrete. The first branches innervate the muscles of the palate, larynx, and pharynx. These muscles are very important to swallowing (deglutition) and to speech and respiration.

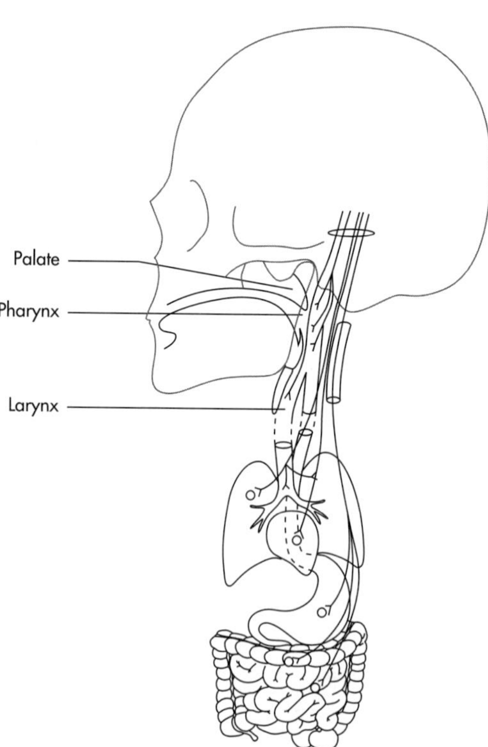

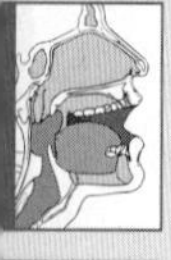

Other parasympathetic fibers run to the viscera of the digestive tract to its smooth muscle and glands to aid in digestion and the passage of food through the tract. Other glands such as the liver and pancreas are regulated by the ________________.

vagus

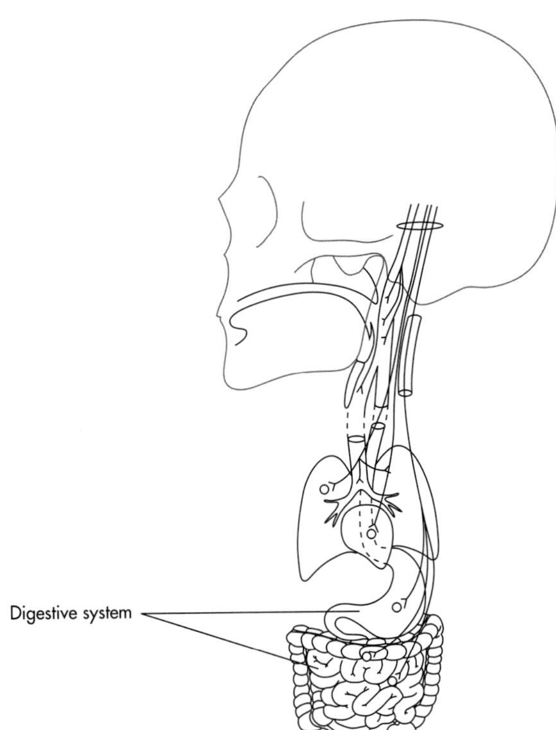

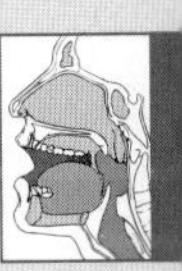

sympathetic

Some of the parasympathetic motor branches run to the bronchi of the lungs and to the heart. These nerves are important to respiration and heartbeat. Parasympathetic nerves, remember, are important to the everyday maintenance of these organs ("slow-down function"), whereas their companion ______________ nerves are called into use in emergencies ("speed-up function").

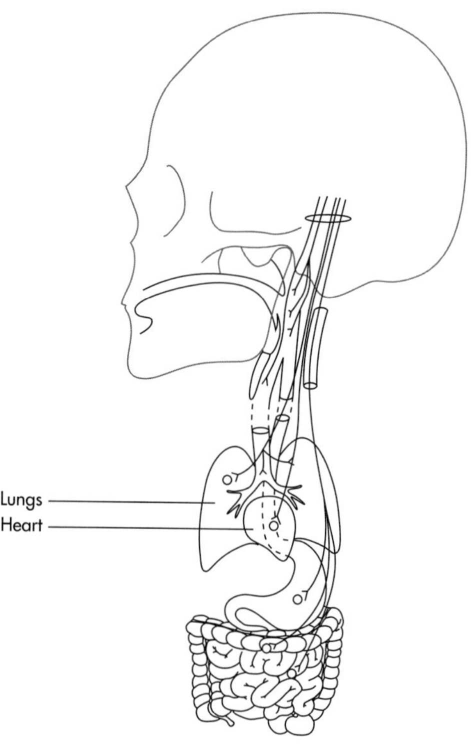

parasympathetic

Sympathetic branches of the nerves come from the **sympathetic chain ganglia** or plexi of the body. They travel with the cranial nerves but do not arise from them. What is the opposite type of nerve?

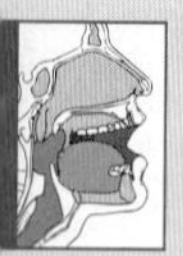

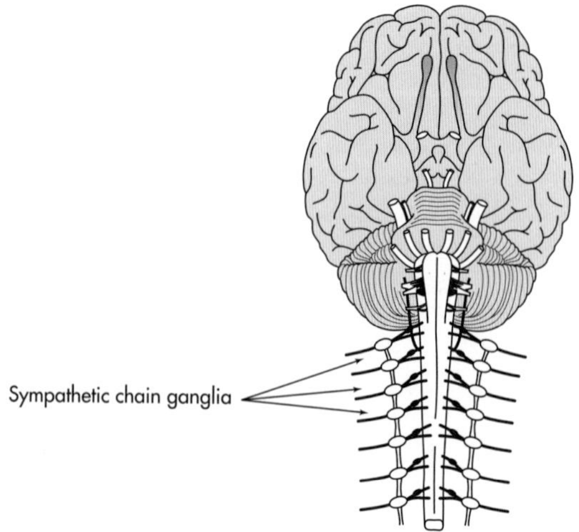

As you can see, the vagus nerve is a very large and important cranial nerve. It is the source of most of the ______________ innervation of the viscera of the body. The nucleus associated with the motor portion of vagus is **nucleus ambiguous.**

parasympathetic

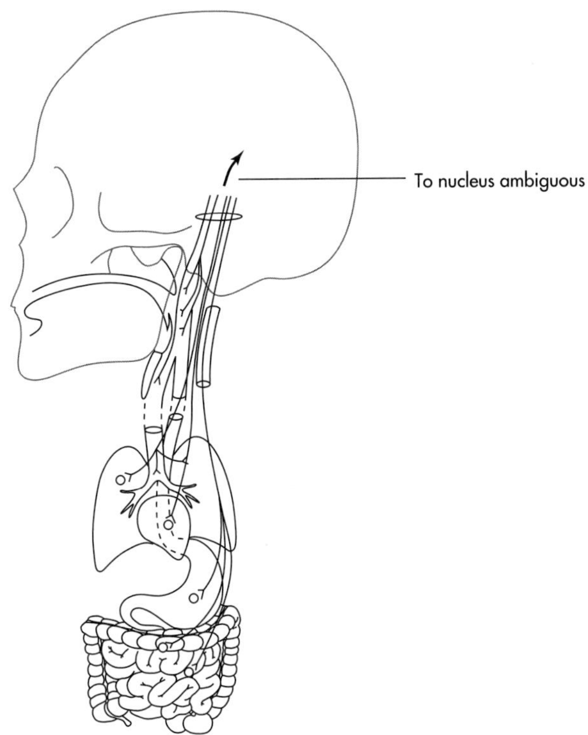

The vagus nerve leaves the brainstem here and then exits the cranium through the jugular foramen. Find it.

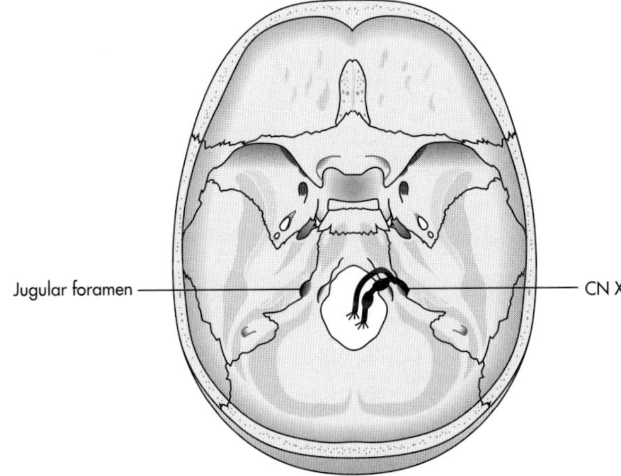

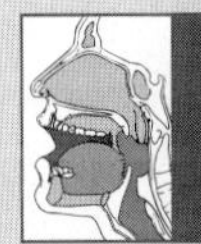

vagus, mixed, jugular foramen; superior, inferior petrosal, IX

Review. Cranial nerve X is the ______________ nerve. It is a ______________ nerve and exits the brainstem through the ______________. The ganglia associated with CN X are the __________ and __________ ganglia (same as for CN ______________!).

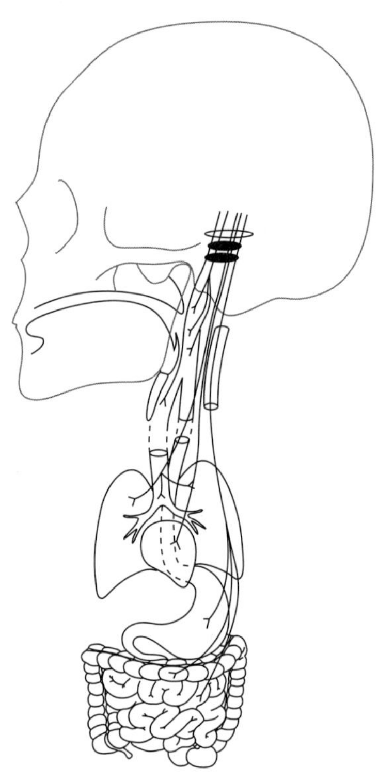

1. outer ear
2. respiratory
3. digestive
4. heart

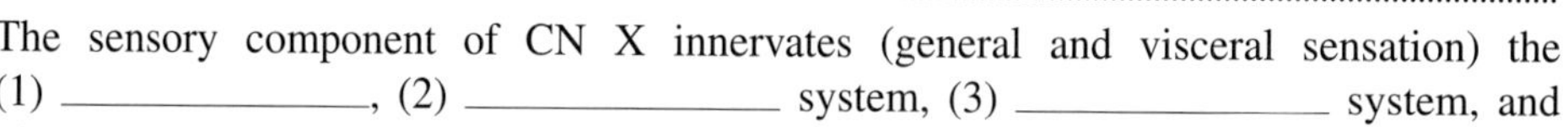

The sensory component of CN X innervates (general and visceral sensation) the (1) ______________, (2) ______________ system, (3) ______________ system, and (4) ______________.

The motor component of the vagus nerve innervates muscles and glands of the (1) ______________ system, (2) ______________ system, and (3) ______________.

1. respiratory
2. digestive
3. heart

It is important to ______________-type innervation of the viscera of the body which regulates the everyday normal functioning of these organs and their muscles and ______________.

parasympathetic, glands

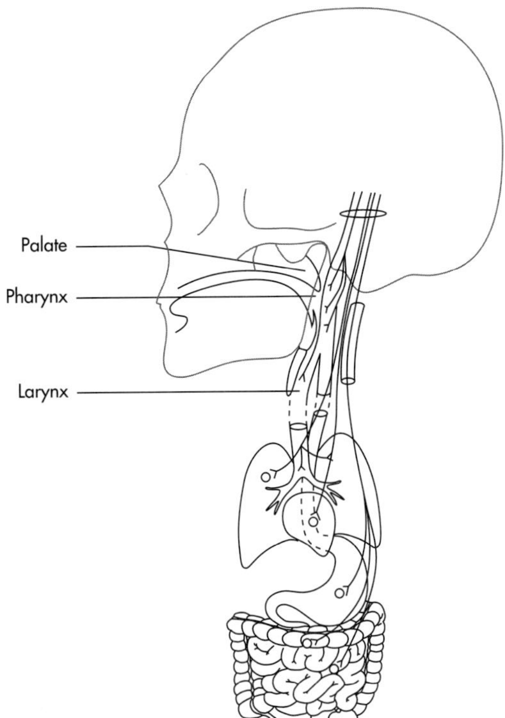

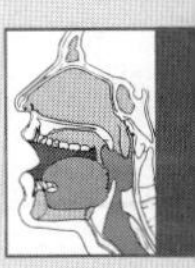

Find the vagus nerve and its associated structures on these drawings. Refer to the preceding frames for your answers.

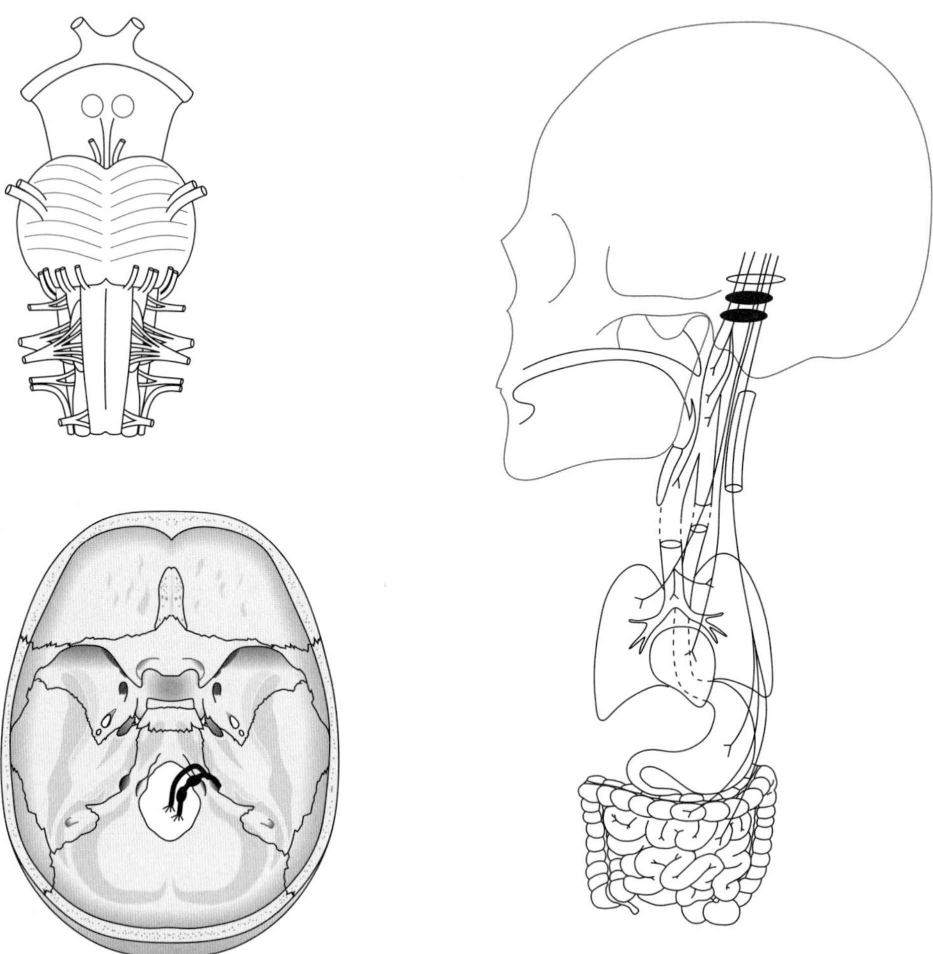

3.8

Cranial Nerve XI: Spinal Accessory Nerve

XI, vagus

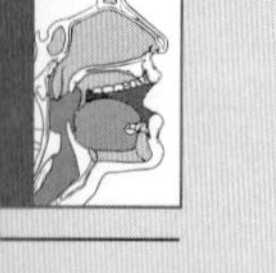

The **spinal accessory nerve,** or CN ______________, is so named because it carries fibers similar to spinal nerves and adds to the fibers of CN X or the ______________ nerve.

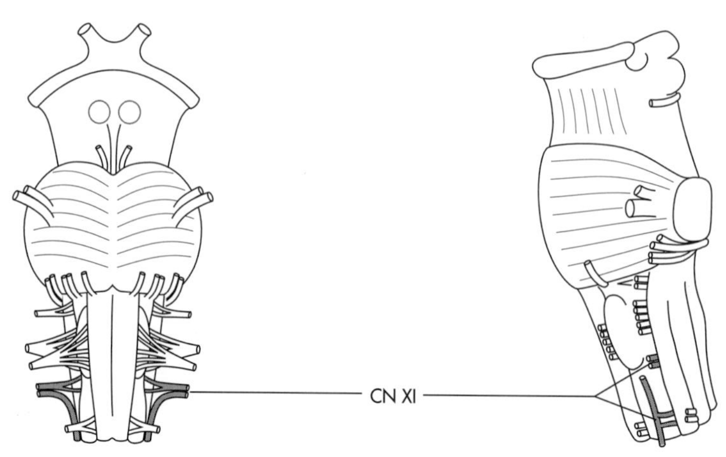

Fibers of the spinal accessory nerve run to the muscles of the larynx with the vagus nerve. These are motor neurons.

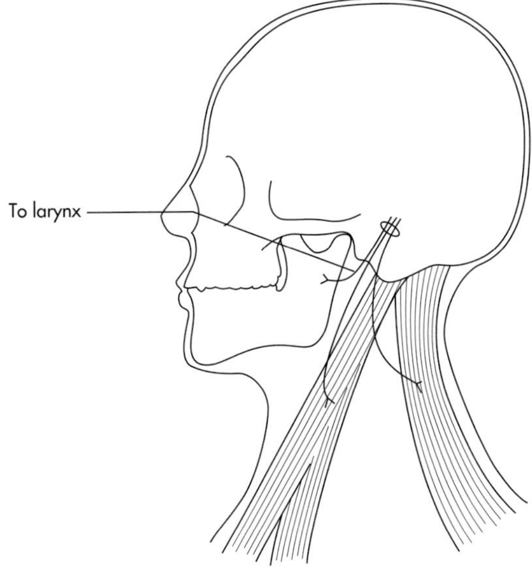

Motor neurons to two large muscles of the neck are part of CN XI. These are fibers to the sternocleidomastoid muscle and the upper portion of the trapezius muscle. These are important muscles for the support of the head and its rotation.

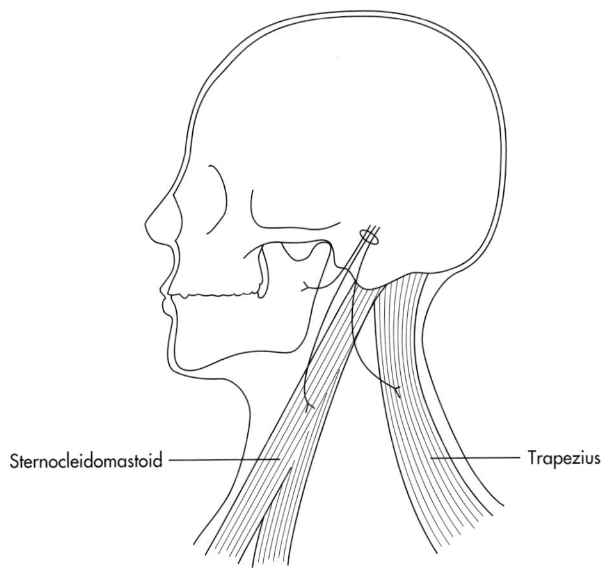

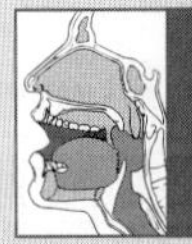

CN XI, motor

Find the sternocleidomastoid and trapezius muscles on the drawing. They are innervated by ______________ and are ______________-type nerves.

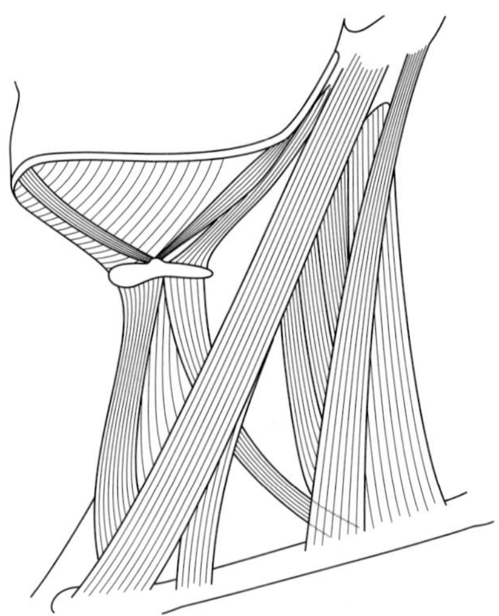

X, IX

The spinal accessory nerve exits the cranium through the jugular foramen with CNs ______________ and ______________, and through foramen magnum.

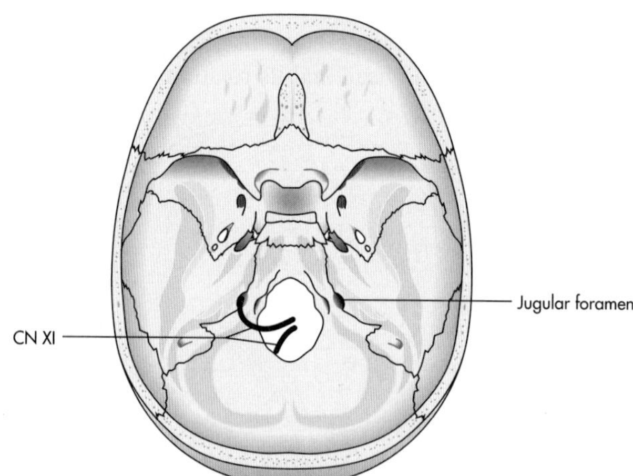

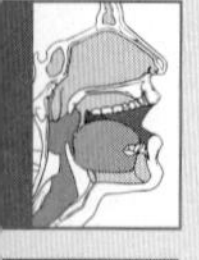

Review. CN XI is the ______________ nerve, a ______________-type nerve that exits the ______________ to innervate the ______________, ______________, and ______________ muscles.

spinal accessory, motor, jugular foramen, larynx, trapezius, sternocleidomastoid

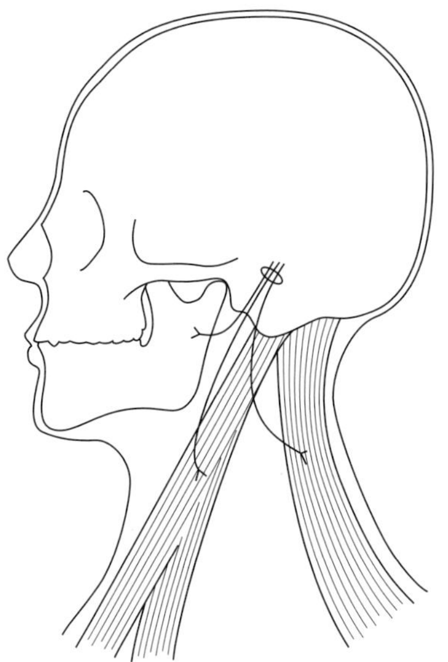

Cranial Nerve XII: Hypoglossal Nerve 3.9

The **hypoglossal nerve,** as the name indicates, runs under the tongue (*glossus* = "tongue").

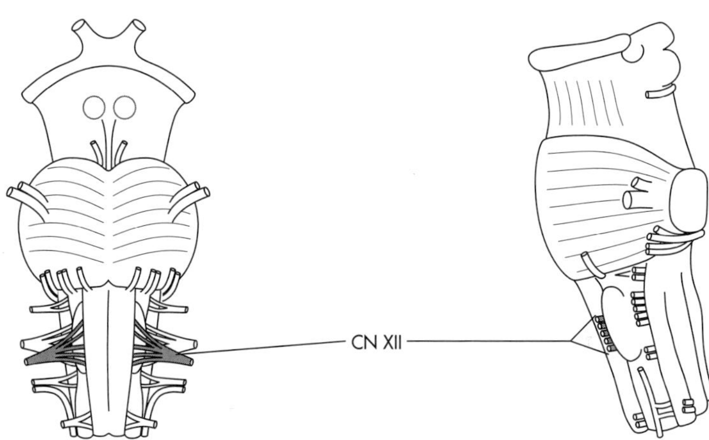

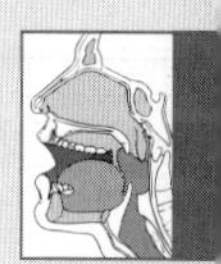

intrinsic, extrinsic

In fact, this nerve runs to all muscles with the suffix *glossus,* or the muscles of the tongue. There are two sets of tongue muscles: muscles within the body of the tongue, the ____________ tongue muscles, and those outside, the ____________ muscles.

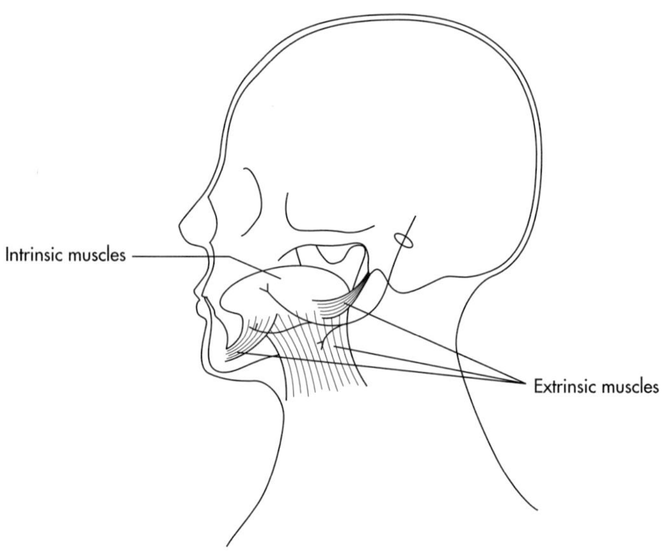

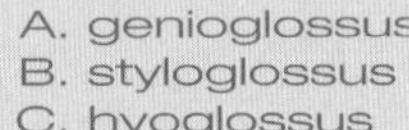

A. genioglossus
B. styloglossus
C. hyoglossus

The extrinsic muscles of the tongue are shown here. Can you name them? Check Chapter Seven for your answers.

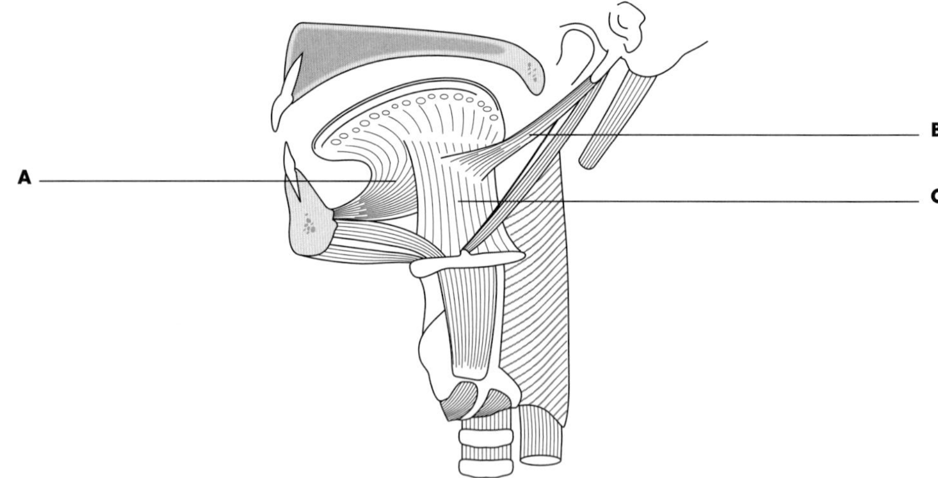

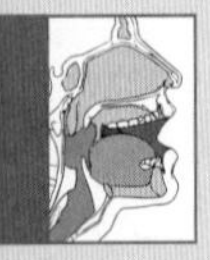

CN XII, the ______________ nerve, innervates the ______________ of the tongue. It exits the brainstem here as a series of merging roots. What type of nerve is it? Which other cranial nerves innervate the tongue?

hypoglossal, muscles; motor; V, VII, and IX—sensory

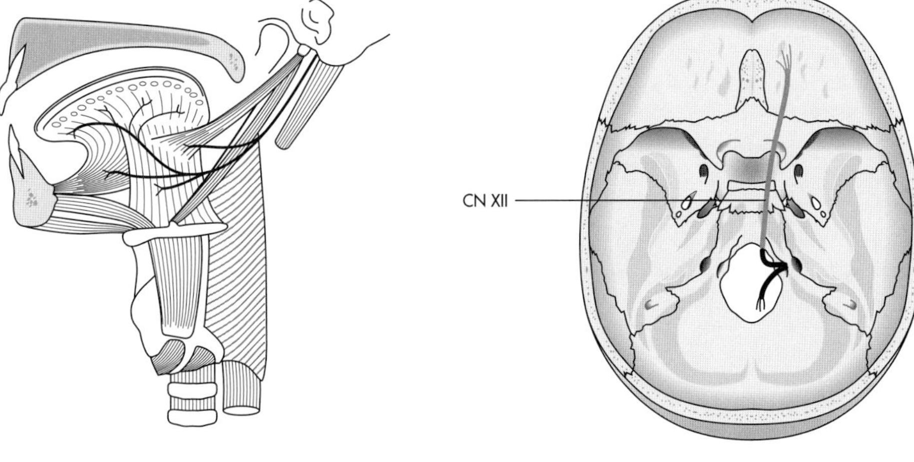

Look at the nerves that innervate the tongue. List them.

	Anterior	Posterior
Sensory		
(General)	1. ______________	4. ______________
(Taste)	2. ______________	5. ______________
Motor	3. ______________	6. ______________

1. V (we haven't discussed this nerve yet)
2. VII
3. XII
4. IX
5. IX
6. XII

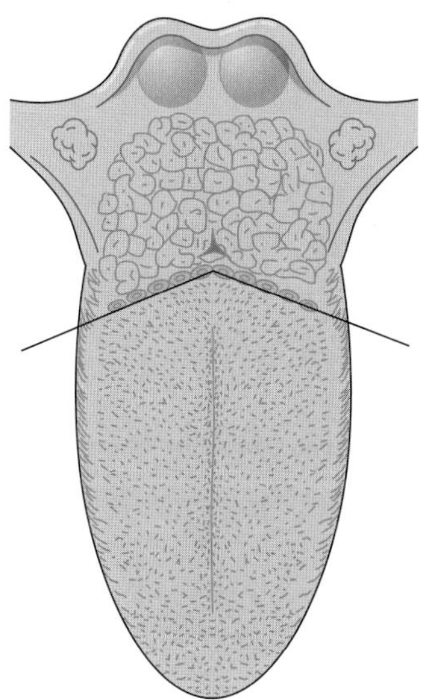

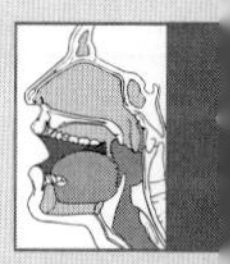

After exiting the brainstem, the hypoglossal nerve leaves the cranium through two small holes adjacent to the foramen magnum called the **hypoglossal canals (foramina).** Find them.

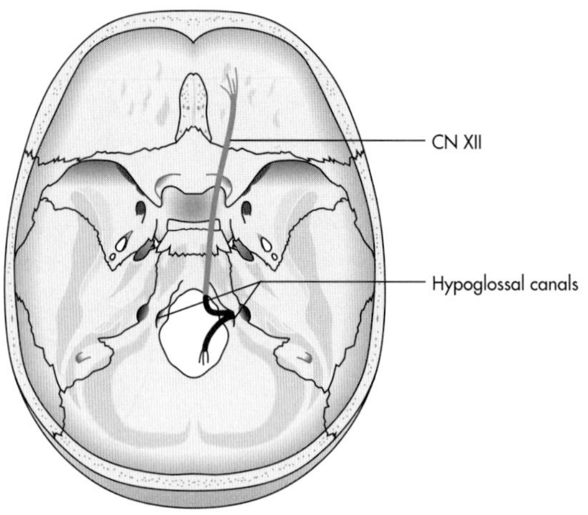

hypoglossal, hypoglossal, motor, muscles of the tongue

Review. The twelfth cranial nerve, or the ______________ nerve, exits the cranium from the brainstem through the ______________ canal. It is a ______________-type nerve, innervating ______________.

Find CN XII on the diagrams. Refer to the preceding frames.

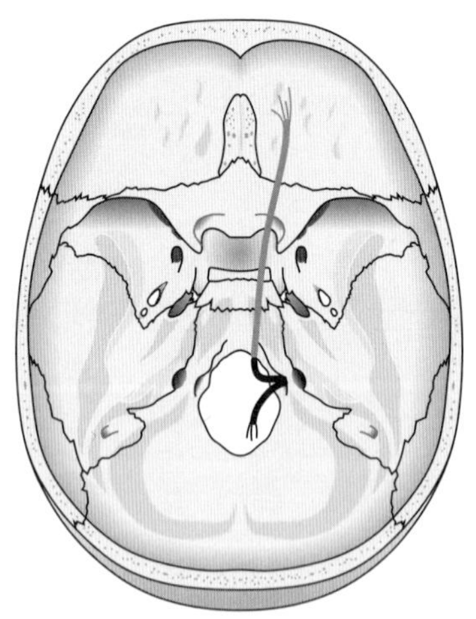

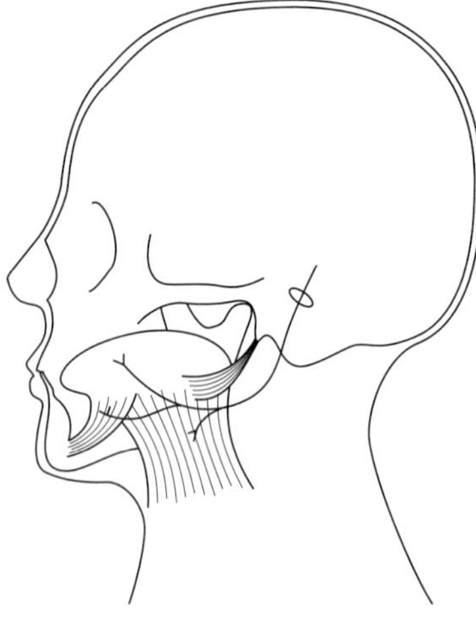

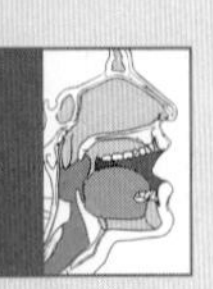

Cranial Nerve V: Trigeminal Nerve

3.10

We have left cranial nerve V, or the **trigeminal nerve,** for last because it is a large, complex nerve with many branches that are important to the oral cavity and face. As its name indicates, the trigeminal nerve comprises three major **divisions.**

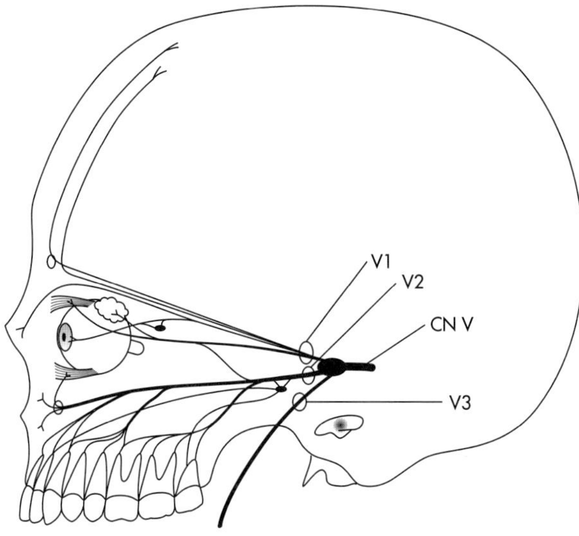

First, let's find the trigeminal as it exits the brainstem in an area known as the **pons.** It is, as all cranial nerves are, a pair of nerves. Find the pons and CN V on the drawing.

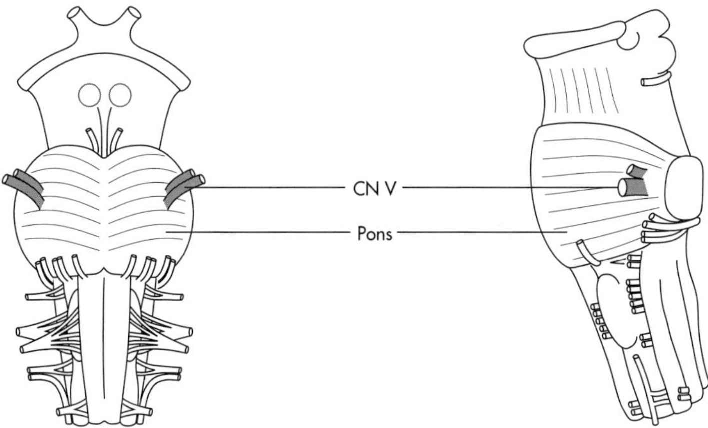

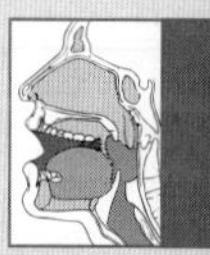

ganglion

Find where CN V exits the pons. Note the large "lump" of tissue that forms after the nerve trunk exits. It is composed of sensory neuron cell bodies and is therefore called a _______________. It is called the trigeminal ganglion.

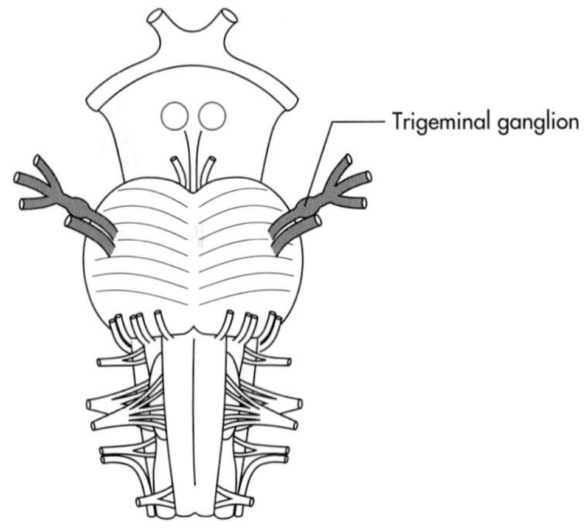

sensory

The trigeminal ganglion is a large ganglion that rests in a fossa in the cranium on either side of the pituitary fossa. It has also, in earlier textbooks, been called the **semilunar ganglion** and the **gasserian ganglion.** It is made up of _______________ cell bodies of CN V.

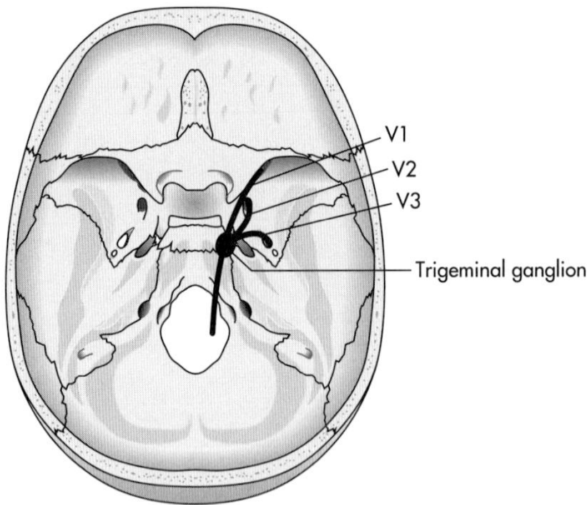

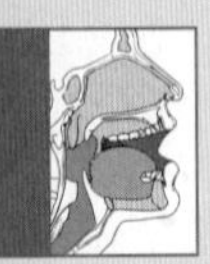

Note how after the ganglion ends, the trigeminal nerve splits immediately into three **divisions.**

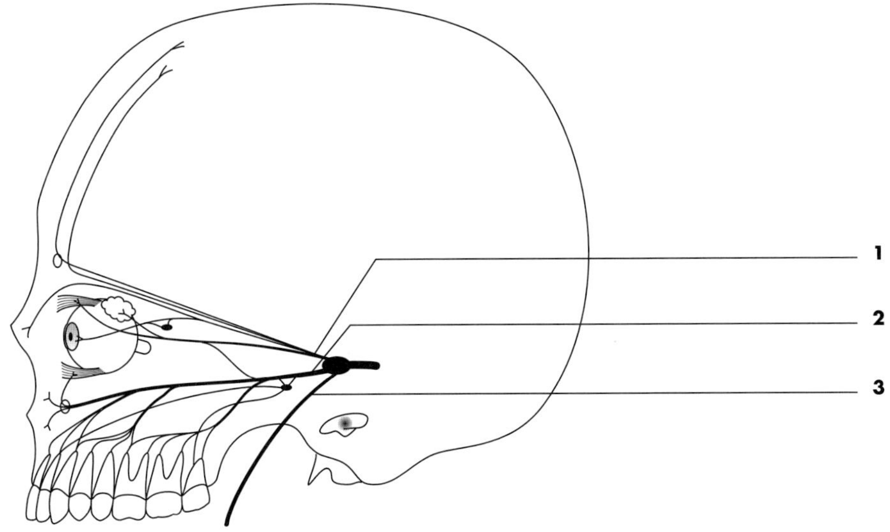

The three divisions of CN V are **V1,** the **ophthalmic division; V2,** the **maxillary division;** and **V3,** the **mandibular division.**

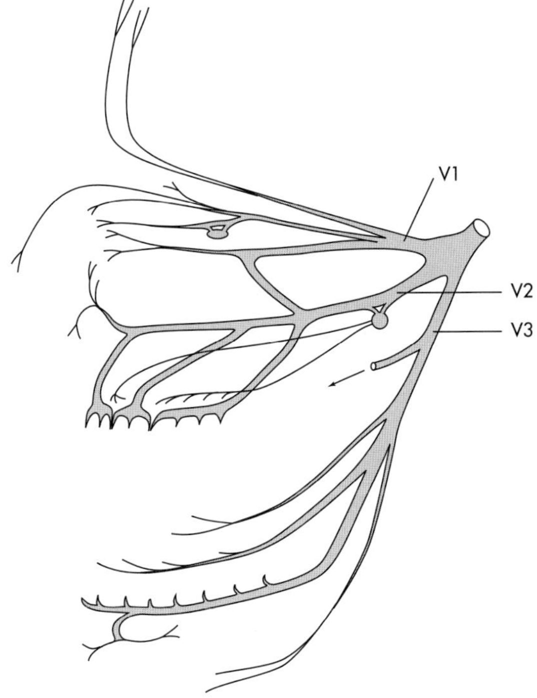

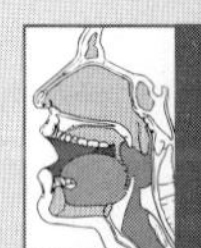

before

Find the three divisions of trigeminal nerve. Does the nerve divide before or after leaving the cranium?

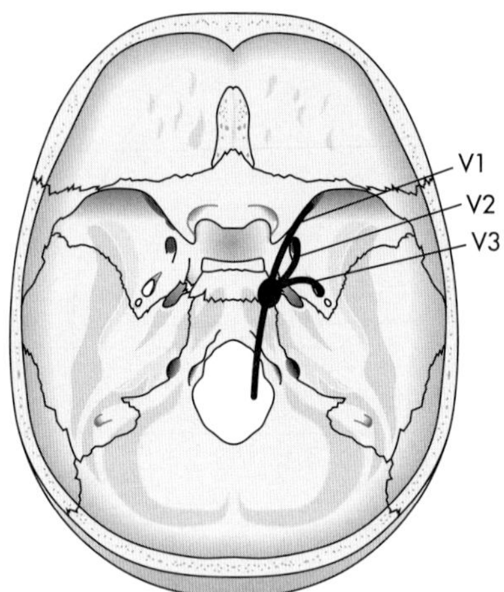

superior orbital fissure

We first show the anatomic divisions of the trigeminal nerve and the branches of each division. Each division of CN V exits the cranium through a different "hole" or foramen. Through which foramen does V1 appear to exit?

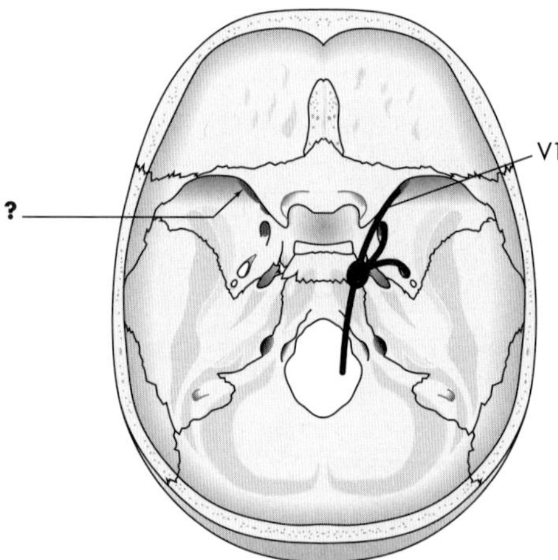

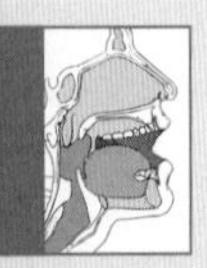

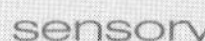

V1, the first division of the trigeminal nerve, is called the **ophthalmic division** because it travels to the region of the eyes and forehead. Find V1 on the drawing. The ophthalmic division is composed of sensory neurons that carry the sensations of touch, pain, and temperature to the CNS. V1 is a _______________ nerve.

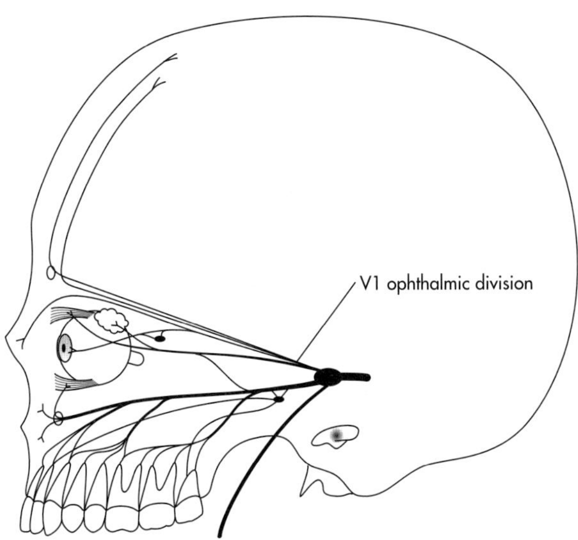

The ophthalmic division branches into three portions: the nasociliary, lacrimal, and frontal nerves. The **nasociliary nerve** connects with the **ciliary ganglion,** sending parasympathetic fibers to the eye and other sensory fibers to the nasal cavity and sinuses, eyeball, and eyelids. The **lacrimal** nerve goes to the lacrimal gland. The **frontal** nerve passes through the supraorbital foramen to become the **supraorbital nerve.**

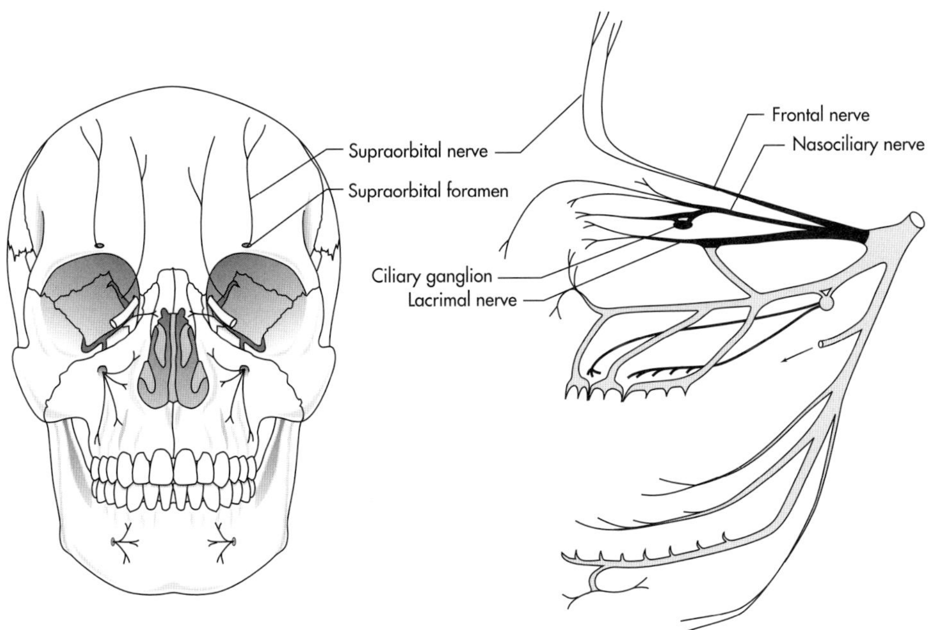

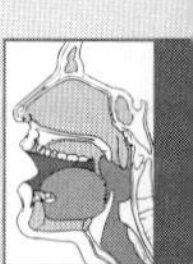

supraorbital nerve, V1

What nerve passes through the supraorbital foramen on the skull? This nerve pair provides sensation to the skin of the forehead as shown by the area shaded. Of what division is this a branch?

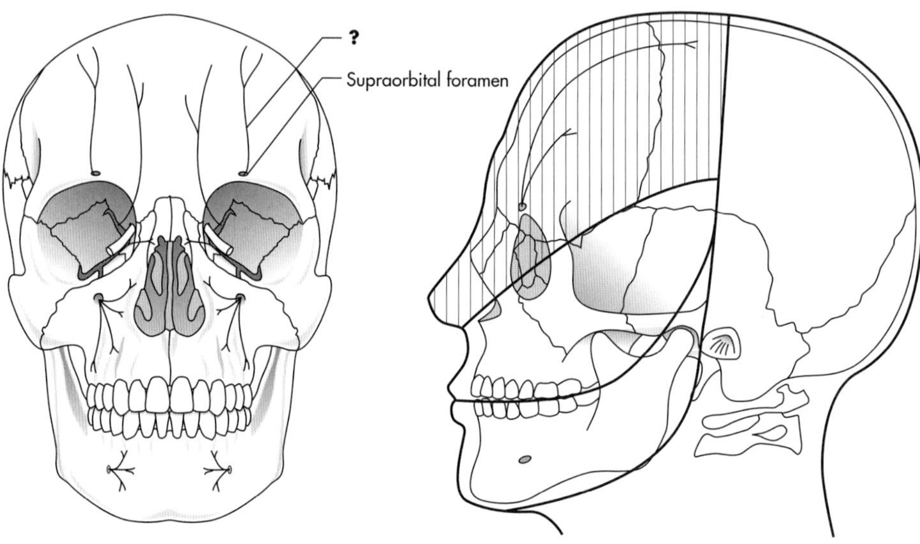

A. supraorbital nerve
B. nasociliary nerve
C. lacrimal nerve
D. frontal nerve
E. ciliary ganglion

Label these branches of V1, the ophthalmic division.

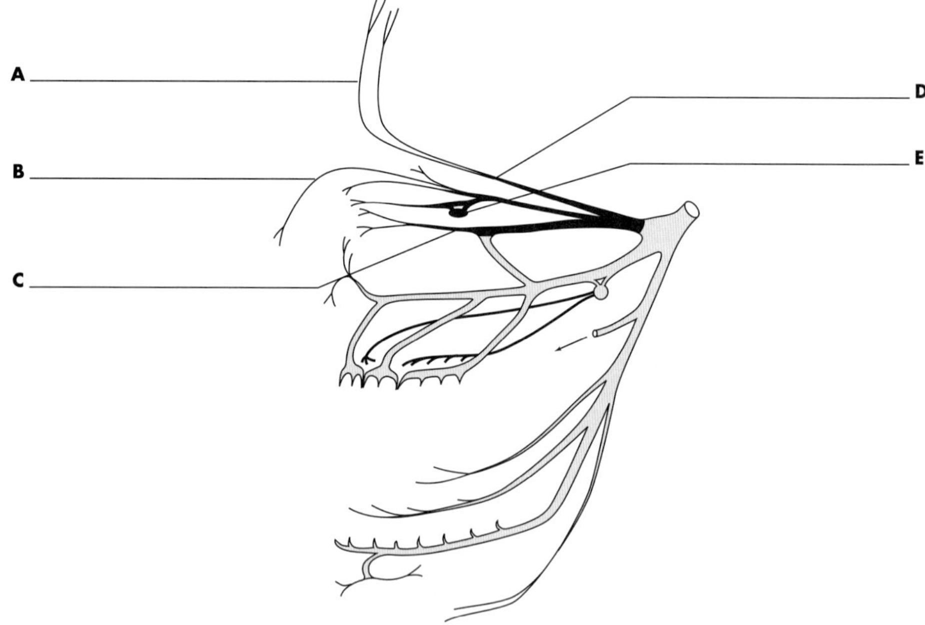

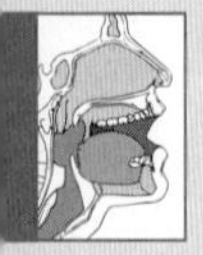

The second division is the **maxillary division** of the trigeminal nerve. It is also a _______________ nerve like the ophthalmic division.

sensory

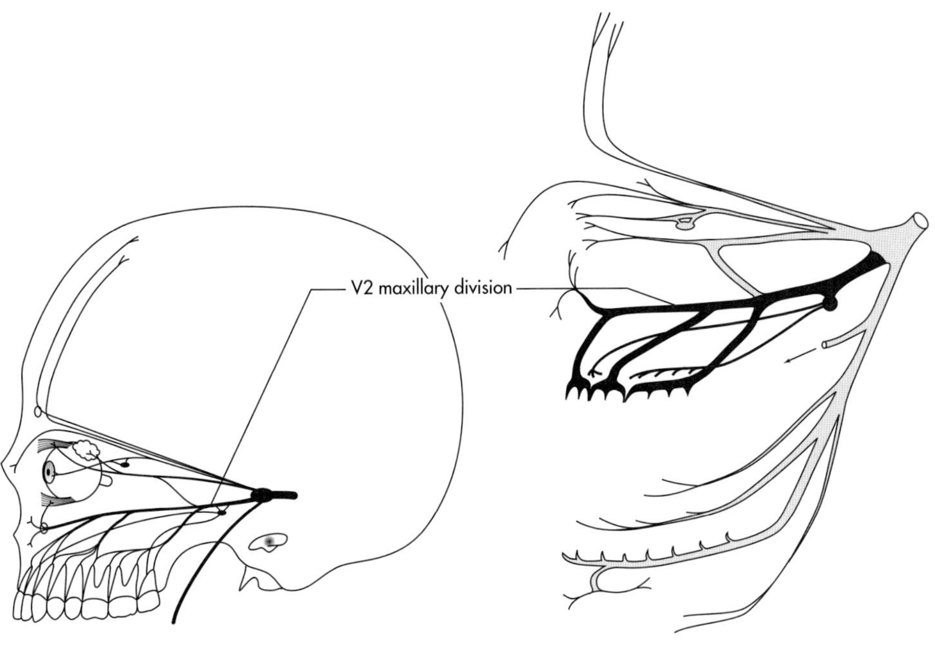

The maxillary division of CN V exits the cranium through which foramen? It travels immediately to the maxilla passing through an area called the **infratemporal fossa.**

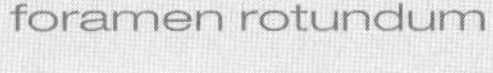
foramen rotundum

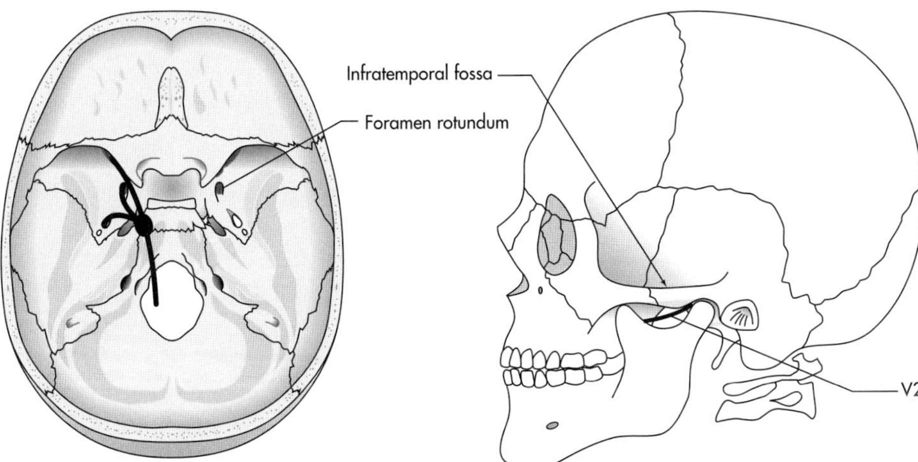

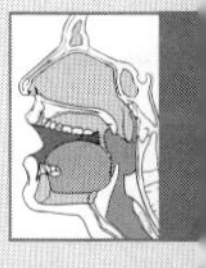

The branches of the maxillary division are many. It first connects with the **pterygopalatine ganglion** for parasympathetic fibers deep within the infratemporal fossa (the pterygopalatine fossa).

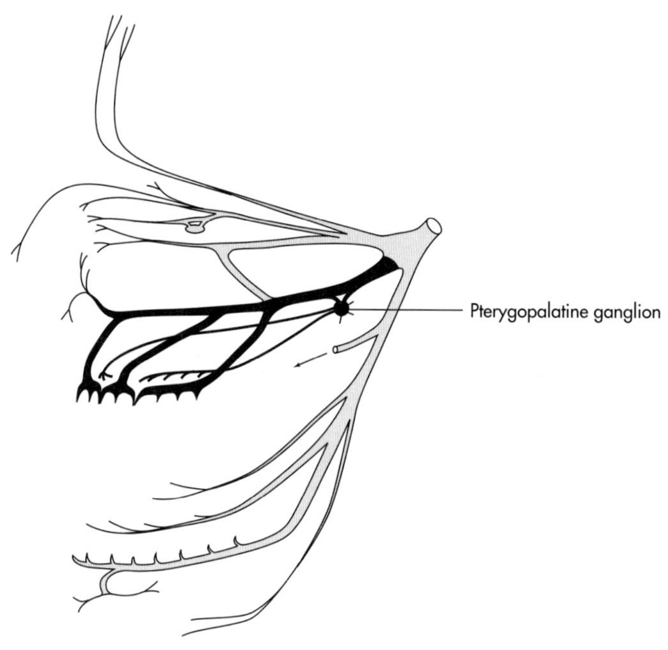

maxillary

There are nasal branches to the floor of the nasal cavity. From these branches arise the **nasopalatine nerve,** which penetrates the incisive foramen and spreads out to the anterior palate. This is a branch of which division?

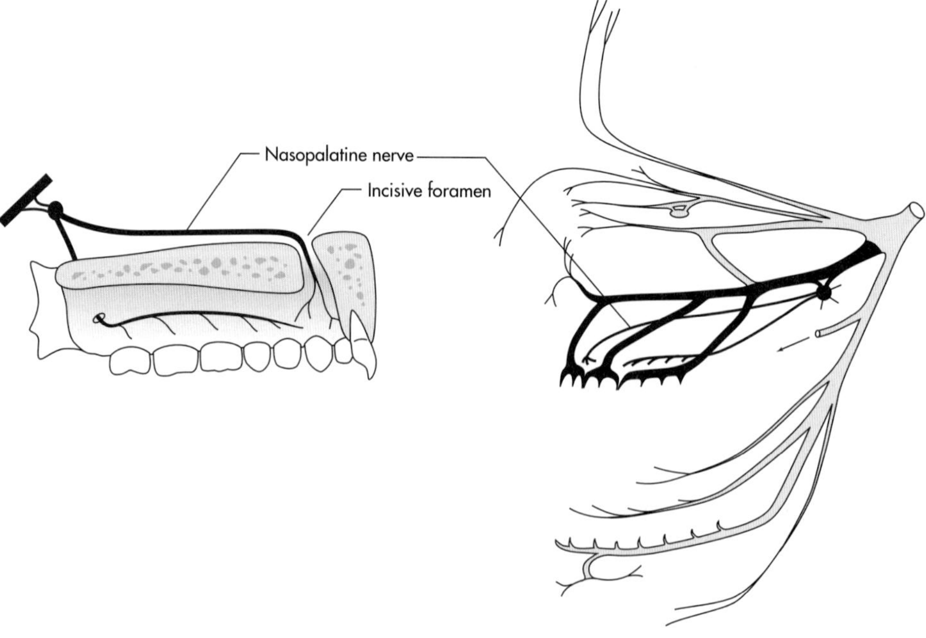

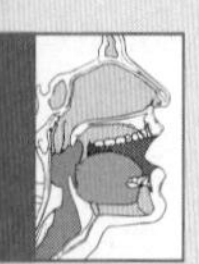

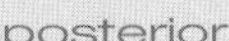

posterior

Other branches of the nasal nerve are the palatine nerves, especially the **greater palatine nerves,** which penetrate the hard palate to innervate its mucosa through foramina of the same name. Which area of the palate do they go to?

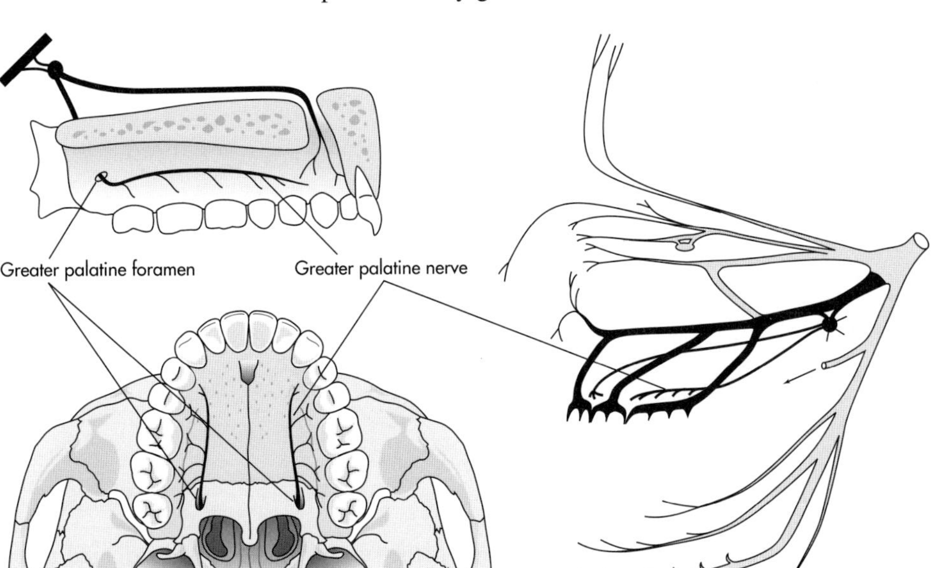

The **superior alveolar nerves** enter the maxillary bone in the area of the roots of the posterior teeth. They begin loops of nerves that innervate all the maxillary teeth on their facial aspects.

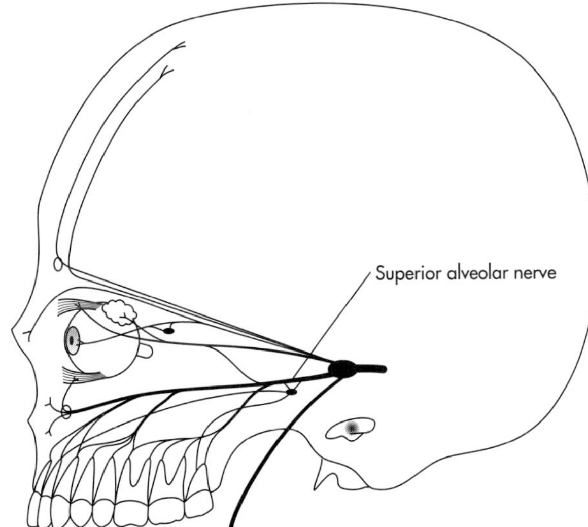

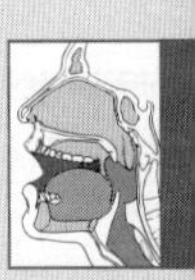

The superior alveolar nerve is divided into three loops or branches: The **posterior superior alveolar (PSA) nerve** spreads in the alveolar bone to innervate the third and second molars and most of the first molar, fascial aspect.

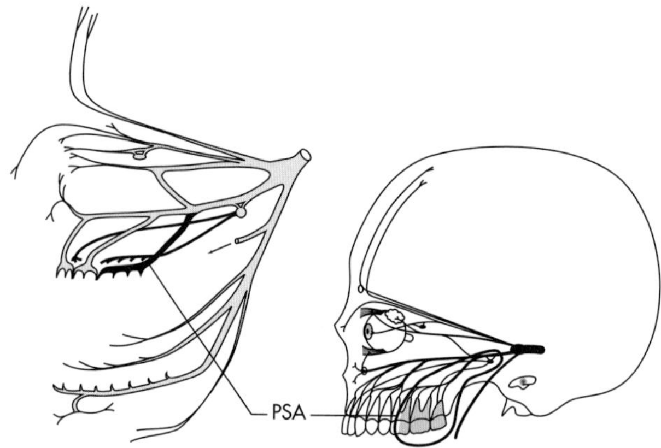

The **middle superior alveolar (MSA) nerve** is the second loop and is distributed to the mesiobuccal cusp of the first molar, the two premolars, and the distal part of the canine, fascial aspect.

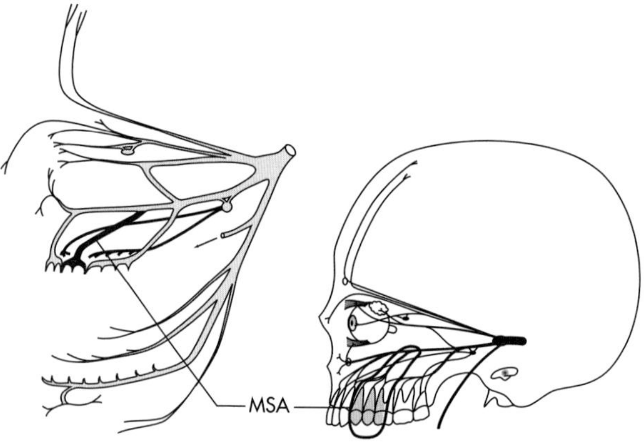

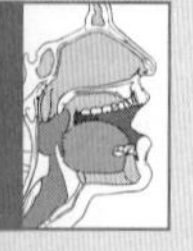

The anterior superior alveolar nerve (ASA) is the last loop of superior alveolar and is distributed to the anterior teeth (except the distal of the canines) of the maxilla, facial aspect.

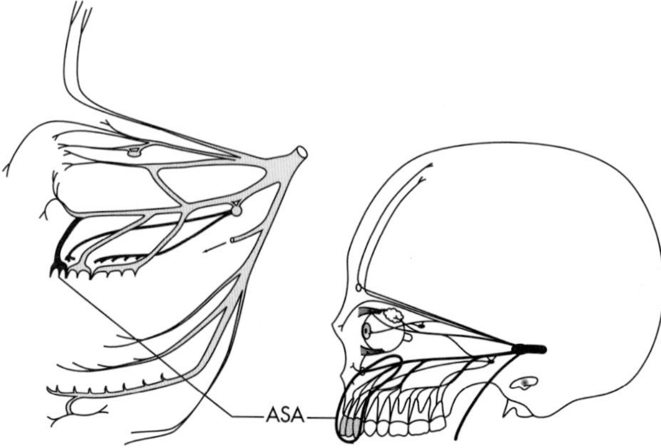

Which portion of the superior alveolar nerve would innervate tooth number 6?

ASA and MSA

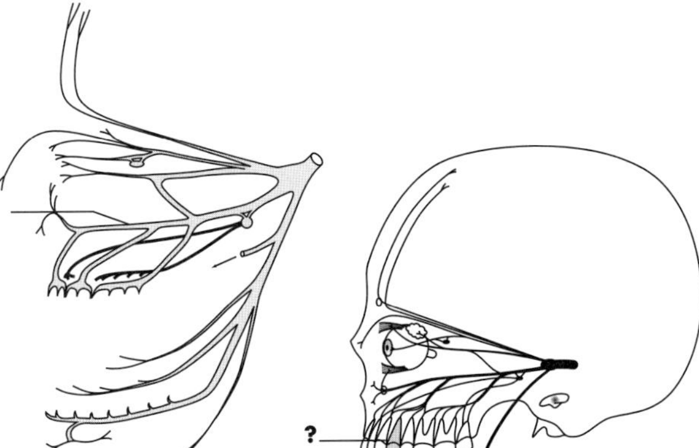

The palatal sides of the maxillary posterior teeth and the distal canine, along with the hard palate itself, are innervated by which branch of V2?

greater palatine

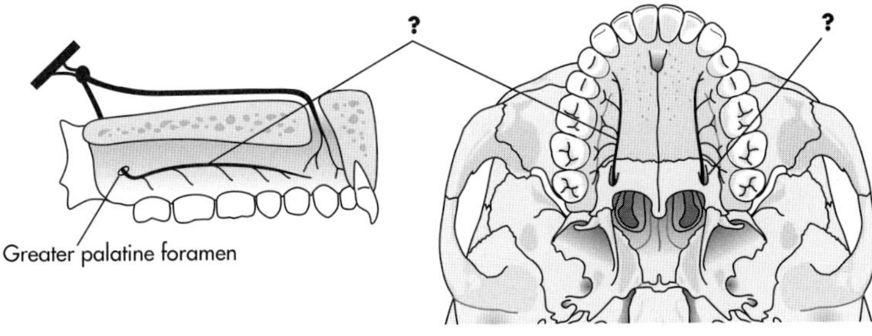

The anterior palate is innervated by which branch?

nasopalatine

The superior alveolar and nasal nerves form a continuous loop as shown in the drawing. The maxillary division is a sensory nerve bringing the senses of touch, pain, temperature, and proprioception to the maxilla and its teeth. Which other branch is sensory?

ophthalmic

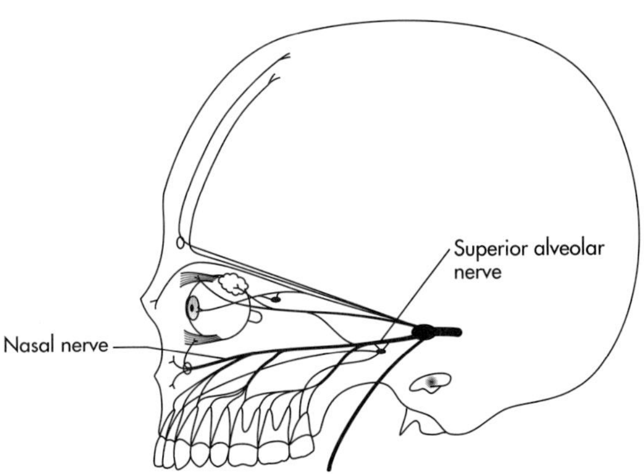

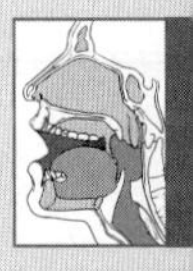

infraorbital foramen, infraorbital nerve

The last portion of V2 exits the skull through a foramen located below the eyes, spreading sensory innervation to the skin of the maxilla or "cheeks." What foramen is this? What nerve is it?

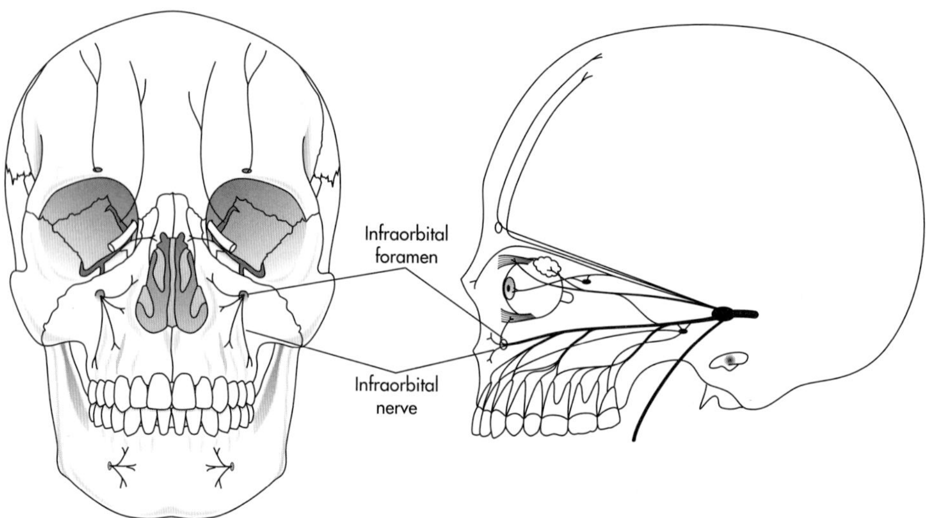

V2

The **infraorbital nerve** branch passes through the infraorbital foramen to spread across the cheeks. Note how the foramen gives a name to things that pass through it? Of what nerve is this nerve a division?

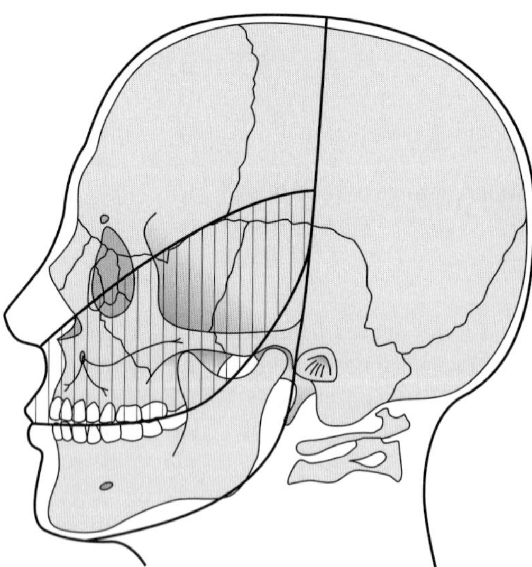

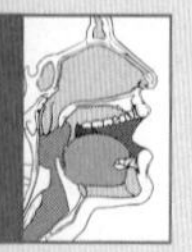

Label these branches of V2, the maxillary division.

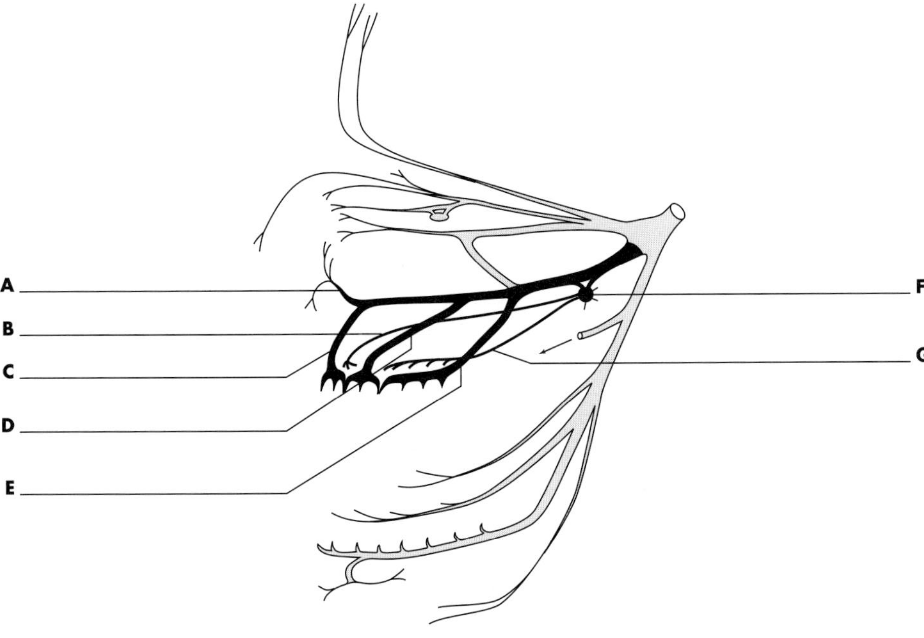

A. infraorbital nerve
B. nasopalatine nerve
C. ASA nerve
D. MSA nerve
E. PSA nerve
F. pterygopalatine ganglion
G. greater palatine nerve

The last division of the trigeminal nerve is the **mandibular division.** Find it.

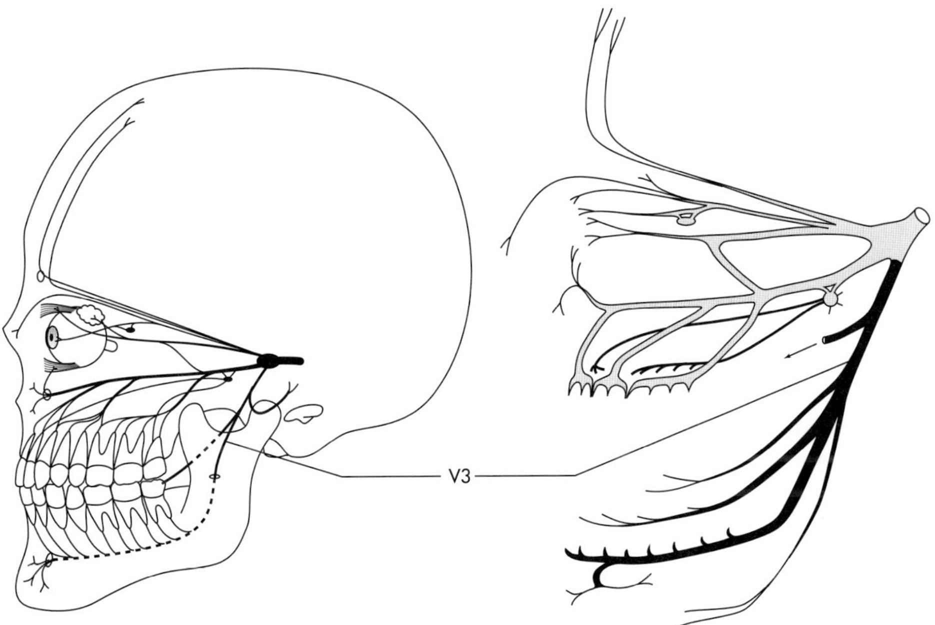

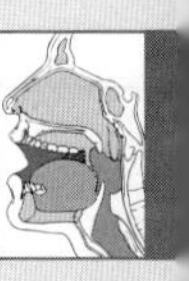

foramen ovale

The mandibular division, or V3, exits the cranium through this foramen. What is it?

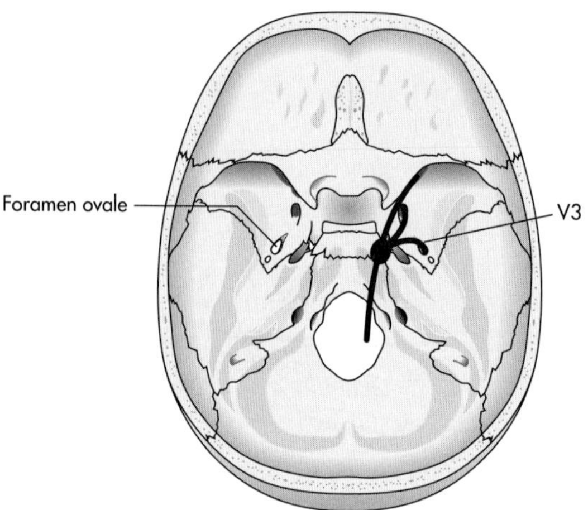

V3 passes through the foramen ovale to turn sharply downward to the mandible. It gives off a few branches to the ear as the **auriculotemporal nerve** and also connects to the **otic ganglion.**

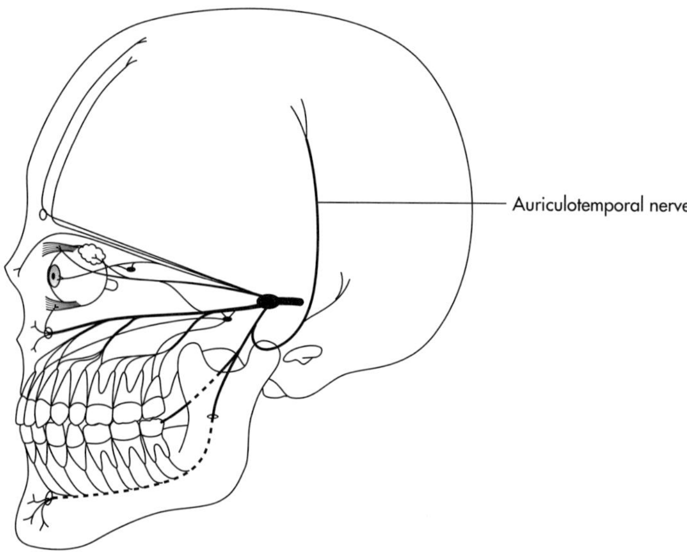

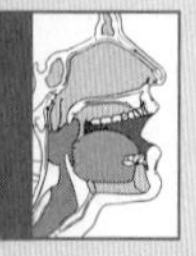

The mandibular division continues down past the condyle and ramus on the medial side, where it divides into two large sensory branches: the lingual nerve and the inferior alveolar nerve. Which nerve goes to the tongue?

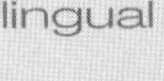

lingual

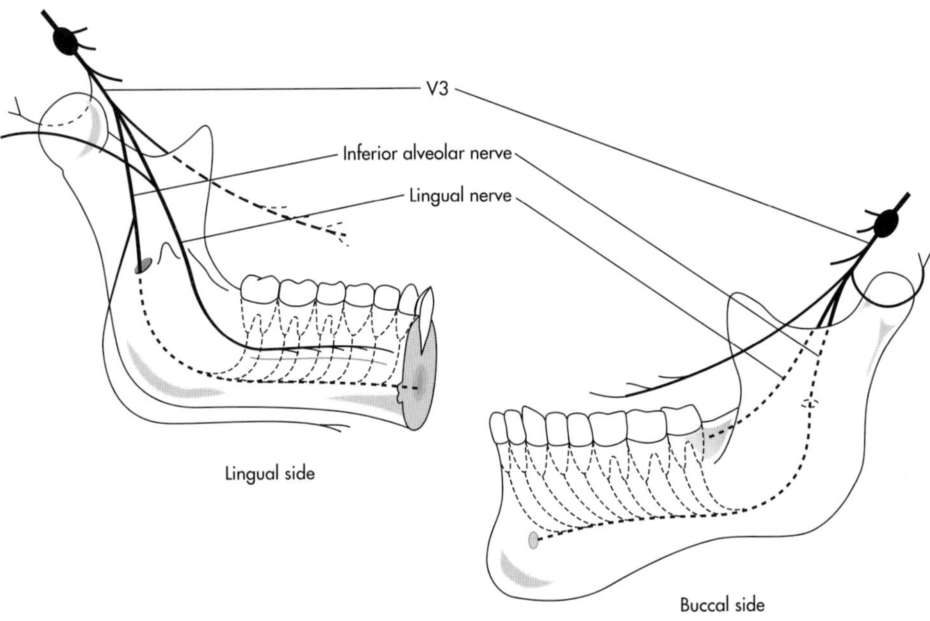

The **lingual nerve** carries general sensory nerves to the anterior two thirds of the tongue mucosa. Another cranial nerve "hitches a ride" on the lingual nerve to bring taste sensation to the anterior tongue. What is it?

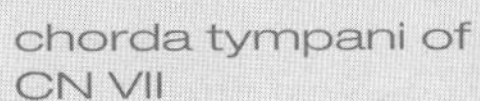

chorda tympani of CN VII

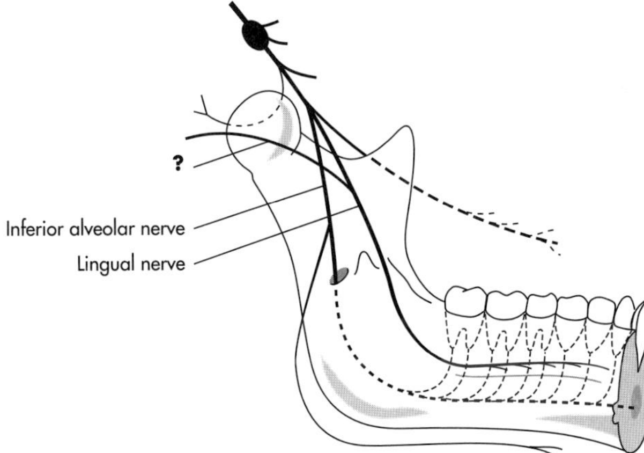

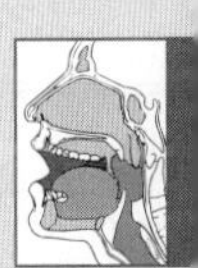

lingual nerve

The facial nerve, via its branch, the **chorda tympani,** travels to the anterior tongue for taste reception by riding on which nerve?

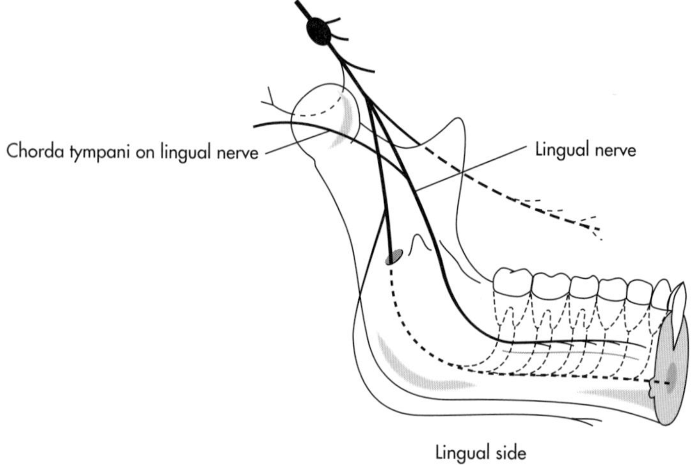

sensory

The **inferior alveolar nerve** dives into the foramen on the medial side of the mandibular ramus called the mandibular foramen. Once inside the mandible, it branches out to each of the mandibular teeth on each right and left side. It picks up the sensations of touch, temperature, proprioception, and pain from the teeth and gingiva. This branch is what kind of nerve?

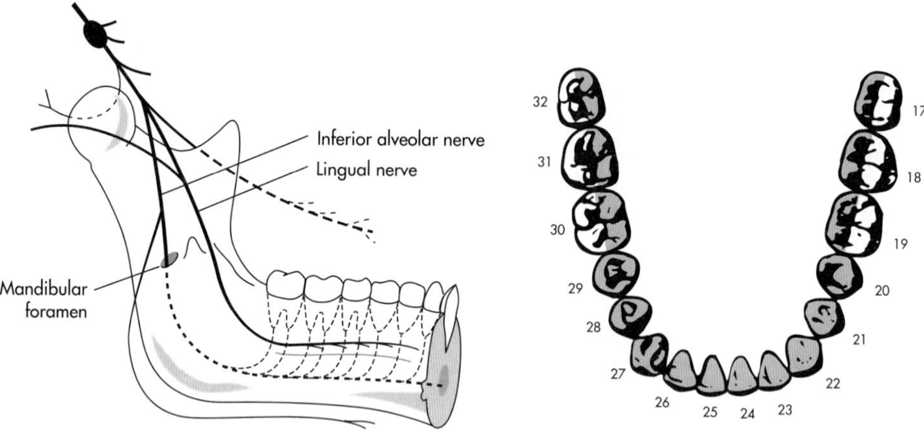

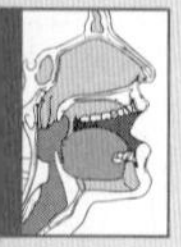

Before the the inferior alveolar branches out to the mandibular teeth, it extends a smaller branch called the **buccal,** which circles around to innervate the buccal side of the mandibular molars. There is no equivalent to the buccal nerve for the anterior teeth.

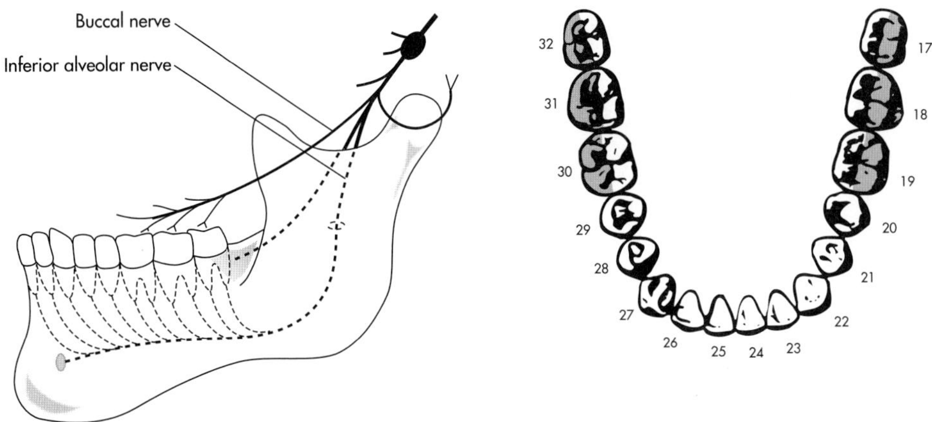

mental foramen

The inferior alveolar nerve continues in the mandibular canal down the length of the body of the mandible, directly inferior to the teeth. It branches upward to each of the mandibular teeth on each side. A portion of the inferior alveolar exits through a foramen on the mandible. What foramen is it?

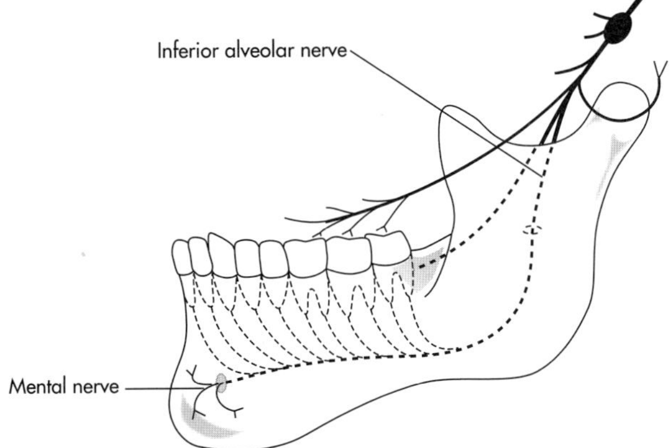

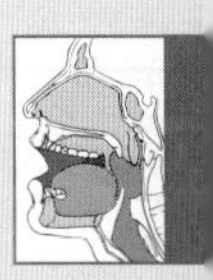

mental foramen

The **mental nerve** is another branch of V3 that spreads out on the skin of the chin to provide its sensation on the area shown. Through what foramen does it pass?

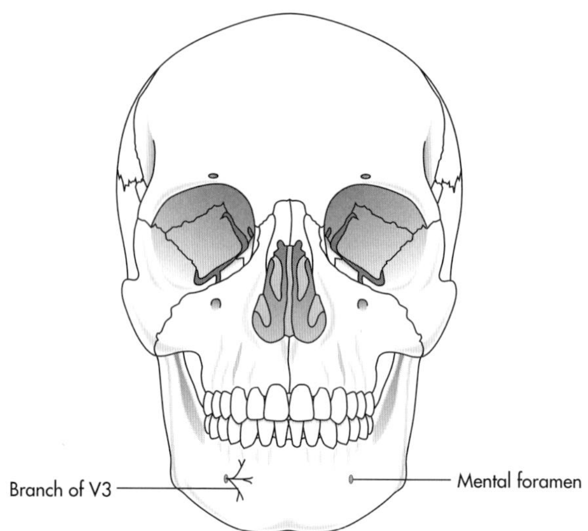

1. nasopalatine nerve
2. greater palatine nerve
3. PSA nerve
4. MSA nerve
5. ASA nerve

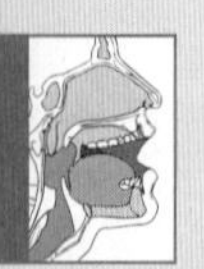

Let's summarize the innervation of the teeth. On the diagram of the maxillary teeth, label the nerves that go to the areas designated.

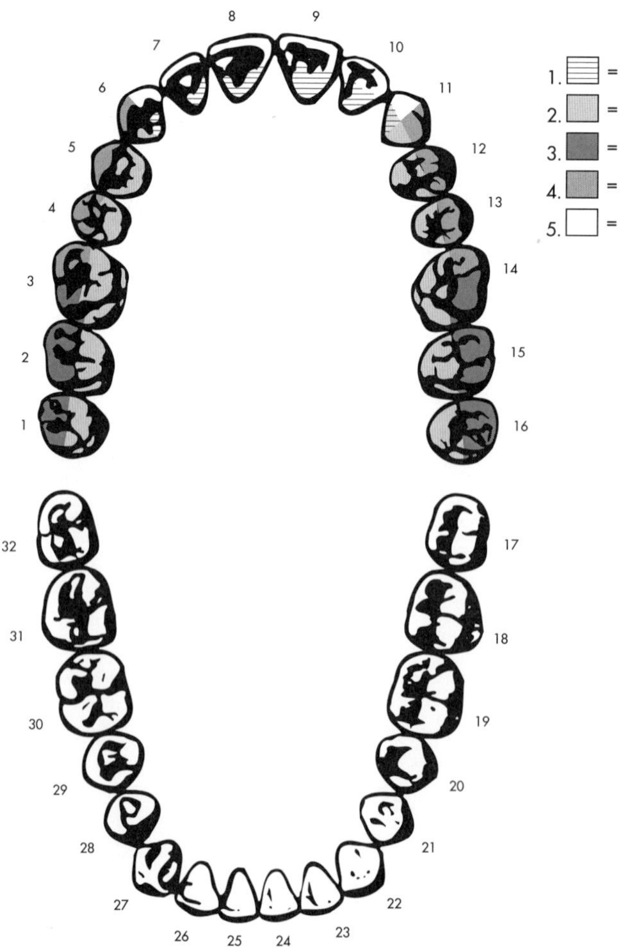

On the diagram of the mandibular teeth, label their innervation.

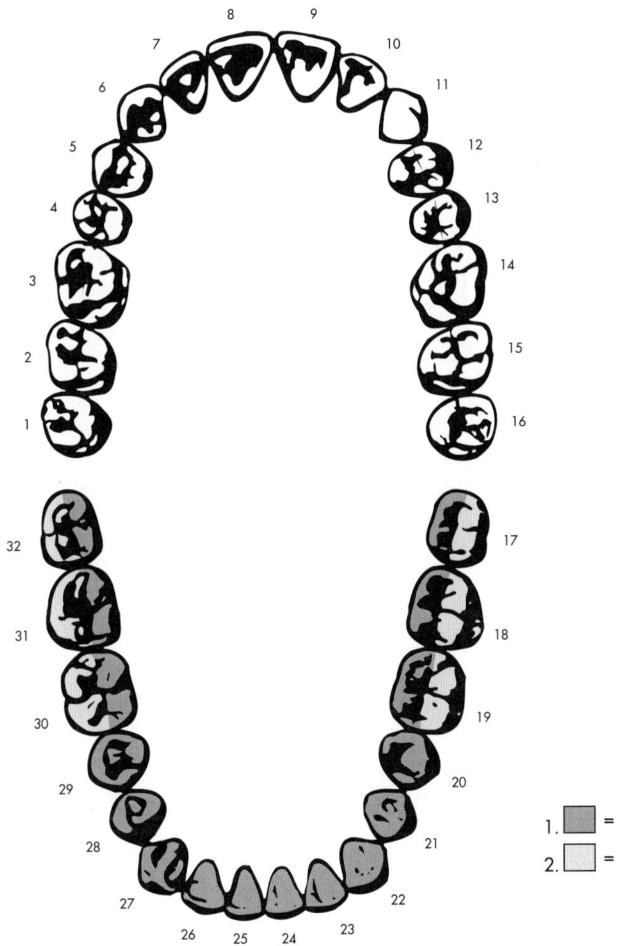

1. inferior alveolar nerve
2. buccal nerve

Lastly, there is a motor branch of the trigeminal nerve. As there are both sensory and motor nerves in CN V, this is a ______________-type nerve.

mixed

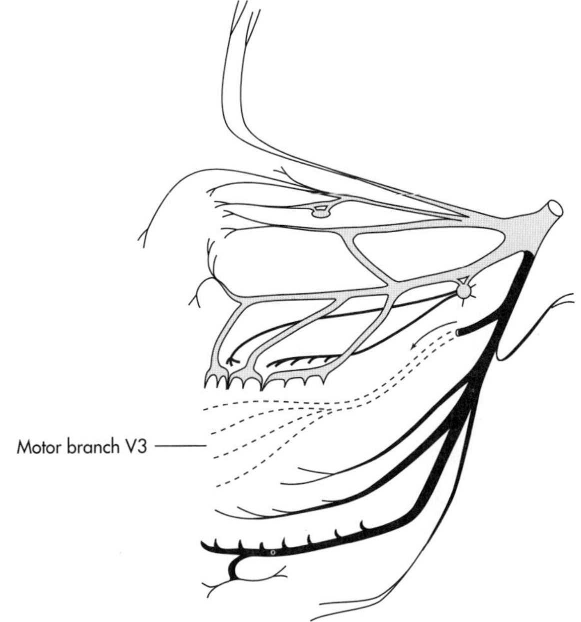

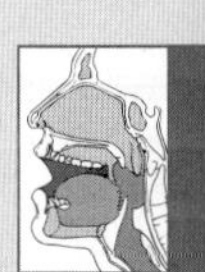

V3

The **motor branch** of the trigeminal nerve rides strictly on the third division or _______________. It branches off immediately into four nerves that each travel to one of the four muscles of mastication. (There is also a small branch to the mylohyoid muscle.)

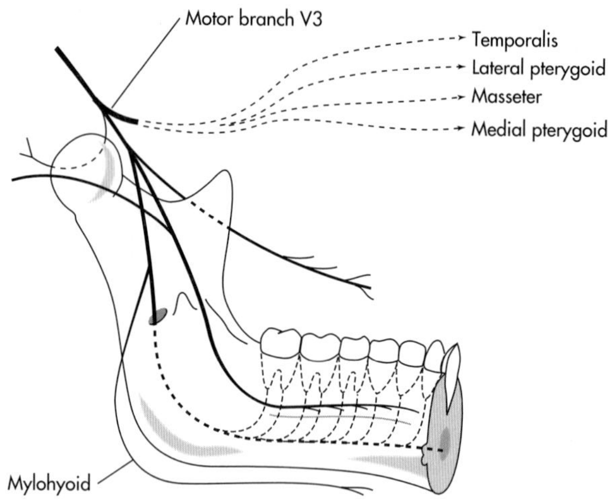

V3; masseter, temporalis, medial, lateral pterygoid, and mylohyoid muscles

Find the motor branch of V3. In which division does it travel? Name the muscles it innervates.

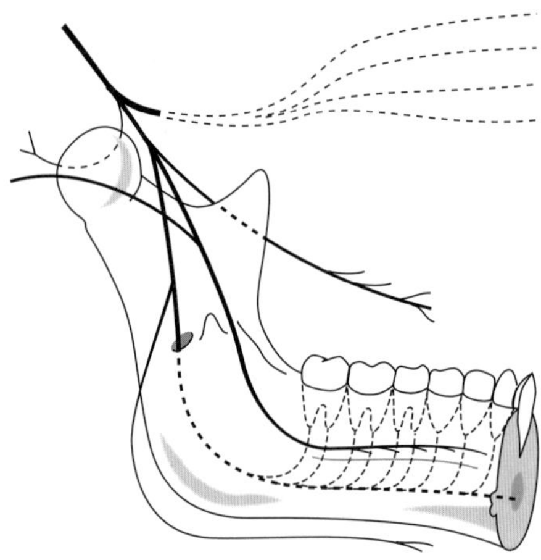

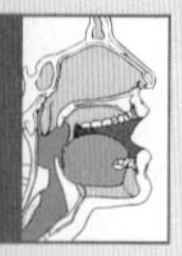

Label the branches of V3, the mandibular division.

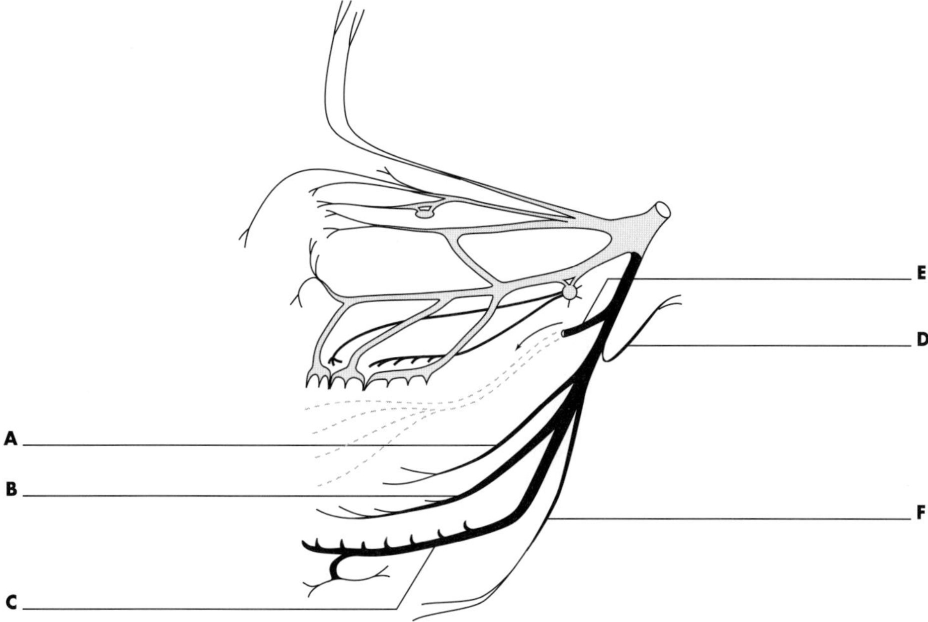

A. buccal nerve
B. lingual nerve
C. inferior alveolar nerve
D. auriculotemporal nerve
E. motor branch
F. mylohyoid nerve

Which cranial nerves innervate the muscles of mastication? The muscles of facial expression? The muscles of the tongue? The sternocleidomastoid muscle? The muscles of the larynx and pharynx?

V, VII, XII, XI, X

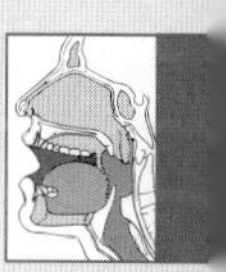

A,B. supraorbital nerve and foramen (V1)
C,D. infraorbital nerve and foramen (V2)
E,F. mental nerve and foramen (V3)

Review the sensory innervation of the face. Which division of CN V innervates each area? Through which foramen does the division exit the cranium? Through which foramen does the branch exit to innervate the skin? Name the branches.

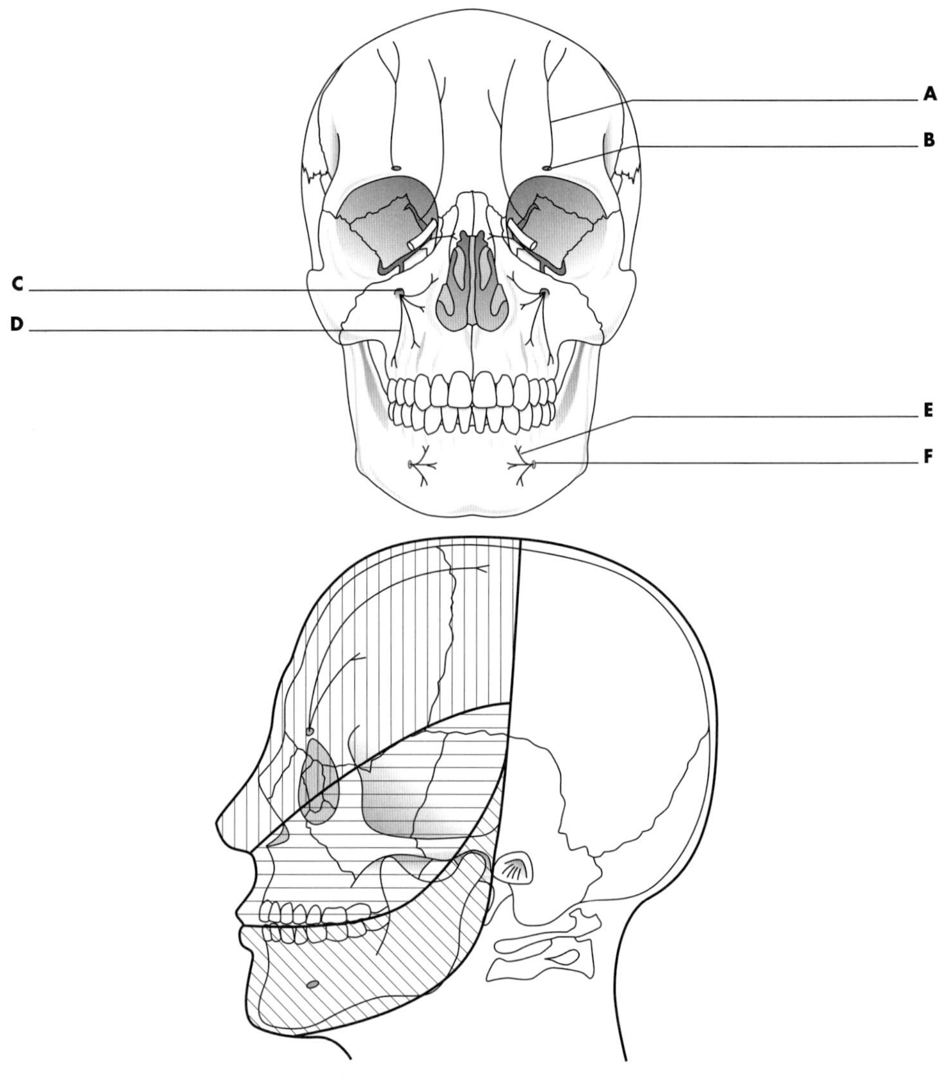

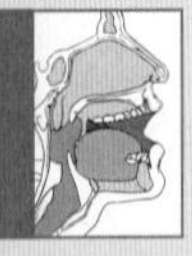

Let us look briefly at the connections of the trigeminal nerve in the brainstem. What was the sensory ganglion outside of the brainstem associated with CN V? **Nuclei** of the trigeminal nerve are within the brainstem.

trigeminal ganglion

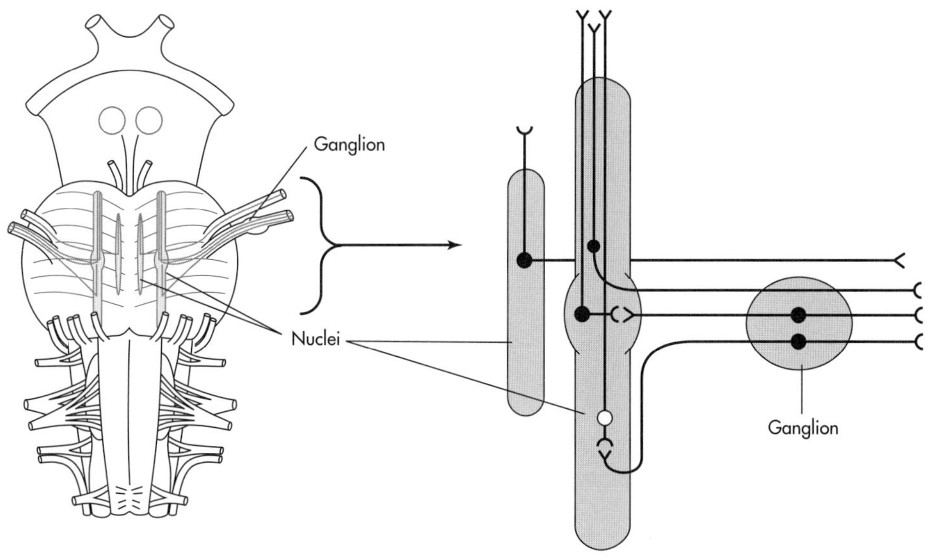

Nuclei of the trigeminal nerve are within the brainstem. CN V has a large nucleus inside of the brainstem called the **chief sensory nucleus of CN V.** Find the chief sensory nucleus and trigeminal ganglion.

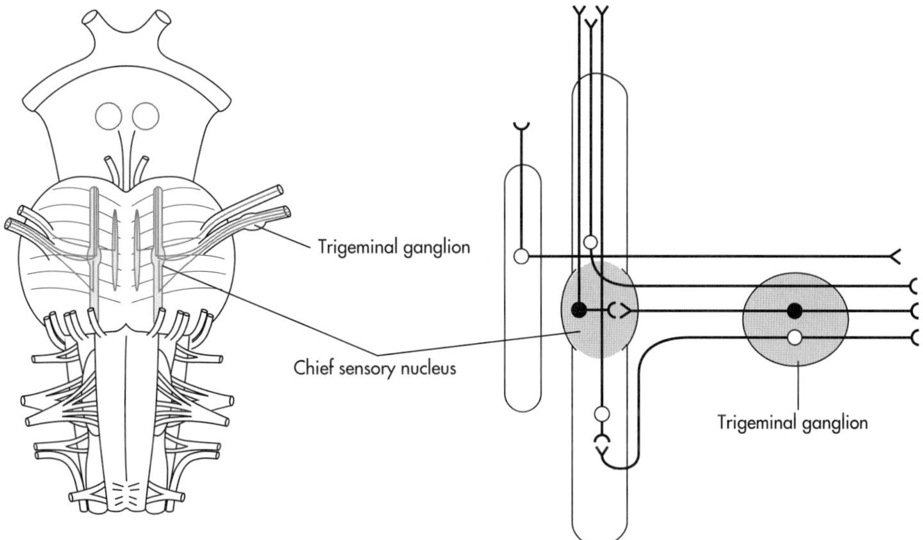

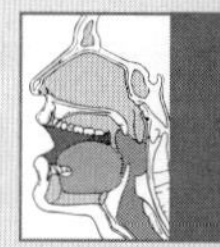

chief sensory nucleus

The caudal portion is called the **spinal nucleus.** Sensory neurons synapse with the cell bodies in this nucleus (pain, touch, temperature) before connecting with higher centers in the thalamus and cerebrum. The spinal nucleus lies below which nucleus?

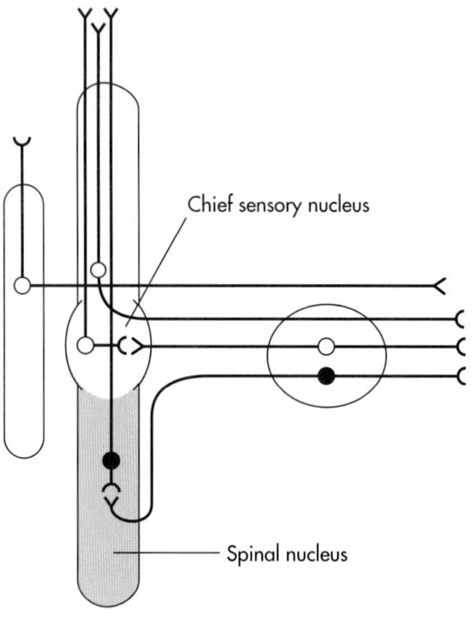

trigeminal ganglion, chief sensory nucleus, mesencephalic nucleus

All sensation, except the sense called **proprioception,** synapses in the spinal and chief sensory nucleus. These neurons, which begin in the periodontal ligament (PDL) and joint, have their cell bodies in a special nucleus (not the trigeminal ganglion) called the **mesencephalic nucleus.** In what three places could you find sensory neuron cell bodies?

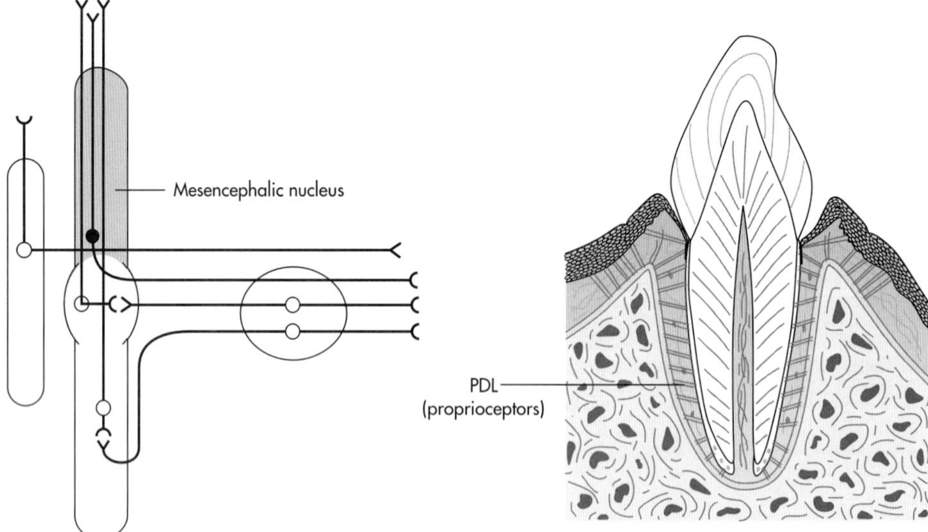

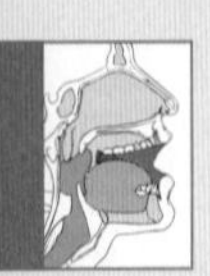

_______________ is position sense, and by bringing the teeth together, we fire neurons that tell us where our jaw is in space. These proprioceptors are located in the _______________ and temporomandibular _______________. Information then travels to the _______________ nucleus.

Proprioception, PDL, joint, mesencephalis

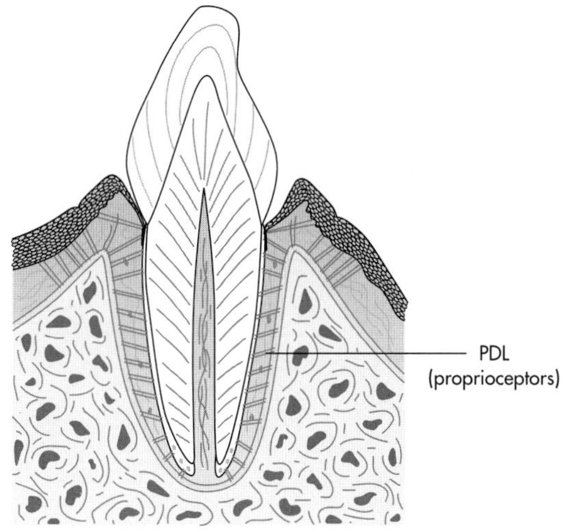

There is also a **motor nucleus** of CN V that lies in the brainstem that contains the cell bodies of the motor neurons that operate the muscles of _______________.

mastication

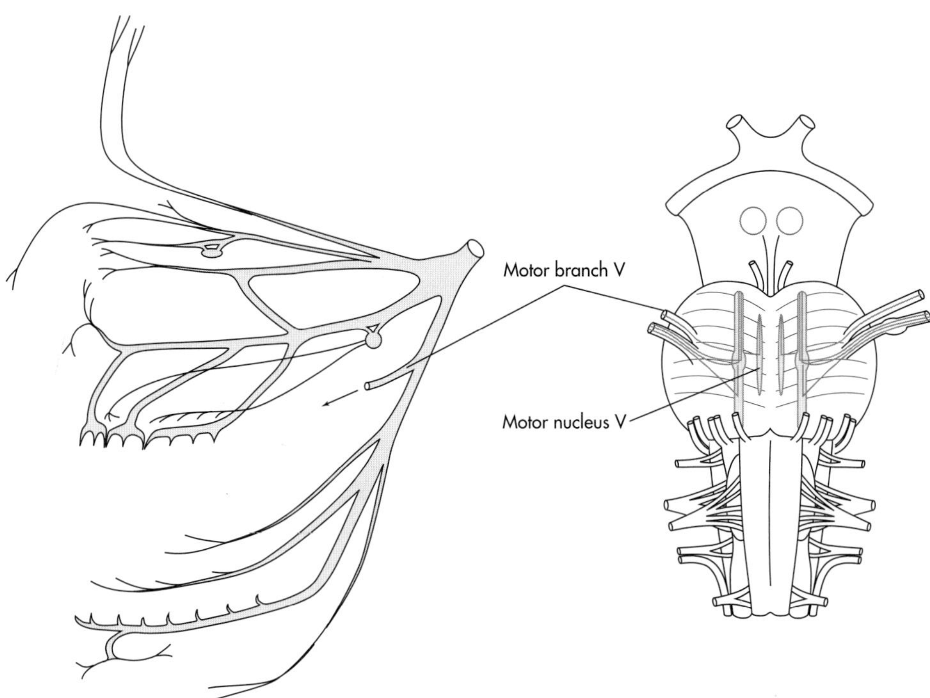

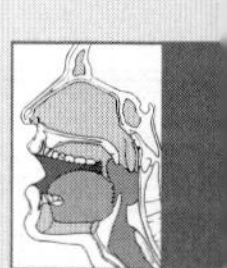

A. motor nucleus
B. chief sensory nucleus
C. spinal nucleus
D. mesencephalic nucleus
E. trigeminal ganglion

Label all of the nuclei associated with the trigeminal nerve and ganglia.

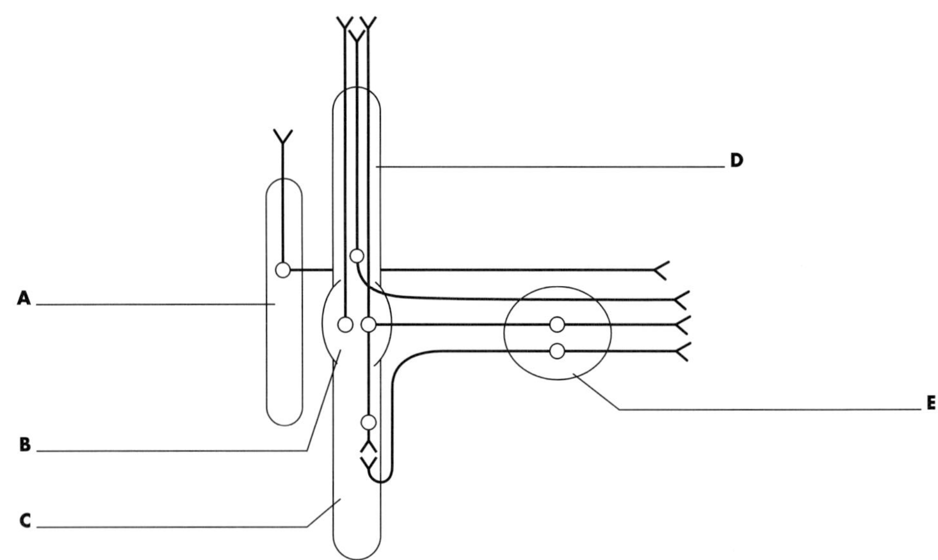

ophthalmic division

A. supraorbital nerve: skin of upper face
B. nasociliary nerve: nasal cavity, eye
C. lacrimal nerve: lacrimal gland
D. frontal nerve
E. ciliary ganglion

Review the divisions and branches of the trigeminal nerve. Tell what each branch innervates.

V1: ______________

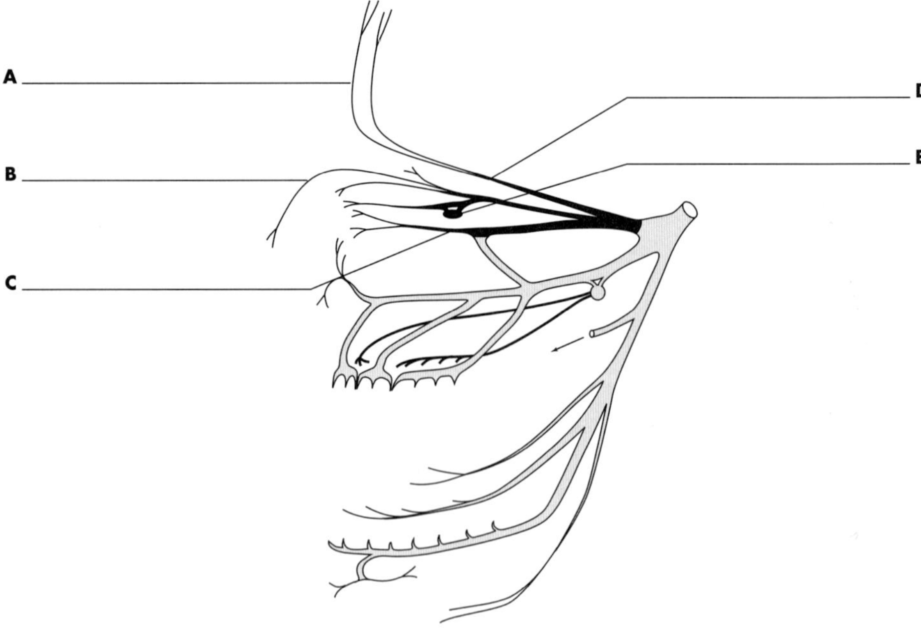

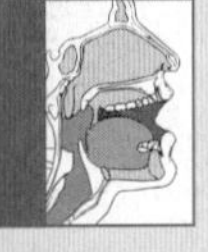

V2: ______________

A
B
C
D
E
F
G

maxillary division

A. infraorbital nerve: skin over maxilla
B. MSA nerve: mesiobuccal cusp of first maxillary molar, premolars, and distal canine
C. PSA nerve: maxillary molars
D. ASA nerve: maxillary incisors and mesial canine
E. pterygopalatine ganglion
F. nasopalatine nerve: lingual maxillary anteriors
G. greater palatine nerve: lingual maxillary posteriors

V3: ______________

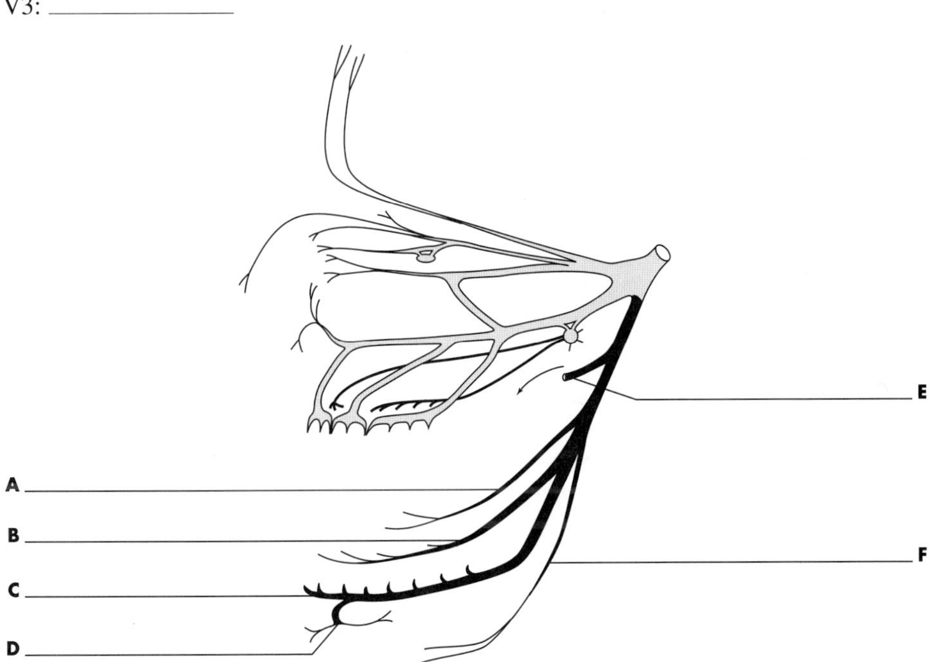

mandibular division

A. buccal nerve: cheek, buccal mandibular molars
B. lingual nerve: anterior two thirds of tongue
C. inferior alveolar nerve: mandibular teeth
D. mental nerve: skin of chin
E. motor branch: muscles of mastication
F. mylohyoid nerve: mylohyoid muscle

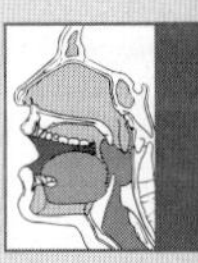

mixed (mostly sensory); trigeminal ganglion, chief sensory nucleus, spinal nucleus, mesencephalic nucleus, motor nucleus; pons

What type of nerve is CN V? Look at the preceding drawings for the areas it innervates. What ganglia and nuclei are associated with it? From what portion of the brain does it originate?

3.11 Summary of Cranial Nerves

Let us now chart all 12 cranial nerves: Draw your information from this chapter. An example is completed for CN I.

CN	Name	Type	Ganglia/Nuclei	Foramen	Innervation
I	Olfactory	Sensory	Optic bulb	Cribriform plate	Nose—smell
II					
III					
IV					
VI					
V1					
V2					
V3					
VII					
VIII					
IX					
X					
XI					
XII					

Find all 12 cranial nerves.

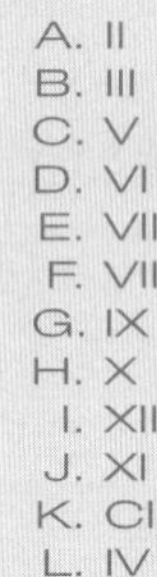

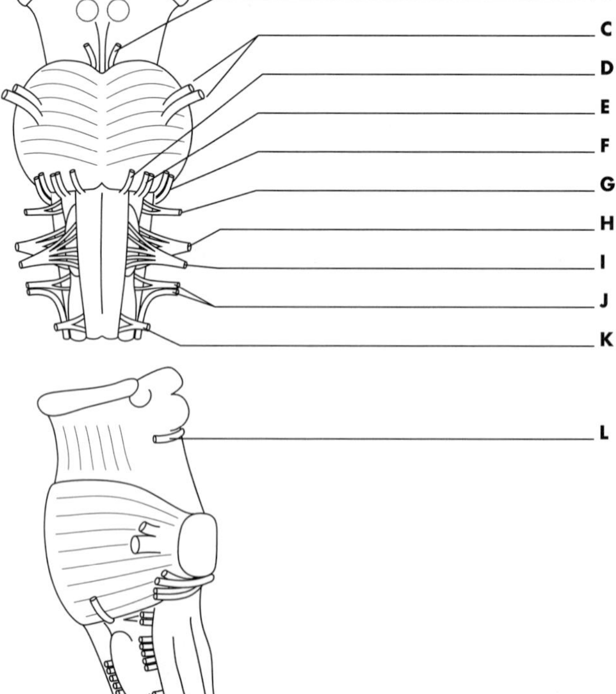

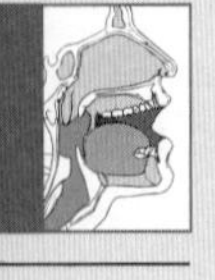

REVIEW TEST 9.1

SELECT OR FILL IN THE CORRECT ANSWER.

1. Neuron processes that receive signals are ________, and those that send signals are ________.

2. Neurons that are used to sense the environment are ________-type neurons, and those that cause a proper response to the sensation are ________-type neurons.

3. The CNS consists of the brain, spinal cord, and spinal nerves. True or false?

4. What is a group of neuron cell bodies found outside of the CNS called?

   a. nucleus b. ganglion
   c. nerve d. cord

5. Sensory and motor neuron processes traveling in the same bundle are called a ________ nerve.

6. The seven pairs of nerves exiting the spinal cord in the neck are called the ________ nerves.

7. The ________ nervous system consists of pathways that control "conscious" bodily functions, whereas the ________ system regulates "unconscious" functions.

8. That part of the autonomic nervous system that regulates body response to stress is the ________ nervous system.

9. C-2 is a ________ and innervates the ________.

10. The telencephalon consists of the ________ and the ________.

11. Name the four anatomic areas (lobes) of the cortex.

12. Which areas in the frontal lobe are involved with voluntary movement? Which area in the parietal lobe controls reception of sensation?

REVIEW TEST 9.2

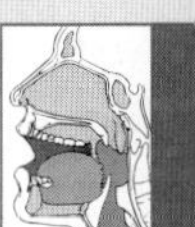

SELECT OR FILL IN THE CORRECT ANSWER.

1. Match the sensation associated with each area of the cortex:

   a. calcarine sulcus ________ 1. vision
   b. lateral sulcus ________ 2. hearing
   c. Wernicke's area ________ 3. speech
   d. Broca's area ________ 4. language comprehension

2. The basal ganglia are groups of nuclei in the telencephalon associated with motor movements. True or false?

3. Which is not a part of the diencephalon?

   a. pineal gland b. subthalamus
   c. basal ganglia d. hypothalamus

4. The sensory relay station of the cerebrum is (are) the ______________
   a. thalami
   b. epithalamus
   c. hypothalamus
   d. basal ganglia

5. The epithalamus contains the ______________ gland, which is associated with biorhythmic signals.

6. Which is not a function of the hypothalamus?
   a. regulation of thirst
   b. regulation of muscle coordination
   c. regulation of hunger
   d. control of endocrine function

7. Which portion of the brain is important to coordination of motor movement and connects to the cerebrum and brainstem?

8. List the three areas of the cerebellum.

9. The large area of the brainstem that serves as a neuronal crossover for pathways is called the ______________.

10. How many pairs of cranial nerves are there?

11. Write the names of the following cranial nerves:
    a. II ______________
    b. V ______________
    c. IX ______________
    d. III ______________
    e. VII ______________
    f. XII ______________

REVIEW TEST 9.3

FILL IN THE CORRECT ANSWER.

1. The olfactory nerve is associated with the sense of ______________.

2. CN I receptor neurons synapse on the neurons located in the ______________ bulbs of the brain.

3. Olfactory nerve neurons pass through the ______________ to enter the cranium.

4. CN II is associated with the sense of ______________.

5. The crossing over of right and left optic nerves occurs in the ______________ in the pituitary fossa.

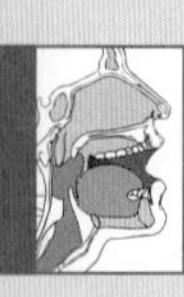

6. Visual pathways end in the visual cortex along the ______________ sulcus of the occipital lobe.

7. Light and images are focused on the ______________ portion of the eye.

8. Two types of receptor neurons are responsible for vision; they are called the ______________ and ______________.

9. CN II passes through the ______________ foramina to enter the cranium.

10. Match the cranial nerve with its number. What do these nerves innervate?

a. trochlear ______________	III
b. abducens ______________	IV
c. oculomotor ______________	VI

11. Through what foramen do CNs II, IV, and VI exit from the cranium?

12. CN VII is called the ______________ nerve, because it spreads across the superficial face to innervate the muscles of ______________.

13. The superficial portion of CN VII exits through the ______________ foramen behind the ear.

14. The deep portion of CN VII gives parasympathetic innervation to which two salivary glands?

15. The ganglia associated with the parasympathetic portion of CN VII are the ______________ and ______________ ganglia.

REVIEW TEST 9.4

SELECT OR FILL IN THE CORRECT ANSWER.

1. The branch of CN VII that picks up the sense of taste sensation is called the ______________, and it "rides" on the ______________ nerve to reach the anterior tongue.

2. The sensory ganglion of the facial nerve is the ______________ ganglion.

3. What is the best name for CN VIII? Why?

4. What are the three ossicles of the ear and what do they do?

5. The ______________ ganglion is the sensory ganglion for the cochlear portion of CN VIII; the ______________ ganglion is for the vestibular portion.

6. ______________ cells are the type of receptor neurons for both hearing and balance.

7. The vestibule is that portion of the inner ear concerned with hearing and the cochlea is used in balance. True or false?

REVIEW TEST 9.5

SELECT OR FILL IN THE CORRECT ANSWER.

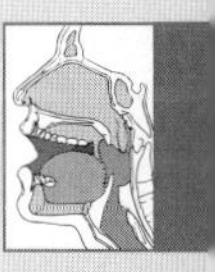

1. The endpoint of the hearing pathway is the auditory cortex, located on the ______________ sulcus of the temporal lobe.

2. The vestibular pathway is concerned with position sense (proprioception) and balance and makes many connections with the brainstem nuclei, cerebellum, and cerebrum. True or false?

3. CN VII passes through the ______________ to reach the cranium and brain.

4. *Glossopharyngeal* means ______________ and pharynx, indicating the destination of CN ______________.

5. CN IX exits the cranium through the ______________ foramen, and the ______________ and ______________ ganglia are associated with its sensory pathways.

6. Which salivary gland(s) does CN IX innervate?

7. The vagus nerve is CN ______________ and is the main ______________ nerve of the body.

8. The motor pathways of CN X are important to

   a. swallowing b. speech
   c. digestion d. heartbeat
   e. respiration f. all of the above

REVIEW TEST 9.6

SELECT OR FILL IN THE CORRECT ANSWER.

1. The nucleus associated with the vagus nerve is the ______________ nucleus. The ganglia associated with its sensory paths are the ______________ and ______________ ganglia.

2. The vagus nerve exits the cranium through the ______________ foramen.

3. The swallowing (and gag) reflex is controlled by the interaction of the sensory paths of CN ______________ and the motor paths of CN ______________.

4. CN IX, the ______________ nerve, is a ______________-type nerve that innervates ______________ and ______________.

5. Which muscle does not receive innervation from CN XII?

   a. hypoglossus b. intrinsic muscles of tongue
   c. stylohyoid d. genioglossus

6. The hypoglossal nerve exits the cranium through which foramina?

REVIEW TEST 9.7

SELECT OR FILL IN THE CORRECT ANSWER.

1. Name the three divisions of the trigeminal nerve and the three foramina through which each enters the cranium.

2. Give two more names for the trigeminal ganglion.

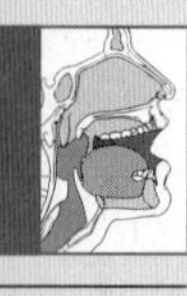

3. From which portion of the brainstem does CN V exit?

4. Match the branch of V1 with the structure it innervates:

   a. frontal ______________ 1. lacrimal gland
   b. nasociliary ______________ 2. skin of forehead
   c. lacrimal ______________ 3. nose, eye (ciliary)

5. In what fossa does CN V2 lie after exiting the foramen rotundum? With what parasympathetic ganglion does it connect here?

6. Match the branch of V2 with its foramen and destination:

   a. greater palatine ______________ 1. incisive foramen
   2. lingual anterior teeth
   b. nasopalatine ______________ 3. lingual posterior teeth
   4. greater palatine for

REVIEW TEST 9.8

SELECT OR FILL IN THE CORRECT ANSWER.

1. Match the three loops of superior alveolar nerve with the teeth they innervate (you may use an answer more than once):

   a. maxillary first molar ______________
   b. maxillary second premolar ______________
   c. maxillary canine ______________
   d. maxillary second molar ______________

   ASA
   MSA
   PSA

2. The following teeth need to be extracted. Which branches of V2 or V3 need to be anesthetized?

   a. tooth 3 ______________
   b. tooth 11 ______________
   c. tooth 13 ______________
   d. tooth 30 ______________
   e. tooth 24 ______________

3. What sensation (besides pain) is unique to the PDL nerve fibers?

4. Through which foramen does V3 pass to enter the mandible?

5. What branch of V2 provides sensation to the skin of the upper cheeks and lips?

REVIEW TEST 9.9

SELECT OR FILL IN THE CORRECT ANSWER.

1. The branch of V3 to the tongue is called the ______________ nerve, and that to the cheek, posterior facial gingiva, and molars is the ______________ nerve.

2. What branch of V3 travels in the mandibular canal? Which part of this nerve pokes out through the mental foramen?

3. What group of muscles does V3 innervate?

4. Which three nerves (branches of trigeminal) provide sensory innervation to the face?

5. Match the nucleus of the trigeminal nerve with the neuron type it receives?

   a. spinal nucleus ______________
   b. motor nucleus ______________
   c. chief sensory ______________
   d. mesencephalic ______________

   1. motor (mastication)
   2. pain
   3. touch, temperature
   4. proprioception

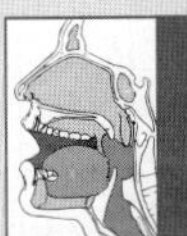

REVIEW TEST 9.10

LABEL THE DIAGRAMS.

1.

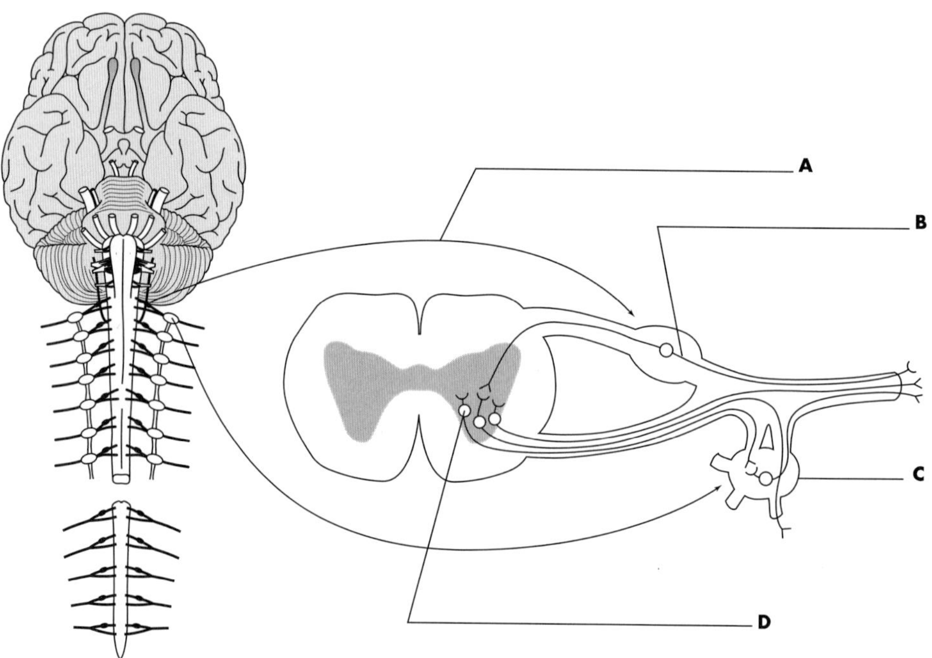

2.

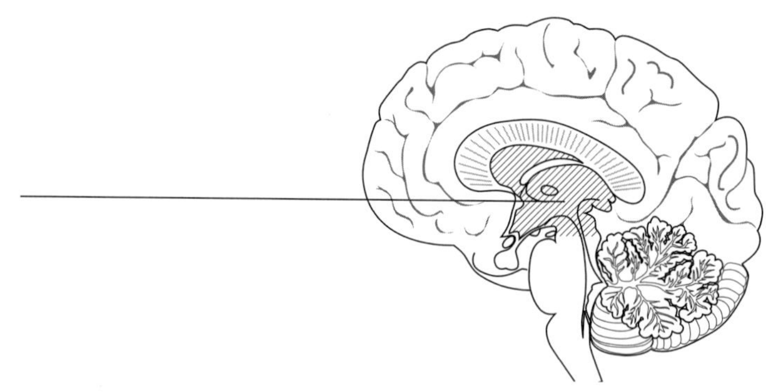

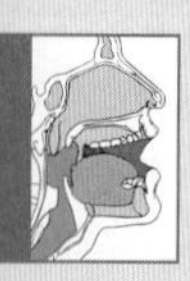

3.

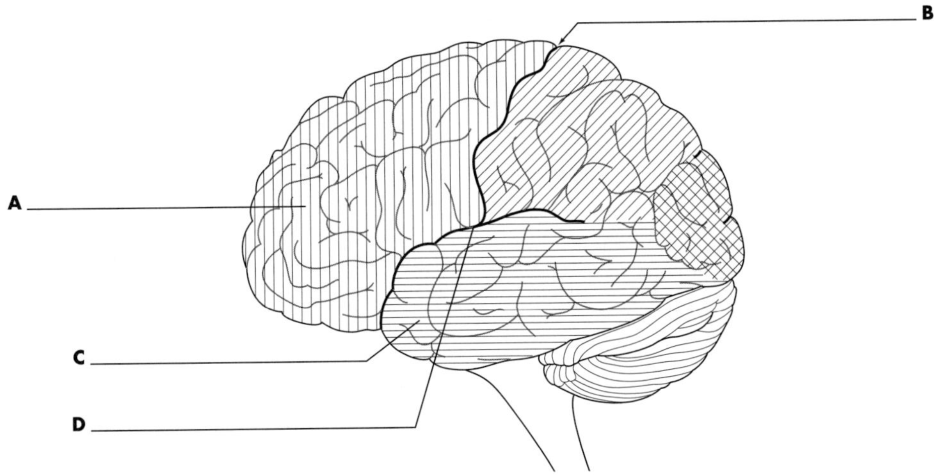

4.

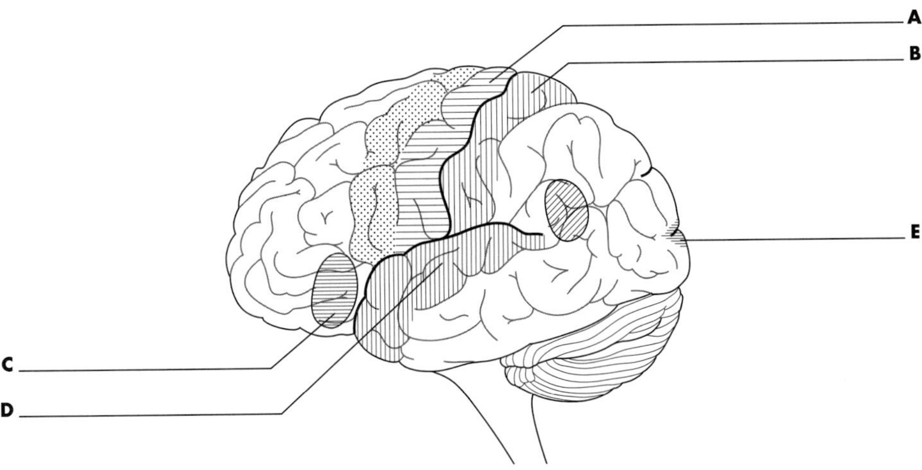

5.

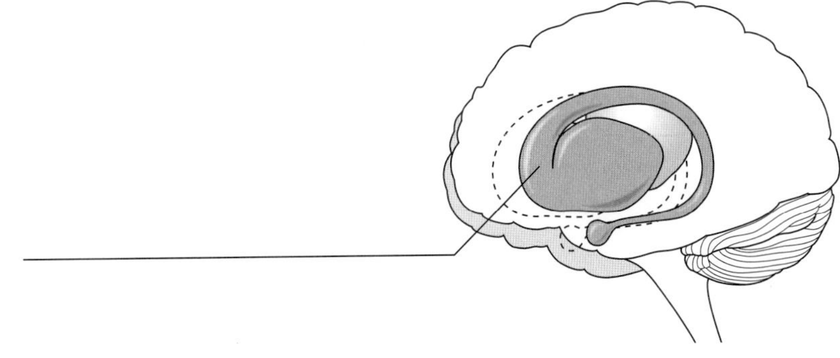

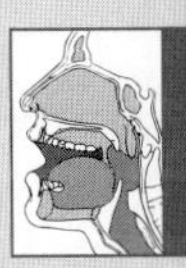

6.

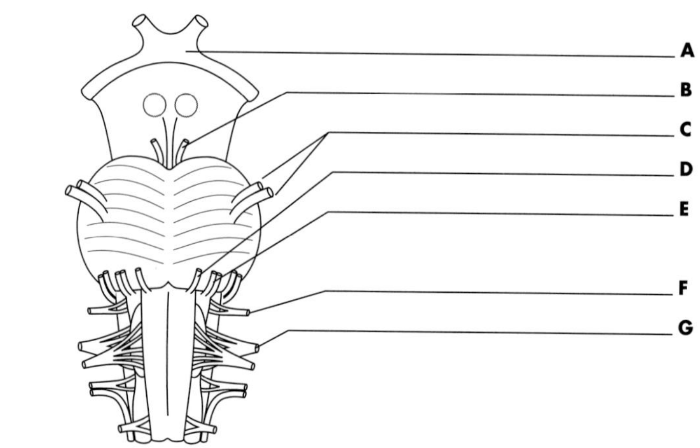

7.

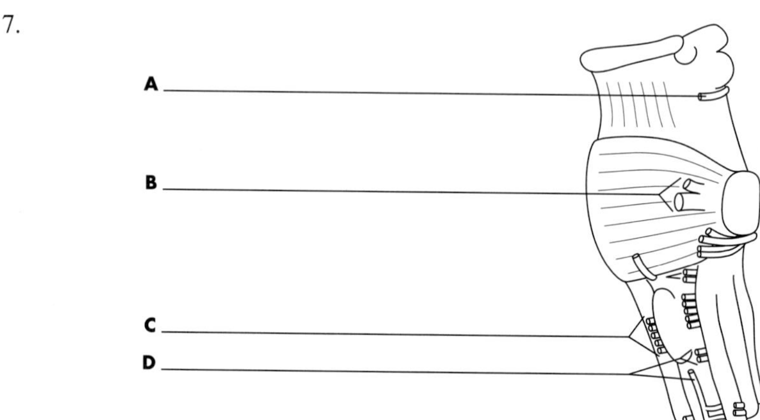

8.

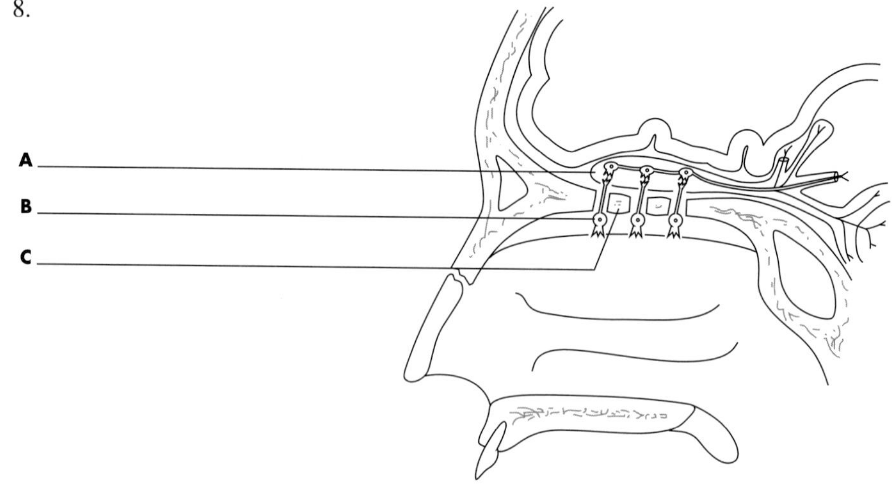

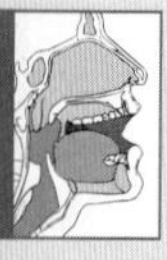

9.

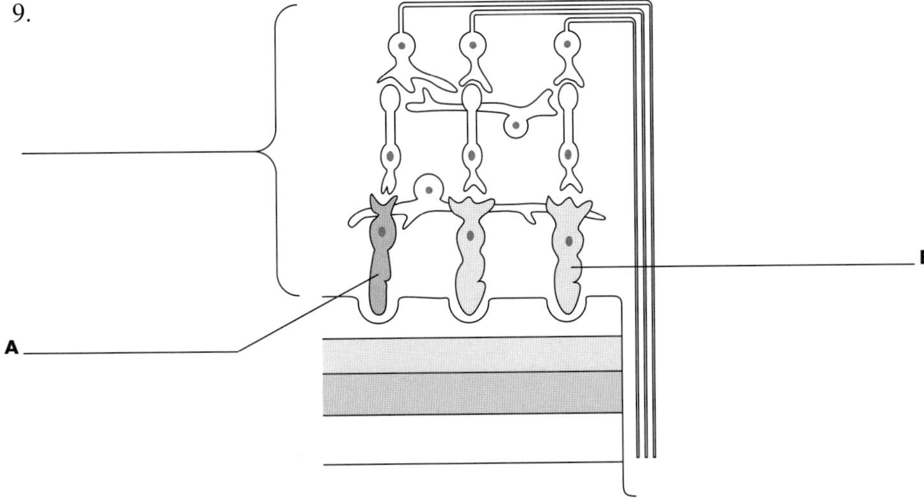

10.

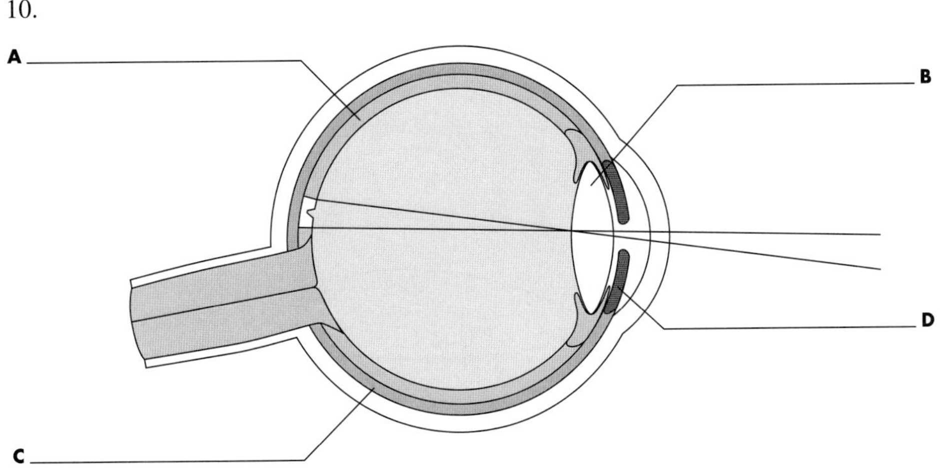

11.

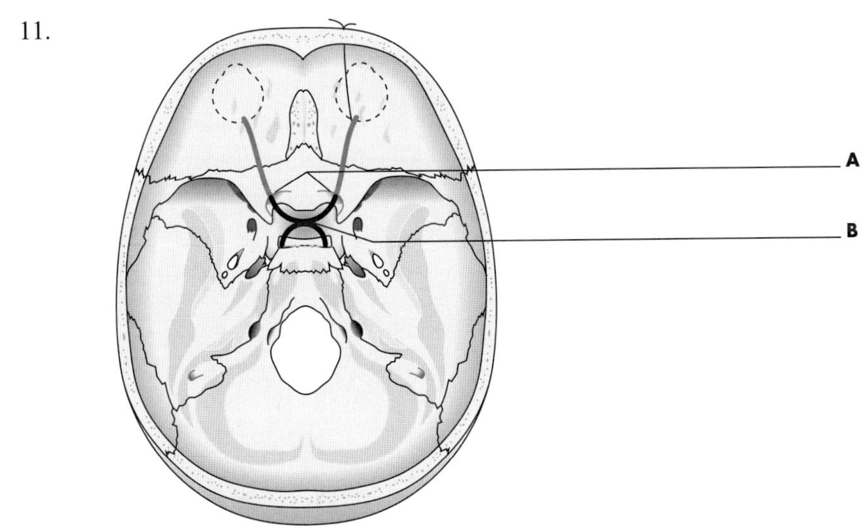

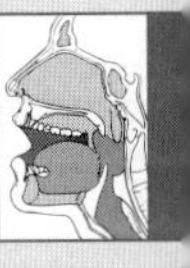

12.

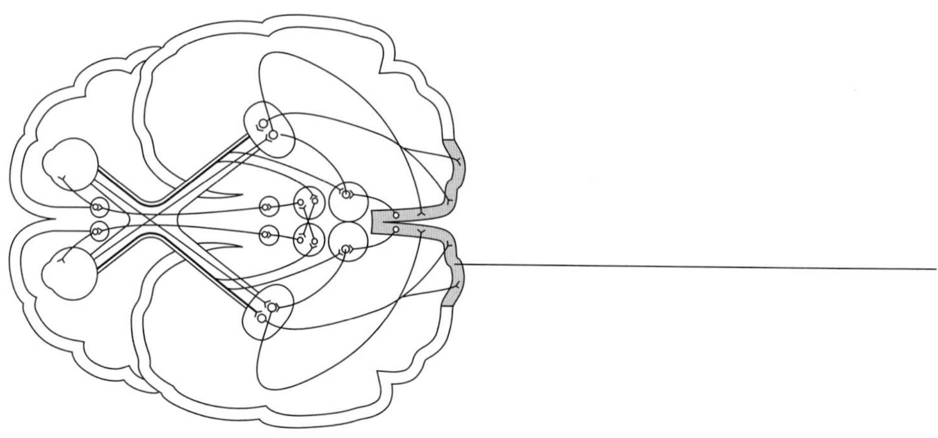

13.

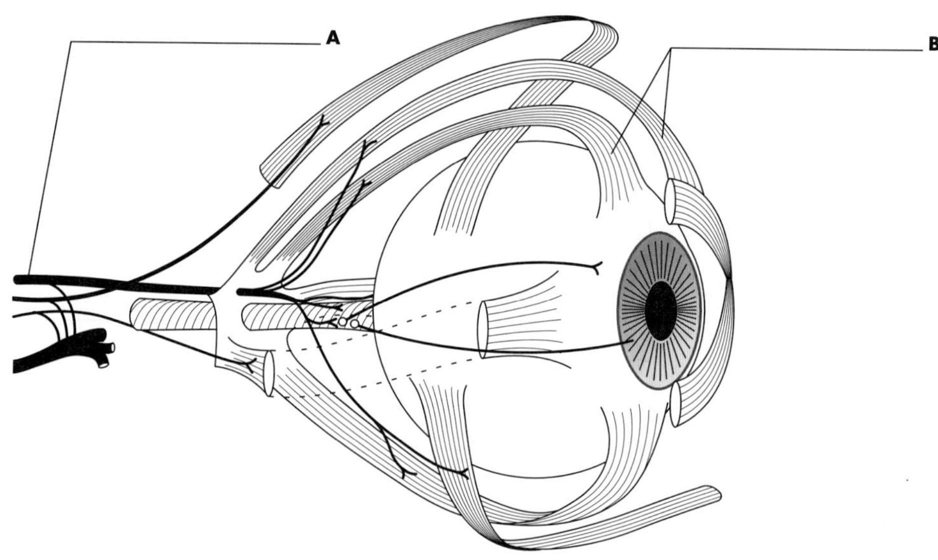

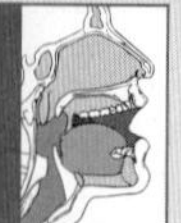

14.

Give the area's innervation:

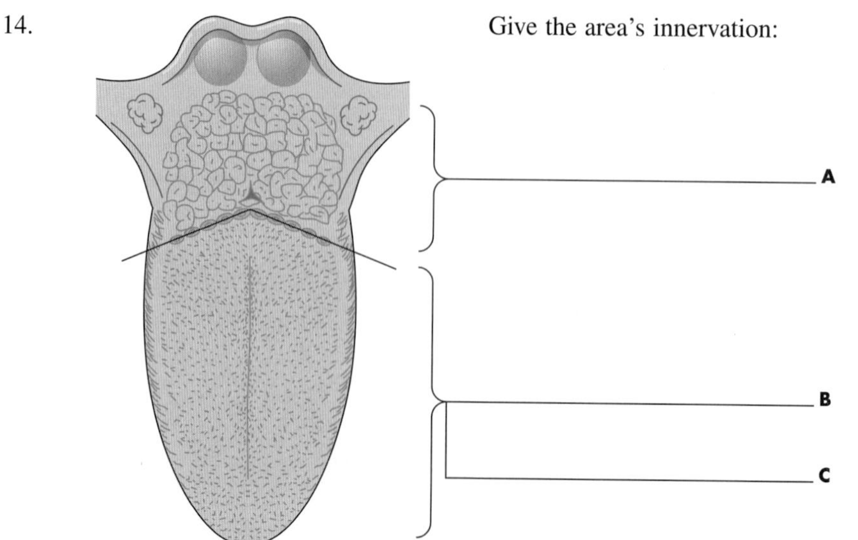

15.

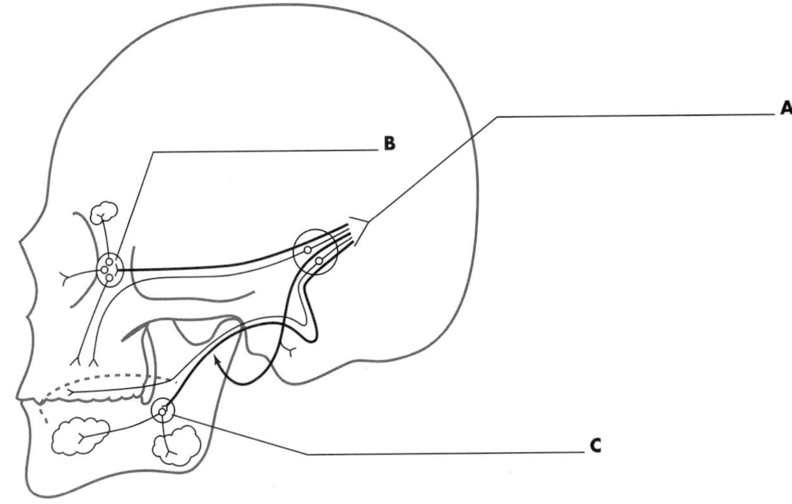

16.

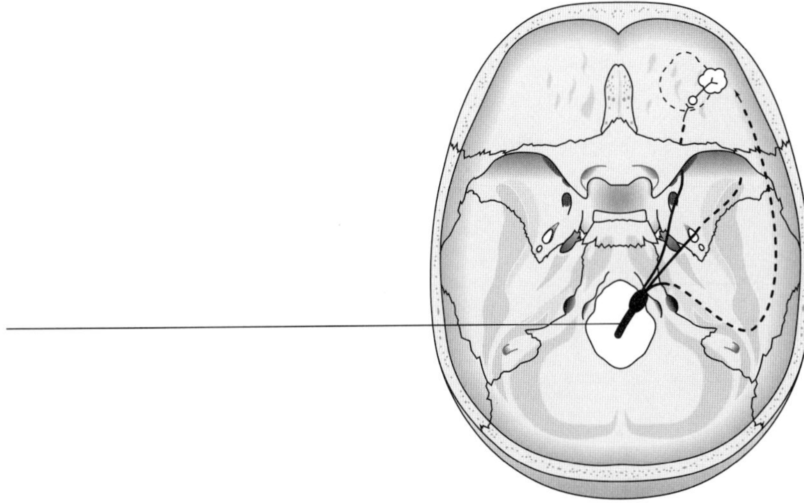

17.

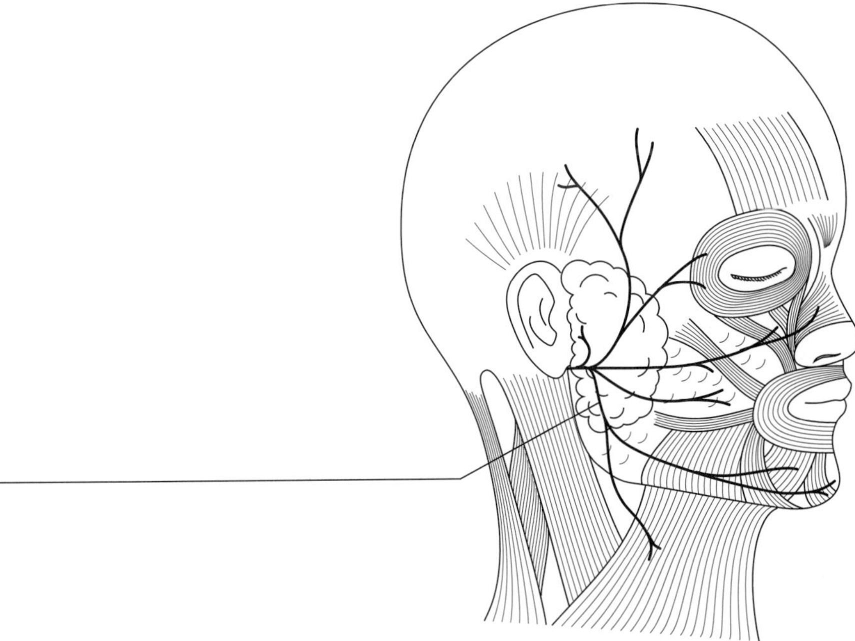

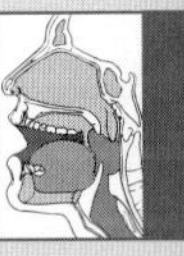

18.

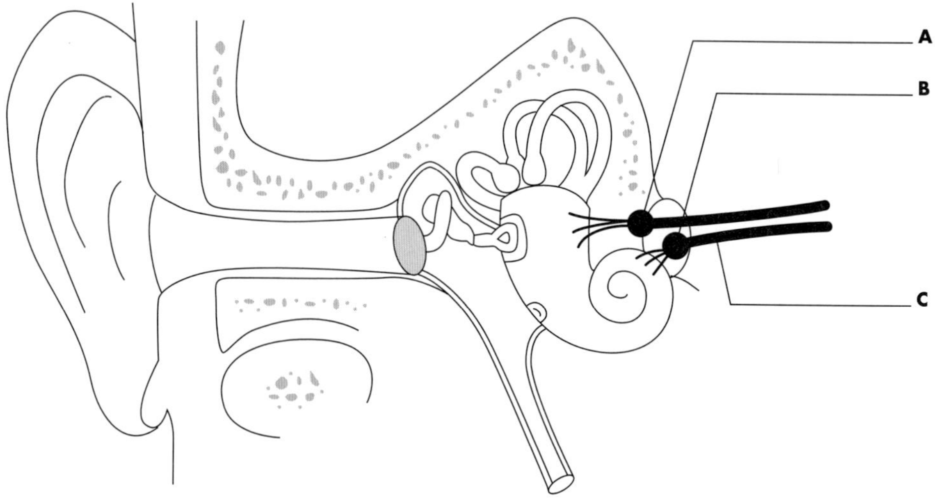

19.

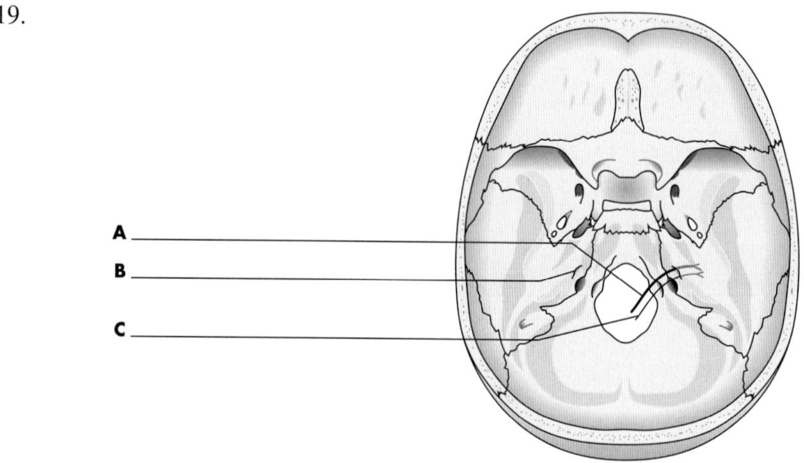

20.

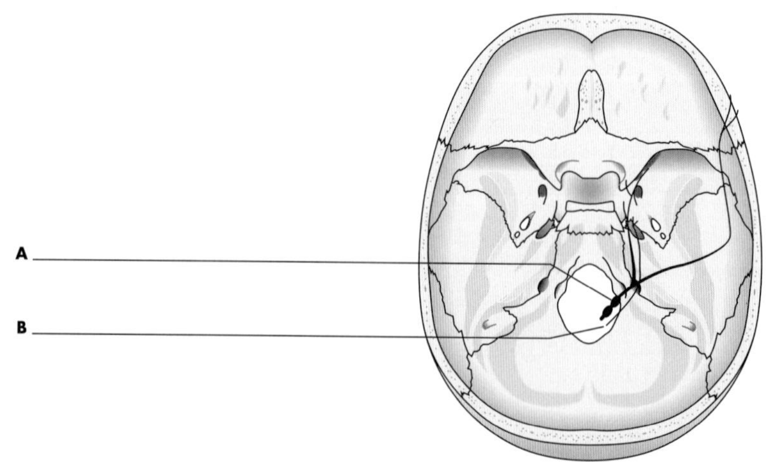

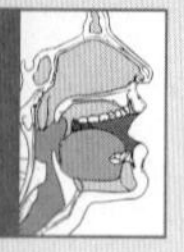

21.

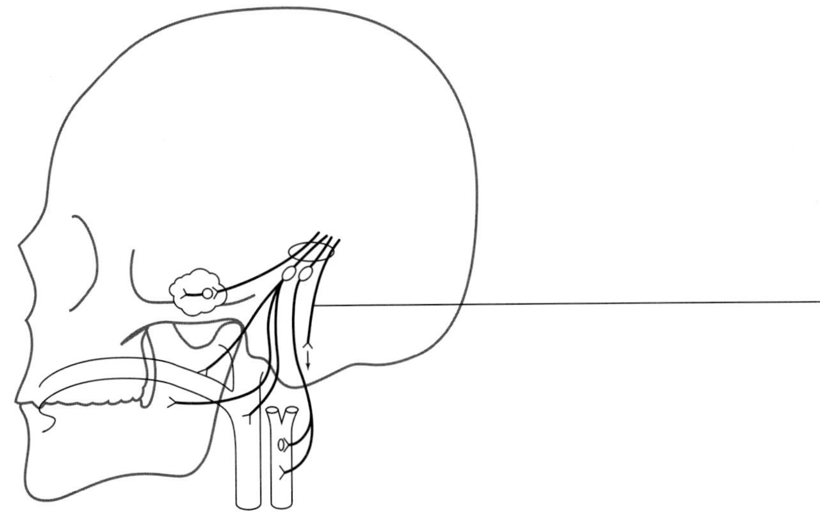

22.

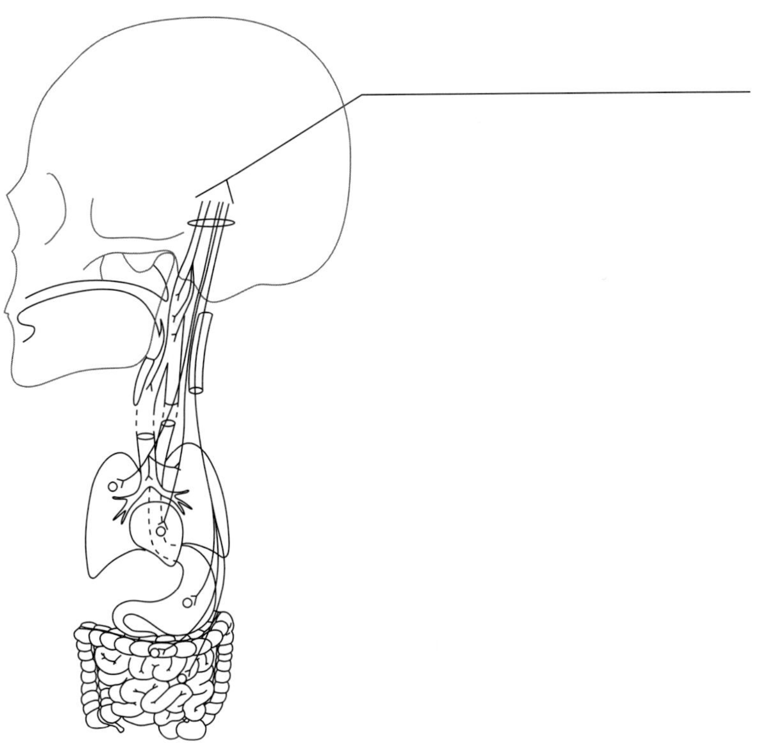

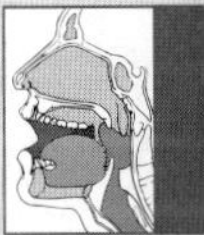

23.

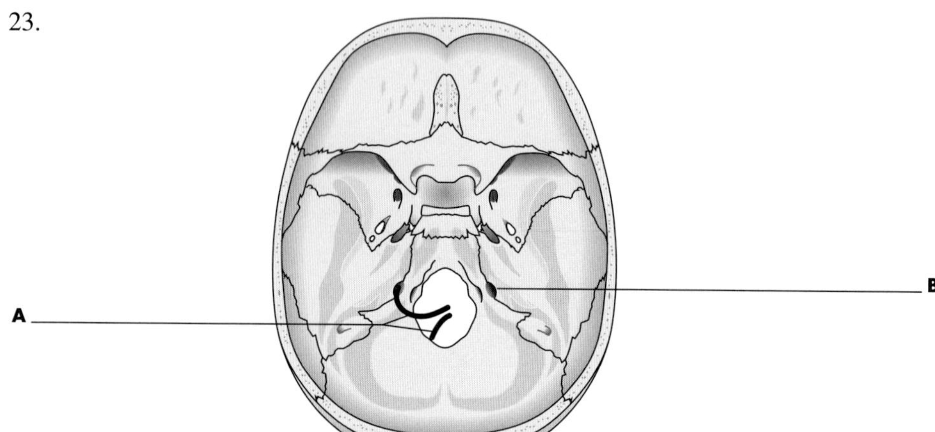

24.

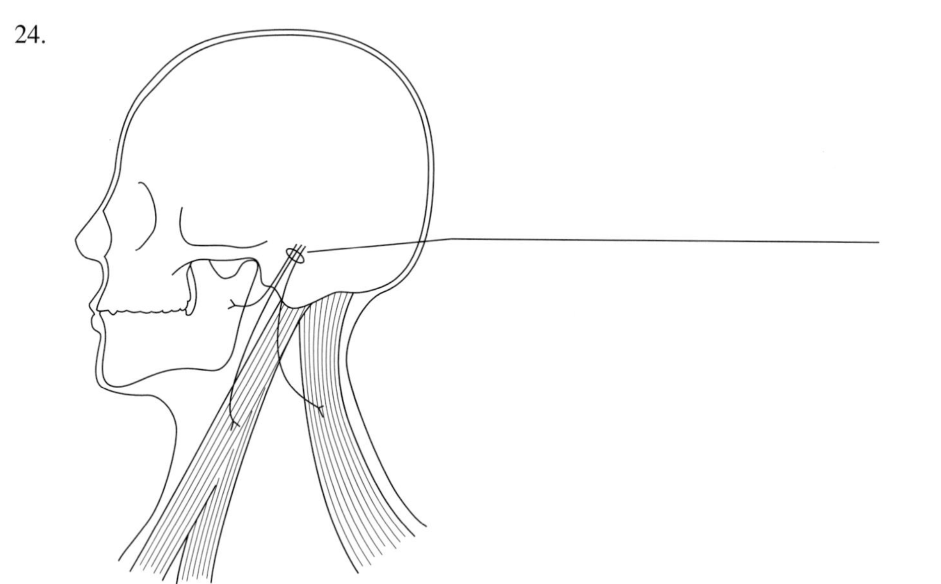

25.

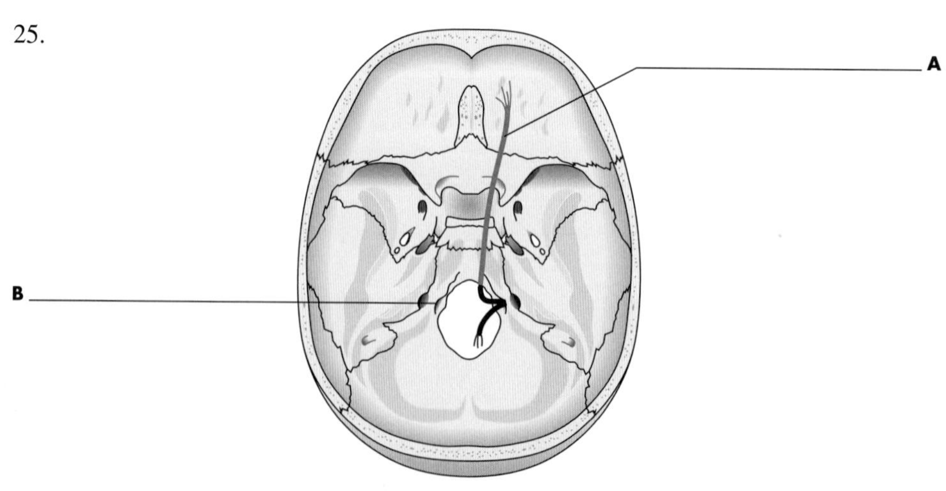

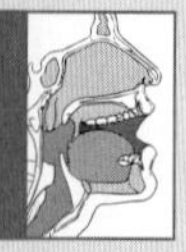

26.

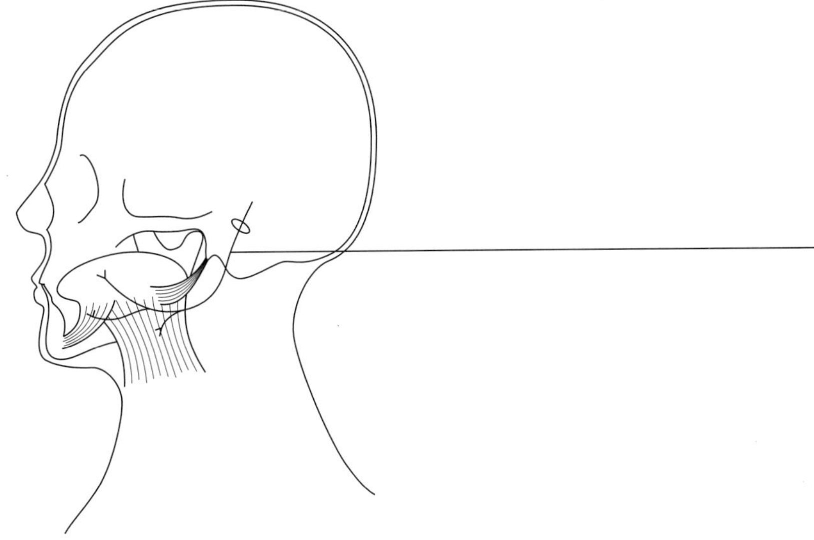

27.

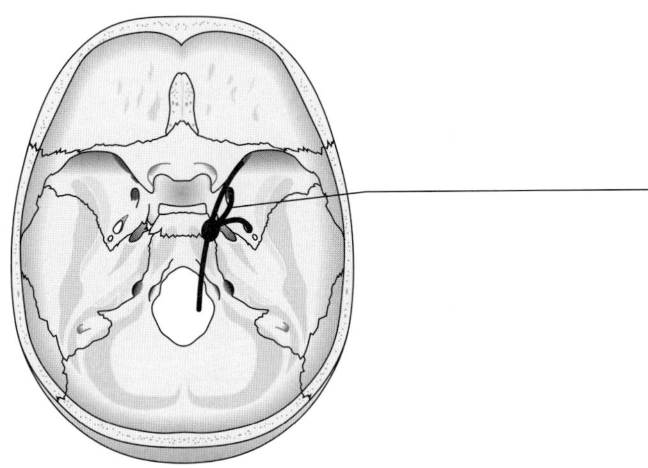

28.

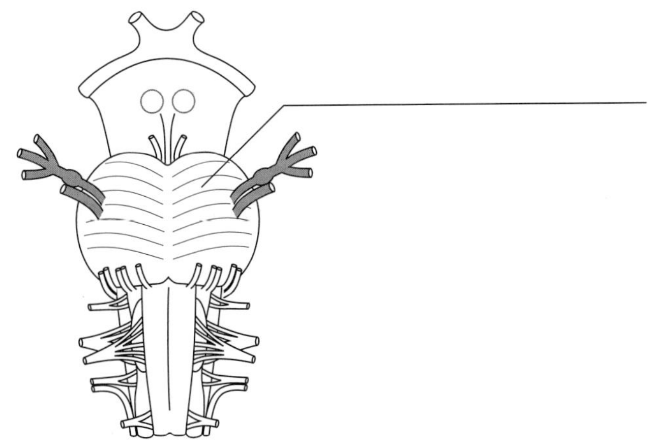

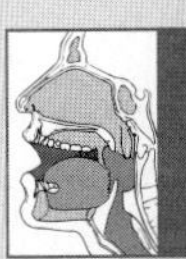

29.

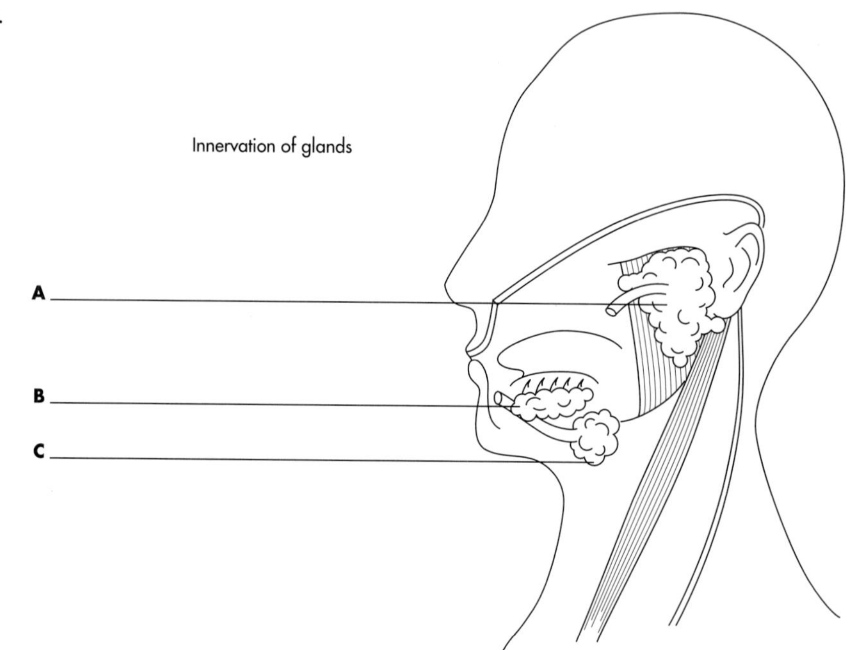

30.

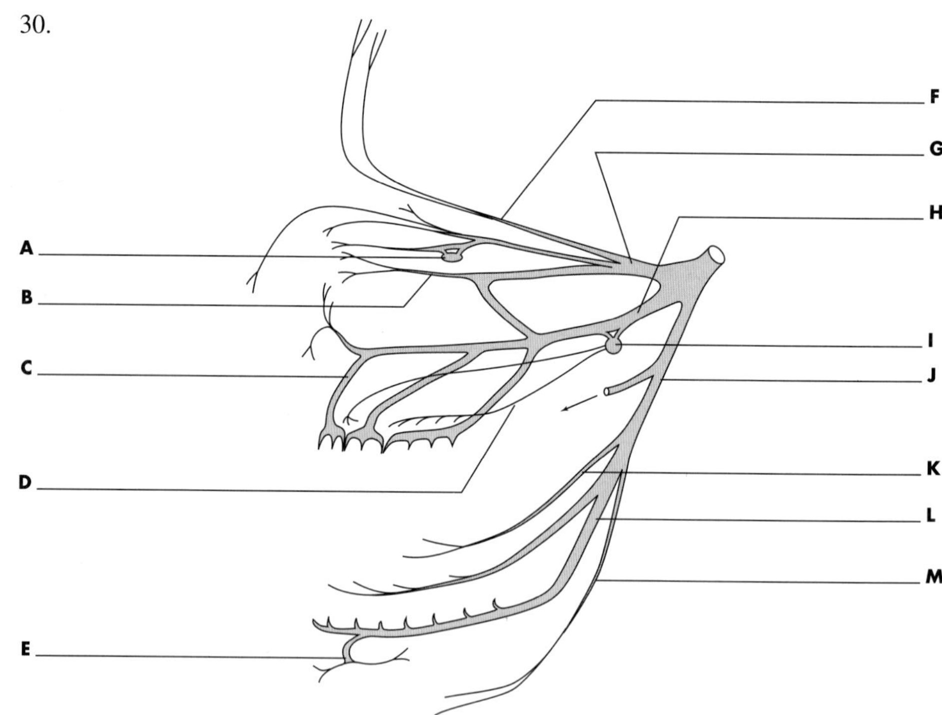

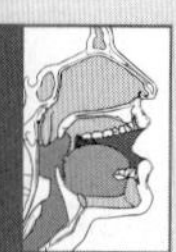

31.

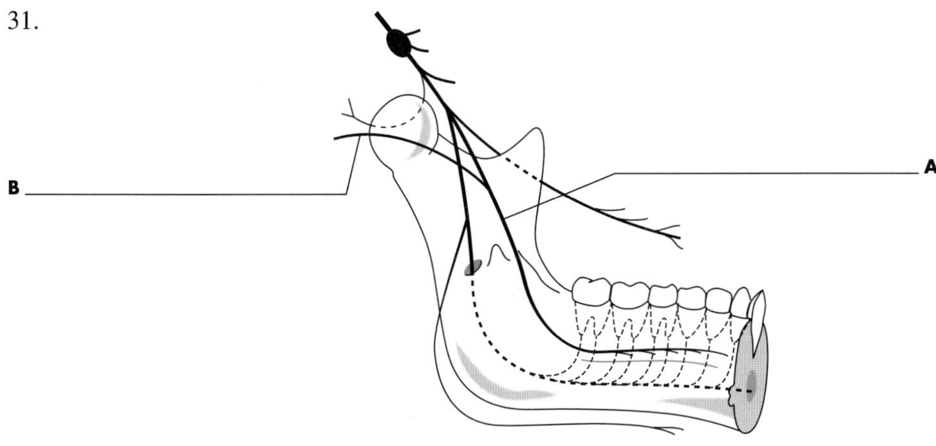

32.

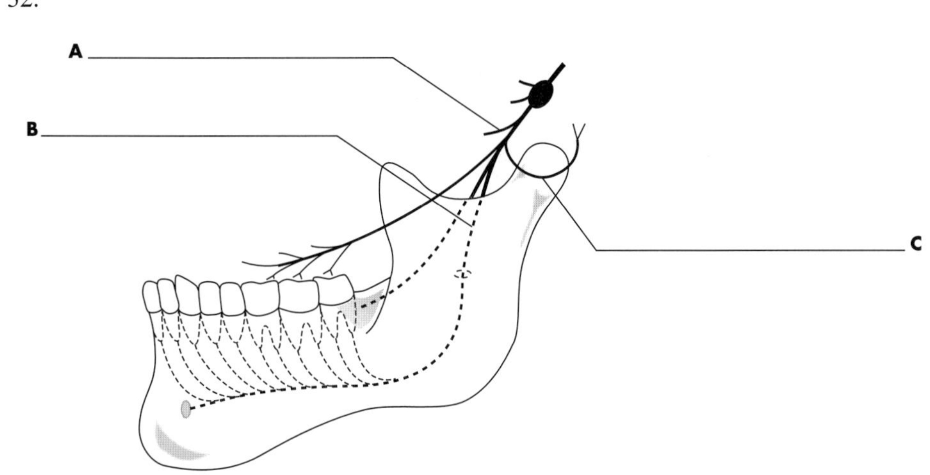

33.

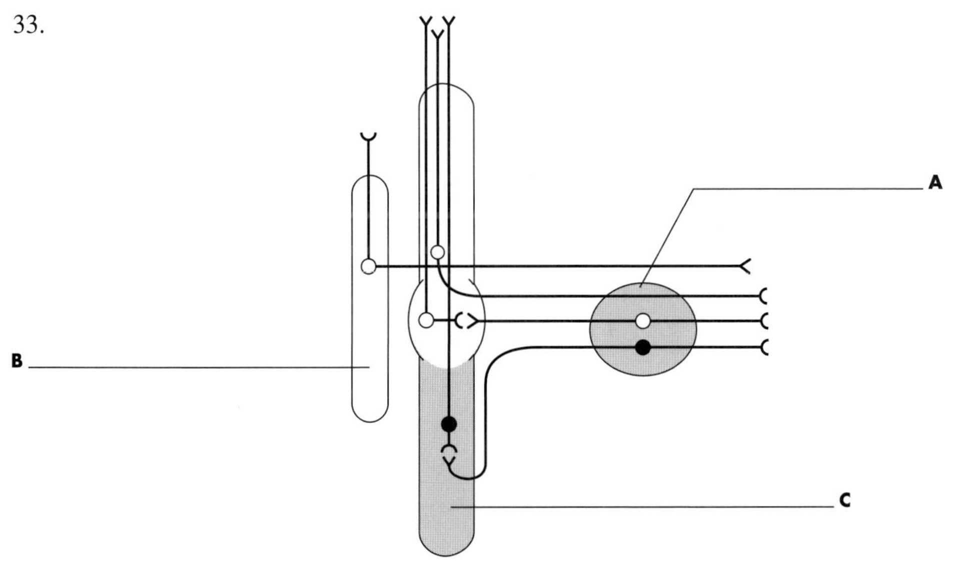

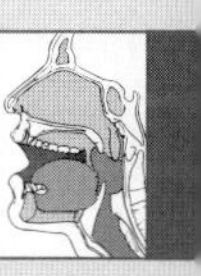

34.

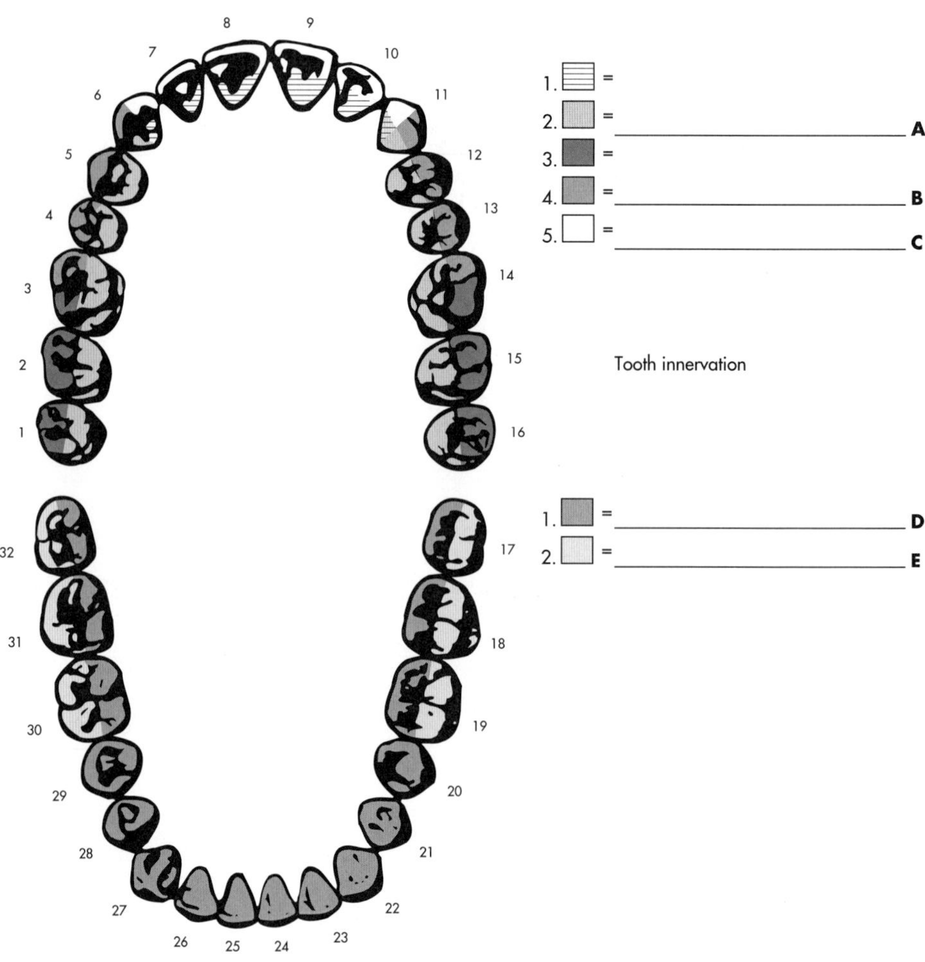
8
9
7
10
6
11
5
12
4
13
3
14
2
15
1
16
32
17
31
18
30
19
29
20
28
21
27
22
26
25
24
23
1. =
2. = A
3. =
4. = B
5. = C
Tooth innervation
1. = D
2. = E

35.

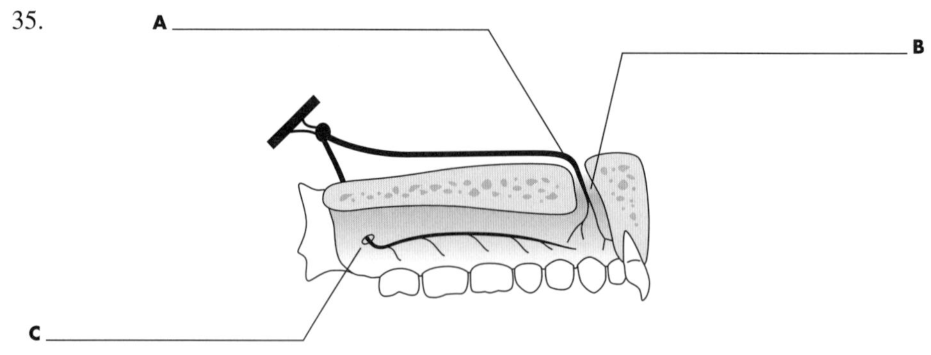
A
B
C

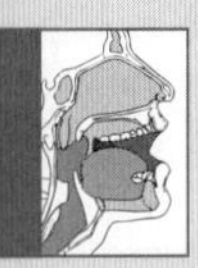

36.

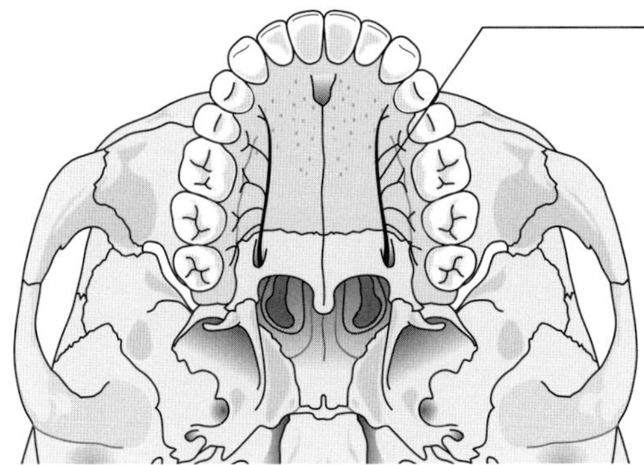

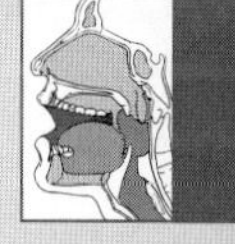

10

Circulatory System

The **circulatory system** consists of a series of tubes (blood and lymph vessels), a pump (heart), and a fluid medium in which nutrients/wastes, blood gases, and cells can be carried to any part of the body.

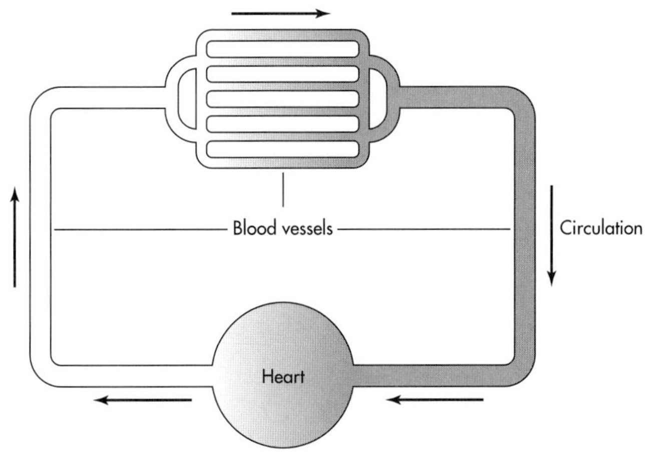

circulatory

The word ______________ means "in a circle." Nutrients and oxygen are picked up in the digestive and respiratory systems and circulated by way of the blood vessels to all the cells of the body.

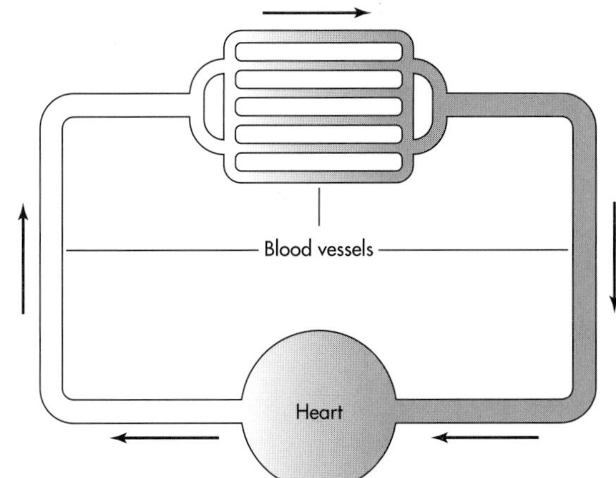

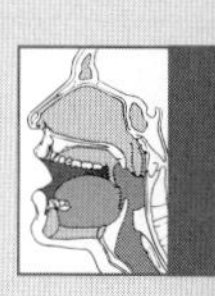

Waste products (including carbon dioxide) are gathered at the cellular level and circulated to the digestive, urinary, and respiratory systems for disposal. These nutrients and waste products are carried in the fluid portion of the circulatory system or blood, which we have seen in histology to be composed of erythrocytes, leukocytes, platelets, and serum.

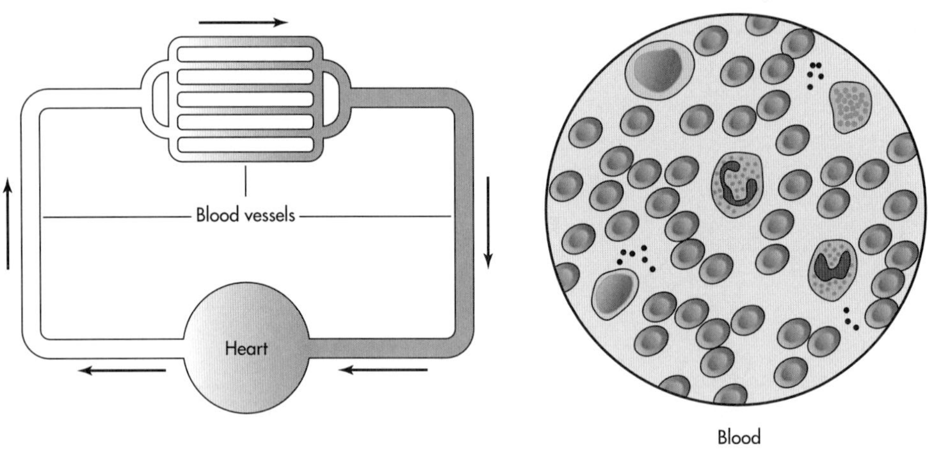

Leukocytes are defensive cells; platelets are for clotting.

Erythrocytes carry oxygen (O_2) and carbon dioxide (CO_2), and the **serum** portion carries nutrients and waste products to the cells. What function do **leukocytes** and **platelets** have?

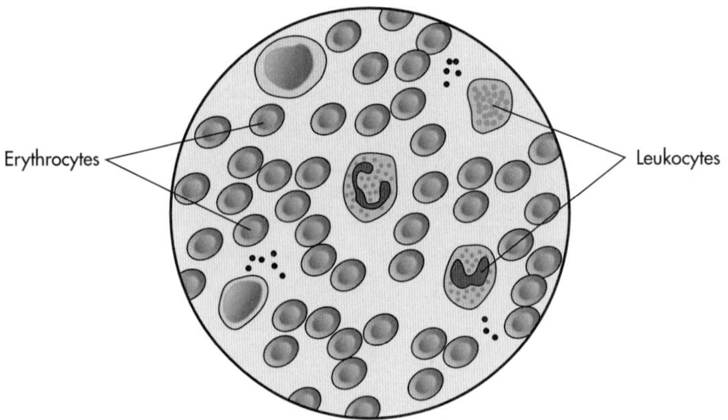

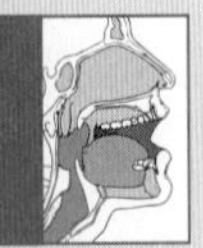

How, then, does the circulatory system get down to the cellular level to deliver and pick up these body products? It does this by transporting the products in smaller and smaller tubes. The largest tubes carrying oxygenated, nutrient-laden blood away from the heart are called **arteries.** They are often colored in red in anatomic drawings but are lighter colored in our drawings. (You may wish to color arteries we study in red and veins in blue, or choose different colors for each branch vessel.)

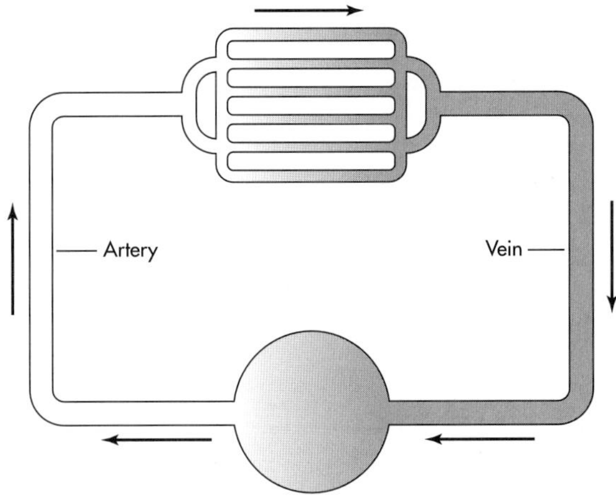

Arteries feed down into small vessels called **arterioles,** and these, in turn, break down into even smaller vessels called **capillaries,** which are the size of cells. Product exchange occurs through the walls of the capillaries: nutrients and O_2 are delivered and wastes and CO_2 are picked up.

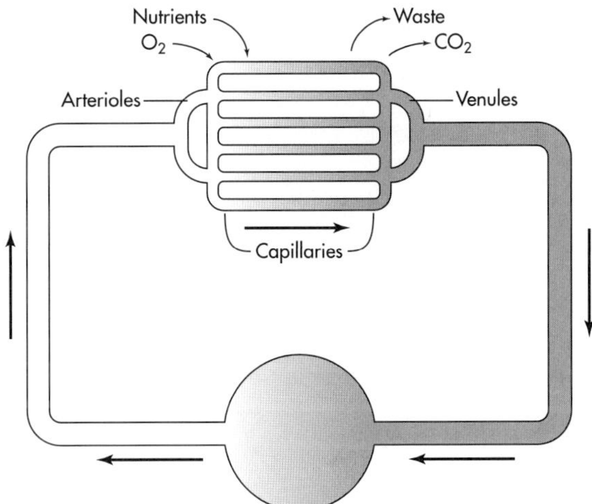

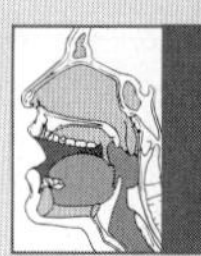

arteries

Pictured here are the vessels called ______________, which transport nutrients and O_2 to the body. Arteries are thick-walled vessels. They feed down into smaller vessels called the arterioles.

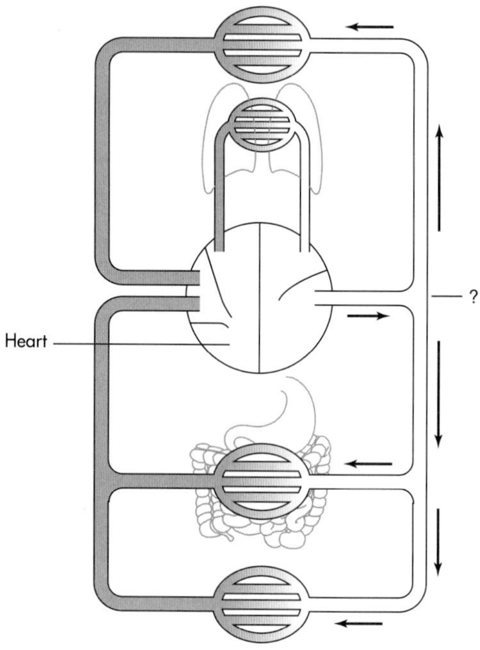

veins

In this drawing are the vessels called ______________. They are thin-walled vessels that carry blood toward the heart. They form larger vessels as they progress toward the heart. The smallest veins are called **venules.**

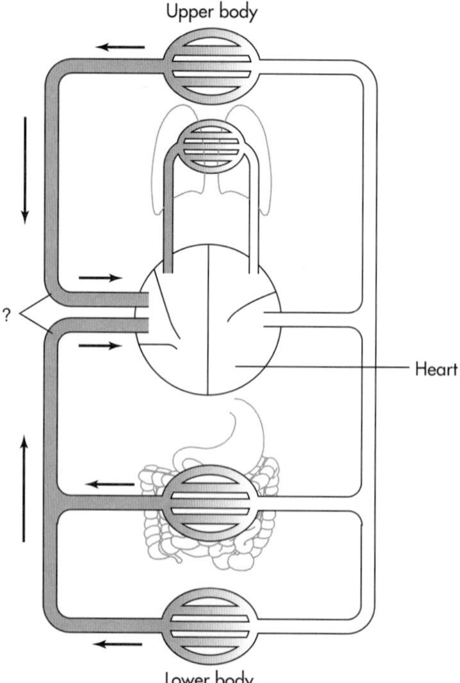

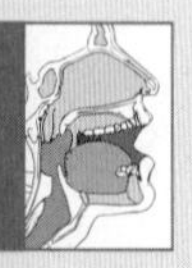

Only the largest vessels, that is, the _______________ and _______________, have names.

arteries, veins

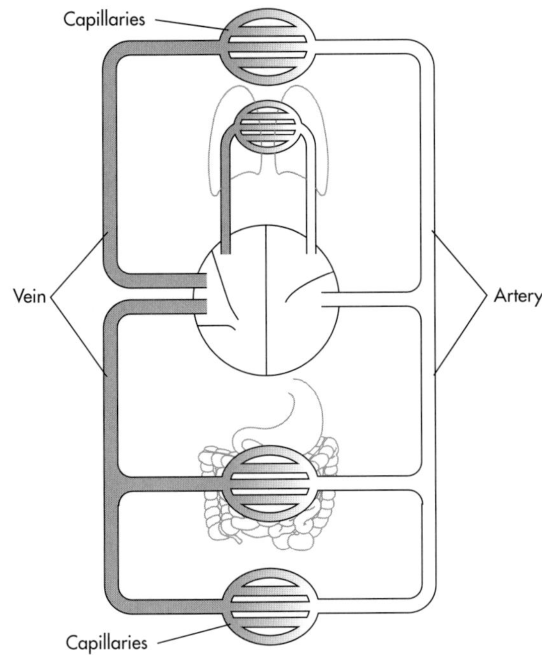

We look briefly at the "pump," that is, the heart. In humans this is a four-chambered heart; the upper chambers are the **atria,** and the lower ones, the **ventricles.** Follow the path of blood flow around the heart.

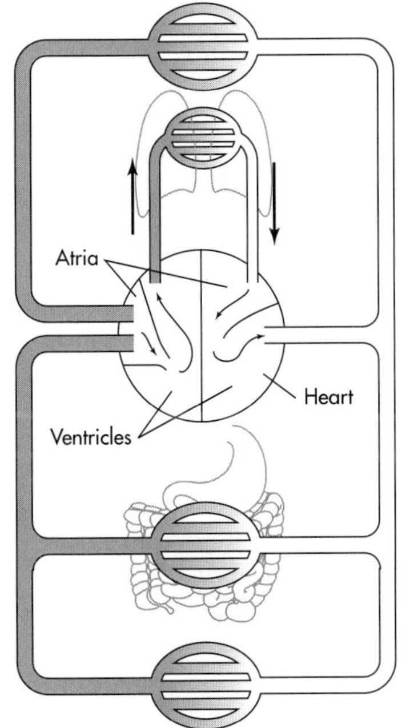

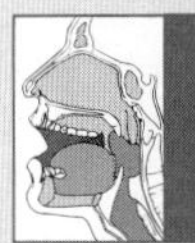

to the lungs

The heart has two jobs: to pump the blood to and from the lungs and to pump the blood to and from the rest of the body. The drawing shows systemic blood flow through the heart and to the lungs and the body. Where does blood first go to after leaving the heart?

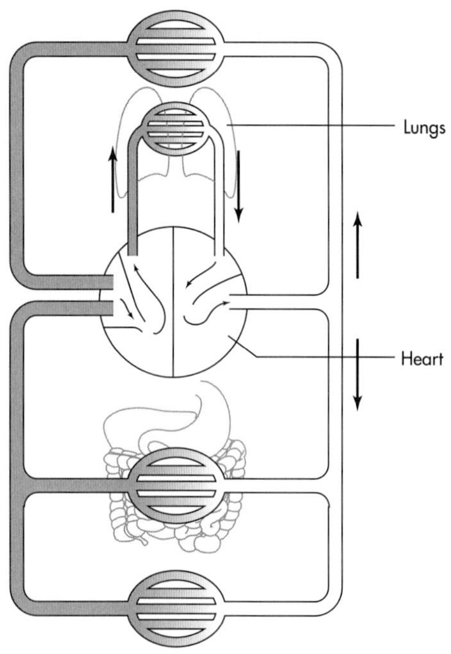

back to the heart via the vena cavae

Also pictured is the digestive system/liver. Blood travels to the body via the aorta. Where does blood go after leaving the digestive system?

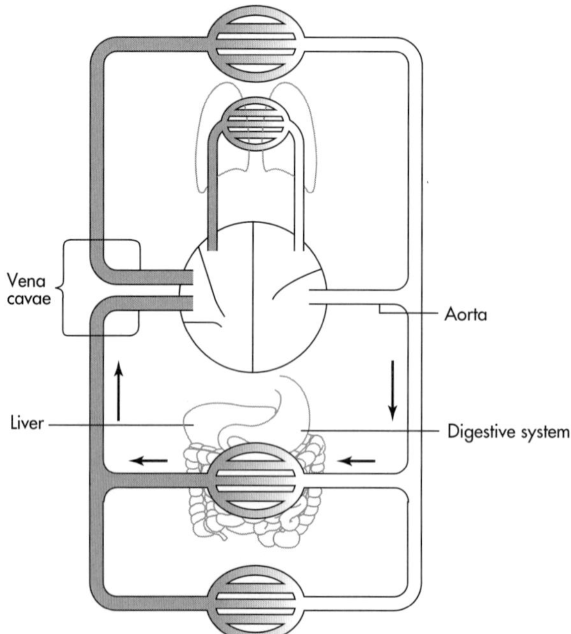

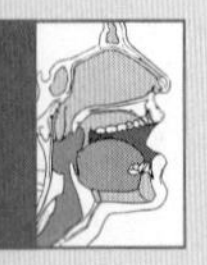

Which portion of the diagram represents the upper body or head and neck? Blood flow to our head and neck region includes vessels that go up the neck to the head, **supplying** blood. These vessels break down into smaller vessels until they become ________________.

the top loop (bracket), capillaries

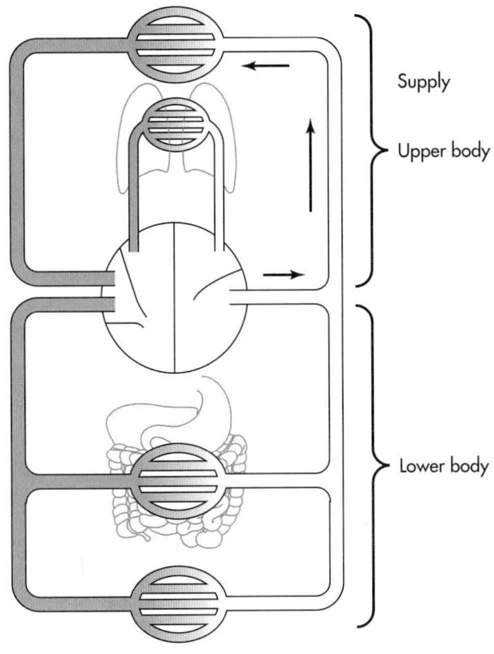

Capillaries gather together, becoming larger vessels known as ________________. These veins **drain** blood from the head and down the neck.

veins

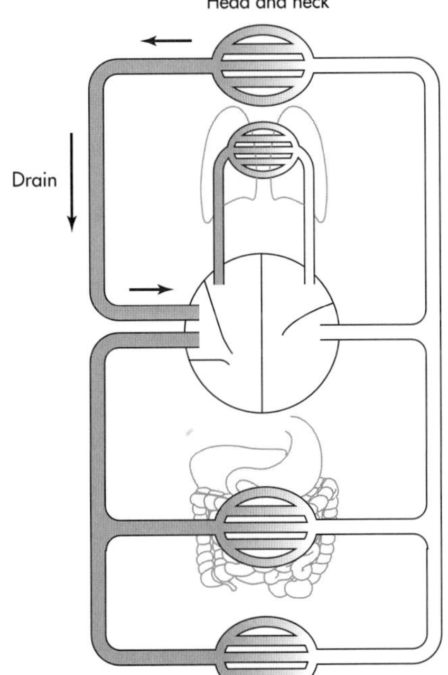

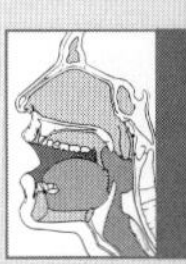

closed

The other portion of the circulatory system is an open system, whereas the **blood-vascular system** portion is a ______________ system of tubes. The **lymphatic system** is composed of lymph vessels, lymph fluid and cells, and lymph nodes.

Lymph vessels collect tissue fluid that bathes the cells of the body (extracellular fluid). It then is called **lymph fluid** once in the system. Lymph cells (lymphocytes) are added to the fluid at the **lymph nodes.**

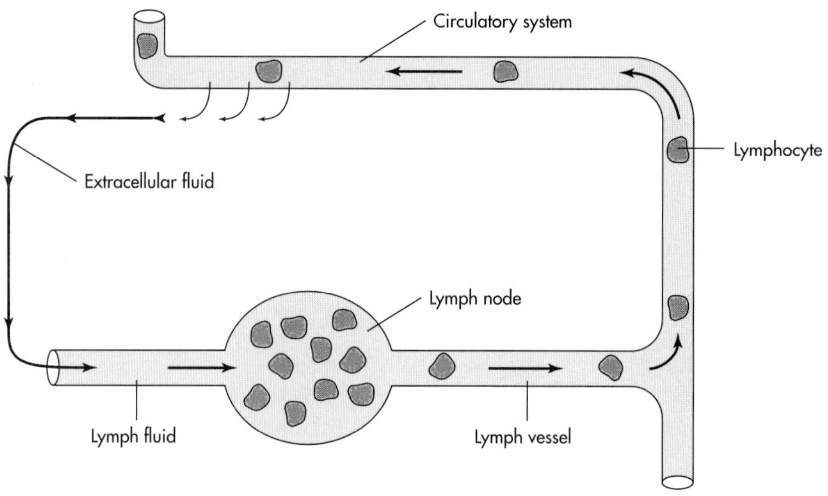

open

Lymph fluid then travels into larger and larger vessels until it empties into the largest vessel, the **thoracic duct,** which empties into the large veins, into the heart, and travels in the vascular system to the capillaries. This is where the fluid "leaks" back out into the body as cellular fluid. What type of system is this?

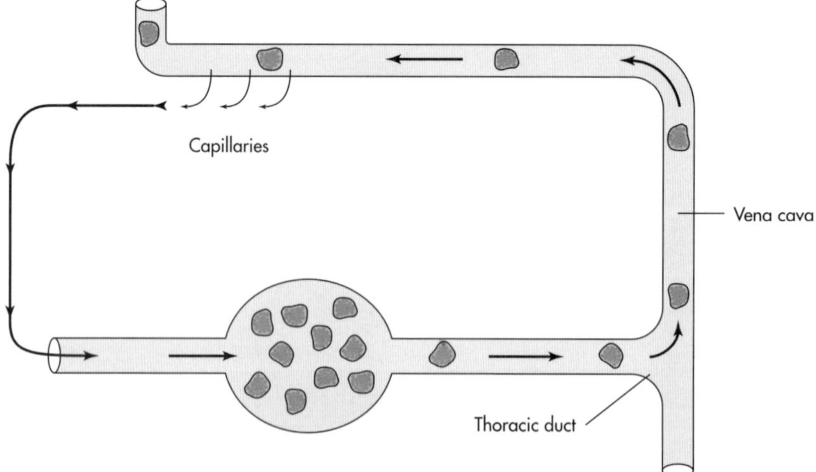

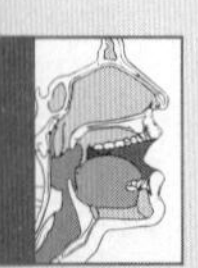

MAJOR ARTERIES

1.0

Arteries of the Neck

1.1

Blood supply to the head is very important, considering that this is where the brain resides! The brain is a high-metabolic organ and needs a rapid source of both nutrients (glucose) and oxygen. This major pathway from the heart to the brain is by way of the large arteries called the **carotid vessels.** Find them.

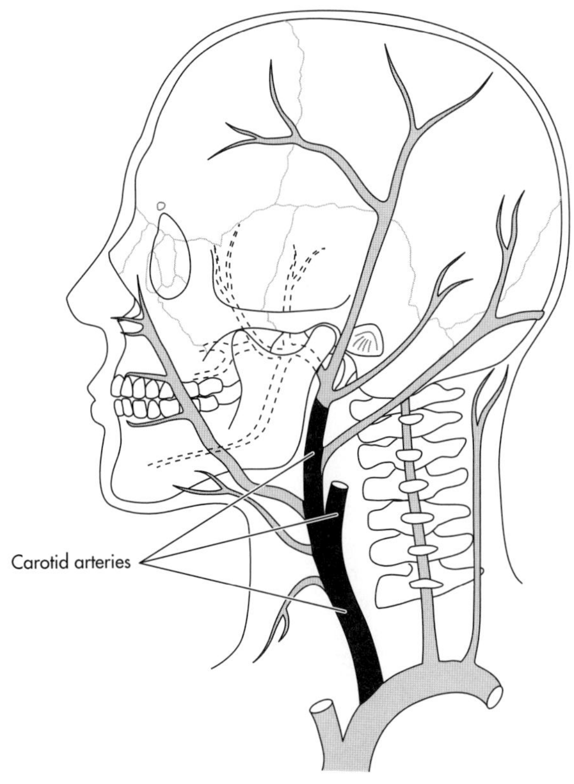

The carotid arteries are paired, right and left, and run along the border of which muscle?

sternocleido-
mastoid

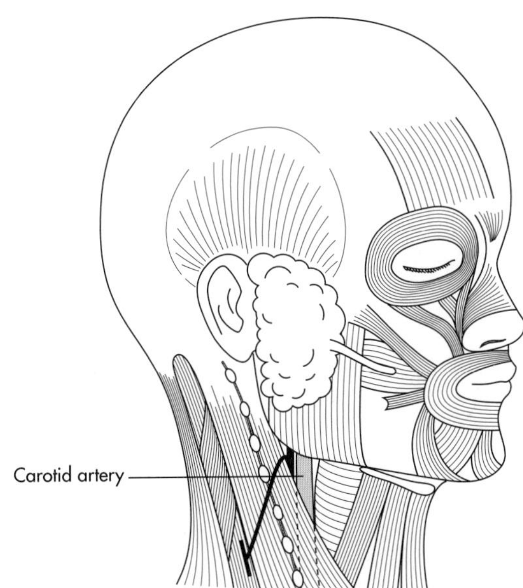

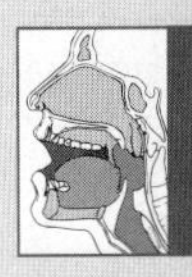

Find the carotid arteries in the drawing. The largest portion of the vessels is called the **common carotid artery,** and this divides below the mandible into the external carotid artery and the internal carotid artery. Find them.

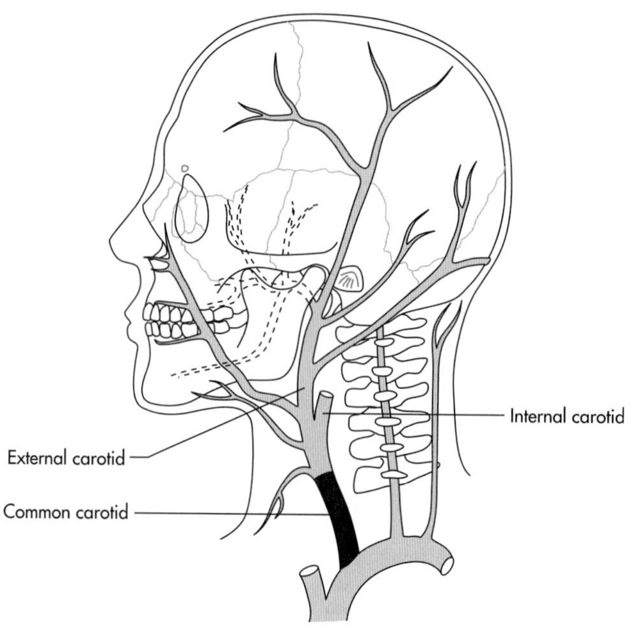

internal

The **external carotid artery** extends many branches to the outside of the face and head. The ______________ **carotid artery** goes into the cranium to supply the brain.

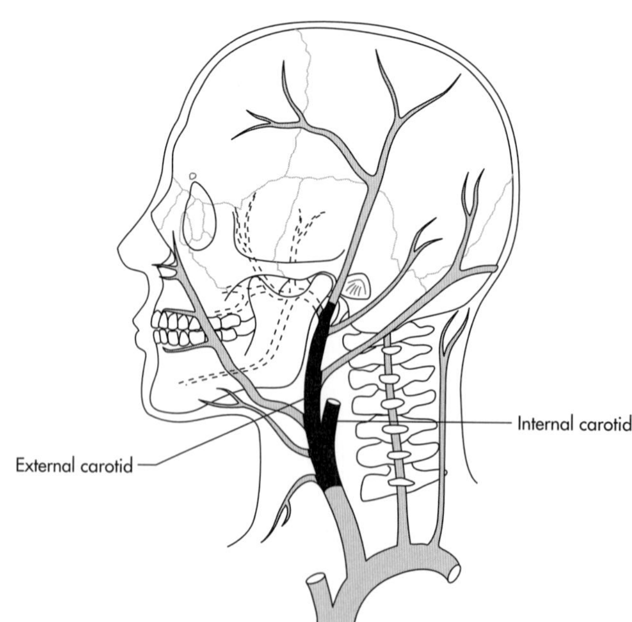

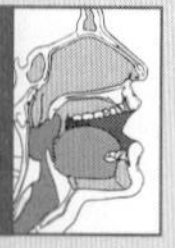

This is the ______________ artery. It supplies the ______________.

external carotid, face and outside of the head

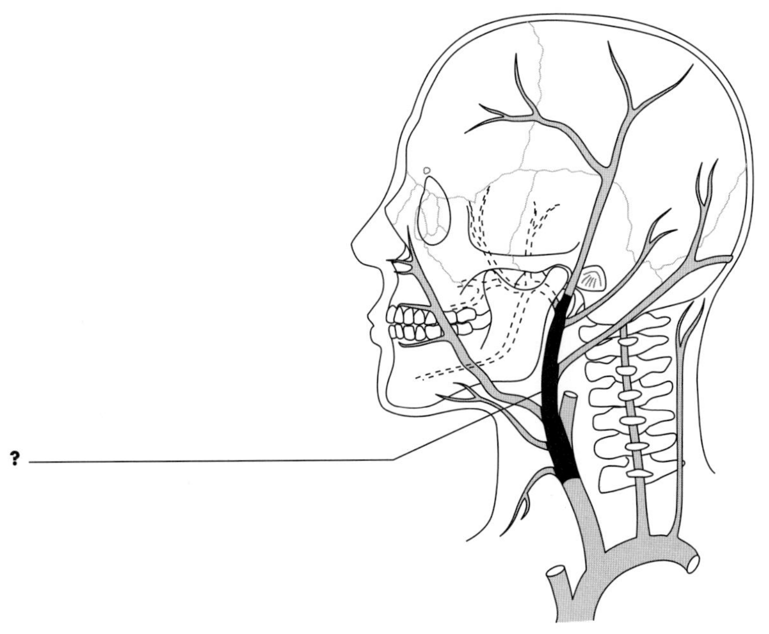

This is the ______________ artery. It supplies the ______________.

internal carotid, brain

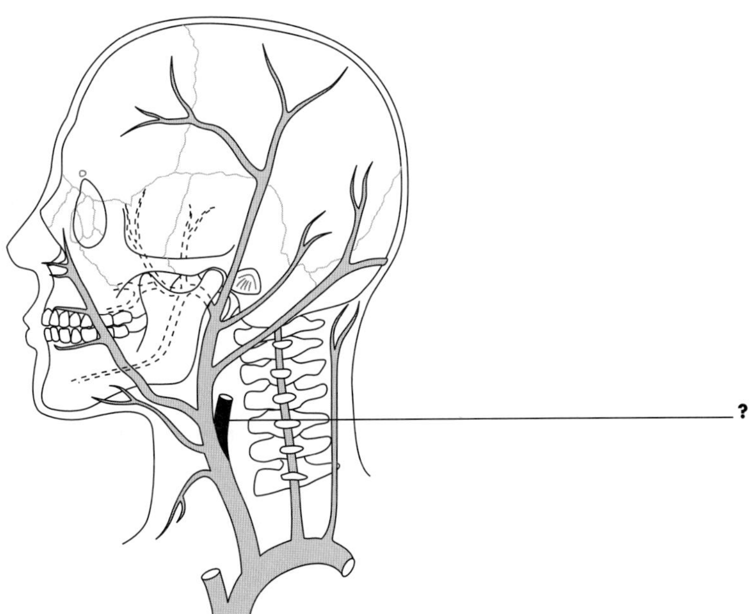

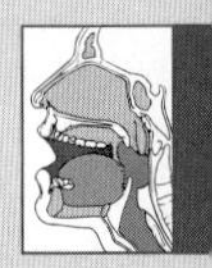

sternocleido-
mastoid muscle

The area where one can find the carotid arteries is along the ______________. A good place to find a pulse is along this muscle and below the mandible. This is called the **carotid pulse.**

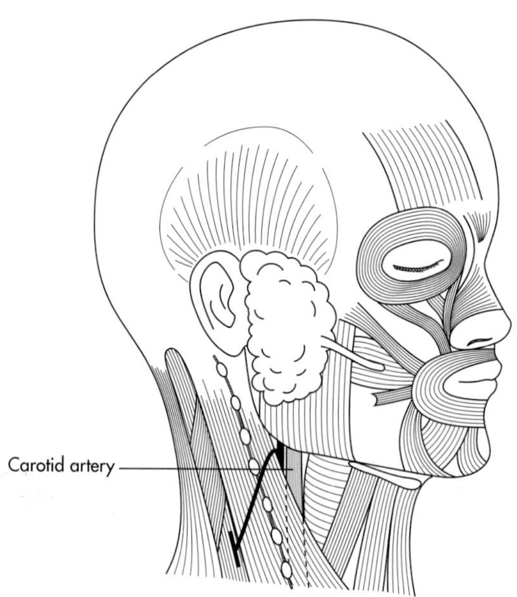

common

Let us look first at the branches of the external carotid and then at those of the internal carotid, which arise from the ______________ carotid artery.

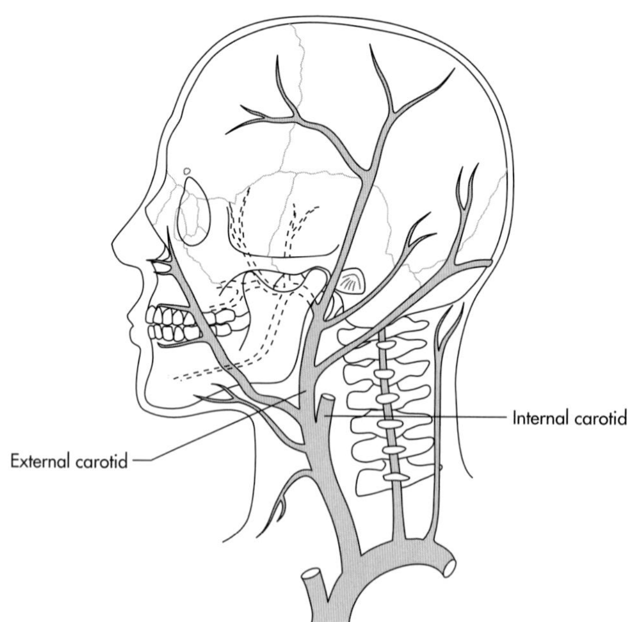

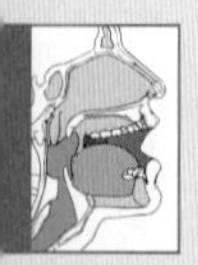

Branches of External Carotid Artery

1.2

The first branch of the external carotid artery we look at is one of the **thyroid arteries,** the superior one. Find it darkened in on the diagram.

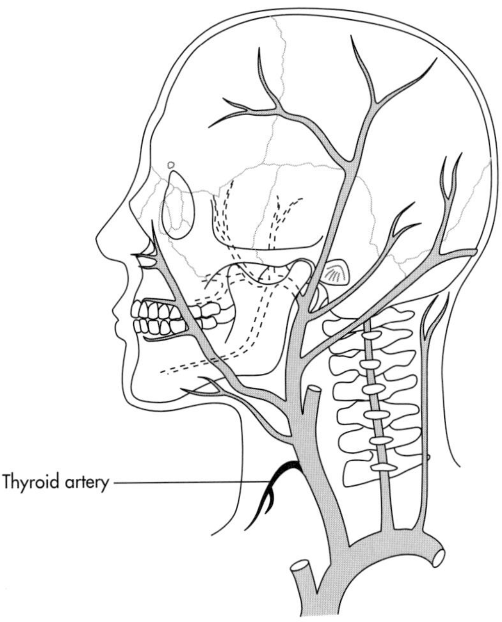

thyroid, two

The second branch of the external carotid lies above the ______________ artery and passes under the mandible to supply the tongue. It is called the **lingual artery** (remember that this occurs on both right and left sides of the head, so there are ______________ lingual arteries). Find it.

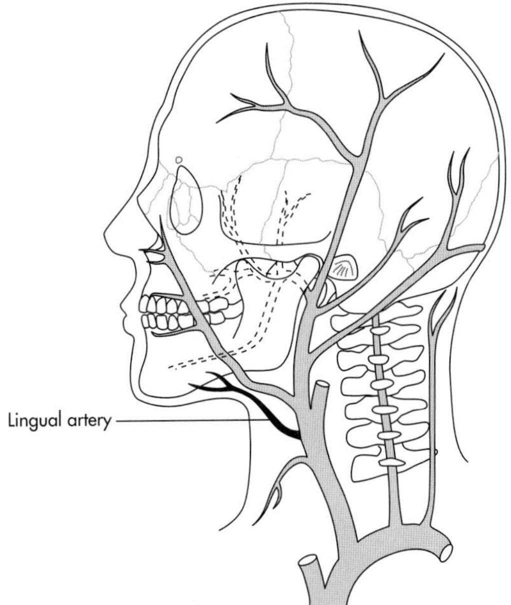

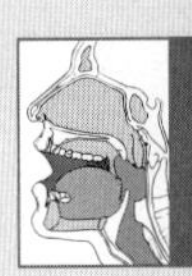

tongue

The lingual artery supplies the ______________ with blood. Superior to it is an artery that passes over the inferior border of the body of the mandible. It is called the **facial artery.** Find it.

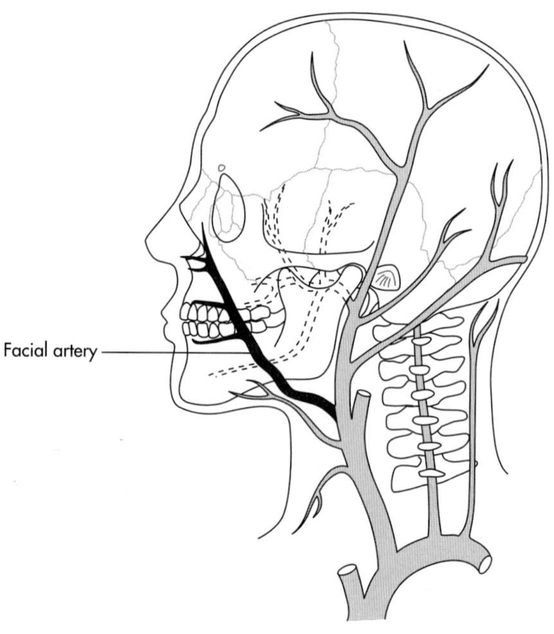

mandible, face

The facial artery can be felt as a pulse along the inferior border of the ______________. It spreads upward across the face to supply the structures of the ______________.

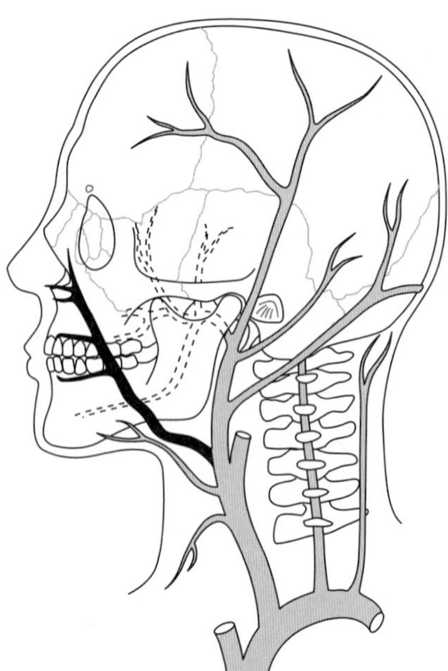

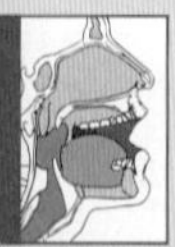

Above the ______________ artery, which goes to the face, is the **occipital artery.** This vessel distributes its branches to the occipital region or the back of the head. Find it.

facial

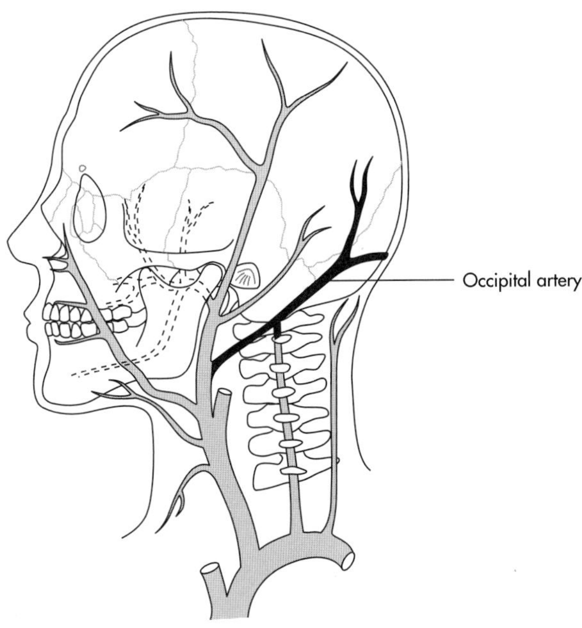

Above the occipital branch is a branch to the posterior ear region, or the **postauricular** branch. Find it.

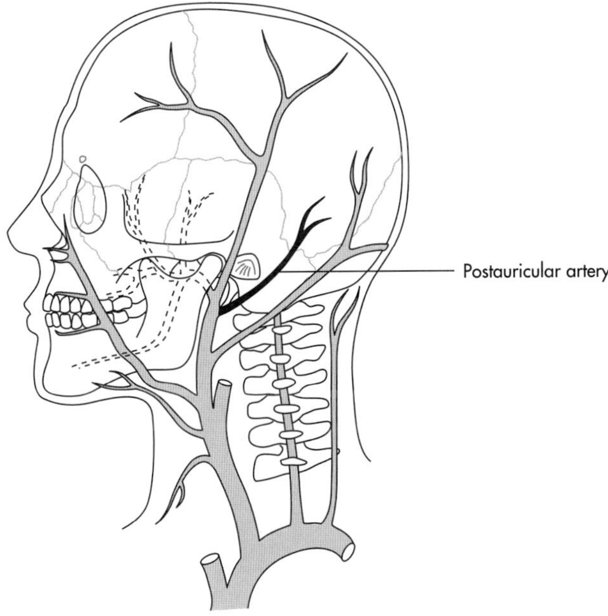

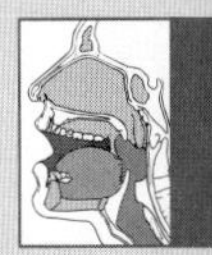

external carotid artery

Above the postauricular branch is a large branch spreading directly below the skin to the side of the head, over temporal and parietal bones. It is called the **superficial temporal artery.** Find this large branch. Of what is the superficial temporal a smaller branch?

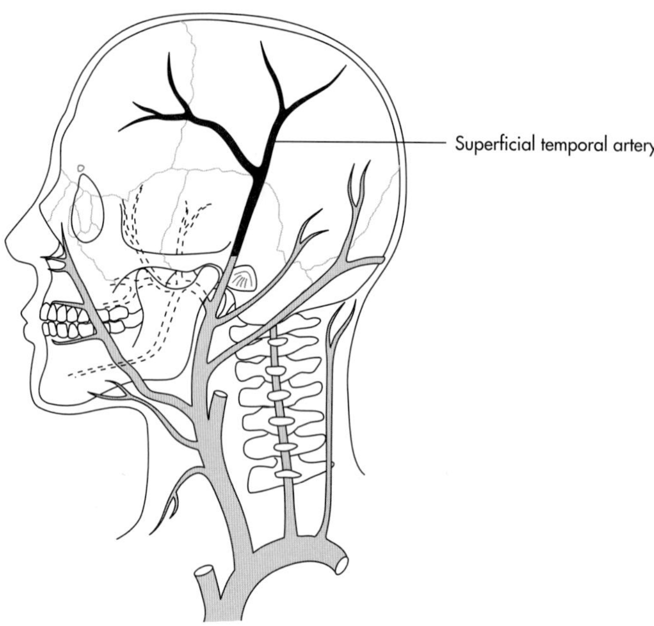

The last major branch of the external carotid is a complex vessel that travels internally to supply the maxilla and mandible and the nasal cavity. We will look at this vessel in more detail. It is called the **maxillary artery.** Find it as it goes behind the neck of the condyle.

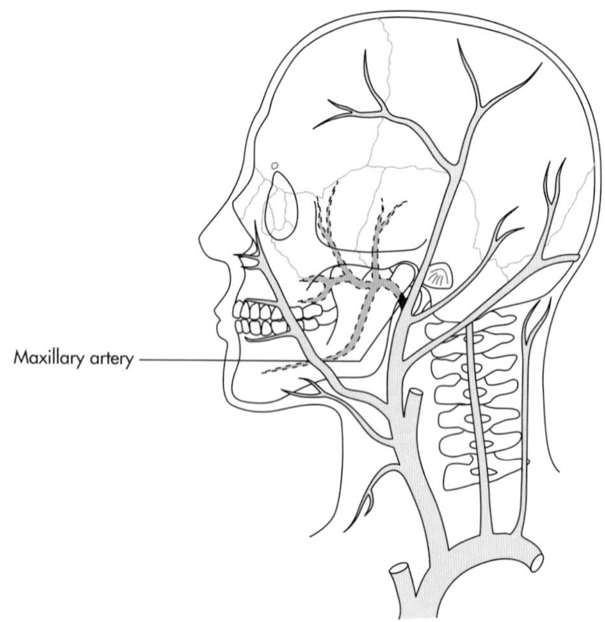

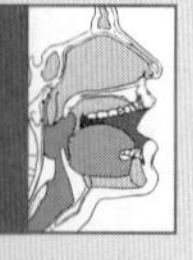

The maxillary artery travels behind the neck of the condyle within the infratemporal fossa. Find this fossa on the drawing. What else travels in this fossa?

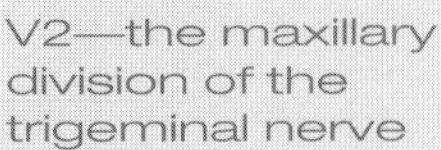
V2—the maxillary division of the trigeminal nerve

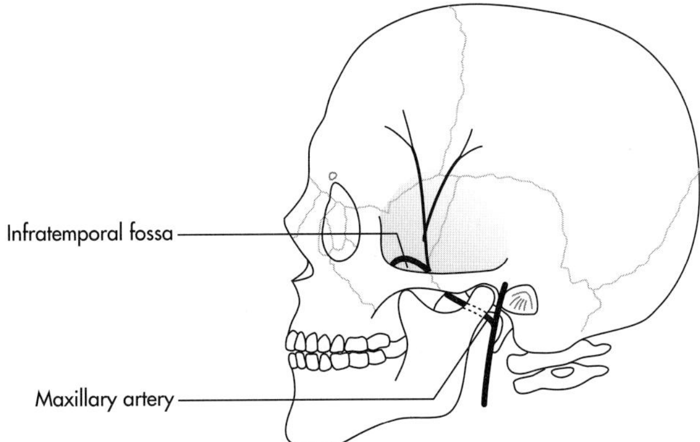

The maxillary artery is a branch of the ______________ artery, which is a branch of the ______________ artery.

external carotid, common carotid

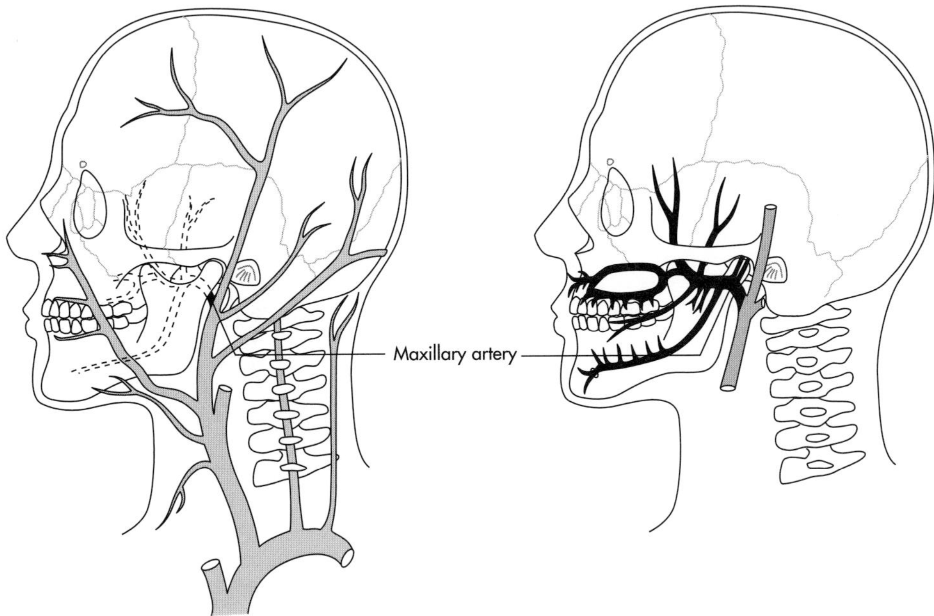

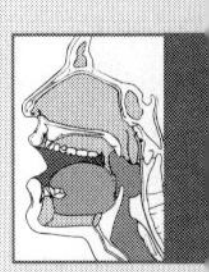

lingual, tongue

This is the ______________ artery. It supplies the ______________.

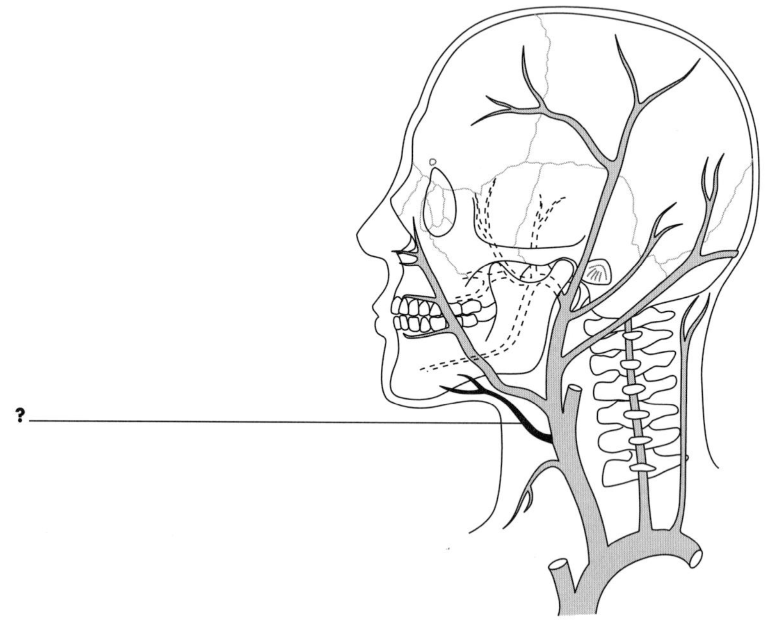

thyroid, thyroid gland

This is the ______________ artery. It supplies the ______________.

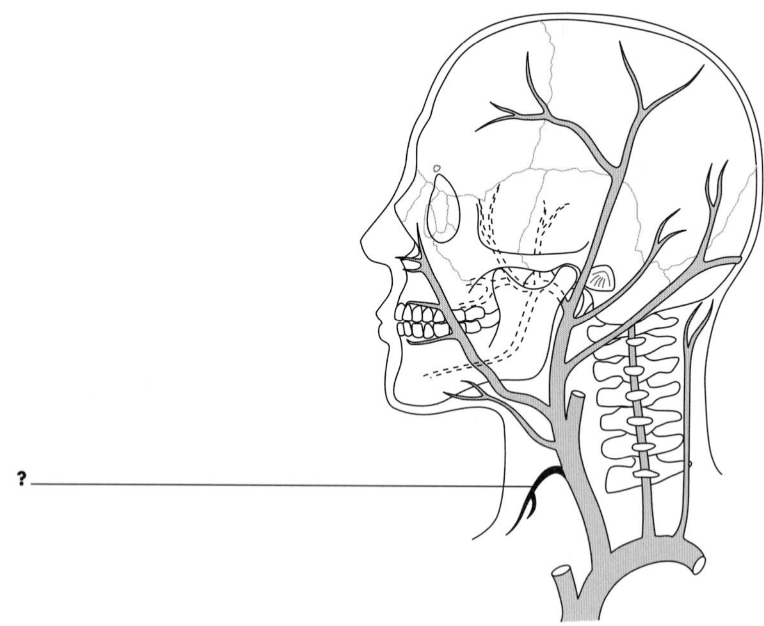

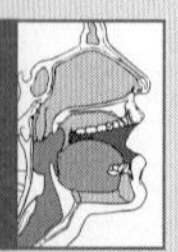

This is the ______________ artery. It supplies the ______________.

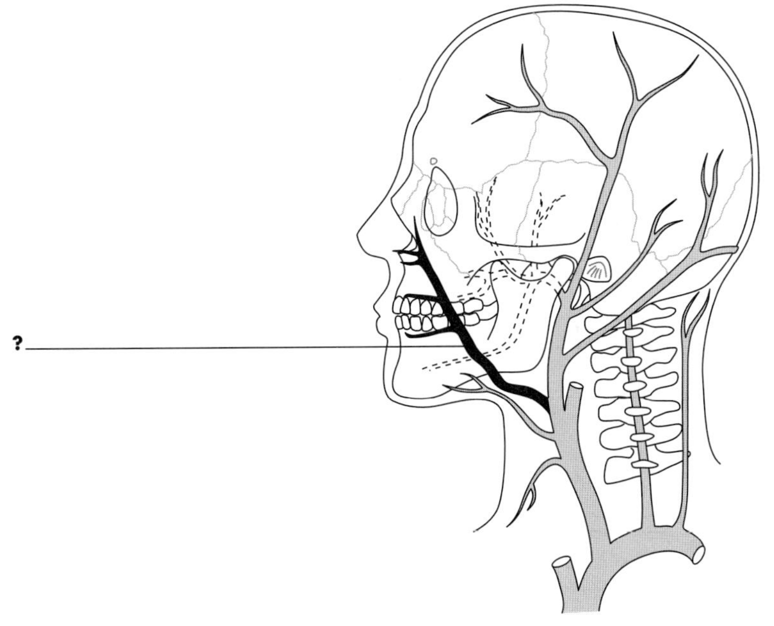

facial, face

This is the ______________ artery. It supplies the ______________.

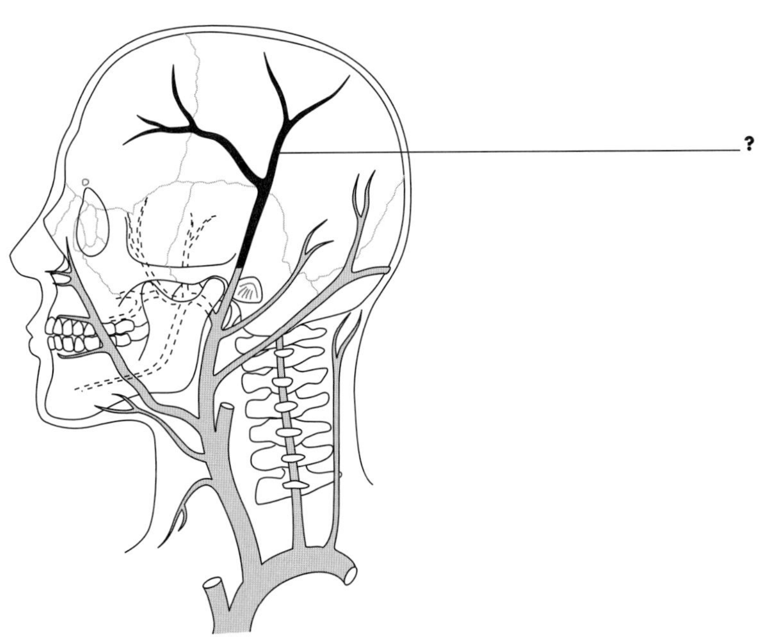

superficial temporal, sides of the head

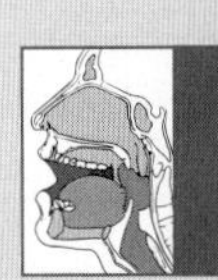

MAXILLARY ARTERY

external, condyle

The **maxillary artery** is a major branch of the ______________ carotid artery. It travels behind the neck of the ______________ to supply structures of the maxilla and mandible. This large artery has many branches. We will not learn all the branches.

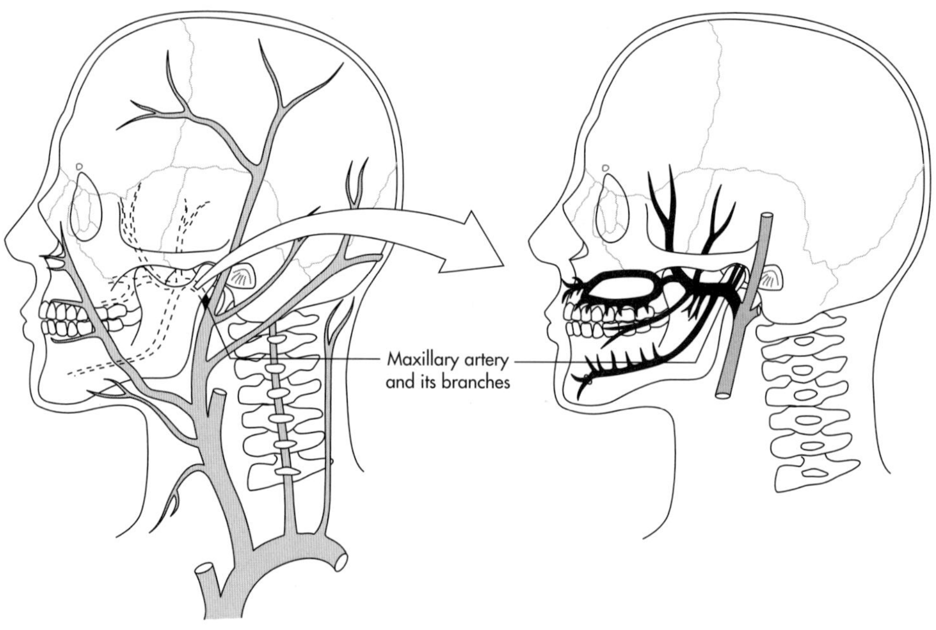

After extending a few small **meningeal** branches, the maxillary artery provides a large branch to the mandible, the **inferior alveolar artery.** Find it.

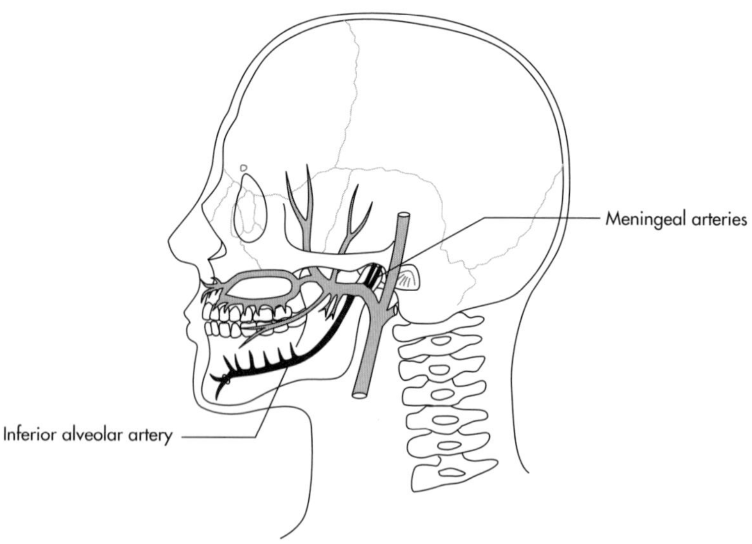

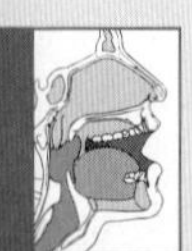

The _______________ artery provides blood to the mandible and to the mandibular teeth, traveling in the **mandibular canal** with the inferior alveolar nerve. Through what foramen does the inferior alveolar artery pass to get into the mandible?

Inferior alveolar, mandibular foramen

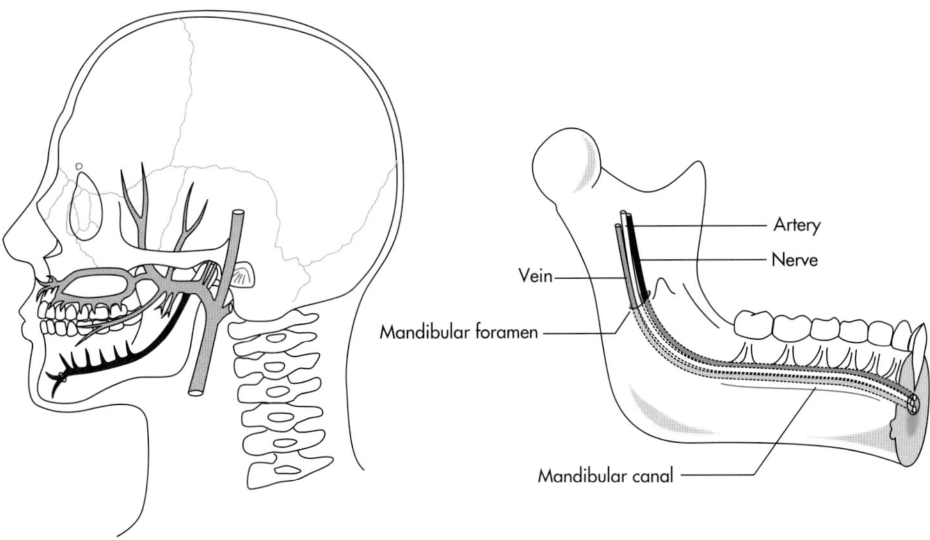

The blood supply and nerve supply to the mandible are a little different. Compare the two. What is different?

The nerve supply has two separate branches to the maxilla and mandible.

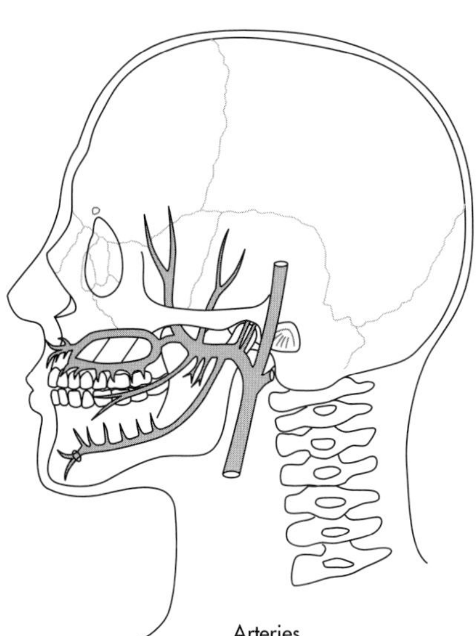
Arteries

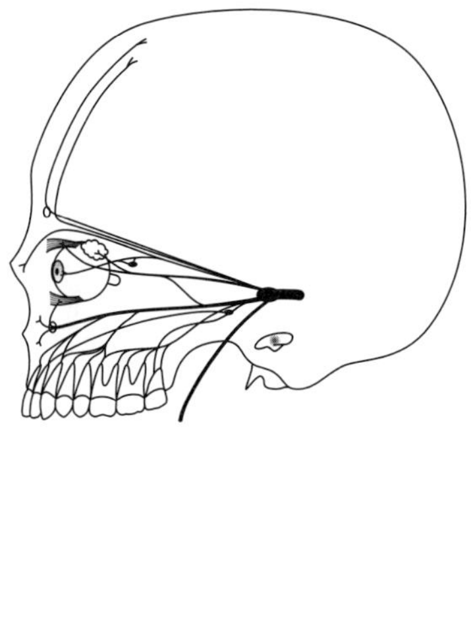
Nerves

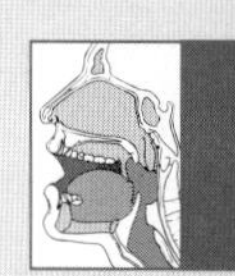

temporalis, masseter, medial and lateral pterygoid muscles

The next small branches represent the **branches to the muscles of mastication.** Three are inferior and one superior. The superior branch is called the **deep temporal artery.** Find them. What are the four muscles they supply?

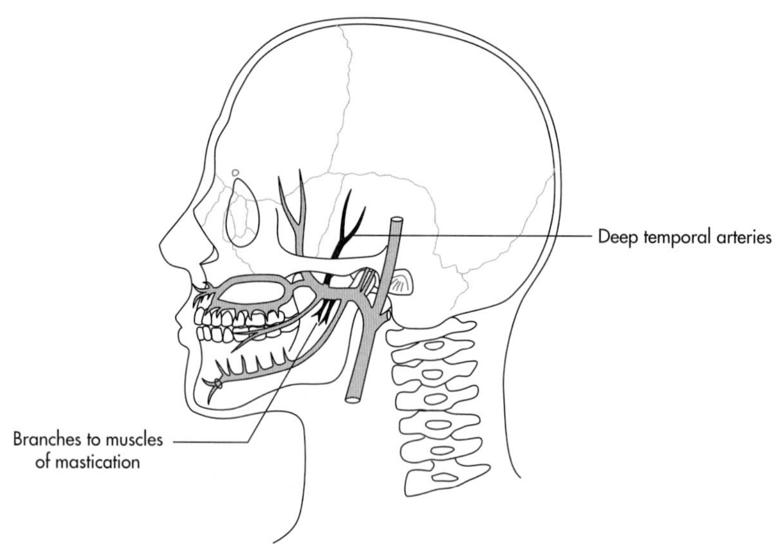

The large branch running directly behind the palate and nasal cavity is the **sphenopalatine artery.** A portion of this artery supplies the palate and sphenoid sinus.

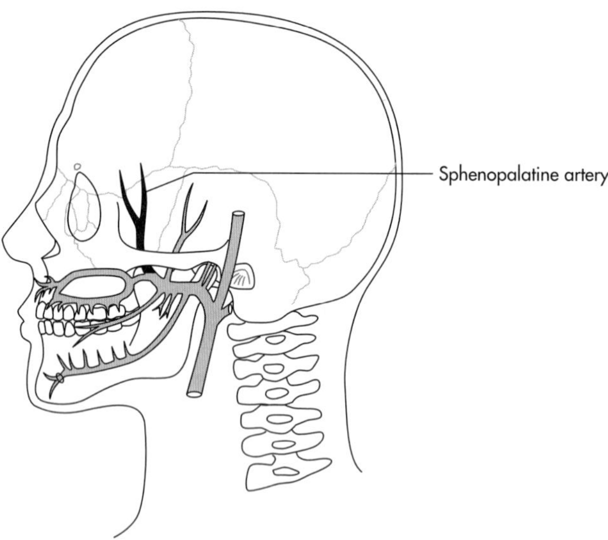

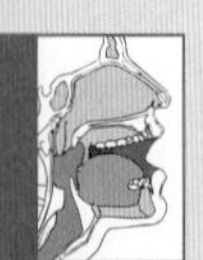

The sphenopalatine artery creates a circular branch or loop of arteries, beginning with the **superior alveolar artery.** Find it. It perforates the posterior portion of the maxilla, where it begins its branches to the maxilla and its teeth.

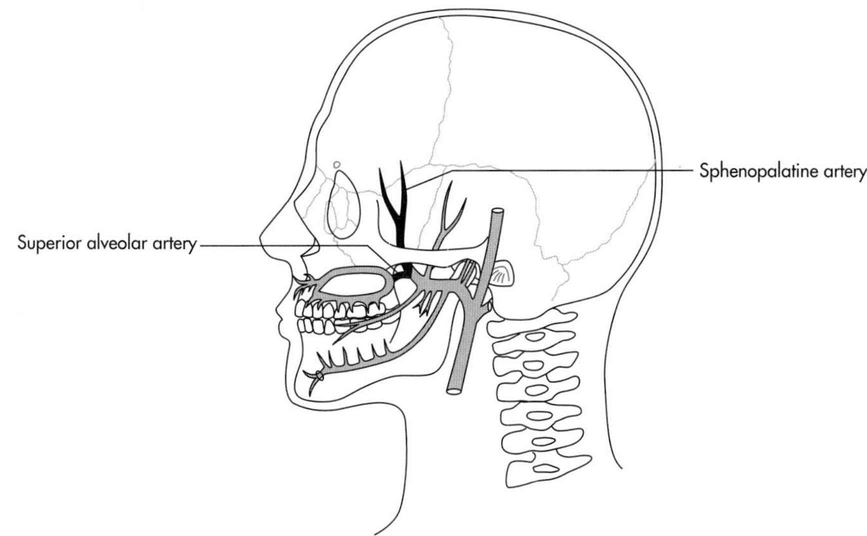

superior alveolar

The superior alveolar artery follows a path of distribution similar to that of the superior alveolar nerve. It divides into three loops, to the posterior, middle, and anterior teeth and periodontium. These are as follows: **posterior superior alveolar (PSA) artery, middle superior alveolar (MSA) artery,** and **anterior superior alveolar (ASA) artery.** These are branches of the ______________ artery.

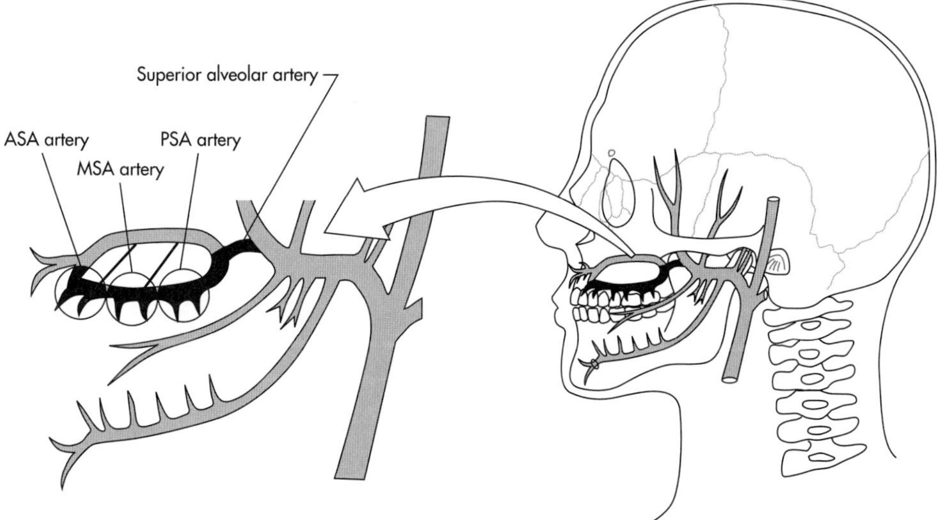

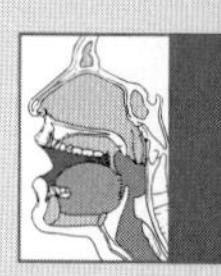

The next branch of the maxillary artery is the superior portion of the sphenopalatine artery as it branches upward to become the **nasopalatine artery.** It goes forward in the nasal cavity to emerge into the oral cavity through the incisive foramen. Find it.

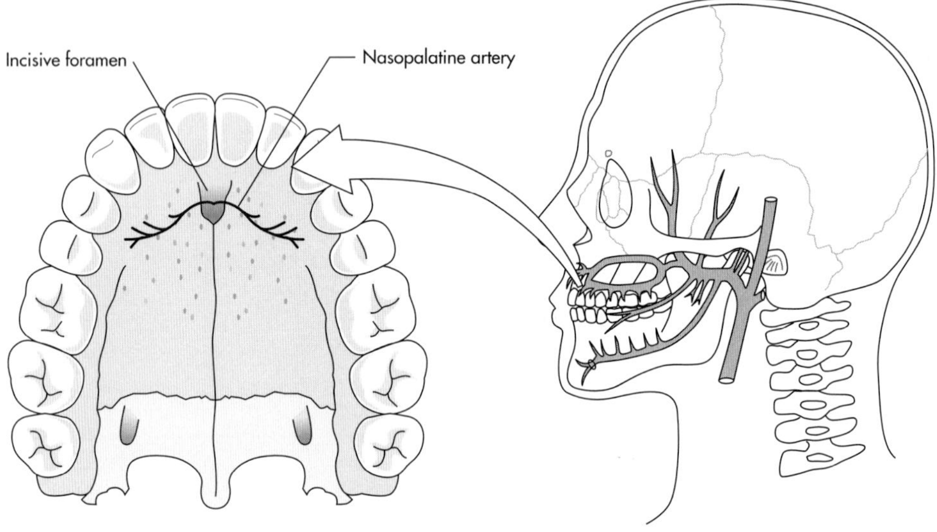

incisive foramen

The nasopalatine artery follows the same distribution as the nerve of the same name to the anterior palate. Through what foramen does it pass with the nasopalatine nerve? (Note: The foramen has a different name than the nerve and artery.)

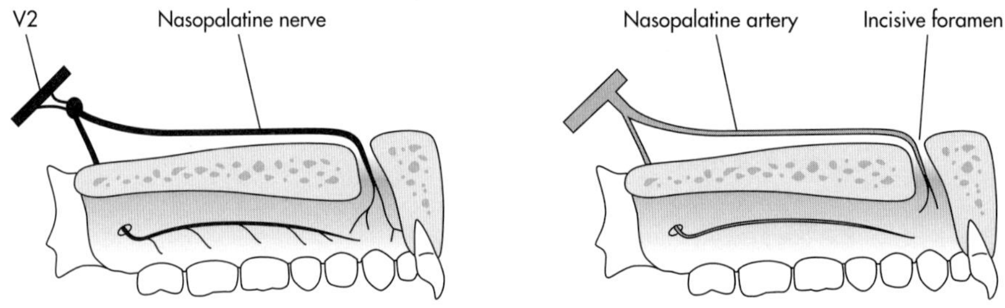

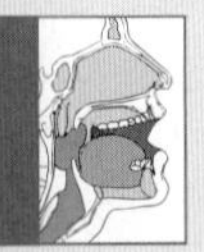

This is the ______________ artery. Its inferior portion becomes the ______________ artery. It then divides into three portions: ______________, ______________, and ______________ arteries.

sphenopalatine, superior alveolar, PSA, MSA, ASA

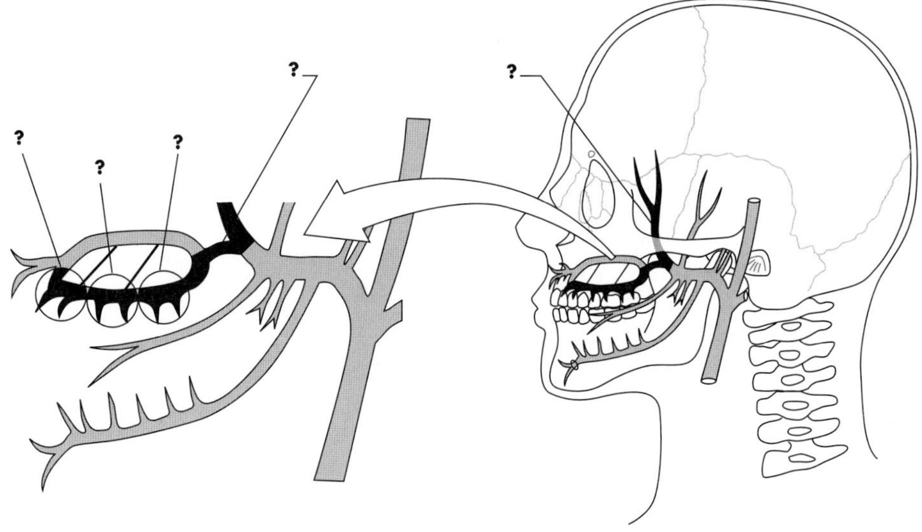

The nerves of the maxilla are branches of which division of cranial nerve V? Note that they follow the same distribution as the arteries. What major artery gives rise to these maxillary vessels?

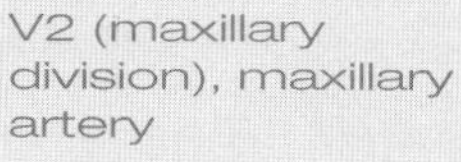

V2 (maxillary division), maxillary artery

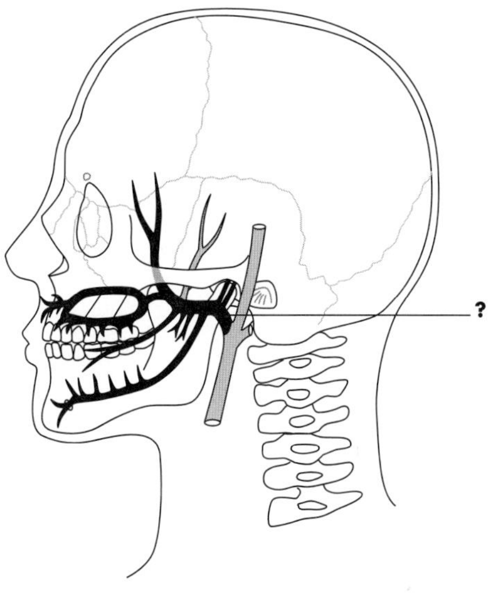

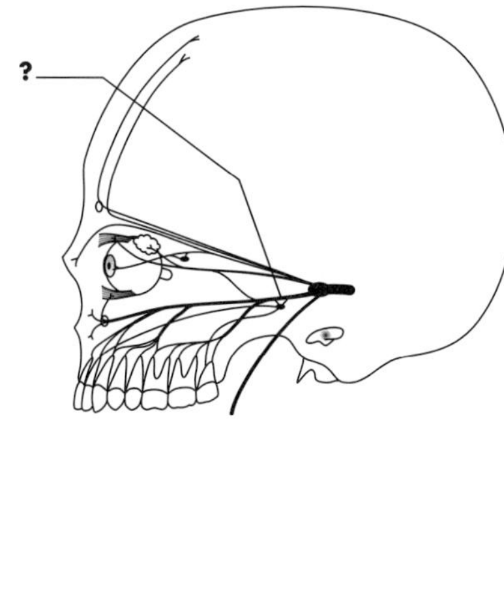

greater palatine artery (and nerve)

Another branch of the sphenopalatine artery goes to the back of the palate, emerging into the oral cavity through two holes: the greater palatine foramina. What artery would you guess travels here with the nerve of the same name?

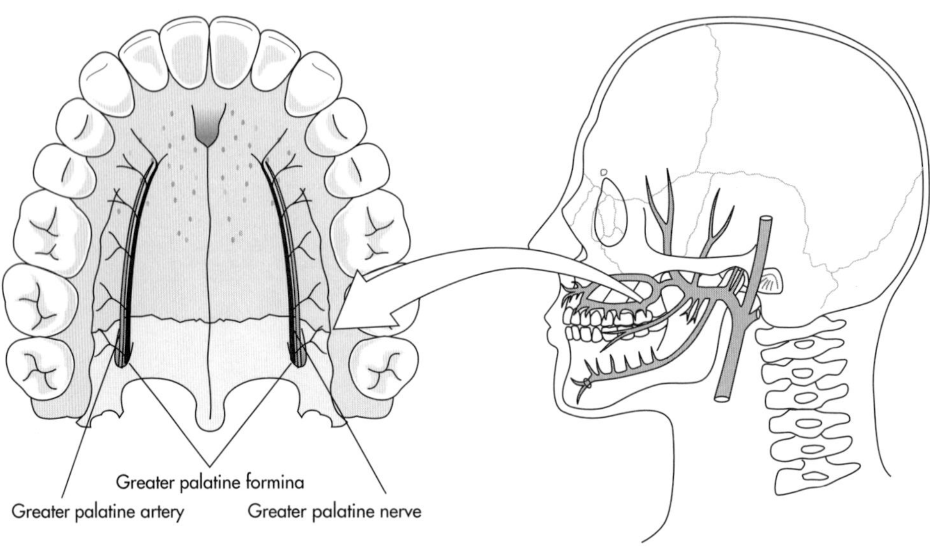

palate, nasopalatine

Greater palatine arteries distribute blood to the posterior ______________. The ______________ artery distributes to the anterior palate.

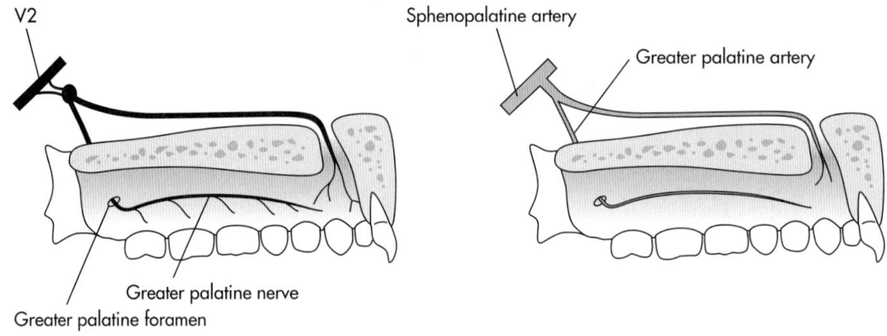

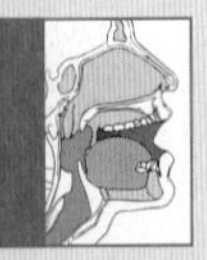

A small branch of this circular loop of blood vessels emerges from the maxilla to the midfacial region, along with a nerve of the same name. This is the **infraorbital artery** and it exits the maxilla through the _______________ foramen. Another exiting branch of the inferior alveolar artery called the **mental artery** is shown here through the _______________ foramen.

infraorbital, mental

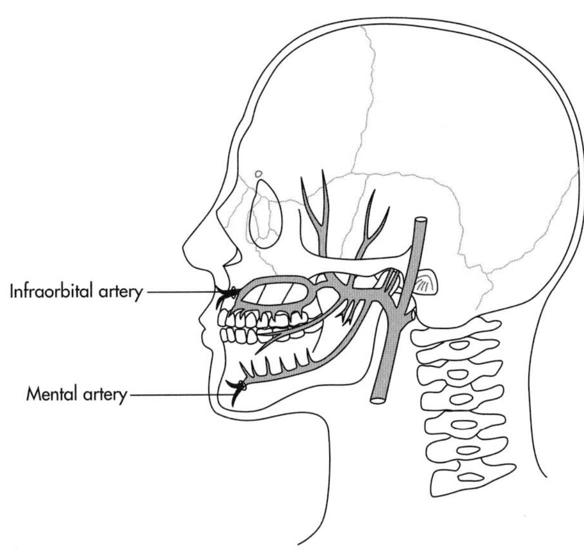

Lastly, a long branch of the maxillary artery spreads across the inner surface of the cheek. It is called the **buccal artery** and it supplies the cheek mucosa and musculature. Find it.

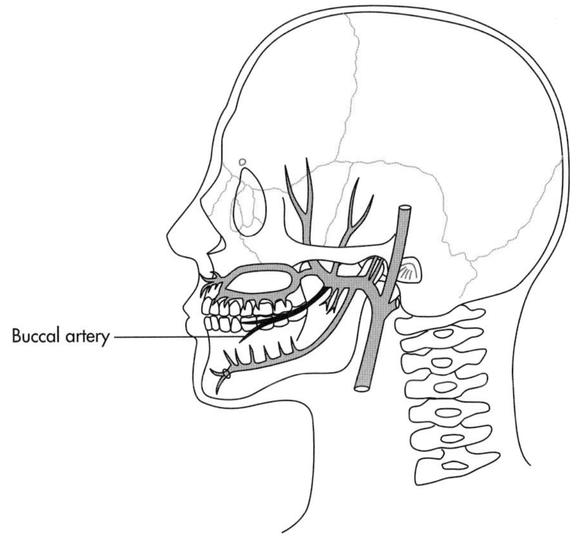

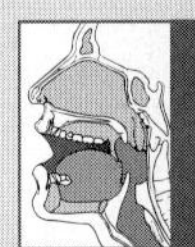

inferior alveolar, mandible

What branch of the maxillary artery is this? What does it supply?

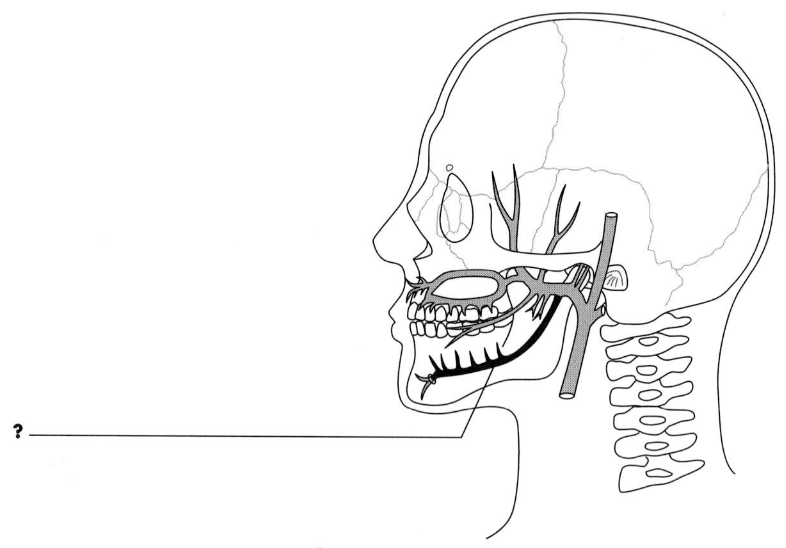

MSA; premolar teeth, distal canine, and periodontium

What branch of the maxillary artery is this? What does it supply?

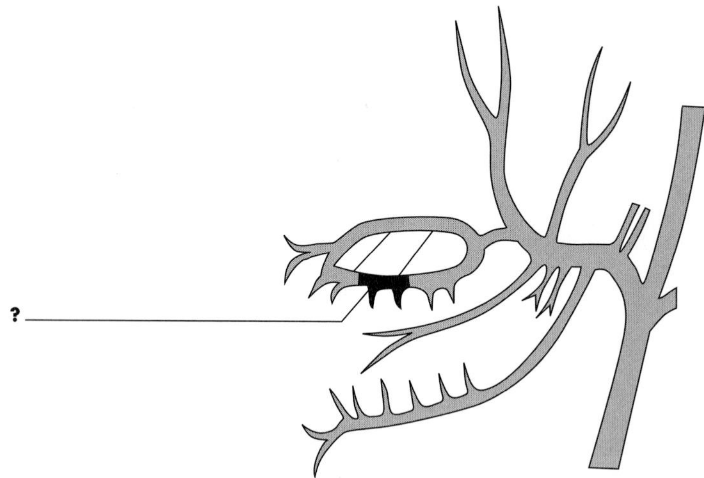

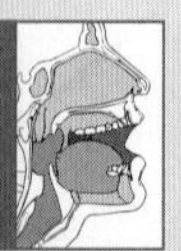

What branch of the maxillary artery is this? What does it supply?

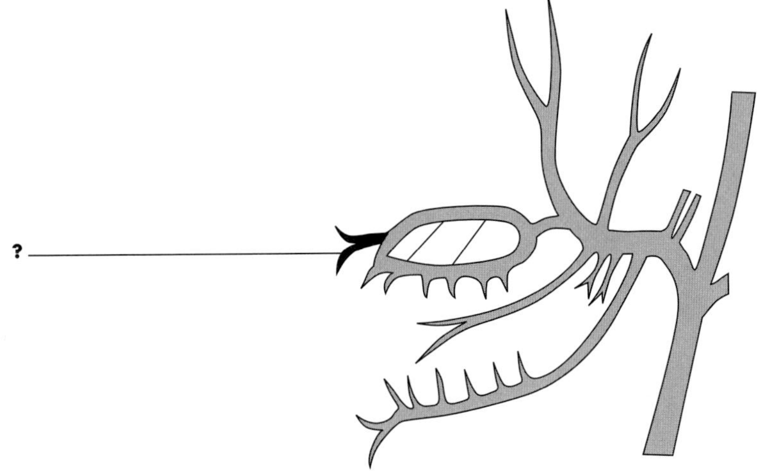

infraorbital, midface

What branch of the maxillary artery is this? What does it supply?

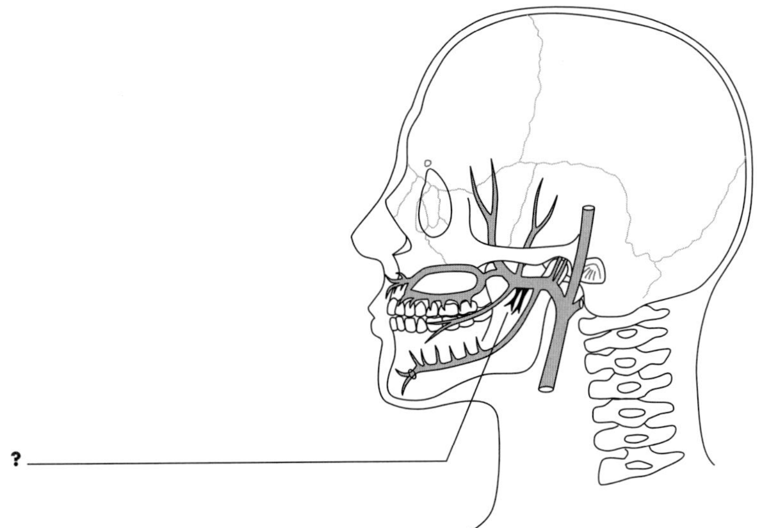

branch to muscles, muscles of mastication

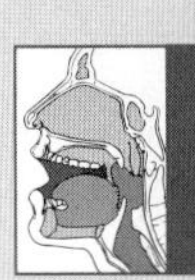

1.3

arteries, internal carotid

Arteries of the Brain

The brain is an organ that needs a rich supply of glucose and oxygen. This supply is delivered by which type of blood vessels? If the external carotid artery supplies the neck and outer surfaces of the head, which major vessel delivers blood to the inside of the cranium?

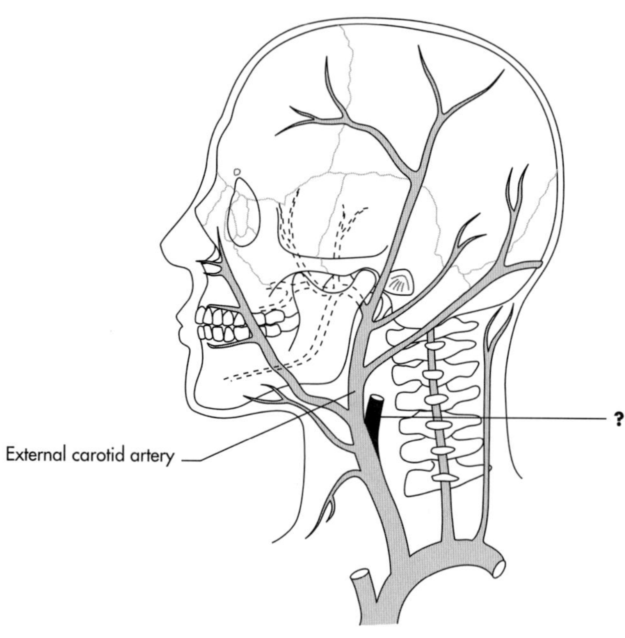

carotid canal

The **internal carotid artery** is the vessel shown cut away. It leads into the cranium through which foramina shown on the right?

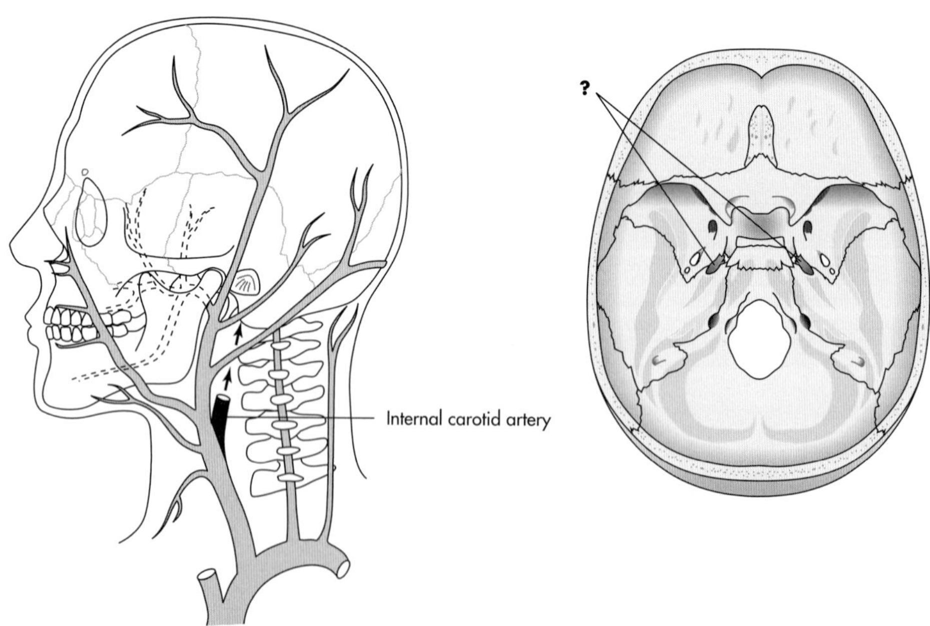

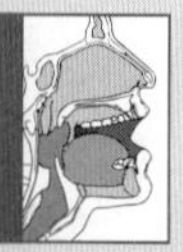

The carotid canals are large tubular foramina that lead the internal carotid arteries in a curved pathway into the cranium. They lie on either side of the pituitary fossa.

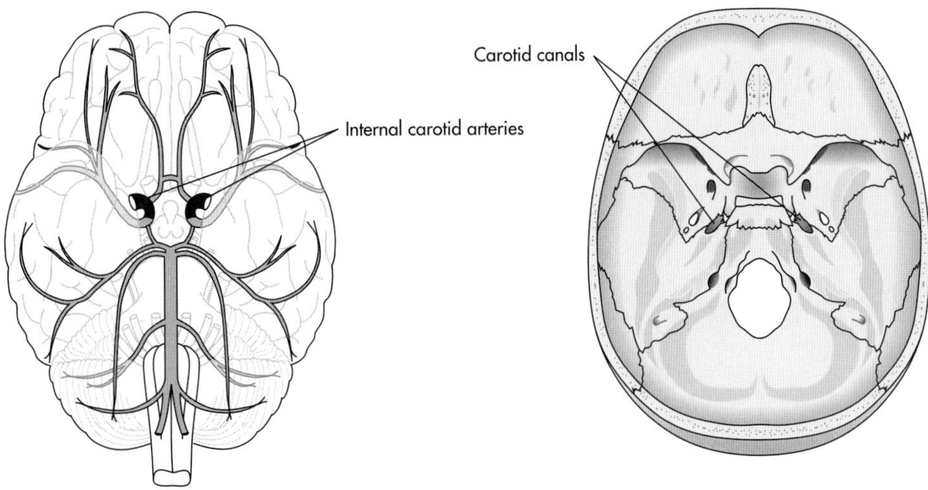

The internal carotid arteries then divide into branches that supply the brain. The first branch is a large one that supplies large areas of the temporal and parietal regions of the cerebrum. It is called the **middle cerebral artery.** Find it.

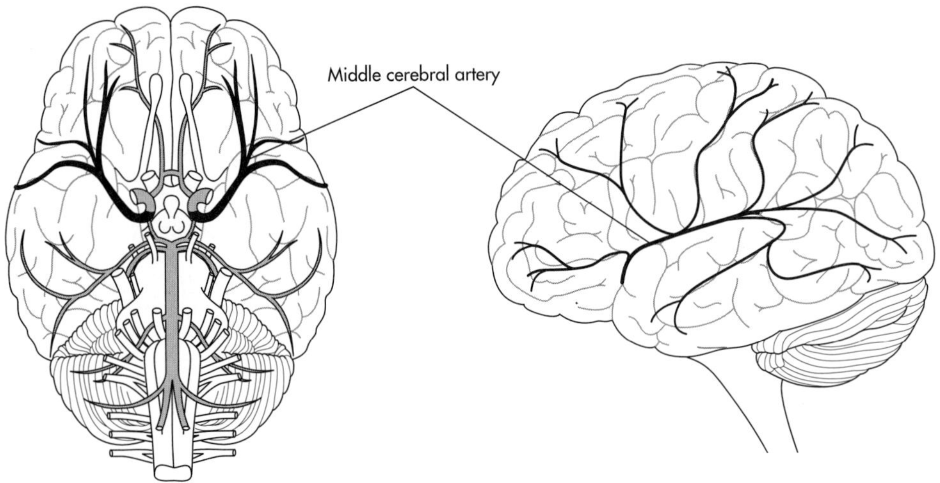

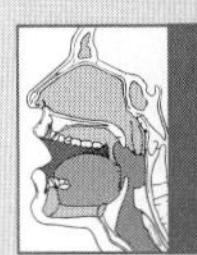

anterior

If the middle cerebral artery supplies the midportion of the cerebrum, then the **anterior cerebral artery** supplies the _______________ portion.

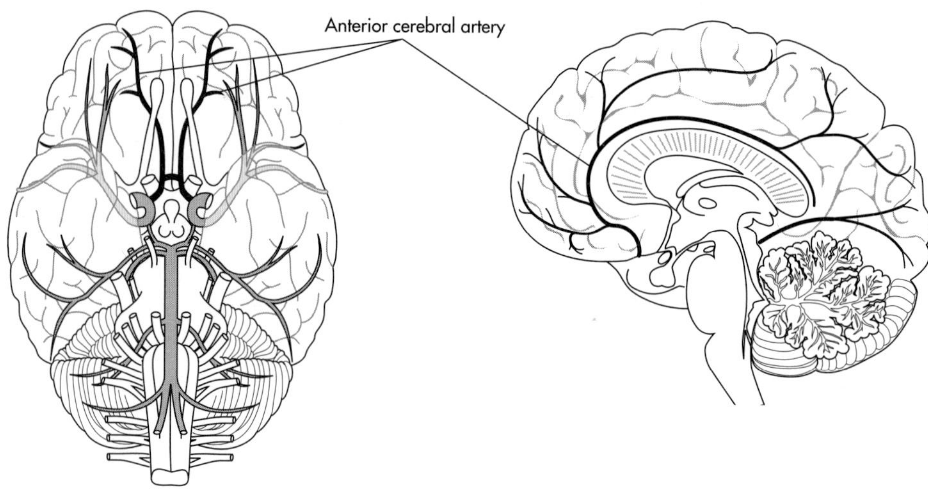

posterior

The _______________ or occipital region of the cerebrum is supplied by the **posterior cerebral artery.**

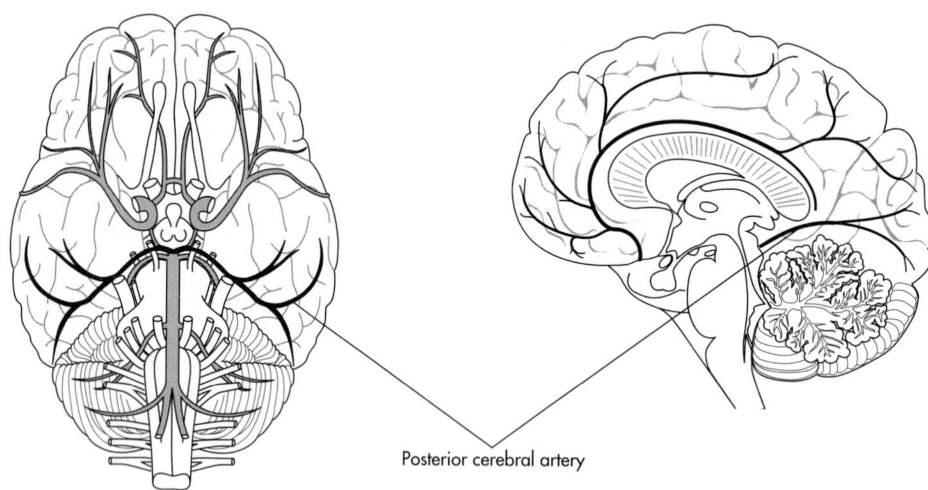

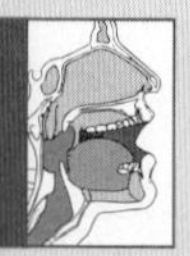

This is the ______________ artery. It supplies the ______________.

middle cerebral, temporal and parietal regions of the cerebrum

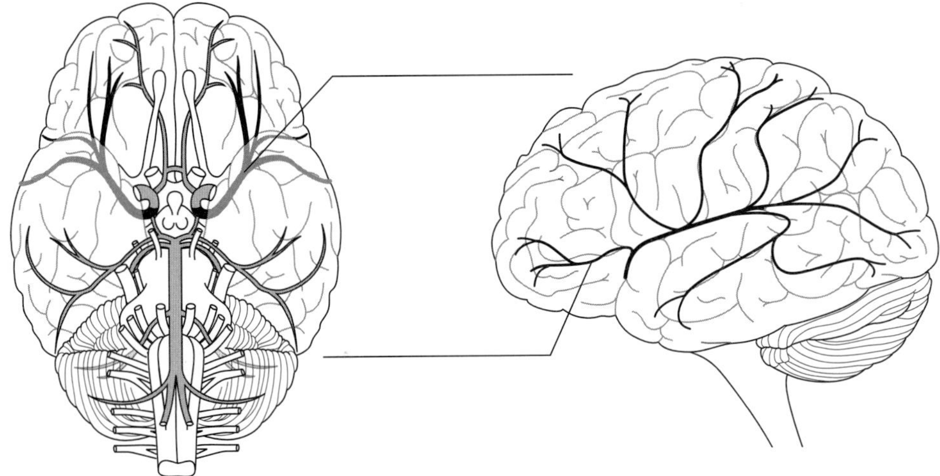

This is the ______________ artery. It supplies the ______________.

internal carotid, brain

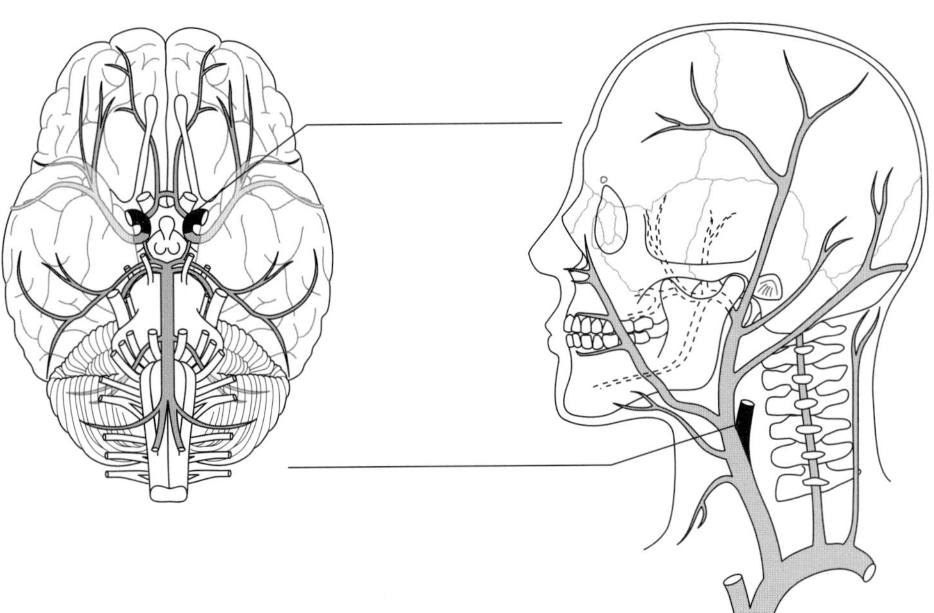

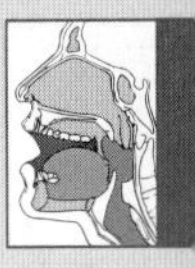

rich, internal carotid

Because the brain needs a _______________ supply of blood, a second system of vessels is brought into the cranium. The brain has, therefore, a dual source of blood. One source is the _______________ arteries. The second source is the **vertebral arteries.**

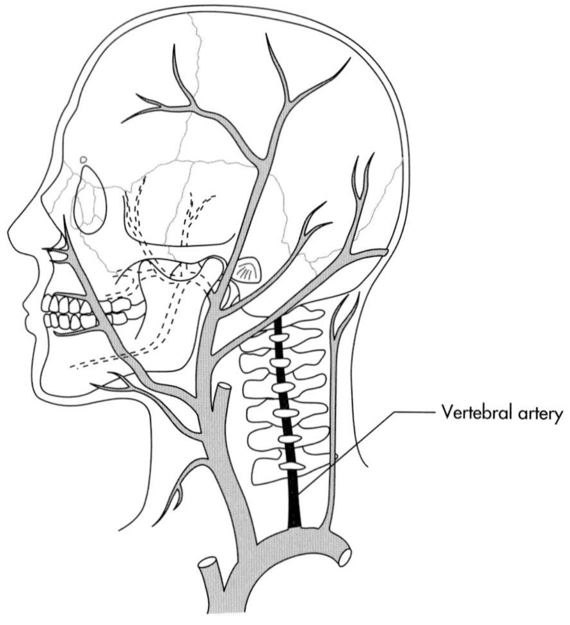

seven

Find the vertebral artery on this drawing. Note how it runs up the cervical vertebrae on either side, within special foramina in the vertebrae. How many cervical vertebrae are there?

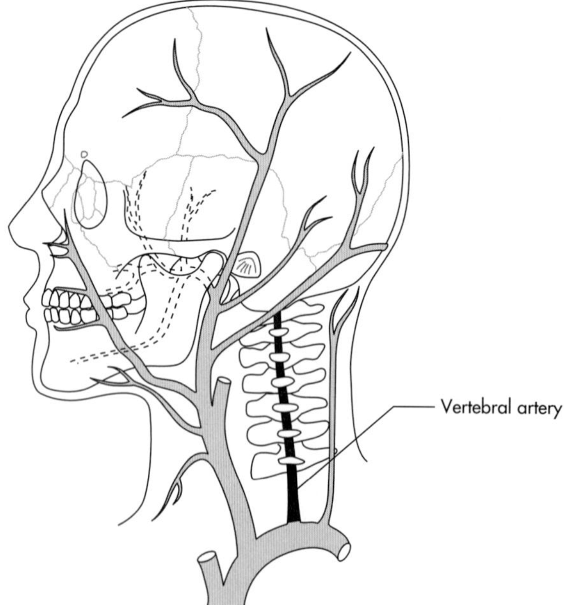

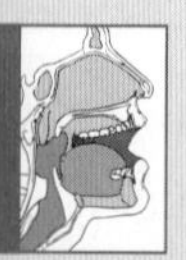

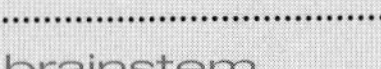

The vertebral arteries enter the cranium along with the spinal cord through foramen magnum. They fuse together to become one vessel on top of the ________, called the **basilar artery.**

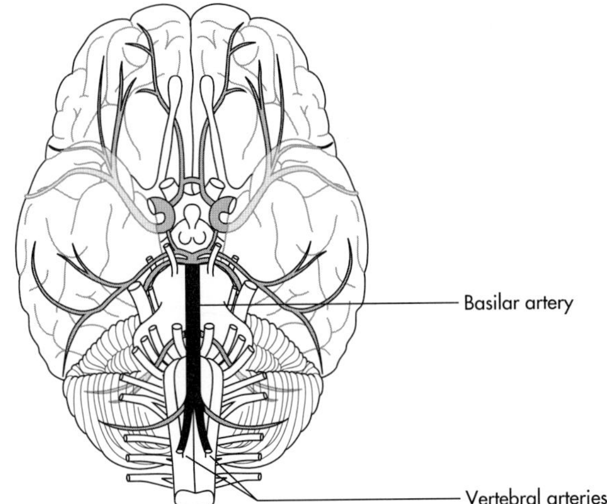

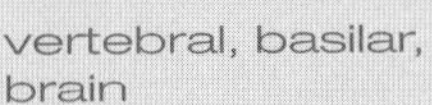

These are the ________ arteries. They fuse together to become the ________ artery. They supply the ________.

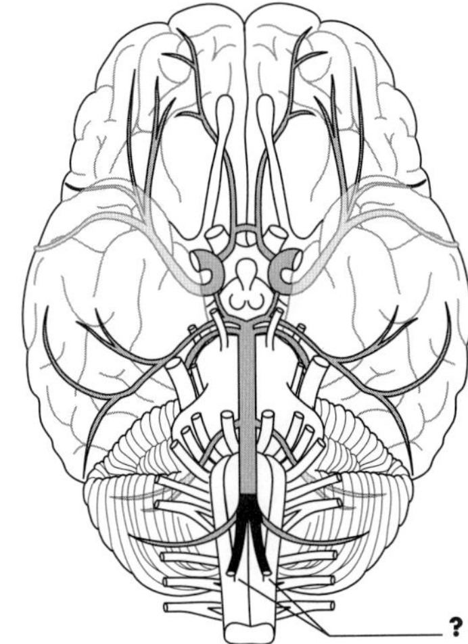

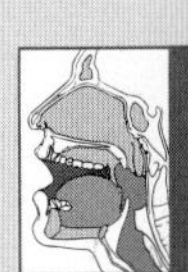

pituitary

Branches of the basilar artery supply the brainstem and cerebellum. The basilar artery then travels to the region of the base of the brainstem near the ______________ fossa to join an unusual group of vessels.

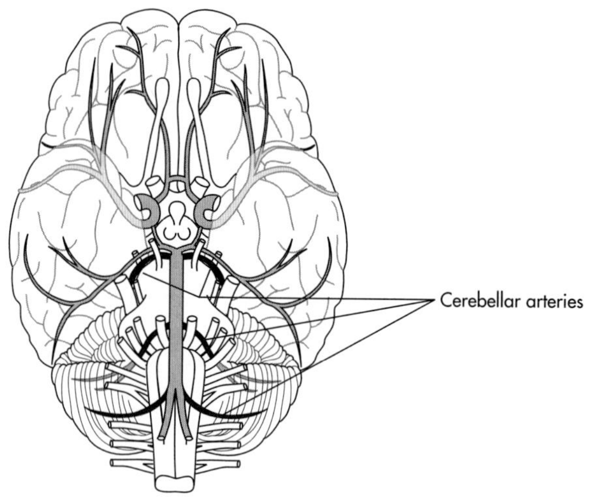

internal carotid, basilar

Note how connecting vessels complete a "circle" around the pituitary gland and connect to the internal carotid arteries. This group of vessels that connects the ______________ arteries with the ______________ artery is called the **circle of Willis.**

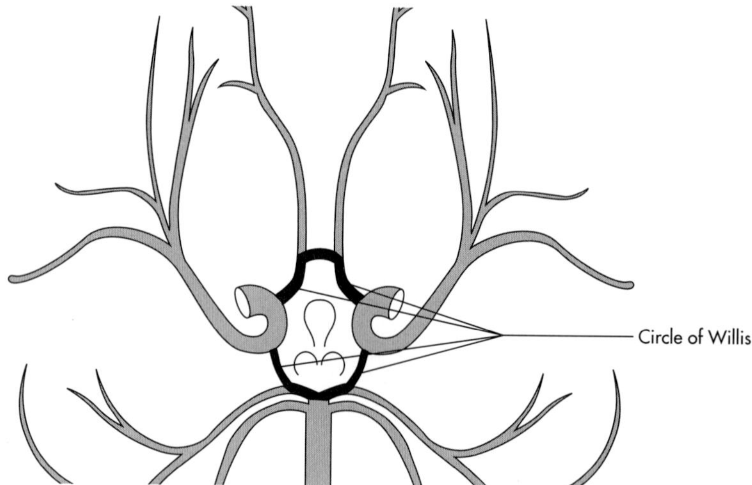

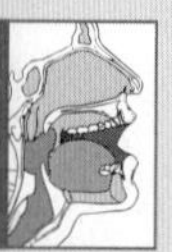

The ______________ is a safety device for blood supply to the brain. In case of damage to one of the vessels along the circle, blood can be rerouted around the blockage. This connection also shows that the brain has a ______________ source of blood.

circle of Willis, dual

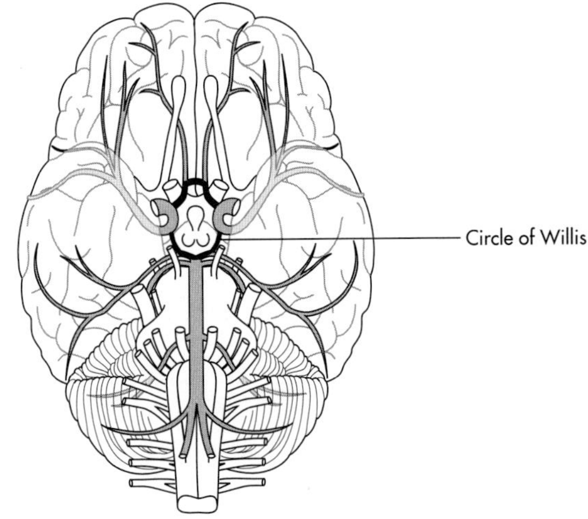

This is the ______________. It connects the two sources of blood supply to the brain.

circle of Willis

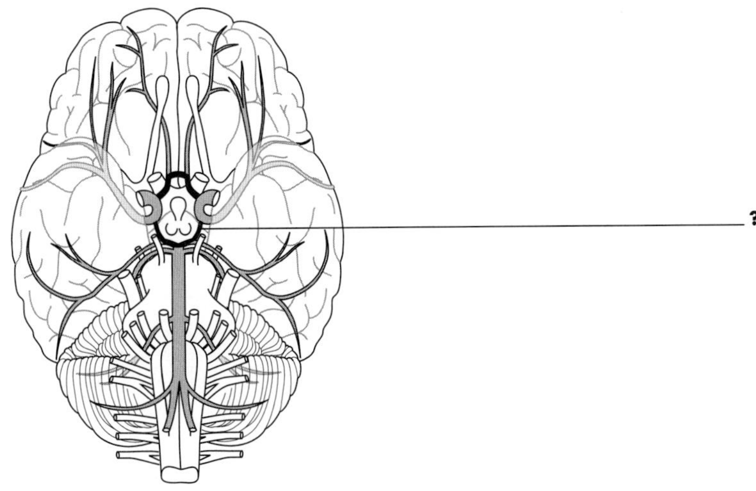

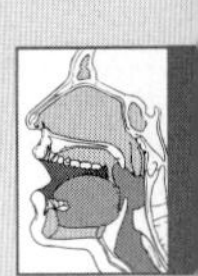

2.0 MAJOR VEINS

veins

The thin-walled vessels that carry blood toward the heart are called ______________. The veins of the head and neck drain blood from this region, carrying metabolic waste products and CO_2 down the neck, back to the heart.

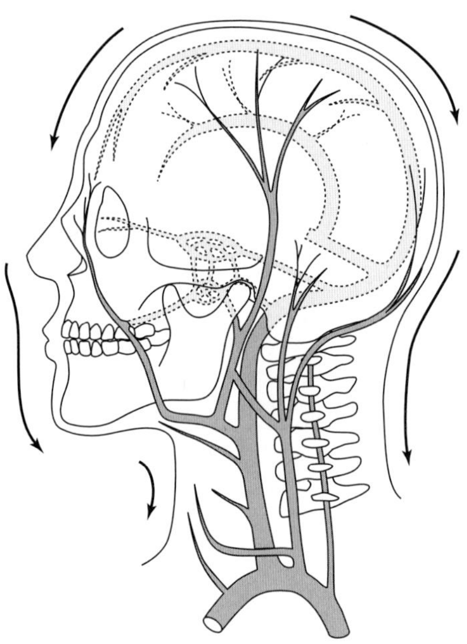

drain

The large major veins that ______________ the head and neck are called the **jugular veins.** They are thinner walled than the carotid arteries and have a more irregular shape.

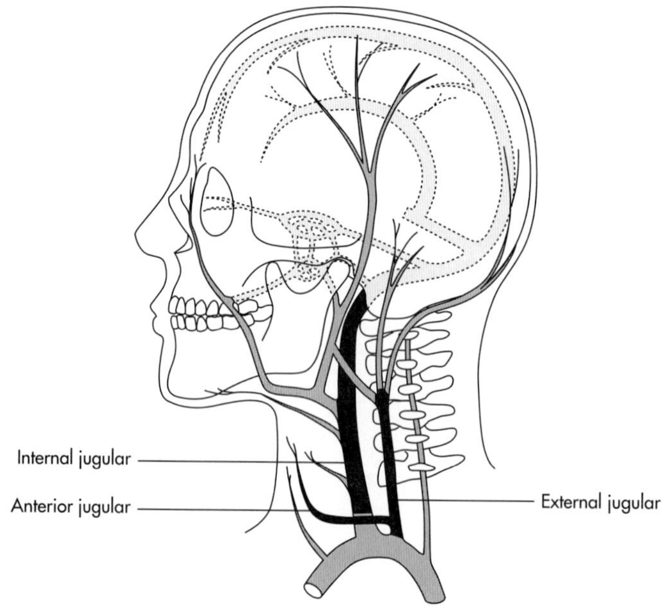

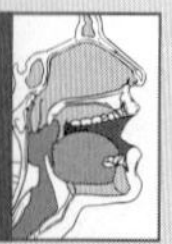

The jugular veins are divided into three divisions: external, internal, and anterior jugular veins. Which areas of the head and neck do you suppose they drain?

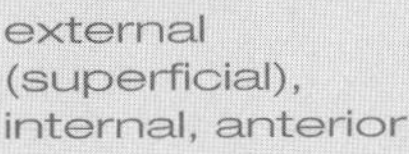
external (superficial), internal, anterior

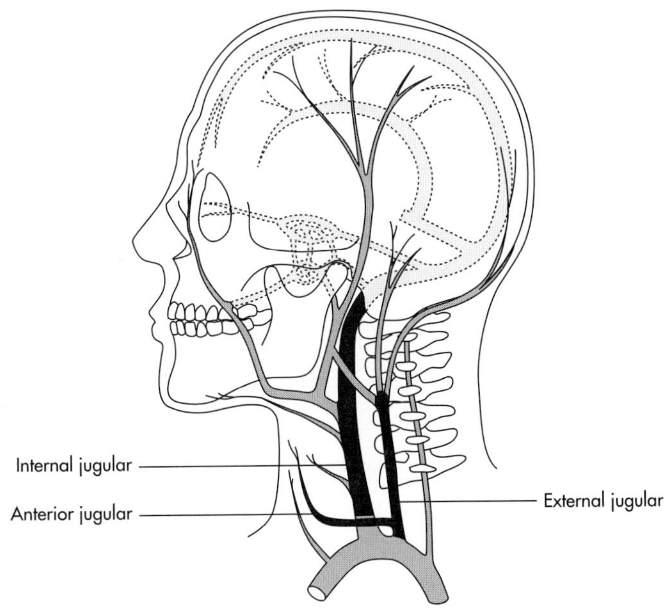

This is the **external jugular vein.** Directly anterior to this vein lies the **anterior jugular vein,** which has contributions from the external jugular and subclavian veins. They blend together and drain the anterior portion of the neck.

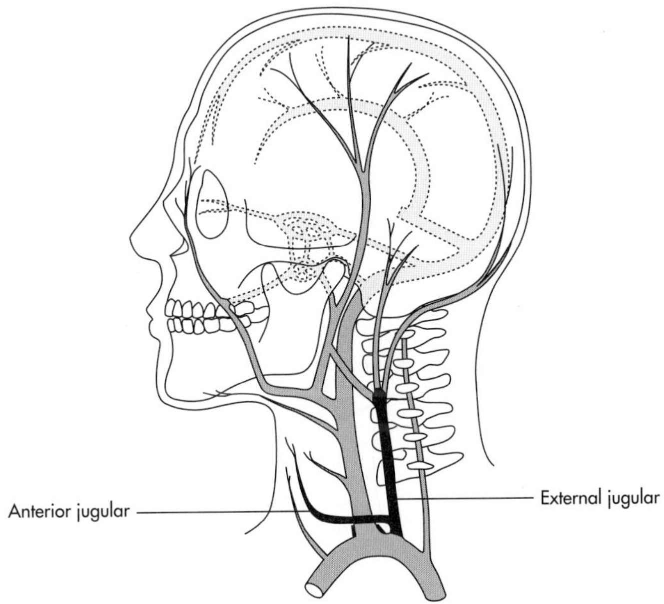

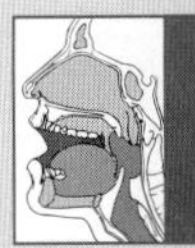

inside

This is the **internal jugular vein.** It is the largest of the three jugulars and travels to the _______________ of the cranium, where it is represented by dotted lines in the drawing on the left and is colored in on the right. The internal jugular drains the brain.

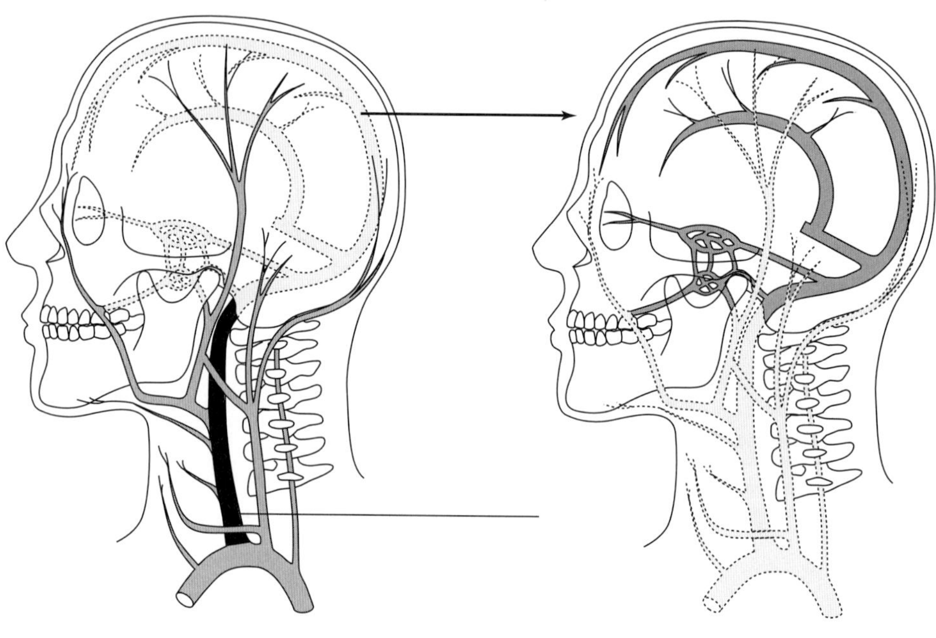

internal jugular, brain

This is the _______________ vein. It drains the _______________. Note the connection between the internal jugular and external jugular near the angle of the mandible.

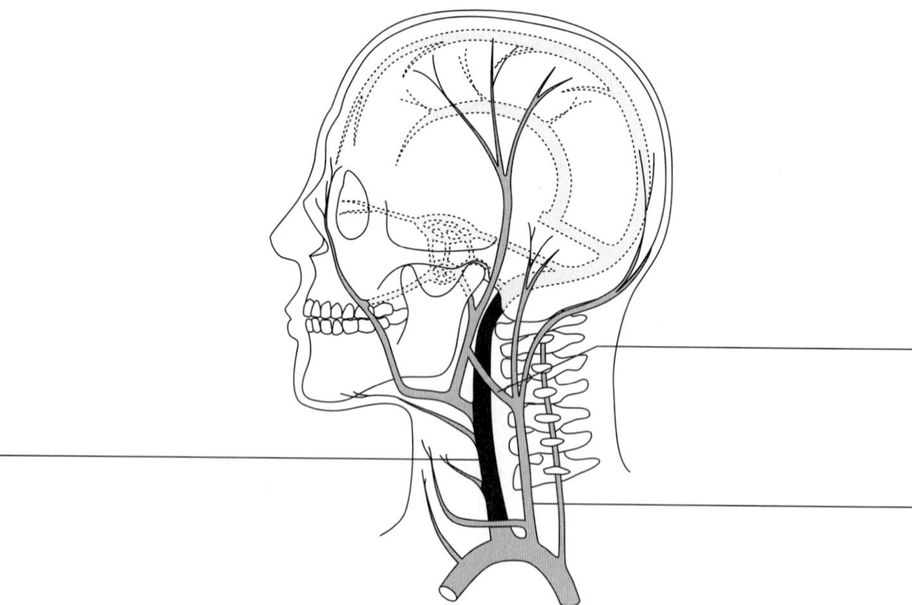

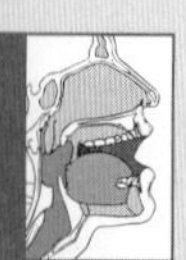

External Jugular Vein

2.1

behind the mandible, in the brain area

The branches of the external jugular run in a path similar to, but not the same as, the branches of the external carotid artery. Find two areas that look different.

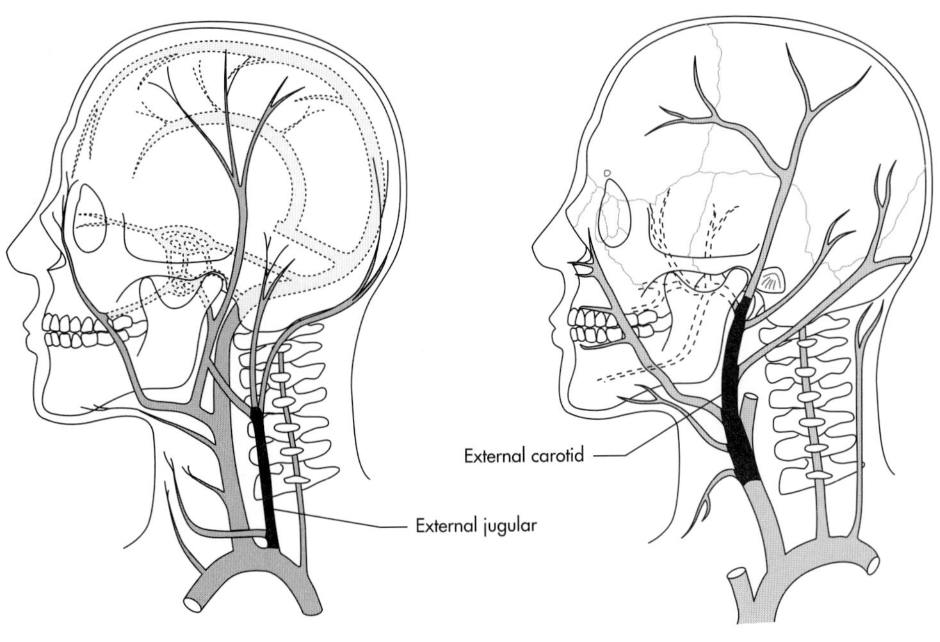

The first branch is actually a connection between the external and internal jugulars known as the **retromandibular vein.** Find it.

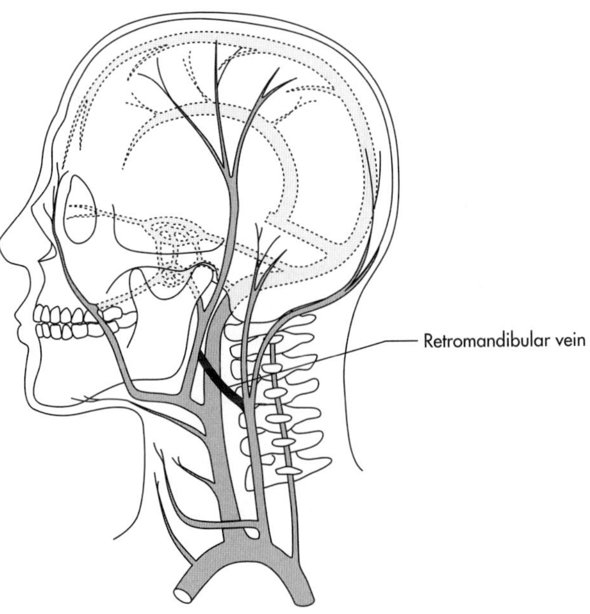

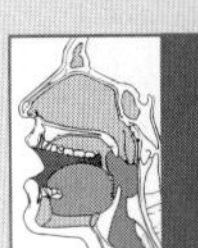

Another branch of the external jugular travels toward the back of the head or occipital region and is called **occipital vein.** Close to it is a **retroauricular branch** behind the ear. Find them.

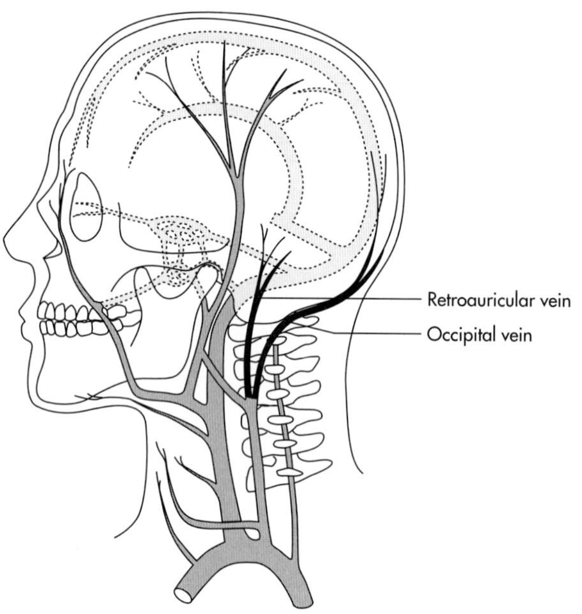

temporal and parietal sides of the head

Proceeding upward is the **superficial temporal vein.** What region does it appear to drain?

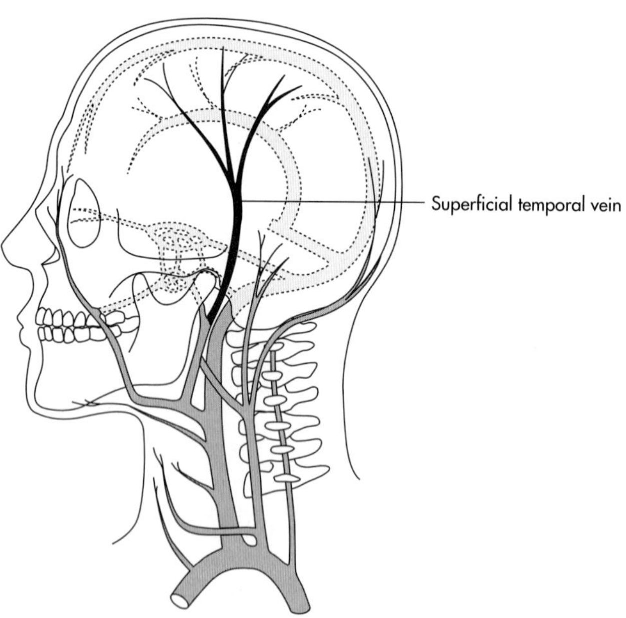

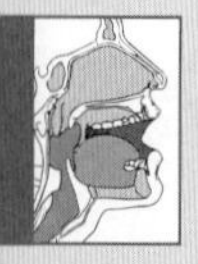

This is the ______________ vein. It drains the ______________.

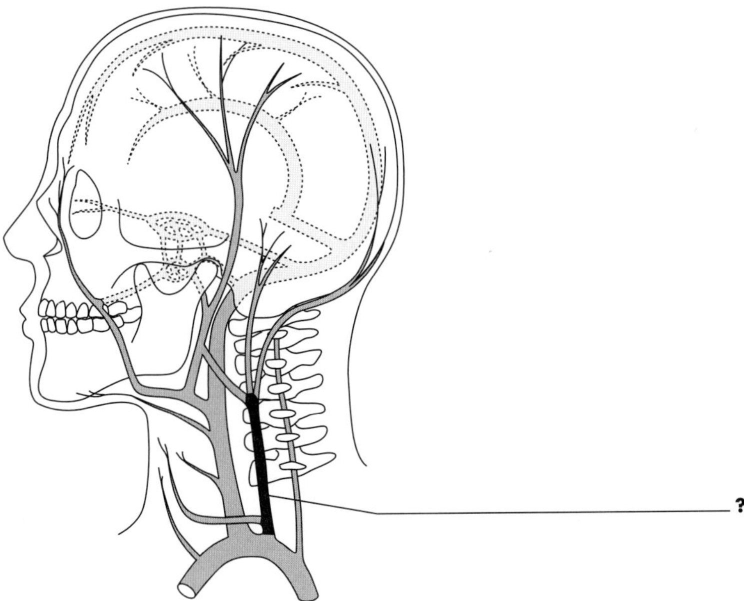

external jugular, superficial head and neck

This is the ______________ vein. It is a connection between the ______________ and ______________.

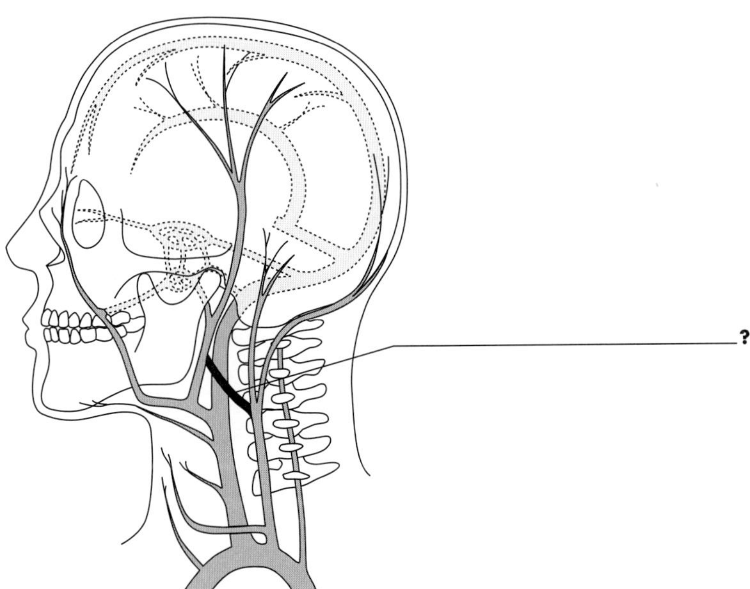

retromandibular, internal jugular, external jugular

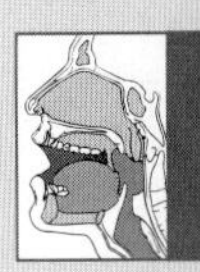

superficial temporal, external jugular vein, temporal and parietal regions

This is the ______________ vein. It is a branch of the ______________ and drains the ______________.

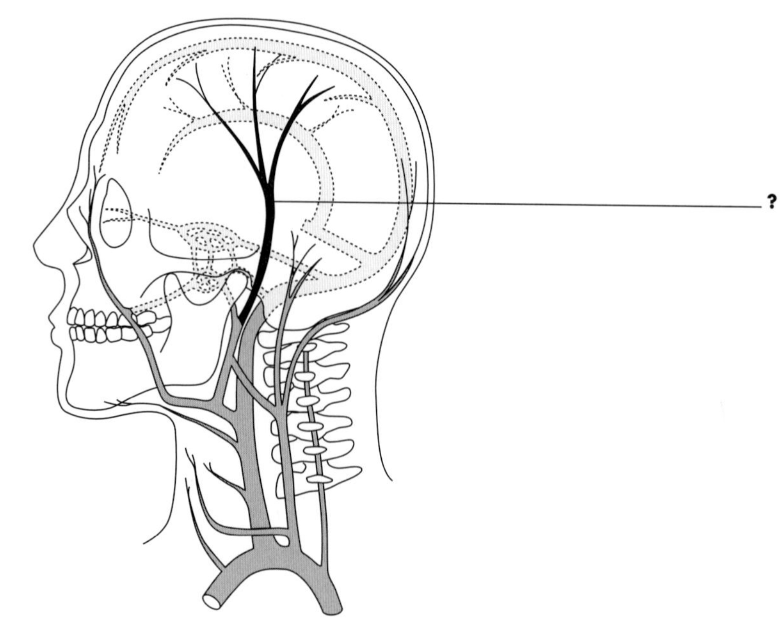

retroauricular, back of ear

This is the ______________ vein. It drains the ______________.

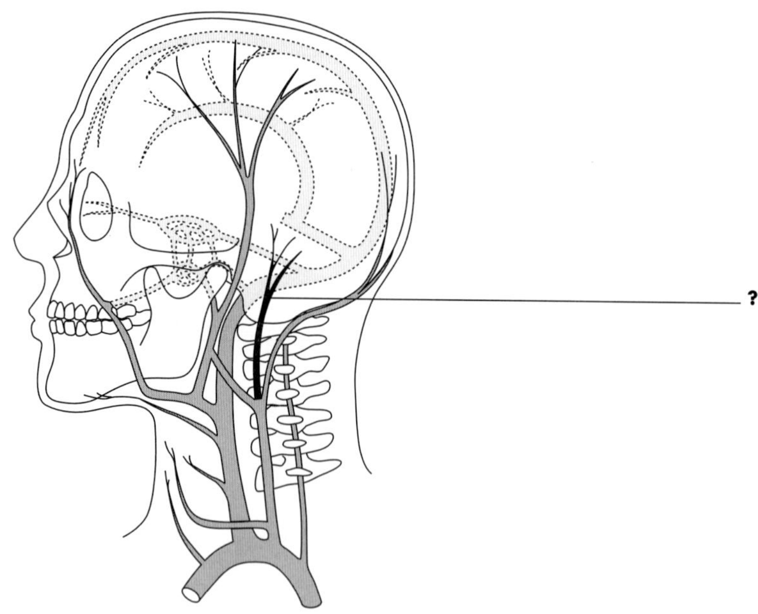

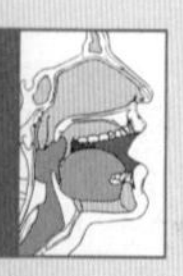

Internal Jugular Vein

2.2

As you can see, it is difficult to distinguish the branches of the internal and external jugular veins because they connect at the ______________ vein behind the ramus of the mandible. There are a few "external" branches of the internal jugular, after it exits the brain. One very large branch is the **facial vein.** Find it.

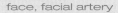

retromandibular

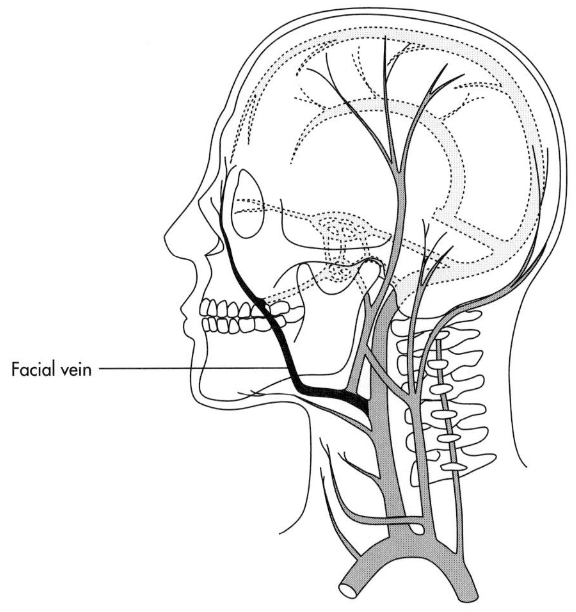

The **facial vein** spreads across the ______________ to drain this large region. Some of its small branches connect with the deeper veins of the face and brain through the orbit, supraorbital, and infraorbital veins. With which artery do you suppose it runs?

face, facial artery

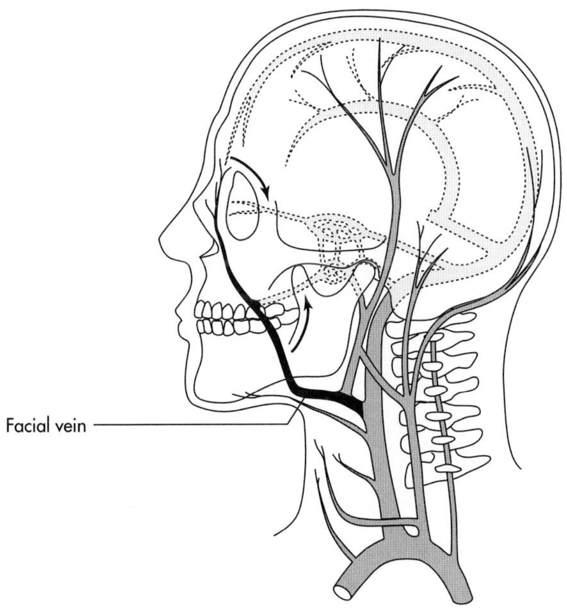

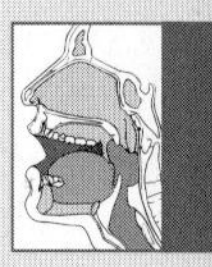

tongue and thyroid gland

Below the facial vein lies the **lingual vein** and the **thyroid veins.** What do these veins drain?

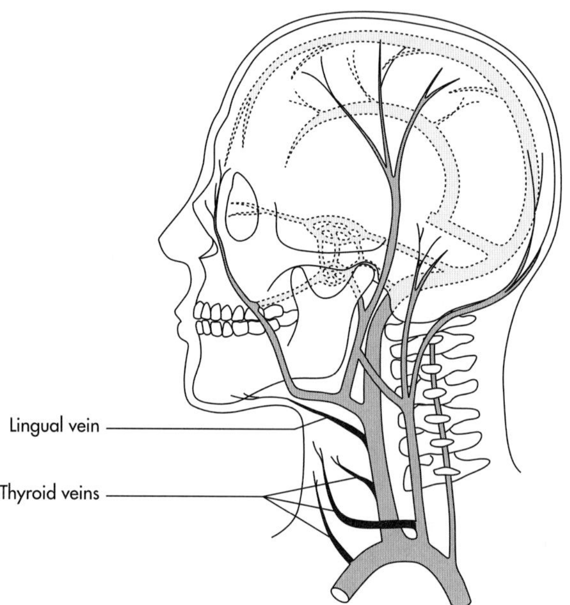

The last major branch is really a branch of both internal and external jugular veins and travels behind the condyle within the infratemporal fossa. It spreads out for a time into a network or plexus of small veins and then regroups as a single vein. The beginning of the vessel is called the **maxillary vein** and it rapidly becomes the **pterygoid plexus.**

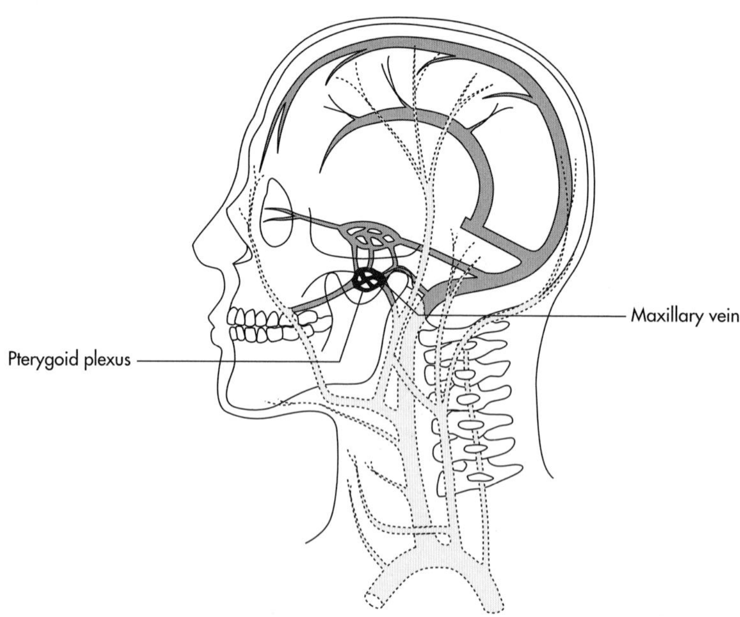

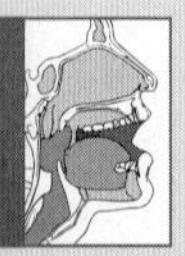

The **pterygoid plexus** is a ______________ of veins, draining the maxilla and nasopalatine areas. It lies in the ______________ fossa, right next to the ______________ artery, which supplies the same area.

network, infratemporal, maxillary

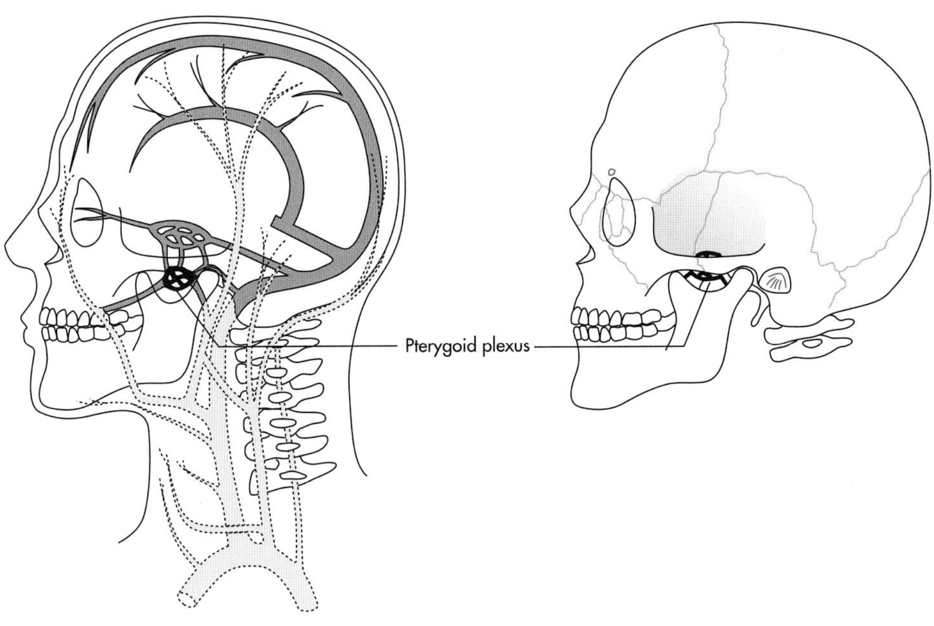

The infratemporal fossa is an area where dental anesthetic injections are given to numb V2 (PSA branch of the maxillary division). Besides the nerve, we now know of two major blood vessels in the area: the maxillary artery and the ______________ plexus. To avoid penetrating them, we use a technique of injection called aspiration.

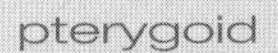

pterygoid

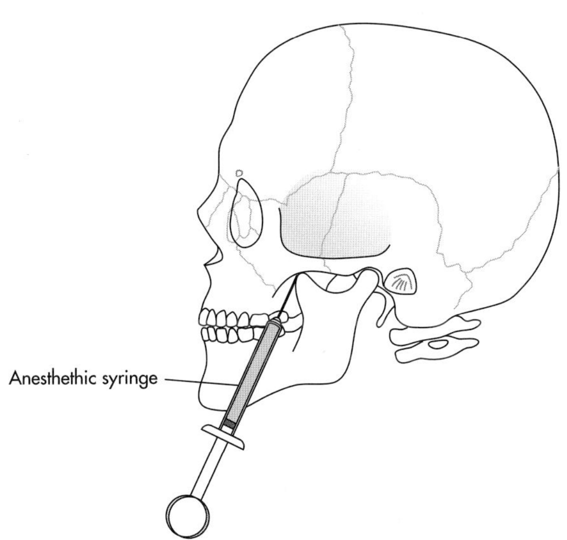

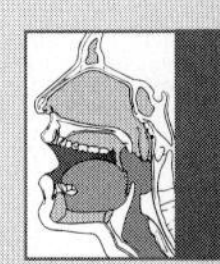

PSA—posterior teeth, MSA—premolars, ASA—anterior, inferior alveolar—mandibular teeth and periodontium

The pterygoid plexus ends as the veins come back together to form the veins of the maxilla. They follow a distribution path equivalent to the arteries, so that there are **PSA, MSA,** and **ASA veins.** There is also an **inferior alveolar vein.** What do they drain?

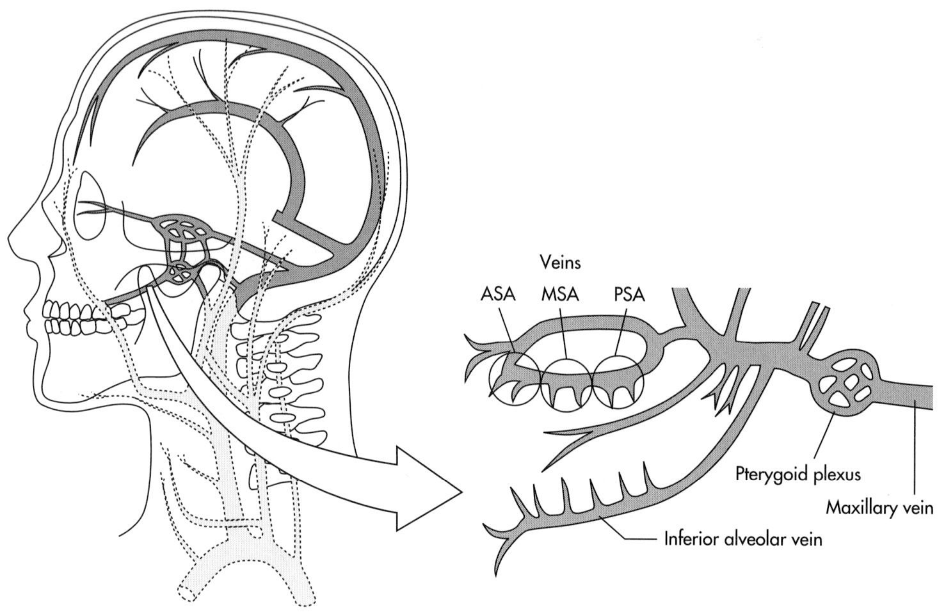

vein

There are also **greater palatine veins** and **nasopalatine veins**. A pattern has been established that you should be able to recognize now: to each organ, structure, or tissue travels a nerve, artery, and ______________. They all bear the same name.

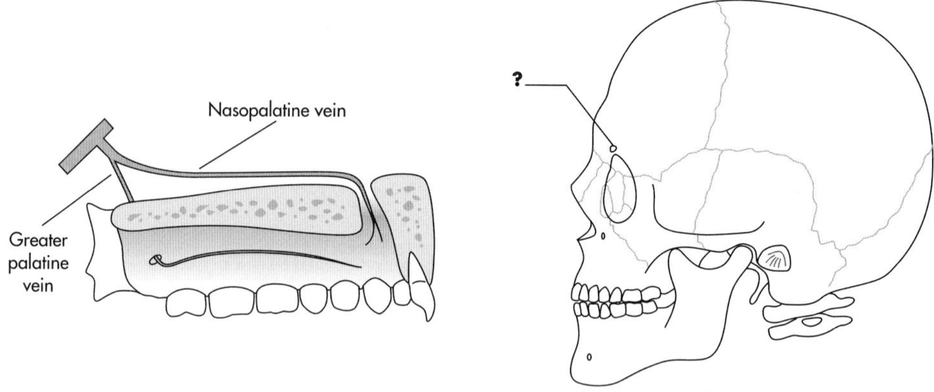

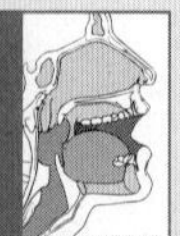

supraorbital artery, vein, and nerve through supraorbital foramen

For example, a PSA nerve (V2), a PSA artery, and a PSA vein supply the maxillary molars (except the mesiobuccal cusp of the first). What would you name the three structures that emerge through this foramen to supply the forehead?

Name the artery, vein, nerve, and foramina shown here.

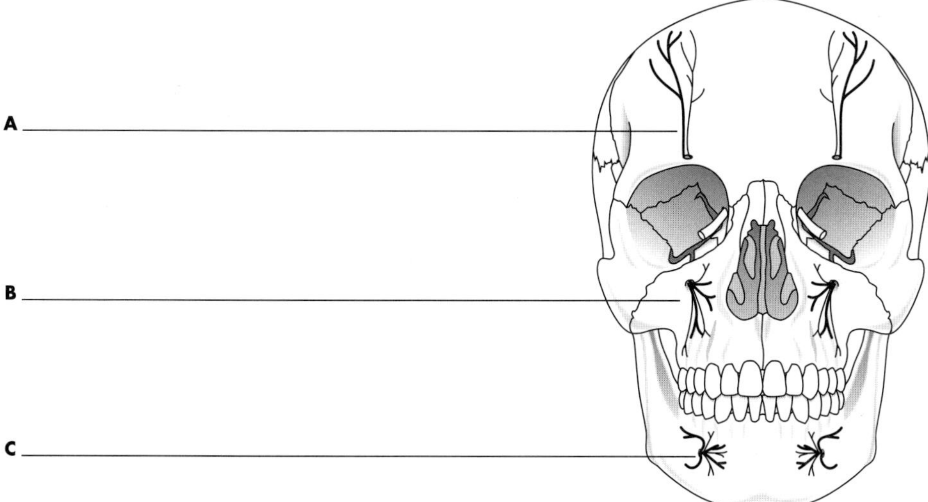

A. supraorbital artery, vein, nerve, and foramen
B. infraorbital artery, vein, nerve, and foramen
C. mental artery, vein, nerve, and foramen

This is a **vertebral vein.** To what artery are its name and position similar? In what does it travel?

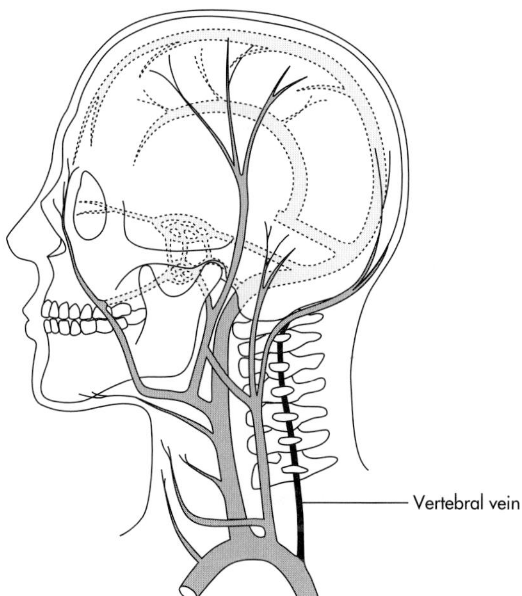

vertebral artery, in the foramina of the cervical vertebrae

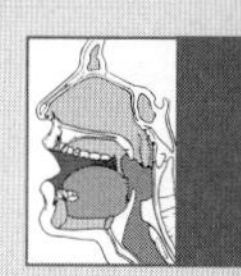

vertebral

The ______________ vein (one of a pair), however, does not go into the brain as does the artery, but, rather, connects with the **occipital veins.**

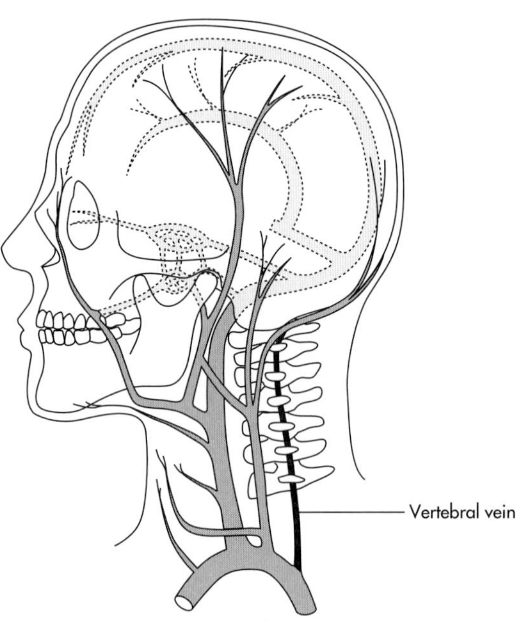

2.3 Vessels of the Brain

The large venous vessels of the brain are not called veins, but, rather, are called **sinuses.** Do not confuse this term with the paranasal sinuses, which are hollowed out areas in the cranial bones.

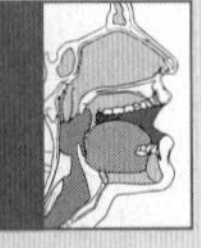

The venous vessels of the brain begin in a single large midline vessel that lies between the cerebral hemispheres. It is inferior to the parietal suture of the skull, where it creates a groove in the bone. This vessel is called the **superior sagittal sinus,** and it is the largest vein, draining the upper portion of the cerebrum. It is not paired like the other veins.

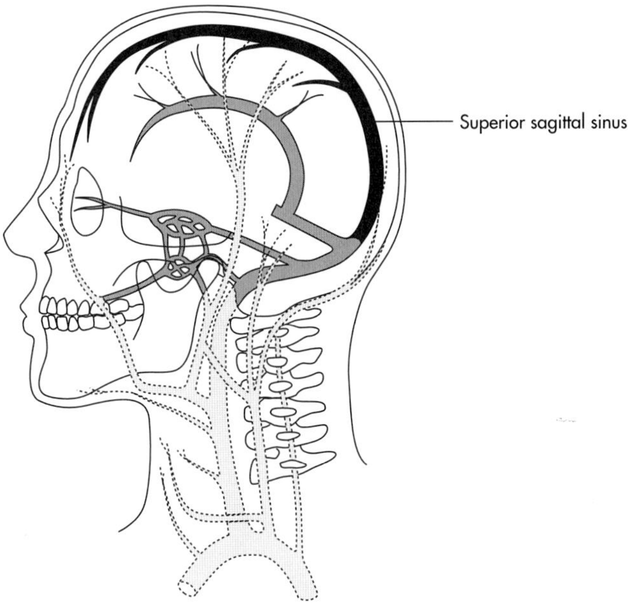

The superior sagittal sinus is also part of the cerebrospinal fluid system by way of small venous extensions off the main vessel that connect with the arachnoid space.

Find the superior sagittal sinus. Near the cerebellum it divides into two sections, the **transverse sinuses,** after picking up drainage from the interior vessel, the **inferior sagittal sinus.** Find them below.

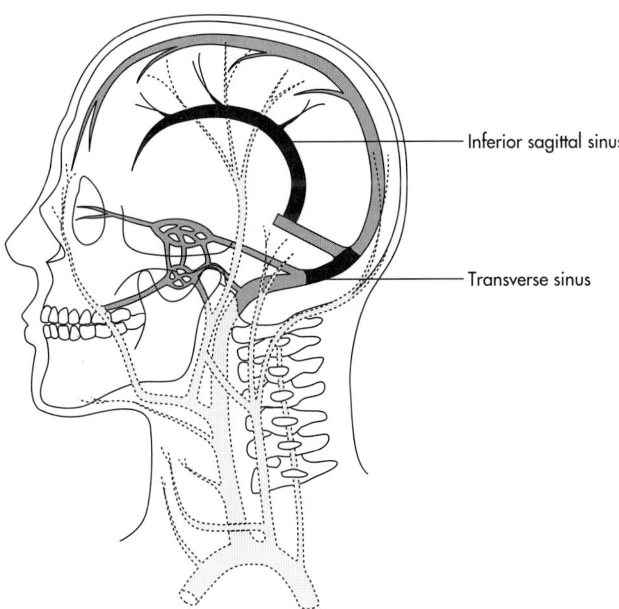

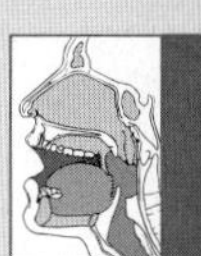

inferior

The ______________ sagittal sinus looks like a mirror image of superior sagittal sinus. It drains the interior surfaces of the brain not serviced by the superior vessel.

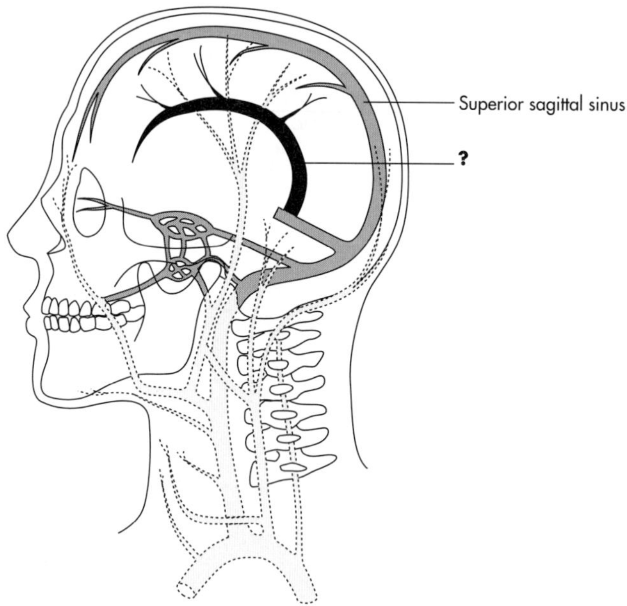

Directly inferior to the inferior saggital sinus is an area of veins—another network—that lies in the pituitary fossa. This is called the **cavernous sinus.** It is a tortuous network of veins, receiving drainage from the orbital areas and base of the brain.

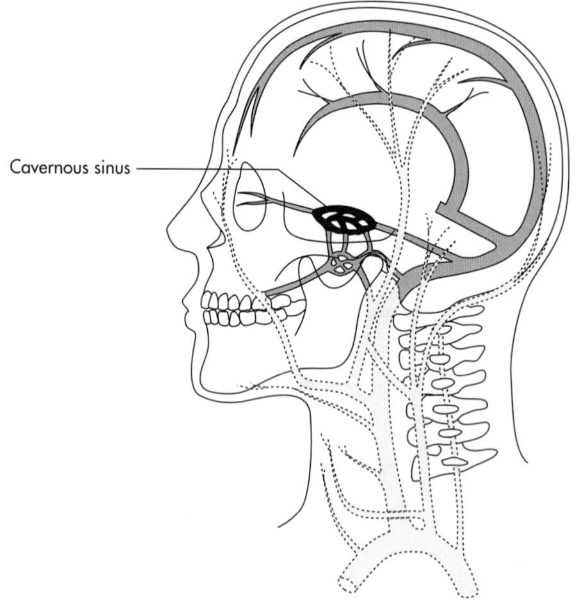

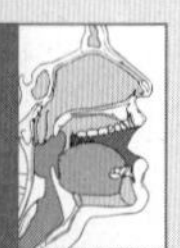

Note how the ______________ sinus connects with drainage from the facial area, or exterior veins, and with drainage from the maxillary region through the pterygoid plexus.

cavernous

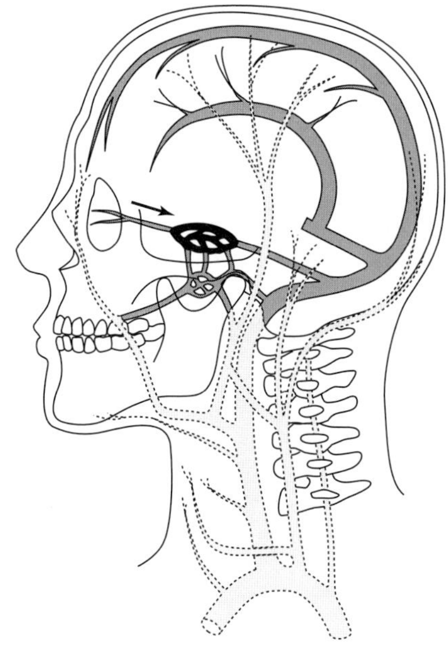

We have found that the pituitary fossa, besides containing the pituitary gland (hypophysis), has a number of important structures running close to it. Name as many as you can remember.

pituitary gland,
internal carotids,
optic chiasm,
branches of CN V,
cavernous sinus,
CN III, IV, and VI

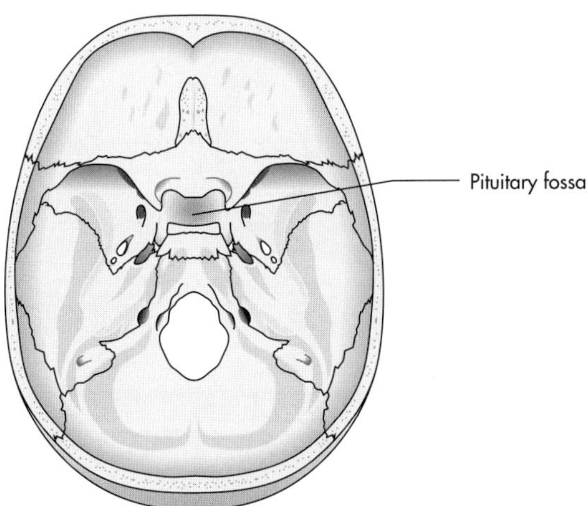

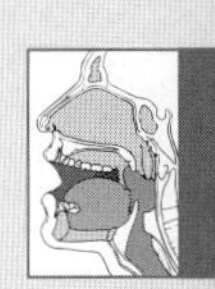

The pituitary fossa has, in its vicinity, the pituitary gland, cavernous sinus, internal carotid arteries, and cranial nerves (CNs) II, V, III, IV, and VI. Look at a slice through this area. A lot of these structures actually run right through the cavernous sinus.

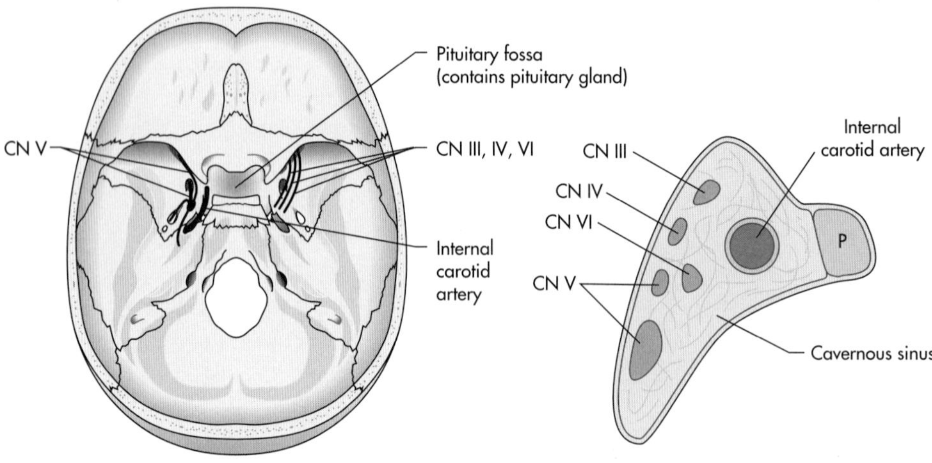

With connections to the facial veins and to the pterygoid plexus, the cavernous sinus becomes a high-risk area if infection enters the venous system. Venous blood tends to pool (is not circulated out swiftly) in plexus areas. So, if veins of the face or maxilla become contaminated they may pass infection to the cavernous sinus, which could be a serious threat to the brain.

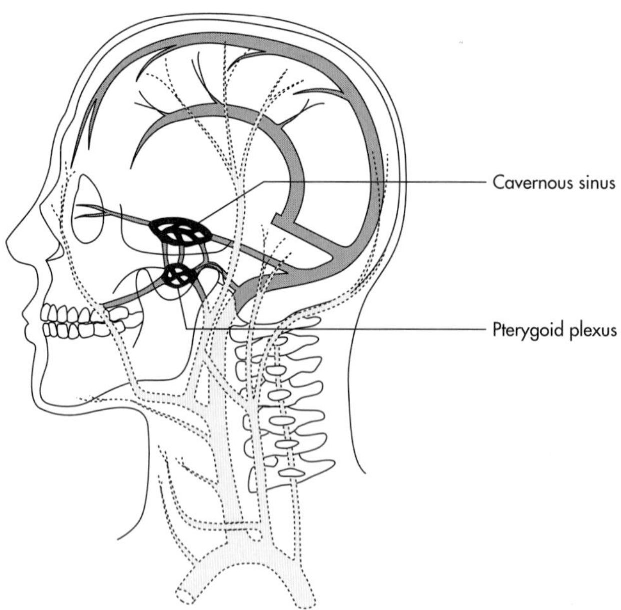

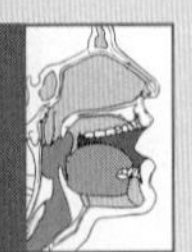

If an infected dental needle were to penetrate the venous vessels, what would happen? What is this area?

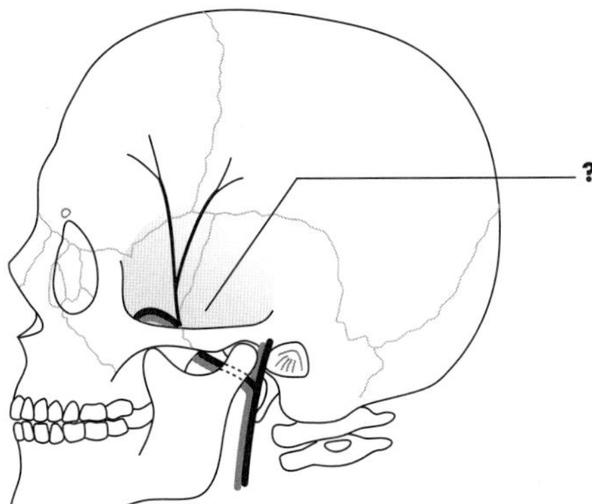

pass infection to the cavernous sinus via pterygoid plexus, infratemporal fossa

This area of the skull is called the ______________ fossa. When dental injections are made to numb the PSA nerve (block injection), the technique of aspiration is used to avoid penetrating what two vessels?

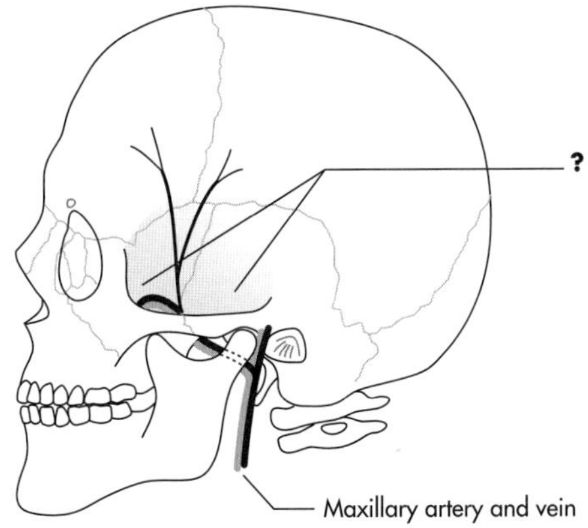

infratemporal, maxillary artery and pterygoid plexus

What three things lie in the infratemporal fossa?

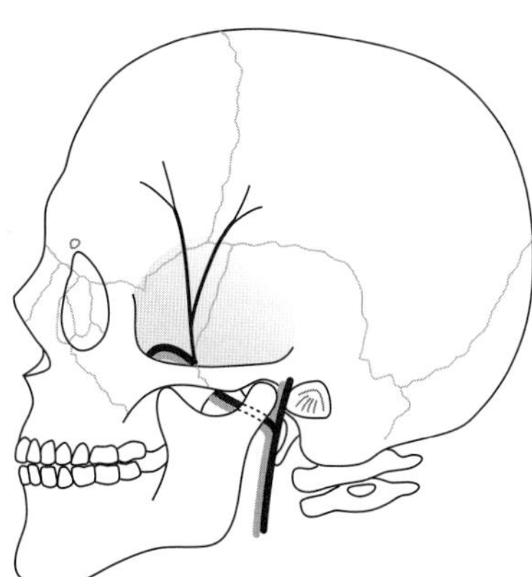

maxillary artery, vein (pterygoid plexus), nerve (V2—PSA)

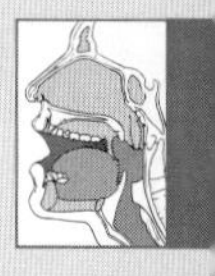

transverse

The ______________ sinuses split off around the cerebellum and become curved on the floor of the posterior cranium.

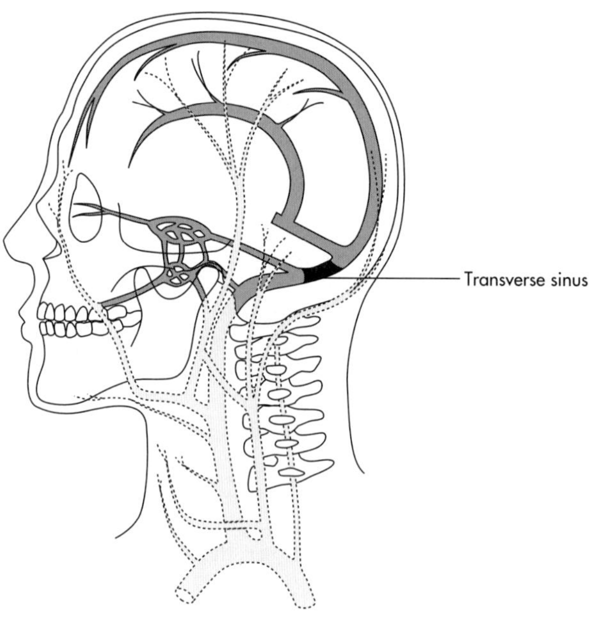

This S-shaped portion of the venous system is called the **sigmoid sinus.** There are two, and they lie in S-shaped grooves in the occipital bone.

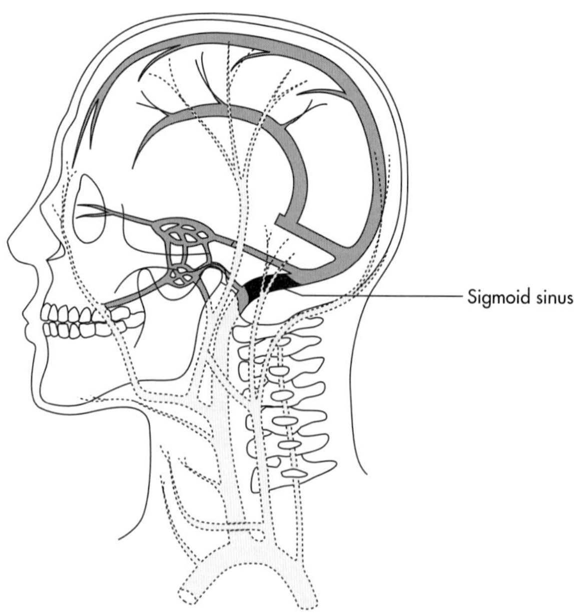

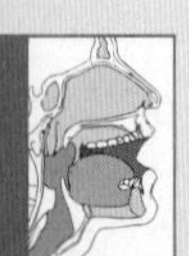

The ______________ sinuses are the last portion of the venous drainage before it exits the cranium through the **jugular foramina.** Find the grooves that hold the sigmoid sinuses and the two jugular foramina.

sigmoid

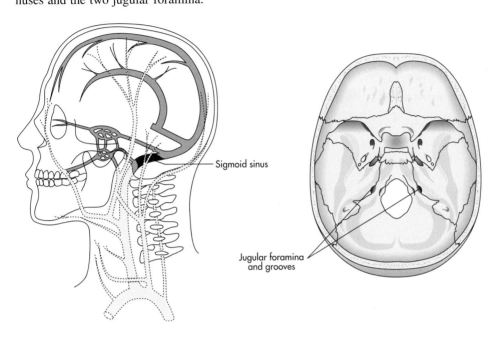

Sigmoid sinus

Jugular foramina and grooves

As the sigmoid sinus leaves the cranium, it becomes the **internal jugular vein,** and the blood from the brain follows the drainage path down the neck and eventually into the vena cava.

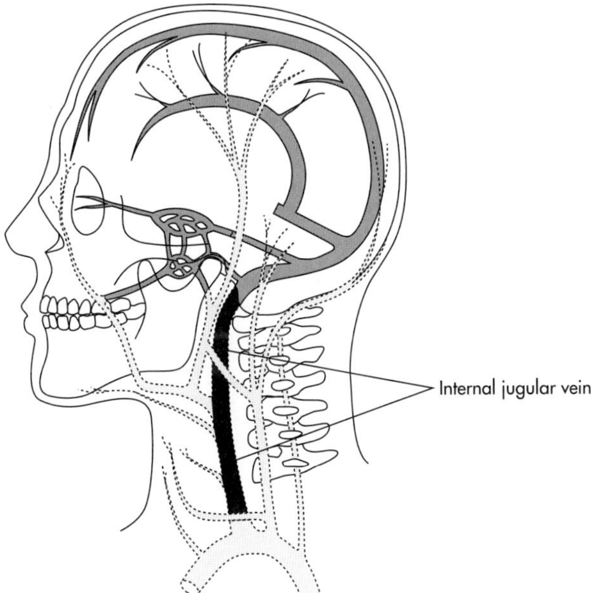

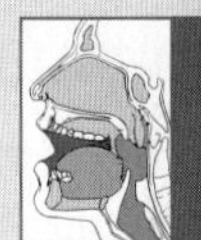

superior sagittal sinus, superior brain

This is the ______________. It drains the ______________.

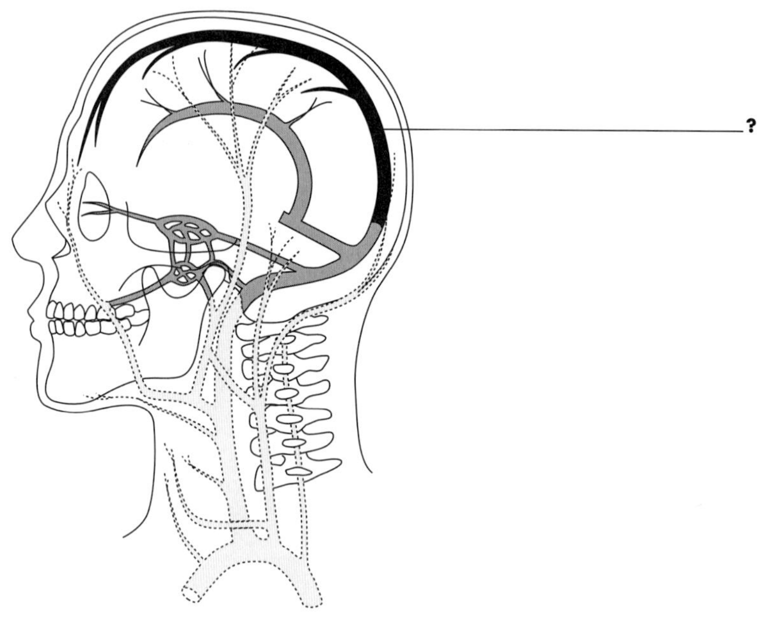

inferior sagittal sinus, inferior brain

This is the ______________. It drains the ______________.

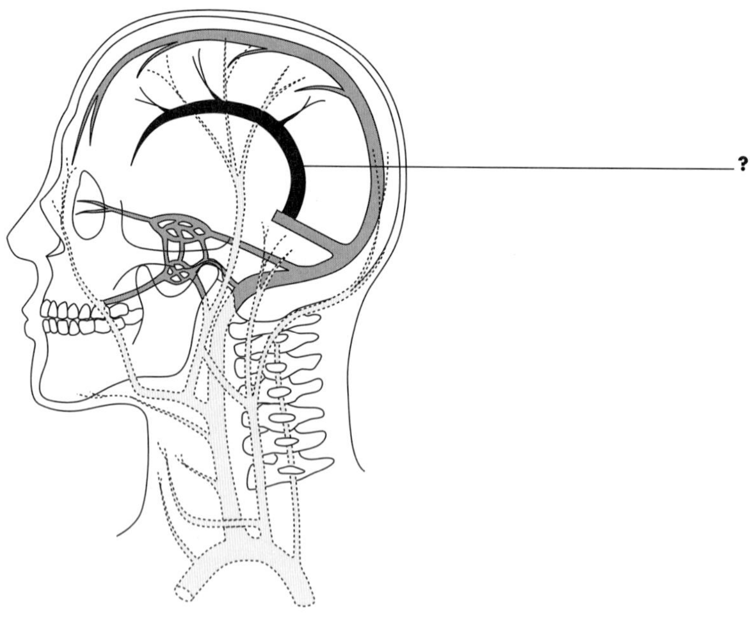

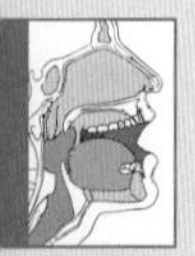

This is the ______________.

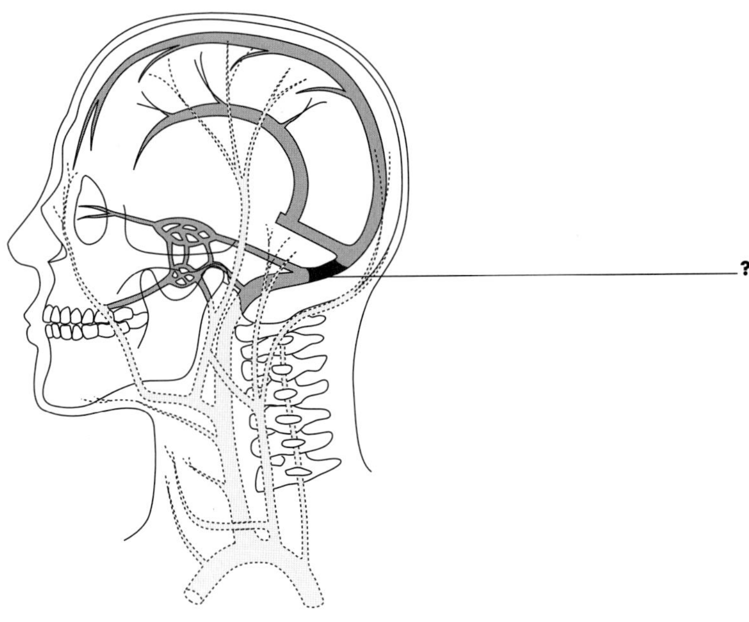

transverse sinus

This is the ______________. It exits through the ______________, and the vessel becomes the ______________.

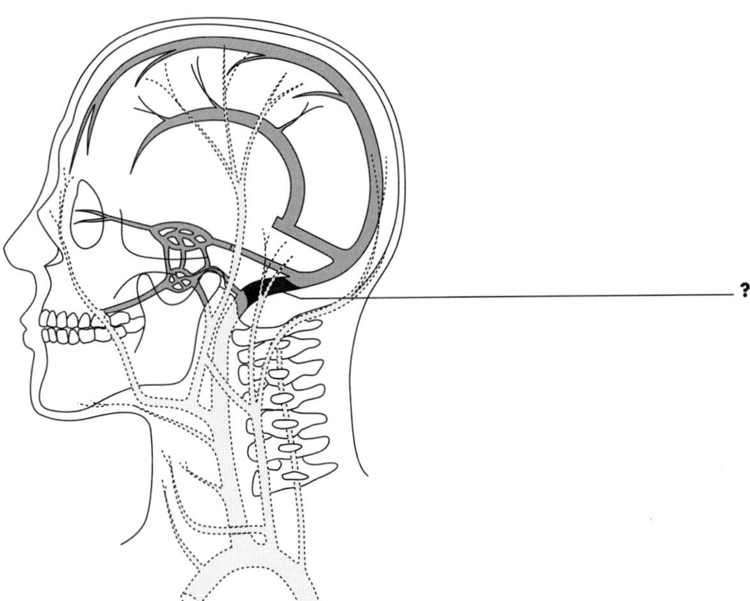

sigmoid sinus,
jugular foramen,
internal jugular vein

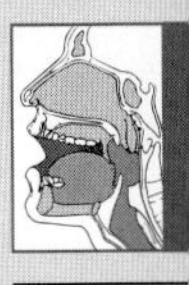

cavernous sinus, facial and maxillary veins, pituitary fossa

This is the ______________. It has connections to the ______________. It lies next to the ______________.

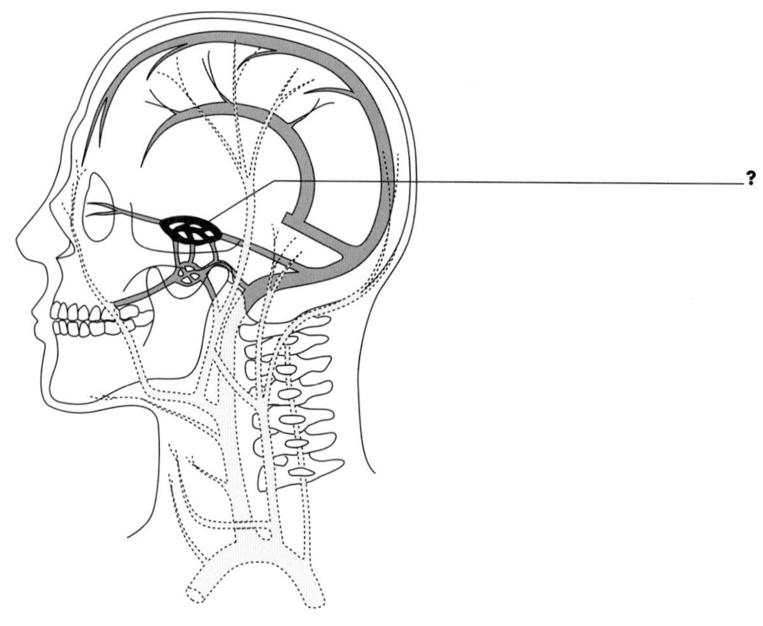

3.0

LYMPHATIC SYSTEM

open, lymph

The lymphatic system is a(an) ______________ system of fluid circulation, as compared with the vascular system, which is a closed system of tubes. Extracellular (tissue) fluid is absorbed into small ______________ vessels, which become increasingly larger.

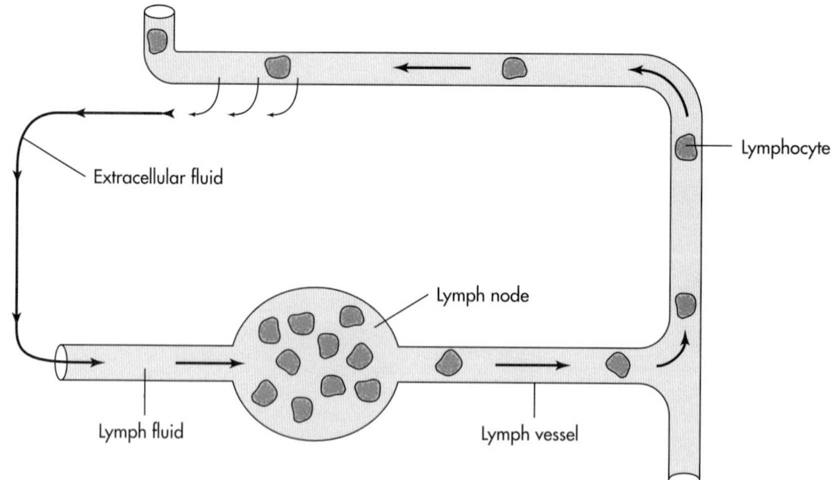

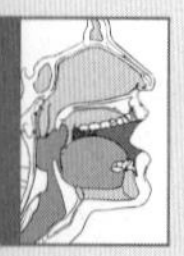

nodes

Along the pathway of lymph vessels toward their connection with the vena cava (and, thus, the vascular system) are the **lymph nodes,** which act as "filters." They add to the body fluids lymphocytes, which combat invaders such as bacteria, viruses, and foreign cells. Note that there are prominent clusters of lymph ______________ in the groin, armpit, and head/neck areas.

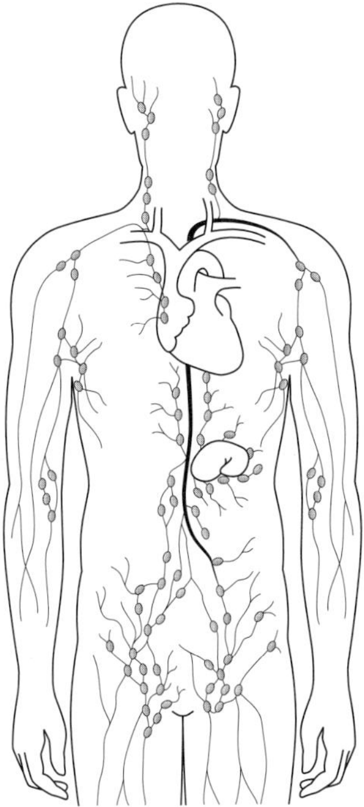

nodes

The lymph ______________ are said to "drain" a particular region of the body, usually near their location. They drain tissue fluids from that area, and if defense action is needed against infection or other disease processes (as cancers), they enlarge because of the increased activity. In the case of infection, lymph nodes become swollen and tender. In response to many cancer processes they become rubbery and nontender.

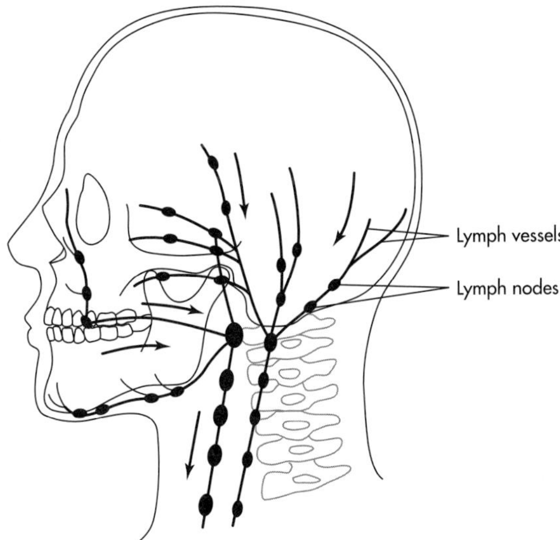

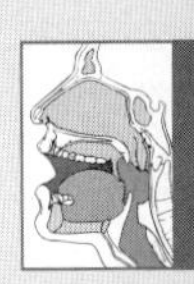

running down the neck

Look at the locations of the lymph nodes and vessels of the head and neck. Where do you see a large concentration of nodes?

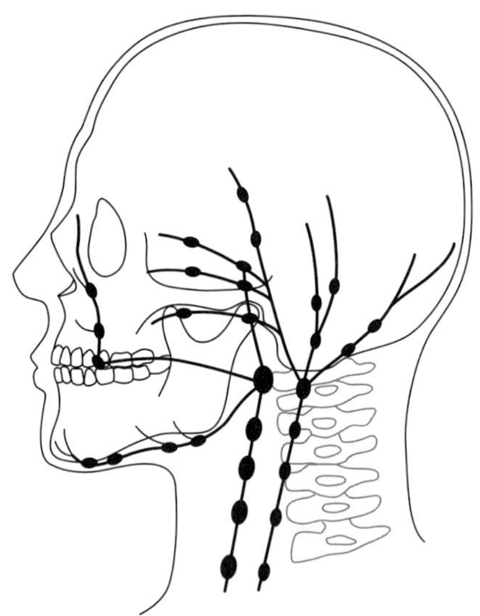

sternocleido-mastoid

A group of interconnected nodes and vessels run along this muscle of the neck. It is ______________. These nodes are called the **cervical lymph nodes** and there are a **deep group** and a **superficial group.**

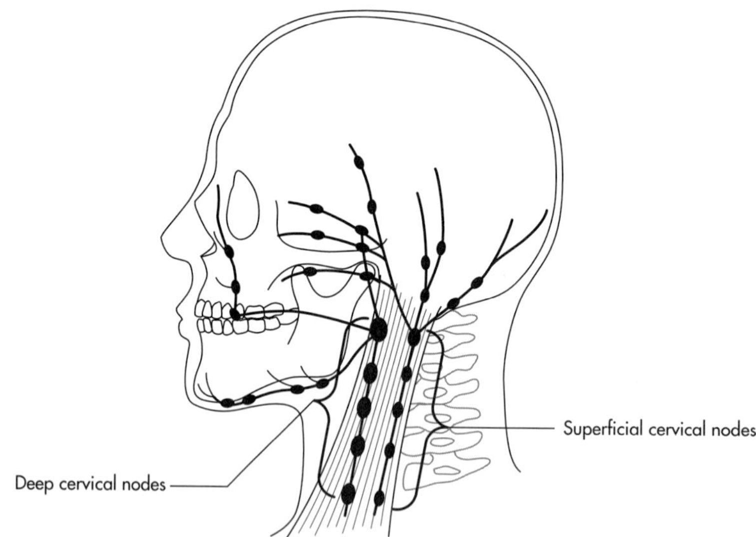

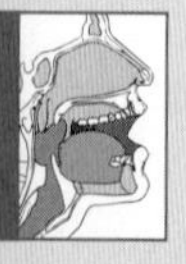

These are the ______________ nodes. They drain the tissue fluids of the head down the neck, toward the heart and thoracic duct. One of the most superior nodes in this cervical chain is a larger node found below the angle of the mandible. It is called **jugulodigastric node** and it can be felt or "palapated" easily by following along the anterior edge of the ______________ muscle.

cervical, sternocleido-mastoid

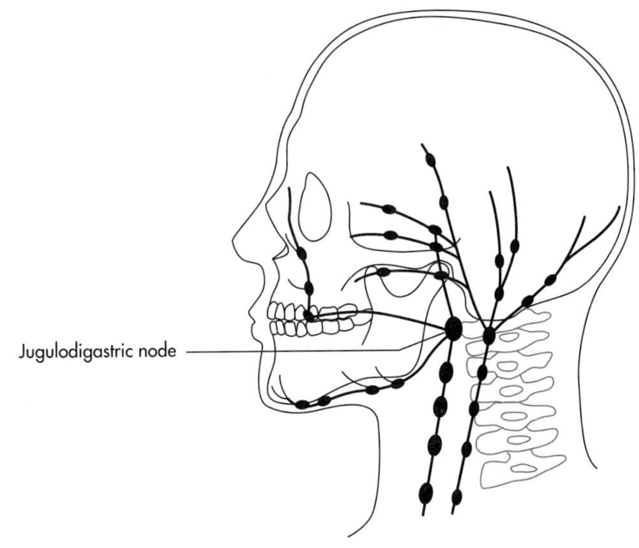

The ______________ node is a large node at the top of the cervical lymph nodes. Note how it connects by lymph vessels to other nodes of the face and jaw.

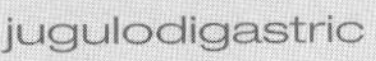
jugulodigastric

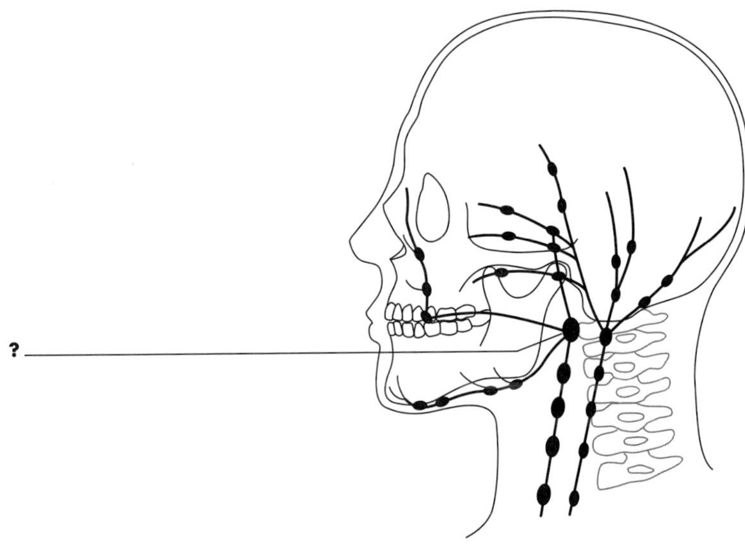

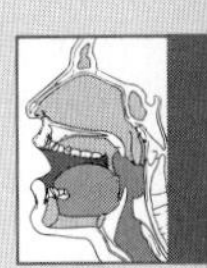

carotid arteries, internal jugular vein

What other structures have we found along the border of the sternocleidomastoid muscle?

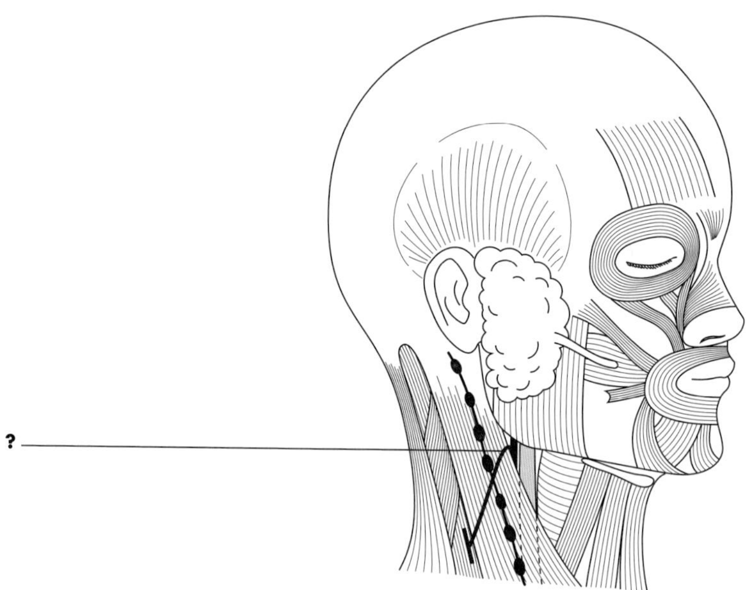

carotid

The sternocleidomastoid muscle is a landmark for locating several structures of the neck, including the major blood vessels and CN X (vagus). The ______________ pulse can be found on its border, directly beneath the mandible.

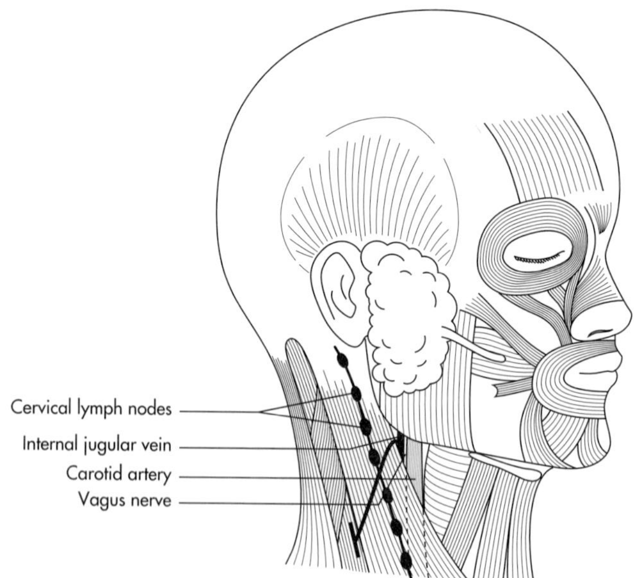

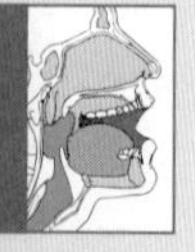

We also know now that we can palpate the _____________ lymph nodes along the sternocleidomastoid muscle.

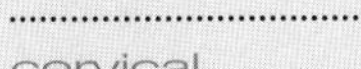

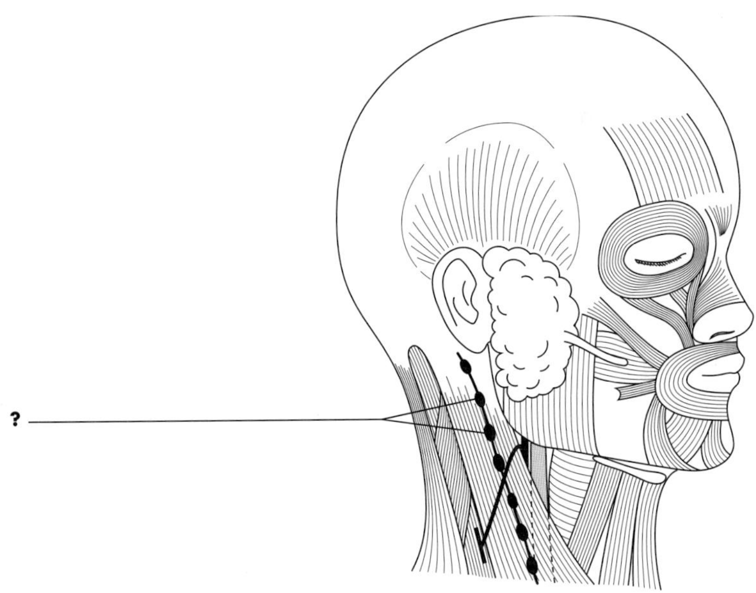

Note the other clusters of lymph nodes of the head. There are **occipital, postauricular, parotid,** and **preauricular nodes.** Find them.

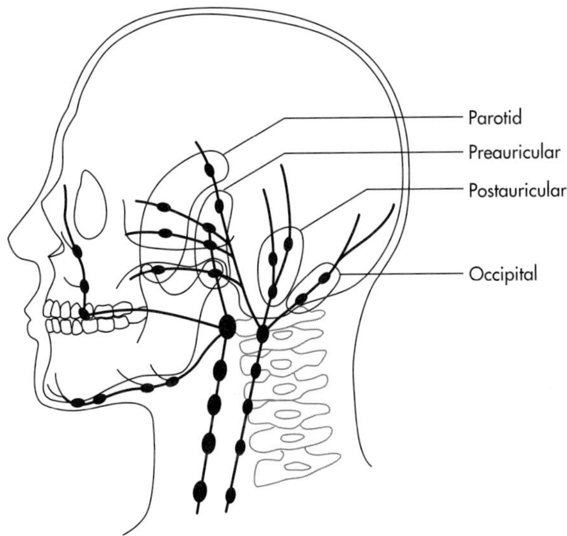

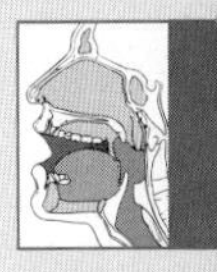

There are also groups of **facial lymph nodes** draining all portions of the face, downward into the cervical nodes and nodes of the lower face.

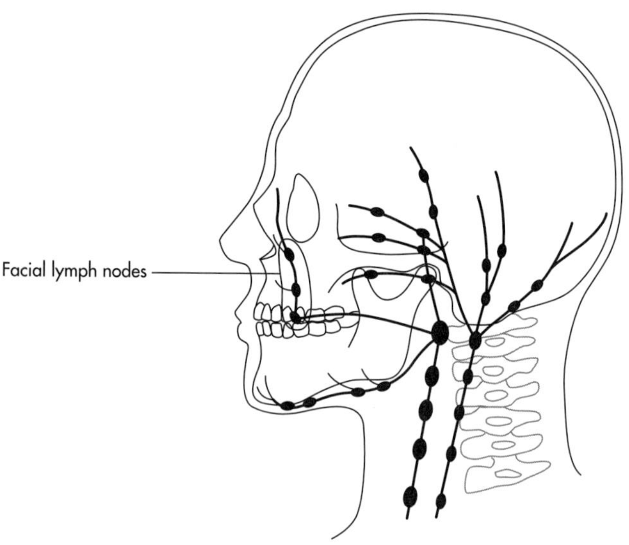

submandibular salivary gland

Two sets of lymph nodes are important to the dental area. Though there are small **maxillary nodes,** most drainage of the dental arches goes through the **submandibular lymph nodes,** located below the skin under the mandible, close to the submandibular salivary gland. Do not confuse the two! Which lies in the submandibular fossa?

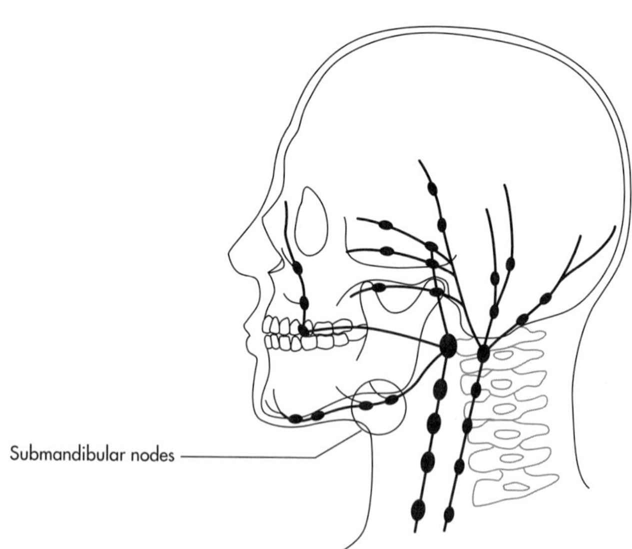

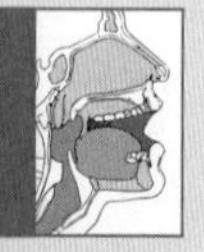

If there were an infection in the maxillary dentition or the mandibular posterior teeth, swelling would occur in the ______________ lymph nodes.

submandibular

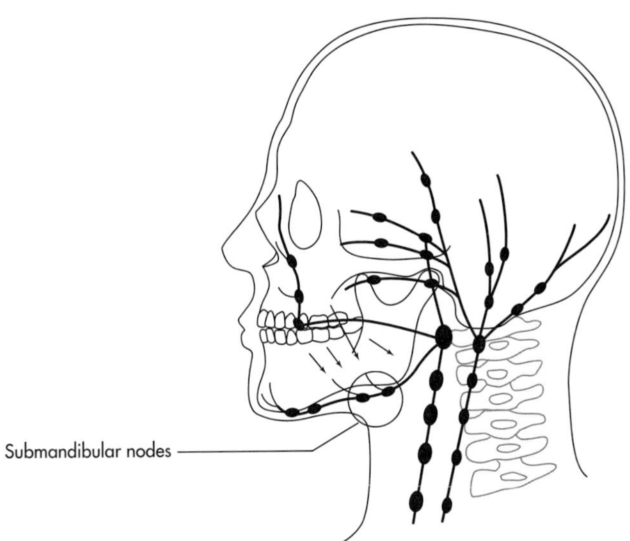

The **submental lymph nodes** are located more anteriorly, below the chin. Find these on the drawing.

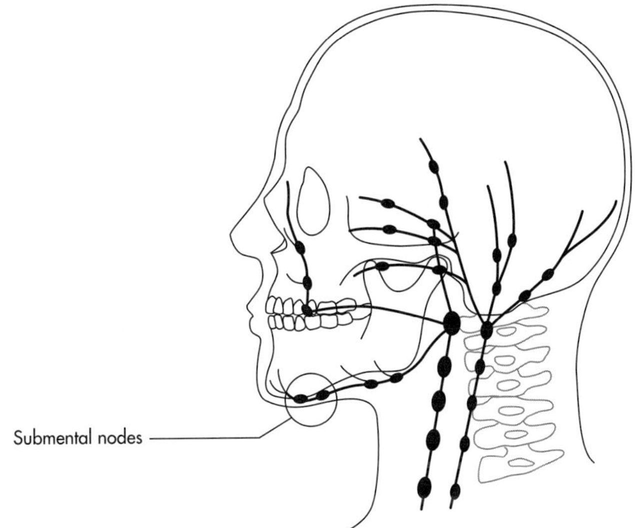

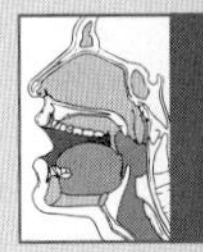

submental

The ______________ lymph nodes drain the lower anterior mandible only.

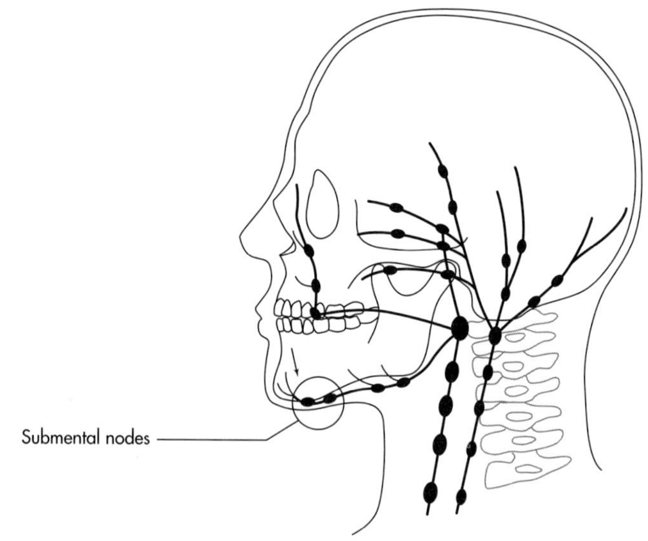

superficial and deep cervical, head and neck

These are the ______________ nodes. They drain the ______________.

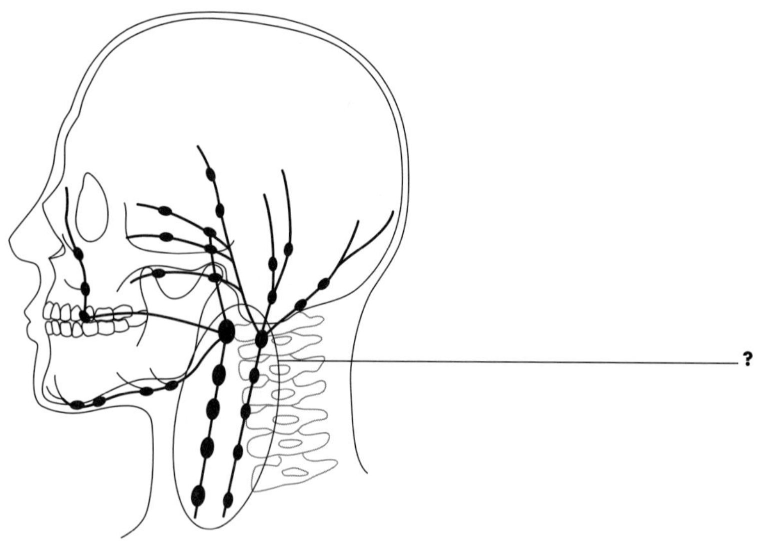

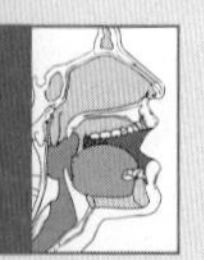

These are the ________ nodes. They drain ________ area.

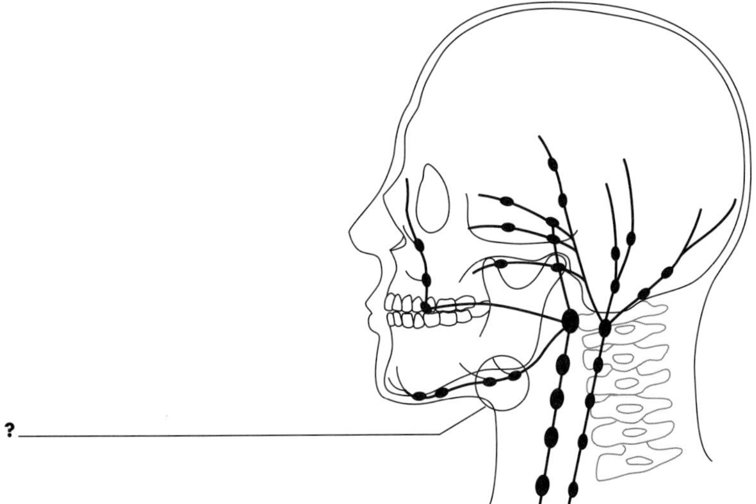

submandibular, most of the maxilla and mandible

These are the ________ nodes. They drain the ________ area.

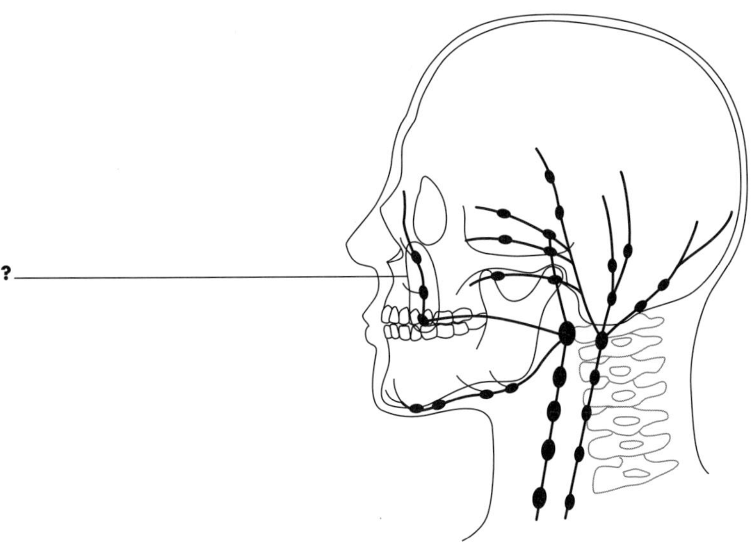

facial, face

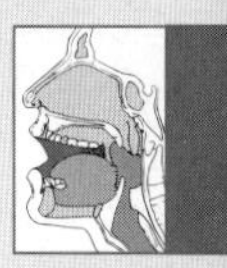

submental, lower anterior mandible

These are the ______________ nodes. They drain the ______________ area.

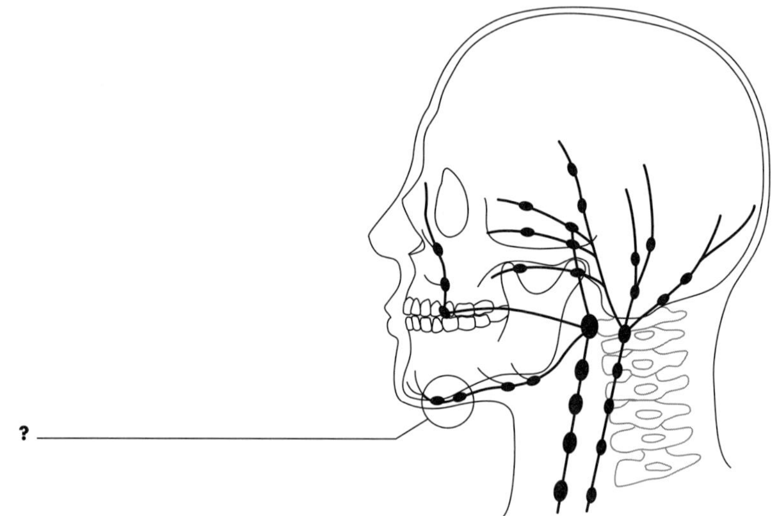

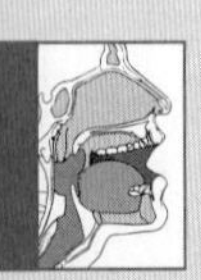

REVIEW TEST 10.1

SELECT OR FILL IN THE CORRECT ANSWER.

1. The name *circulatory system* refers to transportation of a fluid medium through a series of vessels. True or false?

2. ______________ are blood cells that carry O_2/CO_2, and ______________ are defensive cells of the body.

3. The blood vascular system is a(n) ______________-type system; the lymphatic system is an open-type system.

4. ______________ are vessels that supply a body area (such as the head and neck) with blood, and ______________ are vessels that drain an area.

5. What portion of the lymphatic system acts as a "filter," adding lymphocytes and removing foreign substances from the system?

   a. lymph fluid b. lymph nodes
   c. lymph vessels d. thoracic duct

REVIEW TEST 10.2

SELECT OR FILL IN THE CORRECT ANSWER.

1. The main arteries of the neck that supply it and the head are the ______________ arteries.

2. The major veins that drain the head and neck are called the ______________ veins.

3. What structures can be found along the sternocleidomastoid muscle?

   a. carotid arteries b. jugluar veins
   c. CN X d. cervical lymph nodes
   e. all of the above f. none of the above

4. The common carotid artery divides below the mandible into two vessels called the ______________ artery and the ______________ artery.

5. The lingual artery supplies the ______________, and the ______________ vein drains it.

6. The facial artery and vein run over the border of the ______________ to supply the face.

7. The best vessel(s) to use to find a patient's pulse in the head and neck region is the ______________.

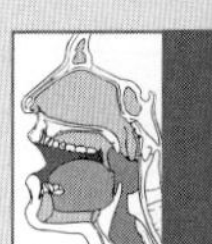

REVIEW TEST 10.3

SELECT OR FILL IN THE CORRECT ANSWER.

1. Which artery is not a branch of the external carotid?

   a. maxillary   b. superficial temporal
   c. vertebral   d. facial

2. Which artery goes behind the neck of the condyle to supply the maxilla and mandible?

3. Match the branch of maxillary artery that supplies each tooth listed.

   a. No. 20 ______________   PSA artery
   b. No. 8 ______________   MSA artery
   c. No. 4 ______________   ASA artery
   d. No. 2 ______________   inferior alveolar artery

4. Which branch of the maxillary artery supplies the posterior palate?

5. Through what foramen does the nasopalatine artery pass?

REVIEW TEST 10.4

SELECT OR FILL IN THE CORRECT ANSWER.

1. What three structures pass through the mandibular foramen into the mandibular canal?

2. The brain has a dual source of blood via which two arteries?

   a. internal and external carotids
   b. internal carotid and vertebral
   c. vertebral and external carotid
   d. jugular and carotid

3. Name the structure created by the connection of the arteries of the brain around the pituitary gland.

4. The "fusion" of the two vertebral arteries creates the ______________ artery.

5. Large venous vessels of the brain are called

   a. sinuses   b. plexus
   c. venules   d. veins

6. The vein connecting the internal and external jugulars, found behind the mandible, is the ______________ vein.

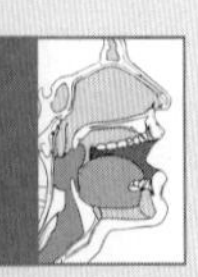

REVIEW TEST 10.5

SELECT OR FILL IN THE CORRECT ANSWER.

1. A network of veins found before the maxillary vein that is one of the hazards for dental PSA block injections is the ______________.

2. A network of veins found at the base of the brain, around the pituitary gland, is the ______________.

3. The cavernous sinus connects with

   a. facial veins b. veins at base of brain
   c. pterygoid plexus d. all of the above

4. What three things pass through the supraorbital foramen?

5. Which sinus lies in the groove between the parietal bones and between the two hemispheres of the brain?

6. Which of these structures is not in or around the pituitary fossa?

   a. pituitary gland b. cavernous sinus
   c. CN V d. CN III
   e. carotid arteries f. CN X

7. Infection could pass from the pterygoid plexus to the cavernous sinus. True or false?

8. Tissue fluid and/or infection drains to which nodes from these areas?

   a. face ______________ facial nodes
   b. mandibular posterior teeth ______________ submandibular nodes
   c. back of ear ______________ submental nodes
   d. mandibular anterior teeth ______________ preauricular nodes
   postauricular nodes

9. Where can you find the cervical lymph nodes?

10. Name three things found in the infratemporal fossa.

11. The major veins that drain the inside of the cranium, exiting through two large, irregular foramina, are called the ______________ veins.

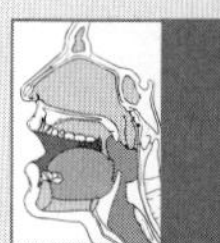

REVIEW TEST 10.6

LABEL THE DIAGRAMS.

1.

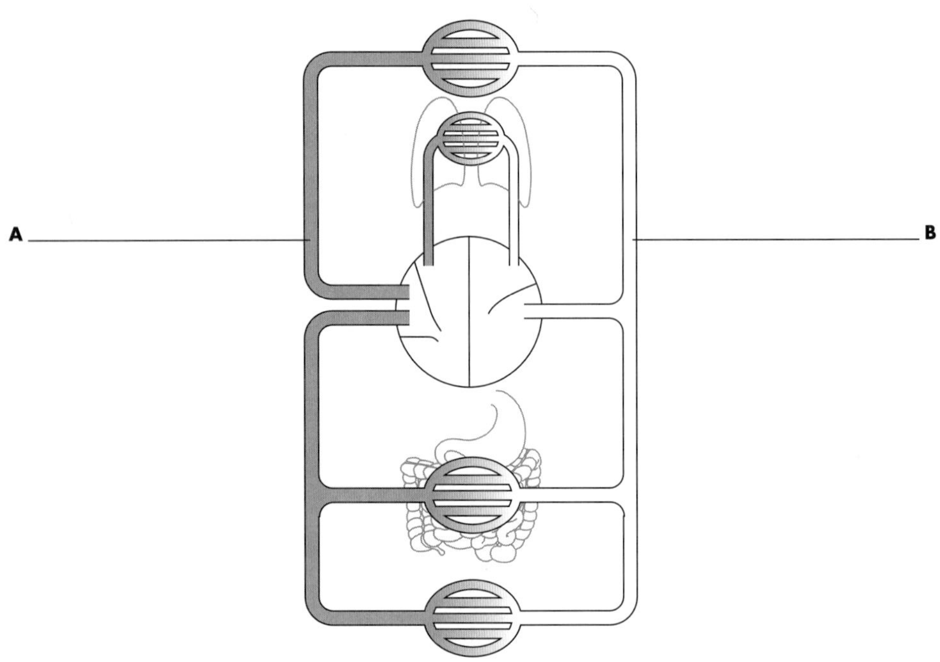

2.

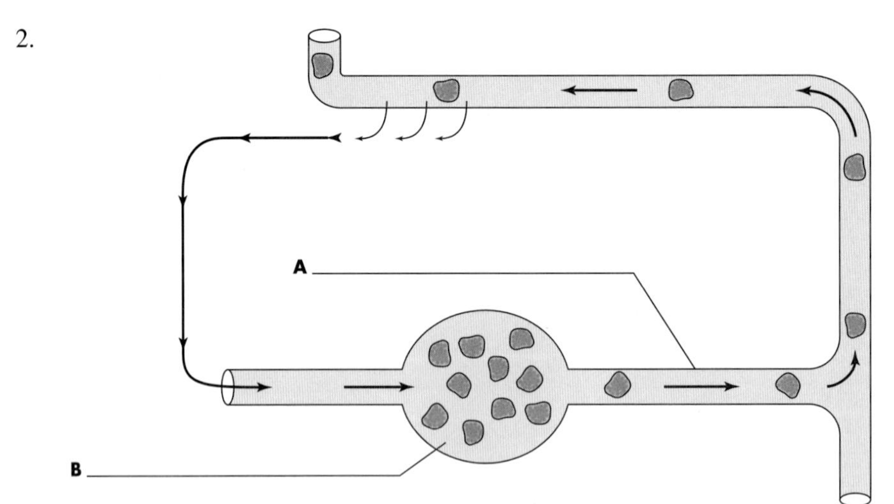

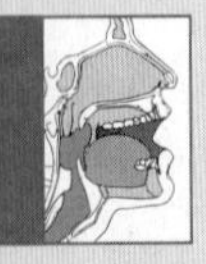

3.

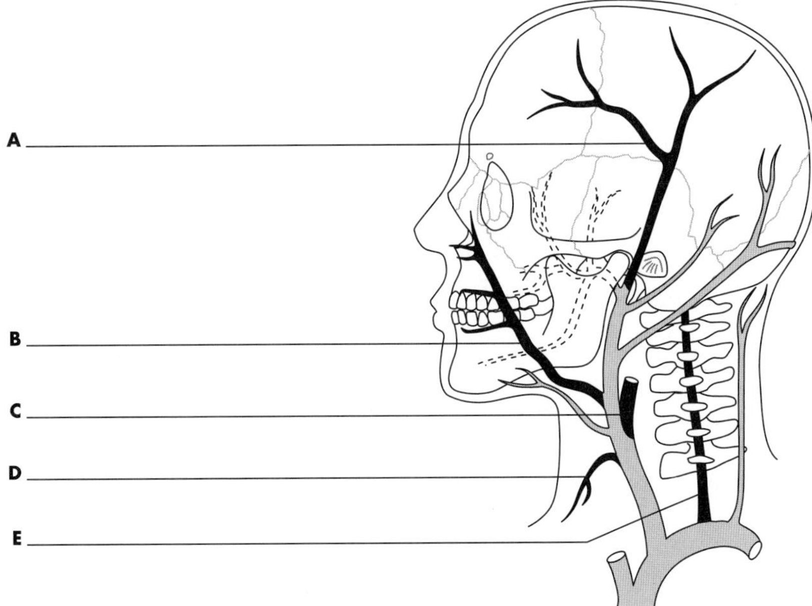

4.

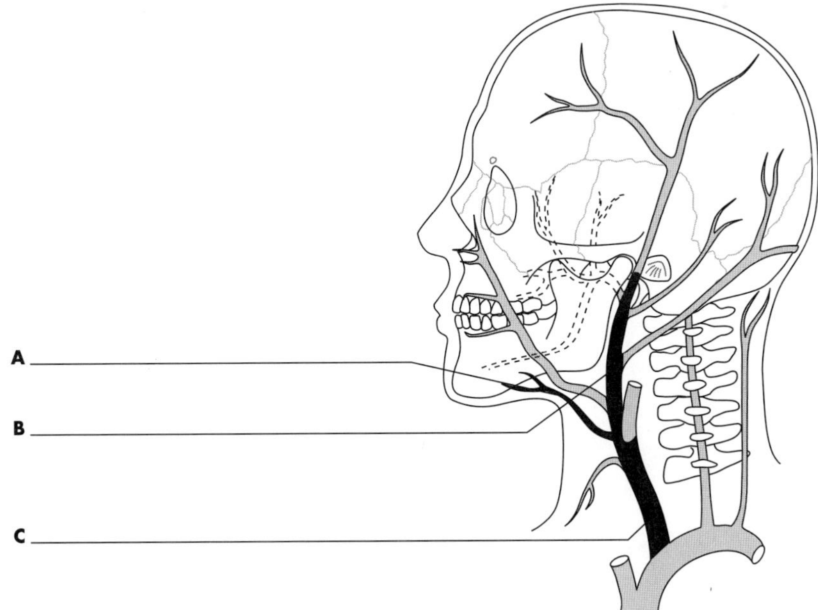

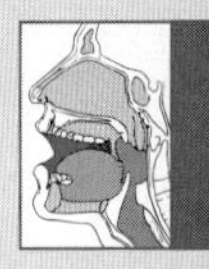

5.

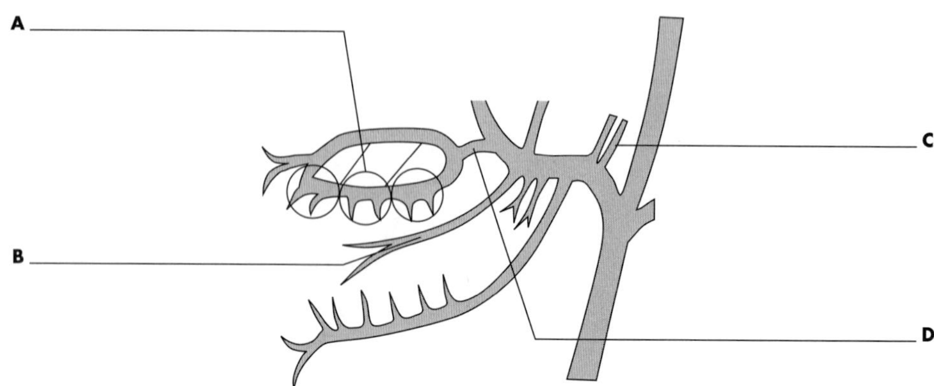

6.

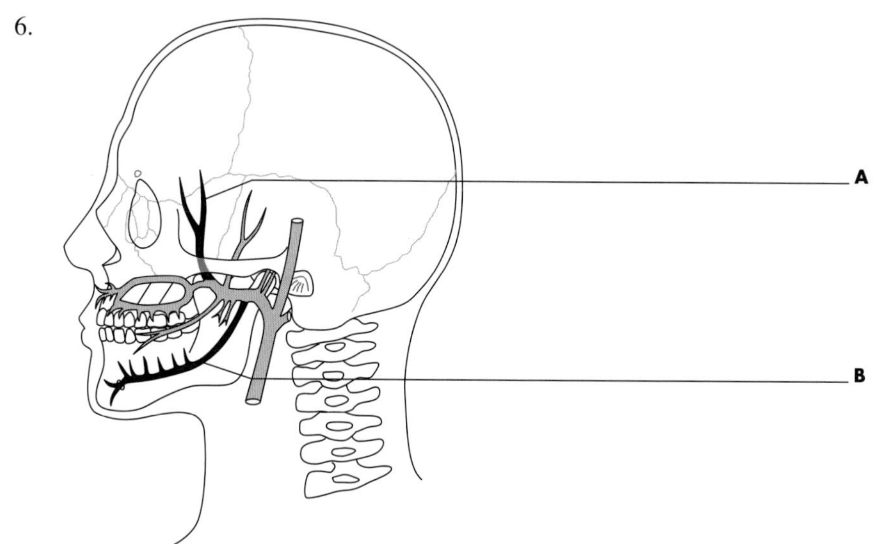

7.

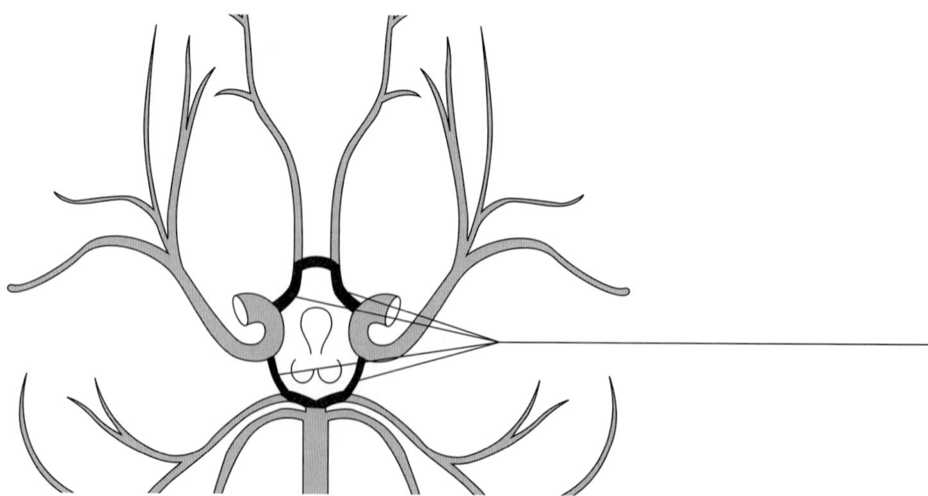

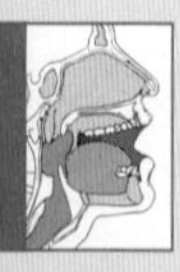

8.

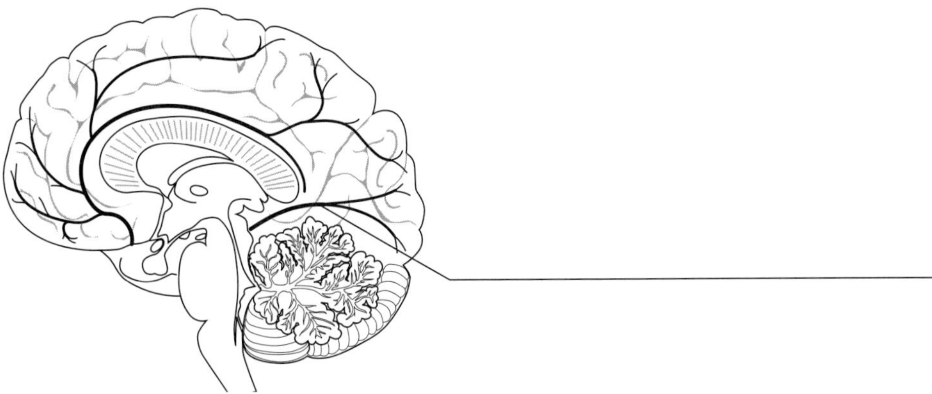

9.

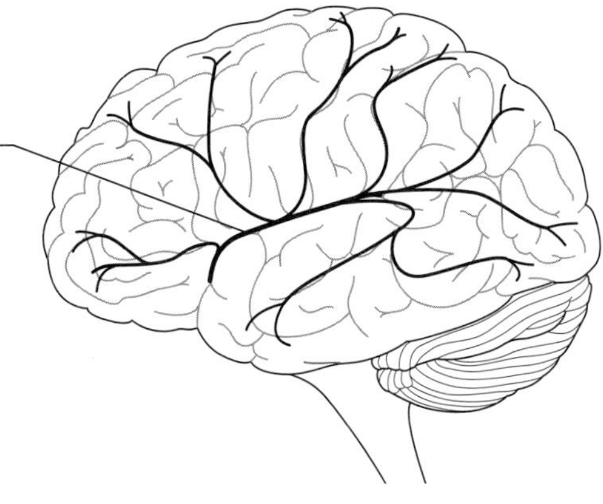

10.

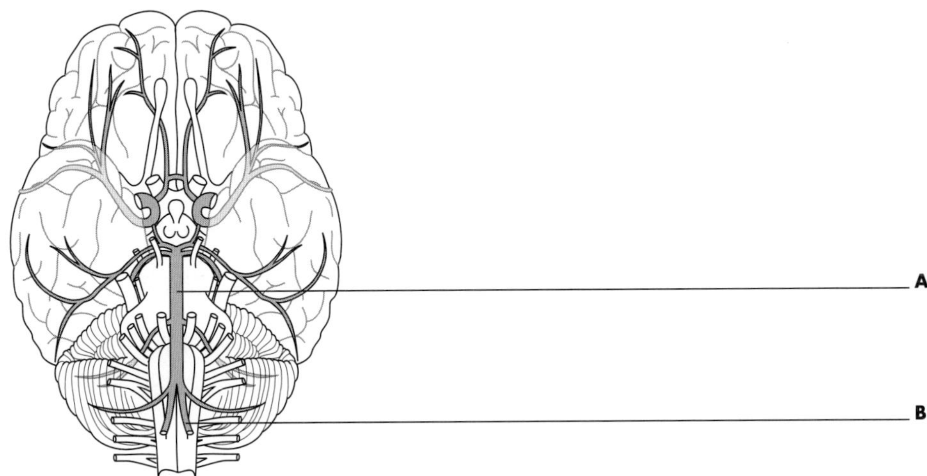

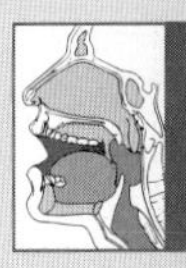

11.

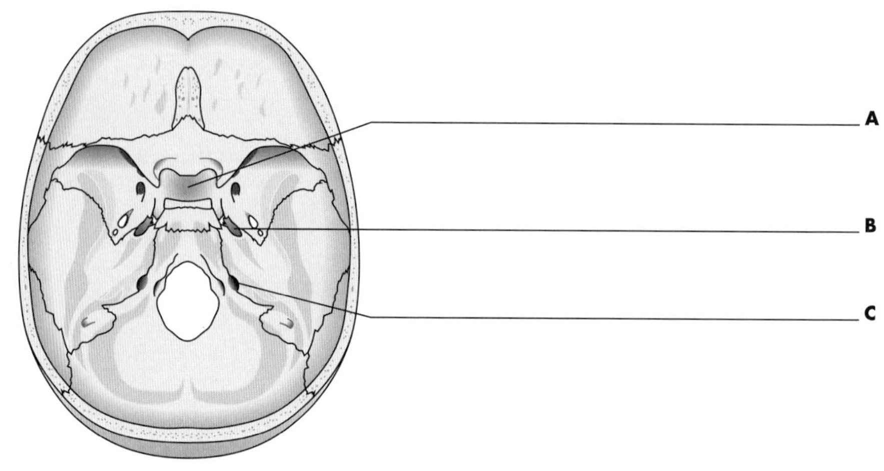

12.

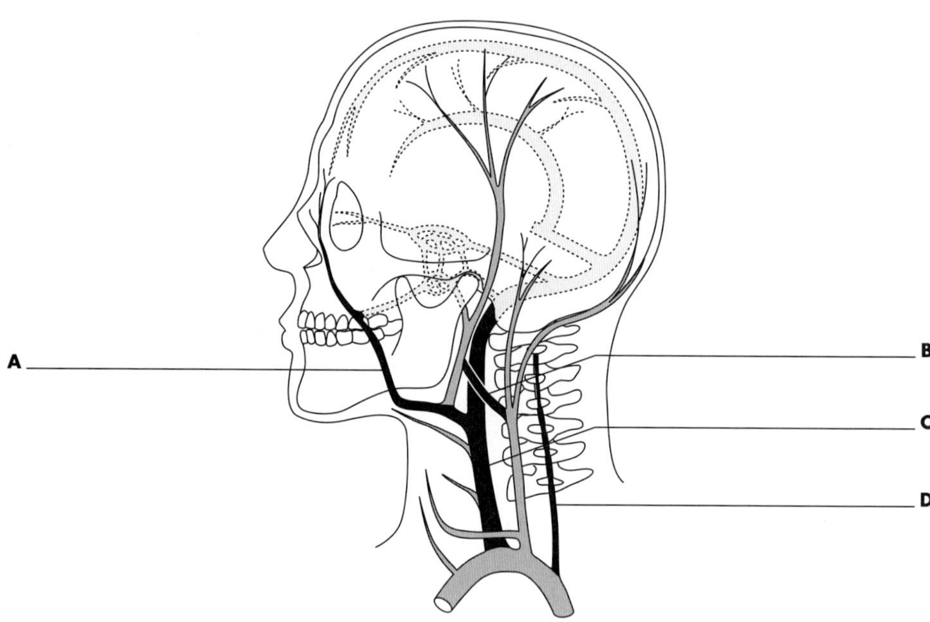

13.

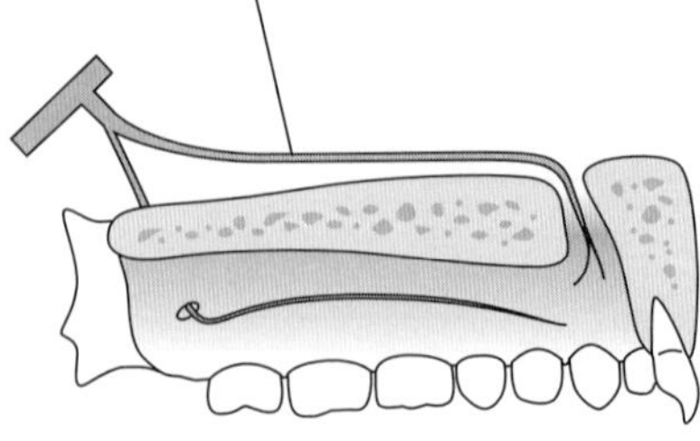

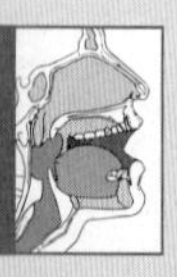

14.

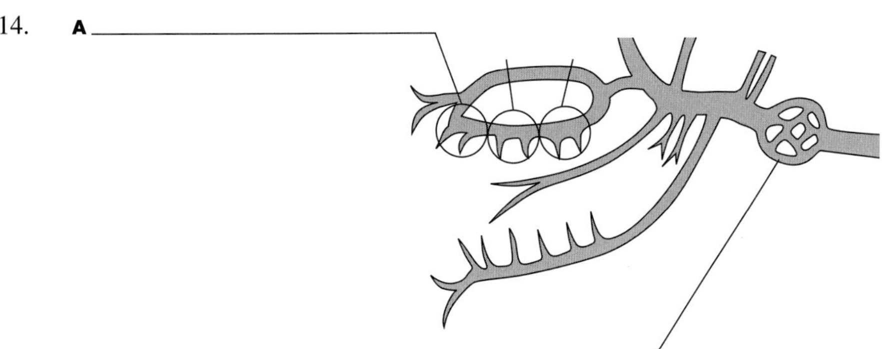

15.

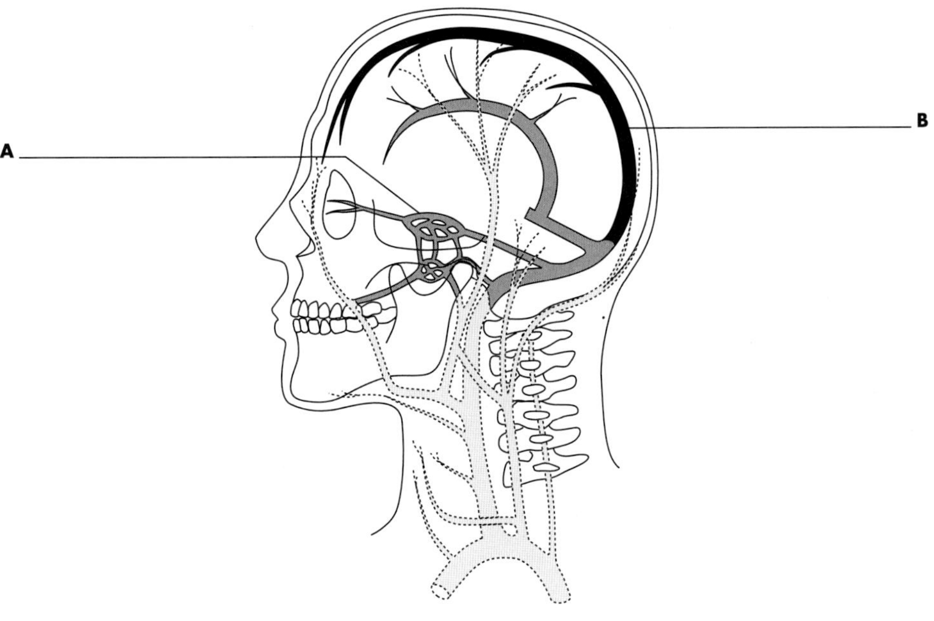

16.

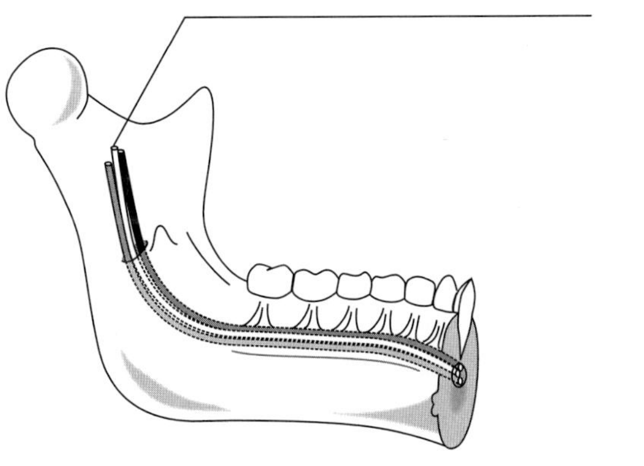

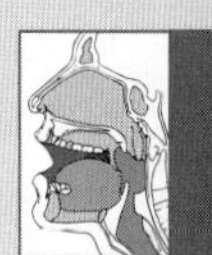

17.

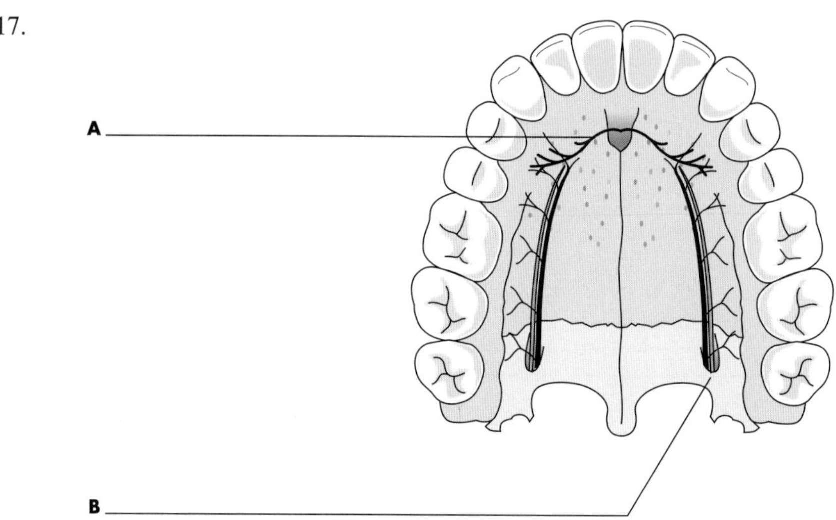

18.

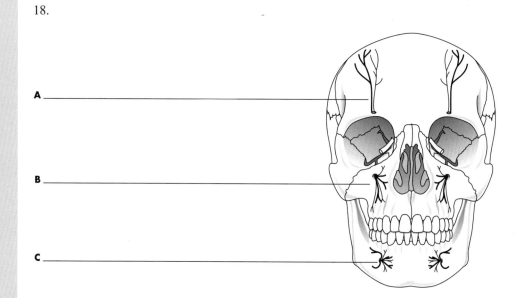

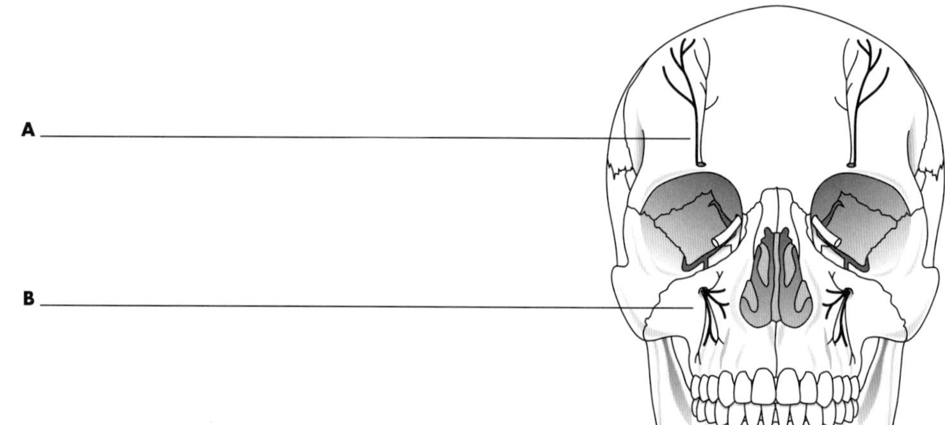

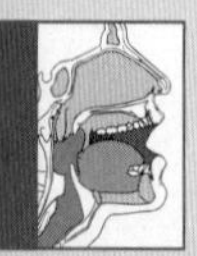

19.

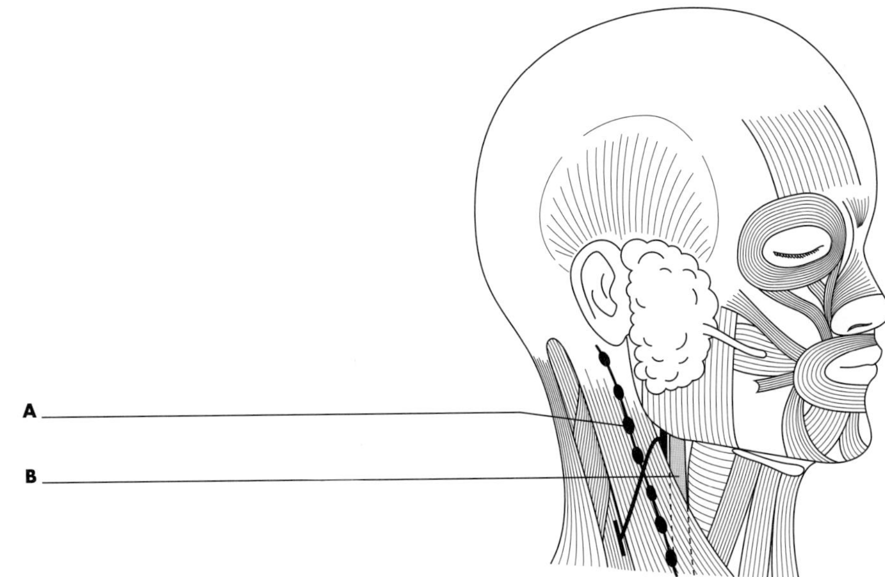

20.

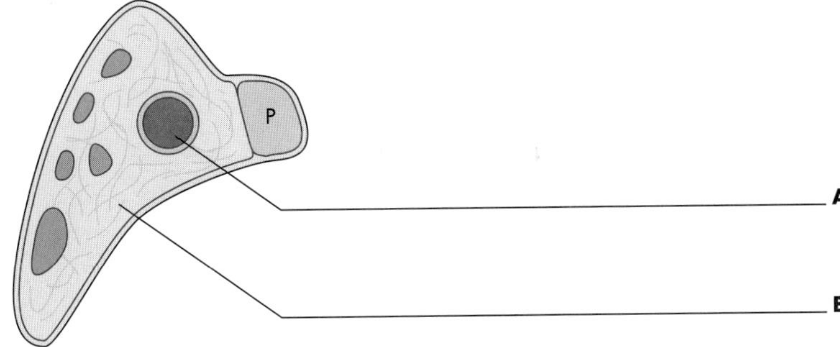

21.

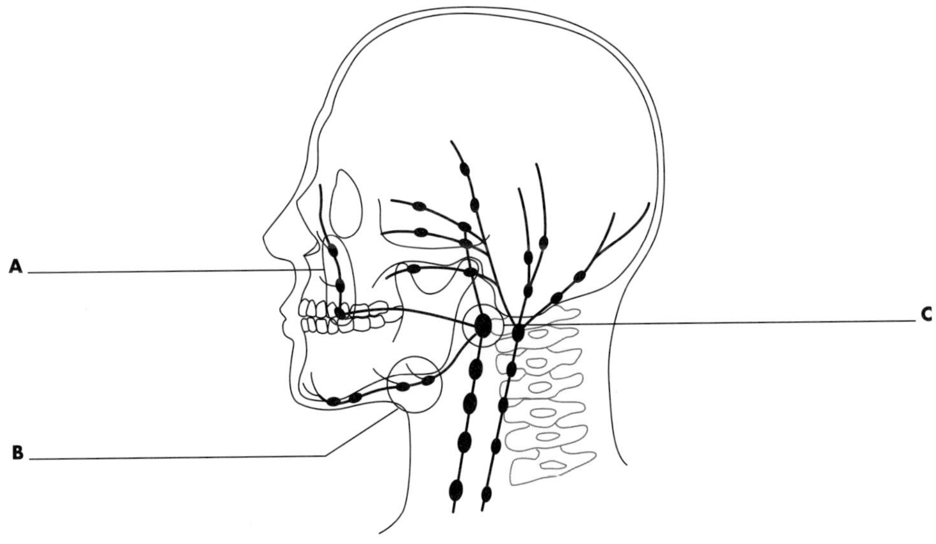

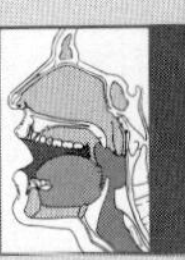

22.

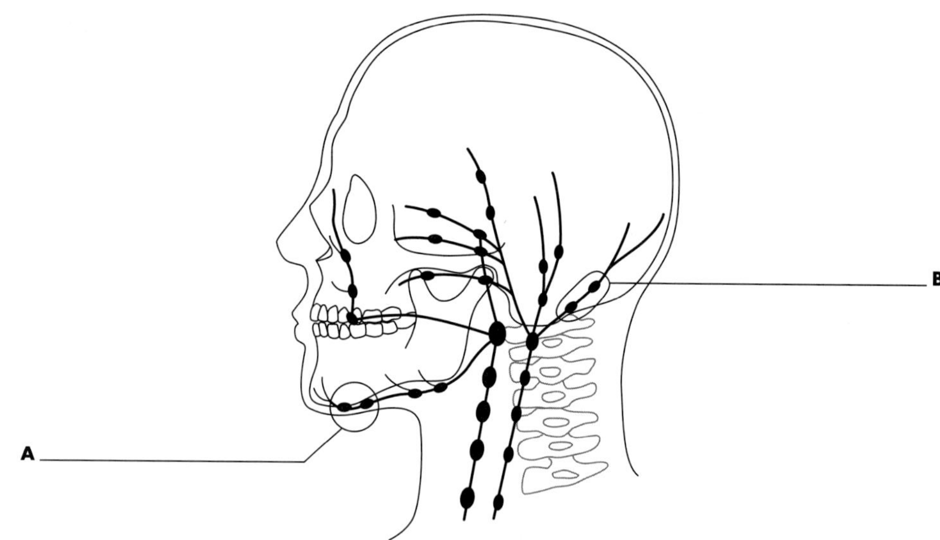

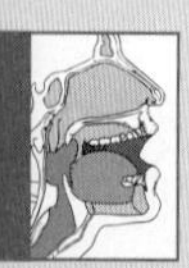

11 Other Systems

Portions of the following systems are also present in the head and neck areas of the body. Let's look at them. We often refer to this drawing, which is a sagittal slice bisecting the head and neck. Can you find the brain and spinal cord, vertebral column, cranium, and hyoid bone?

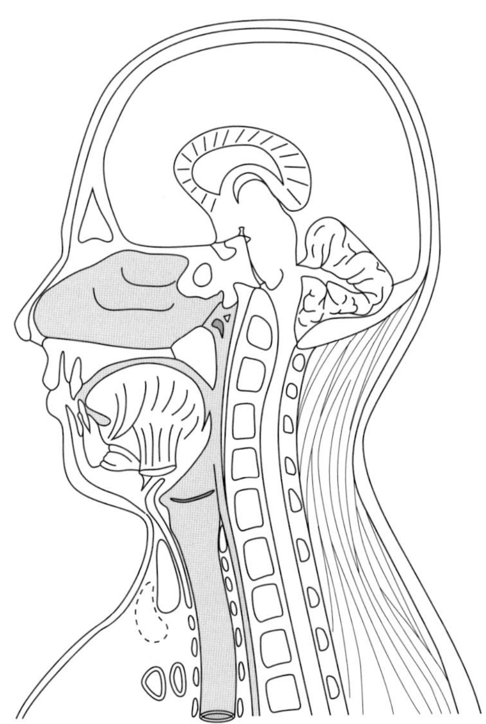

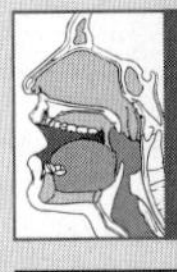

1.0 DIGESTIVE SYSTEM

The beginning of the digestive system lies in the head and neck, commencing with the **oral cavity, pharynx,** and **esophagus.** Find these, as well as the **nasal cavity,** which lies directly above the oral cavity.

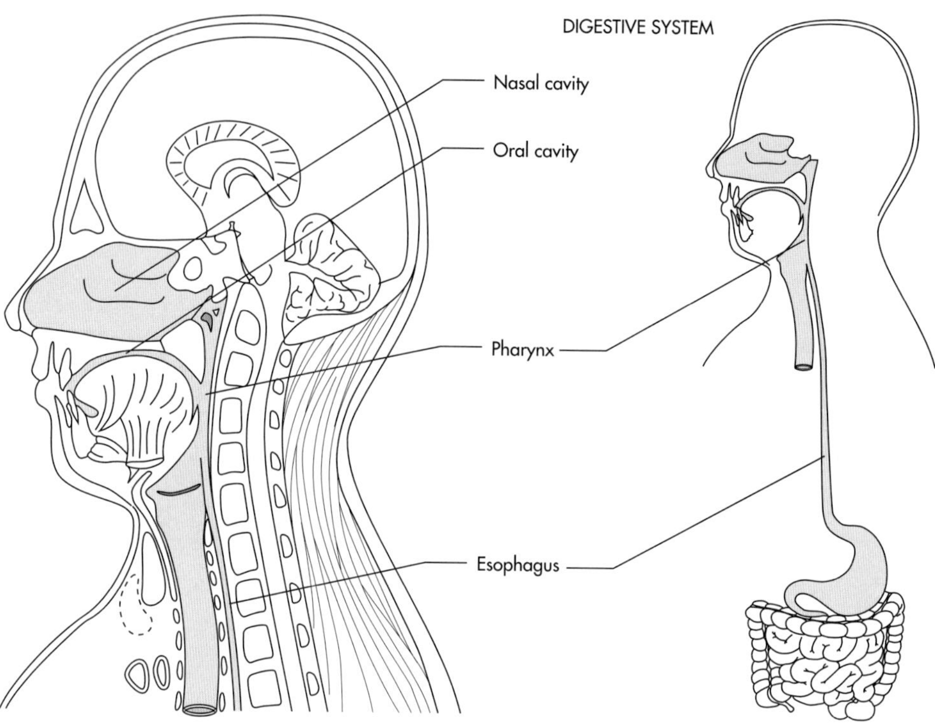

hard and soft palate

What structure separates the oral and nasal cavities?

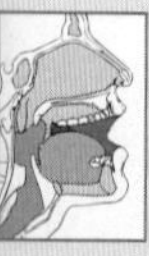

Oral Cavity Landmarks and Anatomy, Pharyngeal Anatomy, and Esophagus

1.1

ORAL CAVITY

Digestion begins in the ______________ cavity, where food is masticated (chewed). After being processed into a **bolus,** food undergoes **deglutition** or swallowing, which begins in the oral cavity and continues in the pharynx and, then, in the esophagus.

oral

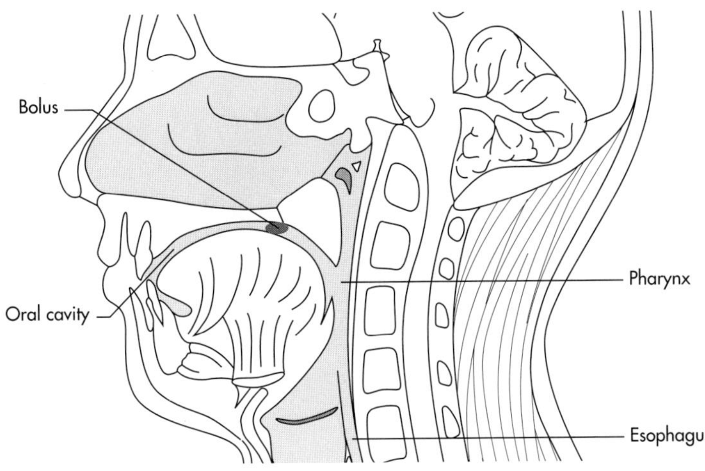

Find the following structures belonging to the digestive system: oral cavity, nasal cavity, palate, pharynx, esophagus.

A. nasal cavity
B. oral cavity
C. pharynx

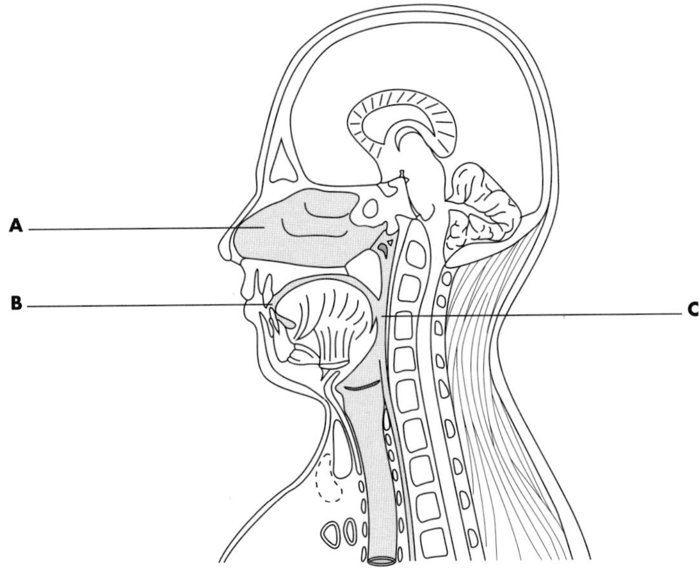

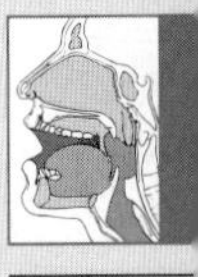

Reviewing Chapter Six on mucosa, please locate these structures found within the oral cavity: maxillary teeth, mandibular teeth, tongue (anterior and posterior), hard and soft palate, buccal mucosa, Stensen's duct, Wharton's duct, sublingual plica, sublingual caruncles, ducts of Rivinus, tonsillar pillars (fauces), palatine tonsils, pharynx, alveolar mucosa and bone, lips. Check the next diagram to test yourself.

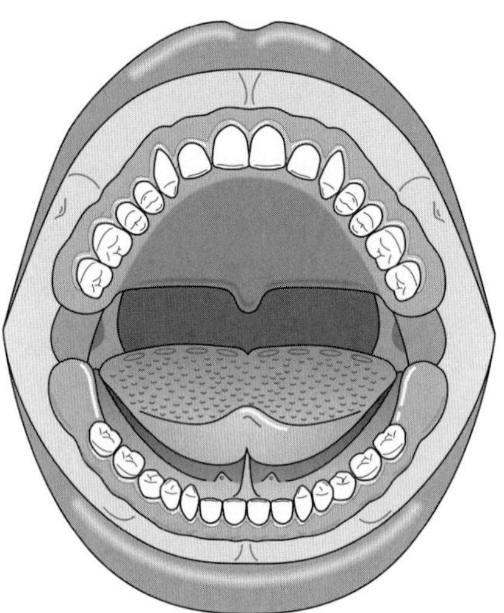

Earlier, we considered these structures as mucosa-covered structures. Now we need to view them as total parts of the functioning oral cavity.

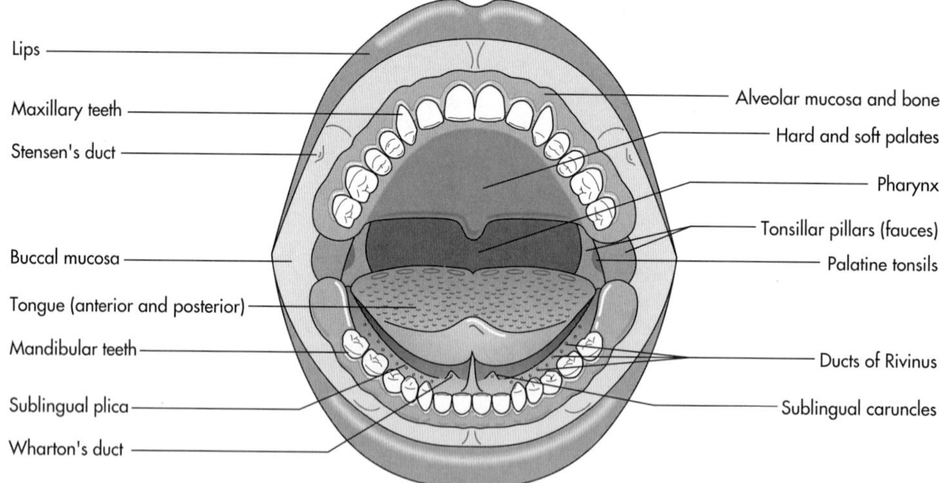

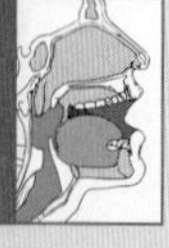

For example, the teeth are essential to the process of breaking down food called **mastication.** ______________ is the process of chewing, which breaks down the food mechanically and adds saliva to create a bolus ready for swallowing. This occurs in the ______________ cavity.

mastication, oral

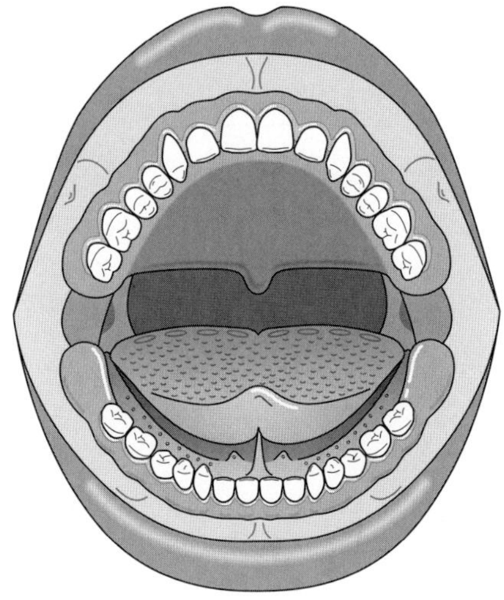

Below the mucosa are muscles and bone of the oral cavity. The bony structure includes the **maxilla** and the ______________.

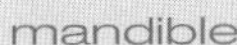

mandible

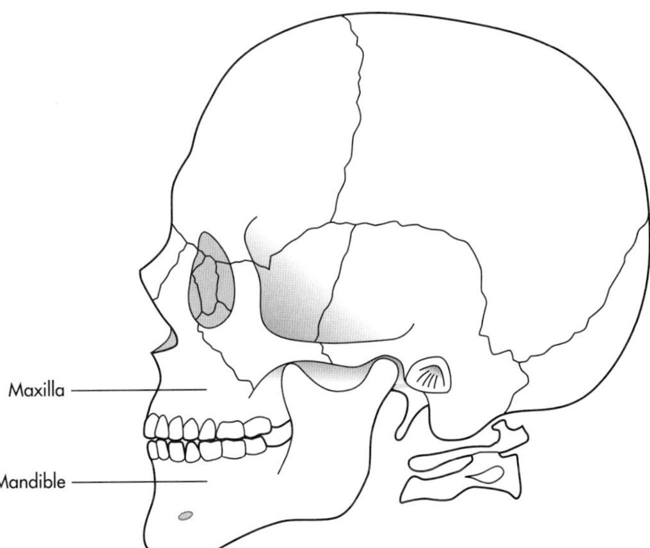

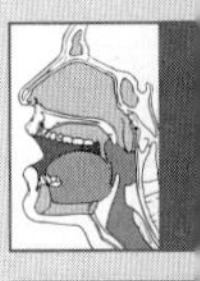

temporo-
mandibular

The joint between the cranium and jaw is known as the ______________ joint or **TMJ.** Review its anatomy. This is a unique joint in the body, in that it is really two joints in one.

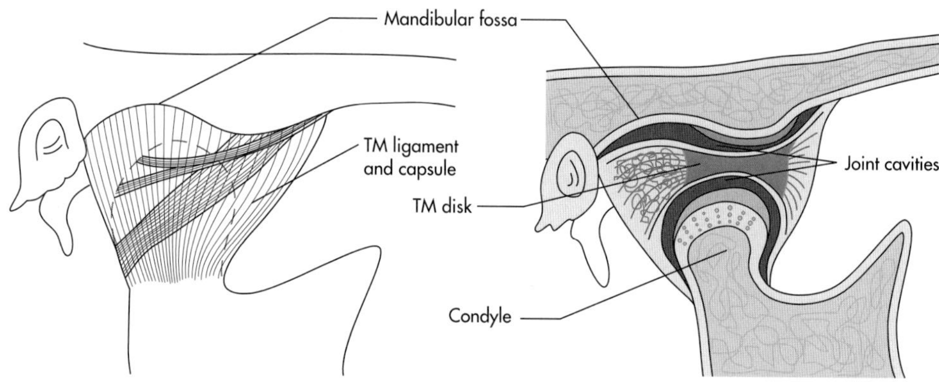

lateral pterygoid

The TMJ is divided into two compartments, **superior** and **inferior joint cavities,** by the **temporomandibular (TM) disk,** a fibrous pad of protective tissue. Which muscle inserts into this disk and is responsible for maintaining it in place?

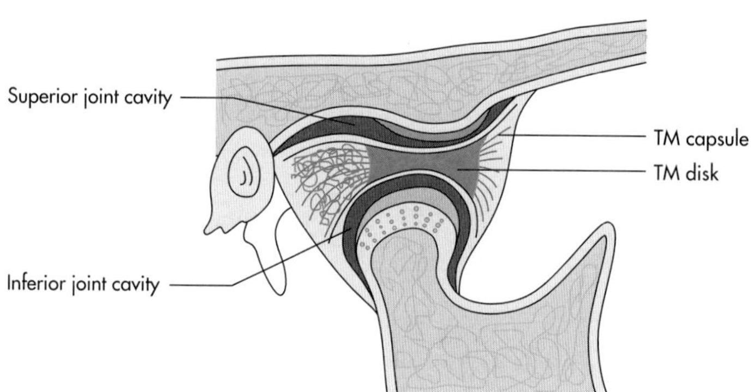

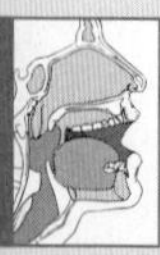

Musculature of the oral cavity includes three of the muscle groups we studied. First are the **muscles of mastication.** Find and name them. What are their origins and insertions?

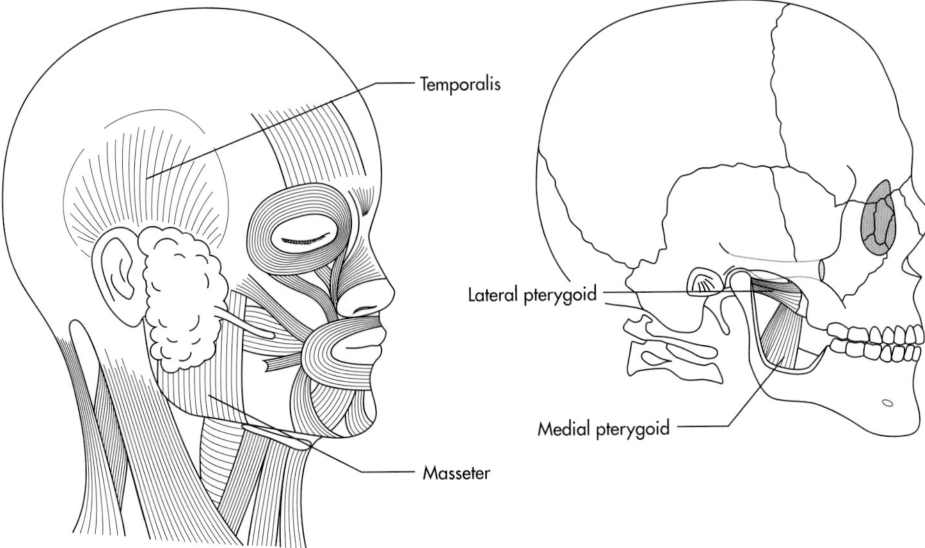

1. temporalis (o-temporal fossa, i-coronoid process)
2. masseter (o-zygomatic arch, i-angle of mandible)
3. medial pterygoid (o-pterygoid plate, i-angle of mandible)
4. lateral pterygoid (o-pterygoid plate, i-neck of condyle, disk)

Which cranial nerve innervates these muscles and what are their actions?

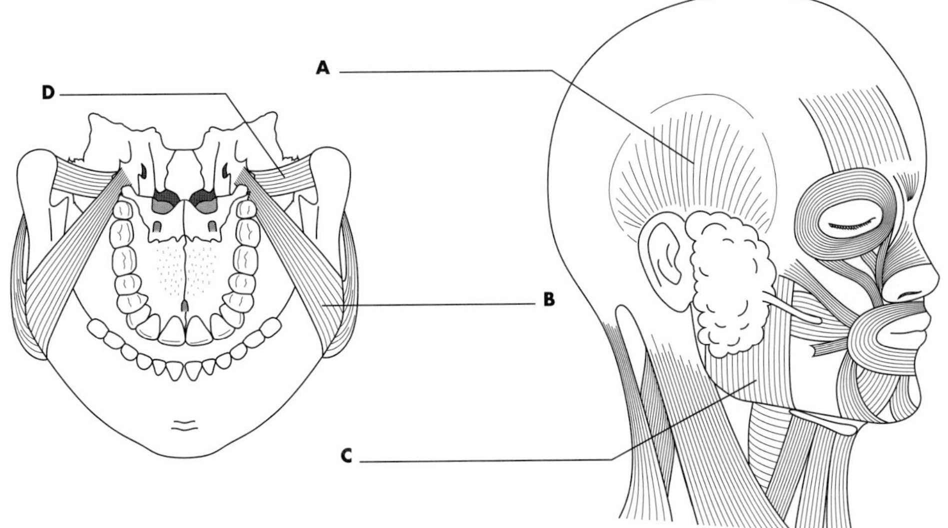

CN—V3; (a)temporalis, (b)medial pterygoid, and (c)masseter are elevators of mandible (d)lateral pterygoid is responsible for lateral and protrusive motion

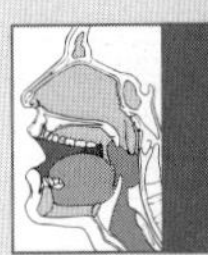

buccinator, suprahyoid

Other muscles that aid in the function of the oral cavity are the muscles of the cheek, or _______________ muscles, and muscles found below the mandible and above the hyoid, known as _______________ muscles.

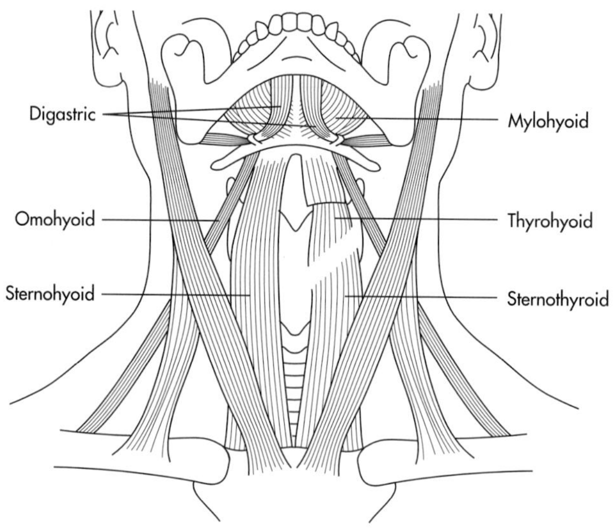

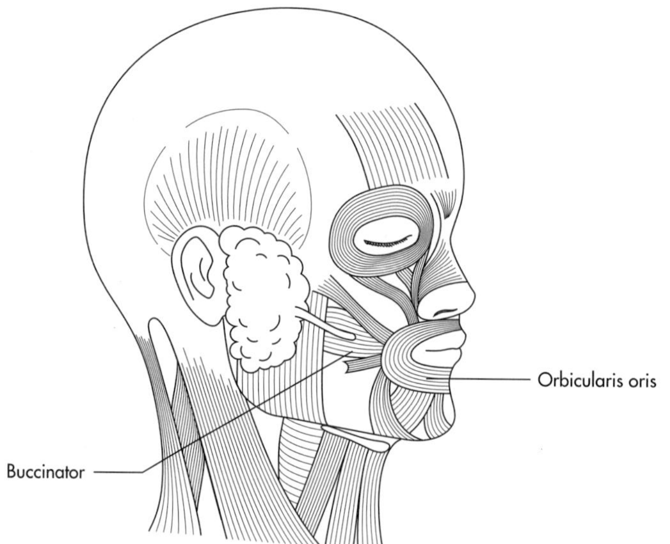

VII

The **buccinator** moves the bolus of food in towards the tongue. This is aided by the lip muscles or **orbicularis oris.** The buccinator muscle is one of the facial expression muscles innervated by CN _______________.

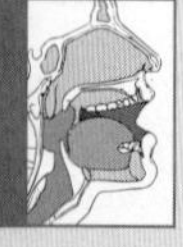

The **suprahyoid muscles** have what action on the mandible? This is the opposite action of what muscles?

depress the mandible, elevators (temporalis, etc.)

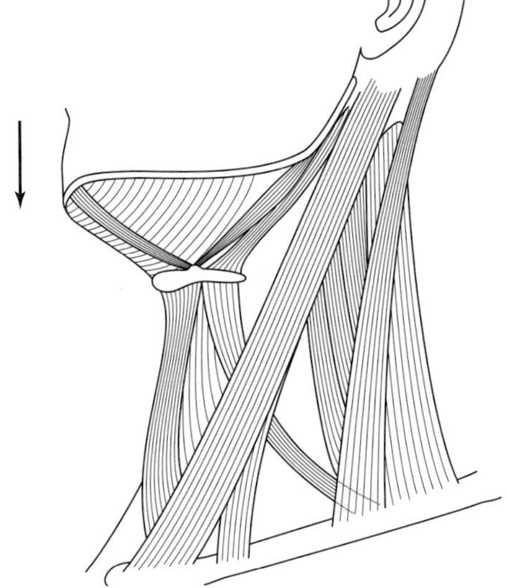

Another group of muscles within the oral cavity are the **tongue muscles.** Review them.

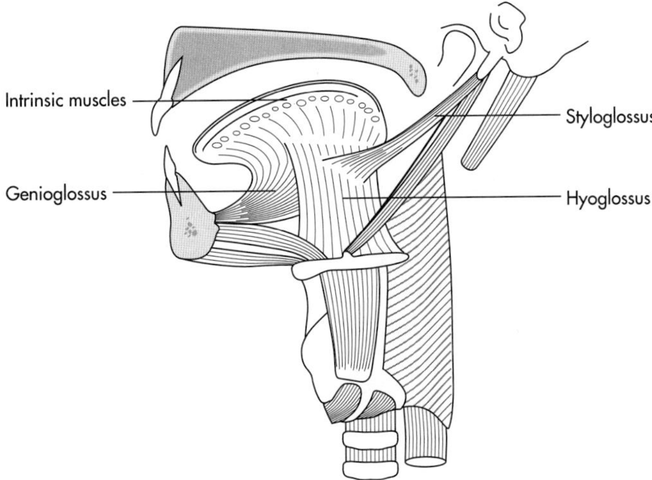

What nerve innervates these muscles?

CN XII

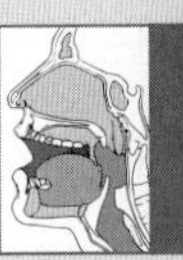

Emptying into the oral cavity are the ducts of the **major salivary glands.** Name those three glands and their ducts. Saliva is used to make the bolus and to begin chemical digestion.

1. parotid gland
2. sublingual gland
3. submandibular gland

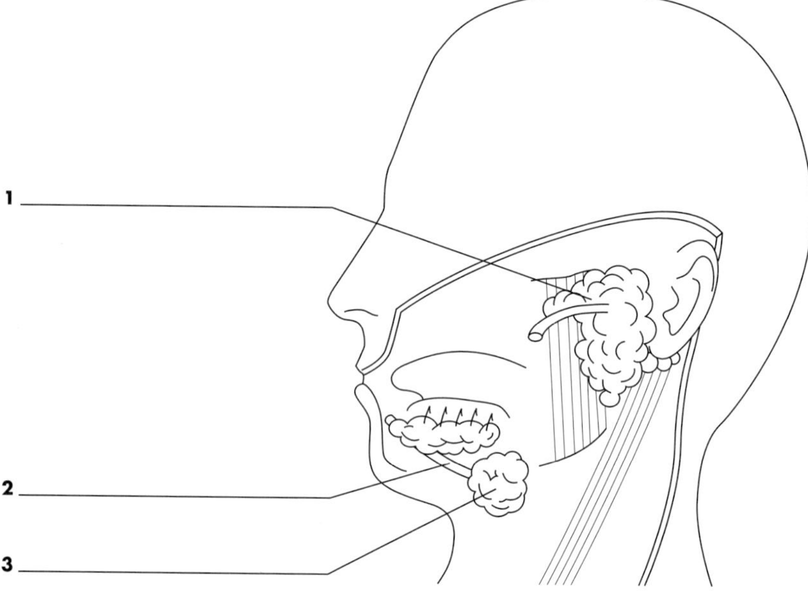

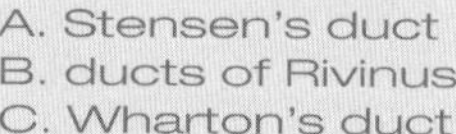

A. Stensen's duct
B. ducts of Rivinus
C. Wharton's duct

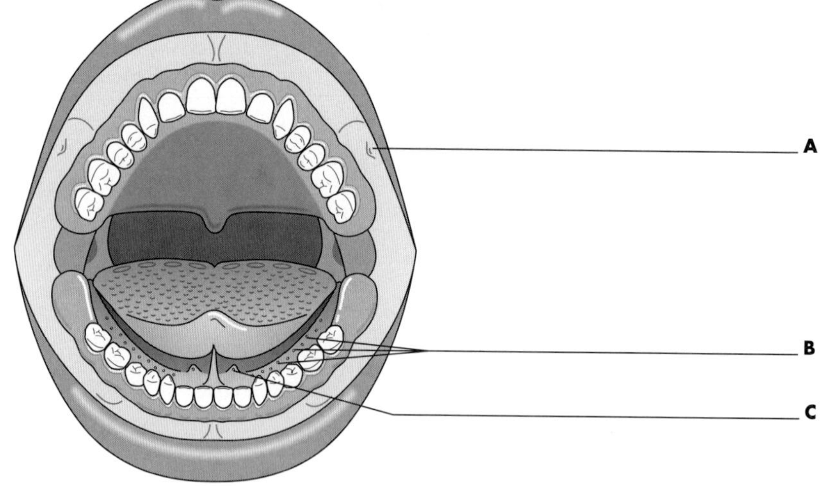

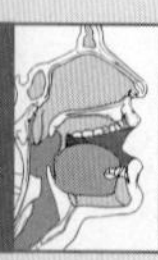

PHARYNX

The next portion of the "food tube" is the **pharynx,** which you see divides into three regions.

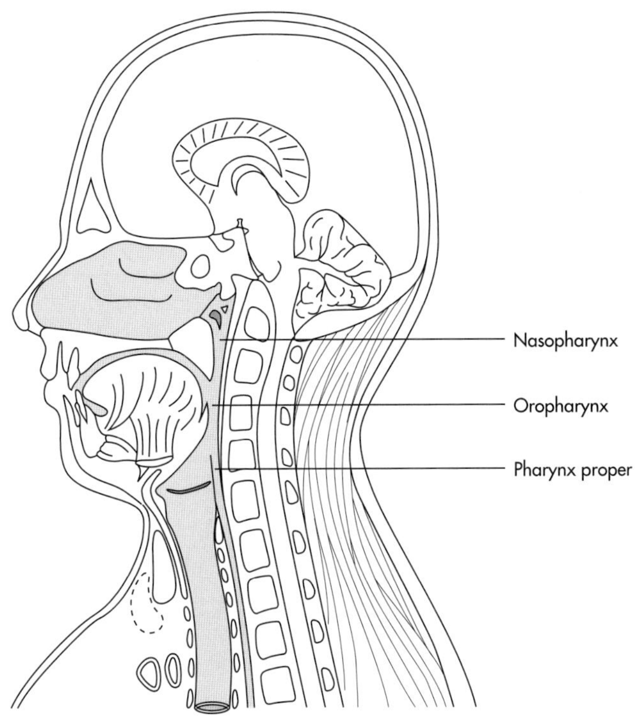

Label the three regions of the pharynx.

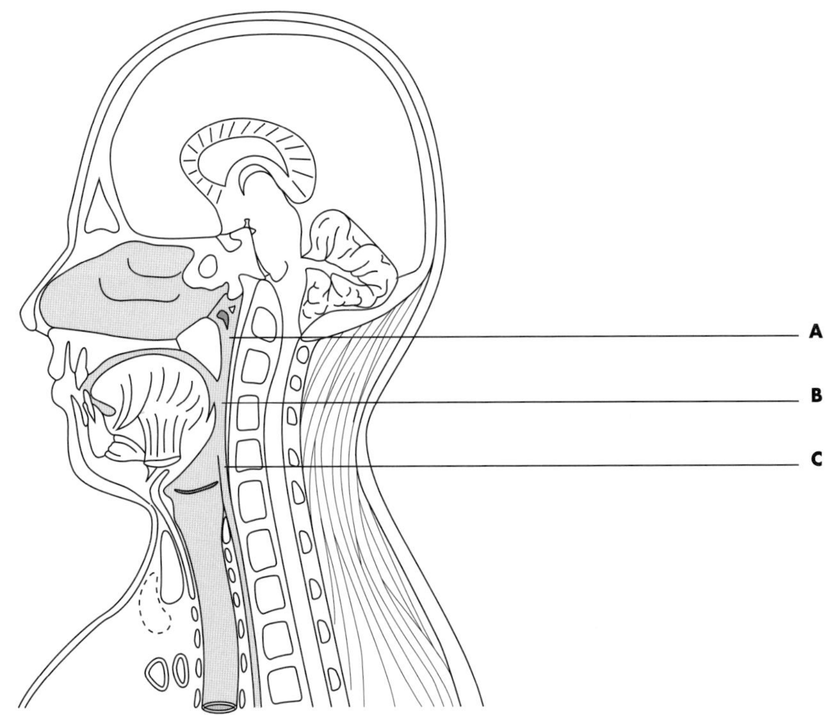

A. nasopharynx
B. oropharynx
C. pharynx proper

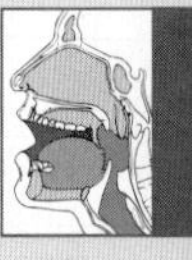

The **oropharynx** is the region directly adjacent to the oral cavity and visible from the open mouth. Find the **hard palate, soft palate, tongue,** and **epiglottis.**

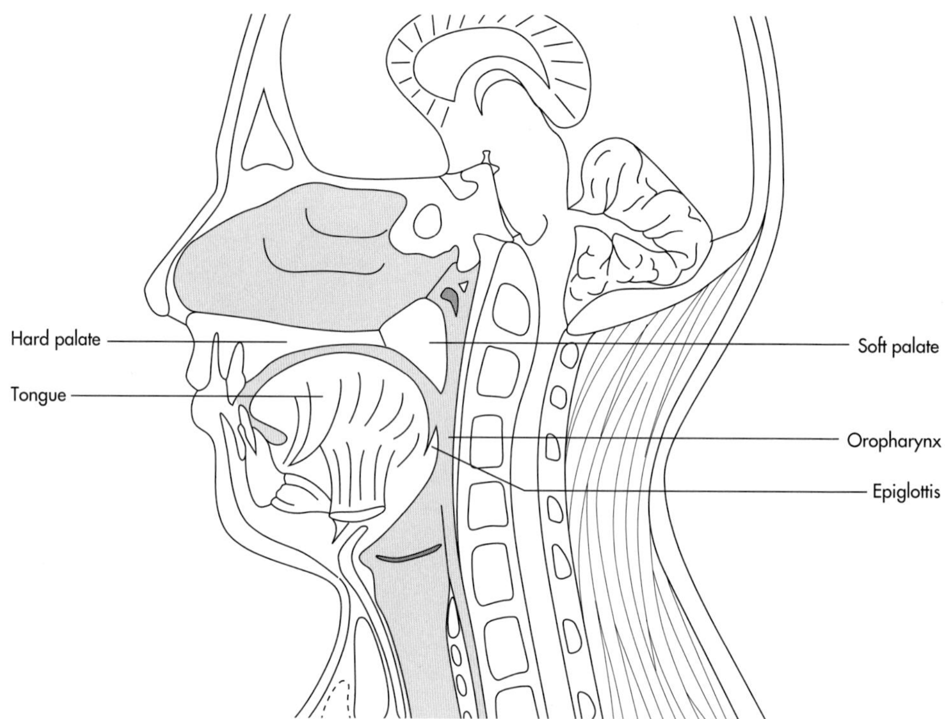

Review the muscles of the oral cavity and oropharynx. Find the **buccinator, pterygomandibular raphe, superior constrictor,** and **Stensen's duct.**

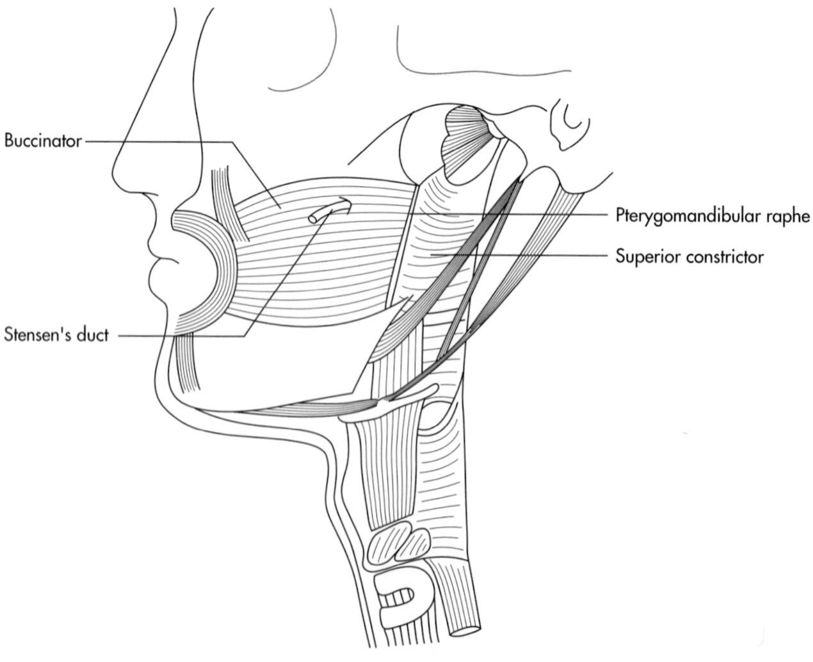

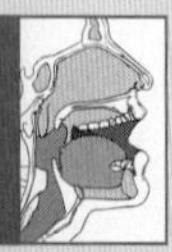

Find the muscles of the palate: **palatoglossus, palatopharyngeus,** tensor veli palatini (TVP), and levator veli palatini (LVP).

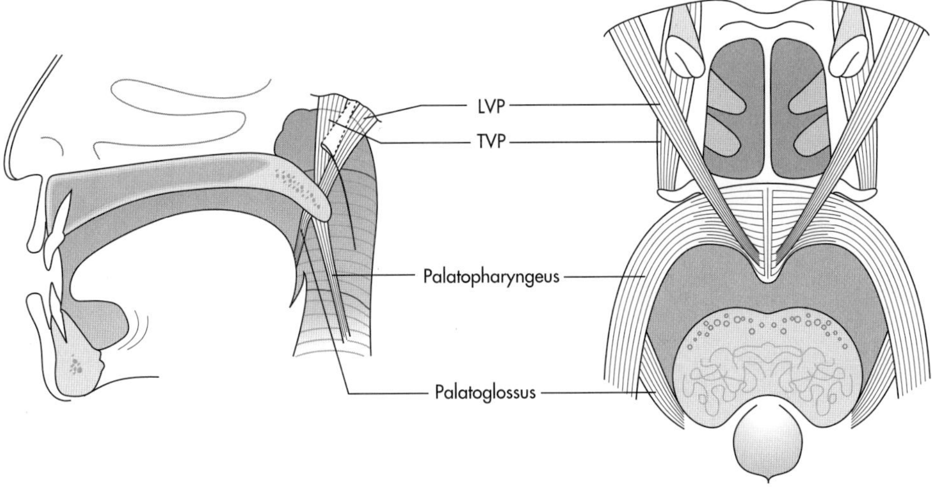

The palatoglossus and palatopharyngeus are covered by oral mucosa and are seen in the mouth as a landmark called the pharyngeal ______________.

pillars

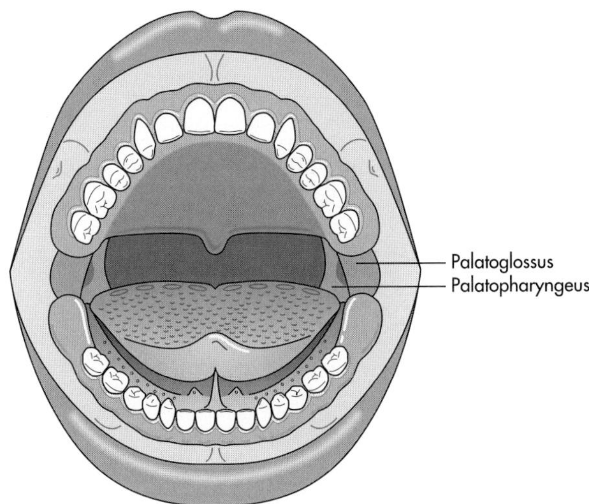

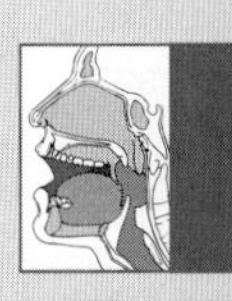

CN X

The **constrictors** act on the pharynx to squeeze the tube from top to bottom. What cranial nerve innervates these muscles? This muscular action is involuntary once initiated at the top of the oropharnx.

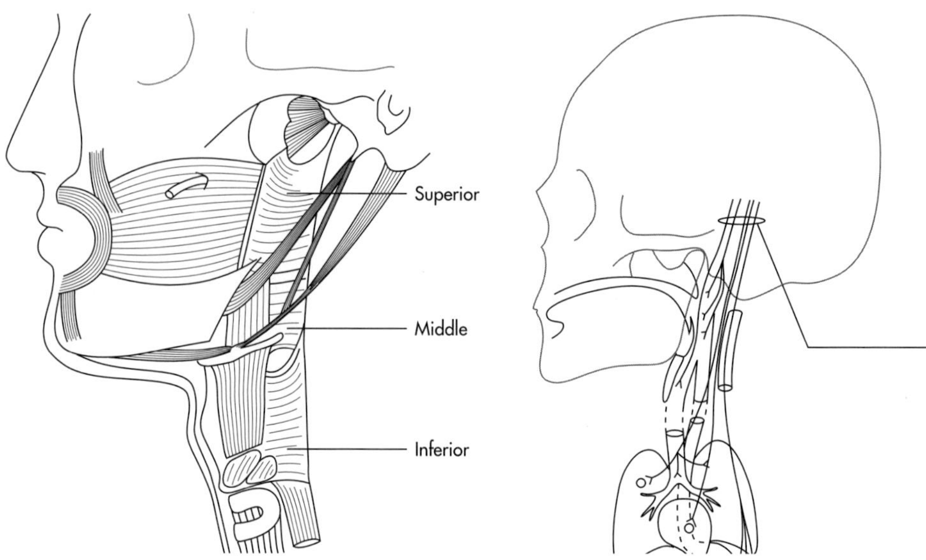

The muscles of the pharynx are a blend of skeletal muscle fibers that make a transition to smooth muscle fibers toward the esophagus.

CN IX

The presence of something (bolus or any object) triggers the sensory nerves of the pharyngeal mucosa. Which cranial nerve is the sensory innervation to the pharynx?

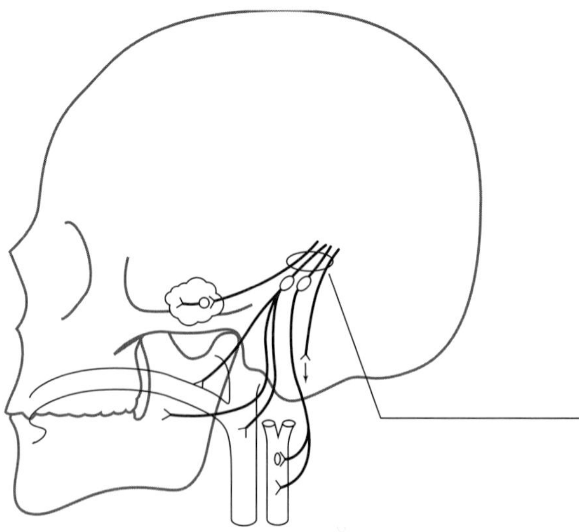

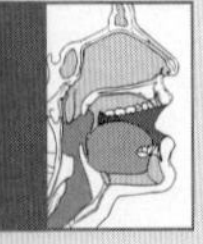

The next portion of the pharynx is the **nasopharynx,** which is directly superior to the oropharynx. It forms the back of what cavity?

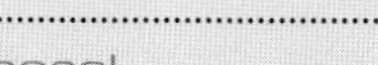

nasal

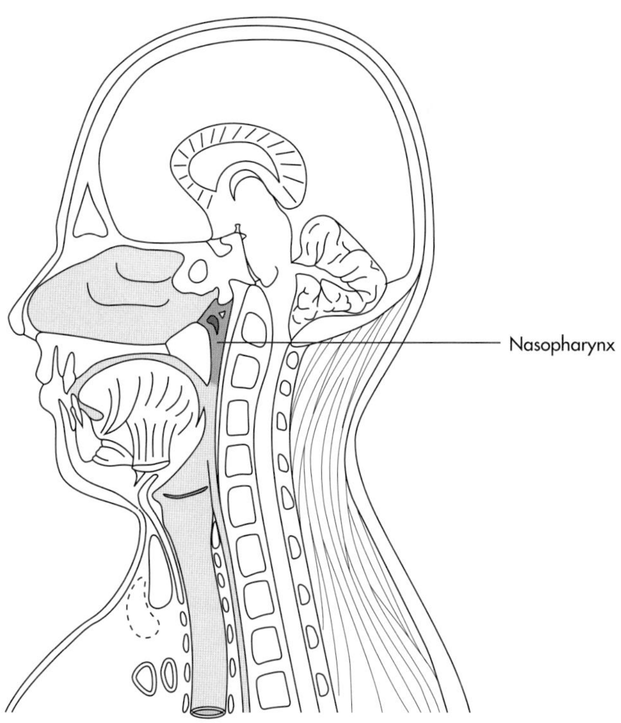

The nasal cavity is separated from the oral cavity by the ______________, but has continuity by way of the nasopharynx. Again, look at the musculature of the palate and nasopharynx.

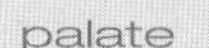

palate

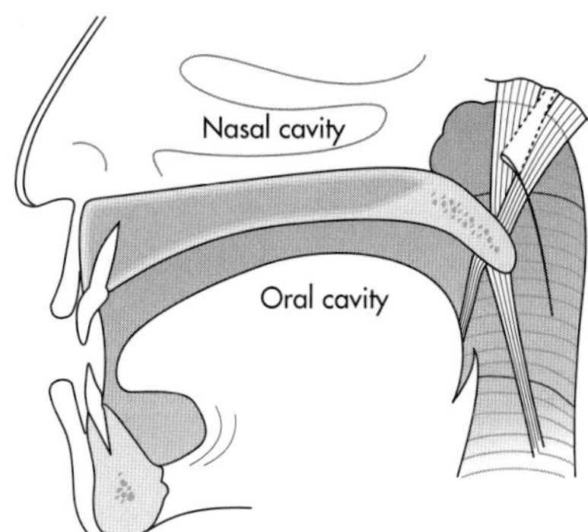

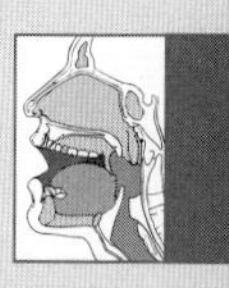

Two structures are found within the nasopharynx. The first is an opening into the middle ear via a tube called the **Eustachian** or **tympanic tube.** Find it.

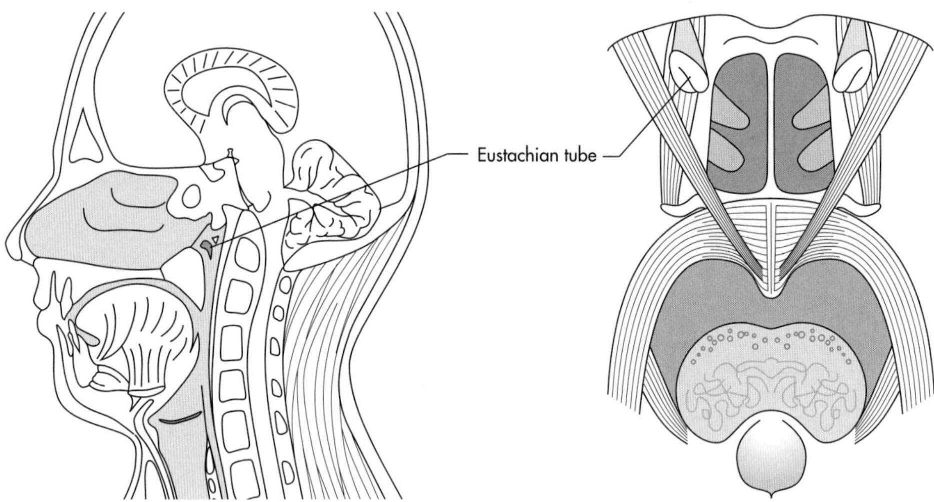

TVP

What palatal muscle regulates the opening of the Eustachian tube?

The second structure is the **pharyngeal tonsil.** Find it.

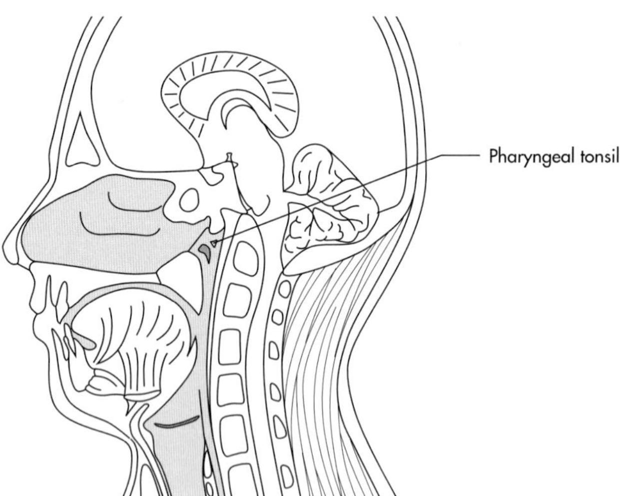

Eustachian tube, pharyngeal tonsil

What two structures are found in the nasopharynx?

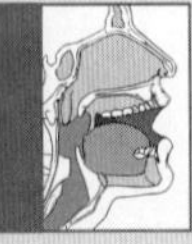

The last portion of the pharynx is the **pharynx proper,** which is below the oropharynx.

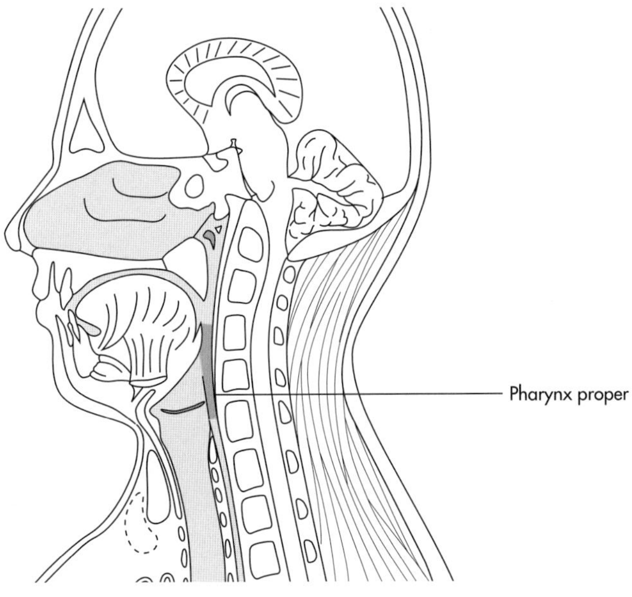

The pharynx is a muscular "tube," with three sets of muscles that wrap around it called the constrictors. They are designated by their position as the **superior, middle,** and **inferior constrictors.** Find them on the drawing.

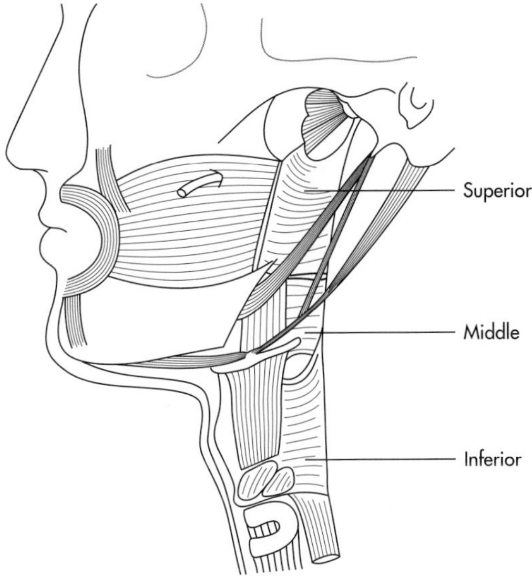

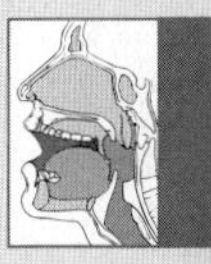

CN IX, CN X; superior, middle, inferior

Innervation of the pharynx is provided by (sensory) ______________ and (motor) ______________. The three muscles of the pharynx are ______________, ______________, and ______________ constrictors.

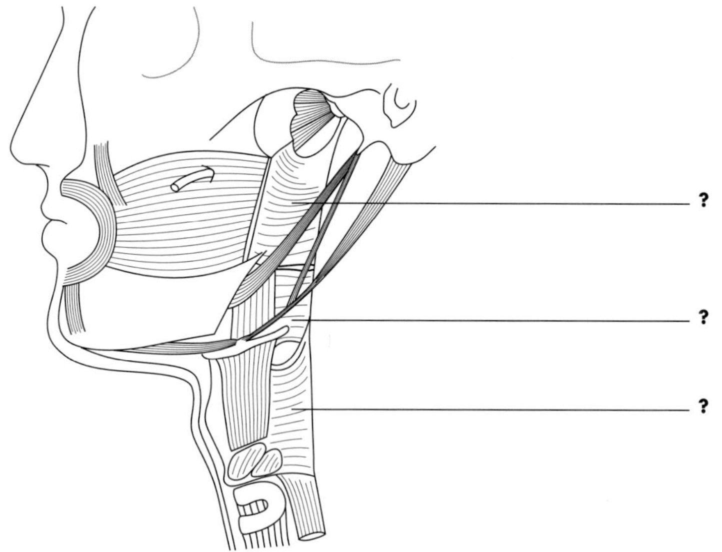

A structure found at the junction of oropharynx and pharynx proper is a mucosa-covered "flap" of cartilage called the **epiglottis.** Find it at the base of the tongue.

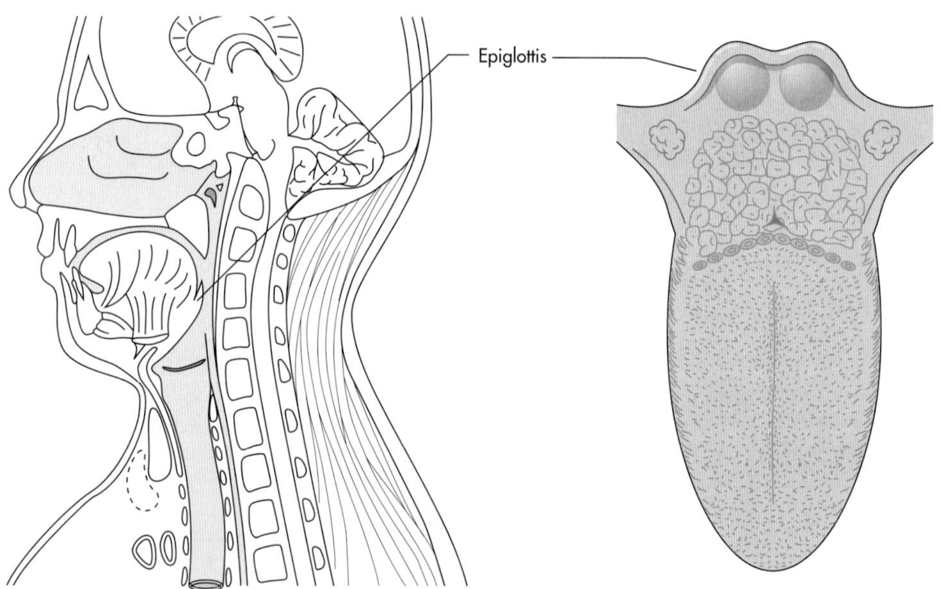

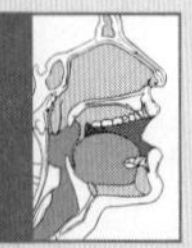

ESOPHAGUS

The last portion of the "food tube" or digestive system present in the neck is the **esophagus.** It is also a continuous muscular tube that connects the pharynx with the ______________.

stomach

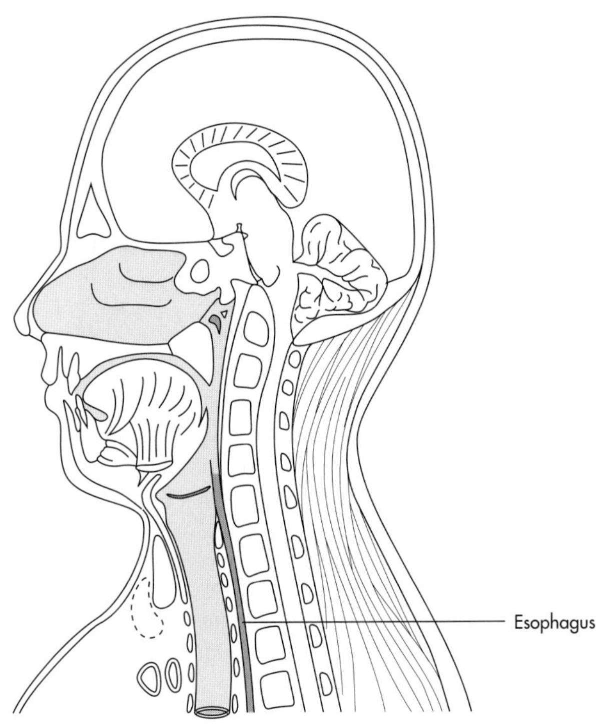

The muscles of the esophagus are incorporated into the layers of the tube and are all involuntary, smooth muscle fibers. What cranial nerve innervates them?

CN X

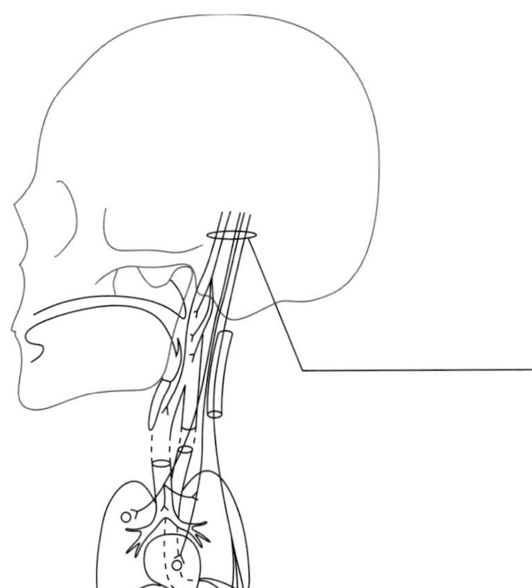

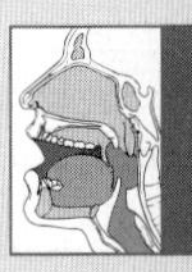

1.2 Mastication

chewing

Now that we have reviewed the anatomy of the oral cavity, pharynx, and esophagus, let us see how they function together. First, we study the action known as mastication, which in simple terms is ______________.

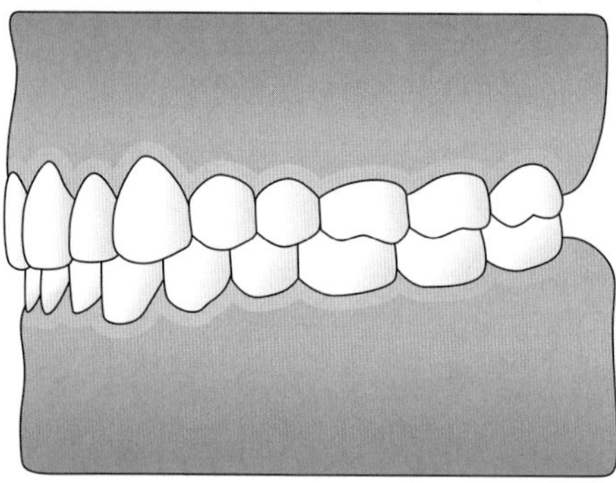

The process by which the oral cavity breaks down food into smaller pieces, moistens it with saliva, and places it onto the back of the tongue in a **bolus** ready to swallow is called **mastication.**

Breakdown is initially caused by the functioning of the teeth; incision, tearing, and grinding **(trituration)** are carried out by the incisors, canines, and premolars/molars, in that order. Each tooth group is built especially for its function and to fit together (occlude) with teeth in its opposing arch. Find each tooth group.

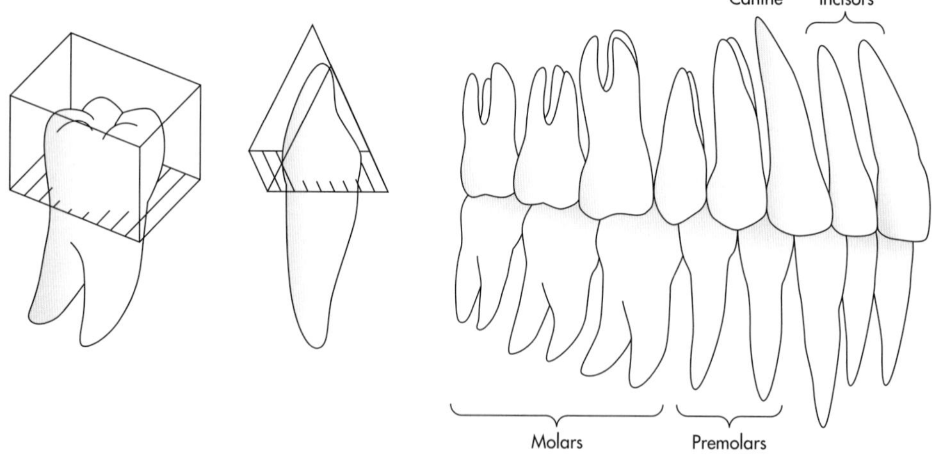

maxilla

In mastication, it is movement of the mandible against the ______________ that produces mastication. The mandible, because of its joint (the TMJ) and the occlusion and anatomy of the teeth, allows a particular range of **mandibular movements.** The mandibular movements are classified as (1) hinge movements—elevation and depression, and (2) gliding movements—lateral movement (protrusion and retrusion).

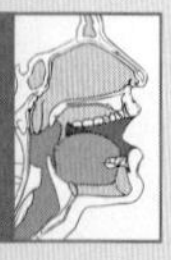

In this illustration of **hinge movement,** is this elevation or depression of the mandible? Which muscle(s) causes this movement? What cranial nerve does this?

elevation; temporalis, medial pterygoid, masseter; CN—V3

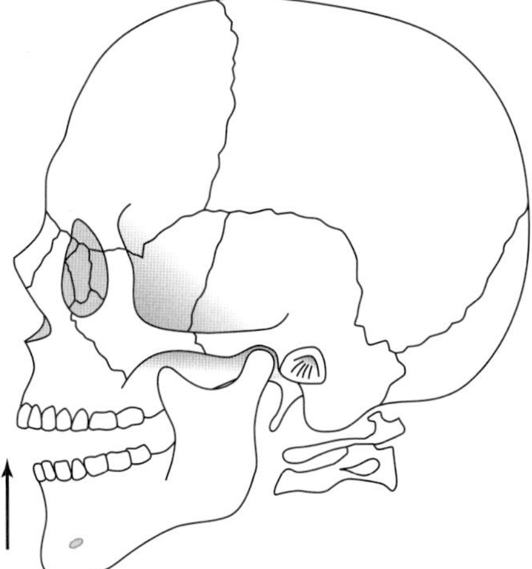

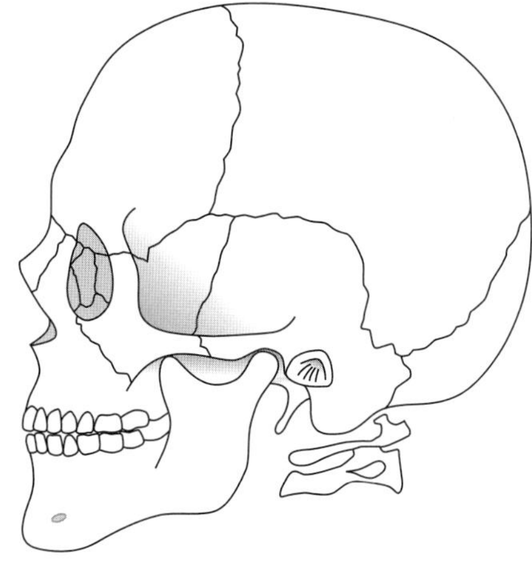

What is this hinge movement? What muscles direct it?

depression, suprahyoids

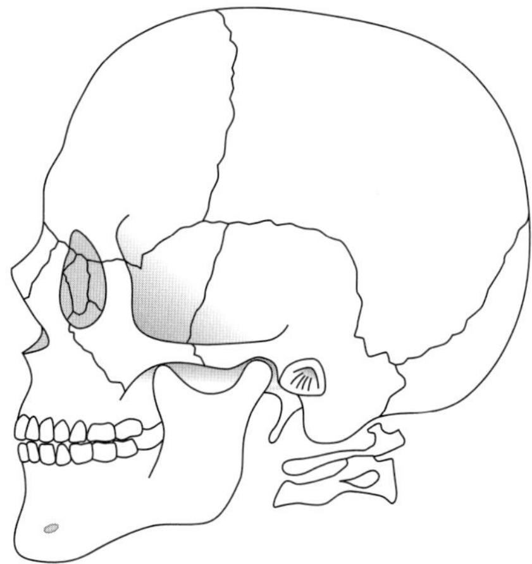

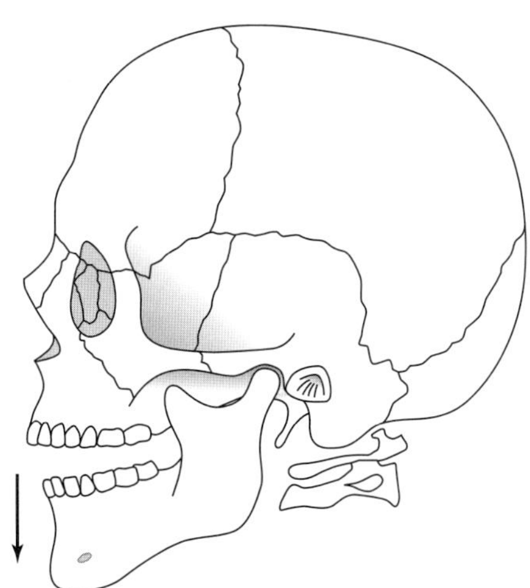

The lower joint cavity of the TMJ allows the hinge movements of the mandible, which are ______________ and ______________. The working cusps of the posterior teeth occlude in their fossae when the mandible is fully elevated into dental occlusion.

elevation, depression

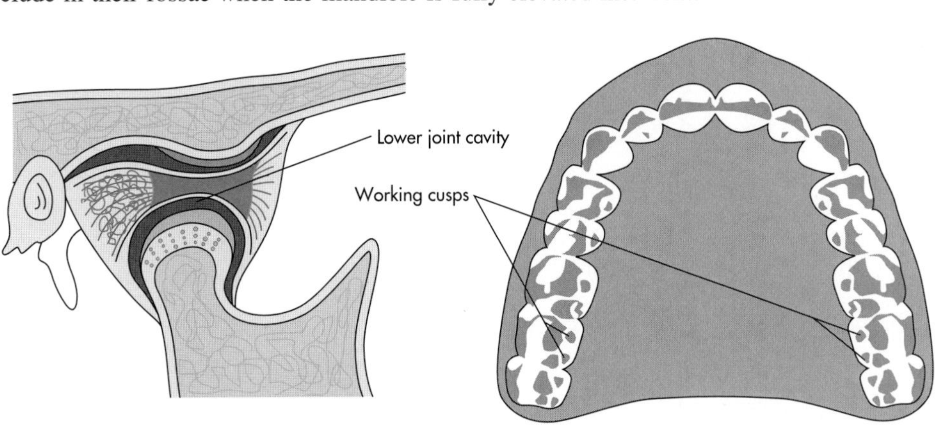

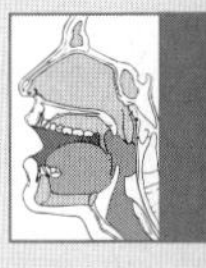

Hinge movements give a vertical component to mastication. This is the only component of the chewing cycle of carnivores or meat eaters. They possess sharp, single-cusp teeth and their mandibles move up and down during mastication.

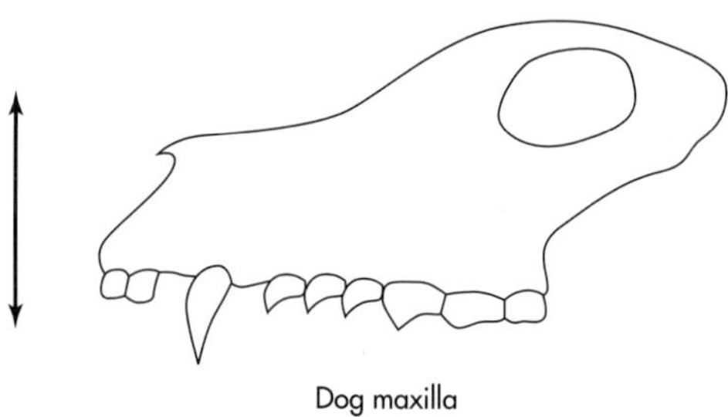

Dog maxilla

lateral, protrusive/retrusive

The gliding movements of the mandible include ______________- and ______________-type movements. The superior joint cavity of the TMJ allows these movements.

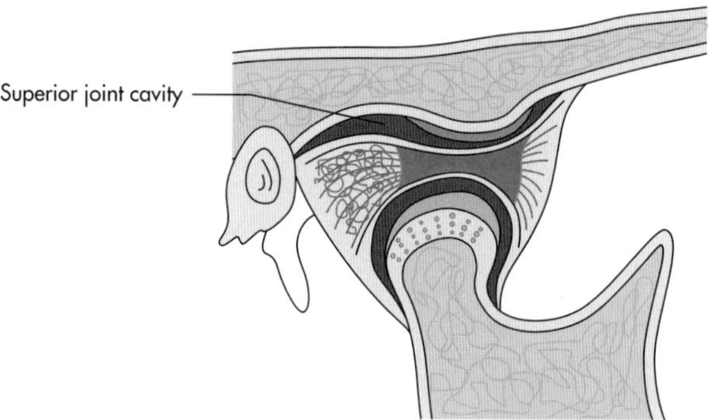

lateral pterygoid, V3

The movement illustrated is **lateral movement,** toward the right. This action is caused by contraction of the left ______________ muscle, innervated by CN ______________.

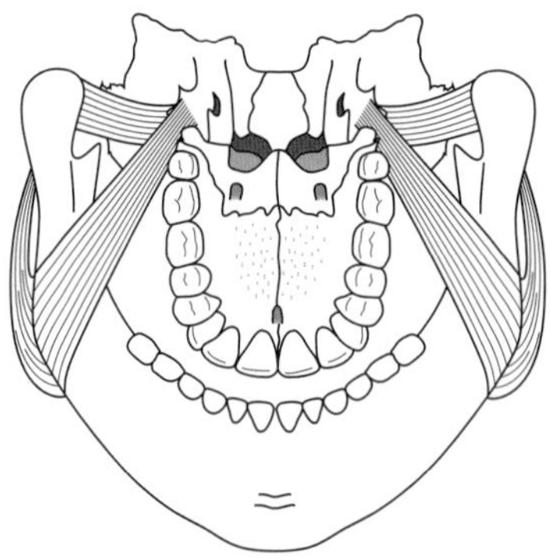

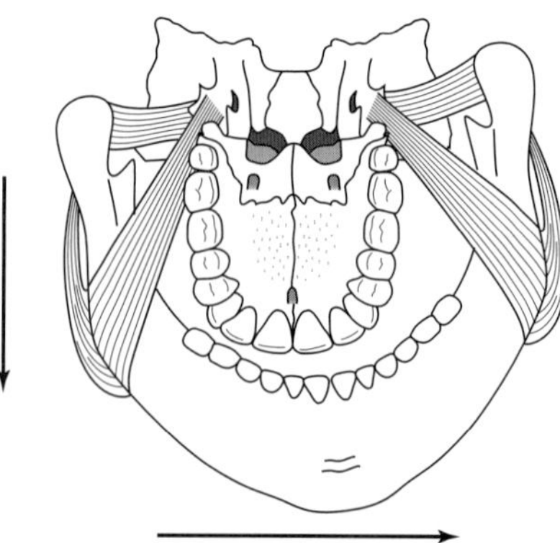

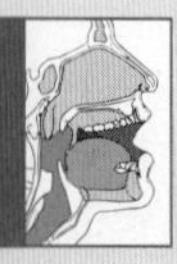

disk

The lateral pterygoid inserts into the neck of the condyle and into the TM _______________. The second insertion allows for tension on the disk during all jaw movements, keeping its proper protective position while the condyle moves.

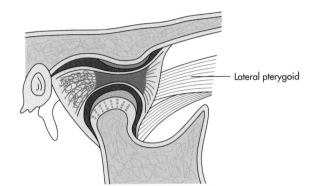

Lateral pterygoid

lateral movement

Contraction of both lateral pterygoids produces the mandibular movement known as **protrusion.** Contraction of one lateral pterygoid is _______________.

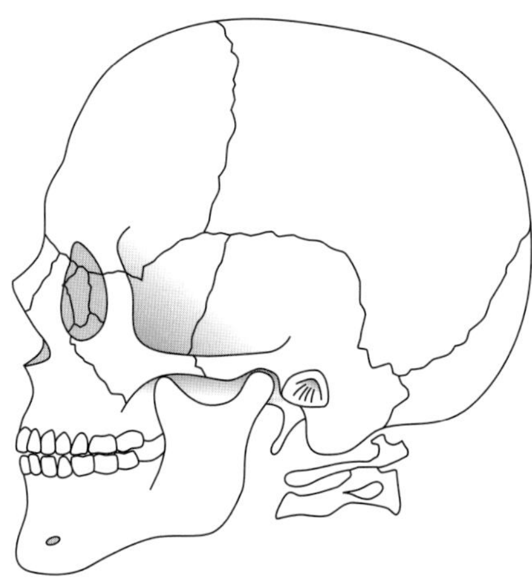

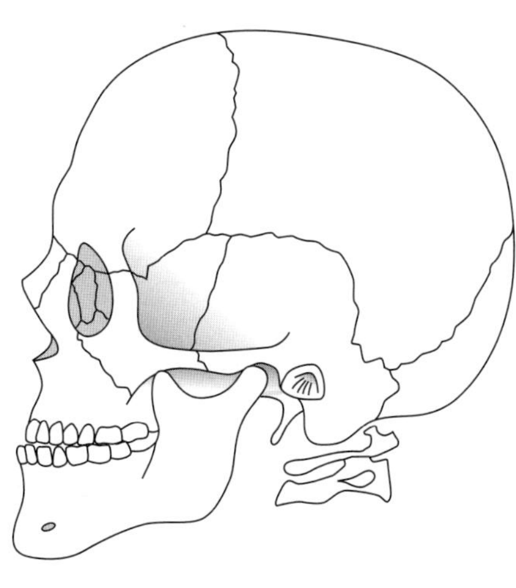

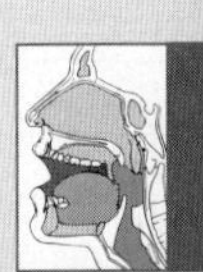

Retrusion is the opposite motion to protrusion. It brings the mandible back into the mandibular fossa. It is accomplished by relaxation of the lateral pterygoids and bilateral masseteric, anterior temporalis, and medial pterygoid action.

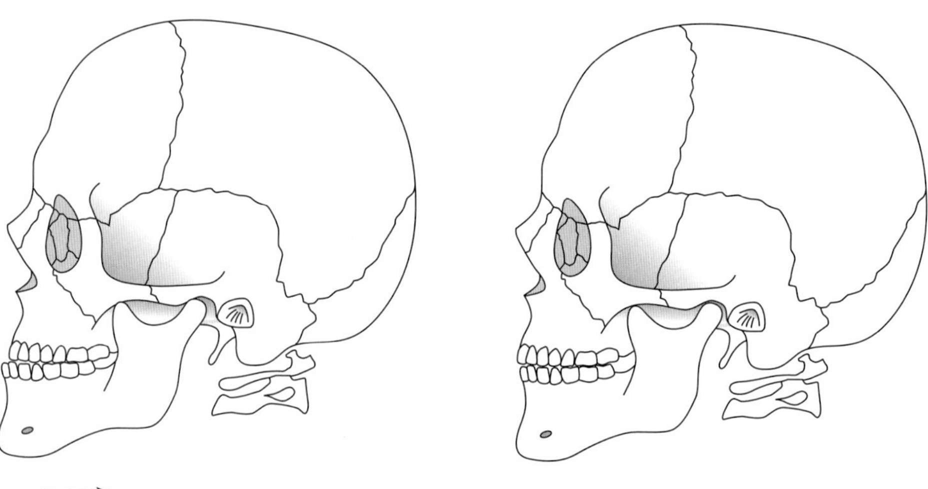

gliding, superior

Lateral movement, protrusion, and retrusion are ______________-type mandibular movements allowed by the ______________ joint cavities. The features of the teeth that allow these movements are the balancing or second set of cusps on the posterior teeth and the occlusal grooves.

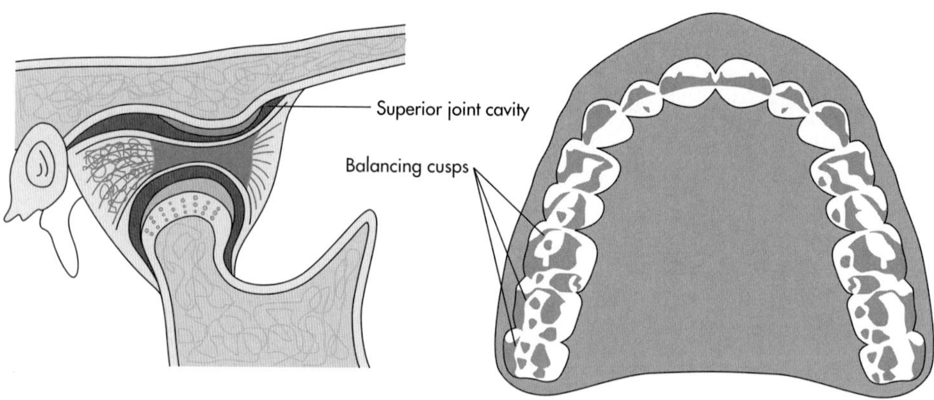

Gliding movements add a horizontal component to mastication. This type of jaw movement is illustrated in herbivores or plant eaters, who possess flat teeth and move their mandibles side to side when chewing.

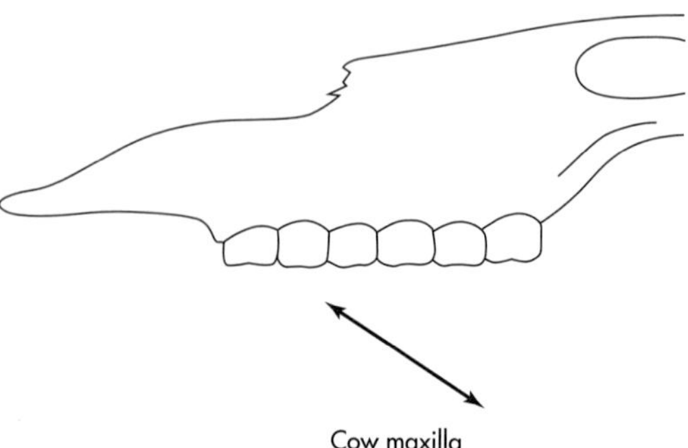

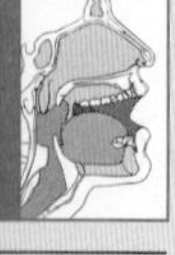

If we put together the vertical and horizontal components of mastication we come up with an **elliptical (masticatory) chewing cycle,** which is typical of omnivores (animals eating meat and plants).

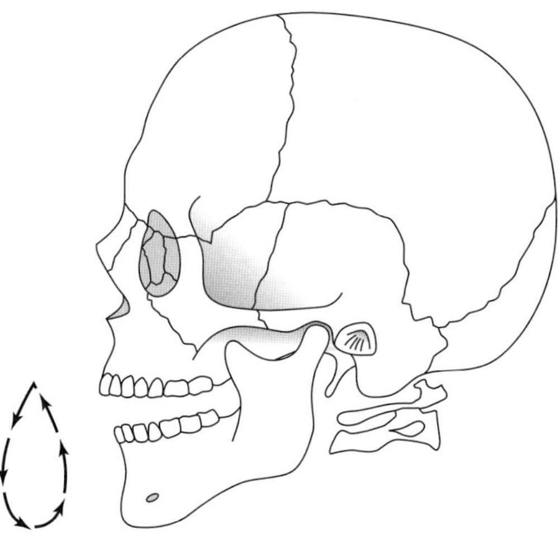

Our masticatory cycle is allowed by two things: the structure of our jaw joint and the structure of our teeth. Explain this.

Dual TMJ and double-cusped teeth allow hinge and gliding motion of the mandible.

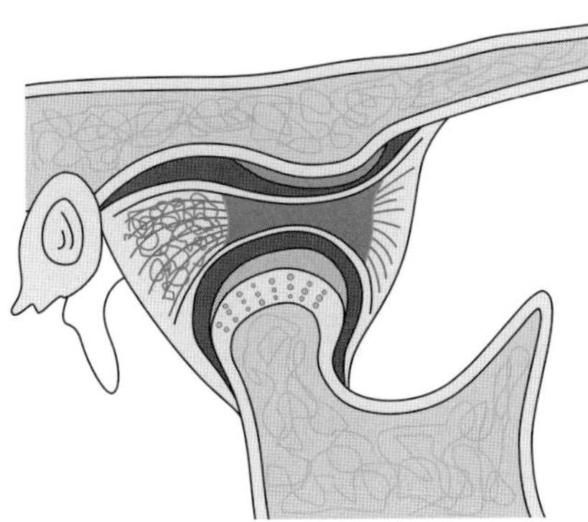

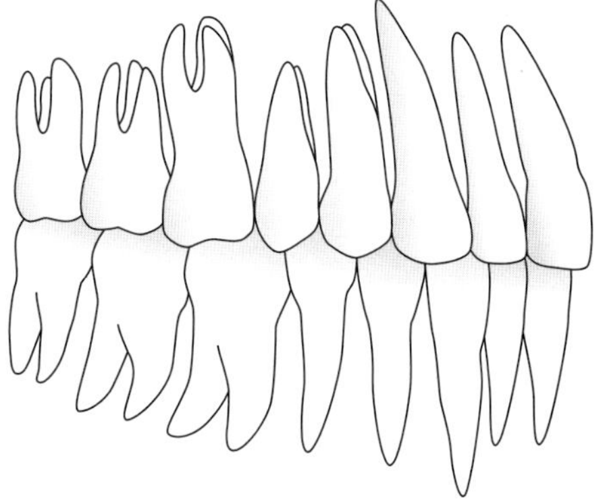

1.3 Deglutition

Swallowing a bolus of food is called **deglutition.** It is divided into **three phases,** beginning in the oral cavity and ending in the pharynx. It begins in the oral cavity as a voluntarily initiated action and ends as a totally involuntary one.

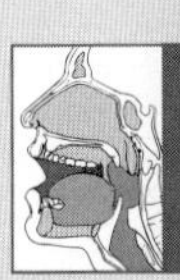

ORAL PHASE

The bolus is gathered together after mastication and the addition of saliva. It is positioned by the buccinator muscle and the intrinsic muscles of the tongue onto the posterior and middle of the tongue to initiate deglutition.

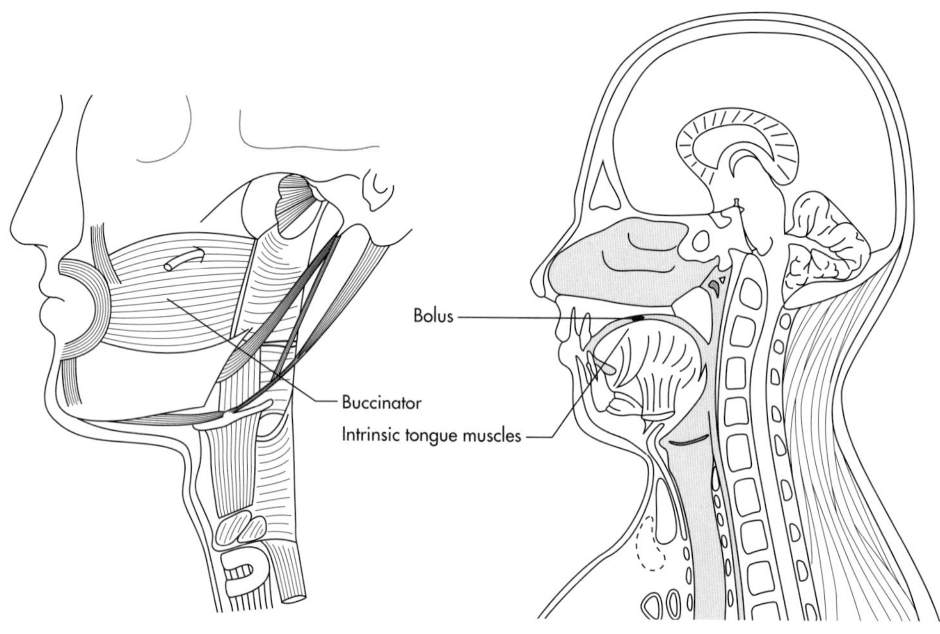

What innervation of muscles is involved in this phase?

buccinator—CN VII, tongue muscles—CN XII

What major salivary glands are involved to moisten the bolus? What innervation causes them to secrete saliva?

parotid—CN IX, submandibular—CN VII; sublingual—CN VII

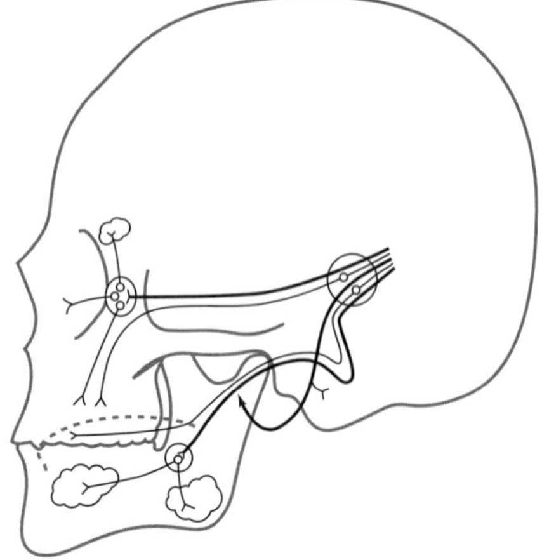

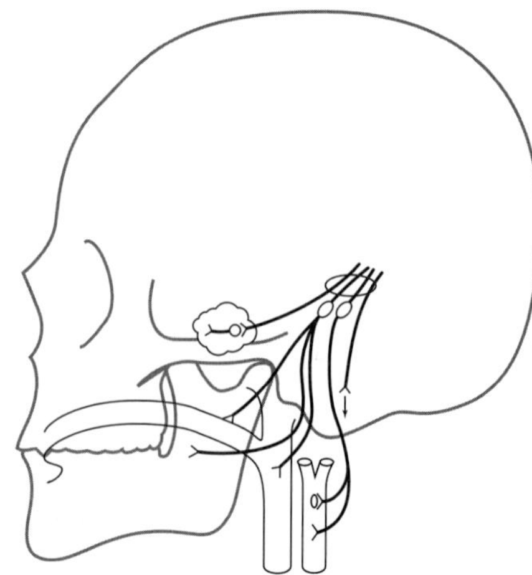

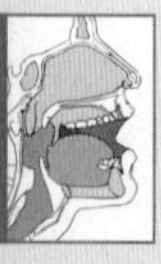

Mucosal sensation in the oral cavity and tongue is carried on three cranial nerves. This would give the brain information on the physical characteristics of the bolus and taste before swallowing—important information in the decision, to swallow or not! What nerves are involved?

general sensation—CNs V and IX (anterior and posterior); taste—CN VII (chorda tympani) and IX (anterior and posterior)

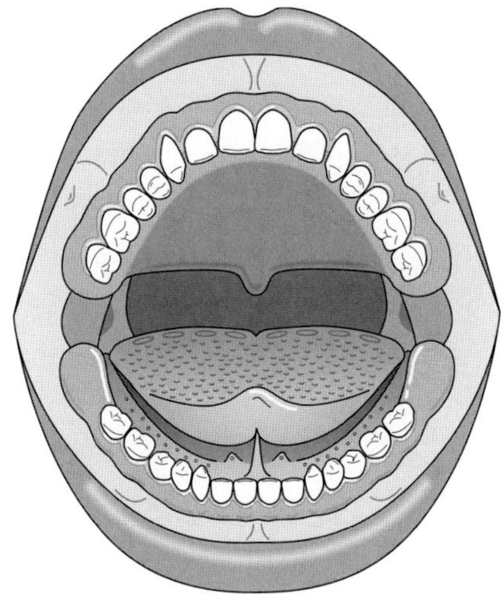

To prevent the bolus from moving upward into the nasopharynx, this portion of the tube must be sealed off. What structure could do this?

soft palate

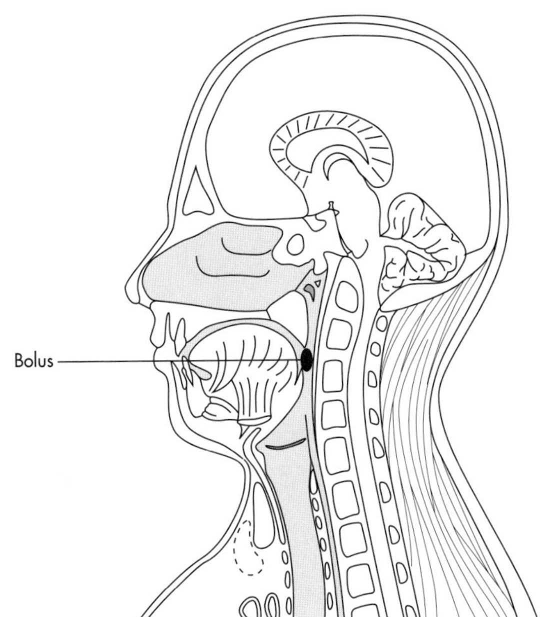

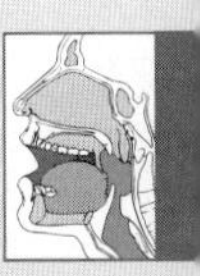

nasopharynx

The muscles of the soft palate are shown again. Their activity during deglutition is to tense and elevate the soft palate up against the posterior wall of the pharynx. When a swallow is initiated, this automatically occurs, sealing off the ______________.

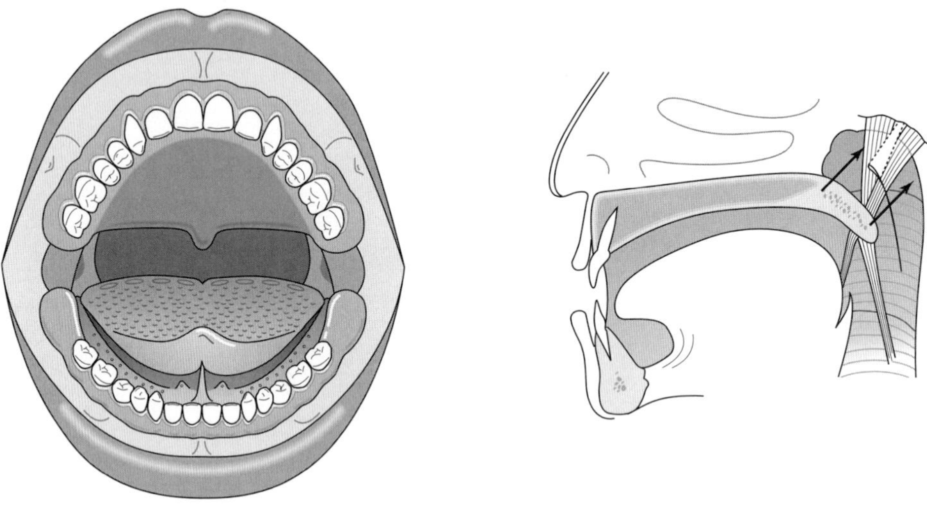

TVP

While deglutition is beginning and as the palate seals off the nasopharynx, another activity is initiated. With each swallow and thus palatal elevation, the Eustachian tube opens, equalizing pressure in the middle ear. What muscle is responsible?

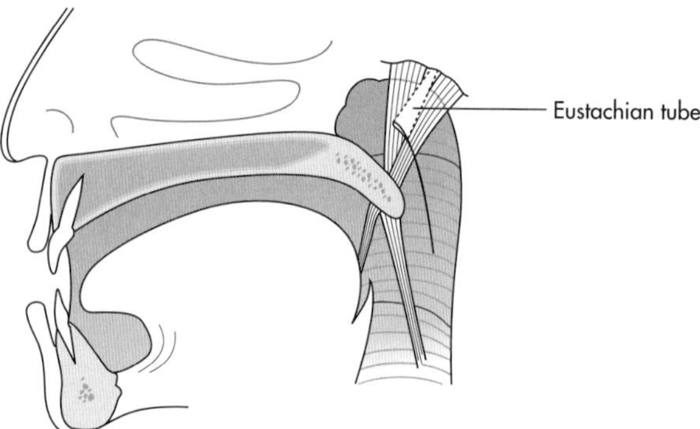

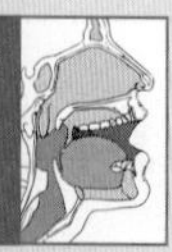

A portion of the TVP contracts to open the ______________ tube during palatal elevation. This muscle is also innervated by CN—V3.

Eustachian

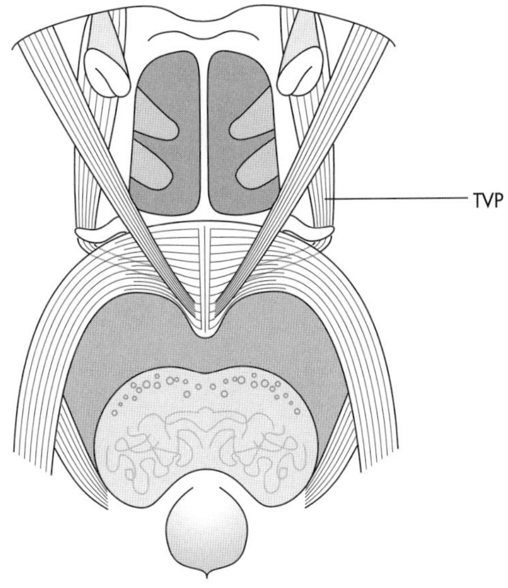

PHARYNGEAL PHASE

The bolus is positioned on the back of the tongue at the beginning of the oropharynx. Sensation picked up by CNs V, VII, and especially IX is used to decide whether to allow the bolus to pass downward. If the decision is "no," the muscles of the pharynx (run by the vagus nerve) rapidly expel the object or bolus. This is called the **gag reflex.**

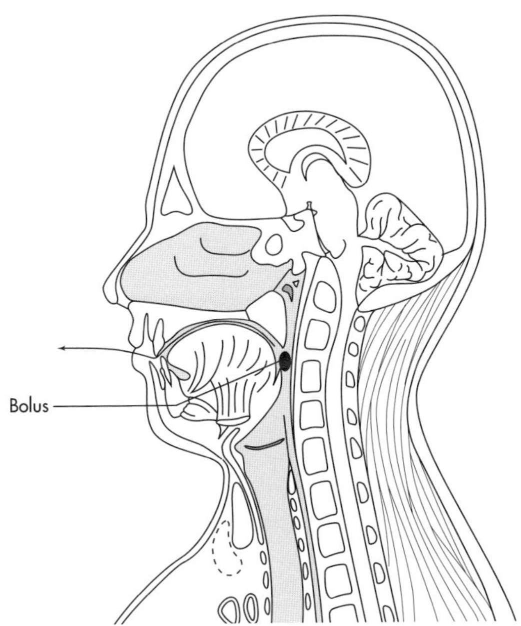

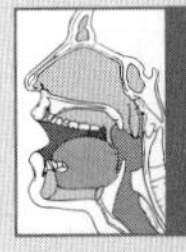

superior, XII

If the answer is "yes," the bolus is propelled downward by the first of the pharyngeal muscles, the ______________ constrictor. This action is aided by the muscles of the tongue, innervated by CN ______________.

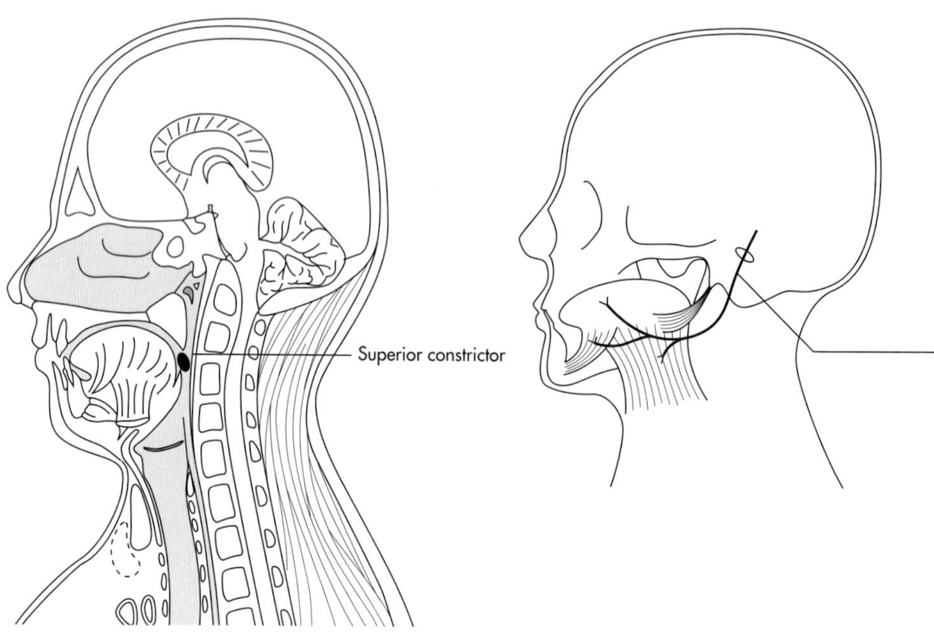

CN X

The superior constrictor squeezes the bolus down the pharynx. This muscular action is innervated by ______________, the vagus nerve. The action continues in a wave through all three constrictor muscles as they pass down the bolus.

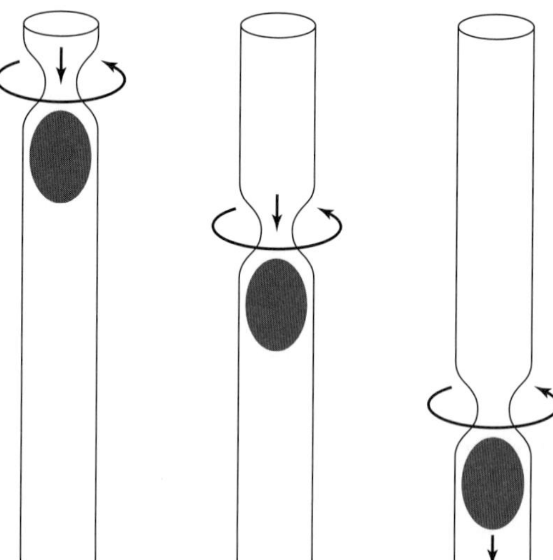

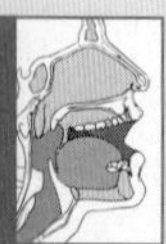

The pharyngeal constrictors are the ______________, ______________, and ______________ constrictors. The constrictors are composed of ever-decreasing amounts of skeletal-type muscle which becomes mixed with smooth muscle cells as it approaches the esophagus. What significance does this have?

superior, middle, inferior

Deglutition becomes involuntary down the tube.

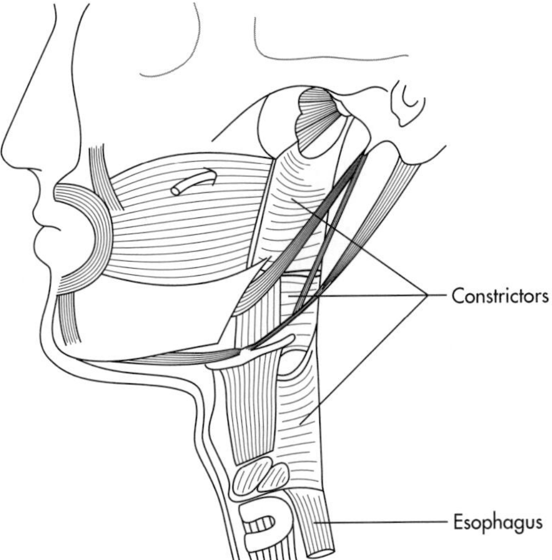

As the bolus travels downward, it can pass into either of two tubes: the pharynx or the larynx. What prevents food or drink from passing into the airway?

epiglottis

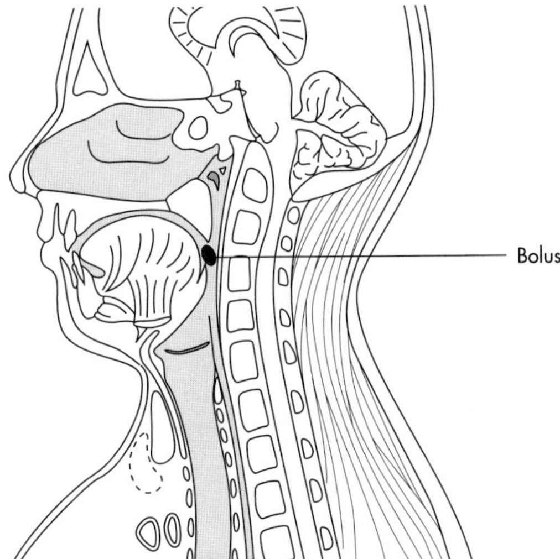

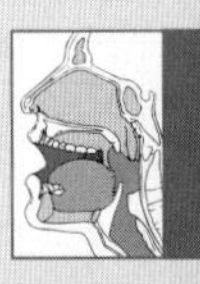

CN X

The epiglottis is a mucosa-covered cartilage flap found at the base or root of the tongue. The epiglottis seals off the larynx while the bolus passes down the pharynx. The larynx is actually lifted up against the epiglottis by the laryngeal muscles. What cranial nerve mediates this action?

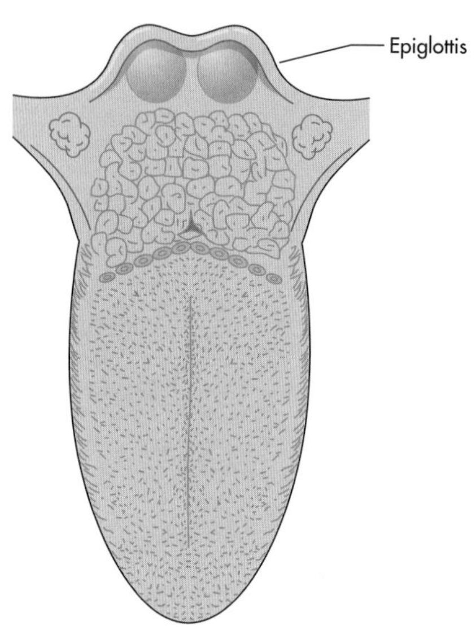

ESOPHAGEAL PHASE

The bolus is now headed inevitably into the digestive system. By now the musculature of the esophagus is purely smooth muscle tissue.

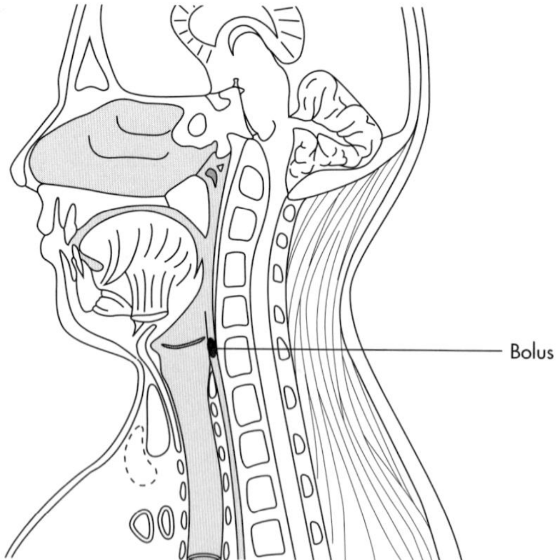

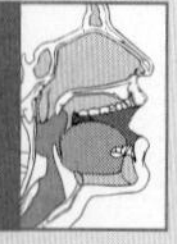

The action of the muscles of the esophagus is to continuously squeeze the bolus toward which organ? This action is called **peristalsis.** It continues down the entire digestive tract and is controlled by CN ______________ up to the last portion of the colon.

stomach, X

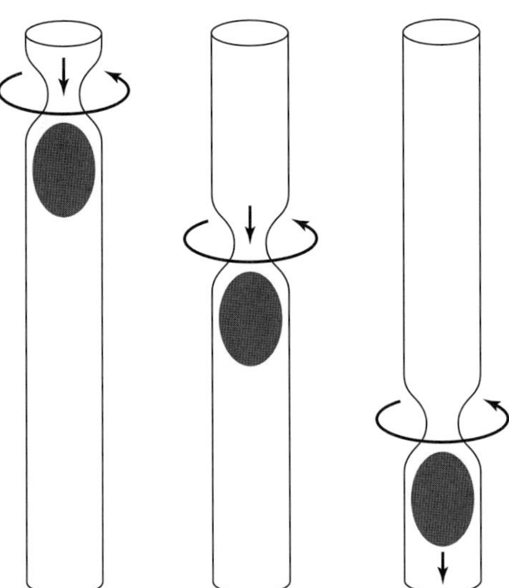

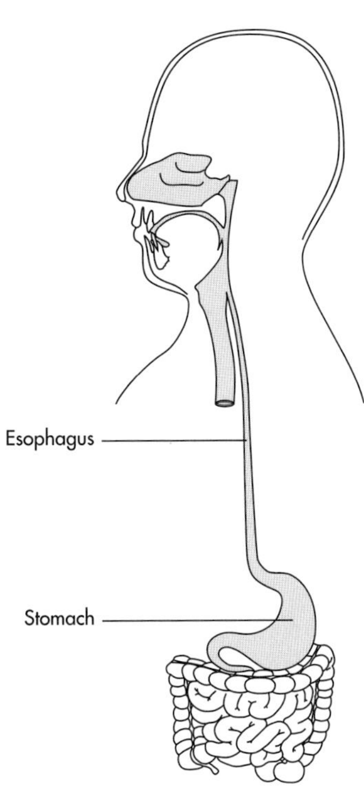

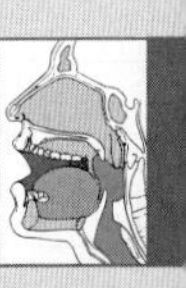

A. esophagus
B. stomach

Review the digestive system in the head and neck. Label these parts of the digestive system.

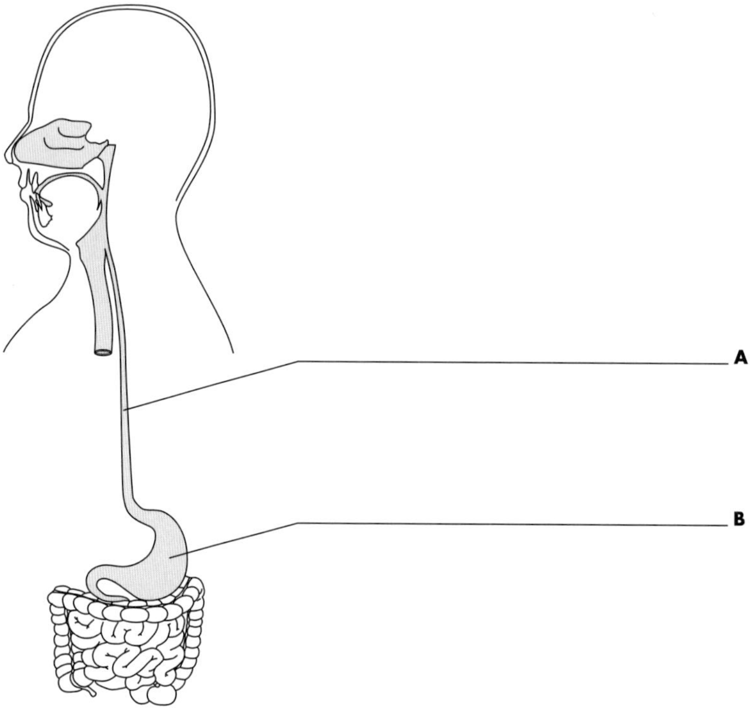

A. oral cavity
B. pharynx proper
C. esophagus
D. nasopharynx
E. oropharynx

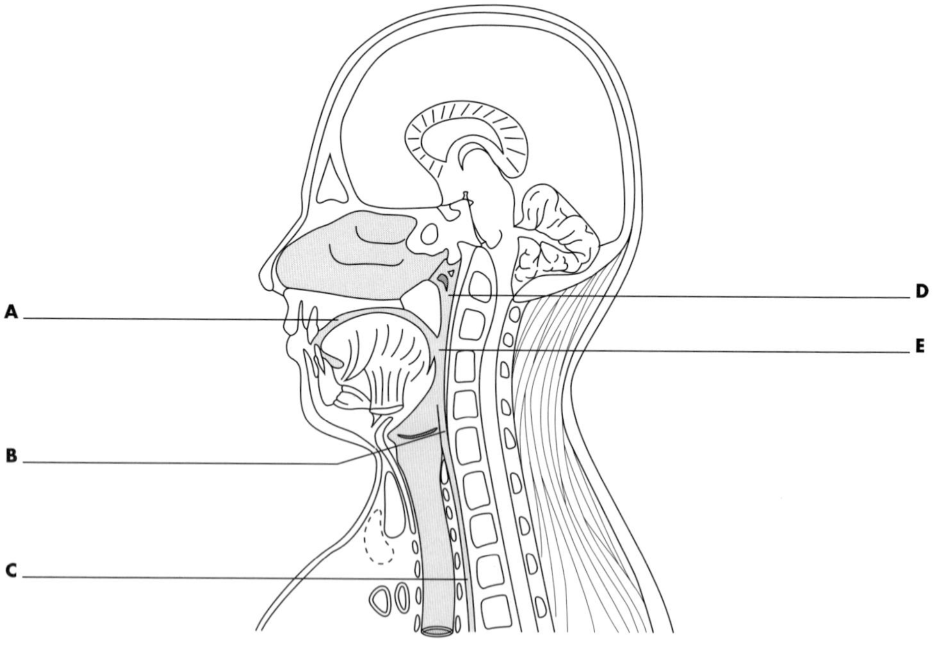

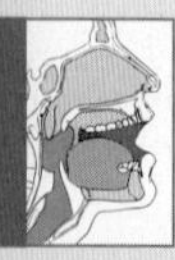

A. List the muscles and their cranial nerves associated with the following actions:

	Muscle(s)	Nerve
Mastication		
1. Elevation of mandible	______	______
2. Depression of mandible	______	______
3. Lateral movement of mandible	______	______
4. Protrusion of mandible	______	______
5. Saliva production	______	______
Deglutition		
1. Tongue movement	______	______
2. Cheek movement	______	______
3. Pharyngeal swallow	______	______
4. Palatal elevation and tension	______	______
5. Epiglottal seal	______	______
6. Esophageal peristalsis	______	______

B. Sensation in the oral cavity and pharynx falls into two categories: taste and general sensation. List the cranial nerves responsible.

	Taste	General
1. Anterior oral cavity	______	______
2. Posterior oral cavity	______	______
3. Oropharynx	______	______

C. List the two things that determine the chewing (masticatory) cycle.

D. What is it about the anatomy of the TMJ that allows the two different mandibular movements?

E. What other action occurs simultaneously with deglutition?

F. List the three phases of deglutition and what occurs during each.

A.
Mastication
1. Temporalis, medial pterygoid, masseter: CN V
2. Suprahyoid: CN V, cervical
3. Lateral pterygoid: CN V
4. Lateral pterygoid: CN V
5. Parotid, submandibular, sublingual: CN IX, CN VII

Deglutition
1. Tongue muscles: CN XII
2. Buccinator: CN VII
3. Constrictors: CN X
4. LVP, TVP, palatopharyngeus, palatoglossus: —
5. Muscles of larynx: CN X
6. Esophageal muscles: CN X

B.

	Taste	General
1.	VII	V
2.	IX	IX
3.	VII	V

C. Tooth structure and joint structure of mandible

D. Dual joint allows hinge and gliding motions

E. Opening of the Eustachian tube

F. oral (positioning of bolus on posterior, middle of tongue); pharyngeal (beginning of involuntary squeezing of bolus down into pharynx); esophageal (further peristalsis of bolus down into digestive tract)

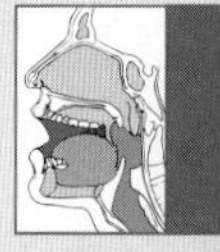

2.0 RESPIRATORY SYSTEM

The system that allows us to take in the oxygen needed for life and eliminate waste carbon dioxide has some representation in the head and neck. It is the beginning of the respiratory system.

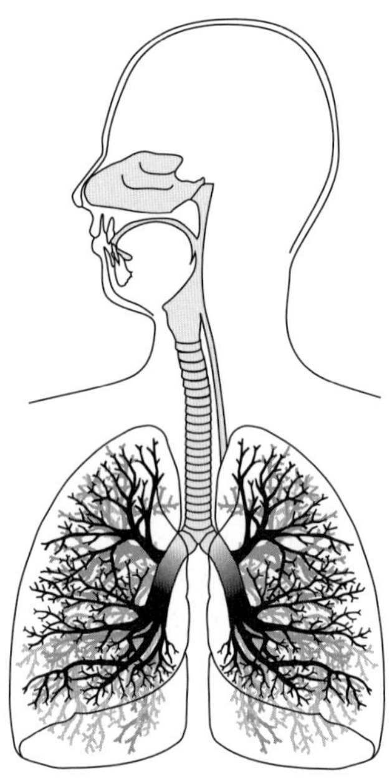

Find the following parts of the respiratory system: nasal cavity, oral cavity, nasopharynx, oropharynx, pharynx proper, epiglottis, larynx, trachea.

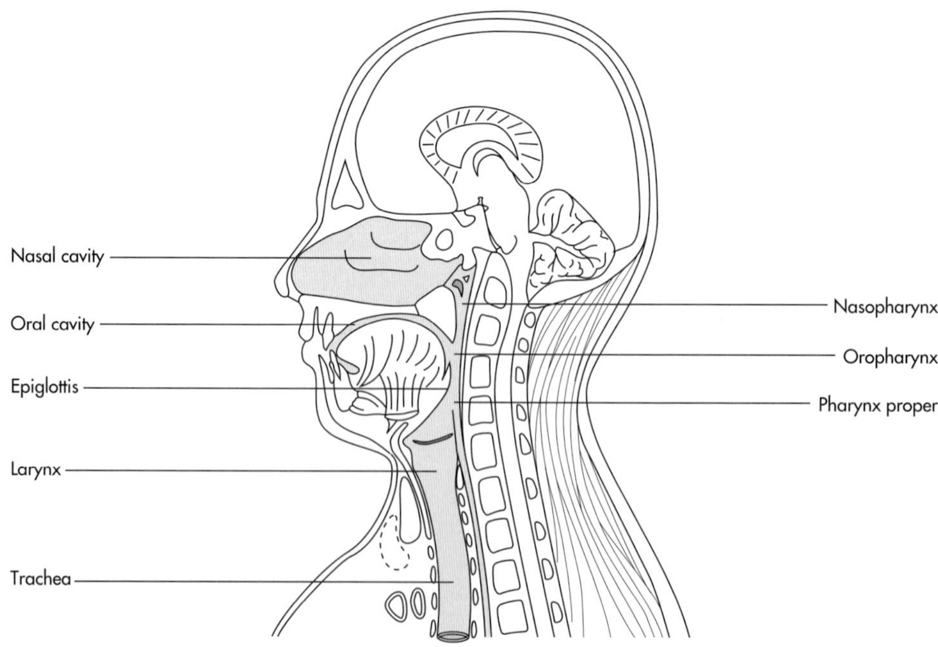

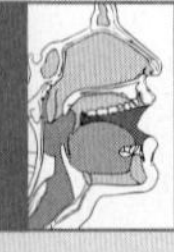

What we need for the respiratory system to work is a patent airway, that is, a tube with no obstructions that leads directly to the lungs. Note, in the drawing, the position of the oral/nasal cavities and the trachea in the body and how they connect via the bronchi to the ______________.

lungs

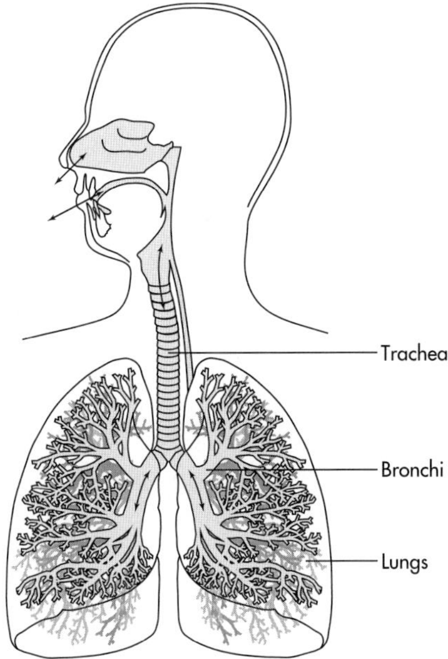

The nasal cavity is the beginning of the respiratory system, although air may come in through the mouth. The ______________ cavity is designed to filter incoming air of particulate matter before it goes to the lungs. For this reason it is lined with respiratory mucosa, a pseudostratified, ciliated mucosa with a mucous coating.

nasal

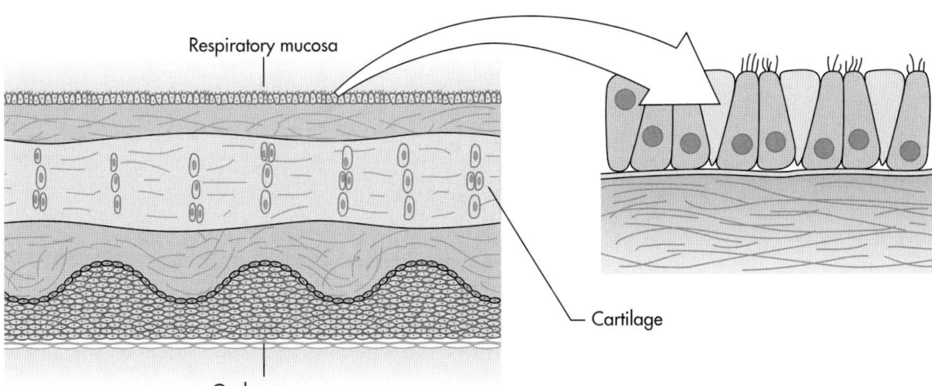

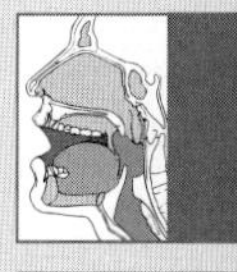

turbinates

Inside the nasal cavity we find three “baffles” or nasal turbinates that warm and moisten the incoming air. Also, located beneath the ______________ are the openings or meatii of the paranasal sinuses, and this is where those sinuses drain.

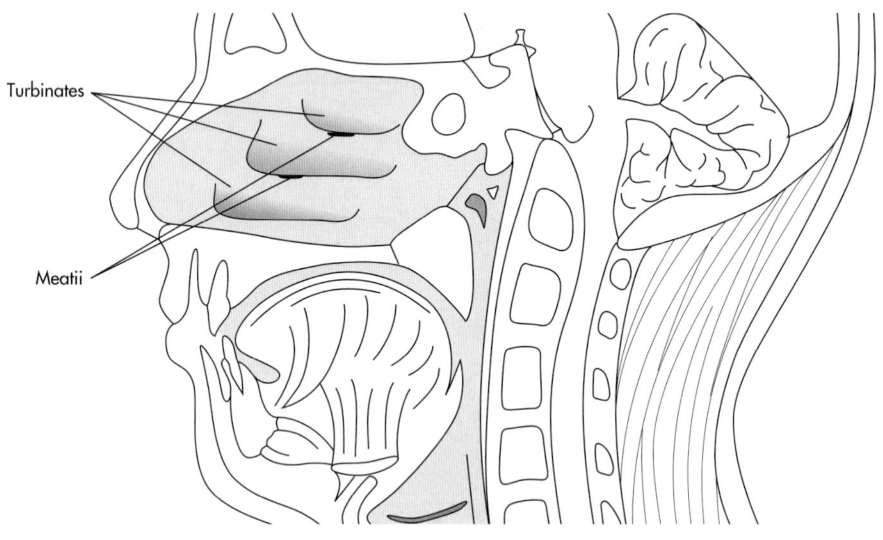

pharynx, palate and epiglottis

Which “tube” in the neck shares the passage of food/drink and air? What anatomic devices are used to make sure the two are not mixed?

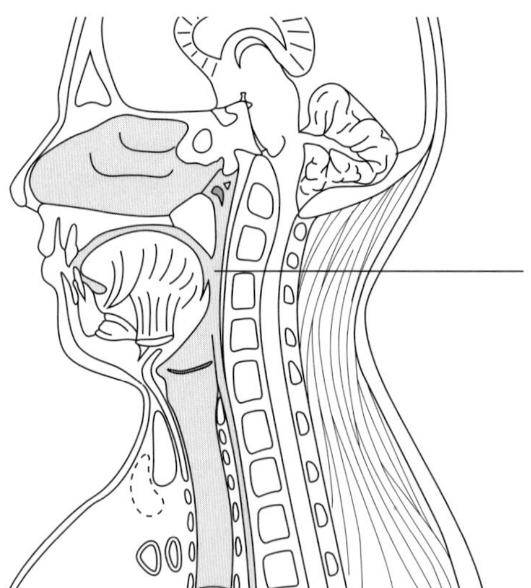

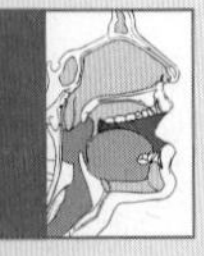

The first problem to solve is sealing off the nasal cavity from the oral cavity, so that food does not pass upward. The muscular "flap" that does this during each swallow (deglutition) is the ______________ palate.

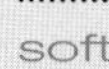

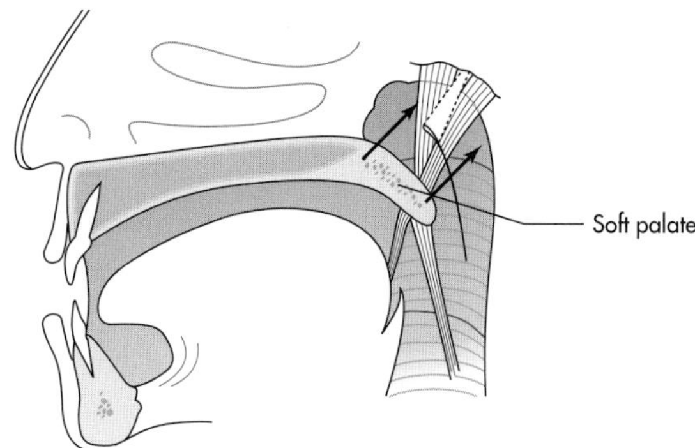

Air may pass through either the nasal or oral cavity into the pharynx. Beyond this point, we need another protective device to prevent food from going down the trachea (larynx). A "flap" of cartilage posterior to the tongue accomplishes this. It is called the ______________.

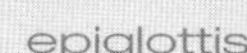

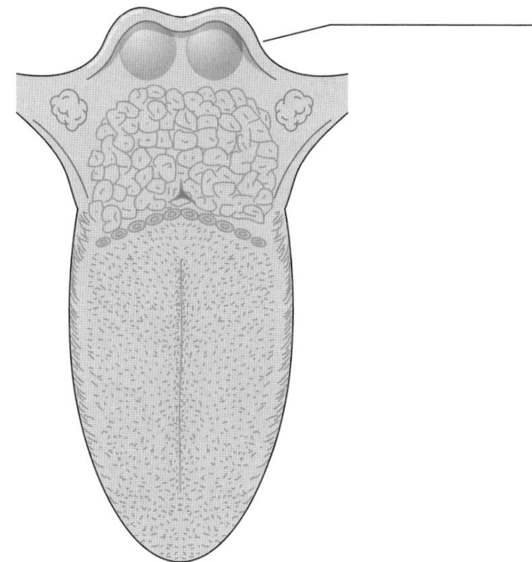

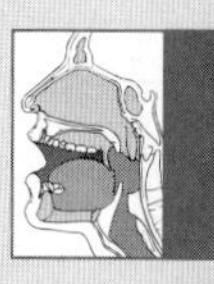

The laryngeal muscles actually pull the larynx up against the epiglottis. This seals off the airway and prevents food/drink from passing down the pharynx and esophagus.

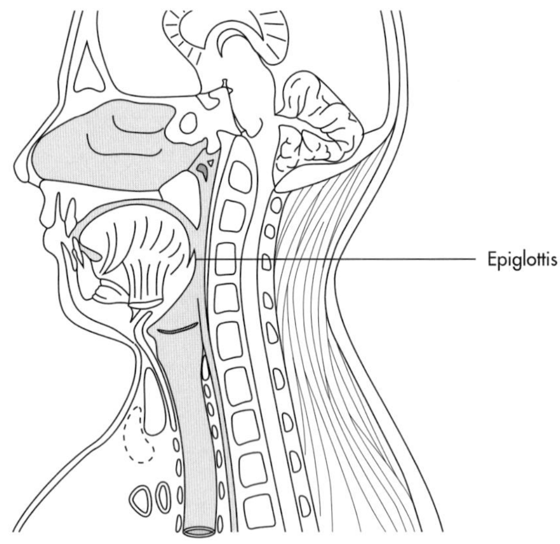

true, larynx

Air passage, thus, cannot occur during deglutition. True or false? What is this structure?

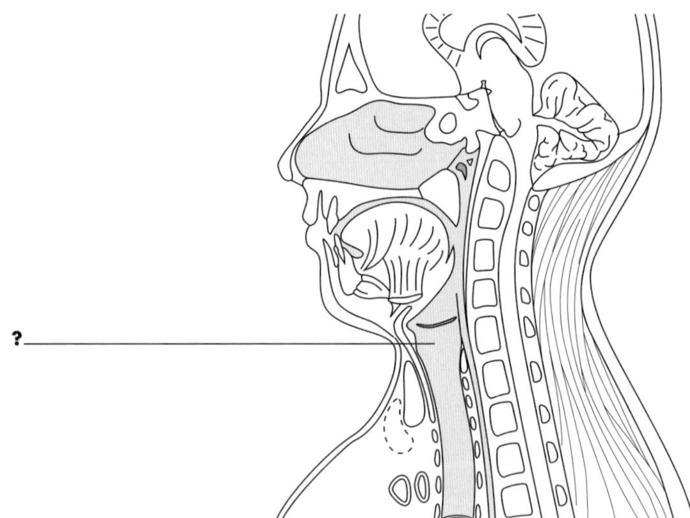

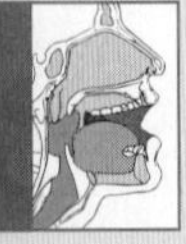

The **larynx** is a mucosal tube with a cartilage shield on its anterior side, called the **thyroid cartilage.** Cartilage is often used in the respiratory system to create rigid tubes that remain open for air passage. Look at the two different views of the larynx.

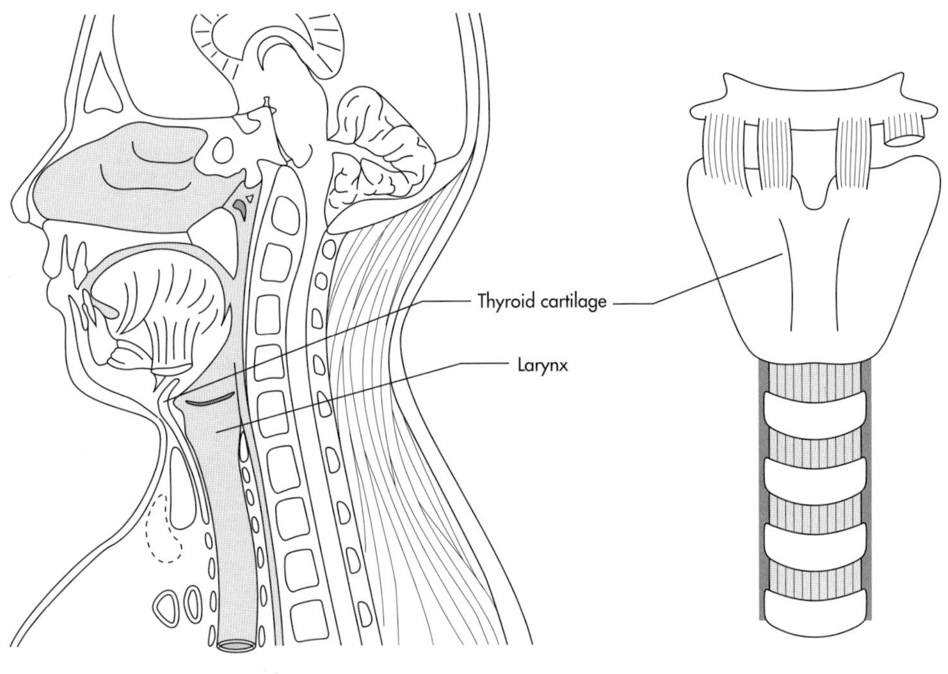

This view of the larynx shows the ______________ cartilage. It is larger in males, often seen in the neck as the "Adam's apple."

thyroid

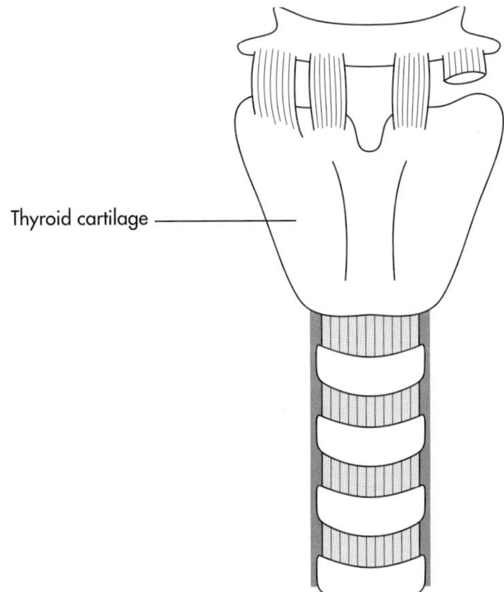

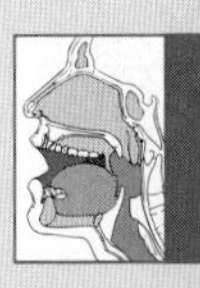

thyroid

Thyroid cartilage is so named because the ______________ gland lies on top of it.

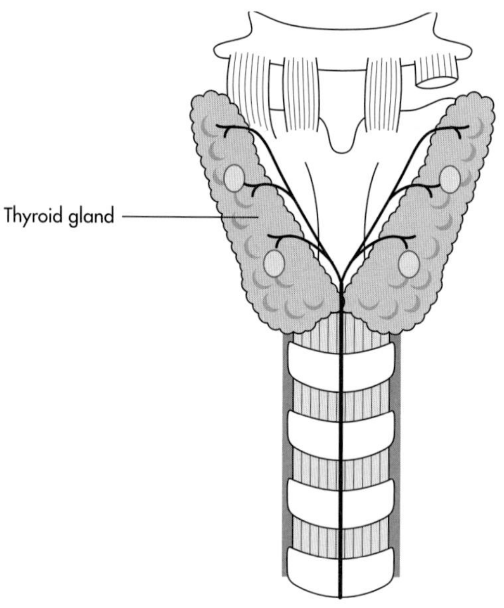

larynx

Inside the ______________ we see two folds of mucosa called the **vocal folds** or **vocal chords.** As air passes through the larynx, they can be made to vibrate and produce sound—the voice.

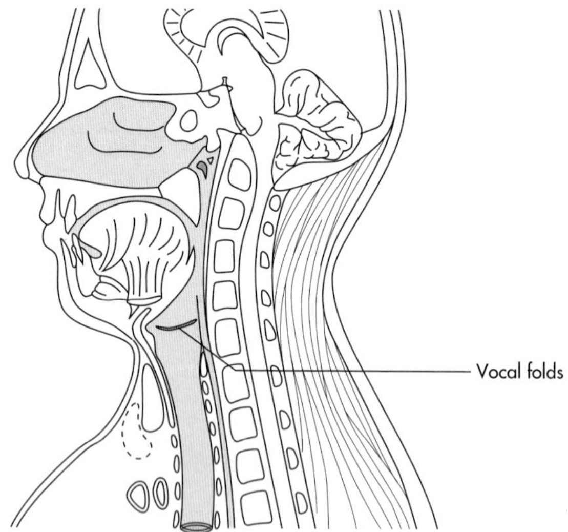

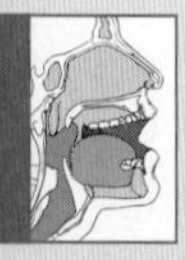

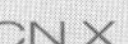

Shown here is a diagram of a cross section through the trachea. By adjusting the vocal folds with muscles, a variety of sounds can be produced. They are altered by the tongue, cheeks, lips, and nasal cavity as they pass from the body as speech. What cranial nerve innervates the muscles of the larynx?

CN X

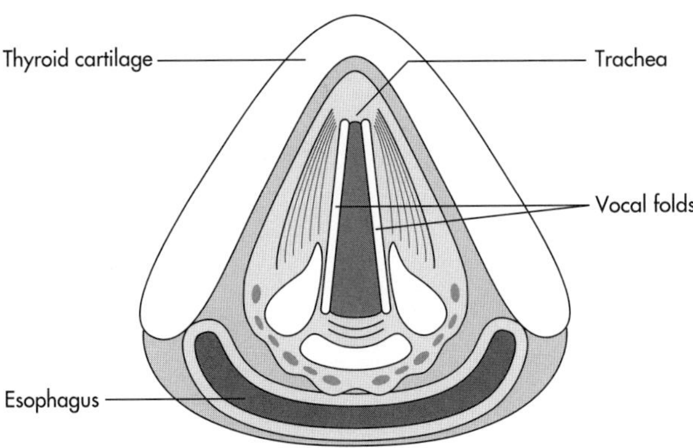

Below the larynx lies a rigid tube that passes down the entire length of the neck, into the chest, where it divides into two. This single tube appears ringed and is called the ________________.

trachea

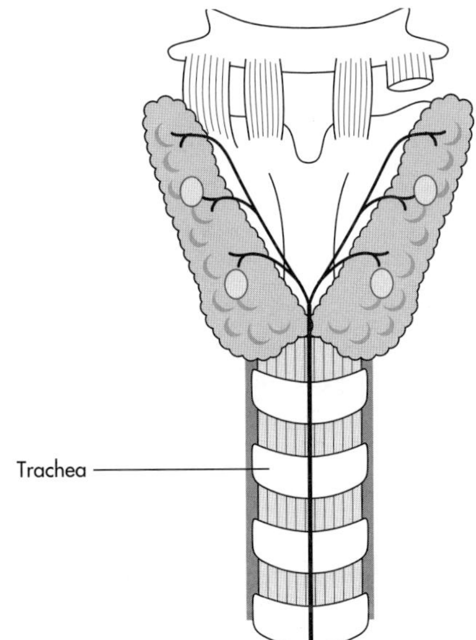

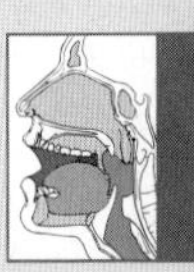

The **trachea** is a mucosal tube, encircled with almost complete cartilaginous rings, the **tracheal rings.** The tracheal rings keep the airway patent during respiration.

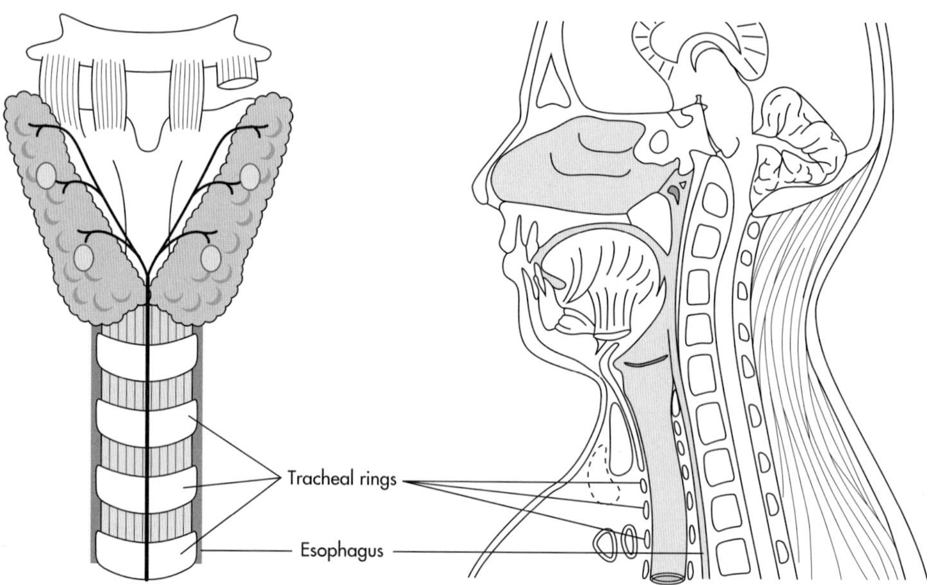

trachea, can be felt on neck

Which tube is more anterior, the esophagus or the trachea?

A. turbinates
B. meatii
C. nasopharynx

Label these anatomic parts of the respiratory system.

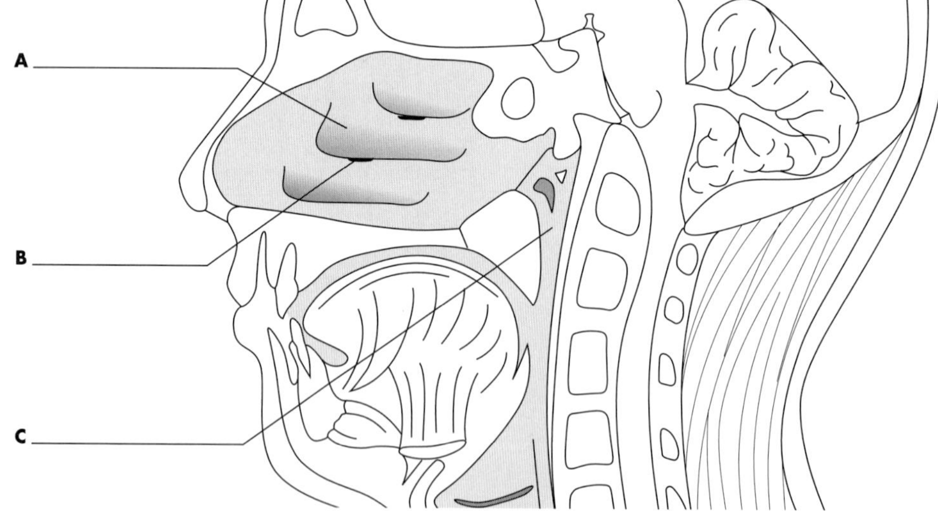

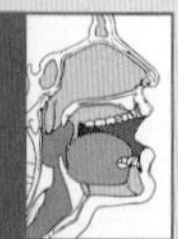

continued

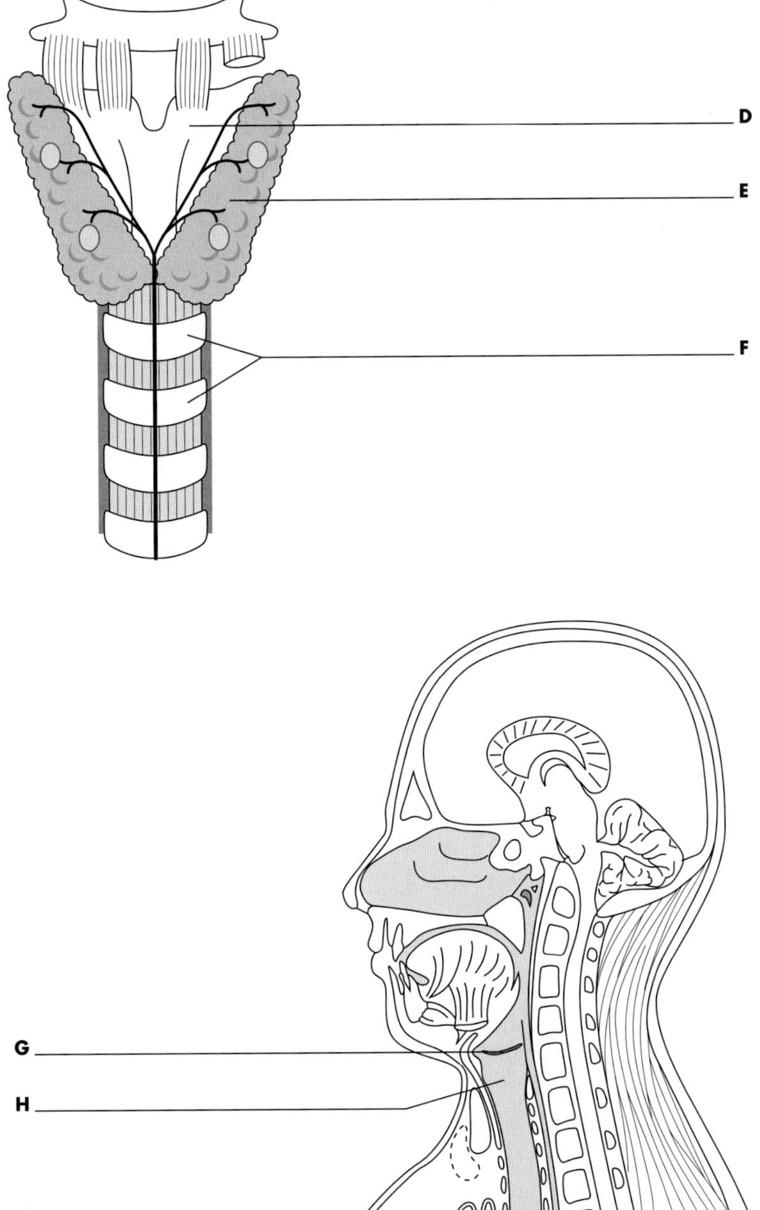

D. thyroid cartilage
E. thyroid gland
F. tracheal rings

G. vocal fold
H. larynx
I. trachea

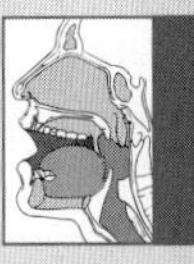

Food travels from the oral cavity to the oropharynx, to the pharynx proper, to the esophagus and into the digestive system. Air travels from the oral/nasal cavities, to the pharynx and to the larynx and trachea, to the respiratory system. The nasopharynx is protected from food passage by the soft palate. The trachea is protected from food passage by the epiglottis.

Explain where air passes and where food passes and why the two do not get mixed?

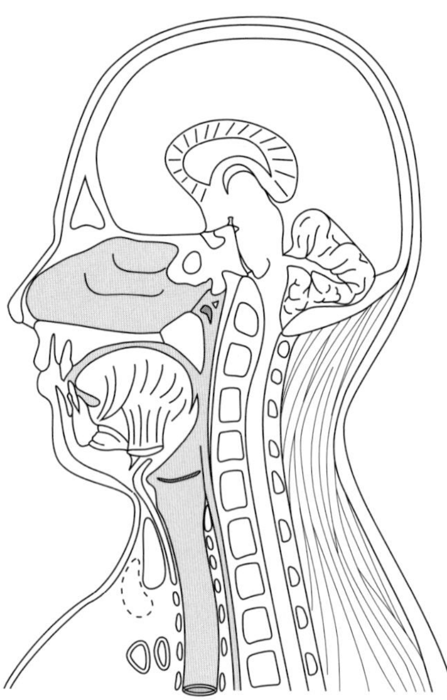

The soft palate prevents food or drink from passing upward into the nasopharynx by sealing it off during a swallow (deglutition). Also, the larynx is lifted up to the epiglottis, thus sealing it off from the passage of food or drink downward.

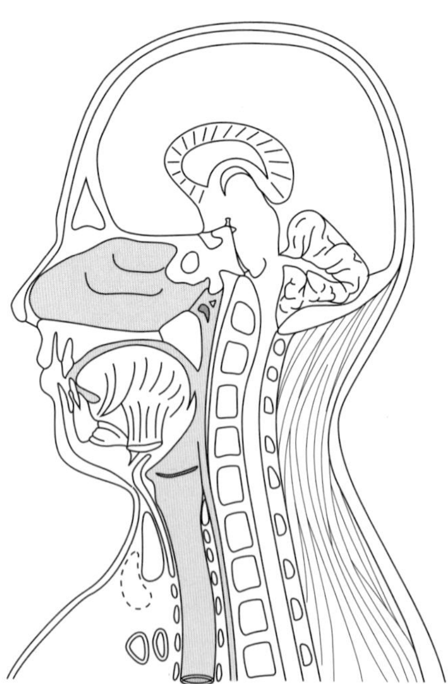

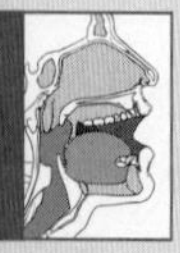

OTHER ANATOMIC STRUCTURES

3.0

Pineal Body (Epiphysis)

3.1

A small neuroepithelial gland, the **pineal body,** or gland, is found in the brain. Find it on the drawing.

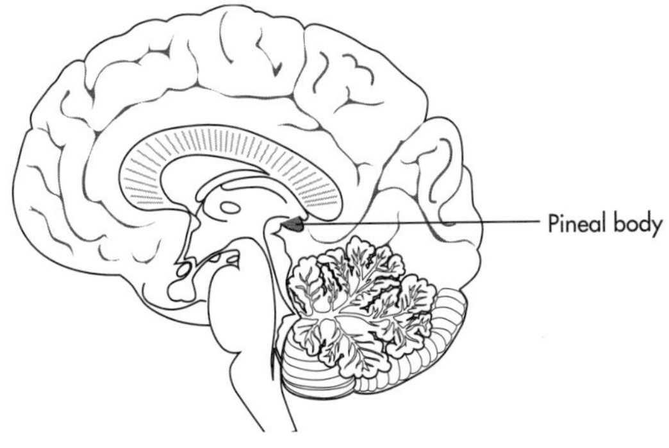

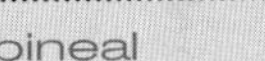

pineal

The ______________ body or gland produces a chemical called **melatonin,** the function of which is not clear. In lower mammals, this area has to do with photo (light) reception. It appears that in humans, secretion of melatonin may have significance in timing the various body cycles, such as sexual development and estrous cycles.

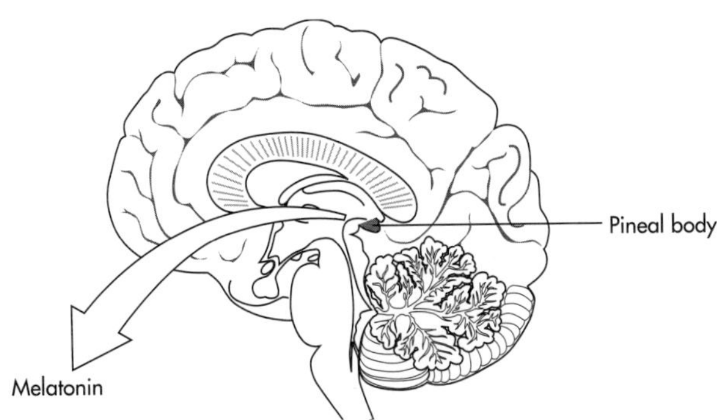

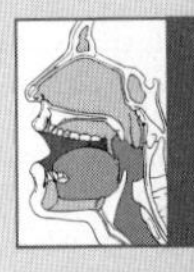

3.2

Pituitary Gland (Hypophysis)

pituitary

The **pituitary gland** lies in the ______________ fossa of the cranium. It is attached to the base of the brain. Find the gland and its fossa.

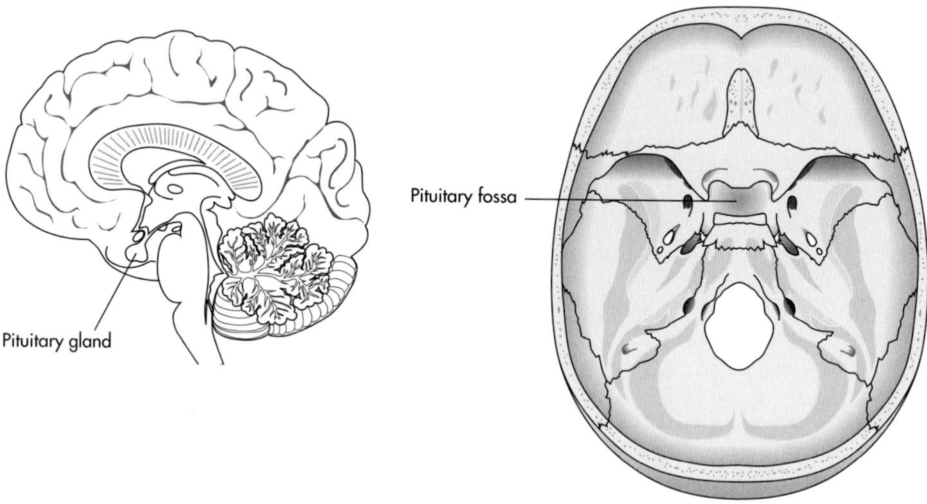

The pituitary is composed of two separate entities: the neurohypophysis and the adenohypophysis.

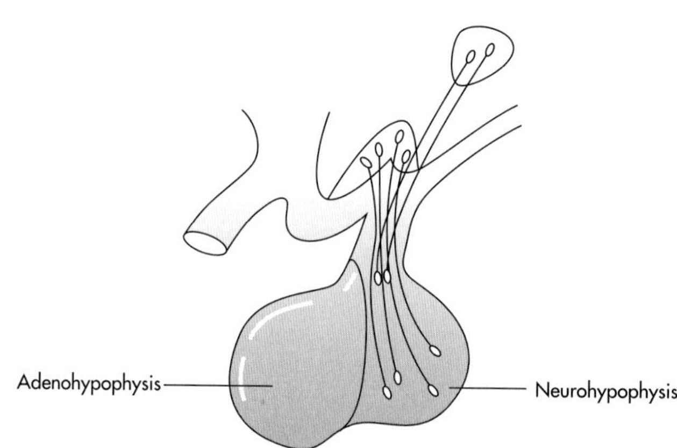

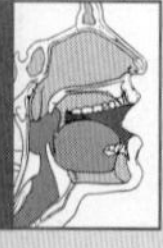

The **neurohypophysis** is composed of the nerve endings of brain cells. Secretion from these neurons may pass into the bloodstream. Find the neurohypophysis.

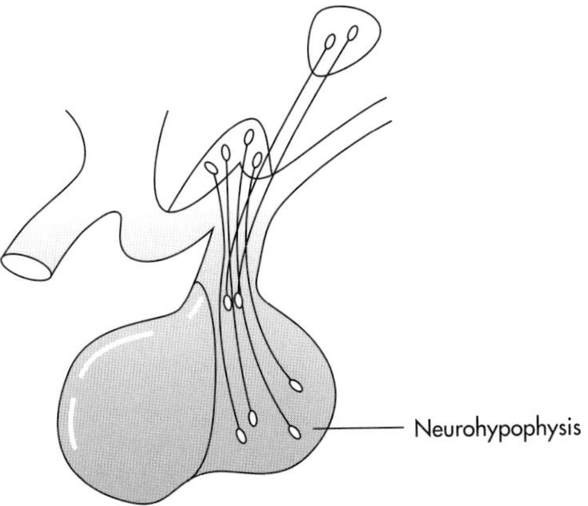

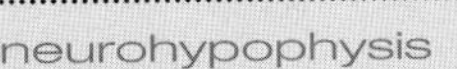

The ______________ portion of the pituitary contains the endings of neurons and secretes two hormones that have influence on the kidneys and the uterus.

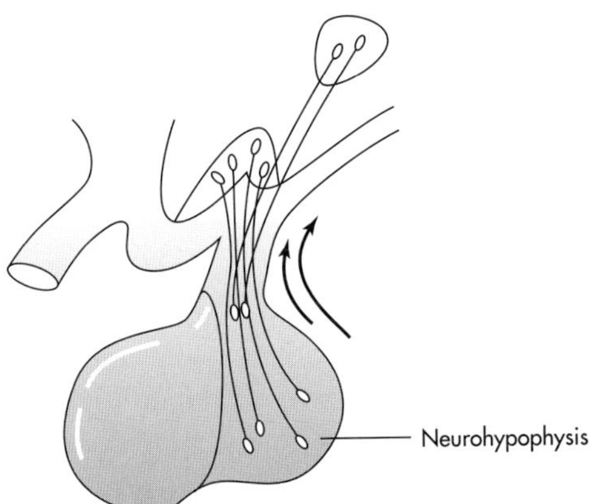

The other portion of the pituitary, the **adenohypophysis,** is composed of glandular-type cells. Find the adenohypophysis.

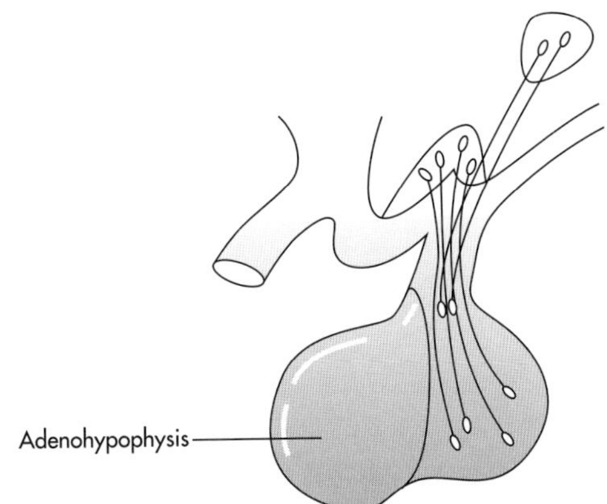

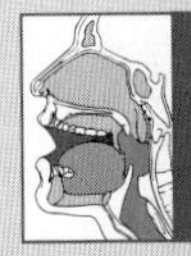

adenohypophysis

The ______________ portion of the pituitary is composed of glandular cells that secrete various hormones. **Hormones** are chemicals carried in the blood that can have an effect on the regulation of body organs.

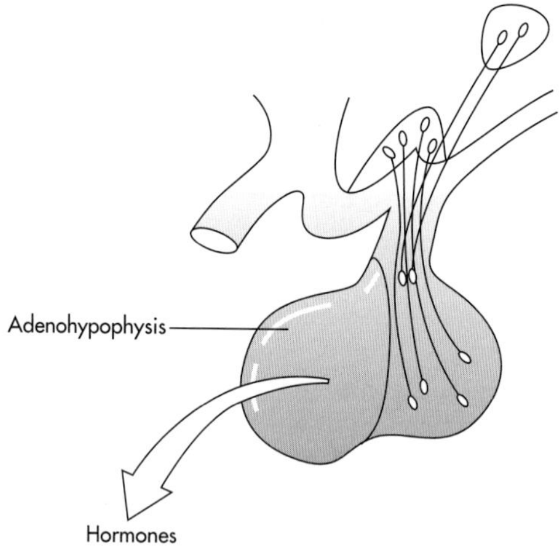

One of the hormones secreted into the bloodstream by the adenohypophysis is **growth hormone (GH)**, which regulates the growth of bones.

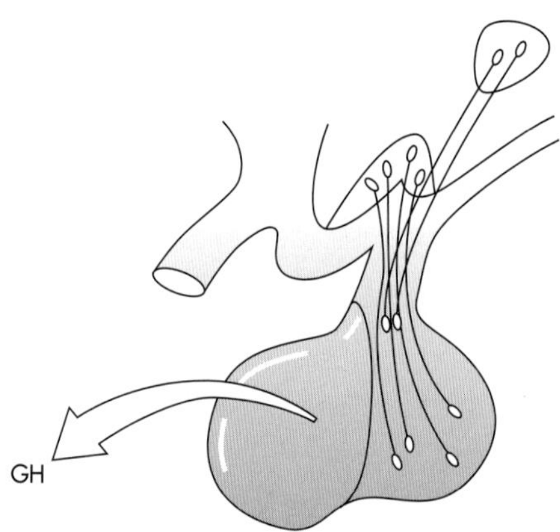

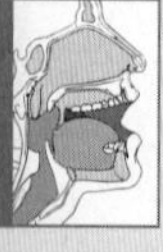

_______________ hormone is produced by the adenohypophysis. Other hormones produced include **lactogenic hormone (LH)**, **thyrotropic hormone (TTH)**, **gonadotropic hormone (GTH)**, and **adrenocorticotropic hormone (ACTH)**. These hormones have varied functions such as regulation of milk production, regulation of metabolism, regulation of the sex organs, and regulation of the adrenal glands.

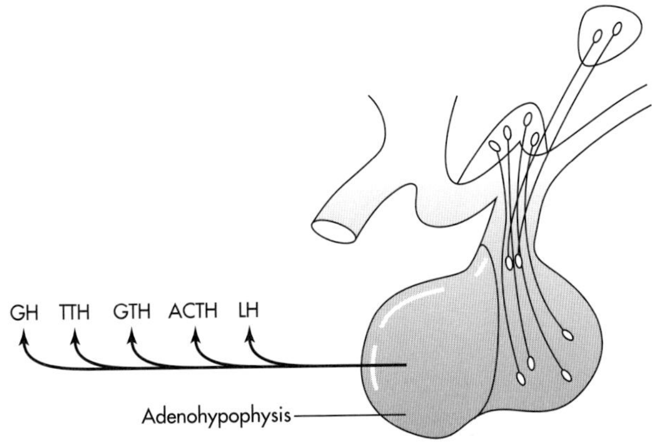

Growth

Find the two portions of the pituitary gland on the drawing.

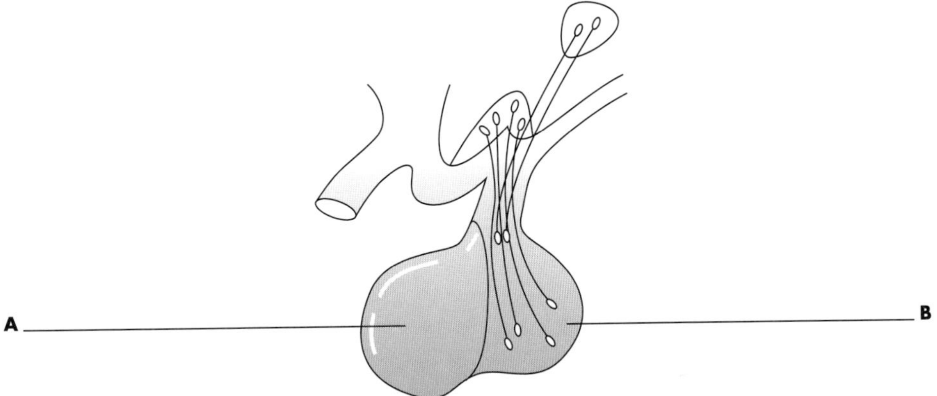

A. adenohypophysis
B. neurohypophysis

What are the functions of the neurohypophysis? What are the functions of the adenohypophysis?

neurohypophysis—regulation of the kidneys and uterus; adenohypophysis—regulation of milk production, metabolism, sex organs, adrenal glands, and growth

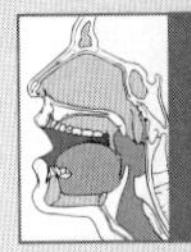

3.3 Thyroid and Parathyroid Glands

thyroid

The **thyroid gland** is a bilobed gland found in the anterior compartment of the neck, on the ______________ cartilage.

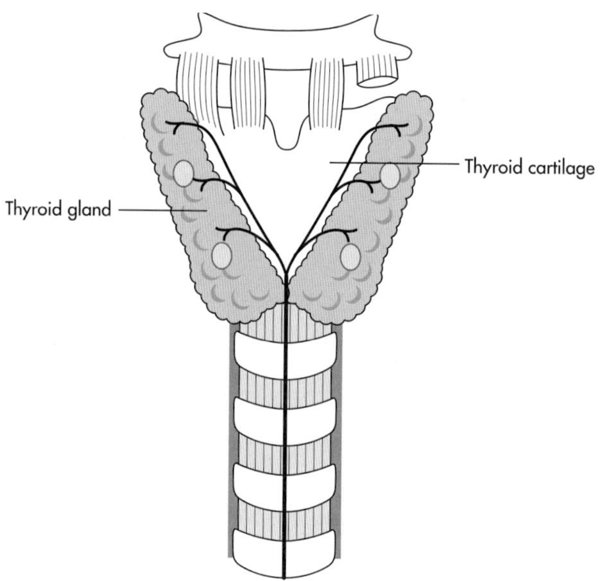

endoderm, tongue

Check back in Chapter Two for the development of this gland. It arose from an outpouching of ______________ from the pharynx, on the back of the ______________.

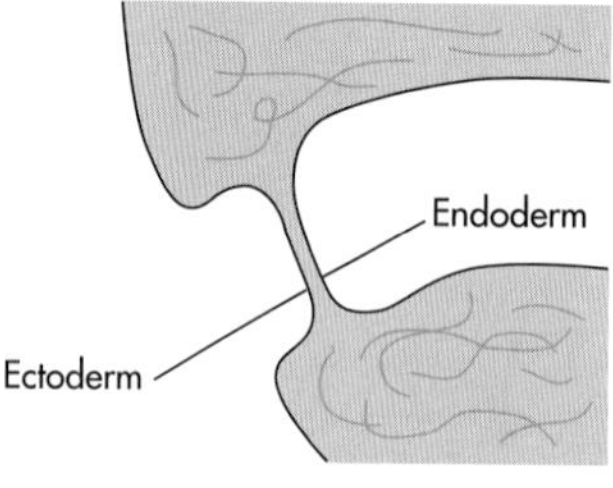

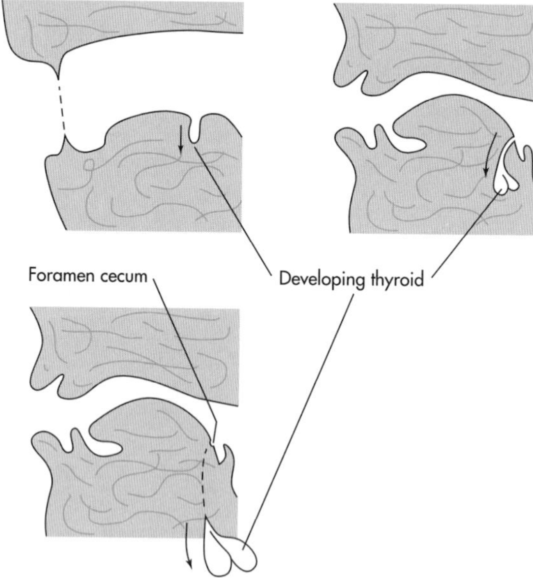

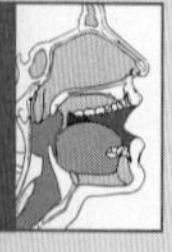

As it grows down into the neck, the developing ______________ gland breaks away from its origin on the tongue. It leaves a remnant on the tongue called the ______________.

thyroid, foramen cecum

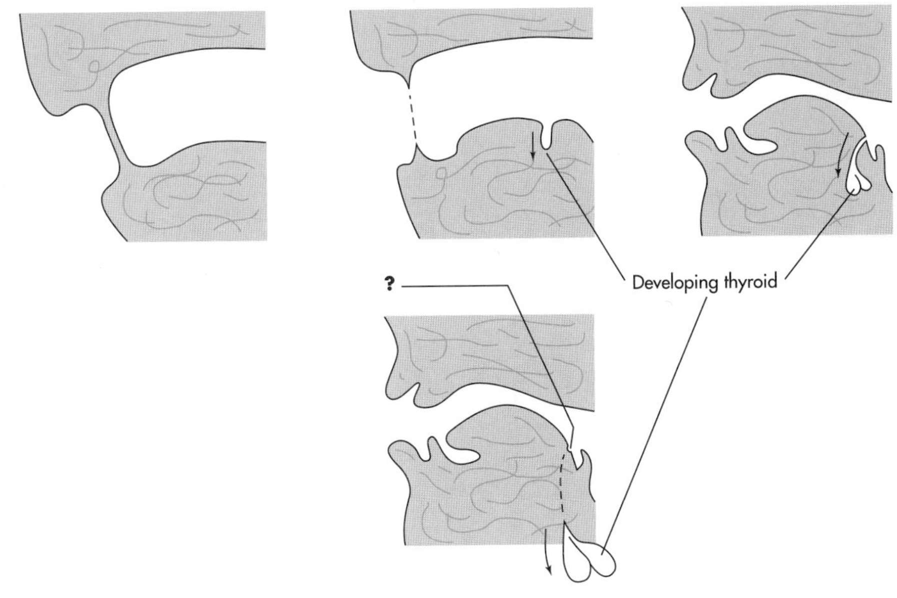

The thyroid gland is an **endocrine gland,** which means a "ductless gland." It pours its hormonal product, **thyroxin,** directly into the bloodstream. Name a gland with a duct; this is an **exocrine gland.**

salivary gland

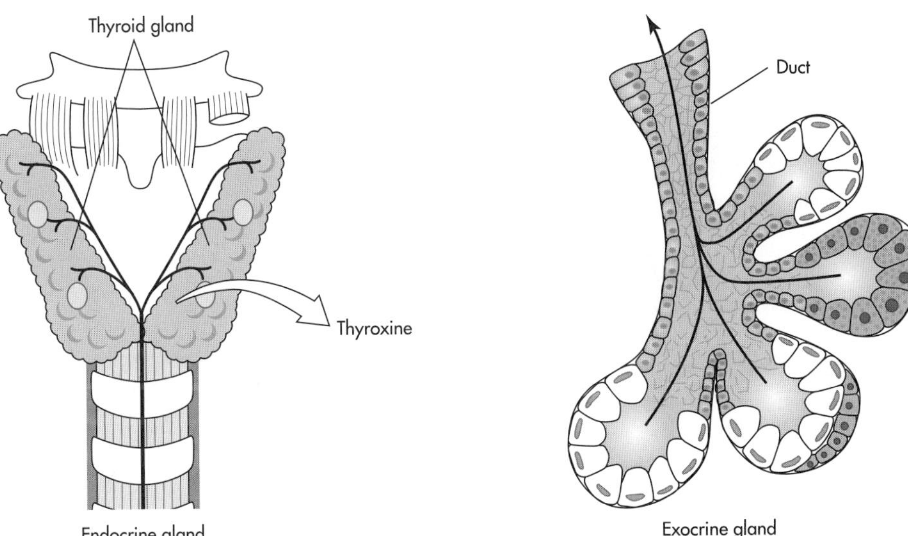

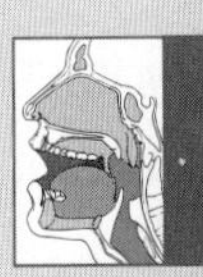

metabolism

Thyroxin controls the metabolic rate of the body as it processes food into energy. The main function of the thyroid gland is the control of ______________.

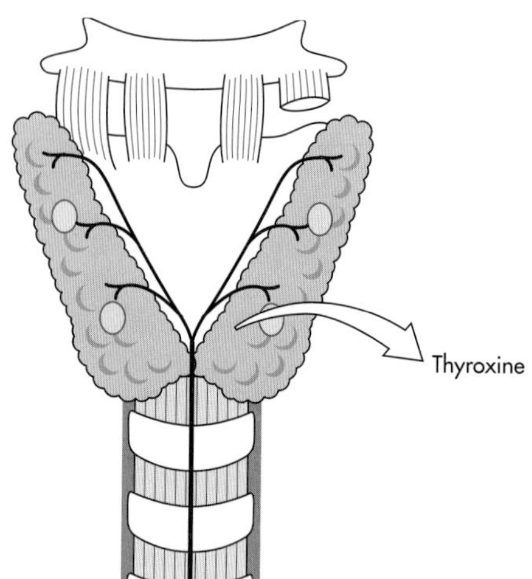

There are other cells within the thyroid gland called C cells that are responsible for the production of **calcitonin.** These cells came from the endoderm of the fourth pouch (see Chapter Two). They help regulate calcium metabolism.

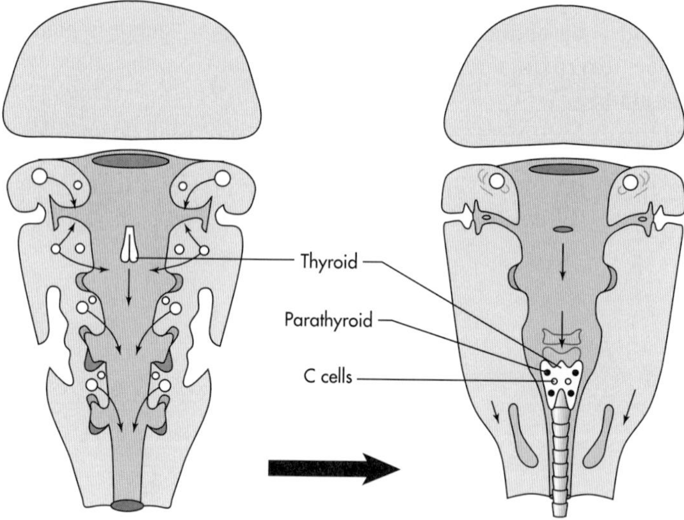

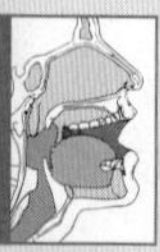

continued

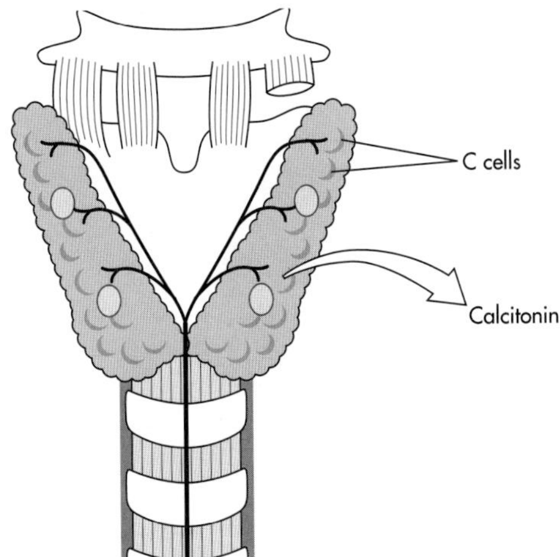

________ cells are found scattered within the body of the thyroid gland. There are other cells gathered in four distinct spherical groups that also take part in calcium metabolism. These are the **parathyroid glands.** Find them embedded within the thyroid gland.

C

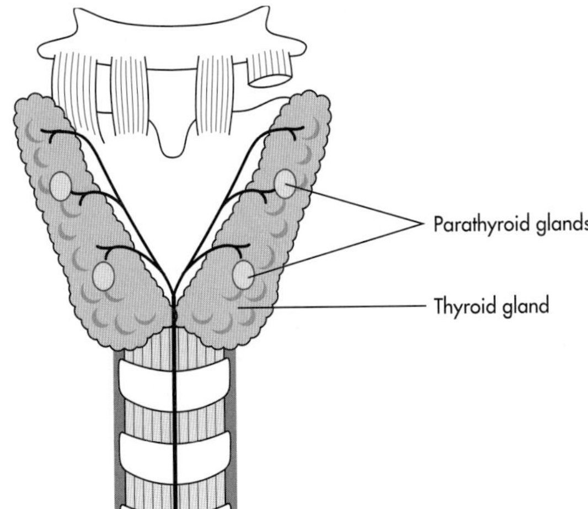

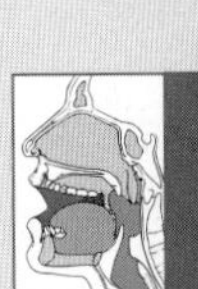

parathyroid, thyroid, calcium, C

The ______________ glands are embedded within the body of the ______________ gland. They help regulate ______________ metabolism along with the ______________ cells of the thyroid gland.

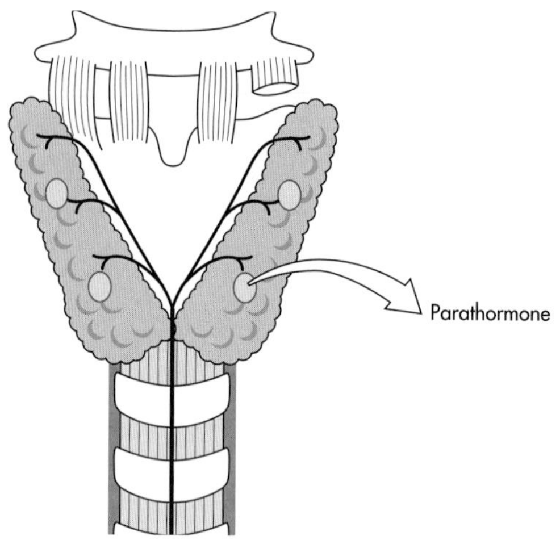

A. thyroid gland, thyroxin
B. C cells, calcitonin
C. parathyroid, parathormone

Label the different glands and write down what each produces.

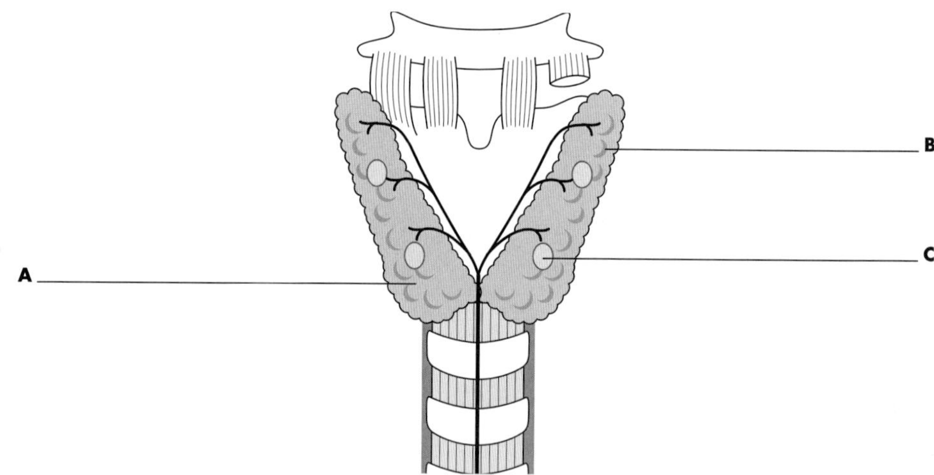

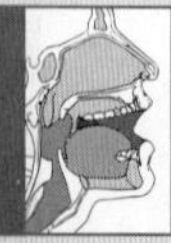

Thymus and Tonsils

3.4

The next group of "glands" does not comprise true glands, in that they do not produce a secretory product. They are, instead, lymphatic tissue and produce lymphocytes. What structure have we already studied that produces lymphocytes?

lymph nodes

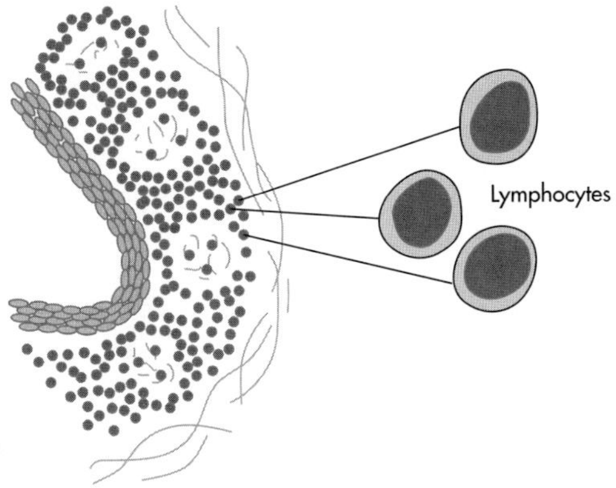

The **thymus** is a bilobed structure found in the anterior neck. Find it as well as the thyroid gland in the drawing.

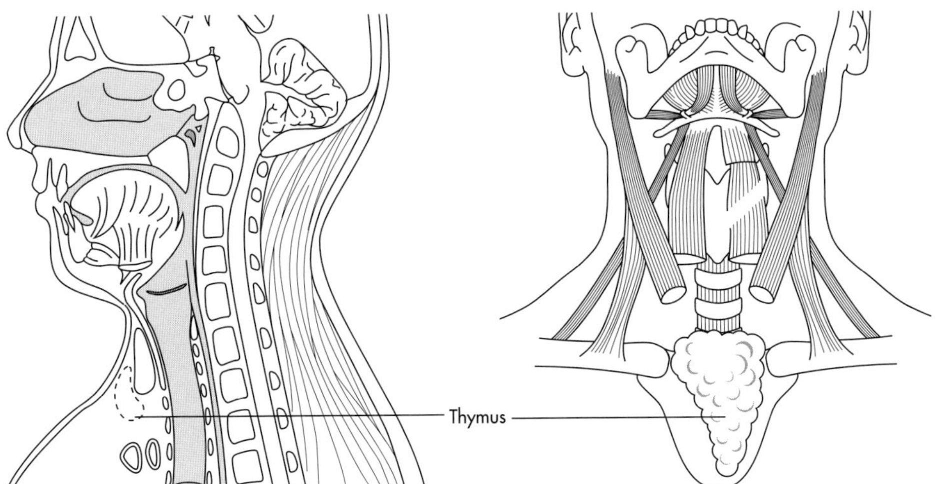

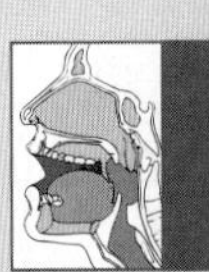

The thymus is a relatively large structure in the child until puberty, when it begins to involute (disappear). All that remains in the adult is a cord of connective tissue.

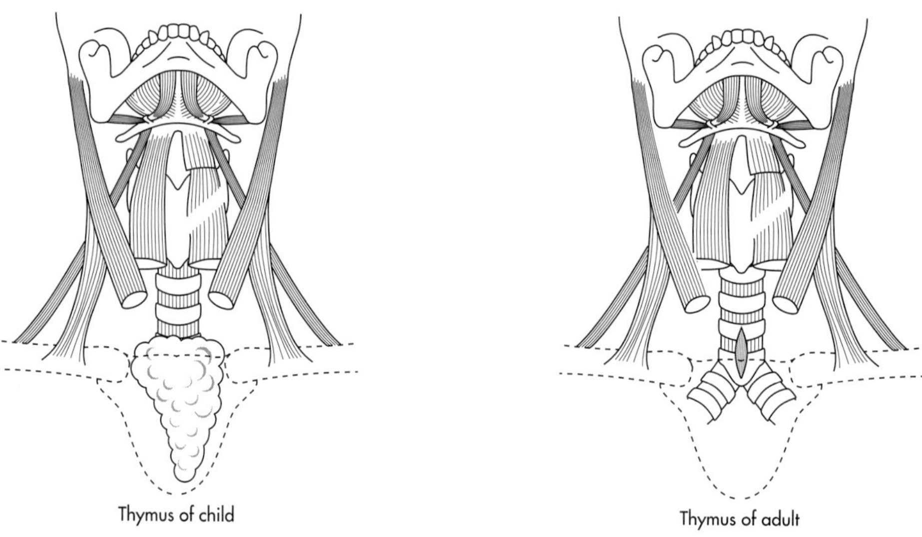

thymus

The ______________ gland is active during childhood, producing T lymphocytes. T lymphocytes are an important part of the body's defensive system and are all produced during childhood. B lymphocytes are produced in other lymphatic tissue.

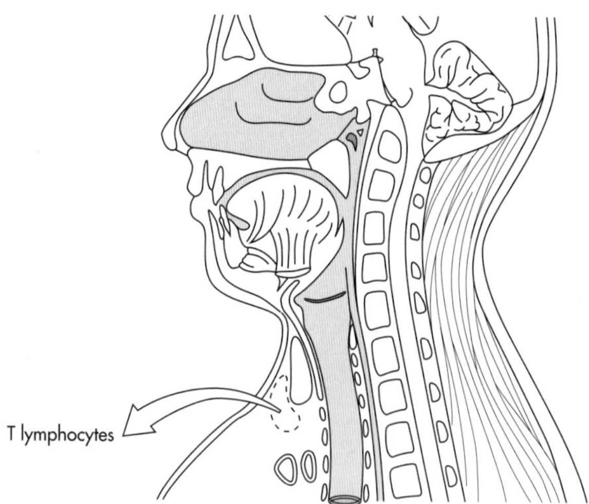

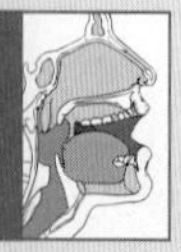

Another lymphatic tissue found in the head and neck is the **tonsils.** Find a pair of tonsils on the drawing.

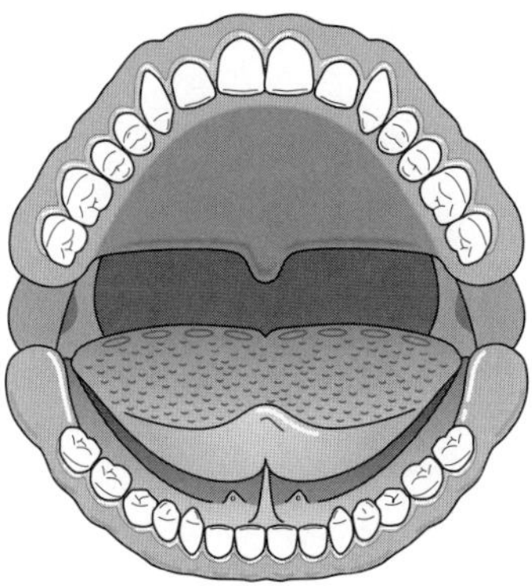

This first pair of tonsils is called the ______________ tonsils. They arose from pouch II in the embryo. Within what muscular structures in the oral cavity/oropharynx are they nestled?

pharyngeal (palatine), pillars

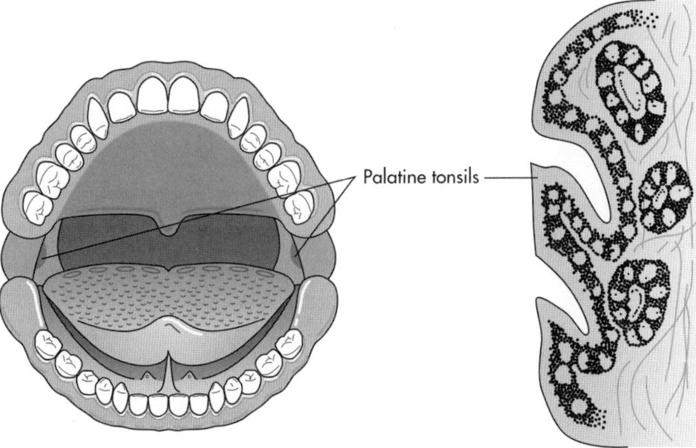

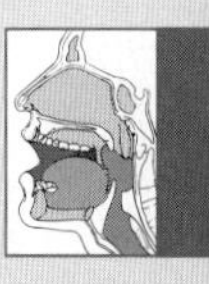

The posterior or root of the tongue houses the next group of tonsils, the **lingual tonsils.**

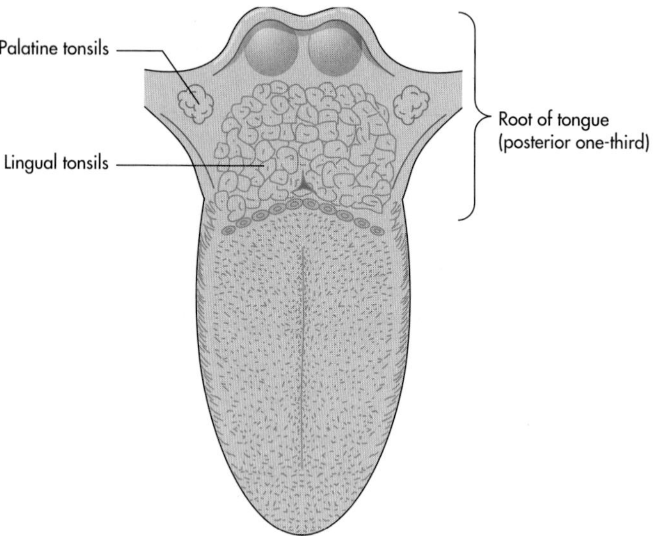

lingual, root, tongue

The ______________ tonsils are located on the ______________ of the ______________.

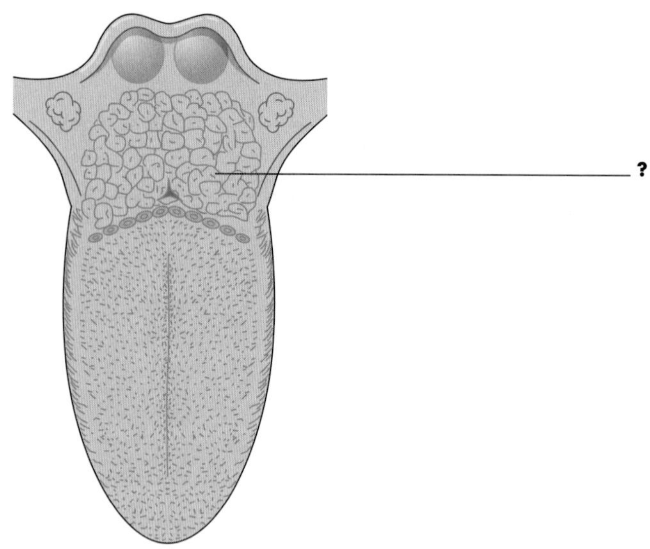

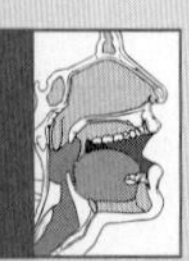

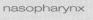

The third and last pair of tonsils is the **pharyngeal tonsils,** which, in the past, have been called the "adenoids." In what portion of the body do these appear to lie?

nasopharynx

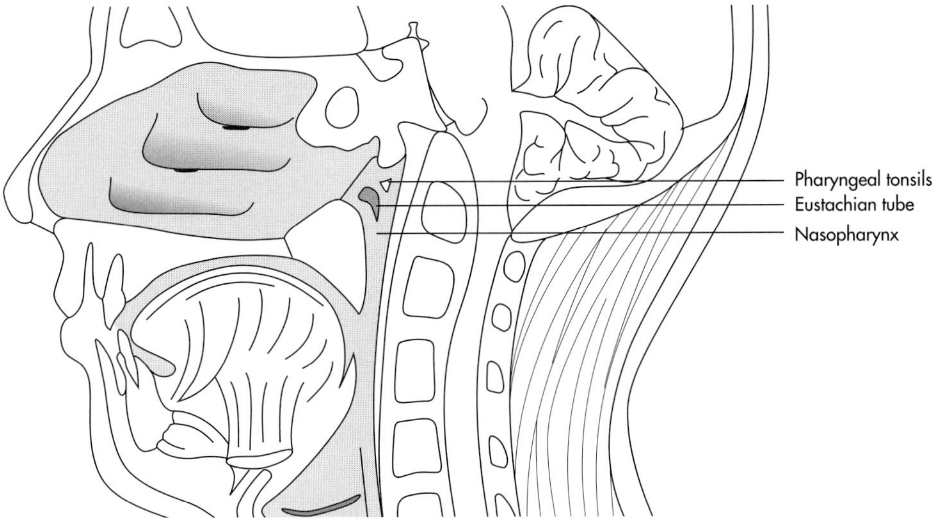

The pharyngeal tonsils lie in the nasopharynx near each Eustachian tube opening. How many are there?

two

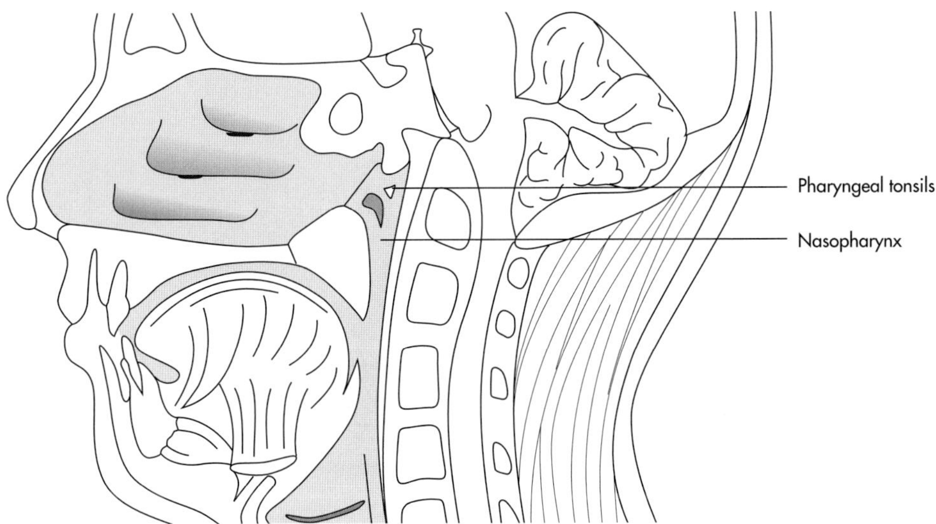

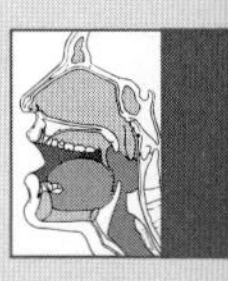

lymphocytes

The palatine, lingual, and pharyngeal tonsils are all located around the opening of the pharynx. They may serve as a protective mechanism, as they all produce ____________, which are defensive cells.

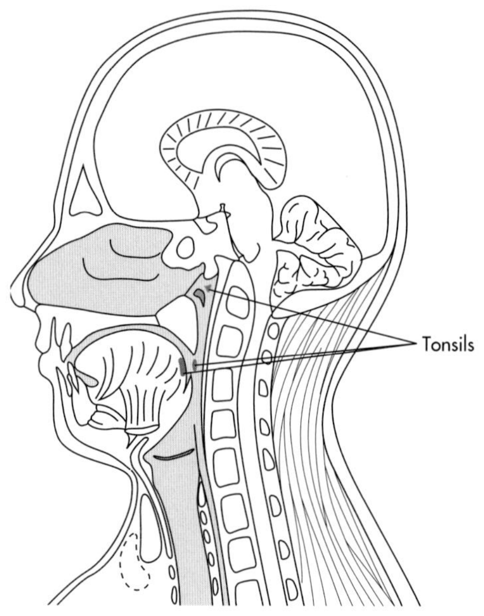

palatine, lingual, pharyngeal

This "ring" around the pharynx in which the tonsils are located is called **Waldeyer's ring.** It consists of which tonsils?

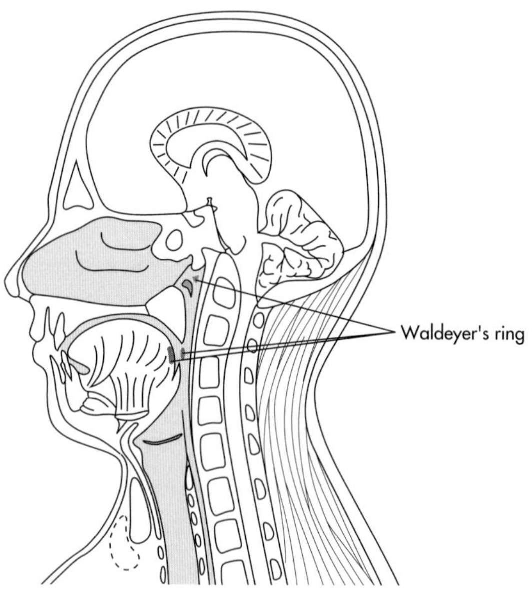

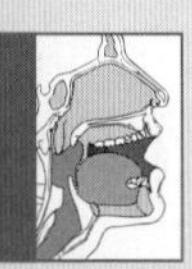

Label these lymphatic structures. What do they produce?

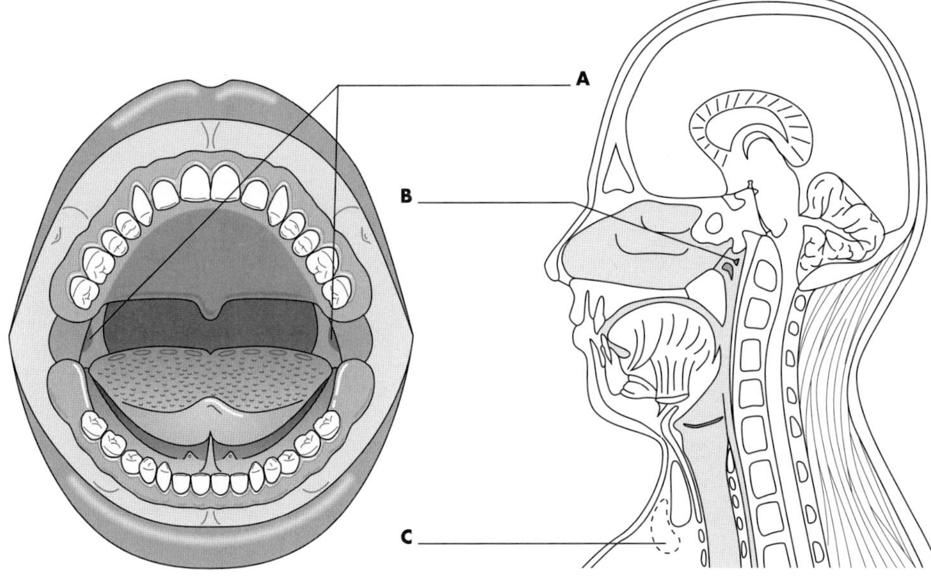

A. palatine tonsils
B. pharyngeal tonsil
C. thymus gland

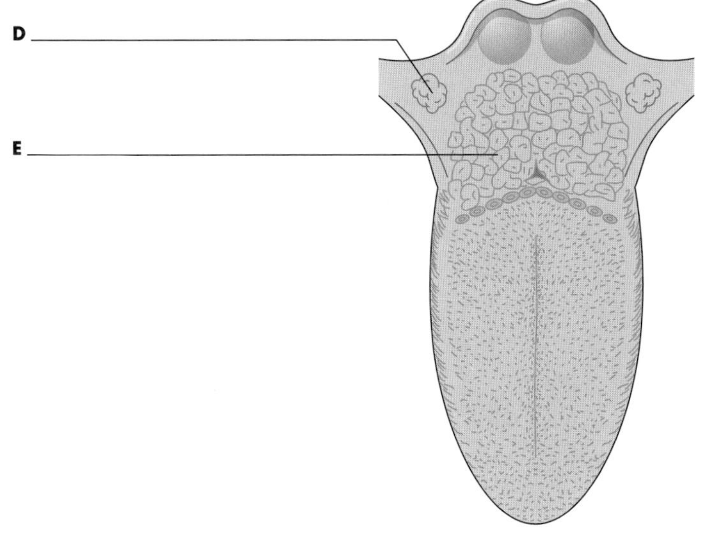

D. palatine tonsil
E. lingual tonsils

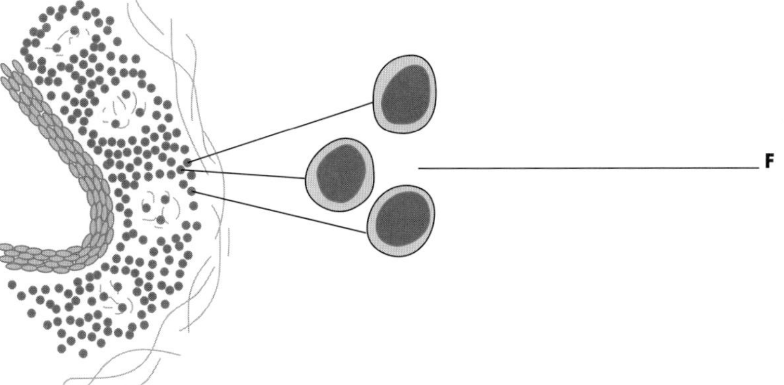

F. lymphocytes
They produce lymphocytes (T lymphocyte = thymus).

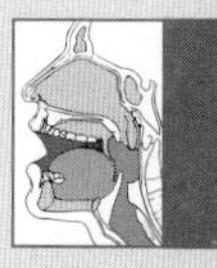

4.0 FASCIA AND SPACES OF THE HEAD AND NECK

Fascia is connective tissue that envelopes the muscles, blood vessels, and organs. It serves as a protective sleeve and allows the various structures to move past each other within the body, because there exists a **space** between each fascia-covered surface that is lubricated by fluid.

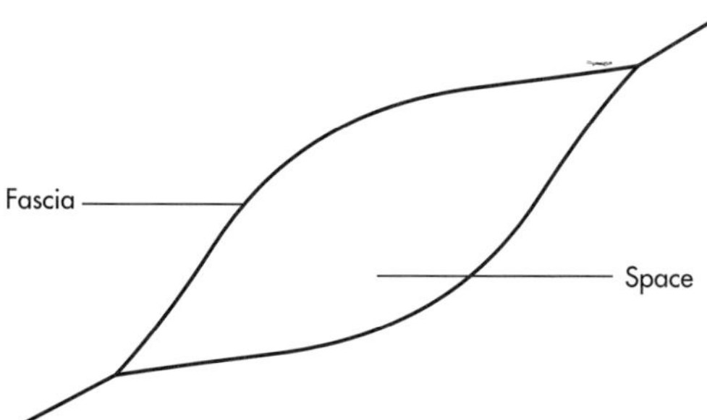

Fascia

______________ is a connective tissue covering of muscles, blood vessels, and organs. Within the head and neck are several fascias that are named, as are the spaces that exist between them.

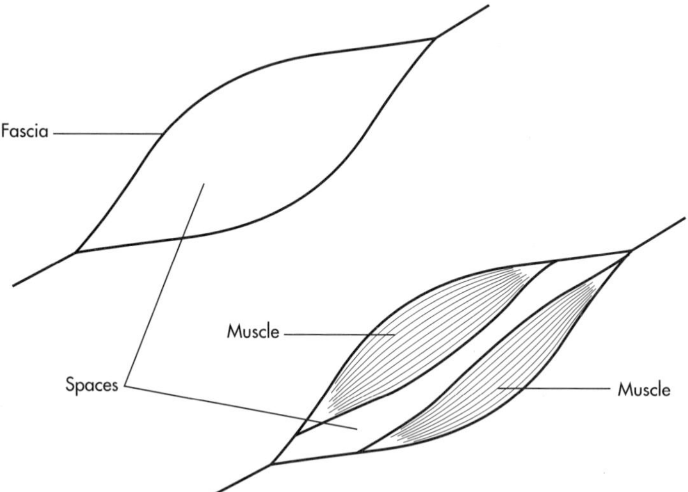

Fascia may cover one or more structures and different fascias connect to each other. The spaces between fascia are important to learn, because they are areas where infection is often isolated and causes swelling.

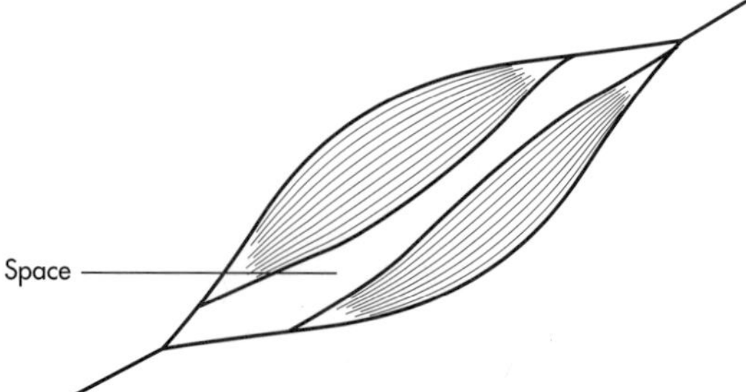

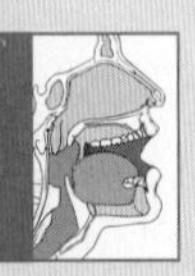

There is **superficial fascia** directly under the skin and investing the muscles of facial expression. **Deep fascia** occurs surrounding the deep structures of the head and neck. Illustrated here is a section through the muscle and its fascia. The fascia appears as a line and the spaces as white spaces. You must remember, however, that these are three-dimensional coverings and spaces.

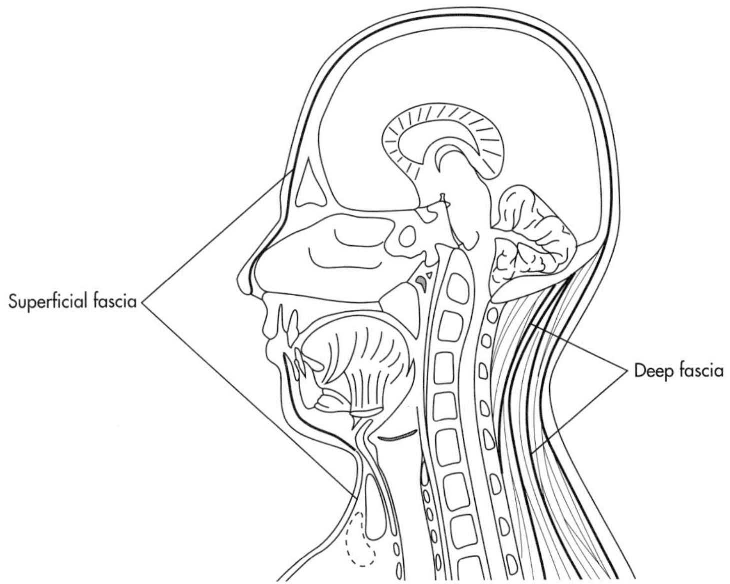

The fascia of the face are the **temporal fascia** and the **parotideomasseteric fascia.** They cover the temporalis muscle, parotid gland, masseter muscle, and zygomatic process. Find them.

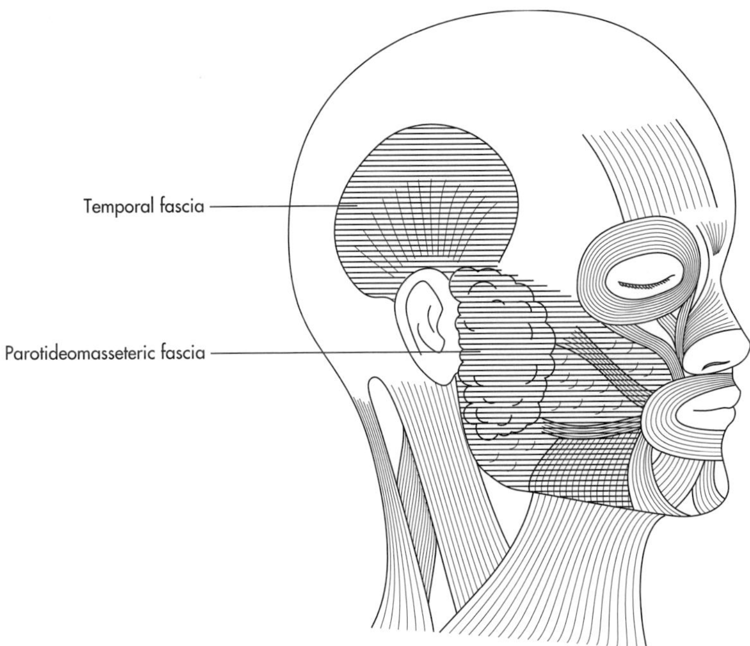

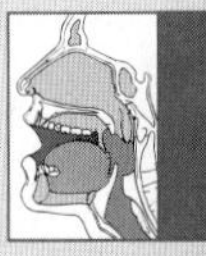

temporal, parotideo-masseteric

These are the ______________ and ______________ fascias.

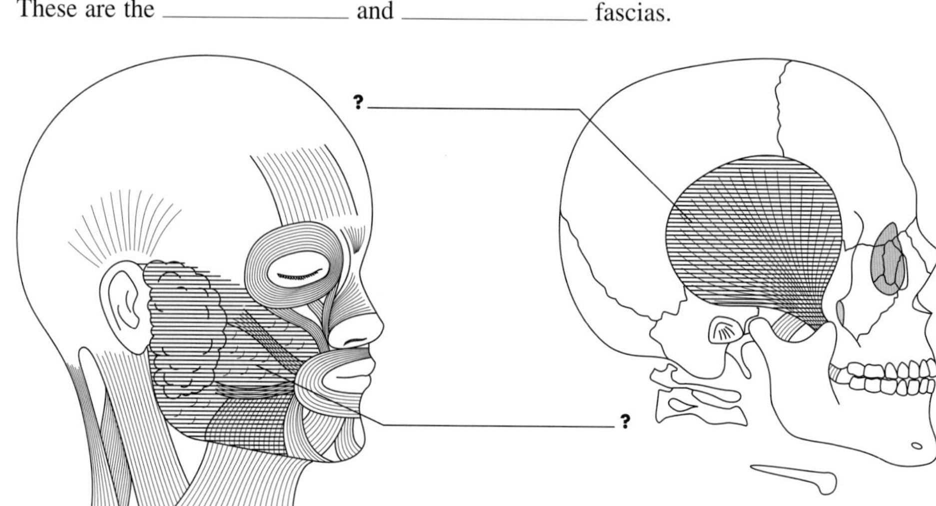

The fascia of the neck is divided into two categories: superficial cervical and deep cervical fascia. The **superficial cervical fascia** covers the platysma. The **deep cervical fascia** is more complex.

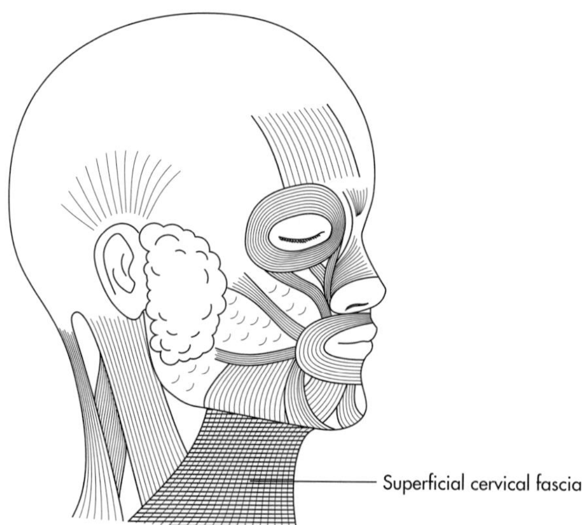

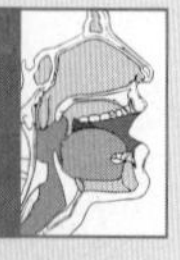

The first portion of the deep fascia covers the **sternocleidomastoid** and **trapezius muscles.** Another portion becomes straplike and is known as the **stylomandibular ligament.** Find it on the drawing.

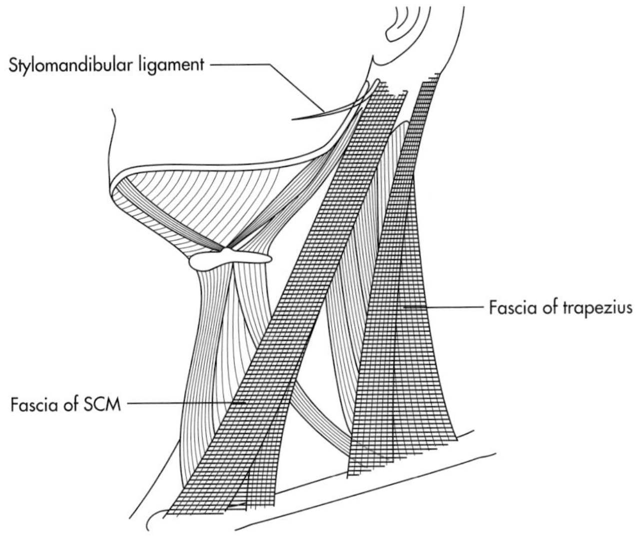

This is the ______________ ligament. It is part of the ______________ cervical fascia.

stylomandibular, deep

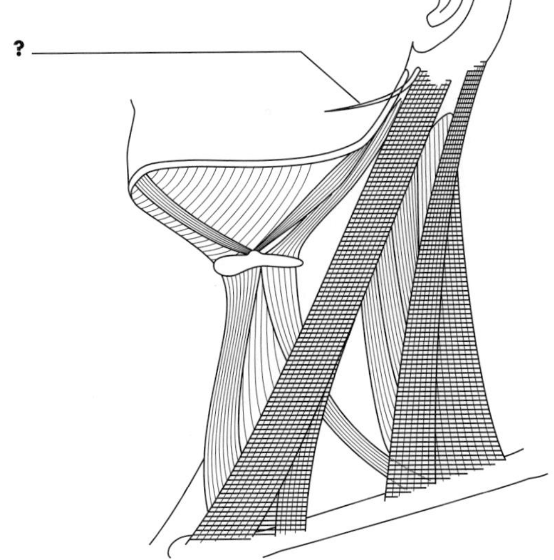

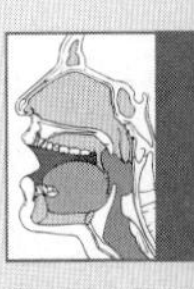

Another portion of the deep cervical fascia covers the **suprahyoid muscles.** Below it, a separate portion covers the infrahyoids and is known as the **middle cervical fascia.**

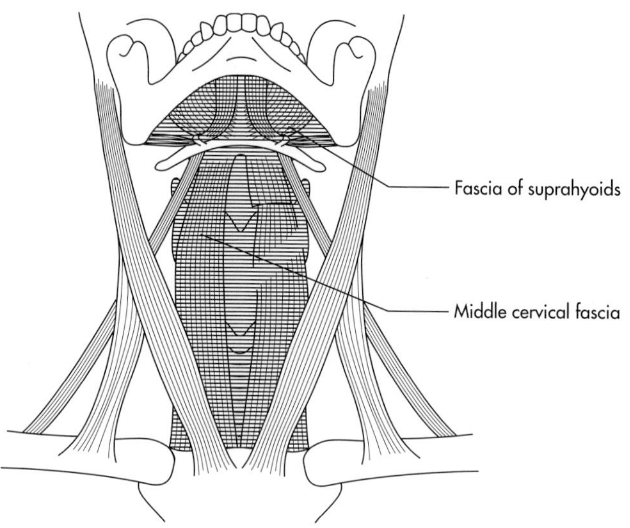

the carotid arteries and internal jugular vein

There are three "tubes" of deep cervical fascia. The first, the **carotid sheath,** is fascia that covers what blood vessels? A second, the **visceral fascia,** covers the trachea and esophagus/pharynx. The connecting strap of fascia between these two is the **alar fascia.**

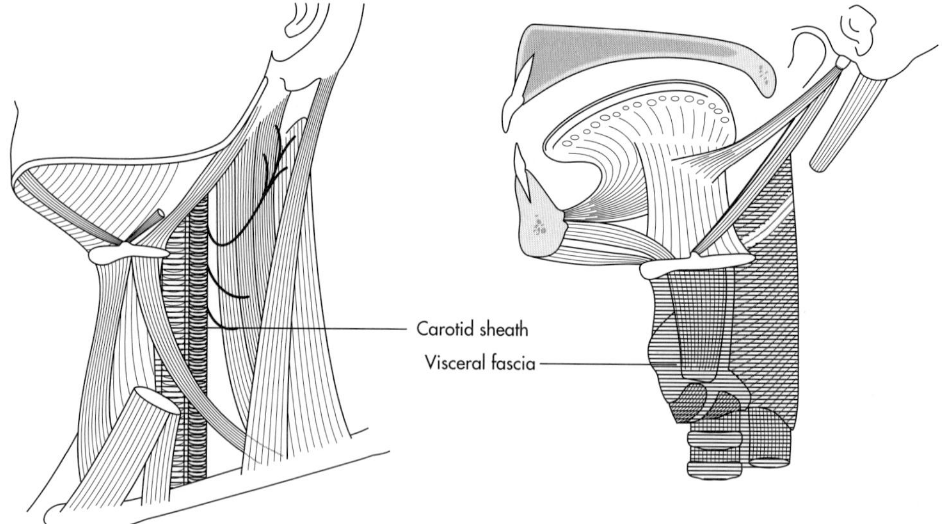

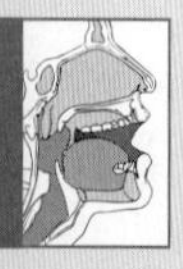

The last deep cervical fascial tube is the **vertebral fascia,** which covers the vertebral column and its muscles. What separates all these fascias?

a space

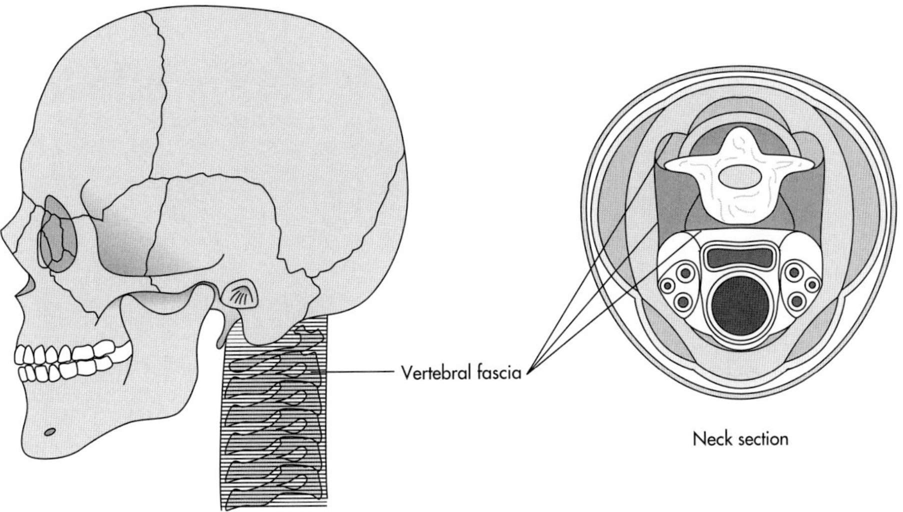

The **spaces of the head and neck** follow. There are three spaces in the neck and eight spaces in the face. A section through the neck illustrates its spaces. What color are they on the drawing? And the fascia?

white are spaces, black lines

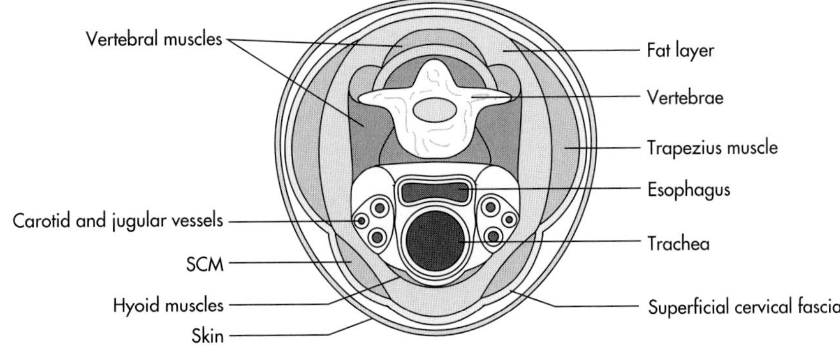

Several of the fascias of the neck are "cut through" and seen as dark lines on this drawing. Find the fascias.

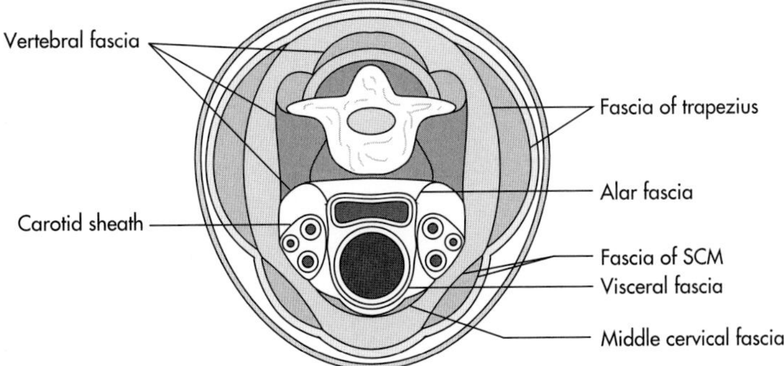

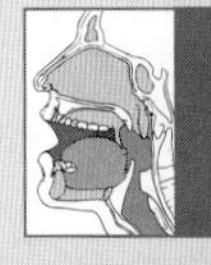

The spaces between the fascia are labeled here. These are the three spaces of the neck: the **lateral pharyngeal space,** the **retropharyngeal space,** and the **pretracheal space.** The pretracheal space is filled with thyroid tissue.

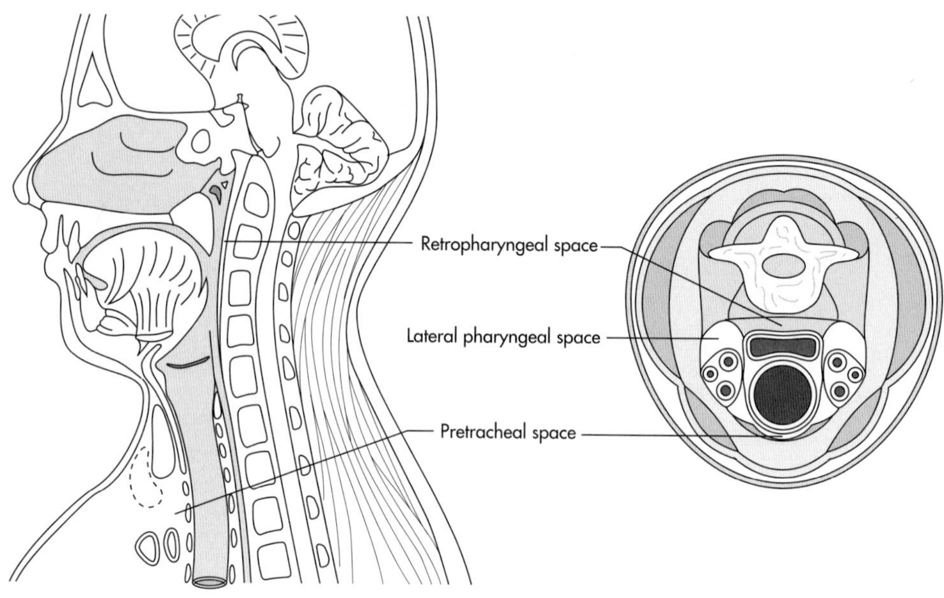

The spaces of the face are many and can be seen in section (below) or in other views. This section is at the level of the oral cavity. Note the landmarks to find where this section was made. Find the **carotid** and **retropharyngeal spaces**, which are continuous from the neck.

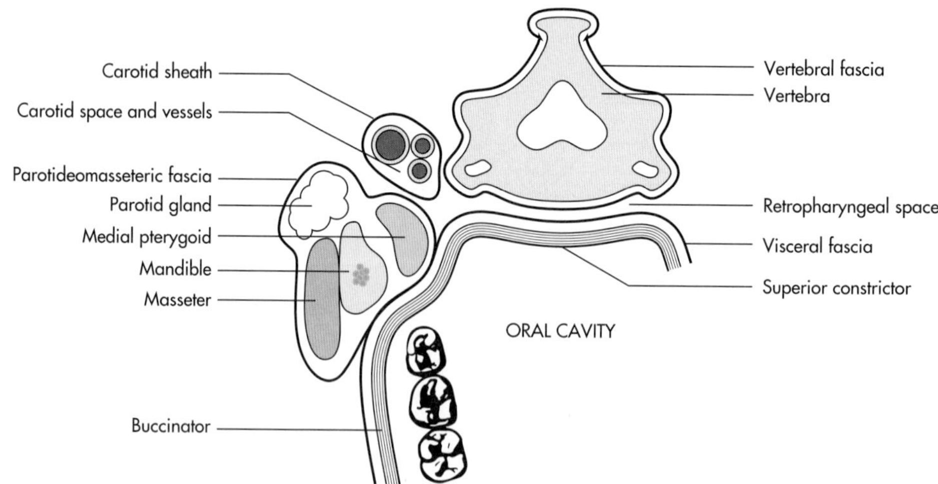

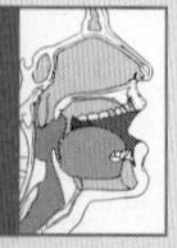

The **masticator space** is a cleft between the parotideomasseteric and pterygoid fascias. The masseter and medial pterygoid muscles lie within this space, as does the mandible. Find this space.

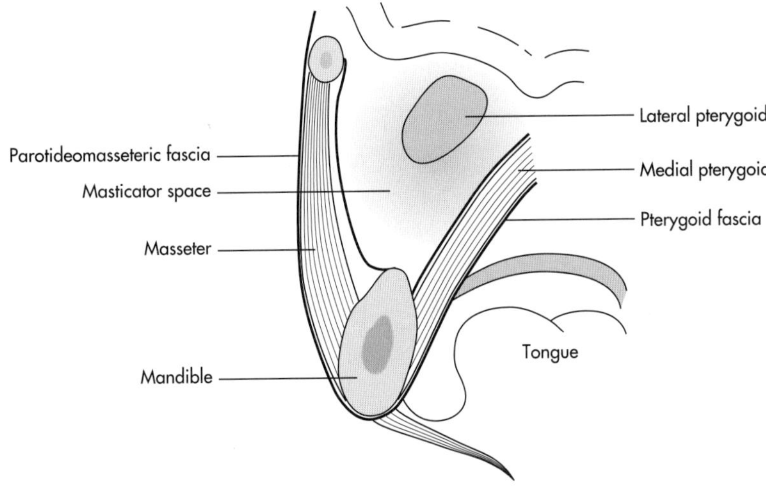

The **pterygomandibular space** is a deeper space containing the inferior alveolar nerve, artery, and vein and is found within the masticator space. What is found in this space?

inferior alveolar nerve and vessels

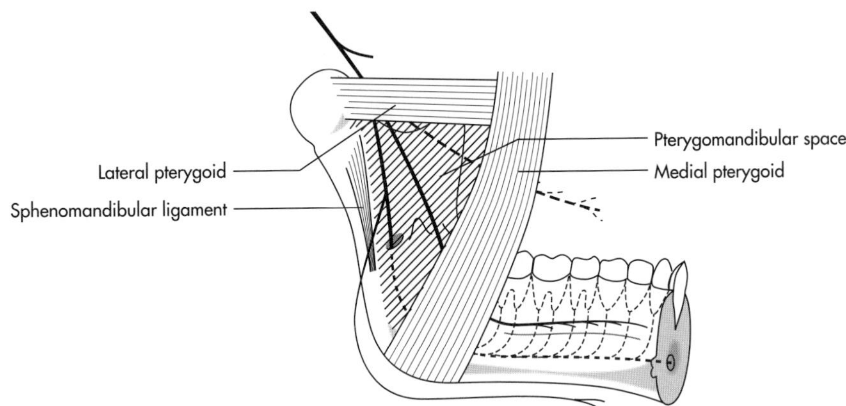

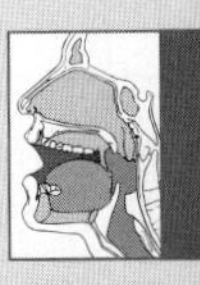

Stensen's

One of the spaces of the face is called the **buccal space.** Find it. The buccal space contains the **buccal fat pad,** which lies anterior to the parotid gland just deep to the skin. What is the duct of that gland? The **canine space** is also shown. The **parotid space** lies around the parotid gland. The **temporal space** lies between the temporal muscle and its envelope of fascias.

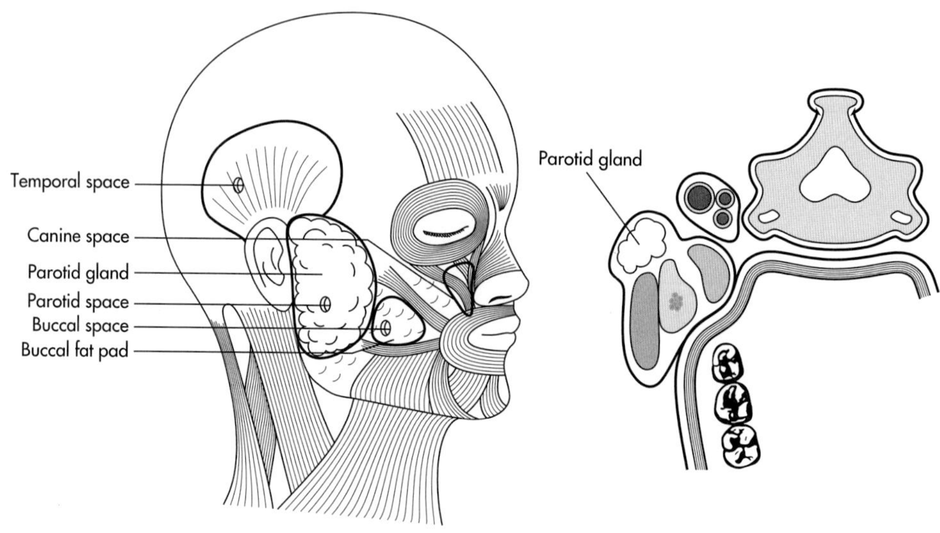

A. masticator space
B. pterygomandibular space
C. retropharyngeal

What are these spaces called?

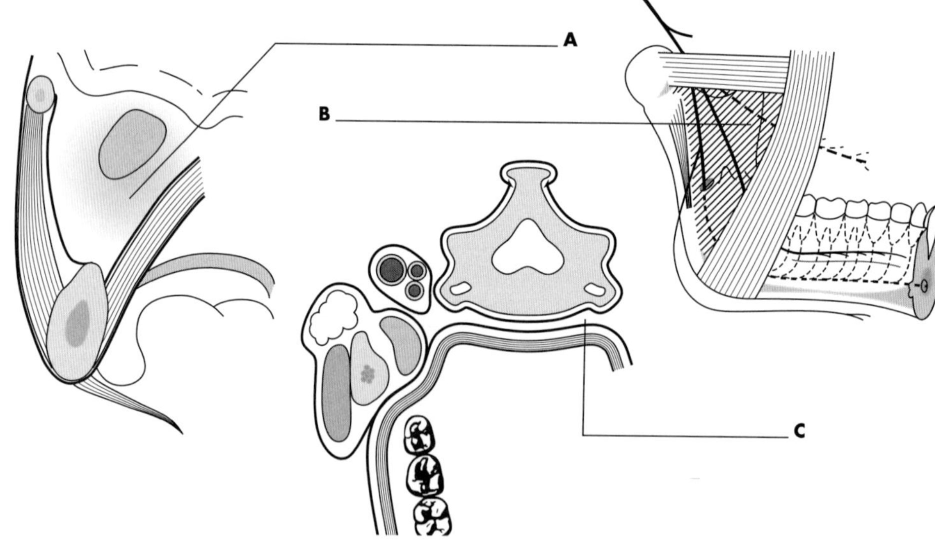

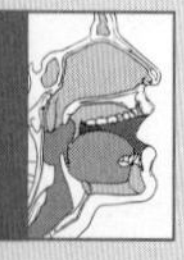

The space of the body of the mandible runs around the mandible as shown. From another view of the mandible, one can see the **submandibular, submental,** and **sublingual spaces.**

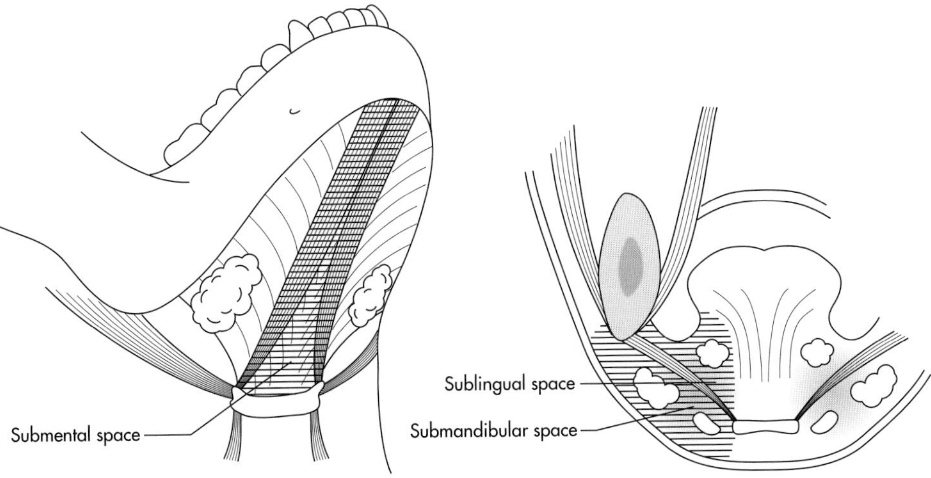

Find the submandibular, submental, and sublingual spaces.

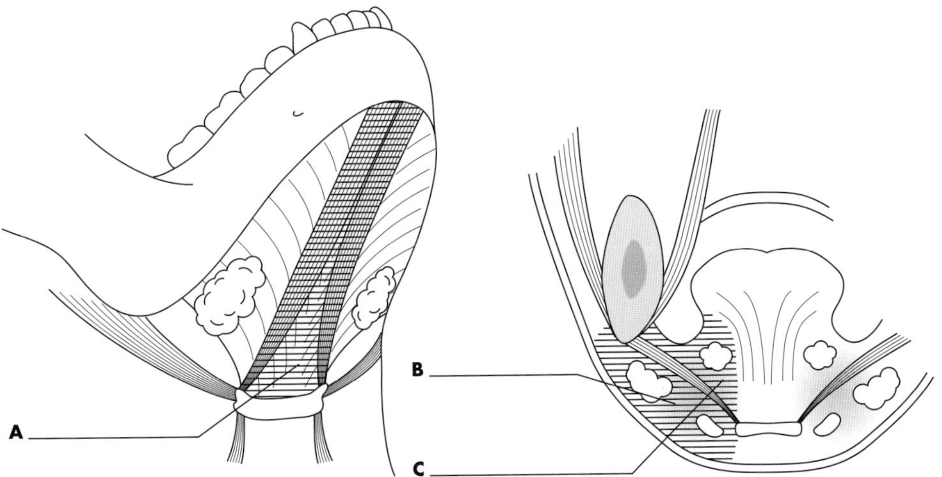

A. submental
B. submandibular
C. sublingual

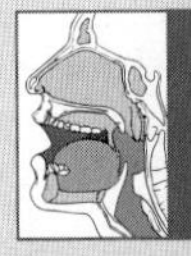

What are these spaces? Check your answers in the preceding text.

A. submental
B. carotid
C. parotid
D. submandibular
E. sublingual

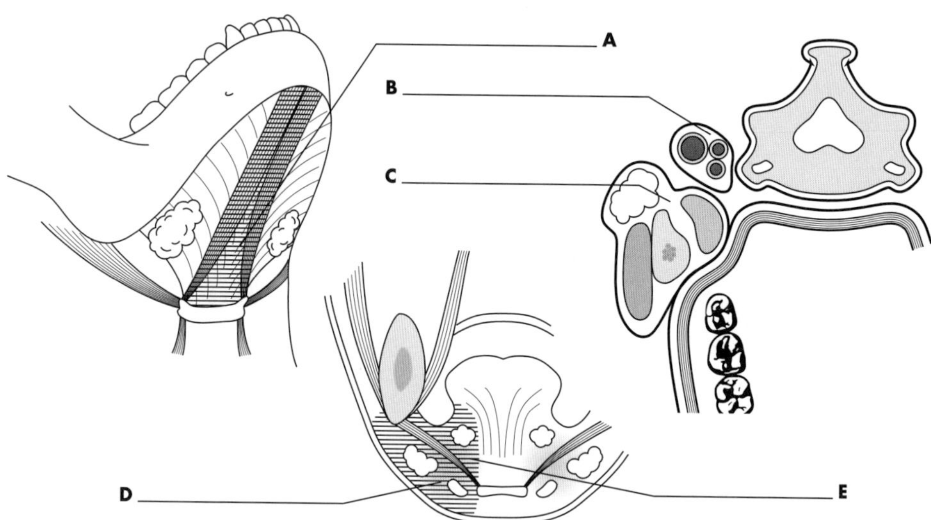

5.0 INJECTION SITES

Review the innervation of the maxillary and mandibular teeth as learned in Chapter Nine. Name the nerve that goes with that portion of the **maxillary teeth** it innervates.

A. nasopalatine nerve
B. greater palatine nerve
C. PSA
D. MSA
E. ASA

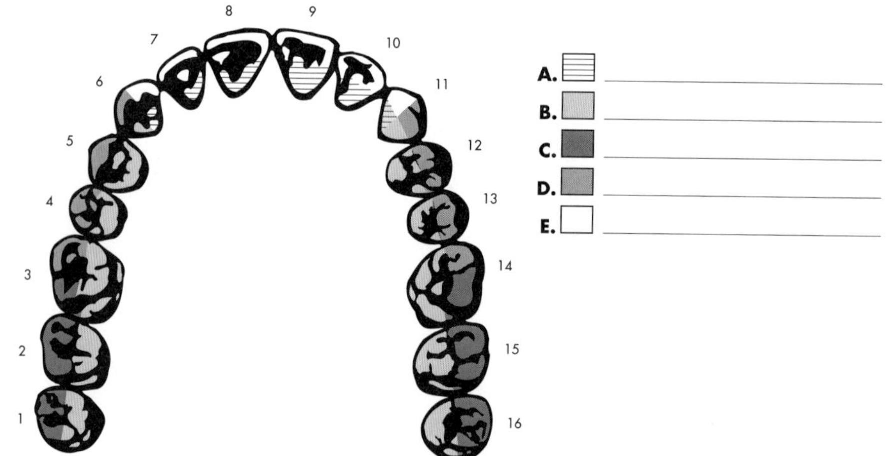

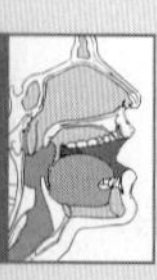

Do the same for the mandibular teeth.

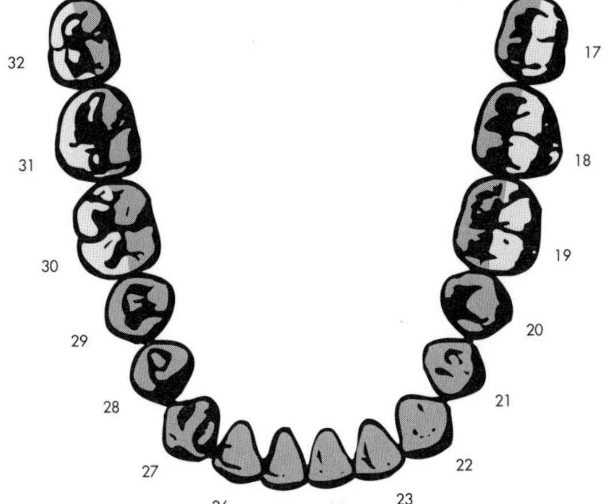

A. buccal nerve
B. inferior alveolar nerve

Anesthesia for the teeth is provided by the injection of an anesthetic solution into the area of the nerve(s) that services that tooth. An injection that deposits the solution near the nerve trunk is called a **block injection.** An injection in which the solution passes through other tissue to get to the nerve branches is called an **infiltration injection.** Which type of injection places anesthetic directly by the nerve trunk going to the tooth (teeth)?

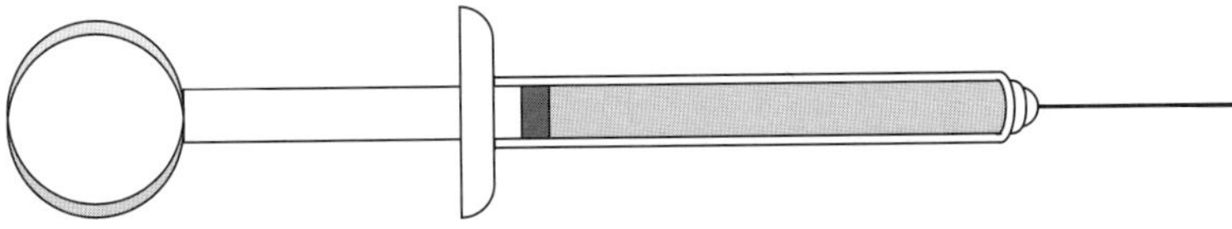

block

Let us see how each of the teeth may be anesthetized. We will be talking about complete anesthesia.

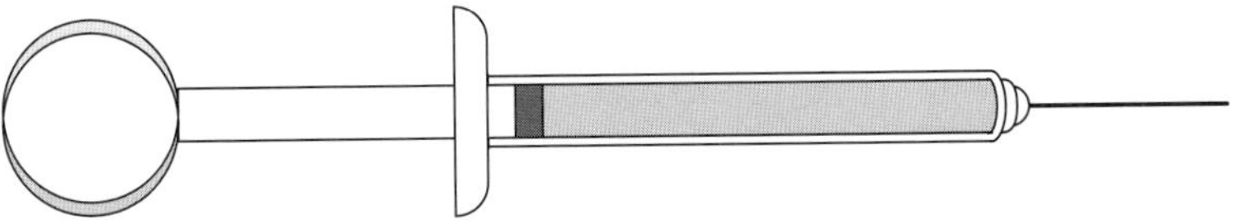

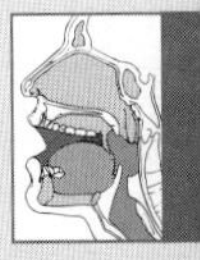

buccal = PSA nerve in pterygomandibular fossa, palatal = greater palatine nerve in hard palate opposite tooth

Beginning with the upper arch and the posterior molars (Nos. 1, 2, 14, and 15), which nerves innervate these teeth? Where do you find them?

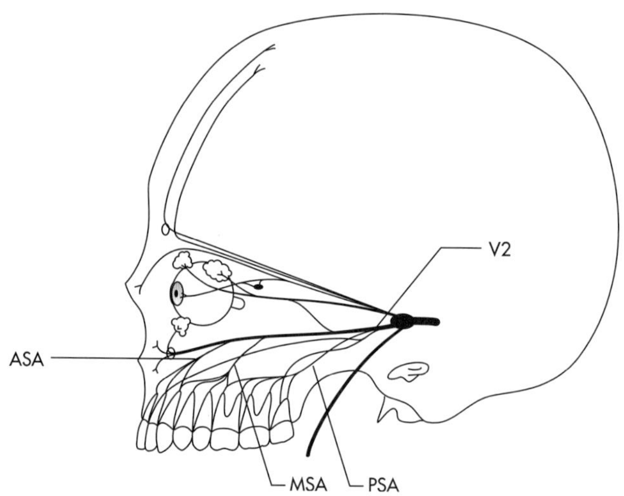

maxillary artery and pterygoid plexus

To anesthetize the maxillary molars, we need to target the PSA nerve with a **PSA block injection.** The operator places the needle up into the pterygomandibular fossa and deposits the solution. You must be careful not to penetrate or damage what two structures that lie alongside this branch of V2?

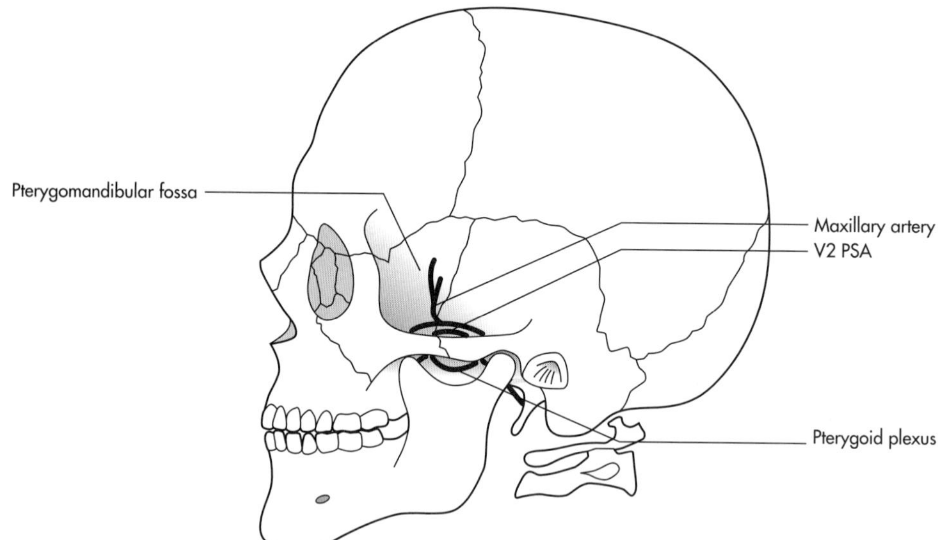

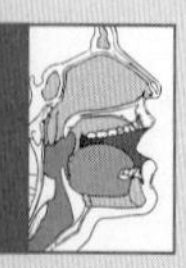

By placing reverse pressure on the syringe (aspirating), one may check if he or she has penetrated the maxillary artery or pterygoid plexus by noting the presence of blood. If so, the needle is moved. What is the name of this injection and what does it numb?

PSA block, buccal maxillary molars

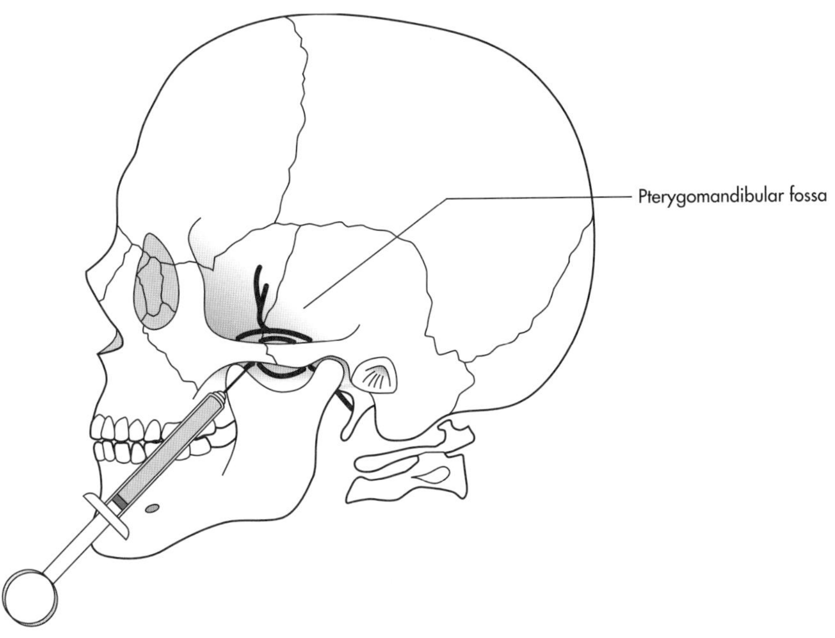

The palatal side of the molars must be reached by infiltrating the ______________ nerve, found directly opposite the tooth on the palate.

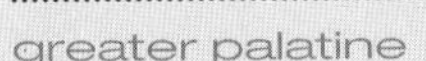
greater palatine

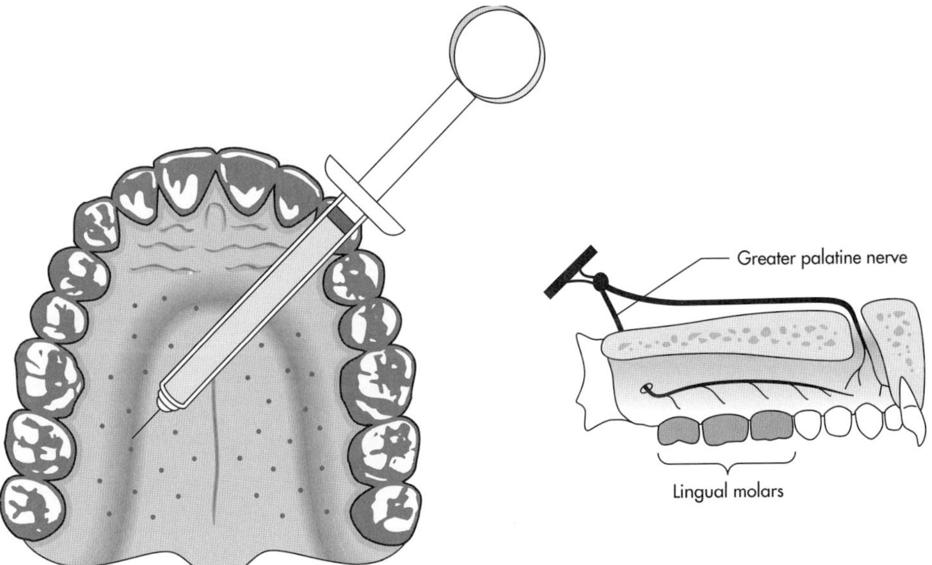

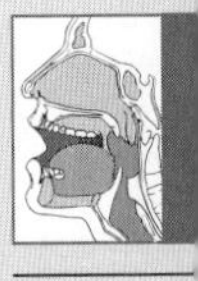

MSA

The exceptions to the maxillary molars are the two first molars, Nos. 3 and 14, for which a third nerve must be numbed. This is the ______________ nerve, which can be infiltrated next to the mesiobuccal cusp of the tooth.

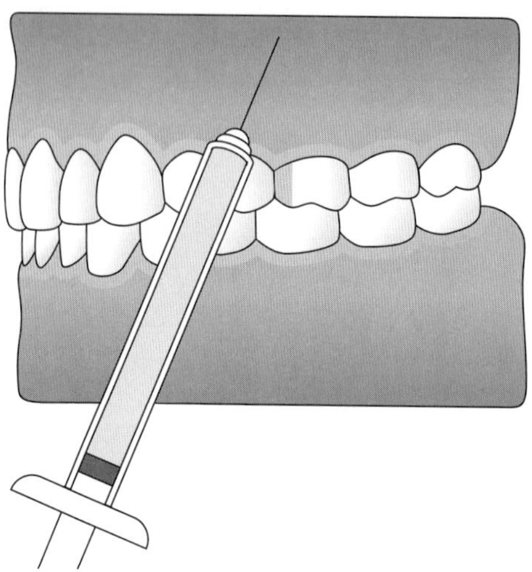

greater palatine

The MSA nerve, the PSA nerve, and the ______________ nerve innervate the maxillary first molars and must be anesthetized separately.

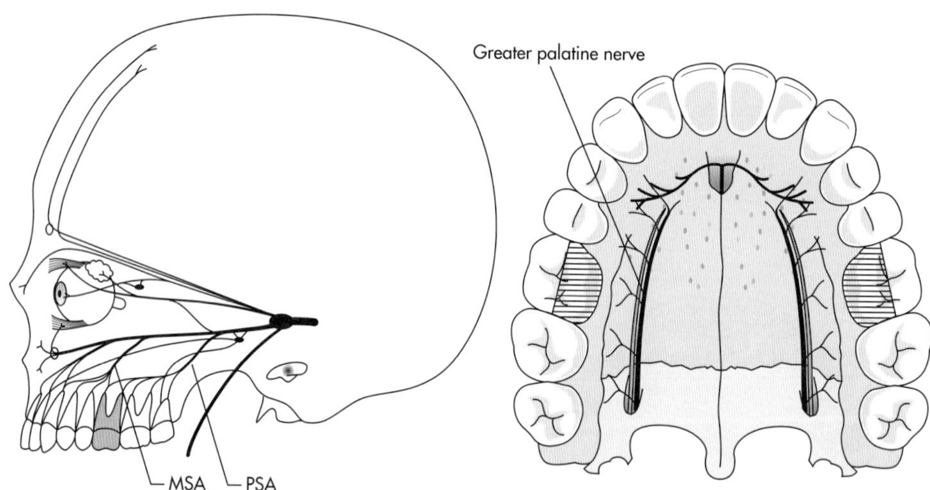

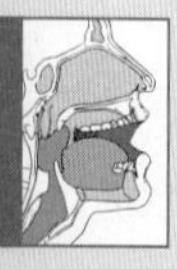

Infiltration can be accomplished by depositing anesthetic solution, with the syringe below the mucosa of the vestibule, directly opposite the tooth to be numbed. Which tooth is being numbed in this picture?

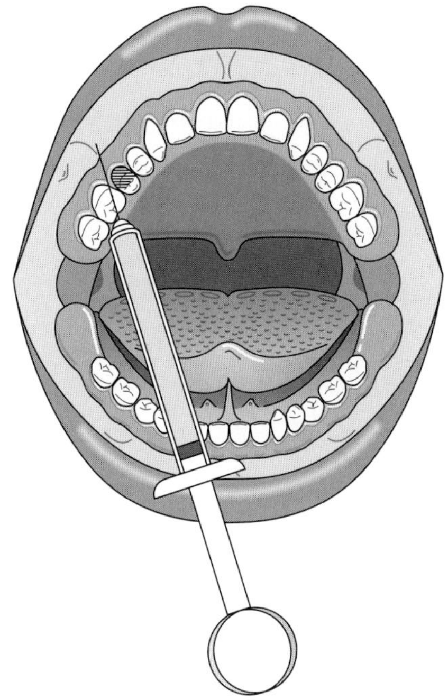

maxillary second premolar

The premolars (Nos. 4, 5, 12, and 13) can be anesthetized on the buccal aspect by infiltrating which nerve?

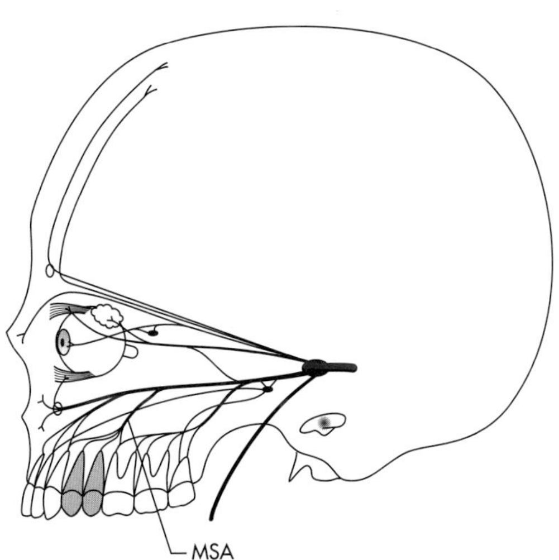

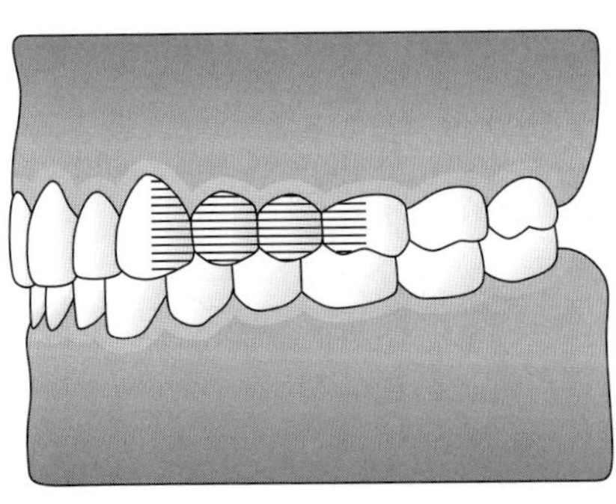

MSA nerve

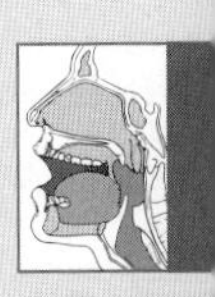

first

The middle superior alveolar nerve innervates the buccal aspect of the premolars, the distal of the canine, and the mesiobuccal cusp of the maxillary ______________ molar.

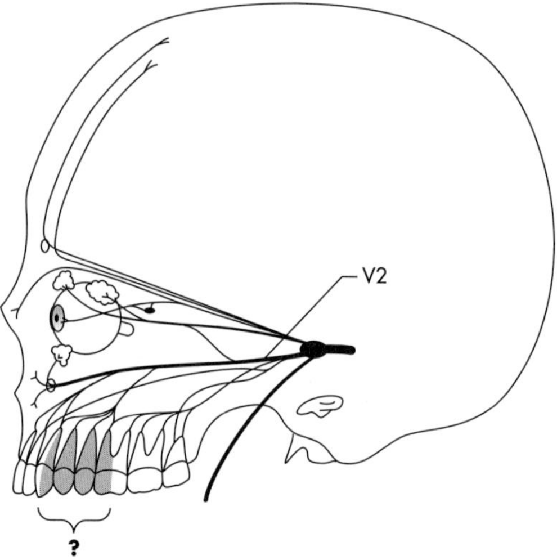

greater palatine

To numb the lingual aspect of the premolars and distal canine, an infiltration directly opposite each tooth is given, numbing what nerve?

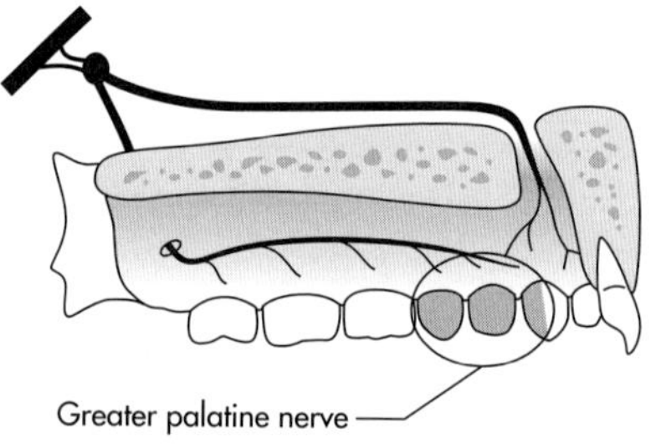

MSA, ASA, greater palatine, nasopalatine

The maxillary canines (Nos. 6 and 11) have multiple innervation. Which four nerves supply them?

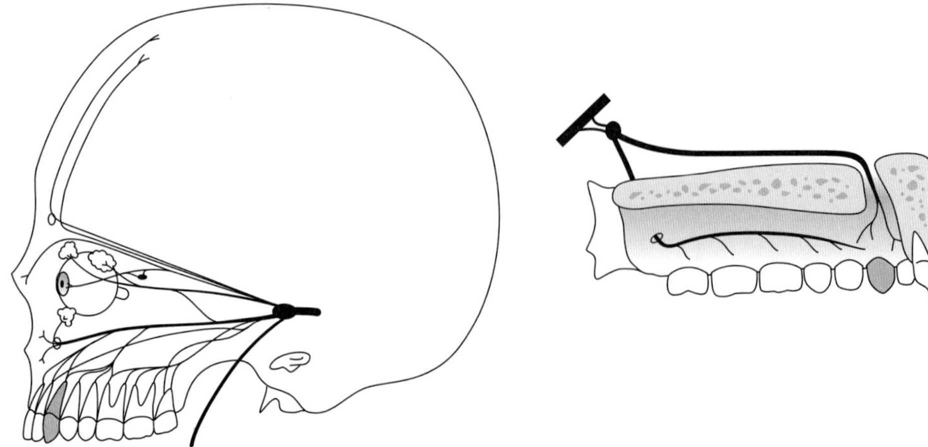

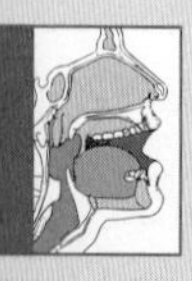

Fortunately, both the MSA and ASA nerves can be targeted by one injection, which numbs the ______________ side of the tooth.

facial

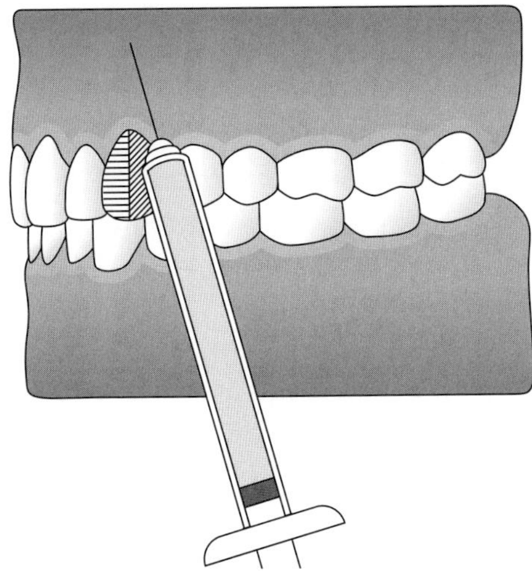

The lingual side of the maxillary canines requires two injections. The first is an infiltration directly behind the tooth, numbing which nerve?

greater palatine

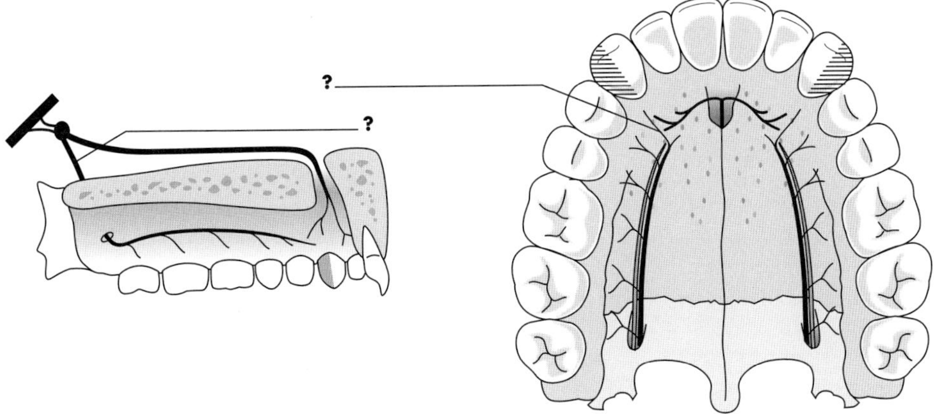

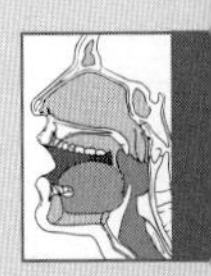

incisive

The second injection is a block injection into a soft tissue structure known as the incisive papilla. Which foramen lies beneath this "bump?"

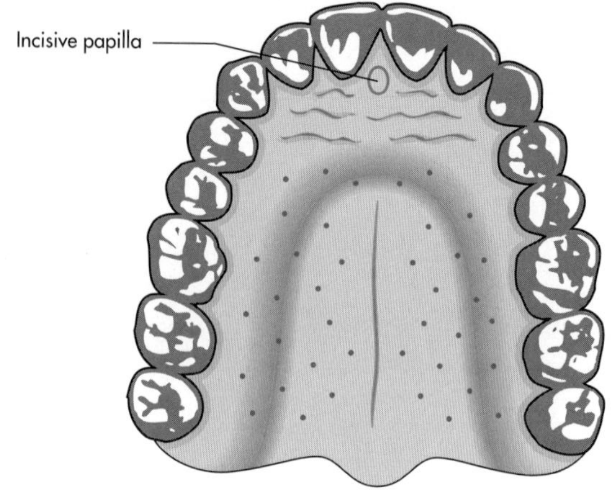

nasopalatine

What nerve exits through the incisive foramen to innervate the lingual sides of the anterior teeth?

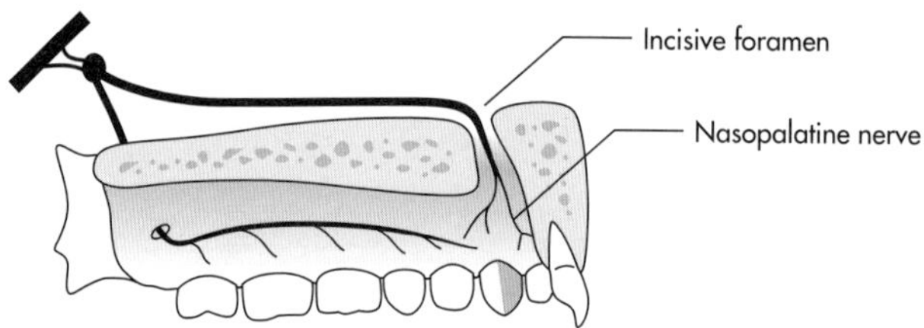

The nasopalatine nerve is numbed by block injection into the incisive papilla, which numbs the mesial side of the maxillary canine.

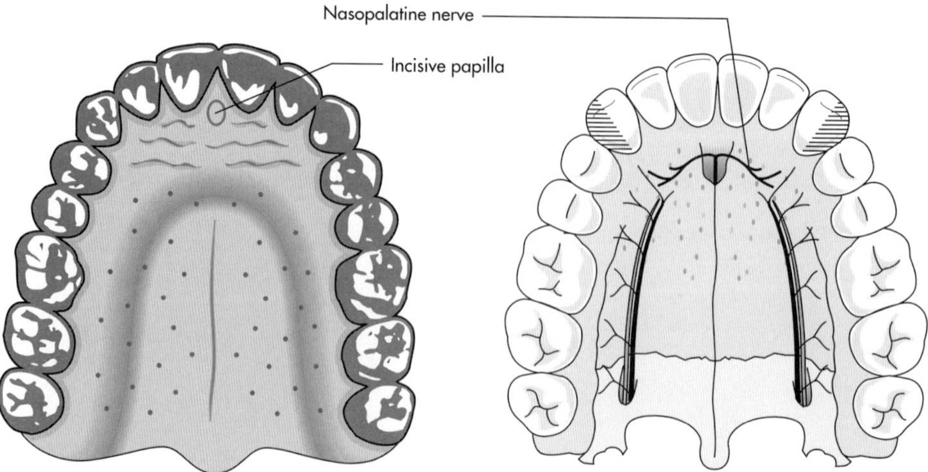

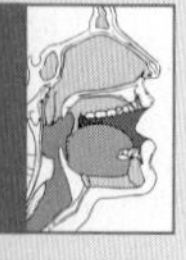

The maxillary incisors (Nos. 7–10) can be anesthetized by an infiltration directly opposite them on the facial side, numbing the ______________ nerve.

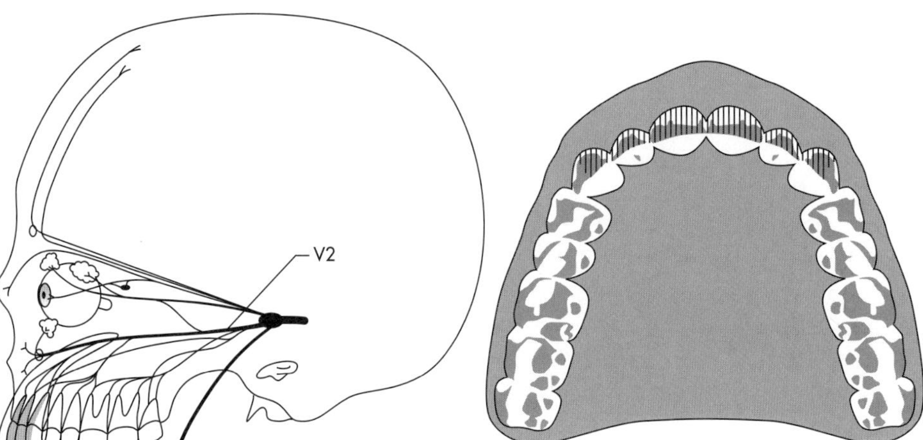

ASA

The lingual side of the incisors is innervated by the ______________ nerve and can be numbed by a block injection into the ______________ papilla.

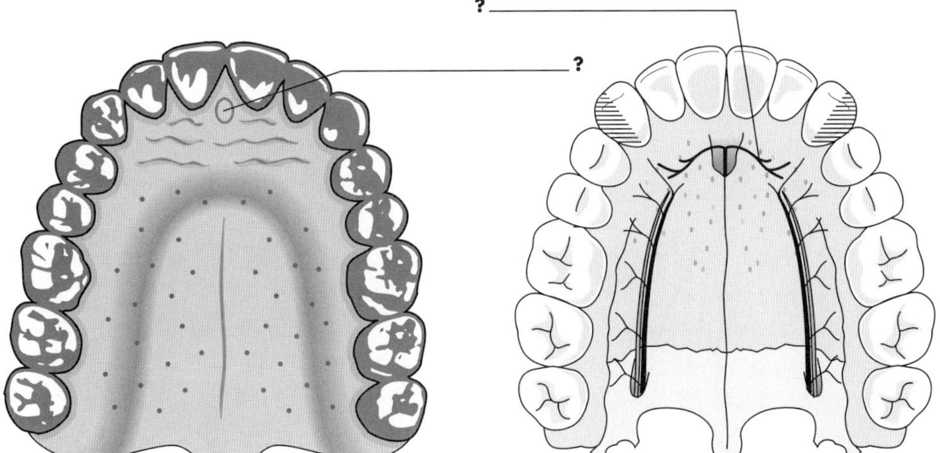

nasopalatine, incisive

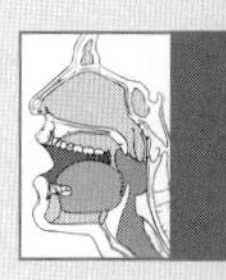

inferior alveolar nerve, mandibular, mandibular

Only two branches of V3 innervate the mandibular teeth, so injections are somewhat simpler. Name this major branch of V3 pointed out. It enters the mandible through the ______________ foramen and travels in the ______________ canal to branch out to the mandibular teeth.

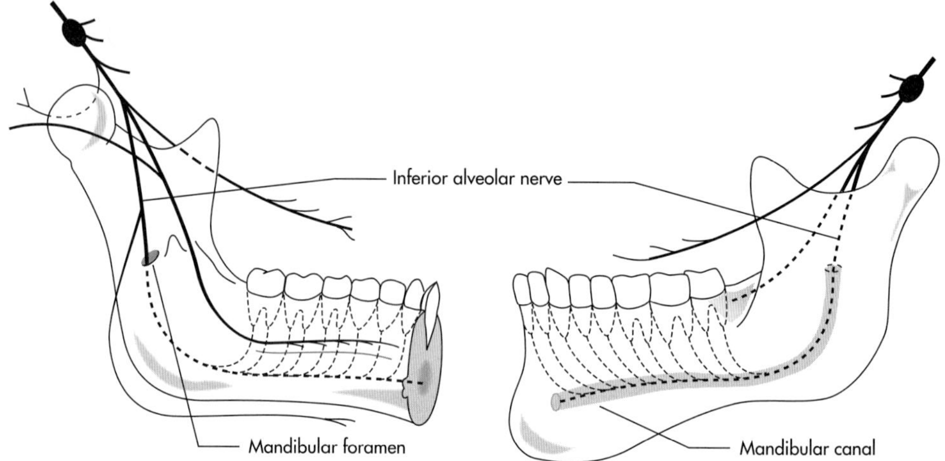

To reach the inferior alveolar nerve, we need to deposit anesthetic solution near where the nerve enters the mandible, in the pterygomandibular space. This can be found by asking the patient to open wide and feeling for his/her coronoid process. Aiming from a point across the arch where the mandibular premolars are, we place the needle into the space. The needle is delivered at the level where the thumb feels the curve of the coronoid.

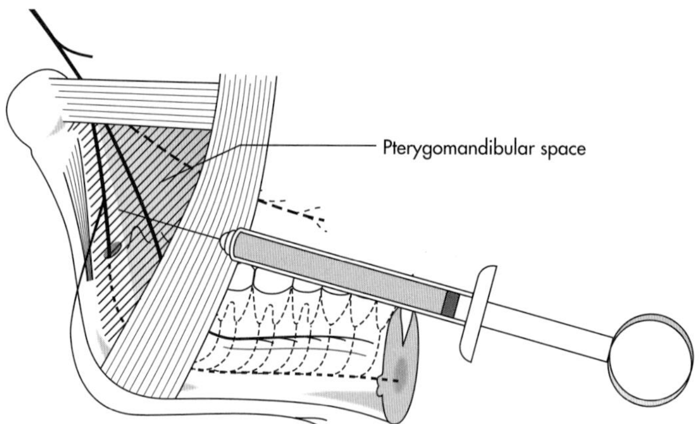

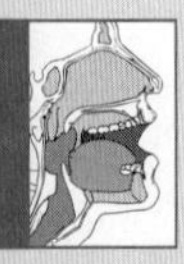

An injection in which anesthetic is delivered this close to the inferior alveolar nerve is a ________________-type injection. It numbs the lingual sides of the molars.

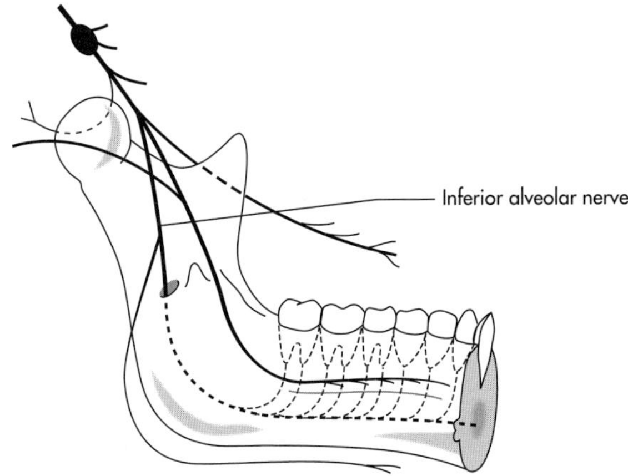

block

An **inferior alveolar block injection** numbs the lingual of the molars and all of the rest of the mandibular teeth on that side where it is given. It has an unfortunate consequence that occurs. That half of the tongue is also numbed. Why?

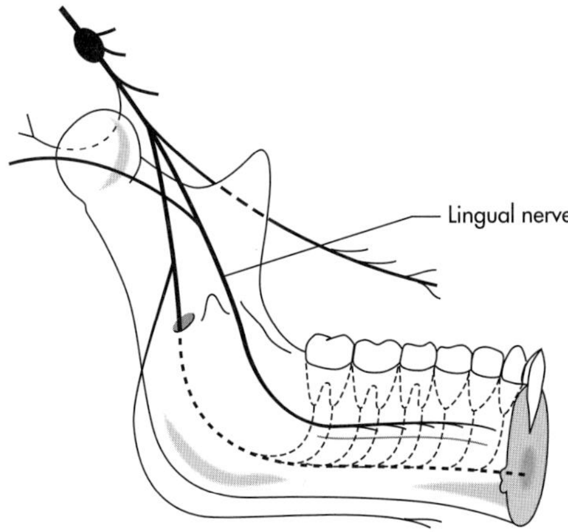

because the lingual nerve is close

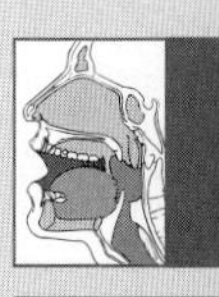

lingual, mandibular

The ______________ nerve branches off of V3 at about the same spot as the inferior alveolar nerve. This is right before the inferior alveolar nerve goes into the ______________ canal. The lingual nerve branches off to innervate half of the tongue.

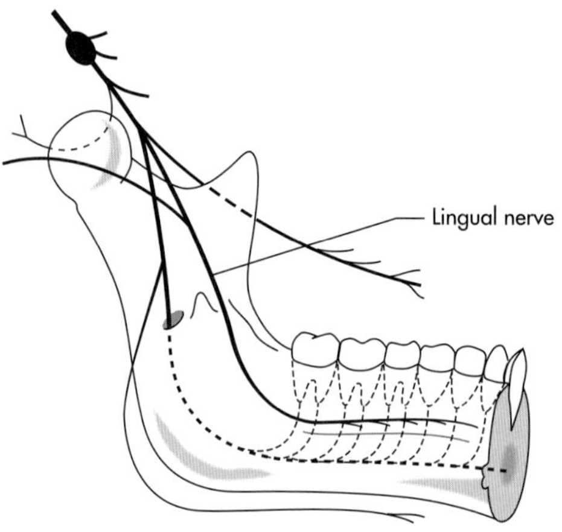

mental, mental

Half of the chin and lip may also be numbed as a consequence of the numbing of a branch of the inferior alveolar nerve. This is the ______________ nerve, which exits the mandible through the ______________ foramen.

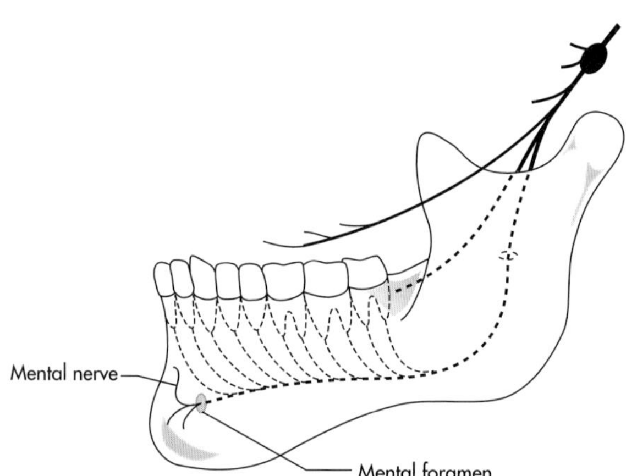

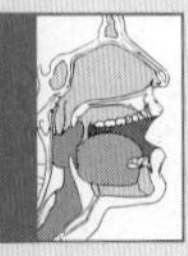

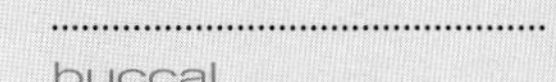

The buccal side of the mandibular molars has a separate innervation. It is the _______________ nerve, another branch of V3 that travels in the mucosa of the cheek.

buccal

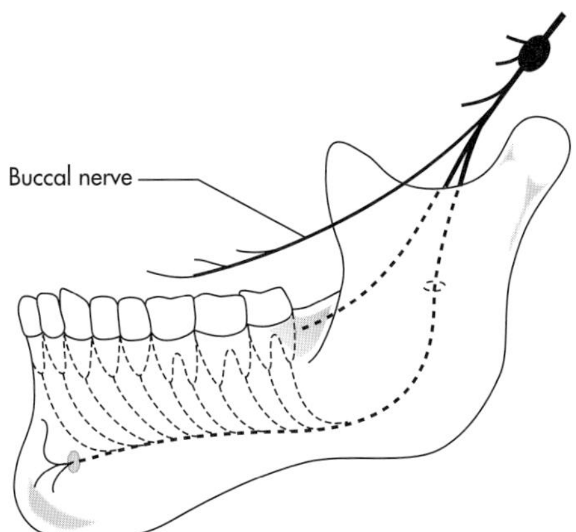

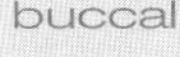

The buccal nerve innervates the _______________ side of the mandibular molars. It can be numbed by an infiltration into the buccal mucosa opposite the molar to be numbed.

buccal

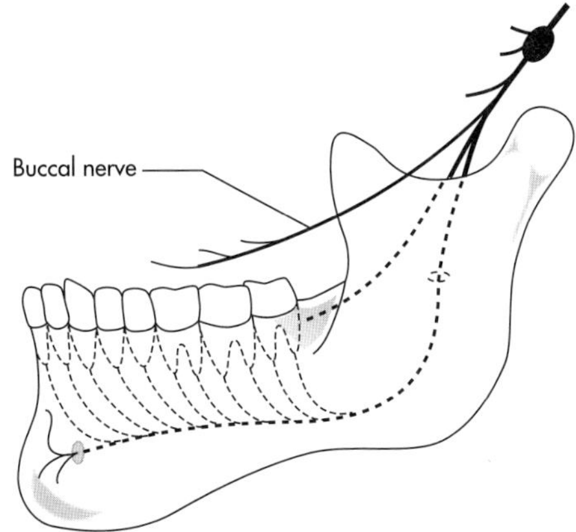

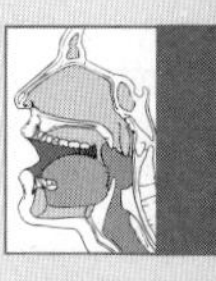

inferior alveolar block, buccal infiltration

A(n) ______________ injection plus a(n) ______________ injection are needed to numb tooth No. 30.

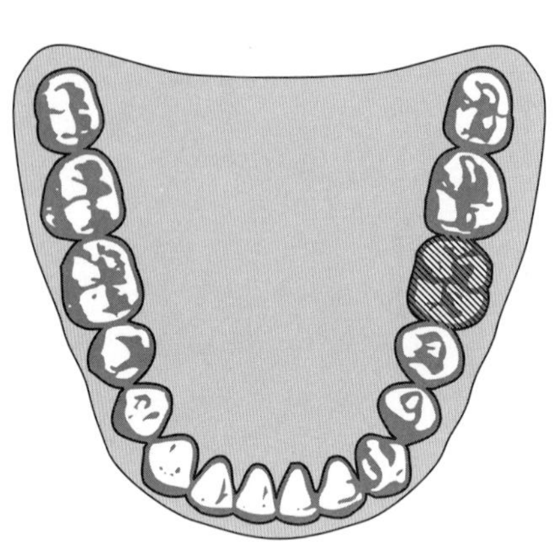

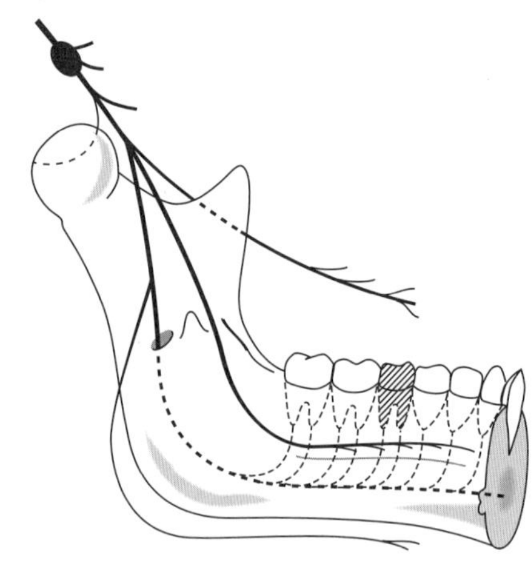

inferior alveolar only

Tooth No. 22 can be numbed by which injection(s)?

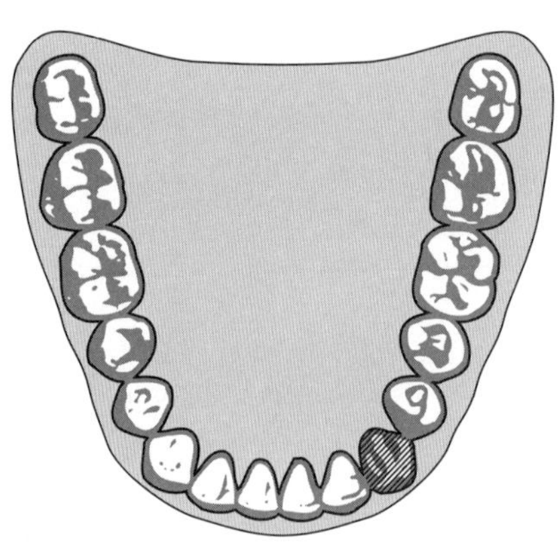

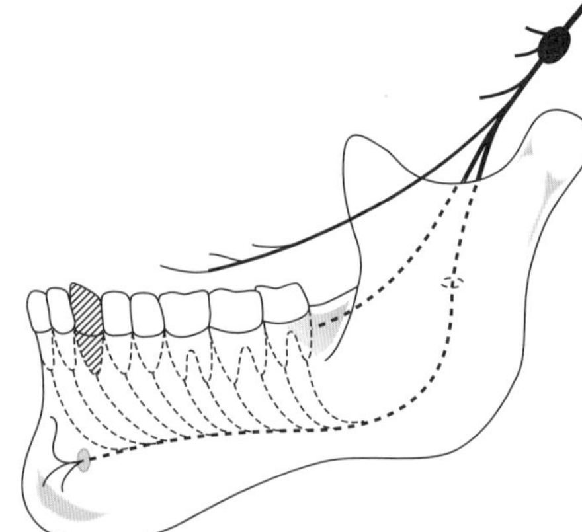

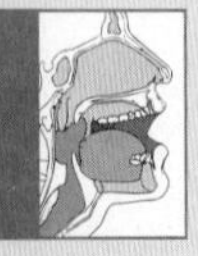

REVIEW TEST 11.1

SELECT OR FILL IN THE CORRECT ANSWER.

1. What structure separates the nasal and oral cavities?

2. Another term for "swallowing" is ______________, and a term for "chewing" is ______________.

3. List the muscles of mastication and their innervation.

4. The TMJ allows what two main types of mandibular movement?

5. Which muscles prepare the food bolus for the initial or oral phase of deglutition, positioning the bolus on the tongue?

   a. buccinator
   b. orbicularis oris
   c. tongue muscles
   d. all of the above
   e. a and b only

6. What function do the teeth serve and how are they built to do this job?

7. List the three regions of the pharynx.

8. There is an opening to a tube that lies within the nasopharynx. Name it.

9. The muscles of the pharynx are called the ______________ and are innervated by CN ______________.

10. The mucosa of the pharynx is sensitive to the presence of a bolus or other object by way of CN ______________. If an inappropriate object is felt, a reverse muscle action called the ______________ reflex occurs.

REVIEW TEST 11.2

SELECT OR FILL IN THE CORRECT ANSWER.

1. Hinge movement of the mandible is caused by the ______________ muscles acting on the ______________ joint cavity of the TMJ.

2. Gliding movement of the mandible is caused by the ______________ muscles acting on the ______________ joint cavity of the TMJ.

3. Humans have an elliptical chewing cycle because of their double-cusped teeth and the dual joint of the mandible, allowing an omnivore diet. True or false?

4. Name the three phases of deglutition.

5. The TVP muscle contracts to open the ______________ during a swallow.

6. The constrictors of the pharynx are composed of skeletal voluntary muscle only. True or false?

7. The system that allows us to take in oxygen and eliminate carbon dioxide is the ______________ system.

8. For respiration to occur, a patent airway is needed. True or false?

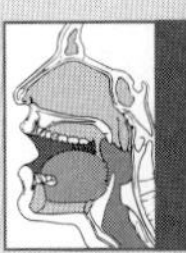

REVIEW TEST 11.3

SELECT OR FILL IN THE CORRECT ANSWER.

1. The pharyngeal muscles pull up on the larynx to seal it against the epiglottis during a swallow. True or false?

2. The thyroid cartilage is part of the

   a. bronchi b. trachea
   c. pharynx d. larynx

3. What structure lies within the larynx and is capable of making sound?

4. The gland responsible for the regulation of body cycles by the production of melatonin is the _______________.

MATCH THE STRUCTURE WITH THE CHEMICAL IT PRODUCES.

5. melatonin _______________
6. parathormone _______________
7. thyroxin _______________
8. calcitonin _______________

a. thymus
b. pineal
c. parathyroid
d. C cells
e. thyroid

REVIEW TEST 11.4

SELECT OR FILL IN THE CORRECT ANSWER.

1. Name the two divisions of the pituitary gland.

2. The neurohypophysis is a collection of nerve endings regulating the kidneys and intestine. True or false?

3. The adenohypophysis does not produce

   a. GH b. TTH
   c. TMJ d. ACTH
   e. LH f. GTH

4. On what structure does the thyroid gland lie?

5. Which gland involutes in adulthood?

6. What three tonsillar groups constitute Waldyer's ring?

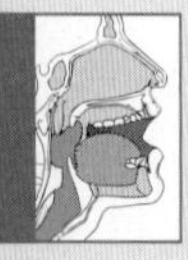

REVIEW TEST 11.5

NAME THE INJECTION(S) NEEDED TO TOTALLY ANESTHETIZE THESE TEETH.

1. No. 30 ______________
2. No. 6 ______________
3. No. 24 ______________
4. No. 13 ______________
5. No. 14 ______________
6. No. 7 ______________

REVIEW TEST 11.6

LABEL THE DIAGRAMS.

1.

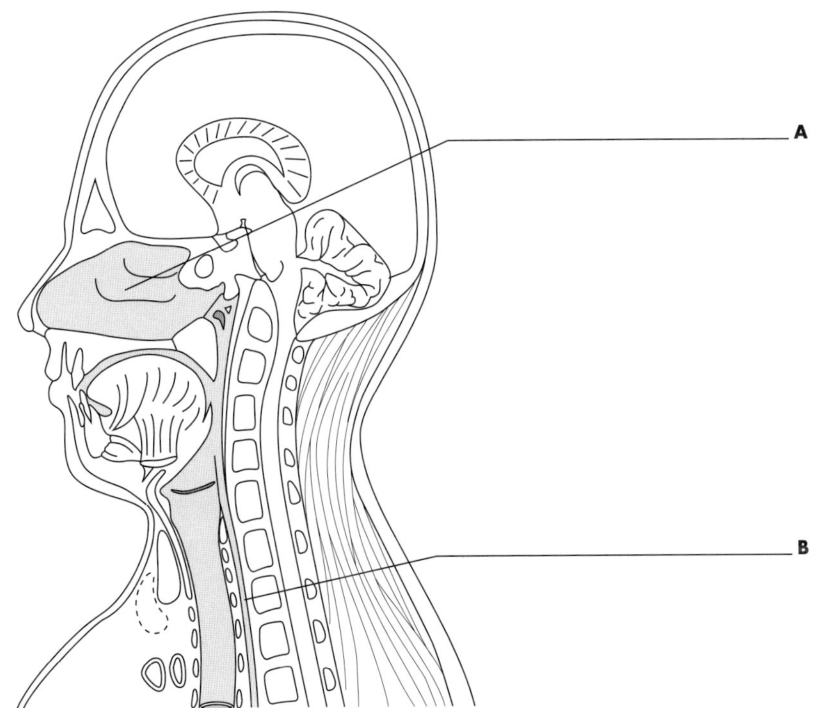

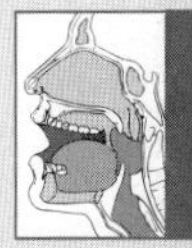

2.

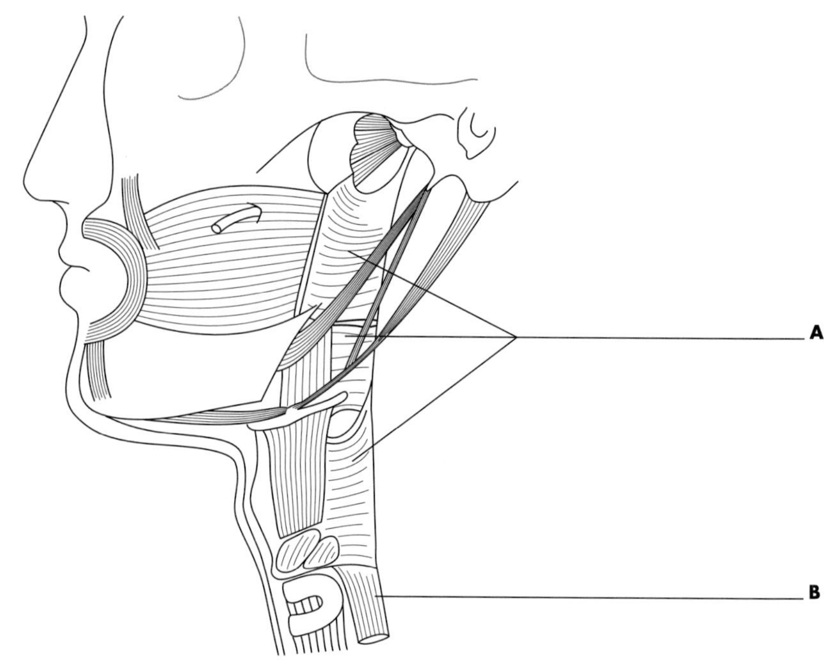

3.

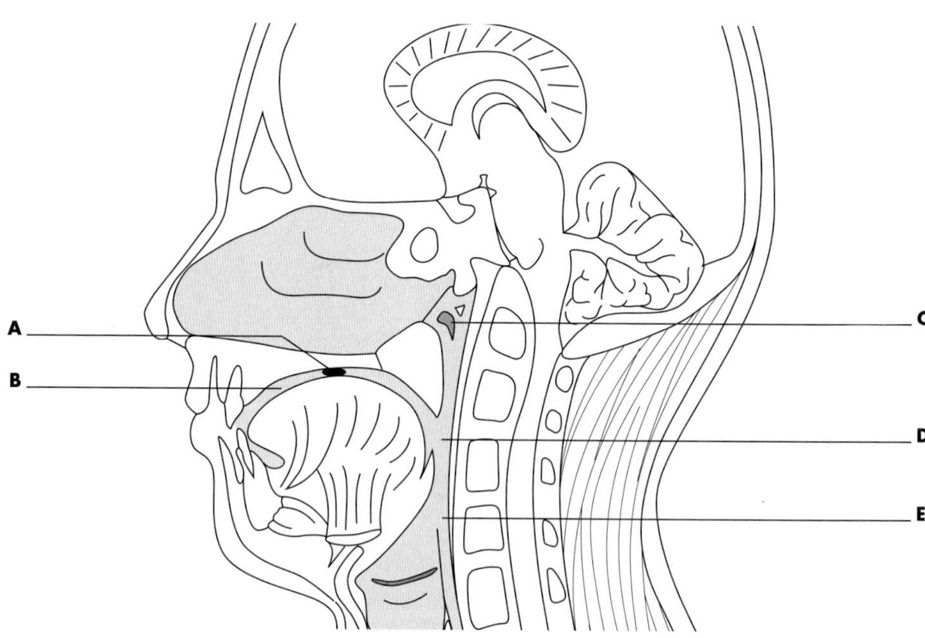

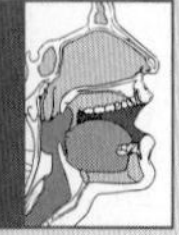

4.

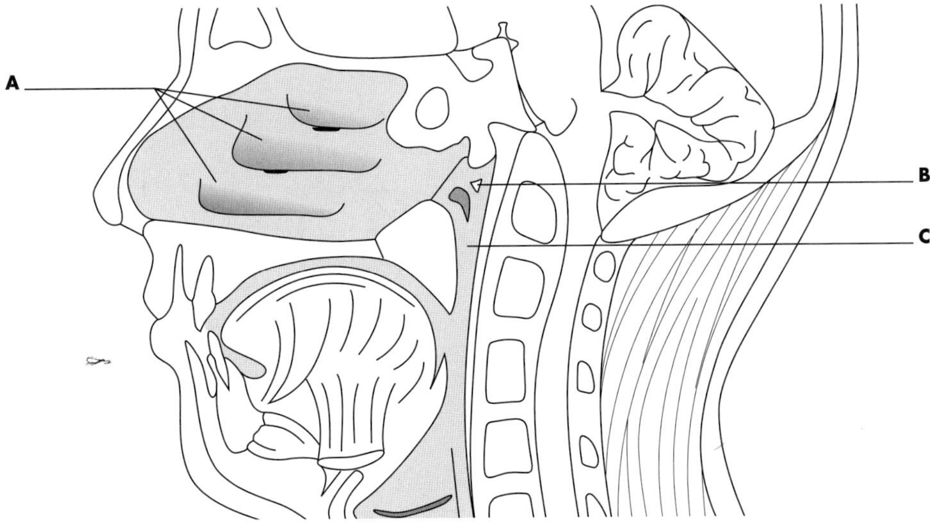

5.

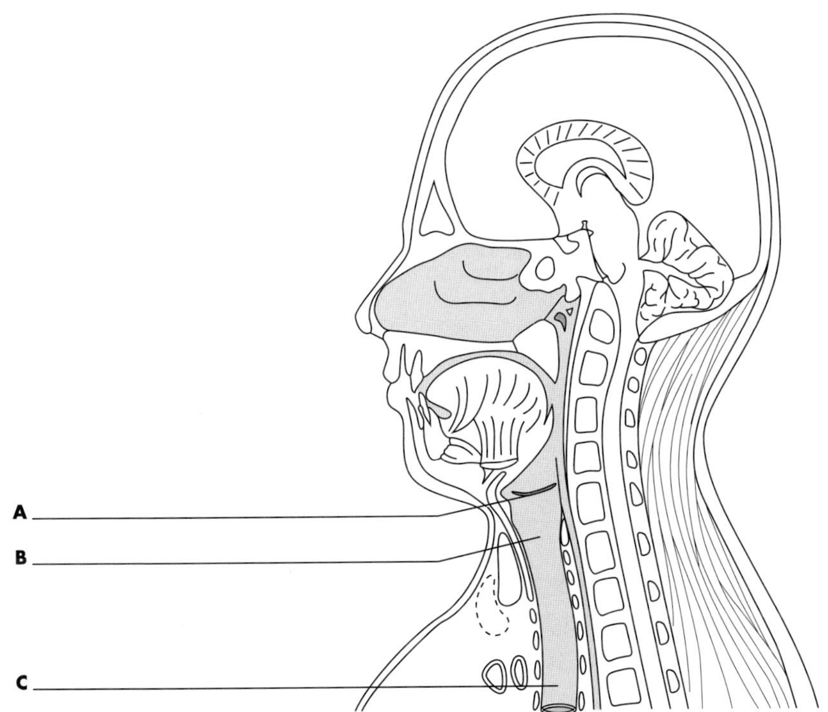

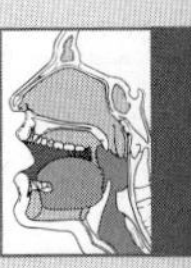

6.

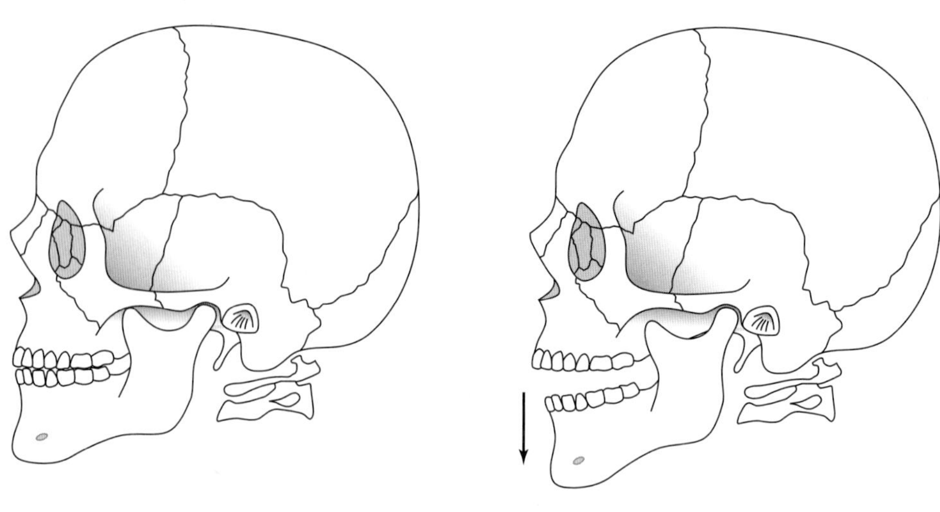

7.

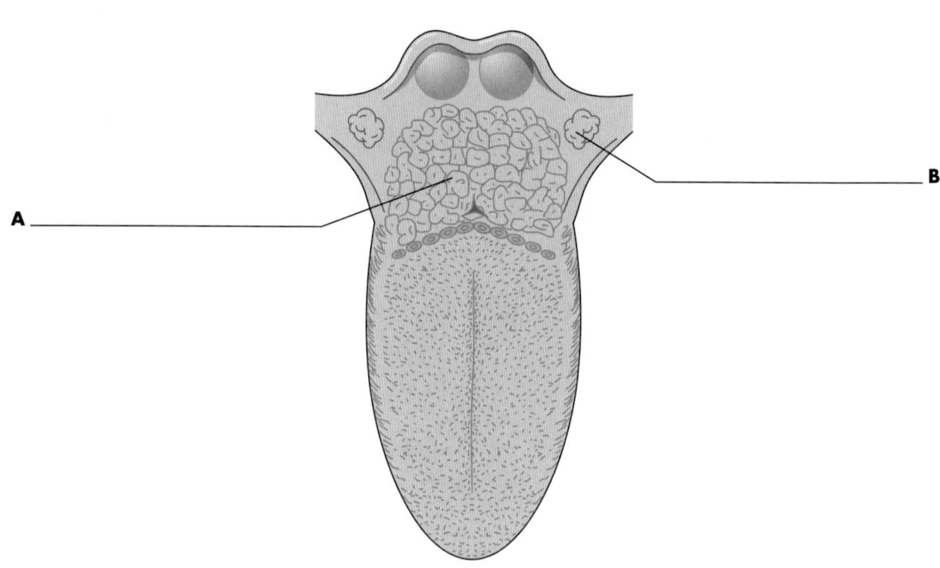

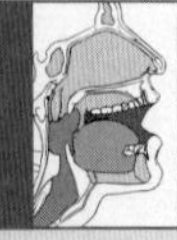

8.

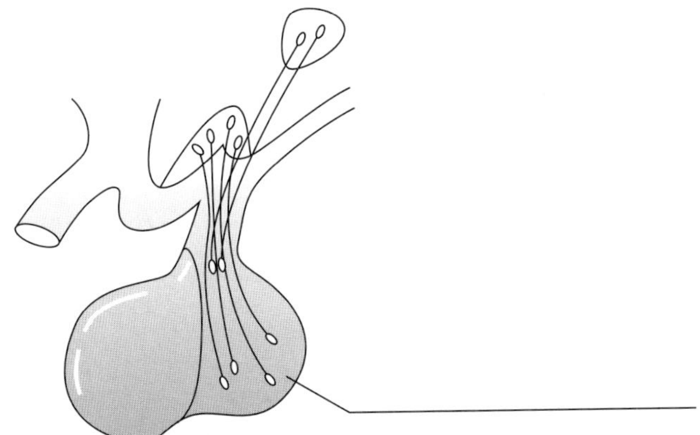

9.

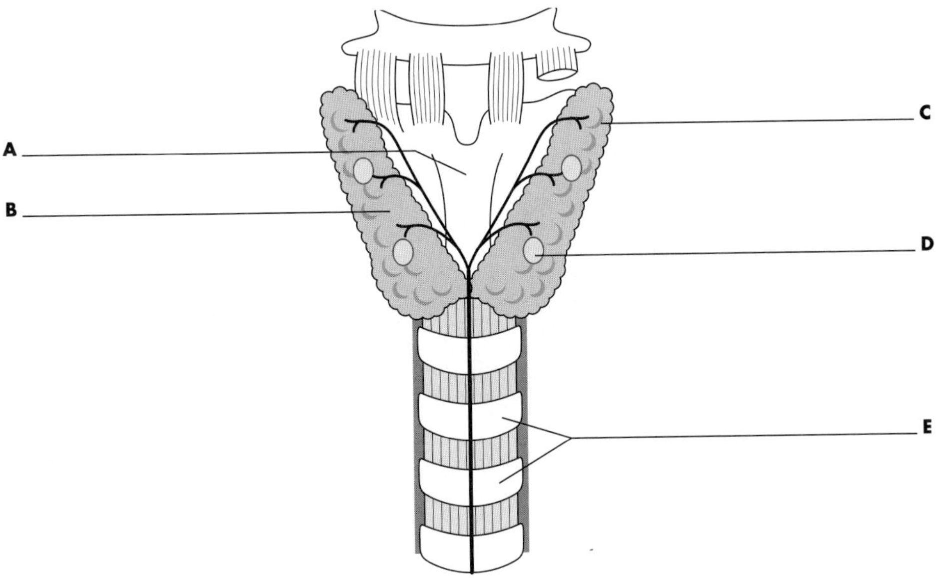

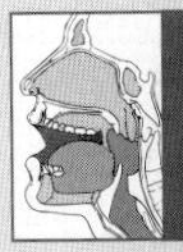

10.

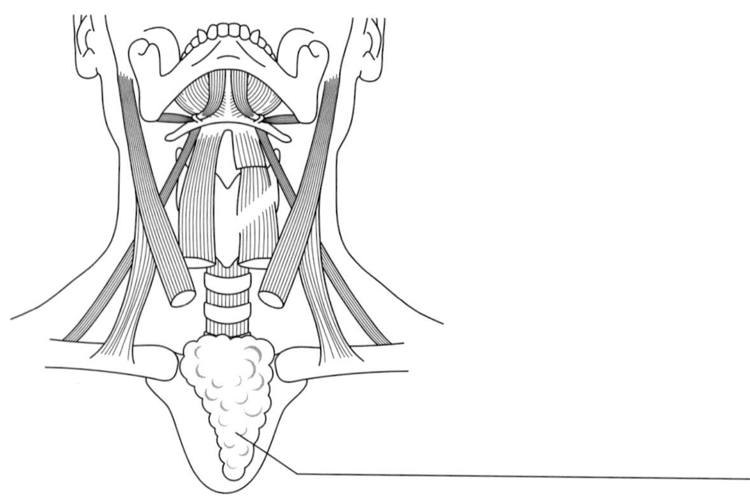

11.

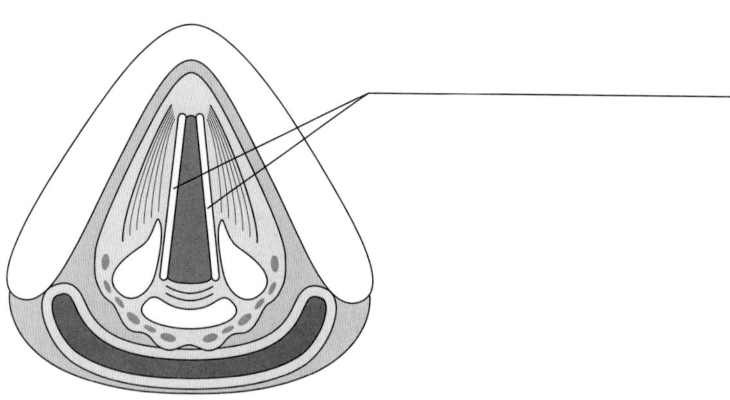

12.

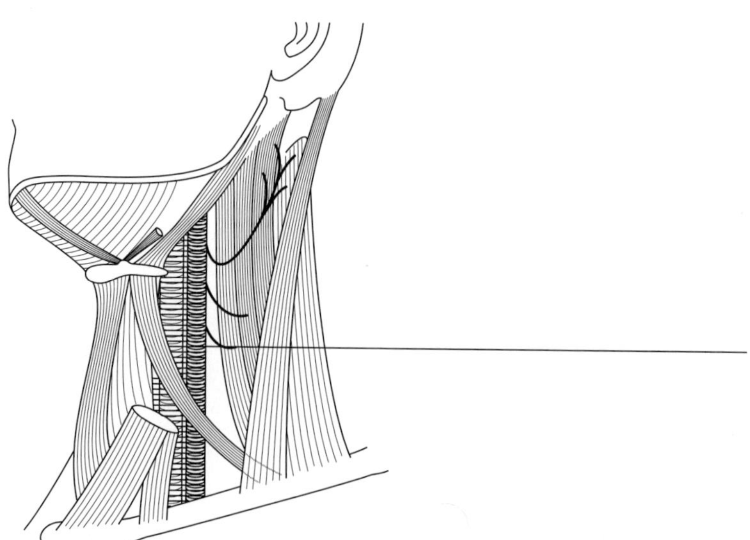

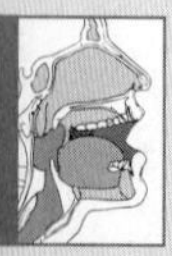

13.

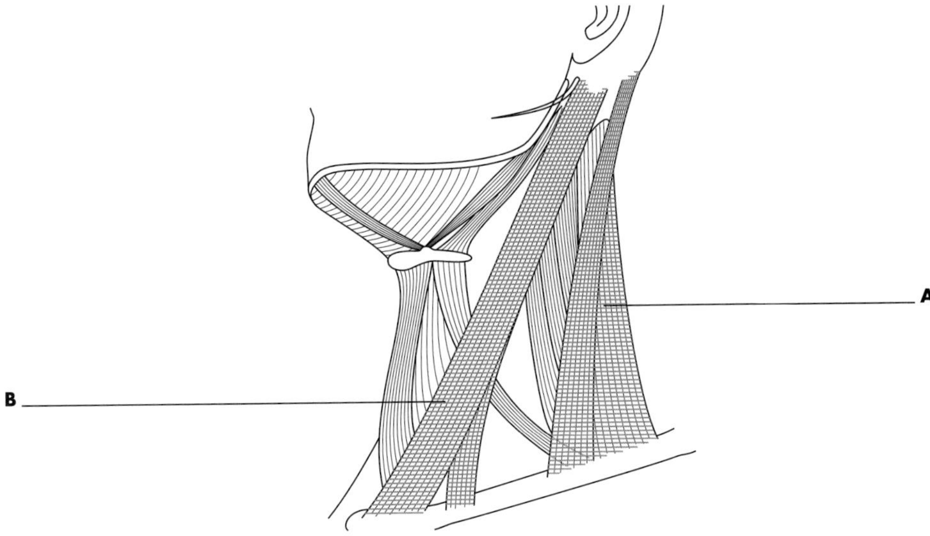

14.

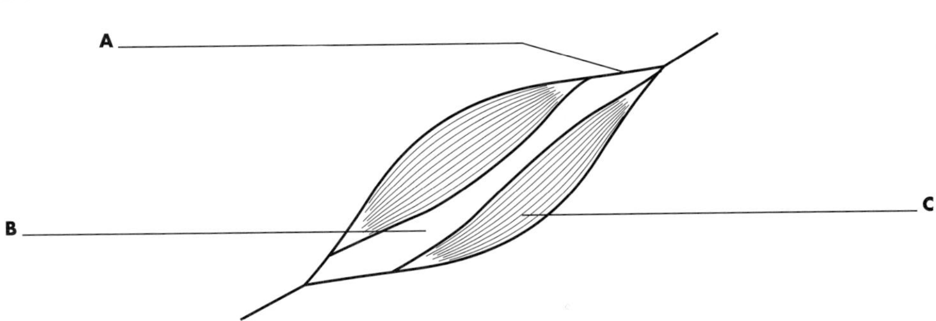

15.

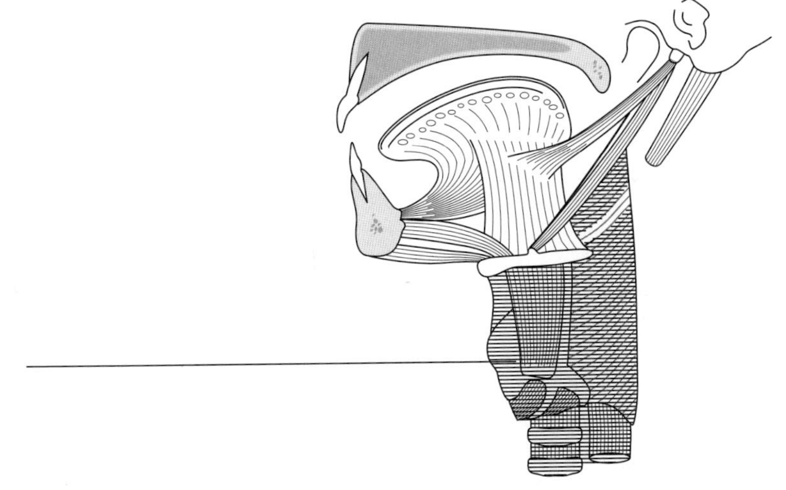

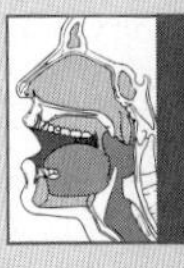

16.

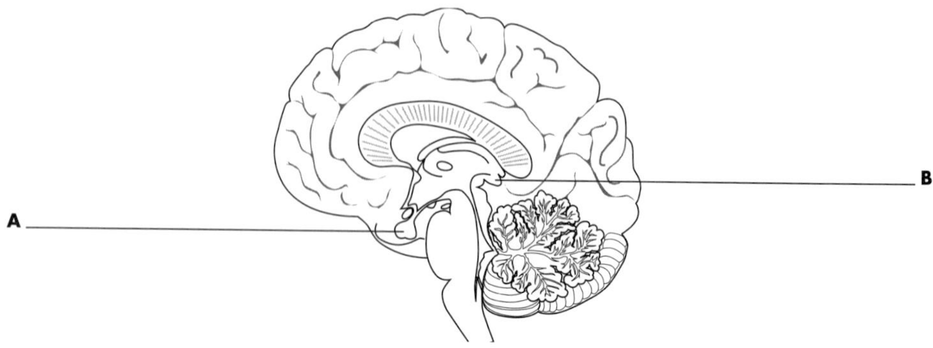

17.

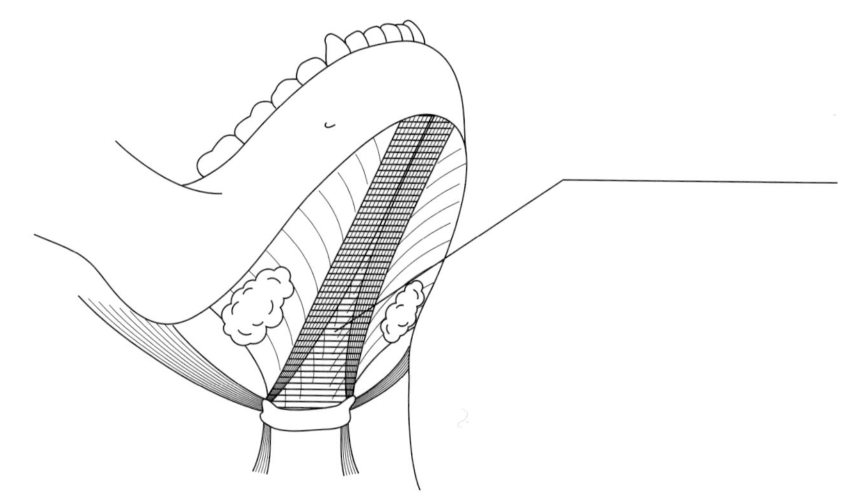

18.

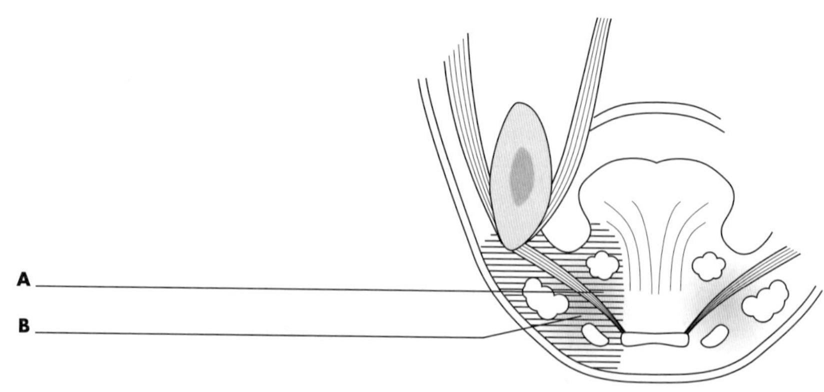

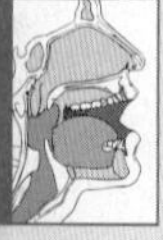

19.

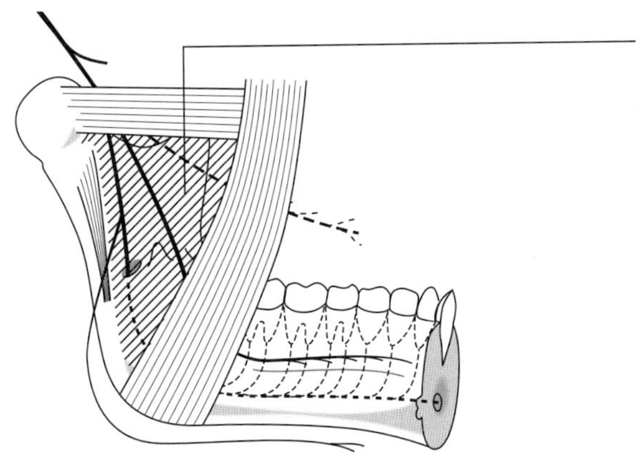

20.

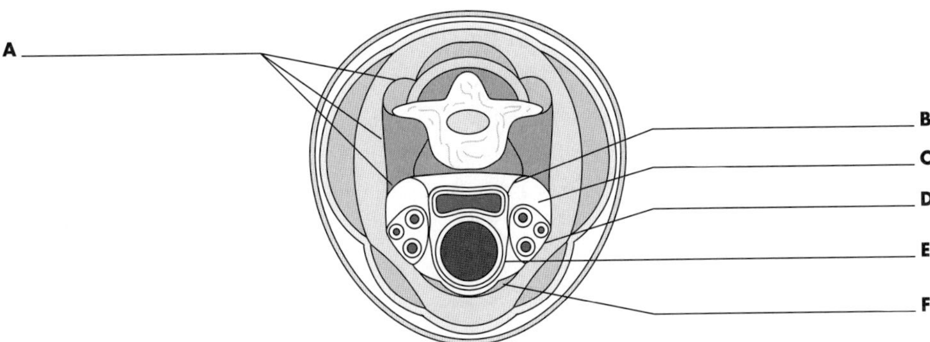

21.

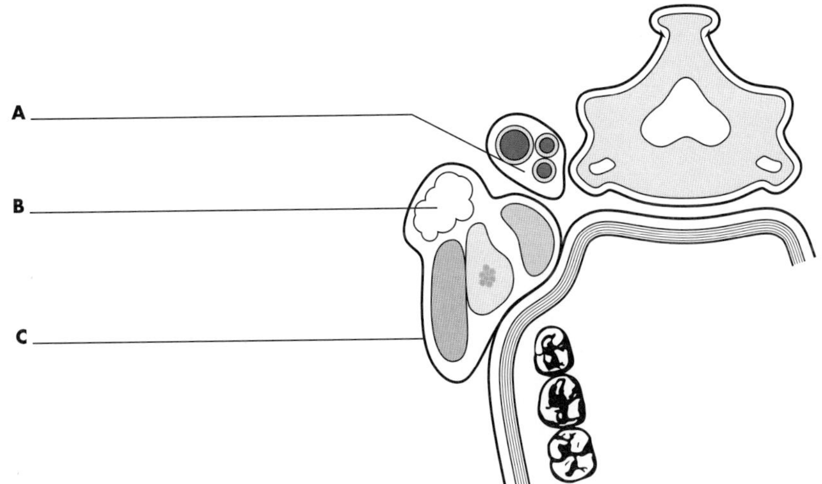

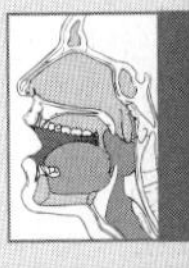

22.

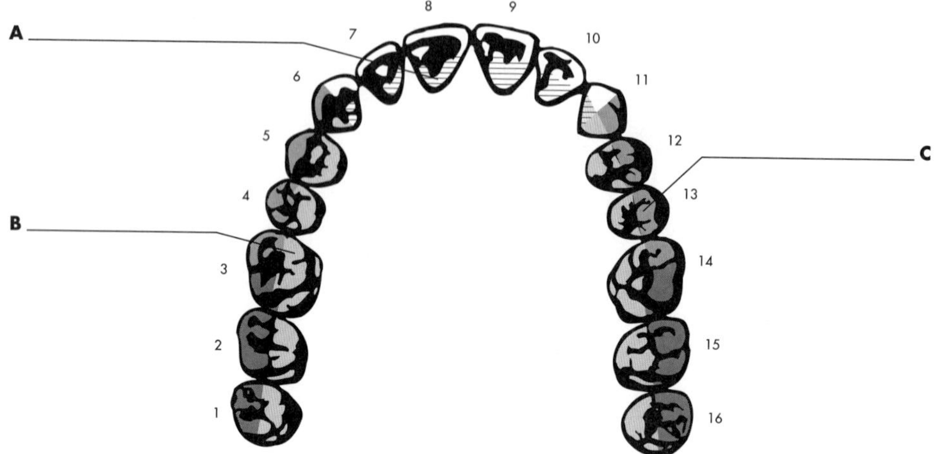
A
B
C
1
2
3
4
5
6
7
8
9
10
11
12
13
14
15
16

23.

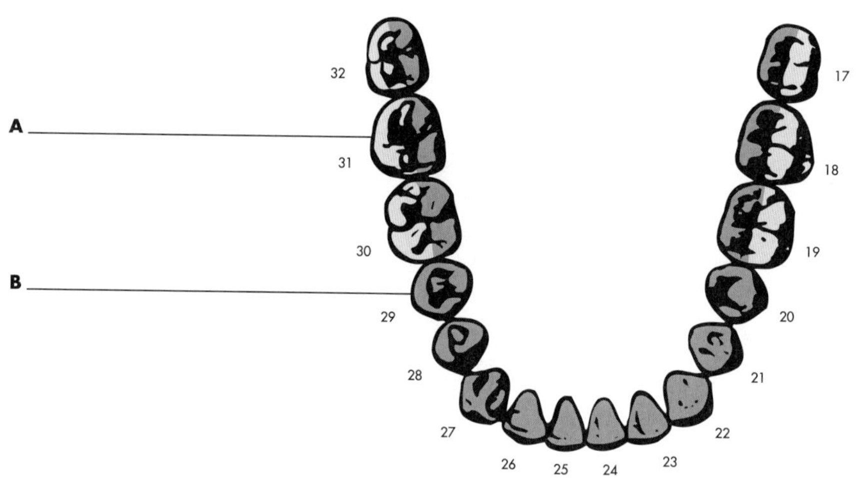
A
B
17
18
19
20
21
22
23
24
25
26
27
28
29
30
31
32

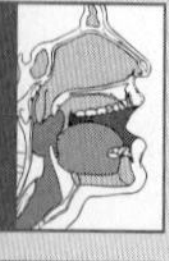

Appendix: Review Test Answers

CHAPTER 1

REVIEW TEST 1.1

1. c
2. a
3. a
4. b
5. c
6. c
7. d
8. b
9. c
10. a

REVIEW TEST 1.2

1. a
2. false
3. d, a, b, c
4. true
5. true
6. false
7. b
8. d
9. d
10. true

REVIEW TEST 1.3

1. nucleus
2. tissue
3. a. epithelium
   b. connective
   c. muscle
   d. nervous
4. stratified squamous
5. ciliated pseudostratified
6. secretory unit
7. a. skeletal
   b. cardiac
   c. smooth
8. synapse
9. a. collagen
   b. elastic
   c. reticular
10. adipose

REVIEW TEST 1.4

1. erythrocytes
2. chondrocytes, chondroblasts
3. osteocytes, osteoclasts
4. cell processes
5. osteons
6. endochondral
7. fontanel
8. stratified squamous
9. a. stratum basale
   b. stratum spinosum
   c. stratum lucidum
   d. stratum corneum
10. keratin

REVIEW TEST 1.5

1. A. villi or cilia
   B. golgi apparatus
   C. nucleus
   D. mitochondrion
2. A. duct
   B. secretory unit
3. A. stratified squamous
   B. pseudostratified
   C. simple squamous
   D. stratified cuboidal
   E. simple columnar
   F. transitional
4. A. collagen fiber
   B. elastic fiber
5. A. dense irregular connective tissue
   B. adipose connective tissue
   C. skeletal muscle
   D. smooth muscle
   E. cardiac muscle
6. A. neutrophil
   B. platelets
   C. monocytes
7. A. dendrite
   B. axon
   C. myelin sheath
8. A. haversian canal
   B. Volkmann's canal
   C. laminae
   D. cell body
   E. lacuna
9. A. blood vessel
   B. salivary/mucous gland
   C. mucosa proper
   D. lamina propria
10. A. stratum corneum
    B. stratum basale
    C. hair follicle and sebaceous gland
    D. epidermis
    E. dermis

CHAPTER 2

REVIEW TEST 2.1

1. c
2. c
3. b
4. a
5. a
6. c
7. c
8. b
9. b

REVIEW TEST 2.2

1. b
2. d
3. b
4. a
5. c
6. c
7. false
8. a
9. c

REVIEW TEST 2.3

1. false
2. a
3. c
4. b
5. false
6. d
7. a
8. a
9. true

REVIEW TEST 2.4

1. fertilization
2. implantation
3. true
4. supporting tissues
5. true
6. yolk
7. endoderm, mesoderm, ectoderm
8. yellow
9. neural, neural
10. brain, spinal cord
11. spinal
12. false
13. nervous
14. blue
15. digestive, respiratory

REVIEW TEST 2.5

1. red
2. skeletal, muscular
3. remnant
4. stomodeum, buccopharyngeal membrane
5. Meckel's
6. Reichert's
7. six
8. foramen cecum
9. frontal
10. primary palate, lateral palatine
11. yes, in posterior palate
12. cleft
13. Meckel's cartilage

REVIEW TEST 2.6

1. c
2. c
3. a
4. b
5. a
6. b
7. c
8. a

REVIEW TEST 2.7

1. d
2. f
3. b
4. e
5. a and d
6. a

REVIEW TEST 2.8

1. e
2. a
3. f
4. c
5. b
6. e
7. b

REVIEW TEST 2.9

1. A. morula
   B. sperm
   C. egg
   D. blastula
   E. uterus
2. A. gametes
   B. zygote
   C. morula
   D. blastula/gastrula
3. A. yolk sac
   B. amnion
   C. umbilical
   D. ectoderm
   E. neural groove
   F. endoderm
4. A. neural groove (blue)
   B. neural tube (blue)
   C. neural crest (blue)
   D. spinal nerve (blue)
   E. neural crest cells
5. A. neural groove
   B. heart bulge
   C. somites
   D. umbilical
   E. ear
   F. eye
   G. pharyngeal arches
   H. limb bud
   I. placenta
   J. umbilical cord
6. A. lateral lingual processes (blue)
   B. circumvallate papillae
   C. tuberculum impar (blue)
   D. foramen cecum
   E. copula (yellow)
   F. epiglottis (yellow)
7. A. somites (red)
   B. sclerotome (red)
   C. GI tube (yellow)
   D. circulatory tubes (red)
8. A. lungs (endoderm: yellow)
   B. brain (ectoderm: blue)
   C. intestines (endoderm: yellow)
9. A. frontal process (blue: outside; red: inside)
   B. arch I
   C. external auditory meatus (blue)
   D. palatine tonsil (yellow)
   E. groove II (blue)
   F. pouch III (yellow)
   G. cartilage IV (red)
   H. parathyroid gland (yellow)
10. A. arch III
    B. stomodeum
    C. maxillary process
    D. median nasal process
    E. globular process
    F. lateral nasal process
    G. lateral nasal process
    H. mandibular process
    I. lateral palatine process

CHAPTER 3

REVIEW TEST 3.1

1. b
2. b
3. c
4. a
5. ameloblasts
6. odontoblasts
7. c
8. a
9. a

REVIEW TEST 3.2

1. b
2. c
3. c
4. d
5. d
6. c
7. true

REVIEW TEST 3.3

1. ectoderm
2. true
3. secondary lamina
4. inner enamel epithelium, stratum intermedium, stellate reticulum, outer enamel epithelium
5. false
6. odontoblastic process
7. pulp, dentin
8. calcification
9. 'blast, 'clast
10. dentinal tubules
11. rests of Malassez
12. enamel rods
13. predentin

REVIEW TEST 3.4

1. c
2. a
3. b
4. b
5. b

1. a
2. b
3. b
4. a

REVIEW TEST 3.5

1. A. dental lamina
   B. oral ectoderm
   C. dental papilla
   D. dental sac
   E. outer enamel epithelium
   F. stellate reticulum
   G. stratum intermedium
   H. inner enamel epithelium
2. A. dental sac
   B. dental papilla
   C. Meckel's cartilage
   D. enamel
   E. eruption
   F. attachment epithelium
   G. resorption
3. A. secondary lamina
   B. enamel
   C. alveolar bone
   D. PDL
   E. diaphragm
   F. Hertwig's epithelial root sheath
   G. odontoblasts
   H. cementoblast
4. A. ameloblast
   B. fibrous matrix
   C. enamel rods
5. A. dentin
   B. predentin
   C. odontoblast
6. A. resorption
   B. reduced enamel epithelium
7. A. cementoblast
   B. cementocyte
   C. cementum
8. A. dentinal tubule
   B. odontoblastic process
9. A. lines of Retzius
   B. rests of Malassez

CHAPTER 4

REVIEW TEST 4.1

1. enamel
2. lines of Retzius
3. ameloblasts
4. interrod substance
5. Hunter–Schreger bands
6. hypocalcified
7. enamel tufts, spindles

REVIEW TEST 4.2

1. odontoblasts
2. dentin
3. dentinal tubules
4. odontoblastic process
5. globular
6. primary
7. secondary
8. Tome's granular layer
9. cementum
10. lacunae
11. cellular
12. odontoblastic
13. pulp horns

REVIEW TEST 4.3

1. false
2. true
3. d
4. b
5. d
6. e

REVIEW TEST 4.4

1. d
2. d
3. a
4. true
5. c
6. false

REVIEW TEST 4.5

1. A. lines of Retzius
   B. Hunter–Schreger bands
2. enamel rod
3. A. mamelons
   B. developmental line
   C. perikymata
4. enamel tufts and spindles
5. A. cementum
   B. Tome's granular layer
6. A. predentin
   B. dentin
7. A. enamel rods
   B. interrod substance
8. A. odontoblast
   B. sclerotic dentin
   C. dead tract
   D. reparative dentin
9. A. odontoblastic process
   B. dentinal tubule
10. A. pulp
    B. odontoblast
11. A. enamel
    B. cementum
12. A. pulp horn
    B. wall
    C. pulp chamber
13. hypercementosis
14. A. cementocyte cell process
    B. canaliculus
    C. lacuna
15. A. primary dentin
    B. secondary dentin
16. A. line of Retzius
    B. dentinal tubule
    C. globular dentin
    D. pulp
    E. developmental lines
    F. Tome's granular layer
    G. odontoblasts
    H. CEJ
    I. acellular cement
    J. cellular cement

CHAPTER 5

REVIEW TEST 5.1

1. c
2. d
3. d
4. true
5. false

REVIEW TEST 5.2

1. d
2. b
3. c
4. a
5. d

REVIEW TEST 5.3

1. alveolus
2. periodontal ligament
3. crestal
4. lamina dura
5. principal
6. Sharpey's
7. elastic
8. fibroblasts
9. gingiva
10. free
11. attached
12. b
13. sulcular
14. attachment

REVIEW TEST 5.4

1. A. periodontal ligament
   B. sulcus
   C. alveolar bone
2. lamina dura
3. coll
4. A. Sharpey's fibers
   B. principal fibers
5. attachment epithelium
6. A. lamina dura
   B. crestal bone
7. A. papilla
   B. free gingiva
   C. attached gingiva
8. A. salivary gland
   B. mucosa proper
   C. lamina propria
9. A. alveolo-gingival fibers
   B. alveolar crest fibers
   C. horizontal fibers
   D. oblique fibers
   E. apical fibers
10. interradicular fibers
11. transseptal fibers

CHAPTER 6

REVIEW TEST 6.1

1. b
2. d
3. b
4. false
5. c
6. c
7. a

REVIEW TEST 6.2

1. c
2. b
3. a
4. false
5. e
6. masticatory
7. false
8. c
9. true
10. b

REVIEW TEST 6.3

1. a
2. parotid papilla
3. Stensen's duct
4. linea alba
5. pterygomandibular raphe
6. vermillion
7. true
8. ducts of Rivinus
9. Wharton's duct
10. oropharynx

REVIEW TEST 6.4

1. pseudostratified
2. Eustachian, pharyngeal
3. goblet
4. tonsilar (pharyngeal) pillars
5. lymphoid
6. Waldeyer's ring
7. dorsal
8. filiform
9. circumvallate
10. circumvallate

REVIEW TEST 6.5

1. foramen cecum
2. respiratory
3. mucous, serous, serous
4. serous
5. sublingual caruncle
6. parotid papilla
7. fibrous, fibrous
8. hinge, gliding

REVIEW TEST 6.6

1. c
2. b
3. a

REVIEW TEST 6.7

1. sublingual caruncle
2. A. foramen cecum
   B. epiglottis
   C. lingual tonsils
3. A. filiform papilla
   B. fungiform papilla
   C. foliate papilla
4. A. circumvallate papilla
   B. taste cells
5. A. free gingiva
   B. attached gingiva
   C. sulcular epithelium
   D. attachment epithelium
6. A. circumvallate papillae
   B. retromolar pad
   C. ducts of Rivinus
   D. maxillary buccal frenum
   E. maxillary tuberosity
   F. lingual frenum
   G. mandibular labial frenum
7. A. incisive papilla
   B. midpalatine suture
   C. uvula
8. A. parotid papilla
   B. maxillary tuberosity
   C. pharyngeal pillars
   D. maxillary labial frenum
   E. palatine tonsil
   F. pterygomandibular raphe
9. A. Eustachian tube
   B. soft palate
   C. nasopharynx
10. A. parotid gland
    B. Stensen's duct
    C. ducts of Rivinus
    D. sublingual gland
    E. Wharton's duct
    F. submandibular gland
11. goblet cells
12. A. superior joint cavity
    B. bilaminar zone
    C. fibrous covering, condyle
    D. temporomandibular disk
    E. lateral pterygoid
13. A. mandibular fossa
    B. lateral ligaments
    C. articular eminence
    D. temporomandibular capsule
    E. condyle
14. A. duct
    B. serous unit
    C. mucous unit

CHAPTER 7

REVIEW TEST 7.1

1. d
2. c
3. suture
4. fontanel
5. atlas, axis
6. seven
7. anterior, middle, posterior
8. hyoid

REVIEW TEST 7.2

1. supraorbitals
2. b
3. false
4. c
5. spinal cord, occipital
6. pituitary
7. styloid process
8. true

REVIEW TEST 7.3

1. maxilla, temporal, zygoma
2. false
3. optic
4. orbits
5. A. V2
   B. V3
   C. V1
6. superior orbital
7. A. V2
   B. V1
   C. V3
8. maxilla, palatine

REVIEW TEST 7.4

1. hamuli
2. pterygoid plates
3. coronoid
4. jugular, carotid
5. submandibular
6. body
7. b
8. false

REVIEW TEST 7.5

1. A. frontal bone
   B. supraorbital foramen
   C. optic foramen
   D. superior orbital fissure
   E. infraorbital foramen
   F. zygoma bone
   G. maxillary bone
   H. mental foramen
2. A. parietal bone
   B. nasal bone
   C. lacrimal bone
   D. temporal bone
   E. styloid process
   F. occipital bone
3. A. cribriform plate of ethmoid bone
   B. pituitary fossa
   C. carotid canal
   D. ear
   E. anterior cranial fossa
   F. optic foramen
   G. superior orbital fissure
   H. foramen rotundum
   I. foramen ovale
   J. foramen spinosum
   K. jugular foramen
   L. hypoglossal foramen
   M. foramen magnum
4. A. condyle
   B. coronoid process
   C. mandibular foramen
   D. lingula
   E. genial tubercles
   F. mylohyoid line
   G. submandibular fossa
   H. mental foramen
   I. mental fossa
   J. superior oblique line
5. A. incisive foramen
   B. palatine bone
   C. greater palatine foramen
   D. hamulus
   E. pterygoid plates
   F. vomer bone
6. A. articular eminence
   B. zygomatic process
   C. mastoid process
7. A. ethmoid bone
   B. vomer bone
   C. maxillary bone
   D. palatine bone
8. nasal turbinates

CHAPTER 8

REVIEW TEST 8.1

1. origin
2. false
3. a
4. d
5. b
6. d
7. platysma
8. temporal
9. mylohyoid
10. digastric

REVIEW TEST 8.2

1. facial, VII
2. b
3. lateral pterygoid
4. c and e
5. lateral pterygoid
6. lateral, protrusive
7. turns to side
8. true
9. d
10. suprahyoid, infrahyoid

REVIEW TEST 8.3

1. d
2. e
3. b
4. a
5. c

REVIEW TEST 8.4

1. d
2. c
3. a
4. b

REVIEW TEST 8.5

1. a
2. c
3. b
4. d

REVIEW TEST 8.6

1. c
2. a
3. d
4. e
5. b

REVIEW TEST 8.7

1. mylohyoid
2. styloglossus muscle, stylohyoid muscle, stylohyoid ligament
3. genioglossus, geniohyoid
4. SCM, digastric muscles
5. a
6. digastric, omohyoid
7. tongue
8. d

REVIEW TEST 8.8

1. i. a
   ii. b
2. Eustachian (tympanic) tube
3. LVP
4. false
5. superior constrictor, buccinator
6. Stensen's duct
7. TVP

REVIEW TEST 8.9

1. omohyoid muscle
2. A. frontalis muscle
   B. parotid gland
   C. buccinator muscle
   D. mentalis muscle
3. A. orbicularis occuli muscle
   B. levator muscles
   C. orbicularis oris muscle
   D. platysma muscle
   E. nasalis muscle
   F. depressor muscles
4. temporalis muscle
5. masseter muscle
6. A. lateral pterygoid muscle
   B. medial pterygoid muscle
7. A. lateral pterygoid muscle
   B. masseter muscle
   C. medial pterygoid muscle
8. A. digastric muscle
   B. mylohyoid muscle
   C. thyrohyoid muscle
   D. sternothyroid muscle
   E. sternohyoid muscle
   F. sternocleidomastoid muscle
9. A. sternocleidomastoid muscle
   B. trapezius muscle
10. A. Eustachian tube
    B. LVP muscle
    C. TVP muscle
11. A. palatoglossus muscle
    B. palatopharyngeus muscle
12. trapezius muscle
13. A. styloglossus muscle
    B. stylohyoid ligament
    C. genioglossus muscle
    D. geniohyoid muscle
    E. hyoglossus muscle

CHAPTER 9

REVIEW TEST 9.1

1. sensory, motor
2. sensory, motor
3. false
4. b
5. mixed
6. cervical
7. somatic, autonomic
8. sympathetic
9. cervical nerve, neck
10. cortex, basal ganglia
11. frontal, temporal, parietal occipital
12. primary motor area, premotor area, primary sensory area

REVIEW TEST 9.2

1. A. 1
   B. 2
   C. 4
   D. 3
2. true
3. c
4. a
5. pineal
6. b
7. cerebellum
8. vestibulo-, ponto-, and spinocerebellum
9. pons
10. 12
11. A. optic
    B. trigeminal
    C. glossopharyngeal
    D. oculomotor
    E. facial
    F. hypoglossal

REVIEW TEST 9.3

1. smell
2. olfactory
3. cribriform plate
4. sight
5. optic chiasm
6. calcarine
7. retinal
8. rods and cones
9. optic
10. A. IV
    B. VI
    C. III
11. superior orbital fissure
12. facial, facial expression
13. stylomastoid
14. submandibular, sublingual
15. submandibular, pterygomandibular

REVIEW TEST 9.4

1. chorda tympani, lingua
2. facial
3. vestibulocochlear; it describes both pairs
4. malleus, incus, stapes; pass sound vibration mechanically to inner ear
5. spiral, vestibular
6. hair
7. false

REVIEW TEST 9.5

1. lateral
2. true
3. foramen: ovale, superior orbital fissure, and internal auditory meatus
4. tongue
5. jugular foramen, superior and inferior petrosal
6. parotid
7. X, parasympathetic
8. f

REVIEW TEST 9.6

1. ambiguous, superior and inferior petrosal
2. jugular
3. IX, X
4. glossopharyngeal, mixed, posterior tongue and pharynx
5. c
6. hypoglossal foramen

REVIEW TEST 9.7

1. A. V1, ophthalmic superior orbital fissure
   B. V2, maxillary foramen rotundum
   C. V3, mandibular foramen ovale
2. semilunar, gasserian
3. pons
4. A. 2
   B. 3
   C. 1
5. pterygopalatine
6. A. 3, 4
   B. 1, 2

REVIEW TEST 9.8

1. A. PSA, MSA
   B. MSA
   C. MSA, ASA
   D. PSA
2. A. PSA, MSA, GP
   B. MSA, ASA, GP, NP
   C. MSA, GP
   D. IA, buccal
   E. IA
3. proprioception
4. mandibular foramen
5. infraorbital

REVIEW TEST 9.9

1. lingual, buccal
2. inferior alveolar nerve, mental nerve
3. muscles of mastication
4. supraorbital, infraorbital, mental
5. A. 2
   B. 1
   C. 3
   D. 4

REVIEW TEST 9.10

1. A. sensory ganglion
   B. sensory neuron
   C. sympathetic chain
   D. motor nucleus
2. diencephalon
3. A. frontal lobe
   B. central sulcus
   C. temporal lobe
   D. lateral sulcus
4. A. primary motor cortex
   B. primary sensory cortex
   C. Broca's area
   D. auditory cortex
   E. calcarine sulcus
5. basal ganglia
6. A. CN II
   B. CN III
   C. CN V
   D. CN VI
   E. CN VII
   F. CN IX
   G. CN X
7. A. CN IV
   B. CN V
   C. CN XII
   D. CN XI
8. A. olfactory bulb
   B. smell receptor neurons
   C. cribriform plate
9. A. rod
   B. cone
10. A. retina
    B. lens
    C. choroid
    D. iris
11. A. CN II
    B. optic chiasm
12. visual cortex
13. A. CN III
    B. muscles of eye
14. A. CN IX
    B. CN V
    C. CN VII
15. A. CN VII
    B. ciliary ganglion
    C. submandibular ganglion
16. facial nerve CN VII
17. facial nerve CN VII
18. A. vestibular ganglion
    B. vestibular nerve
    C. cochlear nerve
19. A. vestibular nerve
    B. cochlear nerve
    C. internal auditory meatus
20. A. inferior petrosal ganglion
    B. superior petrosal ganglion
21. CN IX
22. CN X
23. A. CN XI
    B. jugular foramen
24. CN XI
25. A. CN XII
    B. hypoglossal foramen
26. CN XII
27. trigeminal nerve
28. pons
29. A. CN IX
    B. CN VII
    C. CN VII
30. A. ciliary ganglion
    B. lacrimal nerve
    C. ASA nerve
    D. greater palatine nerve
    E. mental nerve
    F. frontal nerve
    G. V1, ophthalmic division
    H. V2, maxillary division
    I. pterygopalatine ganglion
    J. V3, mandibular division
    K. buccal nerve
    L. inferior alveolar nerve
    M. mylohyoid nerve
31. A. lingual nerve
    B. chorda tympani
32. A. motor branch
    B. inferior alveolar nerve
    C. auriculotemporal nerve
33. A. trigeminal ganglion
    B. motor nucleus
    C. spinal nucleus
34. A. greater palatine nerve
    B. MSA nerve
    C. ASA nerve
    D. inferior alveolar nerve
    E. buccal nerve
35. A. nasopalatine nerve
    B. incisive foramen
    C. greater palatine foramen
36. greater palatine nerve

CHAPTER 10

REVIEW TEST 10.1

1. false
2. erythrocytes, leukocytes
3. closed
4. arteries, veins
5. b

REVIEW TEST 10.2

1. carotid
2. jugular
3. e
4. internal carotid artery
   external carotid artery
5. tongue, lingual
6. mandible
7. carotid artery

REVIEW TEST 10.3

1. c
2. maxillary
3. A. inferior alveolar artery
   B. ASA artery
   C. MSA artery
   D. PSA artery
4. greater palatine artery
5. incisive foramen

REVIEW TEST 10.4

1. inferior alveolar nerve, artery, and vein
2. b
3. circle of Willis
4. basilar artery
5. a
6. retromandibular vein

REVIEW TEST 10.5

1. pterygoid plexus
2. cavernous sinus
3. d
4. supraorbital nerve, artery, and vein
5. superior sagittal
6. f
7. true
8. A. facial nodes
   B. submandibular nodes
   C. postauricular nodes
   D. submental nodes
9. along SCM muscles
10. maxillary V2, pterygoid plexus, maxillary artery
11. internal jujular

REVIEW TEST 10.6

1. A. veins
   B. arteries
2. A. lymph vessel
   B. lymph node
3. A. superficial temporal artery
   B. facial artery
   C. internal carotid artery
   D. thyroid artery
   E. vertebral artery
4. A. lingual artery
   B. external carotid artery
   C. common carotid artery
5. A. MSA artery
   B. buccal artery
   C. meningeal arteries
   D. superior alveolar artery
6. A. sphenopalatine artery
   B. inferior alveolar artery
7. circle of Willis
8. posterior cerebral artery
9. middle cerebral artery
10. A. basilar artery
    B. vertebral artery
11. A. pituitary fossa
    B. carotid canal
    C. jugular foramen
12. A. facial vein
    B. retromandibular vein
    C. internal jugular vein
    D. vertebral vein
13. nasopalatine vein
14. A. ASA vein
    B. pterygoid plexus
15. A. cavernous sinus
    B. superior sagittal sinus
16. inferior alveolar nerve, artery, and vein
17. A. nasopalatine artery, vein, and nerve
    B. greater palatine
18. A. supraorbital artery, vein, nerve, and foramen
    B. infraorbital artery, vein, nerve, and foramen
    C. mental artery, vein, nerve, and foramen

19. A. cervical nodes
    B. carotid and jugular vessels
20. A. internal carotid artery
    B. cavernous sinus
21. A. facial nodes
    B. submandibular nodes
    C. jugulodigastric node
22. A. submental nodes
    B. occipital nodes

CHAPTER 11

REVIEW TEST 11.1

1. palate
2. deglutition, mastication
3. masseter, medial, and lateral pterygoids, temporalis, CN V
4. gliding and hinge
5. d
6. incise (incisors), tear (canines), grind (molars)
7. nasopharynx, oropharynx, pharynx proper
8. Eustachian (tympanic) tube
9. constrictors, CN X
10. IX, gag

REVIEW TEST 11.2

1. elevators (temporalis, masseter, medial pterygoid) and depressors (suprahyoids), inferior
2. lateral pterygoid, superior
3. true
4. oral, pharyngeal, esophageal
5. Eustachian (tympanic) tube
6. false
7. respiratory
8. true

REVIEW TEST 11.3

1. false
2. b
3. vocal folds
4. pineal gland
5. b
6. c
7. e
8. d

REVIEW TEST 11.4

1. neurohypophysis, adenohypophysis
2. false
3. c
4. trachea (thyroid cartilage)
5. thymus
6. palatine, lingual, pharyngeal tonsils

REVIEW TEST 11.5

1. IA, buccal
2. MSA, ASA, GP, NP
3. IA
4. MSA, GP
5. PSA, ASA, GP
6. ASA, NP

REVIEW TEST 11.6

1. A. nasal cavity
   B. esophagus
2. A. pharyngeal constrictors
   B. esophagus
3. A. bolus
   B. oral cavity
   C. Eustachian tube
   D. oropharynx
   E. pharynx proper
4. A. turbinates
   B. pharyngeal tonsil
   C. nasopharynx
5. A. vocal fold
   B. larynx
   C. trachea
6. hinge movement
7. A. lingual tonsils
   B. palatine tonsils
8. neurohypophysis
9. A. thyroid cartilage
   B. thyroid gland
   C. C cells
   D. parathyroid glands
   E. tracheal rings
10. thymus gland
11. vocal folds
12. carotid sheath
13. A. fascia of trapezius
    B. fascia of SCM
14. A. fascia
    B. space
    C. muscle
15. visceral fascia
16. A. pituitary gland
    B. pineal gland
17. submental space
18. A. sublingual space
    B. submandibular space
19. pterygomandibular space
20. A. vertebral fascia
    B. retropharyngeal space
    C. lateral pharyngeal space
    D. carotid space
    E. visceral fascia
    F. middle cervical fascia
21. A. carotid space
    B. parotid space
    C. parotideomasseteric fascia
22. A. nasopalatine nerve
    B. greater palatine nerve
    C. MSA nerve
23. A. buccal nerve
    B. inferior alveolar nerve

SOURCES

Arey LB. *Developmental Anatomy.* Saunders, Philadelphia, 1965.

Barr ML, Kiernan JA. *The Human Nervous System,* 4th ed. Harper & Row, Philadelphia, 1983.

Bell W. *Temporomandibular Disorders,* 2nd ed. Year Book *Medical,* Chicago, 1986.

Capit W, Elson LM. *The Anatomy Coloring Book.* Harper & Row, Philadelphia, 1977.

Clemente CD. *Anatomy: A Regional Atlas of the Human Body,* 3rd ed. C. D. Clemente, Urban & Schwarzenberg, Baltimore, 1987.

Diamond MC, Scheibel AB, Elson LM. *The Human Brain Coloring Book.* Barnes & Noble, New York, 1985.

Grant JCB. *Grant's Atlas of Anatomy,* 6th ed. Williams & Wilkins, Baltimore, 1975.

Hollinshead WH, Rosse C. *Textbook of Anatomy,* 4th ed. Harper & Row, Philadelphia, 1985.

Jungeira LC, Carneiro J, Long JA. *Basic Histology,* 5th ed. Lange, Los Altos, CA, 1986.

Leeson CR, Leeson TS, Paparo AA. *Textbook of Basic Histology,* 5th ed. Saunders, Philadelphia, 1985.

Melfi RC. *Permar's Oral Embryology and Microscopic Anatomy,* 7th ed. Lea & Febiger, Philadelphia, 1982.

Moore KL. *The Developing Human,* 3rd ed. Saunders, Philadelphia, 1982.

INDEX

NOTES

NOTES

NOTES

NOTES

NOTES

NOTES

NOTES